BRAIN TUMORS

A Comprehensive Text

NEUROLOGICAL DISEASE AND THERAPY

Series Editor

WILLIAM C. KOLLER

Department of Neurology
University of Kansas Medical Center
Kansas City, Kansas

BRAIN TUMORS

A Comprehensive Text

edited by

Robert A. Morantz

*University of Kansas School of Medicine
and University of Missouri — Kansas City
Kansas City, Missouri*

John W. Walsh

*Hermann Hospital
and University of Texas Health Sciences Center at Houston
Houston, Texas*

Marcel Dekker, Inc.   **New York • Basel • Hong Kong**

Library of Congress Cataloging-in-Publication Data

Brain tumors: a comprehensive text / edited by Robert A. Morantz, John W. Walsh.
    p.   cm. — (Neurological disease and therapy; 20)
  Includes bibliographical references and index.
  ISBN 0-8247-8826-5 (alk. paper)
  1. Brain—Tumors. I. Morantz, Robert A. II. Walsh, J. W. III. Series: Neurological
disease and therapy; v. 20.
  [DNLM: 1. Brain Neoplasms. W1 NE33LD v.20   1993 / WL 358 B81346 1993]
RC280.B7B724 1993
616.99'281—dc20
DNLM/DLC
for Library of Congress
                                               93-20607
                                                 CIP

The publisher offers discounts on this book when ordered in bulk quantities. For more information, write to Special Sales/Professional Marketing at the address below.

This book is printed on acid-free paper.

Marcel Dekker, Inc.
270 Madison Avenue, New York, New York 10016

Current printing (last digit):
10 9 8 7 6 5 4 3 2 1

PRINTED IN THE UNITED STATES OF AMERICA

We dedicate this book to our wives,
Marsha Murphy and Ruth G. Kirsch, who have
been so supportive during this
challenging endeavor

Series Introduction

The biology and clinical management of brain tumors is a complex subject that transverses almost all disciplines of basic science and clinical medicine. Brain tumors can be a devastating medical illness. However, our knowledge of the basic mechanisms of brain tumors has dramatically increased in recent years. The molecular biologists and the clinicians have contributed to the improved prognosis of patients with brain tumors. Technological advances such as neuro-imaging, which allows rapid diagnosis and microsurgical instrumentation, and novel pharmacological approaches have provided improved treatment.

In keeping with the goal of the Handbook Series on Neurological Disease, Drs. Morantz and Walsh have provided a comprehensive review of all aspects of brain tumors for both the basic and clinical scientist.

William C. Koller

Preface

This book is a direct outgrowth of the tremendous increase in information that has been gathered over the past decade about brain tumors, their molecular biology and modes of growth and spread, and the identification and treatment of patients harboring them. It is a compilation and distillation of that information and, as such, aims to provide an overview of neuro-oncology as it exists in the 1990s.

After the pioneering work of Cushing and others in the early 1900s, very little new data about brain tumor structure and growth were reported for more than half a century, and relatively little progress was made in prolonging and improving the quality of life for the brain tumor patient. This was due primarily to the fact that the laboratory tools necessary for the study of brain tumor biology had not been developed, and modern diagnostic and surgical instrumentation and adjunctive forms of treatment were not yet available. In recent years, however, there have been dramatic changes in molecular biological techniques and state-of-the-art imaging capabilities (CT, MR, DSA, PET, and ultrasound). In addition, we have seen the introduction of the surgical microscope and microsurgical instrumentation, as well as radiosurgery, brachytherapy, and innovative approaches to adjunctive radiation, chemotherapy, and immunotherapy. With some tumors, such as germinoma and medulloblastoma, a significant improvement in prognosis has been achieved; unfortunately, this has not yet been the case with malignant gliomas. These new advances are the focus of this book and are reviewed, along with other background material, by the authors of each chapter.

Our goal in compiling this book was to provide, in a single source, a relatively comprehensive overview of neuro-oncology. A number of books have recently been published that address specific types of brain tumor, such as malignant glioma, meningioma, or pituitary adenoma, or particular brain tumor topics, such as stereotactic techniques, skull base surgery, or radiosurgery, but a comprehensive text that covers all these areas is not currently available. With this in mind, we made a concentrated effort to select topics that address neuro-oncology as broadly and completely as possible; and we asked each author to represent his or her topic generally, but with sufficient detail to enable readers to provide the most up-to-date care for their patients.

We are aware that such an approach has led to a slight degree of overlap between the chapters, whereby a given topic may be discussed in great detail in one chapter, and then alluded to briefly in several others. In addition, authors may have slightly different approaches to the management of a problem that might arise in a patient having a particular type of tumor. Rather than edit the text so that an artificial "party line" is given throughout the book, we decided to leave intact slightly differing viewpoints; this reflects the lack of unanimity that exists within the contemporary neurosurgical community.

Although much of this work will be useful and of interest to a wide variety of readers, we are specifically targeting this book for the neurosurgeon *not* specializing in tumor surgery, as well as for neurologists, radiation and medical oncologists, and internists and family practitioners who care for brain tumor patients. We believe that it will also be of great value to neurosurgery residents.

We are indebted to all the authors for their contributions to this text.

Robert A. Morantz
John W. Walsh

Contents

Contributors

Nayef R. F. Al-Rodhan, M.D., Ph.D.   Department of Neurosurgery, Mayo Clinic and Mayo Graduate School of Medicine, Rochester, Minnesota

Brian T. Andrews, M.D.   Department of Neurological Surgery, School of Medicine, University of California, San Francisco, California

Daniel L. Barrow, M.D.   Associate Professor and Vice Chairman, Department of Neurosurgery, Emory University School of Medicine, Atlanta, Georgia

Solomon Batnitzky, M.D.   Professor of Diagnostic Radiology, and Chief, Section of Neuroradiology, Department of Diagnostic Radiology, University of Kansas Medical Center, Kansas City, Kansas

James Baumgartner, M.D.   Department of Neurological Surgery, School of Medicine, University of California, San Francisco, California

Nicolaas I. Bohnen, M.D., Ph.D.   Department of Health Sciences Research, Section of Clinical Epidemiology, Mayo Clinic and Mayo Foundation, Rochester, Minnesota

Dennis E. Bullard, M.D.   Chief, Department of Surgery, Rex Hospital and Raleigh Neurosurgical Clinic, Raleigh, North Carolina

Kym L. Chandler, M.D.   Division of Neuro-oncology, Department of Neurosurgery, University of California, School of Medicine, San Francisco, California

Yuan Chang, M.D.   Assistant Professor, Division of Neuropathology/Department of Pathology, Columbia University College of Physicians and Surgeons, New York, New York

Stephen W. Coons, M.D. Staff Neuropathologist, Department of Neuropathology, Barrow Neurological Institute of St. Joseph's Hospital and Medical Center, Phoenix, Arizona

Donald A. Eckard, M.D. Assistant Professor, and Chief, Interventional Neuroradiology, Department of Radiology, University of Kansas Medical Center, Kansas City, Kansas

Fred J. Epstein, M.D. Professor and Director, Department of Pediatric Neurosurgery, New York University Medical Center, New York, New York

Richard G. Evans, Ph.D., M.D., F.A.C.R. Professor and Chairman, Department of Radiation Oncology, University of Kansas Medical Center, Kansas City, Kansas

Arnold I. Freeman, M.D. Professor and Chief, Section of Pediatric Hematology Oncology, Children's Mercy Hospital, Kansas City, Missouri

Floyd H. Gilles, M.D. Burton E. Green Professor of Pediatric Neuropathology, Children's Hospital of Los Angeles, and Professor of Pathology (Neuropathology), Neurosurgery, and Neurology, University of Southern California School of Medicine, Los Angeles, California

Roberta P. Glick, M.D. Associate Professor, Department of Neurosurgery, University of Illinois Medical Center and Cook County Hospital, Chicago, Illinois

Ziya L. Gokaslan, M.D. Department of Neurosurgery, University of Texas M.D. Anderson Cancer Center, Houston, Texas

Wesley E. Griffitt, M.D. University of Kansas Medical Center, Kansas City, Kansas

Mary Katherine Gumerlock, M.D. Associate Professor, Department of Neurosurgery, University of Oklahoma Health Sciences Center, Oklahoma City, Oklahoma

Barton L. Guthrie, M.D. Assistant Professor, Department of Surgery/Neurosurgery, University of Alabama, and Associate Scientist, U.A.B. Comprehensive Cancer Center, Birmingham, Alabama

Philip H. Gutin, M.D. Departments of Neurological Surgery and Radiation Oncology, University of California, School of Medicine, San Francisco, California

Avery Hart, M.D. Senior Attending Physician, Department of Medicine, Cook County Hospital, Chicago, Illinois

Frank P. Holladay, M.D. Assistant Professor, Department of Surgery, Neurosurgery Section, University of Kansas Medical Center, Kansas City, Kansas

Dikran S. Horoupian, M.D. Professor, Division of Neuropathology, Department of Pathology, Stanford University Medical Center, Stanford, California

Peter C. Johnson, M.D.   Chairman, Division of Neuropathology, Barrow Neurological Institute of St. Joseph's Hospital and Medical Center, Phoenix, Arizona

Patrick J. Kelly, M.D.   Professor, Department of Neurological Surgery, Mayo Clinic and Mayo Graduate School of Medicine, Rochester, Minnesota

Bruce F. Kimler, Ph.D.   Professor, Department of Radiation Oncology, University of Kansas Medical Center, Kansas City, Kansas

Paul L. Kornblith, M.D.   Professor of Neurosurgery and Director of Neuro-Oncology, Department of Neurosurgery, University of Pittsburgh School of Medicine, Presbyterian University Hospital, Pittsburgh, Pennsylvania

Mark J. Kotapka, M.D.   Assistant Professor, Department of Neurosurgery, Hospital of the University of Pennsylvania, Philadelphia, Pennsylvania

Diana L. Kraemer, M.D.   Instructor, Section of Neurosurgery, Department of Surgery, Yale University School of Medicine, New Haven, Connecticut

Leonard T. Kurland, M.D., Dr.P.H.   Professor of Epidemiology and Senior Consultant, Health Sciences Research, Section of Clinical Epidemiology, Mayo Clinic and Mayo Foundation, Rochester, Minnesota

Edward R. Laws, Jr., M.D., F.A.C.S.   Professor, Department of Neurosurgery, University of Virginia Health Sciences Center, Charlottesville, Virginia

James G. Lemons, Ed.D.   Director, Pain Management Center, Research Medical Center, Kansas City, Missouri

Robert A. Morantz, M.D.   Clinical Associate Professor of Neurosurgery, University of Kansas School of Medicine and University of Missouri—Kansas City, and Clinical Professor of Radiation Oncology, University of Kansas School of Medicine, Kansas City, Kansas

Edward A. Neuwelt, M.D.   Professor of Neurology and Associate Professor of Neurosurgery, The Oregon Health Sciences University, Portland, Oregon

Roy A. Patchell, M.D.   Chief of Neuro-Oncology, Department of Neurology and Neurosurgery, University of Kentucky, Lexington, Kentucky

Don Penny, M.D., M.Sc.   Assistant Professor, Department of Neurosurgery, University of Illinois Medical Center, Chicago, Illinois

Michael D. Prados, M.D., F.A.C.P.   Associate Professor, Department of Neurosurgery, University of California, School of Medicine, San Francisco, California

Kurupath Radhakrishnan, M.D.   Research Associate, Health Sciences Research, Section of Clinical Epidemiology, Mayo Clinic and Mayo Foundation, Rochester, Minnesota

Mark L. Rosenblum, M.D.   Chairman, Department of Neurological Surgery, and Director, Midwest Neuro-Oncology Center, Henry Ford Health Sciences Center, Detroit, Michigan

Gail L. Rosseau, M.D.   Director of Cranial Base Surgery, Chicago Neurosurgical Center, Chicago, Illinois

Michael Salcman, M.D.   Clinical Professor, Department of Neurosurgery, George Washington University, Washington, D.C.

Raymond E. Sawaya, M.D.   Professor and Chairman, Department of Neurosurgery, University of Texas M.D. Anderson Cancer Center, Houston, Texas

Henry H. Schmidek, M.D.   Marion, Massachusetts

Luis Schut, M.D.   Professor of Neurosurgery, University of Pennsylvania and Children's Hospital of Philadelphia, Philadelphia, Pennsylvania

Laligam N. Sekhar, M.D.   Professor and Chairman, Department of Neurosurgery, George Washington University Medical Center, Washington, D.C.

Peggy Ward Smith, R.N., M.S.N., M.S.   Manager, The Brain Tumor Institute of Kansas City, Research Medical Center, Kansas City, Missouri

Penny K. Sneed, M.D.   Assistant Professor, Department of Radiation Oncology, University of California, School of Medicine, San Francisco, California

Alex J. Tikhtman, M.D.   Department of Neurology, University of Kentucky, Lexington, Kentucky

George T. Tindall, M.D.   Professor and Chairman, Department of Neurosurgery, Emory University School of Medicine, Atlanta, Georgia

John W. Walsh, M.D., Ph.D.   Professor of Neurosurgery and Director of Gamma Knife Radiosurgery, Department of Neurosurgery, Hermann Hospital and the University of Texas Health Sciences Center at Houston, Houston, Texas

Ronald E. Warnick, M.D.   Director, Division of Neuro-Oncology, Department of Neurosurgery, University of Cincinnati Medical Center, Cincinnati, Ohio

William C. Welch, M.D.   Assistant Professor, Department of Neurosurgery, Albert Einstein College of Medicine, Bronx, New York

Jeffrey H. Wisoff, M.D.   Assistant Professor, Division of Pediatric Neurosurgery, Department of Neurosurgery, New York University Medical Center, New York, New York

Gary W. Wood, Ph.D.   Professor, Department of Pathology, University of Kansas Medical Center, Kansas City, Kansas

Byron Young, M.D.   Johnston-Wright Chair, Department of Surgery, University of Kentucky, Lexington, Kentucky

1

Epidemiology of Brain Tumors

Kurupath Radhakrishnan, Nicolaas I. Bohnen, and Leonard T. Kurland
Mayo Clinic and Mayo Foundation, Rochester, Minnesota

I. INTRODUCTION

Epidemiology deals with the distribution and determinants of disease in populations (1). Whereas the clinician is concerned with disease in the individual patient, the epidemiologist is interested in the occurrence of the disease within a defined community or region. Epidemiology may be *descriptive*, providing incidence, prevalence, mortality, and survivorship data; *analytic*, being either hypothesis-generating or hypothesis-testing, or both; and of medicolegal and economic interest with application to health care utilization issues (1,2).

Common indices relevant to brain tumor epidemiology are *incidence* and *mortality rates*. An *incidence rate* is the number of new cases of a given disease per 100,000 persons at risk of having the disease per year. A *mortality rate* is analogous to an incidence rate, but is limited to the number of deaths from a given disease. Usually, incidence rates are preferred as a measure of disease impact, since death rates reflect changes in both incidence and survival. However, in highly fatal diseases, such as malignant brain tumors, mortality data are used because they can be readily obtained on a nationwide basis (3). Incidence and mortality rates can be presented in a standardized way after adjustment for the age and sex distribution in the population (4). The *adjusted rates* allow an overall comparison between different populations because the rates are standardized for dissimilarities in the age and sex distribution.

Brain tumors are second only to stroke as the leading cause of death from neurological disease. It is estimated that about 11,000 United States' residents die from primary nervous system tumors annually (5). Most of the earlier reports dealing with the frequency of neoplasms of the nervous system have been based on the experience of individual neurosurgeons, autopsy series, or proportionate rates of hospital admissions. These data do not necessarily reflect an accurate picture of the true incidence of brain tumors. In this chapter we will review the population-based data concerning primary and secondary brain tumors, as well as many of the methodological problems associated with studying their epidemiological characteristics.

Ascertainment of intracranial tumors is influenced by the degree of medical sophistication, the autopsy rate, and the availability of medical care in a given population at a specific time. All these factors have to be considered when comparing rates between different countries. Furthermore, these factors have changed considerably over the last two decades, with increasing availability of medical care and noninvasive neuroimaging techniques, such as computed tomography (CT) and magnetic resonance imaging (MRI), but with decreasing autopsy rates.

It will be clear that epidemiological studies of brain tumor are beset with many methodological problems. Different sources of bias can seriously flaw the reported outcome of many studies. In particular, the following problems of studying brain tumors epidemiologically warrant emphasis:

1. *Diagnosis*: It has been demonstrated that a significant number of brain tumors remain undiagnosed during life. Percy et al. (6) found that 37% of brain tumors in their Rochester, Minnesota, series were first diagnosed at autopsy, and only one-third of these were symptomatic during life. It seems that clinical misses are unlikely to be reduced to less than 10% even with recent advances in neuroimaging techniques.

2. *Classification*: Most primary intracranial tumors fit into one of two histological categories. The first category represents neoplasia of the primary supporting elements of the central nervous system (gliomas), the second category concerns the usually benign tumors of the dural covering of the brain (meningiomas). Although some epidemiological studies of gliomas use the classification of Kernohan and Sayre (7), others use the three-tiered schemes of Ringertz (8), the World Health Organization (WHO; 9), or Burger (10). Many authors these days use the term *primitive neuroectodermal tumor* (PNET) to refer to a group of highly malignant tumors in children, including medulloblastomas (11). The multiplicity of classification systems hinders a valid comparison of different epidemiological studies.

3. *Crude (unadjusted) data*: The Rochester, Minnesota, data (12) demonstrate that the annual brain tumor incidence per 100,000 persons increases steadily with advancing age from 4.0 at 12 years, 6.5 at 35 years, 18.0 at 55 years, to over 70.0 at 75 years. It is obvious that the incidence of brain tumors will be influenced by the age-specific distribution of the population; hence, no valid comparison can be made between crude epidemiological indices of brain tumors.

4. *Effect of noninvasive neuroimaging techniques*: The introduction of CT in 1973 and its widespread use a decade later increased the ease with which the presence of a brain tumor could be diagnosed. However, neither CT nor MRI can produce images that are distinctly tumor-specific (13,14). This remains one of the crucial problems in the descriptive epidemiology of malignant brain tumors, particularly in the elderly, in whom the proportion with histological verification falls as age increases. At advanced ages, when the frequency of metastases to the brain is highest, a proportion of brain tumors diagnosed as primary, in actuality, may well be secondary.

II. PRIMARY BRAIN TUMORS

A. Incidence Data

While bearing in mind the potential problems complicating the comparison of the incidence rates of primary brain tumors between different populations, we would like to analyze and compare average annual age-adjusted incidence rates of primary brain tumors for several geographic regions.

There is a marked geographic variation in the incidence rates of primary brain tumors. Figures 1 and 2 illustrate the average annual age-adjusted incidence rates of primary brain tumors for different countries worldwide computed by calculating the mean of different reported rates available from each country. The more socioeconomically developed countries have higher incidence rates, for either sex, than the less-developed nations. When all histological types of primary brain tumors are combined, Sweden has the highest rate of 10:100,000 per year, closely

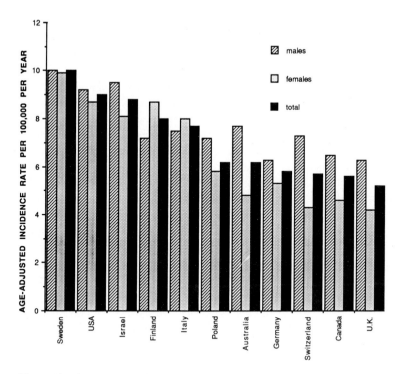

Figure 1 Average annual age-adjusted incidence of primary brain tumors among countries with total rates of more than 5:100,000 population.

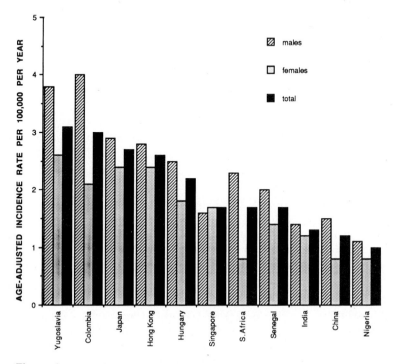

Figure 2 Average annual age-adjusted incidence of primary brain tumors among countries with total rates of fewer than 5:100,000 population.

followed by the United States and Israel. The Asian and African groups and a few of the developing nations report lower rates.

The marked geographic variation in the incidence of primary brain tumors may be a reflection of the differences in the quality of medical practice, availability of diagnostic facilities, and the level of organization of registries for data collection and coding. In addition, improved medical services for the elderly, in whom age-specific rates of primary brain tumors are highest, partly explain the higher rates found in many socioeconomically advanced societies.

However, the observed differences in the incidence rates of primary brain tumors among different world population groups may not be completely artifactual. For example, among countries with low rates are highly developed regions such as Japan, Singapore, and Hong Kong, although the availability and acceptance of the most modern technology may be limited to a segment of the total population. Furthermore, different racial or ethnic groups living in the same region may have markedly different incidence rates. Among Israelis, Jewish immigrants born in Europe and America have higher rates than those born in Asia and Africa (15). In general, Caucasians have higher rates compared with other races. The reported incidence rates for blacks in the United States are generally lower than for their white counterparts residing in the same region (15–17); for example, recent data from Los Angeles County for all types of brain tumors combined indicated that blacks, Asians, and Latinos have lower rates than whites (18).

Most registries report a higher brain tumor rate in males than in females. A comparison using international data on the incidence of primary brain tumors of all histological types combined found an average male/female sex ratio of 1.4 (range: 0.9–2.6) across geographic areas (19).

1. United States Studies

There has been a wealth of information about the incidence of primary brain tumors in the United States from the following sources: The Connecticut Tumor Registry, dating back to 1935 (20); the Rochester, Minnesota, Epidemiological Program Project data on brain tumors (1935–1977) (6,12); the Third National Cancer Survey (1969–1971), which included only neoplasms considered to be malignant (21); the National Survey, which analyzed all intracranial tumors, primary and secondary, based on a probability sample of inpatients in 157 U. S. hospitals during 1973–1974 (22); the National Cancer Institute's *S*urveillance, *E*pidemiology and *E*nd *R*esult (SEER) program, which provided data on malignant brain tumors for about 10% of the U. S. population beginning in 1973 (23); and the Los Angeles County Cancer Surveillance Program (1972–1985) (18,24).

Table 1 summarizes brain tumor incidence rates in four United States surveillance systems. The annual age-adjusted incidence rate per 100,000 population for primary brain tumors ranges from 5.0 in Connecticut to 14.1 in Rochester, Minnesota, with a mean of 9.0 (9.2 for males and 8.7 for females) and a sex ratio of 1.2. The age-specific incidence peaked in the age group 65–75 years; gliomas constituted 50% and meningiomas 28% of the primary brain tumors.

Rochester Data. The population of Rochester, Minnesota, has been the basis for several epidemiological studies of primary brain tumor for the period from 1935 through 1977 (6,12,25). Rochester is unique as a population in that all medical records for the community, including those kept by private physicians, nursing homes, and chronic care facilities, are identifiable through a centralized diagnostic index, the medical records-linkage system of the Mayo Clinic (26). In addition, the autopsy rate for local residents has been about 60%.

Of the 223 primary brain tumors diagnosed between 1935 and 1977, 145 (65%) were diagnosed during life, the remaining 35% being initially diagnosed at autopsy. Of the glioma group, 19% were diagnosed at autopsy, whereas two-thirds of the meningiomas were undetected until autopsy. These were largely asymptomatic tumors in the elderly population. Histological confirmation was available in 96% of gliomas, 97% of meningiomas, and 91% of all tumors.

In comparing the data on primary brain tumor incidence from Rochester, Minnesota, with that

Table 1 Epidemiological Data from Four United States Studies

Study/period (Ref.)	No. of cases	Percentage of pathological verification	Percentage of Incidence per 100,000 per year				
			Glioma	Meningioma	Male	Female	Total
Rochester MN 1935–1977 (12)	233	91	34.9	39.4	14.0	14.2	14.1
Connecticut Tumor Registry 1955–1964 (20)	1731	76	65.0	18.0	5.4	4.5	5.0
National Survey 1973–1974 (22)	1060	74	57.8	19.5	8.5	7.9	8.2
Los Angeles County Cancer Surveillance Program 1972–1985 (18)	8612	90	41.6	35.7	8.9	8.1	8.5

from other populations, the following features are observed: (1) the Rochester population has the highest age-adjusted incidence rate for primary brain tumor reported to date, 14.1 for the period 1935–1977 and 14.7 for the period 1950–1977; (2) the age-specific incidence rates for primary brain tumor in Rochester show a continuous rise with age, in contrast with other surveys that generally show a small peak in childhood, with a second more dramatic increase in the 55- to 75-year-old group, followed by a decrease thereafter (Fig. 3); and (3) a much higher proportion of diagnosed meningiomas in Rochester (see Fig. 5).

These differences are attributed to more complete case ascertainment and the high autopsy rate in Rochester. Thus, when only the cases diagnosed before death were included, the age-adjusted incidence rate for primary brain tumor in Rochester would fall to 10:100,000 per year (27,28). The incidence rates reported from the National Survey (22), Los Angeles County Cancer Surveillance Program (18), and Trento, Italy (29), are lower than the Rochester age-adjusted rate calculated by excluding cases diagnosed initially at autopsy. The study by Joensen (30) from an isolated population of the Faroe Islands, yielded a similar rate of 10.2:100,000 per year for primary brain tumors diagnosed during life.

The incidence rates reported from recent surveys from central Finland (31), 12.3:100,000 per year, and Bolzano City, Italy (32), 13.6:100,000 per year, represent studies with more complete case ascertainment.

2. *Incidence by Histological Type of Primary Brain Tumor*

The SEER network of cancer registries provides incidence data for malignant brain tumors for about 10% of the U. S. population, with a histopathological verification rate of 85% (23,33). Data obtained from the population-based cancer registries in Connecticut; San Francisco, California; Detroit, Michigan; Hawaii; Iowa; New Mexico; Seattle, Washington; Utah; and Atlanta, Georgia are depicted in Figure 4. The overall average annual age-adjusted incidence rates per 100,000 white males and females of 8.8 and 5.8, respectively, from the SEER data are much higher than the 5.3 and 3.9 reported for primary malignant brain tumors from the Swiss Canton of Vaud (34).

In general, gliomas account for 40–67% and meningiomas 9–27% of the primary tumors in population-based studies (35,36). In Rochester, Minnesota, gliomas constituted 35% and meningiomas accounted for 40% of the primary brain tumors (12) (Fig. 5). This unusual distribution is probably attributable to the high autopsy rate in Rochester, particularly for the detection and recording of asymptomatic meningiomas in the elderly.

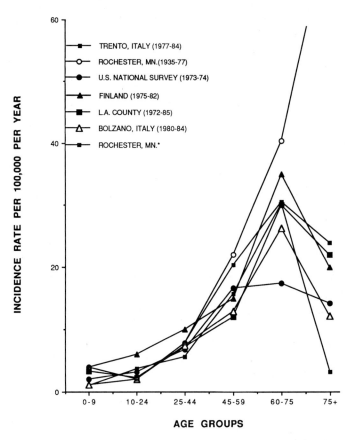

Figure 3 Average annual age-specific incidence rates of primary brain tumors in different populations. Rochester rates, marked with an asterisk [*] do not include disease diagnosed at autopsy.

The sex ratio (SR) varies considerably by histological type. Gliomas are higher in males (SR = 1.5), and meningiomas are higher in females (SR = 0.6) (18). The male/female sex ratio in the SEER registry averaged 1.69 for oligodendroglioma, 1.61 for glioblastoma, 1.45 for astrocytoma, and 1.03 for malignant meningioma (33). In Los Angeles County, black men and women had higher rates of meningiomas than their white counterparts (18) (Fig. 6). In some African populations, meningioma is the most common type of brain tumor reported (37). However, this may be partly a distortion, because patients with a rapidly progressing tumor, such as a glioma, may die before they reach the hospital, or are more likely to be misdiagnosed as stroke or encephalitis.

Gliomas. The annual incidence of gliomas from major studies varies from 2.1:100,000 to 7.1:100,000, being highest in more recent studies. The average annual incidence rate of 5.2:100,000 from Rochester, Minnesota (28,35), is remarkably similar to the figure of 5.6 from southern Finland (38), and 5.4 from Los Angeles County (18). The incidence rate of 7.0 for gliomas from the SEER registry (33) compares with the Swedish rate of 7.1:100,000 per year (39). The age-specific incidence for gliomas was the highest in the 50- to 59-year-old group in Finland and in the 70- to 79-year-old one in Sweden. This difference in age-specific incidence has been attributed mainly to the completeness of case ascertainment and differences in autopsy rate.

Meningiomas. Community-based studies on the incidence of meningiomas are few and most predate the introduction of CT and MRI (17,40–42). They report a variable incidence for symptomatic meningiomas ranging from 1.0:100,000 to 2.8:100,000 per year. The Rochester,

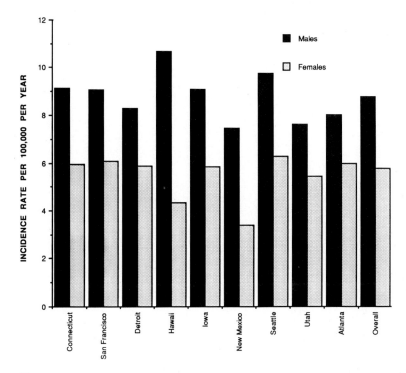

Figure 4 Average annual age-adjusted incidence rates of primary malignant brain tumors for white men and women, aged 35–64 years, by SEER Registry, diagnosed during 1973–1982.

Minnesota, study found an incidence rate of 5.5:100,000 per year for meningiomas, which included cases initially observed at autopsy (35). It seems the availability of CT and MRI has not had the anticipated effect on meningioma ascertainment (18,43). Recent data from Manitoba, Canada, for the period 1980 through 1987, revealed an incidence rate of 2.3:100,000 per year for all meningiomas, and 0.17:100,000 per year for malignant meningiomas (43). The age-specific incidence rate for meningiomas in Manitoba increased with age to the eighth decade, at which it peaked at 8.4:100,000 per year.

The declining incidence of meningiomas after the seventh decade, as observed in Manitoba and other studies, probably reflects a less aggressive investigative approach and lower autopsy rate

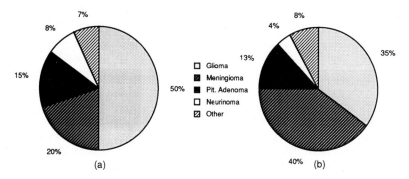

Figure 5 Comparison of the percentage distribution of primary brain tumors by histological type, between (a) population-based studies in general and (b) Rochester data.

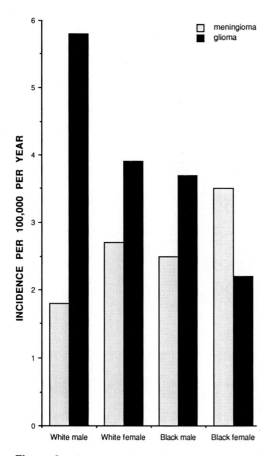

Figure 6   Average annual incidence of meningiomas and gliomas by sex and race in Los Angeles County.

in the elderly. In an autopsy study from New York, Nakasu et al. found that the frequency of incidental meningiomas at autopsy increased with age, and was the highest in people 80 years of age and older (44).

Pituitary Adenomas.   The incidence rate for pituitary adenomas before 1970 is reported as fewer than 1.0:100,000 per year (45). In Olmsted County, Minnesota, the incidence of pituitary adenomas in women aged 15 through 44 years was 7.1:100,000 per year during the period 1970–1977, after being 0.7 through the years 1935–1969 (46). The striking increase in pituitary adenomas diagnosed in women of childbearing age is largely related to the improved diagnostic techniques in neuroradiology and endocrinology, resulting in the identification of heretofore undiagnosed prolactin-secreting and nonfunctional microadenomas (45). In an unselected autopsy series, 27% of the subjects had microadenomas of the pituitary, 41% of which had prolactin-secreting cells (47). If these results can be generalized, nearly one in ten persons of the general population die with a clinically silent prolactinoma (47).

A report from the United Kingdom, based on numerous cases of pituitary adenomas, showed a constant and sizable excess of females for all time periods and age groups (48). In Olmsted County, Minnesota, the age-specific incidence of pituitary adenoma among women declined after age 45 years (46). The observed excess of pituitary adenomas in women in the reproductive age group has generated considerable interest in the possible association with the prior use of oral contraceptives. The frequency of antecedent use of oral contraceptives by patients with pituitary adenomas has been reported to range from 70 to 84% (49,50). However, in a comparison of the women with pituitary adenoma from Olmsted County, Minnesota, with age and time-matched controls, no association was found between the use of oral contraceptives before diagnosis and the onset of symptoms (51).

Primary Brain Lymphoma. Primary non-Hodgkin's lymphoma of the brain (previously designated as reticulum cell sarcoma or microglioma) is a rare malignancy that represents a fraction of all brain tumors (0.5–1.2%) (52). From the data of the SEER program, the average annual incidence of primary brain lymphoma for the years 1973 through 1984 in the United States is 5.4:10 million population (53).

There has been a recent dramatic rise in the incidence of primary brain lymphoma both in individuals who are immunosuppressed and in immunologically normal persons (52). The SEER data disclosed that primary brain lymphoma incidence increased from 2.7:10 million per year in 1973–1975 to 7.5:10 million per year in 1982–1984, and this increase involved both men and women (53). Although part of the increase may be an artifact related to improvement in diagnostic technology and practice, most of the observed increase seems to have antedated the widespread use of new technologies (52,53).

B.   Mortality Data

Mortality rates and their temporal trends are difficult to compare because of the many potentially confounding factors, such as changes in the coding and classification of brain tumors, major advances in diagnostic technologies, variation in autopsy rates, and differences in the adequacy of information available in death certificates.

Goldberg and Kurland (54) analyzed mortality data from 28 countries for primary neoplasms of the nervous system for 1951 through 1958 and found wide geographic variations. Behemuka et al. (55) calculated mortality rates for primary brain tumors from death data of 30 countries for the period 1967 through 1973 and compared these with the available data for the 1951–1958 period. For 1951–1958 the average annual age-adjusted mortality rate ranged from 1.1 to 6.8, whereas for 1967–1973 the range was 4.2:100,000 (Chile) to 10:100,000 (Germany) population. The increase in rates for each country in the intervening 15-year period varied from 12% for Australia, 190% for Japan, to 350% for Mexico. The absolute values, as well as the temporal trends, correlated with the quality and availability of health care and the level of socioeconomic development. More recently, the annual death data due to malignant brain tumors were analyzed for the period 1968 through 1986/1987 for Italy, France, the United States, Germany, and the United Kingdom by Davis et al. (56). An increasing trend in mortality, males experiencing a higher increase than females, was observed.

C.   Is the Incidence of Primary Brain Tumor
in the Elderly Increasing?

Several investigators have reported that the frequency of brain cancer has increased rapidly over the past two decades in persons over the age of 65 years in the United States and elsewhere (56–58). Greig et al. (57) analyzed the data from the SEER program for 1973–1985 and concluded that, between the two periods, there was an increase of 187% for the 75- to 79-year age group, 394% for 80- to 84-year age group, and 501% for the group 85 years and older (Fig. 7). The most common histological type of primary brain tumor in the elderly was glioblastoma.

However, for a comparable period, no significant increase in the incidence rate for brain tumor, even in the older age group was observed in Denmark (58). Furthermore, the trends over time for all ages have been relatively stable from areas such as Rochester, Minnesota (35), Switzerland (59), and Sweden (60), reflecting a constant high level of case ascertainment, diagnostic accuracy, and autopsy rate.

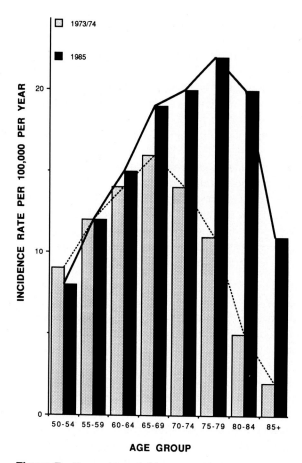

Figure 7 Comparison of the age-specific incidence rates of primary malignant brain tumors in 1973/1974 and 1985 from SEER data.

In our opinion, the reported increase in brain tumors in the elderly seems to be largely artifactual, resulting from a combined effect of the availability of sophisticated diagnostic technology, a change in the definition of an elderly person, with a greater willingness to investigate these persons with less invasive diagnostic procedures, and the introduction of the Medicare program that facilitates access to medical care in the United States.

D. Brain Tumors in Children

Primary tumors of the central nervous system constitute the most common type of solid tumor in childhood. About 1500 children in the United States receive a diagnosis of brain tumor each year (11). In recent years, the prognosis for children with brain tumor has improved remarkably.

Although brain tumors, as a group, are a relatively common form of childhood cancer, the number of children with any single tumor type, such as medulloblastoma or craniopharyngioma, is small. This prevents ascertainment of a sufficient number of patients to derive reliable epidemiological patterns. However, the Third National Cancer Registry (61), SEER data (62), and the Manchester, England, Childhood Tumor Registry (63) contained substantial population-based data on pediatric brain tumors.

The general incidence of brain tumor from birth to 12 years is 2:100,000 to 4:100,000 per year (64,65). In the Third National Cancer Registry, brain tumors were more frequent in white than in black children (61). The boy/girl sex ratio in children under age 15 years is 1.2 for all tumor types combined; in contrast, medulloblastoma, a tumor that occurs almost exclusively in children, has a sex ratio near 2 (66).

The general distribution of brain tumors in children by histological type is depicted in Figure 8. Duffner et al. (62) examined the SEER data for the interval 1973–1980 and found that in children younger than 15 years of age at diagnosis, 23% of brain tumors are medulloblastoma, 25% low-grade astrocytoma, 12% cerebellar astrocytoma, 11% high-grade supratentorial astrocytoma, 9% brain stem glioma, and 8% ependymoma. Brain stem gliomas and cerebellar astrocytomas are rare before the age of 2 years, but low-grade astrocytomas of the hypothalamus, optic tract, and thalamus are relatively common in this age group (67).

E. Analytic Epidemiology of Primary Brain Tumors

Very little is known about the etiology of brain tumors. However, several associations with genetic, occupational, and other environmental factors have been reported.

The evidence for a genetic etiology comes from familial aggregation of brain tumors, the occurrence of primary brain tumors in persons with known genetic disorders, and a suspected association with certain ABO blood groups. There are numerous reports in the literature of individual families with two or more members with intracranial tumors (68–70). However, such reports should be interpreted with caution because familial aggregation may be the result of a high index of suspicion in relatives of the proband, may be related to common environmental factors, or may simply be due to chance. Genetic disorders that have been reported most frequently with primary brain tumor include neurofibromatosis (71), tuberous sclerosis (72), and Werner's syndrome (73) (see Chap. 18). Selversten and Cooper (74) found an association between blood group A and glioma, which was not corroborated in other studies (75,76).

Some blue-collar occupational groups, including workers in rubber and polyvinyl chloride

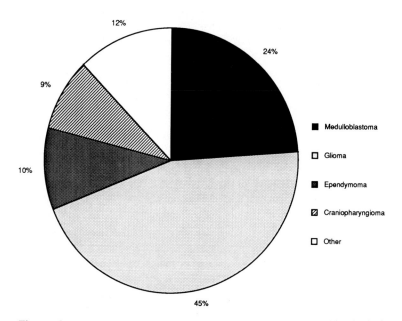

Figure 8 Percentage distribution of pediatric brain tumors by histological type.

plants, machinists (77), and farmers (78), have been reported to have an elevated risk of brain tumors. Since most of the workers are potentially exposed to multiple chemicals, it is difficult to be certain of any specific chemical risk factor. Furthermore, one can speculate on the role of a "diagnostic sensitivity bias," as an explanation for the observed high incidence rate of primary brain tumor among blue-collar workers. This phenomenon, which is due to the fact that blue-collar workers are likely to have more thorough diagnostic studies and more frequent confirmation by histological examination of neoplasms, has been well described by Greenwald et al. in their study of Kodak Company employees (79).

Scientific interest in parental occupation as a risk factor for childhood cancer dates back to the early 1970s (80); however, results of studies in this area since then have generally been inconsistent. An interesting situation occurred in a rural county in Ohio, in which primary intracranial tumor was diagnosed in six genetically unrelated children in a recent 2.4-year period; each child had one parent employed by the same company (81). However, cancer-cluster evaluation is difficult because of the few cases, limited availability of complete records, lack of a priori hypotheses, absence of plausible etiological exposures, and highly charged emotional climates.

Reports on the development of gliomas (82) and meningiomas (83) after administration of radiation suggest a possible relation. Ten out of 468 children with acute lymphoblastic leukemia treated with cranial irradiation and intrathecal methotrexate developed central nervous system malignancies (84). Farwell et al. noted an increased incidence of medulloblastoma in the offspring of women who received polio vaccine contaminated with papovavirus SV40 (85). Considering that SV40 is known to cause central nervous system neoplasms in animals, the finding may be relevant.

Associations of adult glioblastoma with a history of head trauma (86) and those childhood brain tumor with either intrauterine or childhood exposure to barbiturates (87) have been suggested.

Central nervous system infections reported to be associated with increased risk of brain tumor include toxoplasmosis (76), tuberculosis (88), and viral infections, such as those with adenovirus, papovavirus, and retroviruses (89). There is a markedly increased frequency of primary brain lymphoma in patients with acquired immune deficiency syndrome (AIDS) and those receiving prolonged immunosuppression therapy (52). However, case–control and cohort studies from Rochester, Minnesota, failed to reveal any significant association of primary brain tumors with head trauma (90,91), childhood exposure to barbiturates (92), family history, psychiatric disorders, central nervous system infections, and cardiovascular, respiratory, or gastrointestinal disorders (93).

II. SECONDARY BRAIN TUMORS

Metastasis to the brain is the most common structural neurological complication of systemic cancer and is second only to metabolic encephalopathies as a cause of central nervous system dysfunction in cancer patients (94). Approximately 80% of the brain metastases are found in the cerebral hemispheres, 10–15% in the cerebellum, and 2–3% in the brain stem (95). With modern neuroimaging techniques and more careful autopsy studies of cancer patients, it is becoming clear that brain metastases as a group are actually the most common intracranial tumors and slightly outnumber primary brain tumors in the population (22). In addition, the frequency of brain metastasis may be increasing because of longer survival of cancer patients in general.

The National Survey conducted during 1973–1974 remains the most comprehensive data available on brain metastasis (22). This study provided an average annual incidence rate of 8.3:100,000 (9.7 for men and 7.1 for women). The age-specific incidence rapidly rose after 35 years and was more precipitous in men than in women (Fig. 9). Metastasis from bronchogenic carcinoma, the most common primary source, represented an annual incidence rate of 6.1 for men

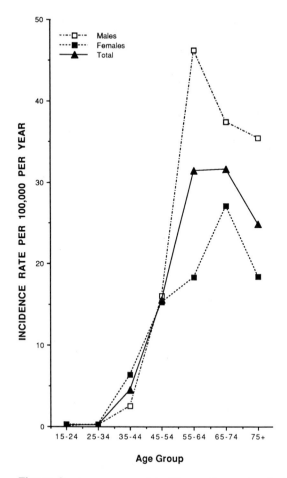

Figure 9   Average annual incidence of secondary brain tumors by age and sex in the National Survey.

and 2.2 for women per 100,000 population. Excluding a large number of unspecified primary sites, the percentage distribution of brain metastases by site of primary neoplasm, based on the data from the National Survey (22), is shown in Figure 10.

III. SUMMARY

There has been a wealth of information concerning the epidemiology of brain tumors in the last three decades. The average annual age-adjusted incidence rate of primary brain tumor is about 10:100,000 per year. For all the histological types combined, males outnumber females; however, meningiomas are more frequent in females. The annual incidence of gliomas is 6–7:100,000 and of meningiomas is 3–4:100,000 population. The age-specific incidence of primary brain tumors increases steadily with age. The reported decline in the age-specific incidence after 75 years probably reflects an underascertainment of these lesions in the very elderly.

The recently reported increase in the incidence of primary brain tumors, especially in the elderly, may be largely related to the emergence of noninvasive neurodiagnostic techniques and better medical care for the elderly population. Primary brain tumors constitute the most common type of solid tumor in the pediatric age group. Case–control studies have shown inconsistent results

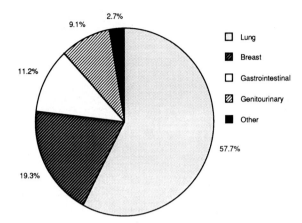

Figure 10 Percentage distribution of brain metastases by site of primary neoplasm from the National Survey.

for the association of genetic, occupational, and other environmental factors associated with primary brain tumors.

Although brain metastases outnumber primary brain tumors in the population, epidemiological data on metastatic intracranial tumors are sparse.

REFERENCES

1. Kurtzke JF, Kurland LT. The epidemiology of neurologic disease. In: Joynt RJ, ed. Clinical neurology, vol. 4. Philadelphia: JB Lippincott, 1983:1–143.
2. Schoenberg BS. Neuroepidemiology. Incidents, incidence, and coincidence. Arch Neurol 1977; 34:261–265.
3. Kurland LT. Geography of neural tumors. In: Minckler J, ed. Pathology of the nervous system, vol 3. New York: McGraw-Hill, 1972:2803–2808.
4. Bourke GJ, McGilvray J. Interpretation and uses of medical statistics. London: Blackwell Scientific Publications, 1975:125–129.
5. Cancer Statistics, 1988. CA-A 1988; 38:5–22.
6. Percy AK, Elveback LR, Okazaki H, Kurland LT. Neoplasms of the central nervous system: epidemiologic considerations. Neurology 1972; 22:40–48.
7. Kernohan JW, Sayre GP. Tumors of the central nervous system. Washington DC: Armed Forces Institute of Pathology, 1952.
8. Ringertz N. Grading of gliomas. Acta Pathol Microbiol Scand 1950; 27:51–64.
9. Zulch KJ. Histological typing of tumors of the central nervous system. Geneva: World Health Organization, 1979.
10. Burger PC. Malignant astrocytic neoplasms: classification, pathological anatomy and response to treatment. Semin Oncol 1986; 13:16–26.
11. Geyer JR, Berger M. Central nervous system malignancies in children. NY State J Med 1990; 90: 601–608.
12. Annegers JF, Schoenberg BS, Okazaki H, Kurland LT. Epidemiologic study of primary intracranial neoplasms. Arch Neurol 1981; 38:217–219.
13. Kinkel W. Computerized tomography in clinical neurology. In: Joynt RJ, ed. Clinical neurology, vol. 1. Philadelphia: JB Lippincott, 1991:1–115.
14. Bronen RA, Sze G. Magnetic resonance imaging contrast agents: theory and application to the central nervous system. J Neurosurg 1990; 73:820–839.

15. Bahemuka M. Worldwide incidence of primary nervous system neoplasms. Geographical, racial and sex differences, 1960–1977. Brain 1988; 111:737–755.
16. McLendon RE, Robinson JS, Chambers DB, Grufferman S, Burger PC. The glioblastoma multiforme in Georgia, 1977–1981. Cancer 1985; 56:894–897.
17. Heshmat MY, Kovi J, Simpson C, Kennedy J, Fan K-J. Neoplasms of the central nervous system: incidence and population selectivity in the Washington, DC, metropolitan area. Cancer 1976; 38:2135–2142.
18. Preston-Martin S. Descriptive epidemiology of primary tumors of the brain, cranial nerves and cranial meninges in Los Angeles County. Neuroepidemiology 1989; 8:283–295.
19. Velema JP, Walker AM. The age curve of nervous system tumor incidence in adults: common shape but changing levels by sex, race and geographical location. Int J Epidemiol 1987; 16:177–183.
20. Schoenberg BS, Christine BW, Whisnant JP. The descriptive epidemiology of primary intracranial neoplasms: the Connecticut experience. Am J Epidemiol 1976; 104:499–510.
21. Biometry Branch, National Cancer Institute. Third National Cancer Survey: incidence data. National Cancer Institute monograph 41. [DHEW publication no. (NIH)75-787]. Bethesda MD: National Institutes of Health, 1975:17,21,25.
22. Walker AE, Robins M, Weinfeld FD. Epidemiology of brain tumors: the national survey of intracranial neoplasms. Neurology 1985; 35:219–226.
23. Surveillance Epidemiology End Results (SEER). Incidence and mortality data, 1973–1977. National Cancer Institute monograph 57. [DHEW publication no. (NIH)81-2330]. Bethesda MD: National Institutes of Health, 1981:158,305,1036,1042.
24. Preston-Martin S, Henderson BE, Peters JM. Descriptive epidemiology of central nervous system neoplasms in Los Angeles County. Ann NY Acad Sci 1982; 381:202–208.
25. Kurland LT. The frequency of intracranial and intraspinal neoplasms in the resident population of Rochester, Minnesota. J Neurosurg 1958; 15:627–641.
26. Kurland LT, Molgaard CA. The patient record in epidemiology. Sci Am 1981; 245(4):54–63.
27. Schoenberg BS, Christine BW, Whisnant JP. The resolution of discrepancies in the reported incidence of primary brain tumors. Neurology 1978; 28:817–823.
28. Kurland LT, Schoenberg BS, Annegers JF, Okazaki H, Molgaard CA. The incidence of primary intracranial neoplasms in Rochester, Minnesota, 1935–1977. Ann NY Acad Sci 1982; 381:6–16.
29. Lovaste MG, Ferrari G, Rossi G. Epidemiology of primary intracranial neoplasms. Experiment in the province of Trento (Italy), 1977–1984. Neuroepidemiology 1986; 5:220–232.
30. Joensen P. Incidence of primary intracranial neoplasms in an isolated population (the Faroese) during the period 1962–1975. Acta Neurol Scand 1981; 64:74–78.
31. Fogelholm R, Uutela T, Murros K. Epidemiology of central nervous system neoplasms. A regional survey in Central Finland. Acta Neurol Scand 1984; 69:129–136.
32. Lona C, Tabiadon G, Dossi BC, Moshenipour I. Incidence of primary intracranial tumors in the province of Bolzano, 1980–1984. Ital J Neurol Sci 1988; 9:237–241.
33. Velema JP, Percy CL. Age curves of central nervous system tumor incidence in adults: variation of shape by histologic type. JNCI 1987; 79:623–629.
34. Levi F, Vecchia CL, Te V. Descriptive epidemiology of malignant brain tumors in the Swiss Canton of Vaud. Neuroepidemiology 1990; 9:135–142.
35. Codd MB, Kurland LT. Descriptive epidemiology of primary intracranial neoplasms. Prog Exp Tumor Res 1985; 29:1–11.
36. Rosenfeld SS, Massey EW. Epidemiology of primary brain tumor. In: Anderson DW, ed. Neuroepidemiology: a tribute to Bruce Schoenberg. Boca Raton: CRC Press, 1991:121–143.
37. Abu-Salih AS, Abdul-Rahman AM. Tumors of the brain in the Sudan. Surg Neurol 1988; 29:194–196.
38. Kallio M. The incidence of intracranial gliomas in southern Finland. Acta Neurol Scand 1988; 78:480–483.
39. Spännare BJ. Supraterritorial astrocytomas grade III and IV in adult patients. A prospective study of incidence, survival, quality of survival (Karnofsky rating), terminal course of the disease and prognostic factors. Acta Univ Ups 1981; 388–397.

40. Barker DJP, Weller RO, Garfield JS. Epidemiology of primary tumors of the brain and spinal cord: a regional survey in southern England. J Neurol Neurosurg Psychiatry 1976; 39:290–296.

41. Cohen A, Modan B. Some epidemiologic aspects of neoplastic diseases in Israeli immigrant populations. III. Brain tumors. Cancer 1968; 22:1323–1328.

42. Gudmundsen KR. A survey of tumors of the central nervous system in Iceland during the 10-year period 1954–1963. Acta Neurol Scand 1970; 46:538–552.

43. Rohringer M, Sutherland GR, Louw DF, Sima AAF. Incidence and clinicopathological features of meningioma. J Neurosurg 1989; 71:665–672.

44. Nakasu S, Hirano A, Shimura T, Llena JF. Incidental meningioma in autopsy study. Surg Neurol 1987; 27:319–322.

45. Gold EB. Epidemiology of pituitary adenomas. Epidemiol Rev 1981; 3:163–183.

46. Annegers JF, Coulam CB, Abboud CF, Laws ER Jr, Kurland LT. Pituitary adenoma in Olmsted County, Minnesota, 1935–1977: a report of an increasing incidence of diagnosis in women of childbearing age. Mayo Clin Proc 1978; 53:641–643.

47. Burrow GN, Wortzman G, Rewcastle NB, Holgate RC, Kovacs K. Microadenomas of the pituitary and abnormal sellar tomograms in an unselected autopsy series. N Engl J Med 1981; 304:156–158.

48. Robinson N, Beral V, Ashley JSA. Incidence of pituitary adenoma in women [letter]. Lancet 1979; 2:630.

49. Chang RJ, Keye WR Jr, Young JR, Wilson CB, Jaffe RB. Detection, evaluation and treatment of pituitary microadenomas in patients with galactorrhea and amenorrhea. Am J Obstet Gynecol 1977; 128:356–363.

50. Davajan V, Kletzky O, March CM, Ray S, Mishell DR Jr. The significance of galactorrhea in patients with normal menses, oligomenorrhea, and secondary amenorrhea. Am J Obstet Gynecol 1978; 130: 894–904.

51. Coulam CB, Annegers JF, Abboud CF, Laws ER Jr, Kurland LT. Pituitary adenoma and oral contraceptives: a case–control study. Fertil Steril 1979; 31:25–28.

52. DeAngelis LM. Primary central nervous system lymphoma: a new clinical challenge. Neurology 1991; 41:619–621.

53. Eby NL, Grufferman S, Flannelly CM, Schold SC, Vogel FS, Burger PC. Increasing incidence of primary brain lymphoma in the U.S. Cancer 1988; 62:2461–2465.

54. Goldberg ID, Kurland LT. Mortality in 33 countries from diseases of the nervous system. World Neurol 1962; 3:444–465.

55. Bahemuka M, Massey EW, Schoenberg BS. International mortality from primary nervous system neoplasms: distribution and trends. Int J Epidemiol 1988; 17:33–38.

56. Davis DL, Ahlbom A, Hoel D, Percy C. Is brain cancer mortality increasing in industrial countries? Am J Ind Med 1991; 19:421–431.

57. Greig NH, Ries LG, Yancik R, Rapoport SI. Increasing annual incidence of primary malignant brain tumors in the elderly. JNCI 1990; 82:1621–1624.

58. Boyle P, Maisonneuve P, Saracci R, Muir CS. Is the increased incidence of primary malignant brain tumors in the elderly real? JNCI 1990; 82:1594–1596.

59. Levi F, LaVecchia C. Trends in brain cancer [letter]. Lancet 1989; 2:917.

60. Ahlbom A, Redvall Y. Brain tumor trends [letter]. Lancet 1989; 2:12–72.

61. Young JL, Miller RW, Incidence of malignant tumors in U.S. children. J Pediatr 1975; 86:254–258.

62. Duffner PK, Cohen ME, Myers MH, Heise HW. Survival of children with brain tumors: SEER program, 1973–1980. Neurology 1986; 36:597–601.

63. Pearson D, Steward JK. Malignant disease in juveniles. Proc R Soc Med 1969; 62:685–688.

64. Schoenberg BS, Schoenberg DG, Christine BW, Gomez MR. The epidemiology of primary intracranial neoplasms of childhood. A population study. Mayo Clin Proc 1976; 51:51–56.

65. Lannering B, Marky I, Nordborg C. Brain tumors in childhood and adolescence in West Sweden, 1970–1984. Epidemiology and survival. Cancer 1990; 66:604–609.

66. Preston-Martin S. Epidemiology of childhood brain tumors. Ital J Neurol Sci 1985; 6:403–409.

67. Jooma R, Hayward RD, Grant DN. Intracranial neoplasms during the first year of life: analysis of one hundred consecutive cases. Neurosurgery 1984; 14:31–41.

68. Kjellin K, Muller R, Astrom KE. The occurrence of brain tumors in several members of a family. J Neuropathol Exp Neurol 1960; 19:528–537.
69. Chadduck WM, Netsley MG. Familial gliomas: report of four families with chromosome studies. Neurosurgery 1982; 10:445–449.
70. Challa VR, Goodman HO, Davis CH. Familial brain tumors: studies of two families and review of recent literature. Neurosurgery 1983; 12:18–23.
71. NIH Conference. Neurofibromatosis 1 (Recklinghausen disease) and neurofibromatosis 2 (bilateral acoustic neurofibromatosis). Ann Intern Med 1990; 113:39–52.
72. Huttenlocher PR. Tuberous sclerosis. In: Matthews WB, Glaser GH, eds. Recent advances in clinical neurology, no 4. Edinburgh: Churchill-Livingstone, 1984:281–298.
73. Herrero FA. Neurological manifestations of heritable connective tissue disorders. In: Vinken PJ, Bruyn GW, eds. Handbook of clinical neurology, vol 39. Amsterdam: North-Holland Publishing, 1980:379–481.
74. Selversten B, Cooper DR. Astrocytoma and ABO blood groups. J Neurosurg 1961; 18:602–604.
75. Garcia JH, Okazaki H, Aronson SM. Blood-group frequencies and astrocytoma. J Neurosurg 1963; 20:397–399.
76. Choi CW, Schuman LM, Gulen WH. Epidemiology of primary central nervous system neoplasms. II: Case–control study. Am J Epidemiol 1970; 19:467–485.
77. Thomas TL, Waxweiler RJ. Brain tumors and occupational risk factors. Scand J Work Environ Health 1986; 12:1–15.
78. Musicco M, Sant M, Molinari S, Filippini G, Gatta G, Berrino F. A case–control study of brain gliomas and occupational exposure to chemical carcinogens: the risk to farmers. Am J Epidemiol 1988; 128:778–785.
79. Greenwald P, Friedlander BR, Lawrence CE, Hearne T, Earle K. Diagnostic sensitivity bias: an epidemiologic explanation for an apparent brain tumor excess. J Occup Med 1981; 23:690–694.
80. Fabia J, Thuy TD. Occupation of father at time of birth of children dying of malignant diseases. Br J Prevent Soc Med 1974; 28:98–100.
81. Wilkins JR III, McLaughlin JA, Sinks TH, Kosnik EJ. Parental occupation and intracranial neoplasms of childhood: anecdotal evidence from a unique occupational cancer cluster. Am J Ind Med 1991; 19:643–653.
82. Liwnicz BH, Berger TS, Liwnicz RG, Aron BS. Radiation-associated gliomas: a report of four cases and analysis of postradiation tumors of the central nervous system. Neurosurgery 1985; 17:436–445.
83. Rubinstein AB, Shalit MN, Cohen ML, Zandbank U, Reichenthal E. Radiation-induced cerebral meningioma: a recognizable entity. J Neurosurg 1984; 61:966–971.
84. Miller DR, Abo V, Leiken S, et al. Brain tumors in survivors of childhood acute lymphoblastic leukaemia. In: Proceedings of the International Society of Pediatric Oncology, 17th annual meeting. Budapest, Hungary, 1986:77.
85. Farwell JR, Dohrmann GJ, Flannery JT. Meduloblastoma in childhood: an epidemiological study. J Neurosurg 1984; 61:657–664.
86. Hochberg F, Toniolo P, Cole P. Head trauma and seizures as risk factors of glioblastoma. Neurology 1984; 34:1511–1514.
87. Gold E, Gordis L, Tonascia J, Szklo M. Increased risk of brain tumors in children exposed to barbiturates. JNCI 1978; 61:1031–1034.
88. Ward DW, Mattison ML, Finn R. Association between previous tuberculous infection and cerebral glioma. Br Med J 1973; 1:83–84.
89. Walsh JW, Zimmer SG, Perdue ML. Role of viruses in the induction of primary intracranial tumors. Neurosurgery 1982; 10:643–662.
90. Annegers JF, Laws ER Jr, Kurland LT, Grabow JD. Head trauma and subsequent brain tumors. Neurosurgery 1979; 4:203–206.
91. Codd MB, Kurland LT. Head trauma and seizures as risk factors in tumors of the glioma group [letter]. Neurology 1985; 35:1532–1533.
92. Annegers JF, Kurland LT, Hauser WA. Brain tumors in children exposed to barbiturates [letter]. JNCI 1979; 63:3–64.

93. Codd MB, Kurland LT, O'Fallon WM, Beard CM, Cascino TL. Case–control study of neuroepithelial tumors in Rochester, Minnesota, 1950–1977. Neuroepidemiology 1990; 9:17–26.
94. Patchell RA. Brain metastases. Neurol Clin 1991; 9:817–824.
95. Delattre JY, Krol G, Thaler HT, Posner JB. Distribution of brain metastases. Arch Neurol 1988; 45:741–744.

2

Pathology of Benign Brain Tumors

Yuan Chang
Columbia University College of Physicians and Surgeons,
New York, New York

Dikran S. Horoupian
Stanford University Medical Center, Stanford, California

I. INTRODUCTION

In this chapter, we will limit our descriptions to benign tumors of the central nervous system and some of the non-neoplastic masses that may present as space-occupying lesions. Therefore, we will discuss only the benign meningiomas and hemangiopericytomas, the benign schwannian and choroid plexus tumors, the paragangliomas, the capillary hemangioblastomas, and tumors of developmental origin such as lipomas and various types of cysts.

II. TUMORS OF LEPTOMENINGEAL ORIGIN

A. Meningioma

Meningiomas are the most common benign brain tumors and comprise approximately 15–20% of all intracranial neoplasms (1–3). These tumors originate from the arachnoid cap cells of the leptomeninges and, therefore, can develop wherever leptomeningeal tissue is found in the central nervous system. They have a propensity for location along major sinuses, where arachnoid villi are found in abundance. The most frequent sites of occurrence include the parasagittal region, the sphenoid ridge, and the convexity (Figs. 1–3). Other important, but less common, locations include the sellar region, the cerebellopontine angle, the olfactory groove, the optic nerve sheath, and the foramen magnum. Intraventricular meningiomas are derived from arachnoid cap cells found within the stroma of the choroid plexus or in the tela choroidea.

Meningiomas have a proclivity for the fifth and sixth decades. In this age group, there is a definite female preponderance, with the female/male ratio approaching 2 : 1 (4). However, in the very young and the very elderly, the sex distribution is even. The increased frequency of meningiomas in women in the middle age group has been postulated to be the result of a sustained and prolonged hormonal effect. Such conjecture is supported by some of the clinical features of meningiomas, in that they grow or display increased symptomatology during pregnancy and are associated with breast carcinoma (5–8). In addition, experimental studies demonstrate the presence

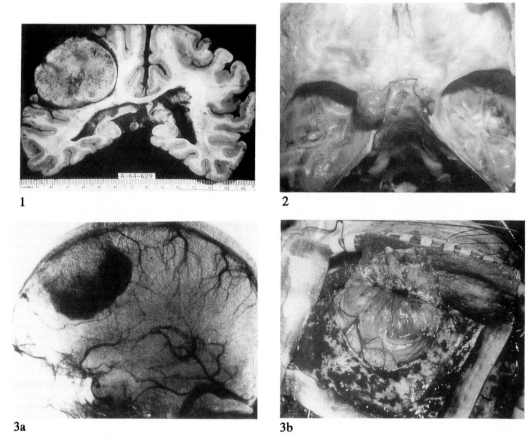

1   2

3a   3b

Figure 1   Large convexity meningioma with variegated cut surface indenting into the compressed parietal lobe.

Figure 2   Small meningioma at medial portion of the sphenoid ridge, found incidentally at autopsy.

Figure 3   (a) Angiogram of frontal parasagittal meningioma. (b) Intraoperative appearance of this meningioma showing broad-based attachment to dura. (Courtesy Dr. G. Steinberg)

of functional progesterone and estrogen receptors in meningiomas (9,10). Predisposing factors, such as trauma and radiation to the skull, have also been related to the development of meningiomas. Finally, genetic abnormalities are implicated in the pathogenesis of some meningiomas: tumor cells frequently have partial or complete deletion of chromosome 22 (11). Furthermore, meningiomas are included in the diagnostic criteria for neurofibromatosis 2, a genetic disorder (12).

Characteristically, meningiomas are well-circumscribed globoid masses with bosselated surfaces (Fig. 4). They are tenaciously adherent to the dura by a broad base and derive their vascular supply from dural vessels (Fig. 5). Meningiomas usually indent or compress the underlying brain tissue, causing pressure atrophy. True invasion into neural parenchyma with breaching of the pial membrane is not seen except with malignant transformation. On the other hand, infiltration into dura and dural sinuses is very common. Even extension into overlying bone and into subcutaneous soft tissues can occur and is not a harbinger of poor outcome (Figs. 6,7). Occasionally, meningiomas can be flat, with a planar growth pattern, and are referred to as *meningioma en plaque*. These tumors are usually found in the lateral third of the sphenoid ridge and have a

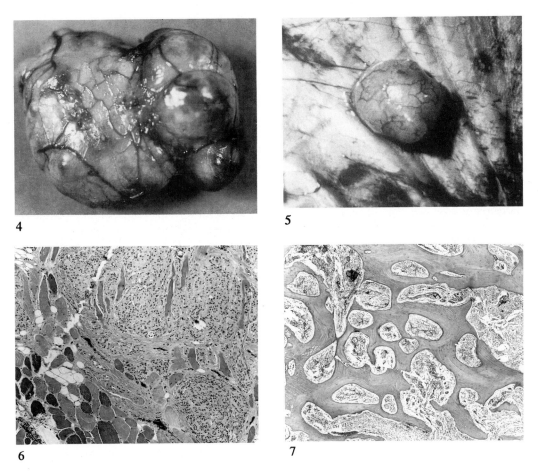

Figure 4 Bosselated, irregular surface of excised meningioma.
Figure 5 Small, incidental meningioma removed with the dura at autopsy.
Figure 6 Cytologically benign meningioma infiltrating the temporalis muscle.
Figure 7 Marrow space of bone infiltrated by meningioma, with associated fibrous reaction.

particular tendency to develop in women. Multiple meningiomas may be seen, frequently associated with neurofibromatosis 2.

Meningiomas are firm, solid tumors, with a gray, lobulated surface on cut section. Increased vascularity results in an accentuated red-brown hue and the presence of psammoma bodies imparts a gritty consistency. Metaplastic or degenerative changes occurring within the tumor result in a variegated gross appearance, with areas of red-brown representing hemorrhage, or with streaks of yellow, indicating lipidization. Cystic change is uncommon, but may also be encountered. Necrosis is not seen, unless the tumor has become so large that it focally outgrows its blood supply, or in the event of malignant transformation.

Historically, numerous schema have been used for the classification of meningiomas. In 1931, Bailey and Bucy first proposed dividing meningiomas into nine subgroups (13). Then in 1938, Cushing and Eisenhardt expanded the subgroups to 22 (14). More recently, in 1979, the World Health Organization (WHO) reduced the subgroups again to nine (15). Recognition that meningiomas can present a myriad of appearances, which may create diagnostic difficulties, underlies the lengthier classification schemata. However, no correlation between clinical prognosis and any particular histological subgroup has been found, except for what has traditionally been referred to as the angioblastic meningioma. These have an aggressive clinical behavior and are set apart by their exuberant vascular component, which ranges from networks of small vessels to large sinusoidal channels.

The benign meningiomas can be divided into three major histological patterns: syncytial (meningothelial), fibroblastic, and transitional. These subdivisions are not mutually exclusive and, in reality, represent a continuous spectrum of histological patterns that may be intermingled in the same tumor. Syncytial meningiomas consist preponderantly of polygonal cells, having abundant cytoplasm and indistinct cell boundaries arranged in sheets or whorls (Fig. 8). This propensity for whorl formation is a distinguishing hallmark of meningothelial cells, whether in cell culture or in normal arachnoidea (Fig. 9). The nuclei, which display delicate chromatin and inconspicuous nucleoli, rarely digress from a regular, round–oval shape. However, they may show pronounced variation in size (see Fig. 9). Reticulin fibers encircle nests of tumor cells and are particularly prominent around vessels. Diagnostically helpful features identifiable in meningiomas are intranuclear pseudoinclusions (Fig. 10) and psammoma bodies. The latter are mineralized, concentric structures of varying sizes that can also be seen in normal arachnoid nests. Meningiomas in which large numbers of these structures are present with only small nests of intervening tumor cells are referred to as *psammomatous*, and this variant is especially common in the spine (Fig. 11).

In the fibroblastic meningiomas, tumor cells have long processes that are aligned in parallel sheaths, fascicles, or storiform patterns, reminiscent of fibrous histiocytic tumors (Fig. 12). Nuclei are elongated and compressed, sometimes forming a palisading pattern similar to that encountered in schwannomas. Psammoma bodies are not as abundant as seen in the syncytial type. The transitional meningioma has features intermediate between the syncytial and fibroblastic types. Characteristic whorls are seen, but the cell processes are longer, and cell borders are more distinct, than in the syncytial type.

A large proportion of the variants represent degenerative or metaplastic change within these three types of meningiomas and include the xanthomatous, microcystic (humid), myxoid, secretory (pseudopsammomatous), lipoblastic, chondroblastic, osteoblastic, and melanocytic (melanoblastic) meningiomas. Xanthomatous change is quite common and, if searched for, can be found at least focally in most meningiomas. It is represented by aggregates of cells, with small, centrally placed nuclei and finely dispersed cytoplasmic lipid, having the appearance of foam cells. The origin of these cells is controversial: do they represent macrophages or lipidized tumor cells? Microcystic meningiomas are made up of tumor cells with stellate morphology and loculated collections of intercellular fluid, imparting a loose, fenestrated appearance to the tumor (16). They sometimes have large, grossly visible intratumoral cavities that result from coalescence of microcysts (Fig. 13). Myxoid variants (Fig. 14) display tumor cells surrounded by a prominent, basophilic matrix that contains hyaluronic acid and chondroitin sulfate (17).

Chondroblastic and lipoblastic variants are examples of meningiomas demonstrating metaplastic change, in which constituent cells show differentiation along various mesenchymal cell lines. The secretory variant may represent a meningioma with differentiation along epithelial cell lines. They have tumor cells that contain round intracytoplasmic, eosinophilic bodies which, by electron microscopy, are composed of fine granular material within intracytoplasmic microvilli-lined lumina (18,19). These structures display a wide range in size, may be multiple, and resemble psammoma bodies (Fig. 15). They are positive with periodic acid–schiff (PAS) and mucicarmine stains (20).

Lymphoplasmacytoid meningiomas contain collections of nonneoplastic lymphocytes and plasma cells, which can be limited to perivascular cuffs or may become so extensive that they obscure the underlying meningeal component (Fig. 16). Russell bodies, germinal centers, and

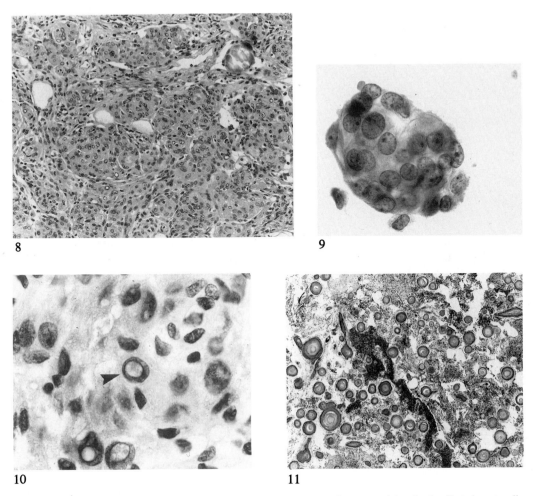

8   9

10   11

Figure 8   Meningiotheliomatous meningioma displaying tumor cells arranged in whorls. Constituent cells appear as syncytium.

Figure 9   Cytological smear preparation of meningioma demonstrating molding of round-to-oval tumor cells to each other in a whorl.

Figure 10   Invagination of cytoplasm into nucleus of meningioma tumor cell (arrow) creating the familiar pseudonuclear inclusion.

Figure 11   Concentric mineralized psammoma bodies found in abundance in an intraspinal meningioma.

amyloid are microscopic features that can be associated with these lymphoplasmacytic infiltrates (21,22). Melanocytic meningiomas are composed of tumor cells that contain melanin pigment, but still display distinguishing characteristics of arachnoidal cells (Fig. 17). These tumors are considered to be different from the benign meningeal melanocytomas, which are derived from leptomeningeal melanophores and are analogous to the cellular blue nevi found in the skin (23).

Immunohistochemically, most meningiomas are positive for epithelial membrane antigen (EMA) and a few show some reactivity to low molecular weight cytokeratin antibodies (24). Vimentin and S-100 protein may also be positive. Leu-7, desmin, neurofilament, and glial fibrillary acidic protein (GFAP) are consistently negative (25,26). The secretory meningiomas may also express carcinoembryonic antigen (CEA) immunogenicity (19). Ultrastructural findings in

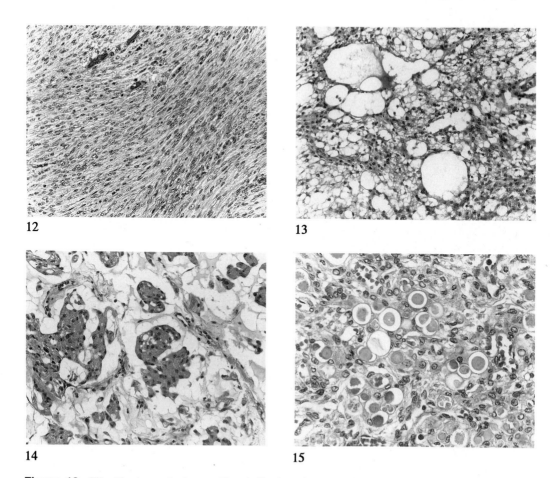

12   13

14   15

Figure 12 Fibroblastic meningioma with spindle-shaped tumor cells arranged in streaming fascicles.
Figure 13 Cysts of various sizes interspersed between tumor cells in a microcystic meningioma.
Figure 14 Islands of myxoid meningioma tumor cells seemingly suspended in basophilic ground substance.
Figure 15 Eosinophilic, spherical material found in the cytoplasm of secretory meningiomas. These structures have a hyalinized appearance and look like psammoma bodies; however, they do not undergo mineralization.

meningiomas are highly characteristic and can be used for diagnostic purposes when light microscopic appearances are atypical. One of the most striking features is the extensive and complex interdigitation of plasma membranes between adjacent cells (Fig. 18). Intercellular connections of various types can be identified, most notably desmosomes, but also gap junctions and tight junctions (27). Tonofilaments and occasional cilia can be identified in the cytoplasm. The intranuclear inclusions seen by light microscopy correspond to membrane-bound cytoplasmic invaginations or pale, chromatin-free areas of loosely floccular nuclear material (2).

Once resected, most meningiomas do not recur. However, in subtotal resection, a variety of histopathological features have been suggested as predictors of recurrence: hypercellularity, necrosis, mitotic activity, nuclear pleomorphism, prominent nucleoli, hemosiderin deposits, hypervascularity, and loss of normal architectural whorling pattern (28). The most important factors in clinical outcome, however, are the localization and resectability of the meningioma.

B. Hemangiopericytoma

Begg and Garrett were the first to report a case of primary intracranial hemangiopericytoma in 1954 (29). Before this time, meningeal hemangiopericytomas were probably categorized as angioblastic meningiomas. Even today, there is still ongoing debate over whether they constitute a distinct entity in the classification of central nervous system neoplasms, or merely represent an aggressive variant of meningioma. Morphological, immunohistochemical, ultrastructural, and tissue culture characteristics have been used on both sides of the argument.

Meningeal hemangiopericytomas have been postulated to arise from a variety of cells including (1) pericytes, which are mesenchymal cells with smooth muscle-like contractile properties located external to endothelial cells in the walls of capillaries and postcapillary venules; (2) arachnoid cap cells, with pericytic divergent differentiation; or (3) multipotential precursor cells, with the capability of giving rise to both meningeal and pericytic tumors. Regardless of exact histogenesis, these tumors recapitulate features attributable to the pericyte and behave clinically in ways that distinguish them from ordinary meningiomas. Hemangiopericytomas are more common in males than in females, present earlier in life than meningiomas, have a significantly shorter duration of symptoms before diagnosis, and have a propensity for local recurrence even with complete resection (30–32). Relative to similarities, hemangiopericytomas occur with a distribution comparable with meningiomas. Most are supratentorial and located parasagittally.

Grossly, hemangiopericytomas are lobulated and vary from pink-gray to red, as a result of their prominent vascularity. Indeed, at surgery, they are remarkable for their tendency to bleed. Their texture is usually firm, but they may occasionally be soft. Histologically, these tumors are highly vascular and exhibit a prominent network of normal-appearing, thin-walled capillaries of varying sizes, with a characteristic staghorn appearance. These channels are lined by flat endothelial cells and are surrounded by masses of closely packed round to oval pericytic-like cells (Fig. 19). The vascular network is particularly pronounced and well outlined by reticulin, which also tends to envelope individual tumor cells. Mitoses can be seen. Whorls and psammoma bodies are absent.

Some of the strongest evidence for separating hemangiopericytomas from meningiomas is based on immunohistochemical studies. Comparisons between central nervous system and extracranial hemangiopericytomas have repeatedly revealed an identical profile, whereas comparison with typical meningiomas have highlighted important differences. Hemangiopericytomas are consistently negative for epithelial membrane antigen and cytokeratins (33). They are positive for vimentin and negative for S-100 protein and GFAP. Occasional tumors are desmin- or actin-positive, reflecting the smooth muscle-like features of pericytes. Factor VIII and *Ulex* stain only the endothelial cells lining the vascular spaces found within these tumors, but never the tumor cells themselves (26,34).

Ultrastructural features of pericytes that are seen in hemangiopericytomas include prominent basal lamina, which may be continuous or interrupted; irregular, long interdigitating cell processes; prominent pinocytic vesicles; poorly formed intercellular junctions; and cytoplasmic filaments (35,36).

C. Meningioangiomatosis

Meningioangiomatosis is a rare malformative lesion characterized by a proliferative process composed of an angiomatous component and a perivascular cellular component (Fig. 20). It is most commonly seen in, but not restricted to, patients with neurofibromatosis 1 (37–39). Patients usually present in the second or third decade with seizures, which resolve following resection of the lesion (40). Grossly, affected areas of the brain show involvement of the leptomeninges by a sharply demarcated plaquelike lesion that is frequently calcified and extends into the underlying cortex (Fig. 21). The latter is firm, rubbery, and may be compressed. Microscopically, a spectrum of histological changes are seen that range between a predominantly angiomatous-like lesion,

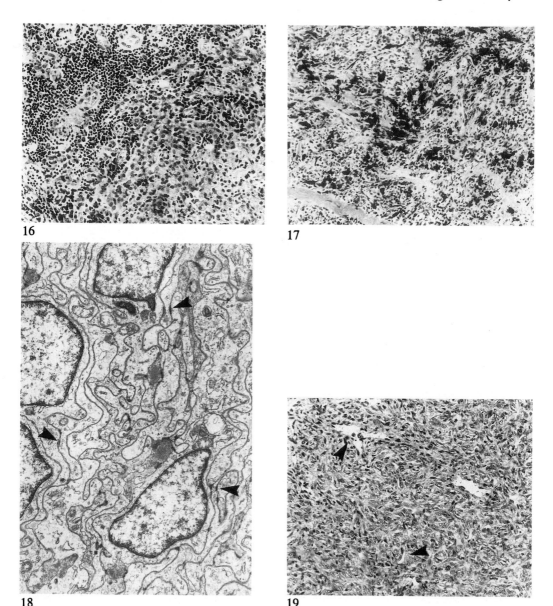

Figure 16   Small lymphocytes and larger plasma cells all but obliterate features of underlying meningioma.
Figure 17   Abundant melanin pigment found in melanocytic meningioma.
Figure 18   Characteristic ultrastructural appearance of meningioma demonstrating intricately interdigitating plasma membranes of tumor cells and intercellular junctions (arrows).
Figure 19   Densely packed, overlapping tumor cells with irregular nuclei in hemangiopericytoma. Vascular channels of various sizes (arrows) are abundantly dispersed throughout the tumor.

containing numerous thick-walled capillaries, and a predominantly cellular lesion, with a proliferation of cells that may form cellular whorls and contain psammoma bodies reminiscent of meningioma. This cellular component has been interpreted as being derived from arachnoid cap cells or, alternatively, from fibroblasts of blood vessel walls. Immunostaining shows that these cells are positive for vimentin, but negative for S-100, GFAP, desmin, factor VIII-related antigen, and low molecular weight keratins (41). In one report, the use of epithelial membrane antigen, a reliable marker for arachnoid cap cells, resulted in negative staining in the perivascular cells (42). Ultrastructural studies have not resolved the issue, since cells with features consistent with both arachnoid cap cells as well as fibroblasts are identifiable.

III. TUMORS OF NERVE SHEATH ORIGIN

A. Schwannoma

Schwannomas, also known as neurilemmomas, are tumors derived from Schwann cells. Intracranially, they account for approximately 7% of all primary tumors (4) and usually originate distal to the glial–schwannian junction of cranial nerves. Almost all arise from the vestibular portion of the eighth nerve. These have been designated as "acoustic" schwannomas and take their origin from within the internal auditory meatus, which becomes enlarged and eroded by the neoplasm. Growth of these schwannomas results in extension into the cerebellopontine angle, where they constitute the bulk of neoplasms found at this site (Fig. 22). Acoustic schwannomas most commonly appear in the fifth and sixth decades, with deafness and tinnitus as the initial symptoms. They occur two to three times more often in women than in men (43). Bilateral occurrence of acoustic schwannomas is diagnostic of neurofibromatosis 2 (44,45). A smaller percentage of intracranial schwannomas originate from the trigeminal and facial nerves and, more rarely, in the oculomotor, trochlear, and hypoglossal nerves (46,47). Infrequently reported intracerebral, intracerebellar, and brain stem examples are believed to arise from ectopic intraparenchymal nests of Schwann cells (48–52). In the spinal cord, they arise from the spinal roots and rarely occur intra-axially. In the peripheral nervous system, they are often solitary and may be present in plexi as well as in cutaneous nerves.

Schwannomas are firm, oval-to-fusiform tumors, with a smooth or bosselated surface. They are eccentrically attached to nerves with adherent fibers stretched over their surface and incorporated into their connective tissue capsule. Small tumors can have a few haphazardly oriented unmyelinated neurites coursing through their substance, which either represent entrapped nerves or regenerating sprouts. Cut surfaces are white to gray and homogeneous; hemorrhages, xanthomatous change, and cystic degeneration may be seen in larger schwannomas.

Microscopically, schwannomas have a distinctive biphasic pattern. These two different histological zones, designated Antoni A and B, are distinguished by differing cytological appearances and architectural arrangement (Fig. 23a). Antoni A regions are populated by compactly grouped, spindle-shaped cells with long, thickly fibrillated processes (See Fig. 23b). These may form sweeping fascicles, interlacing bundles, or even whorls similar to meningiomas. Nuclei are elongated or cigar-shaped and frequently indented. Chromatin is variably dispersed, and nucleoli are not prominent. A characteristic feature, not always found in intracranial schwannomas, is focal alignment of tumor cell nuclei in a linear configuration, referred to as palisading (Fig. 24). Formations made up of anucleated zones of elongated cytoplasmic processes, encircled by these parallel rows of palisading nuclei, are called *Verocay bodies*.

Antoni B regions are looser and contain stellate cells, with round, centrally placed nuclei and vacuolated cytoplasm. These areas are particularly prone to secondary degenerative changes, including xanthomatous transformation, mucoid degeneration, calcification, and cystic replacement of tissues (Figs. 25 and 26). Cysts may attain such large proportions that the actual tumor becomes only a compressed shell surrounding a cavity. These cystic cavities are filled with proteinaceous fluid, which may leak into the cerebrospinal fluid and elevate protein values. Secondary vascular changes are frequent and include hyalinization of vessel walls, sinusoidal dilatation, thrombosis, and hemorrhage, with resultant hemosiderin deposition.

Histological variations on the theme exist. Schwannomas that are composed strictly of Antoni A-type tissue, having densely packed nuclei, are called *cellular schwannomas*. These are not believed to have any higher potential for anaplastic change, which is an exceptional occurrence in

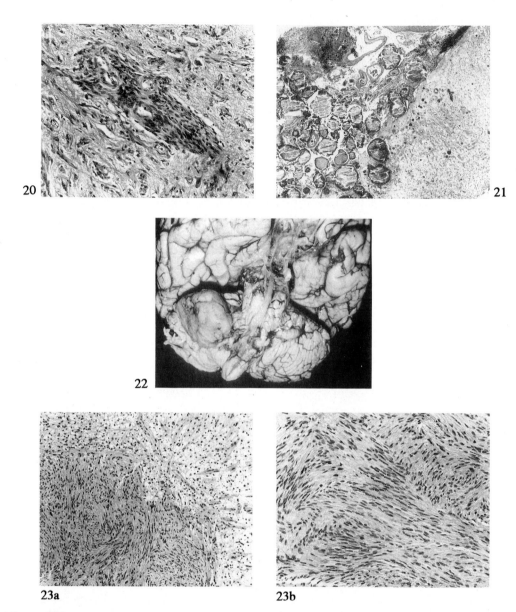

20

21

22

23a   23b

Figure 20 Angiomatous-like array of vessels within cortex in meningioangiomatosis. Some vessels are surrounded by a proliferation of cells thought to be of arachnoidal or fibroblastic derivation.

Figure 21 Meningioangiomatosis with calcified, thick-walled meningeal vessels overlying and extending into cortex.

Figure 22 Large schwannoma of cerebellopontine angle.

Figure 23 (a) Characteristic biphasic appearance of schwannoma, with cellular Antoni A tissue juxtaposed next to loose Antoni B tissue. (b) Compactly arranged spindled cells in Antoni A tissue.

intracranial schwannomas. Some schwannomas can have very pleomorphic nuclei that may be enlarged, hyperchromatic, and even multinucleate. These are referred to as *ancient schwannomas*, and the worrisome cytological features are changes of a degenerative, not malignant, nature. Melanotic schwannomas are distinguished by the presence of intracellular melanin. Despite their varied histological appearances, all schwannomas are immunohistochemically positive for S-100 protein, a property helpful in their differential diagnosis from fibrous lesions (53). Reticulin stains reveal a fine network of positively staining fibers investing each individual cell, a feature that distinguishes them from meningiomas. Mast cells, when identified, can also support the nerve sheath origin of these tumors.

Ultrastructurally, type A tissues show tightly packed, thin cell processes, surrounded by a continuous basal lamina. The stroma contains sparse basement membrane material and long-spacing collagen (Luse bodies), with a banding periodicity of 125–150 nm (54), which differs from that encountered in most connective tissues (Fig. 27). Cell junctions are rare and poorly formed. Cells from type B tissue are also surrounded by a basal lamina, but they have more abundant cytoplasmic organelles. In addition, the extracellular compartment is more prominent. The en-

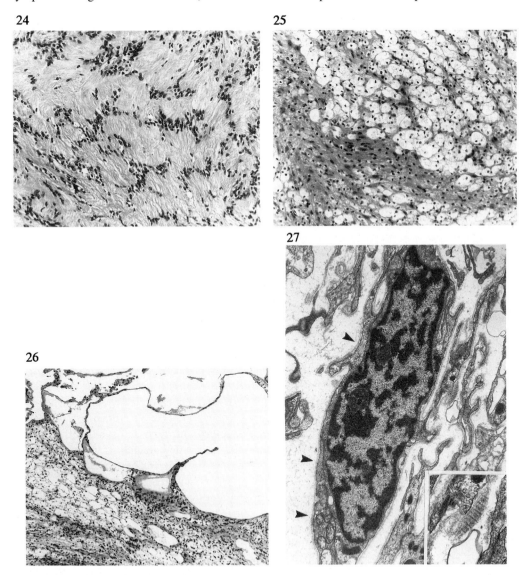

Figure 24 Parallel rows of palisading nuclei in schwannoma.

Figure 25 Focal xanthomatous degeneration in schwannoma. Xanthoma cells have small, centrally placed nuclei and foamy cytoplasm.

Figure 26 Cystic degeneration with replacement of tissue in schwannoma.

Figure 27 Tumor cell from schwannoma demonstrating continuous basal lamina (arrows). Insert shows long-spacing collagen or Luce body, which can be found in these tumors.

dothelial cells in blood vessels of schwannomas, in contrast with the blood vessels of normal peripheral nerves, are fenestrated and lack tight junctions.

Schwannomas are slowly growing tumors that enlarge at an average rate of 0.2 cm/yr. Interestingly, residual tumors appear to have a more indolent growth rate postoperatively, and some even become dormant (55). Microscopic remnants of tumors in cranial nerves do not develop into recurrences, as shown after extended follow-up periods (56). It is thought that this may be due to disruption of the vascular supply as a result of surgery. Thus, although total resection is the operation of choice, subtotal resection may be considered in certain situations for which preservation of nerve function is desired. Recurrences usually declare themselves within 8 years postoperatively (57).

B. Neurofibroma

Neurofibromas show strong association with neurofibromatosis type 1 (45), and are located in small dermal or subcutaneous nerves, major nerve plexi, and spinal nerves. Extension of tumors from the paraspinal nerve roots into the spinal canal results in dumbbell shaped masses that may cause symptoms of cord compression. In contrast with schwannomas, neurofibromas are not well encapsulated and grow in an infiltrative manner into the nerves with which they are associated. Microscopically, wavy cords of spindle-shaped cells, with fine threadlike processes and dark elongated nuclei are loosely arranged in a myxoid stroma containing variable amounts of collagen fibers (Fig. 28). Ultrastructural examination reveals an excess proliferation of a mixture of Schwann cells, perineurial cells, and fibroblasts (58).

IV. TUMORS OF THE CHOROID PLEXUS

A. Choroid Plexus Papilloma

Choroid plexus papillomas (CPP) are rare tumors found preponderantly in the pediatric population, where they account for 3.0–5.0% of intracranial tumors (59–61). With increasing age, there is a sharp dropoff in incidence rates and, in adults, CPP accounts for 0.4–0.6% (59,62,63) of intracranial tumors. These tumors derive from choroid plexus epithelium and may be found anywhere in the ventricular system. There is, however, a peculiar site preference as a function of age. In children, the lateral ventricles are more commonly involved. In contrast, choroid plexus papillomas of adults are found most frequently in the fourth ventricle. The third ventricle is a rare site for both age groups (60,64). Extraventricular CPP are uncommon. Almost all of these are found in adults at the cerebellopontine angle and arise from choroid plexus normally present at the lateral recesses. These cerebellopontine angle tumors present with signs and symptoms similar to other mass lesions found at this site, including cerebellar ataxia and deficits of any of the cranial nerves V through X. Concurrent involvement of multiple sites, extension from one ventricular space to another, as well as seeding from a primary lesion can occur.

Papillomas are soft, friable, pink-gray to red-brown cauliflower-like growths that are frequently pedunculated and have a vascular stalk. Microscopically, papillomas resemble normal choroid, except that they have profuse, delicate papillae. These frondlike projections are lined by simple cuboidal to pseudostratified columnar epithelium, with oval, basally located nuclei (Fig. 29). The epithelial cells are spaced more compactly than in the normal choroid plexus and may contain PAS-positive, diastase-resistant material. Mitoses are absent or very rare. The stromal core of the papillae consists of loose fibrovascular connective tissue that may contain psammoma bodies. In addition to a papillary configuration, CPP can also be focally or predominantly acinar (65). Epithelia may undergo oncocytic transformation (66) or may contain neuromelanin (67).

Immunohistochemical studies show that papilloma tumor cells do not reliably express transthyretin antigenicity, even though the normal choroid epithelium is a site of synthesis for this protein and shows strong immunoreactivity for it (68). The focal anomalous expression of GFAP in some of these tumors has been interpreted as focal glial, perhaps ependymal, divergent differentiation, consistent with the ontogenetic derivation of the choroid plexus (69,70). A subset of papillomas also express low molecular weight cytokeratins (71,72). Ultrastructurally, tumor cells have features similar to normal choroid epithelium. Clusters of microvilli are present at the free surface. The lateral surfaces show interdigitation of membranes and have tight junctions near the luminal end. Nuclei are round to oval, containing fine granular chromatin and small inconspicuous nuclei. Cytoplasmic glycogen is abundant (73,74).

The clinical presentation is most often related to hydrocephalus and increased intracranial pressure. The hydrocephalus has been attributed variably to overproduction of cerebrospinal fluid (CSF) caused by the increased epithelial surface area of papillomas, obstruction of CSF pathways by tumor, and decreased absorption of CSF, secondary to the high protein content or spontaneous hemorrhage associated with these neoplasms (75,76). Although results of a CSF examination may be normal, frequently there is high opening pressure with xanthochromia and high protein content. Recent follow-up of surgical series suggests that total resection alone is adequate to prevent recurrence, with radiation reserved only for recurrent cases (61,77).

B. Choroid Plexus Xanthogranuloma

Xanthogranulomas of the choroid plexus are relatively common findings in the lateral ventricles, and more than half are bilateral. The great majority are small and are discovered as incidental findings at autopsy; however, a few symptomatic cases caused by blockage of the foramen of Monro, with resulting hydrocephalus and increased intracranial pressure, have been reported (78,79). Xanthogranulomas are yellow, rubbery, nodular masses embedded within the choroid plexus. The cut surface shows a thin, circumferential yellow rim surrounding a rust-brown central portion. Microscopically, the yellow rim corresponds to aggregates of xanthoma cells, which have been postulated to develop either from a xanthomatous transformation of invaginating choroid plexus epithelium or from lipid accumulation in the stromal cells of the choroid plexus. Within the central portion of the mass, a granulomatous reaction, with cholesterol clefts surrounded by multinucleated giant cells of foreign-body type, chronic inflammatory cells, fibroblasts, abundant erythrocytes, and hemosiderin, can be identified (Fig. 30). Focal calcification is sometimes seen.

C. Miscellaneous Choroid Plexus Stromal Tumors

Of the choroid plexus stromal neoplasms, the most common is the meningioma, which has features of those found elsewhere in the central nervous system. Other benign neoplasms reported include lipomas and chondromas (80–82). Cysts of the choroid plexus, not associated with any neoplasms, are almost exclusively found in the choroid plexus of the lateral ventricles, where they may be bilateral or multiple. Although they are usually small, they may become large, without causing symptoms. Individual cysts are unilocular and lie within the densely hyalinized and thickened stroma of the glomus. There is no cell lining. The cyst fluid is clear and colorless.

V. MISCELLANEOUS TUMORS OF THE CENTRAL NERVOUS SYSTEM

A. Paraganglioma

Paragangliomas (chemodectomas) of the central nervous system arise from chemoreceptor cells of the intravagal and branchiomeric parasympathetic systems. These include the carotid bodies, the glomus jugulare, the glomus tympanicum, and the vagal body. Paragangliomas usually present between the fourth and sixth decades as isolated lesions; however, multiple as well as familial cases have been reported (83,84). An approximately tenfold increase in prevalence has been found at high altitudes and is attributed to hypoxia-induced hyperplasia of nests of paraganglion cells (84–88).

Paragangliomas are firm, tan-pink, encapsulated tumors that can be intimately attached to adjacent vessels and difficult to excise. Microscopically, they are made up of large monomorphous, round or polygonal cells arranged in a distinctive nesting pattern (*Zellballen*) (Fig. 31). Tumor cells have granular cytoplasms that are positive with the Grimelius stain and immunoreactive with neuron-specific enolase, synaptophysin, and chromogranin. These cytoplasmic granules correspond ultrastructurally to dense-core neurosecretory granules. The nuclei are round and regular; however, nuclear pleomorphism may be seen and is not indicative of malignancy. Mitoses are rare and may presage anaplastic behavior if encountered with any significant frequency. The characteristic architectural nesting pattern is formed by groups of tumor cells surrounded

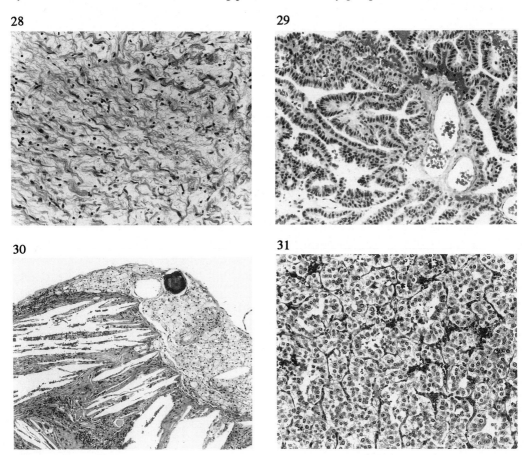

Figure 28   Wavy, spindle-shaped cells loosely arranged in neurofibroma.
Figure 29   Dense papillary fronds in choroid plexus papilloma lined by crowded epithelial cells that still display a sense of polarity. No marked atypical mitotic activity is identifiable.
Figure 30   Choroid plexus xanthogranuloma featuring abundant cholesterol clefts surrounded by giant cells. A rim of xanthoma cells is located peripherally.
Figure 31   Paraganglioma containing round-to-polygonal cells with abundant granular cytoplasm disposed in a characteristic nesting pattern (*Zellballen*).

by richly vascularized fibrous septae containing inconspicuous, spindle-shaped sustentacular cells that are S-100 positive (89).

Although most paragangliomas are benign and not functionally active, symptomatology can arise as the expanding tumor mass encroaches on adjacent structures. Paragangliomas of the glomus jugulare and vagal body can cause 9th, 10th, and 11th nerve palsies (jugular foramen syndrome), as well as invade the labyrinth. Glomus tympanicum tumors occur in the middle ear and usually produce conductive hearing loss, tinnitus, and facial weakness. Aggressive tumors may extend into the posterior fossa, especially in the region of the cerebellopontine angle, and compress the brain stem.

B. Granular Cell Tumor

In the central nervous system, granular cell tumors usually arise in the tuber cinereum and posterior pituitary; however, a few cases have been associated with cranial nerves or described in an intracerebral location, in which case, they are malignant. These tumors have the same light, immunohistochemical, and electron microscopic features of granular cell tumors found elsewhere in the body. They are composed of a uniform population of plump, round-to-polygonal cells with small regular nuclei and abundant, granular eosinophilic cytoplasm. The cytoplasmic granules are PAS-positive, diastase-resistant. With the electron microscope, the granules are seen to be membrane-bound and contain electron-dense amorphous material. Although vimentin, keratin, and S-100 may be variably expressed, peanut lectin appears to be consistently positive in immunohistochemical studies of these tumors (90). The GFAP positivity is seen in the intracerebral granular cell tumors that are malignant (91,92).

As in peripheral granular cell tumors, there has been much speculation concerning cell origin. It appears that these tumors are probably a manifestation of degenerative change that can occur in a variety of cell lines. The intracerebral ones are thought to derive from astrocytes in a gradual process of degradation of intermediate filaments and formation of "autophagic cytosegrosomes" (19). Those that are associated with cranial nerves are thought to derive from Schwann cells (93,94).

VI. BENIGN LESIONS OF VASCULAR ORIGIN

A. Capillary Hemangioblastoma

Capillary hemangioblastomas constitute approximately 1% of all intracranial tumors (4). The vast majority arise in the posterior fossa where they comprise approximately 10% of all primary tumors (95,96). They usually occur in the cerebellum and are paravermal, but about 10–15% are located midline in the vermis (97). In the brain stem, hemangioblastomas commonly arise from the area postrema of the medulla. They can be single or multiple and, if multiple, a genetic background of von Hippel–Lindau syndrome should be considered. They may occur at any age, but are usually found between the third and fifth decades. Children are rarely affected. A male preponderance of 2 : 1 is noted (97). As a neoplasm included in the spectrum of phakomatosis of von Hippel–Lindau syndrome, they can be associated with retinal hemangioblastoma (von Hippel's disease), renal cell carcinoma, pancreatic and renal cysts, cystadenomas of mesosalpinx and epididymis, and adrenal pheochromocytomas (98). (See Chap. 18.)

These tumors have a variable gross appearance. They range from solid neoplasms, with indistinct margins, to cystic lesions, with discrete, small mural nodules (Fig. 32). The solid component is red to yellow as a result of blood and lipid components, whereas cyst fluid, if present, is yellow to brown. The microscopic diagnosis hinges on the identification of a vascular neoplasm with two cellular components (Fig. 33). The first consists of small perivascular endothelial cells with dark, contracted nuclei and sparse cytoplasm. The second consist of "stromal" cells with numerous vacuoles or granular eosinophilic cytoplasm that is usually rich in neutral lipids and may contain glycogen (Fig. 34). These stromal cells may show nuclear pleomorphism; however, mitotic figures are rare. Some difficulty in diagnosing capillary hemangioblastoma arises from the variable proportion of these two cell populations, which can differ markedly from tumor to tumor. Reticulin stain accentuates the sinusoidal spaces and discloses the highly vascular nature of the tumor. Occasionally, extramedullary hematopoeisis can be found within these tumors and is associated with increased levels of erythropoietin.

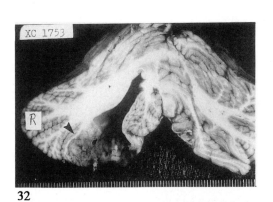

32

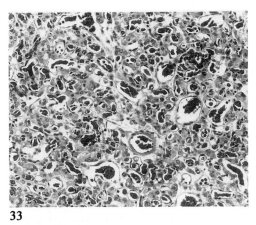

33

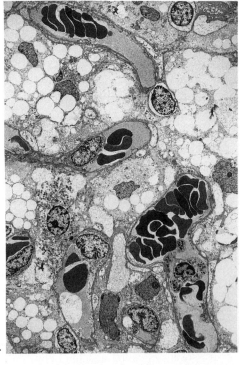

34

Figure 32 Cerebellum, with cystic capillary hemangioblastoma. Mural nodule represents actual tumor.
Figure 33 Capillary hemangioblastoma with plentiful vascular channels and intervening stromal cells.
Figure 34 Ultrastructurally, stromal cells contain abundant lipid droplets.

Immunoperoxidase staining is somewhat variable. There are some consistent findings; namely, the stromal cells are positive for vimentin and negative for cytokeratins and epithelial membrane antigen. S-100 protein can be found, but is a less reliable marker. Glial fibrillary acidic protein (GFAP) is often detected and probably represents antigen ingested by stromal cells or in entrapped astrocytes (99,100). The nature of stromal cells has been difficult to determine. Endothelial, histiocytic, pericytic, astrocytic, neuronal, neuroendocrine, and smooth-muscle derivations, all have been proposed based on immunohistochemical and ultrastructural features.

The duration of symptoms is usually less than 1 year. The symptoms are related to increased intracranial pressure and are manifested by headache and vomiting in up to 80% of patients (97). Other signs include papilledema, dizziness, cranial nerve deficits, nystagmus, and gait problems. Rarely, these neoplasms can cause acute herniation of the cerebellar tonsils and death. In spite of their high vascularity, symptomatic bleeding is uncommon. Polycythemia occurs in approximately 20% of cases and resolves with total resection (101,102).

As this is a benign tumor, complete excision is usually curative. Solid tumors may be more difficult to resect completely, and this is reflected in their greater perioperative mortality. Recurrences and second primaries occur in 15–25% of cases. Clinical correlates of recurrence include young age at diagnosis, von Hippel–Lindau syndrome, and multicentricity at time of diagnosis. Pathological features associated with recurrence include small, solid tumors with few microcysts, and high numbers of eosinophilic stromal cells (103). Rarely, hemangioblastoma may seed along the CSF pathways.

VII. BENIGN LESIONS OF MALDEVELOPMENTAL ORIGIN

A. Cysts of the Central Nervous System

Classification of central nervous cysts has always been a source of controversy. This, in part, is due to the uncertainty of their pathogenesis and, in part, to various terms ingrained as a result of long-term clinical usage. Ultimately, careful pathological examination and well-defined microscopic criteria are required to distinguish between the plethora of grossly similar lesions. True arachnoid cysts have an intra-arachnoid location and are devoid of epithelial lining. Those cysts that are lined by neural elements, such as ependymal or choroidal epithelium, probably arise from embryonic nests and would best be referred to as epithelial cysts. It is unlikely that the arachnoid cells lining intra-arachnoid defects would undergo metaplasia to such an extent that they could produce the well-differentiated mature epithelial lining seen in the epithelial cysts. This difference in pathogenesis would support separation of superficial, fluid-filled epithelial cysts into a category different and distinct from the true arachnoid cysts. Dermoid and epidermoid cysts are well defined clinically and pathologically with little controversy over their identity or classification.

1. Arachnoid Cysts

Arachnoid cysts are circumscribed collections of fluid that have an intra-arachnoid location; they can be congenital or acquired (104). These cysts have thin, delicate membranous walls that collapse easily without the support of overlying dura (Fig. 35). They are unicameral, without septae, and contain watery, clear fluid, with a composition similar to cerebrospinal fluid. This fluid may or may not communicate with the subarachnoid space. The membranous lining of both the superfical and inner surfaces consists of arachnoid cells. At the circumferential edges of the cyst, the two lining surfaces of the cyst join to form a normal, intact arachnoid membrane (105). The subarachnoid space, pia, and leptomeningeal blood vessels lie deep to these cysts. The congenital or primary arachnoid cysts are considered to be benign, developmental lesions; whereas, the acquired cysts are felt to occur as a result of inflammation or trauma which, in many instances, is so minor that it eludes clinical pathological correlation and precludes definitive assessment of origin. A clue to whether a particular cyst is primary or acquired is the presence of inflammatory cells or hemosiderin in the walls of the latter, although congenital cysts may also have these features as a result of spontaneous hemorrhage into the cyst.

Approximately half of the arachnoid cysts are found over the cerebral hemispheres—most frequently in the Sylvian fissure. Partial or total absence of the temporal lobe, not associated with any functional loss and caused by an arachnoid cyst, is referred to as *temporal lobe agenesis syndrome* (106). Posterior fossa locations are not as common as hemispheric sites and include the cerebellopontine angle and vermis. Cysts can also rarely be found in the supracollicular, suprasellar, interhemispheric, and interpeduncular areas (107,108). These cysts compress and indent the adjacent brain tissue; overlying bone deformity may be present. They enlarge progressively and, when of sufficient size, produce signs and symptoms of an expanding mass and increased intracranial pressure (109). Many are detected in childhood; however, some are incidental findings at autopsy.

2. Epithelial Cysts

Colloid Cysts   Colloid cysts are uncommon and represent fewer than 1% of all intracranial neoplasms (110,111). An equal sex distribution is found, and they occur predominantly between the third and fifth decades. They are generally believed to arise from invaginations of neuroepithelium lining the primitive ventricular cavities, although an endodermal origin has also been suggested (112,113). These cysts are spherical and have a thin, smooth fibrous capsule (Fig. 36). The lining epithelium of most colloid cysts is made up of two subpopulations (Fig. 37): ciliated and nonciliated cells containing secretory material (114). The latter, as well as the amorphous cyst contents, are highlighted intensely with PAS stain. Colloid cysts are usually silent, but because of their location near the foramen of Monro, they may cause symptoms related to blockage of CSF, with resultant increase in intracranial pressure and hydrocephalus. Behavioral manifestations have been attributed to compression or vascular compromise of the diencephalon (115). A ball-valve phenomenon between these cysts and the foramen of Monro may manifest in unusual intermittent or episodic symptomatology (116).

Enterogenous Cysts   Enterogenous cysts are congenital and develop as a result of the inclusion of endodermal elements in the central neuraxis. They are usually located ventrally along the spine, preponderantly in the cervical and upper thoracic regions, but cases have been reported intracranially (117–119). They may be intradural, subdural or, less commonly, intramedullary. The cyst wall is lined by columnar epithelium, which may be pseudostratified and ciliated. The presence of goblet cells reflects the intestinal nature of the epithelial lining and confers strong PAS positivity to these cysts (Fig. 38). The cyst fluid is a watery clear-to-viscous, dark brown.

Extraventricular Ependymal Cysts   These fluid-filled cavities are lined by ciliated epithelium resembling ependyma and usually located intraparenchymally. They may be asymptomatic or may present with rapidly progressive symptoms, as a result of expansion secondary to active secretion from the epithelial lining (120).

3. Epidermoid and Dermoid Cysts

Epidermoid and dermoid cysts arise from ectodermal elements displaced during embryogenesis. The dermoid cysts are more commonly found in the midline, can be seen with a variety of dysraphic conditions, and are thought to be associated with defective neural tube closure (121). In contrast, the epidermoid cysts tend to occur laterally and are probably related to events occurring later in embryogenesis than neural tube closure. Epidermoid cysts can also be acquired from repeated lumbar punctures, by the sequestration of implanted epidermal tissue (122). Both these cysts grow slowly and can be located in the skull, epidural, subdural, and subarachnoid spaces, or within neural parenchyma. Microscopically, both have well-differentiated stratified squamous

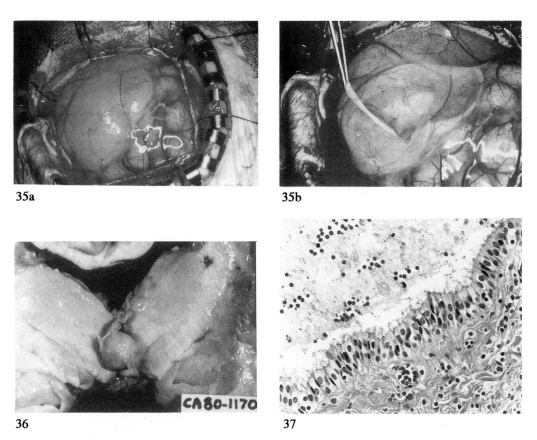

35a 35b

36 37

Figure 35 (a) Intact arachnoid cyst. (b) Unroofing the outer surface of the arachnoid cyst shows cavity filled with clear liquid indenting underlying cortex. (Courtesy Dr. G Silverberg)

Figure 36 Colloid cyst situated in the region of the foramen of Monro. (Courtesy Dr. G. Steinberg)

Figure 37 Pseudostratified, cuboidal and columnar epithelial lining of colloid cyst. Well-preserved specimens may show cilia, as seen here. Lumen contains PAS-positive amorphous secretory material as well as cellular debris.

epithelia; however, the dermoid cysts are distinguished by the presence of a dermal component, underlying the epithelial layer, that contains skin appendages, such as hair follicles and sweat and sebaceous glands (Fig. 39).

Although epidermoid cysts are found throughout the central neuraxis, they occur more commonly intracranially in the petrous bone and in the cerebellopontine angle (Fig. 40). In the latter location, epidermoids are superseded by only schwannomas and meningiomas in frequency. They have a smooth, thin connective tissue capsule that has a characteristic pearly sheen. The cysts contain white, cheesy grumous material made up of desquamated cells. Ruptured cyst contents elicit a marked granulomatous inflammatory response. Epidermoid cysts usually become symptomatic in adulthood. In contrast, dermoid cysts are more common in children, are often associated with a congenital dermal sinus, and display a tendency for the lumbosacral region. The occipital, the orbital, and the suprasellar regions are other sites of involvement (123).

B. Lipoma

Lipomas are rare lesions, considered maldevelopmental in origin, and probably make up no more than 1% of all intracranial tumors. They are present in all age groups and, for the most part, are

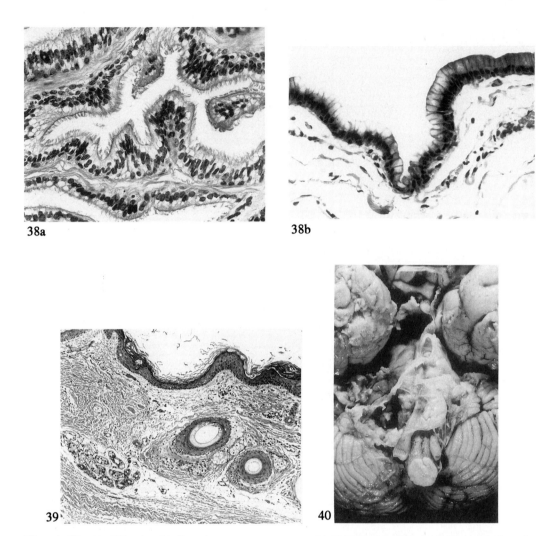

38a   38b

39   40

Figure 38 (a) Ciliated epithelium in enterogenous cyst. (b) Nonciliated goblet cell-like epithelium in enterogenous cyst.
Figure 39 Wall of dermoid cyst lined by stratified squamous epithelium. Underlying dermal components include hair follicles, sweat glands, and sebaceous glands.
Figure 40 Opened epidermoid cyst of cerebellopontine angle, with friable contents.

asymptomatic, detected radiographically or at autopsy. Both sexes seem to be equally affected. There is a pronounced midline proclivity, and 50% of intracranial lipomas are found at the site of the corpus callosum, associated with its partial or complete agenesis. At this site, symptoms are usually nonfocal, frequently the result of associated malformations, including seizures, behavioral changes, and mental retardation (124,125). Other typical locations include the infundibular region, the quadrigeminal plate, between the mammillary bodies, the cerebellopontine angle, the lateral ventricles—attached to the choroid—and the Sylvian fissure (126,127). A third of the intraspinal lipomas are associated with some dysraphic condition.

Lipomas have a distinctive yellow appearance and a soft, greasy consistency. They are encased in thin, fibrous capsules, attached to the meninges by strands of connective and vascular tissue that sometimes penetrate adjacent brain tissue. Microscopically, lipomas are composed of

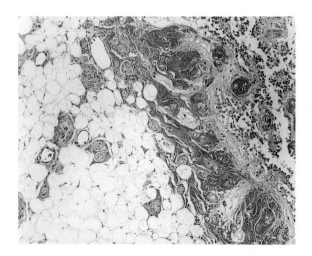

Figure 41 Nerve rootlets embedded in mature adipose fat of cauda equina lipoma.

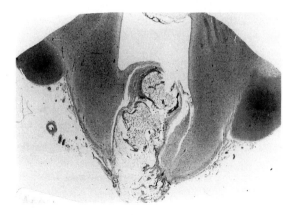

Figure 42 Lipoma of tuber cinereum with peripheral rim of calcification.

mature adipose tissue, traversed by irregular fibrovascular septae (Fig. 41). Neural tissue as well as heterologous mesenchymal elements, including bone, Schwann cells, muscle, and cartilage, have been detected within these lesions. Mineral deposition, when present, collects near the surface, within the capsule, or in adjacent neural tissue, and can be detected radiographically. Bony tissue can also be seen (Fig. 42) and is frequently found with asymptomatic lipomas of the tuber cinereum (128). Those that have a prominent vascular component are designated *angiolipomata* (129).

REFERENCES

1. Boldrey E. The meningiomas. In: Minckler J, ed. Pathology of the nervous system. New York: McGraw-Hill, 1971:2125–2144.
2. Kepes JJ. Meningiomas. Biology, pathology and differential diagnosis. New York: Masson, 1982.
3. Mahaley MSJ, Mettlin C, Natarajan N, Laws ERJ, Peace BB. National survey of patterns of care for brain-tumor patients. J Neurosurg 1989; 71:826–836.
4. Zulch KJ. Brain tumors. Their biology and pathology. New York: Springer-Verlag, 1986:358.
5. Schoenberg BS, Christine BW, Whisnant JP. Nervous system neoplasms and primary malignancies of

other sites. The unique association between meningiomas and breast cancer. Neurology 1975; 25:705–712.

6. Mehta D, Khatib R, Patel S. Carcinoma of the breast and meningioma. Association and management. Cancer 1983; 51:1937–1940.

7. Burns PE, Naresh J, Bain GO. Association of breast cancer with meningioma. A report of five cases. Cancer 1986; 58:1537–1539.

8. Rubinstein AB, Schein M, Reichenthal E. The association of carcinoma of the breast with meningioma. Surg Gynecol Obstet 1989; 169:334–336.

9. Lesch KP, Schott W, Engl HG, Grob S, Thierauf P. Gonadal steroid receptors in meningiomas. J Neurol 1987; 234:328–333.

10. Halper J, Colvard DS, Scheithauer BW, Jiang N-S, Press MF, Graham ML, Riehl E, Laws ER, Spelsberg TC. Estrogen and progesterone receptors in meningiomas: comparison of nuclear binding, dextran-coated charcoal, and immunoperoxidase staining assays. Neurosurgery 1989; 25:546–553.

11. Collins VP, Nordenskjold M, Dumanski JP. The molecular genetics of meningiomas. Brain Pathol 1990; 1:19–24.

12. Parry DM. Gene mapping and tumor genetics, pp 41–42. In: Mulvihill JJ, moderator. Neurofibromatosis 1 (Recklinghausen disease) and neurofibromatosis 2 (bilateral acoustic neurofibromatosis). An update. Ann Intern Med 1990; 113:39–52.

13. Bailey P, Bucy P. The origin and nature of meningeal tumors. Cancer Res 1931; 15:15–54.

14. Cushing H, Eisenhardt L. Meningiomas: their classification, regional behavior, life history and surgical end results. Springfield IL: Charles C Thomas, 1938.

15. Zulch KJ. International histological classification of tumours. 21. Histologic typing of tumours of the central nervous system. Geneva: WHO, 1979:53–58.

16. Kleinman GM, Liszczak T, Tarlov E, Richardson EP Jr. Microcystic variant of meningioma. A light-microscopic and ultrastructural study. Am J Surg Pathol 1980; 4:383–389.

17. Harrison JD, Rose PE. Myxoid meningioma: histochemistry and electron microscopy. Acta Neuropathol (Berl) 1985; 68:80–82.

18. Kepes JJ. The fine structure of hyaline inclusions (pseudopsammoma bodies) in meningiomas. J Neuropathol Exp Neurol 1975; 36:282–289.

19. Alguacil-Garcia A, Pettigrew NM, Sima AAF. Secretory meningioma. A distinct subtype of meningioma. Am J Surg Pathol 1986; 10:102–111.

20. Kepes JJ. Observations on the formation of psammoma bodies and pseudopsammoma bodies in meningiomas. J Neuropathol Exp Neurol 1961; 20:255–262.

21. Stam FC, van Alphen HAM, Boorsma DM. Meningioma with conspicuous plasma cell components. A histopathological and immunohistochemical study. Acta Neuropathol (Berl) 1980; 49:241–243.

22. Horten BC, Urich H, Stefoski D. Meningiomas with conspicuous plasma cell–lymphocytic components. A report of five cases. Cancer 1979; 43:258–264.

23. Lach B, Russell N, Benoit B, Atack D. Cellular blue nevus ("melanocytoma") of the spinal meninges: electron microscopic and immunohistochemical features. Neurosurgery 1988; 22:773–780.

24. Schnitt SJ, Vogel H. Meningiomas: diagnostic value of immunoperoxidase staining for epithelial membrane antigen. Am J Surg Pathol 1986; 10:640–649.

25. Meis JM, Ordonez NG, Bruner JM. Meningiomas. An immunohistochemical study of 50 cases. Arch Pathol Lab Med 1986; 110:934–937.

26. Winek RR, Scheithauer BW, Wick MR. Meningioma, meningeal hemagiopericytoma (angioblastic meningioma), peripheral hemangiopericytoma, and acoustic schwannoma. A comparative immunohistochemical study. Am J Surg Pathol 1989; 13:251–261.

27. Tani I, Ikeda K, Yamagata S, Nishiura M, Higashi N. Specialized junctional complexes in human meningioma. Acta Neuropathol (Berl) 1974; 28:305–314.

28. de la Monte SM, Flickinger J, Linggood RM. Histopathologic features predicting recurrence of meningiomas following subtotal resection. Am J Surg Pathol 1986; 10:836–843.

29. Begg CF, Garret R. Haemangiopericytoma occurring in the meninges. Cancer 1954; 7:602–606.

30. Thomas HG, Dolman CL, Berry K. Malignant meningioma: clinical and pathological features. J Neurosurg 1981; 55:929–934.

31. Guthrie BL, Ebersold MJ, Scheithauer BW, Shaw EG. Meningeal hemangiopericytoma: histopathological features, treatment, and long-term follow-up of 44 cases. Neurosurgery 1989; 25:514–522.

32. Mean H, Ribas JL, Pezeshkpour GH, Cowan DN, Parisi JE. Hemangiopericytoma of the central nervous system: a review of 94 cases. Hum Pathol 1991; 22:84–91.

33. Iwaki T, Fukui M, Takeshita I, Tsuneyoshi M, Tateishi J. Hemangiopericytoma of the meninges: a clinicopathologic and immunohistochemical study. Clin Neuropathol 1988; 7:93–99.

34. Moss TH. Immunohistochemical characteristics of haemangiopericytic meningiomas: comparison with typical meningiomas, haemangioblastomas and haemangiopericytomas from extracranial sites. Neuropathol Appl Neurobiol 1987; 13:467–480.

35. Nunnery EW, Kahn LB, Reddick RL, Lipper S. Hemangiopericytoma: a light microscopic and ultrastructural study. Cancer 1981; 47:906–914.

36. Dardick I, Hammar SP, Scheithauer BW. Ultrastructural spectrum of hemangiopericytoma: a comparative study of fetal, adult, and neoplastic pericytes. Ultrastruct Pathol 1989; 13:111–154.

37. Sakaki S, Nakagawa K, Nakamura K, Takeda S. Meningioangiomatosis not associated with von Recklinghausen's disease. Neurosurgery 1987; 20:797–801.

38. Kunishio K, Yamamoto Y, Sunami N, Satoh T, Asari S, Yoshino T, Ohtuki Y. Histopathologic investigation of a case of meningioangiomatosis not associated with von Recklinghausen's disease. Surg Neurol 1987; 27:575–579.

39. Ogilvy CS, Chapman PH, Gray M, de la Monte S. Meningioangiomatosis in a patient without von Recklinghausen's disease. J Neurosurg 1989; 70:483–485.

40. Liu SS, Johnson PC, Sonntag VKH. Meningioangiomatosis: a case report. Surg Neurol 1989; 31: 376–380.

41. Paulus W, Peiffer J, Roggendorf W. Meningio-angiomatosis. Pathol Res Pract 1989; 184:446–452.

42. Goates JJ, Dickson DW, Horoupian DS. Meningioangiomatosis: an immunocytochemical study. Acta Neuropathol (Berl) 1991; 82:527–532.

43. Kasantikul V, Netsky MG, Glasscock ME, Hays JW. Acoustic neurilemmoma. Clinicoanatomical study of 103 patients. J Neurosurg 1980; 52:28–35.

44. Martuza RL, Eldridge R. Neurofibromatosis 2 (bilateral acoustic neurofibromatosis). N Engl J Med 1988; 318:684–688.

45. Neurofibromatosis conference statement. National Institutes of Health consensus development conference. Arch Neurol 1988; 45:575–578.

46. Dolan EJ, Tucker WS, Rotenberg D, Chui M. Intracranial hypoglossal schwannoma as an unusual cause of facial nerve palsy. J Neurosurg 1982; 56:420–423.

47. Bordi L, Compton J, Symon L. Trigeminal neuroma. A report of eleven cases. Surg Neurol 1989; 31:272–276.

48. Prakash B, Roy S, Tandon PN. Schwannoma of the brain stem. J Neurosurg 1980; 53:121–123.

49. Auer RN, Budny J, Drake CG, Ball MJ. Frontal lobe perivascular schwannoma. Case report. J Neurosurg 1982; 56:154–157.

50. Gokay H, Izgi H, Barlas O, Erseven G. Supratentorial intracerebral schwannomas. Surg Neurol 1984; 22:69–72.

51. Sarkar C, Mehta VS, Roy S. Intracerebellar schwannoma. J Neurosurg 1987; 67:120–123.

52. Tran-Dinh HD, Soo YS, O'Neil P, Chaseling R. Cystic cerebellar schwannoma: case report. Neurosurgery 1991; 29:296–300.

53. Weiss SW, Langloss JM, Enzinger FM. S-100 protein in the diagnosis of soft tissue tumors with particular reference to benign and malignant Schwann cell tumors. Lab Invest 1983; 49:299–308.

54. Erlandson RA, Woodruff JM. Peripheral nerve sheath tumors: an electron microscopic study of 43 cases. Cancer 1982; 49:273–287.

55. Wazen J, Silverstein H, Norrell H, Besse B. Preoperative and postoperative growth rates in acoustic neuromas documented with CT scanning. Otolaryngol Head Neck Surg 1985; 93:151–155.

56. Rosenberg RA, Cohen NL, Ransohoff J. Long-term hearing preservation after acoustic neuroma surgery. Otolaryngol Head Neck Surg 1987; 97:270–274.

57. Beatty CW, Ebersold MJ, Harner SG. Residual and recurrent acoustic neuromas. Laryngoscope 1987; 97:1168–1171.

58. Lassmann H, Jurecka W, Lassmann G, Matras H, Watzek G. Different types of benign nerve sheath tumors. Light microscopy, electron microscopy and autoradiography. Virchows Arch [A] 1977; 375:197–210.
59. Rovit RL, Schechter MM, Chodroff P. Choroid plexus papillomas. Observations of radiographic diagnosis. AJR 1970; 110:608–617.
60. Matson DD, Crofton FDL. Papilloma of the choroid plexus in childhood. J Neurosurg 1960; 17:1002–1027.
61. Spallone A, Pastore FS, Giuffre R, Guidetti B. Choroid plexus papillomas in infancy and childhood. Childs Nerv Syst 1990; 6:71–74.
62. Cushing H. Intracranial tumours. Notes upon a series of two thousand verified cases with surgical mortality percentages pertaining thereto. Springfield, IL: Charles C Thomas, 1932:150.
63. Grant F. Study of results of surgical treatment in 2326 consecutive patients with brain tumor. J Neurosurg 1956; 13:479–488.
64. Bohm E, Strang R. Choroid plexus papillomas. J Neurosurg 1961; 18:493–500.
65. Davis RL, Fox GE. Acinar choroid plexus adenoma. Case report. J Neurosurg 1970; 33:587–590.
66. Stefanko SZ, Vuzevski VD. Oncocytic variant of choroid plexus papilloma. Acta Neuropathol (Berl) 1985; 66:160–162.
67. Reimund EL, Sitton JE, Harkin JC. Pigmented choroid plexus papilloma. Arch Pathol Lab Med 1990; 114:902–905.
68. Albrecht S, Rouah E, Becker LE, Bruner J. Transthyretin immunoreactivity in choroid plexus neoplasms and brain metastases. Mod Pathol 1991; 4:610–614.
69. Rubinstein LJ, Brucher J. Focal ependymal differentiation in choroid plexus papillomas. Acta Neuropathol (Berl) 1981; 53:29–33.
70. Bonnin JM, Colon LE, Morawetz RB. Focal glial differentiation and oncocytic transformation in choroid plexus papilloma. Acta Neuropathol (Berl) 1987; 72:277–280.
71. Kuono M, Kumanshi T, Washiyama K, Sekiguchi K, Saito T, Tanaka R. An immunohistochemical study of cytokeratin and glial fibrillary acidic protein in choroid plexus papilloma. Acta Neuropathol (Berl) 1988; 75:317–320.
72. Miettinen M, Clark R, Virtanen I. Intermediate filament proteins in choroid plexus and ependyma and their tumors. Am J Pathol 1986; 123:231–240.
73. Navas JJ, Battifora H. Choroid plexus papilloma: light and electron microscopic study of three cases. Acta Neuropathol (Berl) 1978; 44:235–239.
74. Matsushima T. Choroid plexus papillomas and human choroid plexus. A light and electron microscopic study. J Neurosurg 1983; 59:1054–1062.
75. Braunstein H, Martin F. Congenital papilloma of choroid plexus. Report of a case, with observations of pathogenesis of associated hydrocephalus. Arch Neurol Psychiatry 1952; 68:475–480.
76. Milhorat TH, Hammock MK, Davis DA, Fenstermacher JD. Choroid plexus papilloma. I. Proof of cerebrospinal fluid overproduction. Childs Brain 1976; 2:273–289.
77. McGirr SJ, Ebersold MJ, Scheithauer BW, Quast LM, Shaw EG. Choroid plexus papillomas: long-term follow-up results in a surgically treated series. J Neurosurg 1988; 69:843–849.
78. Rosner S. Xanthoma of the choroid plexus in a child. J Nerv Ment Dis 1957; 125:339–341.
79. Morello A, Campesi G, Bettinazzi N, Albeggiami A. Neoplastiform xanthomatous granulomas of choroid plexus in a child affected by Hand–Schuller–Christian disease. Case report. J Neurosurg 1967; 26:536–541.
80. Salazar J, Vaquero J, Aranda IF, Menendez J, Jimenez MD, Bravo G. Choroid plexus papilloma with chondroma: case report. Neurosurgery 1986; 18:781–783.
81. Valdueza JM, Freckmann N, Hermann H. Chondromatosis of the choroid plexus: case report. Neurosurgery 1990; 27:291–294.
82. Truwit CL, Williams RG, Armstrong EA, Marlin AE. MR Imaging of choroid plexus lipomas. AJNR 1990; 11:202–204.
83. Kipkie GF. Simultaneous chromaffin tumors of the carotid body and the glomus jugularis. Arch Pathol 1947; 44:113–118.
84. Chedid A, Jao W. Hereditary tumors of the carotid bodies and chronic obstructive pulmonary disease. Cancer 1974; 33:1635–1641.

85. Saldana MJ, Salem LE, Travezan R. High altitude hypoxia and chemodectomas. Hum Pathol 1973; 4:251–263.

86. Arias-Stella J, Valcarcel J. Chief cell hyperplasia in the human carotid body at high altitudes. Physiologic and pathologic significance. Hum Pathol 1976; 7:361–373.

87. Lack E. Hyperplasia of vagal and carotid body paraganglia in patients with chronic hypoxemia. Am J Pathol 1978; 91:497–516.

88. Rodriguez-Cuevas H, Lau I, Rodriguez HP. High-altitude paragangliomas. Diagnostic and therapeutic considerations. Cancer 1986; 57:672–676.

89. Schroder HD, Johannsen L. Demonstration of S-100 protein in sustentacular cells of phaeochromocytomas and paragangliomas. Histopathology 1986; 10:1023–1033.

90. Schwechheimer K, Moller P, Schnabel P, Waldherr R. Emphasis on peanut lectin as a marker for granular cells. Virchows Arch [A] 1983; 399:289–297.

91. Dickson DW, Suzuki K, Kanner R, Weitz S, Horoupian DS. Cerebral granular cell tumor: immunohistochemical and electron microscopic study. J Neuropathol Exp Neurol 1986; 45:304–314.

92. Sakurama N, Matsukado Y, Marubayashi T, Kodama T. Granular cell tumour of the brain and its cellular identity. Acta Neurochir (Wein) 1981; 56:81–94.

93. Chimelli L, Symon L, Scaravilli F. Granular cell tumor of the fifth cranial nerve: further evidence for Schwann cell origin. J Neuropathol Exp Neurol 1984; 43:634–642.

94. Armin A, Connelly EM, Rowden G. An immunoperoxidase investigation of S-100 protein in granular cell myoblastomas: evidence for Schwann cell derivation. Am J Clin Pathol 1983; 79:37–44.

95. Olivecrona H. The cerebellar angioreticulomas. J Neurosurg 1952; 9:317–330

96. Mondkar VP, McKissock W, Russel DS. Cerebellar haemangioblastomas. Br J Surg 1967; 54:45–49.

97. Constans J-P, Meder F, Maiuri F, Donzelli D, Spaziante R, de Divitiis E. Posterior fossa hemangioblastomas. Surg Neurol 1986; 25:269–275.

98. Huson SM, Harper PS, Hourihan MD, Weeks RD, Compston DAS. Cerebellar haemangioblastoma and von Hippel–Lindau disease. Brain 1986; 109:1297–1310.

99. Holt SC, Bruner JM, Ordonez NG. Capillary hemangioblastoma: an immunohistochemical study. Am J Clin Pathol 1986; 86:423–429.

100. Frank TS, Trojanowski JQ, Roberts SA, Brooks JJ. A detailed immunohistochemical analysis of cerebellar hemangioblastoma: an undifferentiated mesenchymal tumor. Mod Pathol 1989; 2:638–651.

101. Palmer JJ. Haemangioblastomas: a review of 81 cases. Acta Neurochir (Wien) 1972; 27:125–148.

102. Jeffreys R. Clinical and surgical aspects of posterior fossa hemangioblastoma. J Neurol Neurosurg Psychiatry 1975; 38:105–111.

103. de la Monte S. Hemangioblastoma: clinical and histopathological factors correlated with recurrence. Neurosurgery 1989; 25:695–698.

104. Naidich TP, McLone DG, Radkiowski MA. Intracranial arachnoid cysts. Pediatr Neurosci 1986; 12:112–122.

105. Schachenmayr W, Friede RL. Fine structure of arachnoid cysts. J Neuropathol Exp Neurol 1979; 38:434–446.

106. Robinson RG. The temporal lobe agenesis syndrome. Brain 1964; 87:87–105.

107. Grollmus JM, Wilson CB, Newton TH. Paramesencephalic arachnoid cysts. Neurology 1976; 26:128–134.

108. Rengachary SS, Watanabe I. Ultrastructure and pathogenesis of intracranial arachnoid cysts. J Neuropathol Exp Neurol 1981; 40:61–83.

109. Choux M, Raybaud C, Pinsard N, Hassoun J, Gambarelli D. Intracranial supratentorial cysts in children excluding tumor and parasitic cysts. Childs Brain 1978; 4:15–32.

110. Batnitzky S, Sarwar M, Leeds NE. Colloid cysts of the third ventricle. Radiology 1974; 112:327–341.

111. Little JR, MacCarty CS. Colloid cysts of the third ventricle. J Neurosurg 1974; 40:230–235.

112. Shuangshoti S, Netsky MG. Neuroepithelial (colloid) cysts of the nervous system. Neurology 1966; 16:887–903.

113. Ghatak NR, Kasoff I, Alexander E. Further observation on the fine structure of a colloid cyst of the third ventricle. Acta Neuropathol (Berl) 1977; 39:101–107.

114. Leech RW, Freeman T, Johnson R. Colloid cyst of the third ventricle. A scanning and transmission electron microscopic study. J Neurosurg 1982; 57:108–113.

115. Lobosky JM, Vangilder JC, Damasio AR. Behavioral manifestations of third ventricular colloid cysts. J Neurol Neurosurg Psychiatry 1984; 47:1075–1080.
116. Malik GM, Horoupian DS, Boulos RS. Hemorrhagic (colloid) cyst of the third ventricle and episodic neurologic deficits. Surg Neurol 1980; 13:73–77.
117. Holmes GL, Trader S, Ignatiadis P. Intraspinal enterogenous cysts: a case report and review of pediatric cases in the literature. Am J Dis Child 1978; 132:906–908.
118. Giombini S. Intracranial enterogenous cysts. Surg Neurol 1981; 16:271–273.
119. Afshar F, Scholtz CL. Enterogenous cyst of the fourth ventricle. Case report. J Neurosurg 1981; 54:836–838.
120. Friede RL, Yasargil MG. Supratentorial intracerebral epithelial (ependymal) cysts: review, case reports, and fine structure. J Neurol Neurosurg Psychiatry 1977; 40:127–137.
121. Fleming R, Botterell JF. Cranial dermoid and epidermoid tumors. Surg Gynecol Obstet 1959; 109:403–411.
122. Blockey NJ, Schorstein J. Intraspinal epidermoid tumors in the lumbar region of children. J Bone Joint Surg 1961; 43-B:558–562.
123. Leech RW, Olafson RA. Epithelial cysts of the neuraxis. Presentation of three cases and a review of the origins and classification. Arch Pathol Lab Med 1977; 101:196–202.
124. Wallace D. Lipoma of the corpus callosum. J Neurol Neurosurg Psychiatry 1976; 39:1179–1185.
125. Suemitsu T, Nakajima S, Kuwajima K, Nihei K, Kamoshita S. Lipoma of the corpus callosum: report of a case and review of the literature. Childs Brain 1979; 5:476–483.
126. Hori A. Lipoma of the quadrigeminal region with evidence of congenital origin. Arch Pathol Lab Med 1986; 110:850–851.
127. Christensen WN, Long DM, Epstein JI. Cerebellopontine angle lipoma. Hum Pathol 1986; 17:739–743.
128. Friede RL. Osteolipomas of the tuber cinereum. Arch Pathol Lab Med 1977; 101:369–372.
129. Wilkins PR, Hoddinott C, Hourihan MD, Davies KG, Sebugwawo S, Weeks RD. Intracranial angiolipoma. J Neurol Neurosurg Psychiatry 1987; 50:1057–1059.

3

Pathology of Primary Intracranial Malignant Neoplasms

Stephen W. Coons and Peter C. Johnson
Barrow Neurological Institute of St. Joseph's Hospital and Medical Center, Phoenix, Arizona

I. INTRODUCTION

Central nervous system (CNS) neoplasms include tumors of the (1) constituent elements of the brain itself; (2) associated organs such as the pineal and pituitary glands; (3) coverings of the brain, spinal cord, and intracranial portions of nerves; and (4) rests of mesenchymal and epithelial cell derivation. This chapter focuses on primary malignant intracranial tumors and will consider all the tumors of glial cells.

The concept of tumor malignancy for primary CNS neoplasms is somewhat different from systemic tumors. In the latter, metastatic potential is often a primary determinant of outcome. Whereas metastasis to the brain is a relatively common occurrence, primary CNS neoplasms rarely metastasize outside the CNS. Factors affecting tumor behavior include location, host defenses, and intrinsic capacity to proliferate, invade, and resist therapy.

Astrocytes, oligodendroglia, ependyma, and choroid plexus share a common glial lineage in their differentiation from the primitive neuroectoderm. *Glioma* is an inclusive term for neoplasms of glial heritage. Although histopathologically they usually reflect only one cell type (e.g., astrocytoma or ependymoma), combinations of two cell types may be seen, most commonly oligodendroglioma and astrocytoma.

An understanding of the special biology of these neoplasms is essential for proper management. As we have indicated, extracranial metastasis is noteworthy only for its infrequent occurrence. Intracranial "metastasis" through cerebrospinal fluid (CSF) pathways is more common and is of particular interest in the management of ependymomas and choroid plexus tumors (CPT). In general, it is the capacity to proliferate and create a space-occupying mass, to infiltrate and injure eloquent and vital structures, and to resist radiation and chemotherapy, that determines glioma behavior and outcome. These properties, and methods to assess them, are explored for the principal tumor types in the next several sections.

II. ASTROCYTOMA

A. Introduction

Astrocytomas constitute the majority of all primary brain tumors and are the most common intracranial neoplasm. They occur throughout the brain, but most are supratentorial and primarily involve the cerebral hemispheres. Astrocytomas occur at any age, but are most common in adults (1).

Astrocytomas are malignant tumors, despite the occasional unfortunate use of the term "benign astrocytoma" to describe low-grade tumors. Survival is affected by several factors. Tumor location plays a dual role: (1) astrocytomas involving the brain stem have an inherently worse prognosis, owing to involvement of the vital structures in this region; (2) astrocytomas involving areas that have a major effect on quality of life, such as the speech and motor centers, often receive less aggressive therapy. Highly aggressive tumors occur at all ages; however, there is a very strong trend toward increasing malignancy with age. The major biological factors affecting an astrocytoma's behavior—proliferative capacity, invasiveness, and resistance to therapy—have already been noted.

Predictive histopathological grading systems have been developed that reflect the varied biology of astrocytomas. The tumor grade is a principal basis for therapeutic decisions. The discussions of tumor pathology and radiology in the remainder of this section are conducted in reference to tumor grade.

B. Histopathological Grading

The foundation of modern histopathological grading was laid by Kernohan, who designed a grading system for astrocytomas that was based on progressive cellular anaplasia and defined several microscopic features that were associated with aggressive behavior (2). These features appear sequentially and with increasing prominence as the degree of malignancy increases (1,3). Cytological atypia and hypercellularity appear first and are present, to some degree, in virtually every tumor. Mitotic figures, indicative of an increased proliferative rate, are seen next. Atypical vascular proliferation and tumor necrosis complete the histological picture of malignancy. These observations are the basis of astrocytoma grading. Current systems differ primarily in the relative importance assigned each feature. The common grading systems are compared in Table 1.

The system of Ringertz (4), as modified by Burger et al., is the most commonly used grading system in the United States (5). It divides astrocytomas into three categories: (low-grade) astrocytoma (LGA), characterized by mild hypercellularity and pleomorphism; anaplastic astrocytoma (AA), with moderate (or greater) pleomorphism, increased proliferative activity, and variable vascular proliferation, but without necrosis; and glioblastoma multiforme (GBM), in which there is tumor necrosis. The system shows excellent overall correlation between grade and outcome, but the use of relative and subjective terms results in problems with inter- and intraobserver reproducibility in the differentiation of LGA and AA. The requirement for tumor necrosis in the diagnosis of GBM makes adequate sampling essential to avoid diagnostic errors resulting from tumor heterogeneity.

The St. Anne–Mayo system, developed recently by Daumas-Duport et al. (6), eliminates subjectivity by determining grade solely on the presence or absence of pleomorphism, mitotic figures, vascular proliferation, and necrosis. Although this is nominally a four-tiered system, grade 1 tumors are negligibly rare. Prediction of outcome is as good as with the Ringertz–Burger classification and most tumors receive equivalent grades. This system is easy to use and is more consistent and reproducible (7). However, reliance on the presence of specific features leaves it more vulnerable to heterogeneity-induced sampling errors.

Table 1 Comparison of Grading Systems for Astrocytomas

Kernohan	Ringertz–Burger	WHO	St. Anne–Mayo
Grades are based on progressive development of anaplasia.	Grades are based on progressive development of anaplasia.	Grade I Pilocytic astrocytoma	Grades are based on presence of specific histological features: pleomorphism, mitoses, vascular proliferation, and necrosis.
Grade 1 Normal-appearing astrocytes without anaplasia.	Astrocytoma: mild pleomorphism and hypercellularity; mitoses and vascular proliferation rare.	II Diffuse growth of well-differentiated astrocytes.	
2 Most cells show mild anaplasia with no mitoses.	Anaplastic astrocytoma: moderate pleomorphism and hypercellularity, increased mitoses; vascular proliferation common.	III Anaplastic features present: pleomorphism, increased mitoses, vascular proliferation.	Grade 1 No features present (negligibly rare) 2 One feature present (pleomorphism)
3 Moderate anaplasia of 50% of cells; mitoses present; vascular proliferation and necrosis may be seen; foci of hypercellularity	Glioblastoma multiforme: features of anaplastic astrocytoma plus zones of necrosis.	IV Undifferentiated or primitive-appearing cells predominate.	3 Two features present (typically pleomorphism and mitoses)
4 Most cells show marked anaplasia; numerous mitoses; vascular proliferation and necrosis may be prominent.			4 Three or four features present (pleomorphism, mitoses, plus vascular proliferation and/or necrosis)

Source: Ref. 312.

The World Health Organization (WHO) system is also nominally a four-tiered system (8). Grade I is reserved for pilocytic astrocytomas. In practice, grades II–IV correspond well with the Ringertz and St. Anne–Mayo classifications. This system is in the process of revision and is expected to incorporate some of the features of the St. Anne–Mayo system.

Figures 1–3 illustrate the features just discussed; the histological grades of each of the major systems is given.

C. Anatomy and Growth Patterns of Astrocytomas

Primary cerebral neoplasms may be characterized as diffusely infiltrating, as expansile, or as having a combination of an expansile core and an infiltrating corona. The margins of diffusely infiltrating tumors (with or without an expansile core), such as astrocytomas and oligodendrogliomas, are not well-defined, making local treatment design problematic (9). Expansile tumors push aside parenchyma as they grow, and there is often only a narrow rim of invasive cells. This usually provides a clear cleavage plane for the surgeon. Ependymomas (9) and malignant CPT (10) typically display this growth pattern.

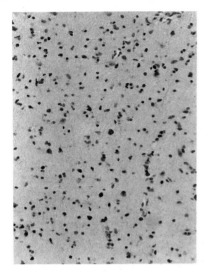

Figure 1 Ringertz–Burger (R/B): (Low-grade) astrocytoma; St. Anne–Mayo (SA/M): grade 2; World Health Organization (WHO): grade 2. Modestly hypercellular proliferation of neoplastic astrocytes that demonstrate little pleomorphism and no mitotic activity (H&E; original magnification × 200).

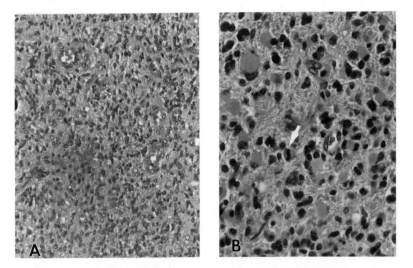

Figure 2 R/B: anaplastic astrocytoma; SA/M: grade 3; WHO: grade 3. (A) Tumor is markedly hypercellular. (B) Moderate pleomorphism is present. Mitotic figures are present (arrow) (H&E; original magnification: A × 200; B × 400).

The gross appearance of gliomas varies with tumor grade (Figs. 4–6). Low-grade astrocytomas tend to infiltrate diffusely and may not form a discrete mass, resulting in only nondestructive expansion of the involved region (9,11) and often limited symptoms. With widespread invasion and pronounced enlargement, the diagnosis of gliomatosis cerebri may be invoked (see Sec. IV). In contrast, AA and GBM form an expanding and infiltrating mass. Although they may appear circumscribed on gross and radiologic evaluation, no cleavage plane is present, and microscopic examination reveals a gradient of infiltrating cells extending away from the main mass (3,9,11).

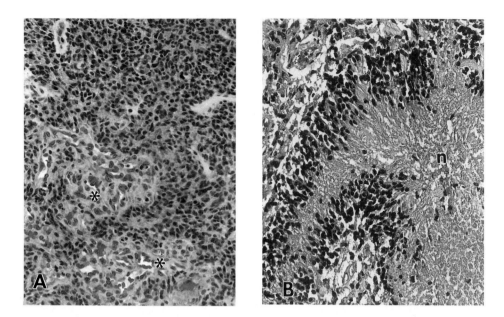

Figure 3 R/B: glioblastoma multiforme; SA/M: grade 4; WHO: grade 4. (A) Atypical vascular proliferation (*) accompanies the pleomorphic, hypercellular tumor. (B) Classic pseudopalisading tumor necrosis is seen: small anaplastic tumor cells delineate an acellular area of necrosis (n) (H&E; original magnification: A × 200; B × 200).

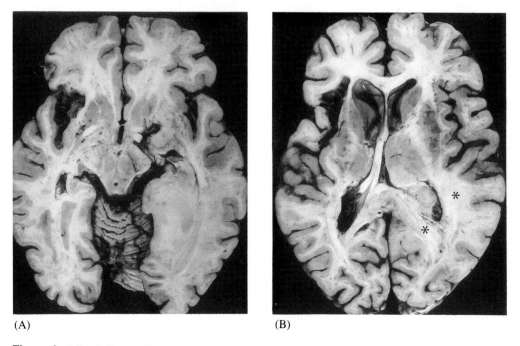

(A)   (B)

Figure 4 Mixed glioma (oligoastrocytoma): untreated. (A) The tumor infiltrates both gray and white matter of medial right temporal lobe without overt parenchymal destruction. Distinction of tumor from white matter is difficult. (B) In low-grade gliomas, the white matter may be expanded by infiltrating tumor cells without a destructive mass lesion (*).

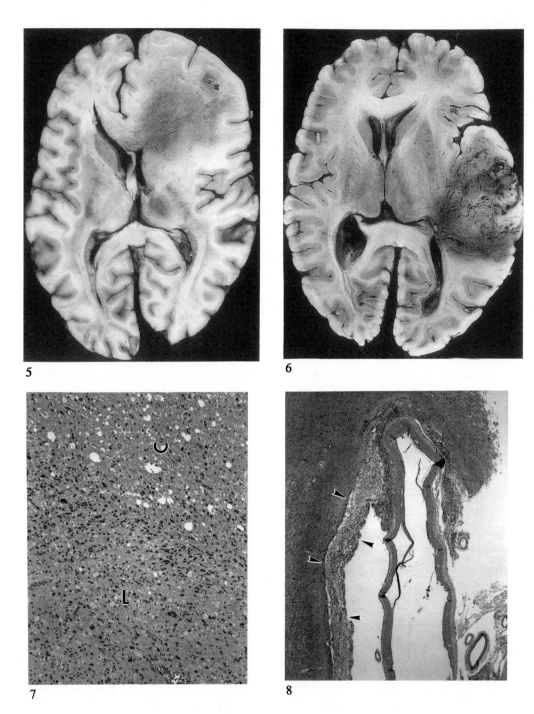

5

6

7

8

High-grade astrocytomas are typically soft and gray, but may be fleshy or myxoid, depending on the expression of astrocytic subtypes and the degree of attendant edema. Areas of hemorrhage, necrosis, cyst formation, and scarring provide a varied appearance, particularly in the aptly named glioblastoma multiforme.

The primary pattern of spread is along the preexisting pathways defined by white matter tracts (Fig. 7) (9,11–13). Gray matter involvement is usually less extensive and may be limited to a few infiltrating cells. Localization of these cells around neurons *(perineuronal satellitosis)* is common (9). Infiltrating tumor cells are usually accompanied by edema, which may facilitate invasion. The extent of infiltration may vary from region to region, and individual cells may infiltrate a long distance from the main tumor mass (9,11,13–14). Subpial spread, over the surfaces of gyri or along blood vessels, and subependymal spread may also be seen (Fig. 8). Proliferation of these remote tumor cells may produce secondary tumor masses that suggest multicentricity in imaging studies (5). At autopsy, the origins of most multicentric astrocytomas can be tracked to the primary tumor mass by following a trail of individual infiltrating cells. Fewer than 10% of high-grade astrocytomas are truly multicentric (15). Anaplastic astrocytomas and GBM may also spread by seeding through the CSF, with the possibility of widespread subependymal and subarachnoid dissemination (1,9). The result is that astrocytomas do not grow as spheres; instead, their contours are highly irregular, as their white matter extensions conform to the barriers of cortical convolutions and deep unclear structures. This growth pattern has important implications in the planning of local therapy.

D. Cytological Features

Astrocytomas demonstrate several distinct cell types (Fig. 9). Some are named after the benign counterparts they most resemble: fibrillary, gemistocytic, protoplasmic, and pilocytic. When one cell type is present to the near exclusion of the others, the tumor is often subclassified, using the morphological term, for example, protoplasmic astrocytoma. A fibrillary or mixed morphologic type is assumed if no modifier is given, and these are, by far, the most common patterns. The various grading systems were designed to evaluate hemispheric "fibrillary astrocytomas," but, except for pilocytic astrocytoma, there is no evidence that these morphological subtypes are predictive of outcome (1).

Two cell types have no correlate in the normal adult brain and are named descriptively as giant cell and small anaplastic cell types. The bizarre nuclear morphologic appearance of giant cells reflects highly aberrant biology that renders them relatively inert. These cells seem to lack significant capacity for effective cell division or infiltration (16,17). However, giant cells are associated with other highly aggressive subpopulations. Tumors in which giant cells are pre-

---

Figure 5   Anaplastic astrocytoma: untreated. The right frontal lobe tumor is homogeneous with ill-defined margins. Centrally, the mass is destructive and the surrounding white matter is thickened by infiltrating tumor cells. Note that the gray matter shows little involvement.

Figure 6   Glioblastoma multiforme: untreated. Variegated tumor mass is present in the right temporal lobe. Cysts and hemorrhage typical of GBM are present. The tumor is destructive of white matter, but a rim of relatively spared gray matter is seen peripherally.

Figure 7   Infiltrating astrocytoma cells tend to follow white matter tracts. The hypercellular lower (L) tract has a much greater concentration of infiltrating tumor cells than the upper tract (H&E; original magnification × 100).

Figure 8   Tumor cell infiltration is seen in the subarachnoid space (arrowheads) (H&E; original magnification × 40).

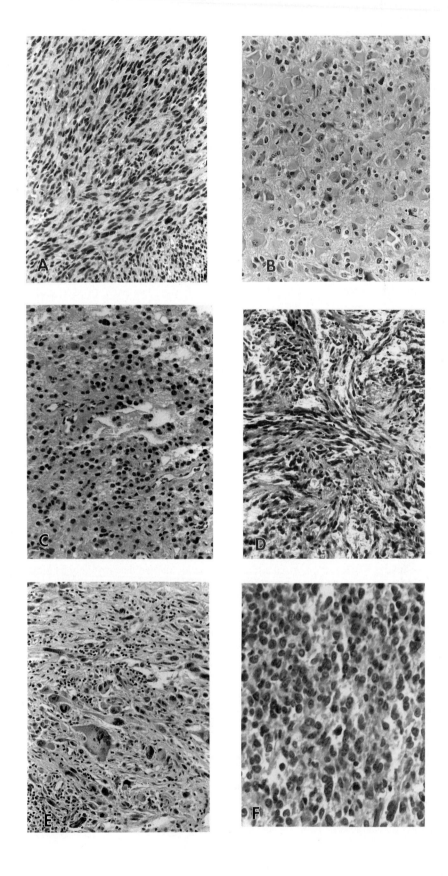

ponderant are almost always GBM, and they have the same grim prognosis. The small anaplastic tumor cell is believed to be a highly undifferentiated astrocyte (16). It is typically found near the infiltrating margin and is often a minor constituent of primary tumors, but occasionally it may be a prominent, diffuse constituent of AA and GBM (9,16,18,19). It is highly invasive (16,18) and proliferative (16). The depletion of small anaplastic cells in early posttreatment-phase tumors suggests that its highly proliferative nature renders it relatively radiosensitive (16). Cell culture studies suggest an enhanced capacity for drug resistance (20,21). Cytogenetic studies, comparing primary and recurrent high-grade astrocytomas, confirm a long-term relative increase in these cells, which often are the ultimate dominant cell type (21,22). This resilient, highly proliferative, and infiltrative cell presents major challenges to improved management of astrocytomas.

E. Imaging Studies: Pathological Correlation

In addition to aiding in diagnosis, magnetic resonance imaging (MRI) and computed tomography (CT) studies are used to define the volume requiring radiation therapy in gliomas. A clear understanding of the relation between the image and the actual tumor extent is critical. In both CT and MRI, contrast enhancement occurs when intravascular contrast material leaks into the parenchyma (11,23). As such, enhancement denotes a failure of the blood–brain barrier, a nonspecific finding that is observed in a variety of conditions, including neoplasm, infection, and infarction. High-grade gliomas enhance owing to absence or deterioration of the blood–brain barrier, whereas well-differentiated tumors generally have intact blood–brain barriers and do not enhance. An important exception is the pilocytic astrocytoma, in which leaky capillaries result in striking uniform enhancement, despite its indolent behavior (24).

The microscopic concomitant of enhancement is a highly cellular and mitotically active neoplasm with proliferating vascular endothelial and stromal cells. Surrounding the area of contrast enhancement is a variably sized region defined by low density in CT images and high T2 signal in MRI images (11–14,19). This zone corresponds to white matter edema. Typically, a decreasing gradient of tumor cells extends away from the enhancing area into the surrounding edema. The vast majority of the cells are within 2 cm of the edge of enhancement, and data show that up to 90% of astrocytomas recur within these 2 cm of the original radiographic lesion (25). In autopsy studies of patients with untreated GBM, the extent of tumor identified by microscopic examination of whole-brain sections was compared with the limits defined by CT scans obtained shortly before death (13,19). The area of enhancement underestimated the extent of tumor in all cases, and in half, tumor was found 2 cm or more from the enhancing rim. Infiltrating cells were found beyond the area of low density in one-third of cases. Studies using CT-guided stereotactic biopsies to define the extent of tumor in vivo had similar findings (11,14).

The MRI is more sensitive to subtle changes in tissue water and generally defines a greater region of edema than does CT. The extent of the T2-signal abnormality is currently the most accurate imaging study of the extent of tumor cell infiltration in primary gliomas (12). Studies of

---

Figure 9 Common histological subtypes of astrocytomas. (A) Fibrillary: spindle cells demonstrate variably prominent glial fiber production. (B) Gemistocytic: large cell body contains a mass of abnormally distributed glial fibers and an eccentrically placed nucleus. (C) Protoplasmic: tumor cells have well-differentiated, round-to-oval nuclei, with scanty cytoplasm and little fiber production. (D) Pilocytic: there is extensive glial fiber production with tapering bundles of glial fibers extending from elongated nuclei. (E) Bizarre giant cells are seen in this GBM. (F) Small anaplastic astrocytes with irregular nuclear contours and chromatin distribution. These undifferentiated tumor cells demonstrate little fiber production (H&E; original magnification: A, C–E × 200; B × 250; F × 400).

MRI-guided stereotactic biopsies of high-grade astrocytomas have shown that tumor cells are typically found throughout, and even slightly beyond, the region of high T2-signal intensity and, thus, beyond the area of CT abnormality (11,14). The area of T2-signal abnormality correlated with the extent of tumor cell infiltration in a study comparing postmortem MRI images and microscopic examination of whole-brain sections from patients with untreated high-grade astrocytomas. Important exceptions were seen in tumors with gray matter infiltration or subarachnoid spread, which were not detected by MRI. It is also clear that isolated tumor cells may infiltrate without eliciting edema, rendering them undetectable by MRI.

The role of MRI contrast agents has not been adequately evaluated, but it appears that studies with contrast enhancement are more sensitive to subarachnoid and subependymal spread than non–contrast-enhanced studies or CT (23). The identification of individual infiltrating tumor cells seems likely to remain beyond the range of detection of any radiologic method for the foreseeable future.

Studies of recurrent tumors are less encouraging: tumor cells typically are present far beyond the CT-predicted limits (19). In a postmortem MRI study of ten recurrent astrocytomas, the T2 signal varied from good correlation with the microscopic extent of disease to significantly over- and underestimating its extent. In two patients with clinical remission, the extent of tumor was greatly overestimated by the T2 abnormality (12). Biopsy of these patients may show only radiation necrosis or gliosis (Fig. 10). A second pattern may show similar changes, but includes foci of less severe reactive changes in which highly atypical cells are scattered. These cells have the appearance of malignant astrocytes, but distinction from radiation-altered reactive astrocytes is difficult. Furthermore, there is evidence that these cells are not proliferative (26). In the absence of obvious tumor regrowth, characterized by confluent nests or sheets of tumor cells, one should be cautious about concluding that a patient has failed therapy. In equivocal cases, an immunohisto-chemical proliferation marker may confirm the presence of actively proliferating tumor

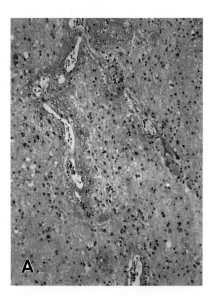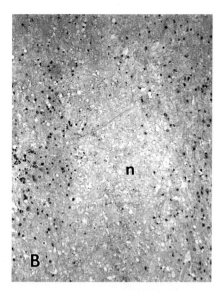

Figure 10 Radiation effect: (A) Loss of endothelial cells is seen and is associated with protein leakage around blood vessels. Atypical reactive or neoplastic astrocytes are present in the surrounding tissue. (B) Scattered atypical astrocytes are present around an acellular area of radiation-induced necrosis (n). Contrast this appearance with the typical pseudopalisading necrosis seen in Figure 3(B) (H&E; original magnification: A, B × 100).

cells (see later discussion). Because radiation necrosis mimics recurrent tumor, imaging studies alone are often insufficient to diagnose recurrent tumor. Positron emission tomography (PET) scanning shows promise here (27). In the absence of new lesions, we have found that a rebiopsy most often shows only radiation necrosis and attendant gliosis and edema, particularly following interstitial radiation.

F. Regional Heterogeneity

Most astrocytomas are believed to begin as LGA, with potential evolution into AA and GBM as the result of progressive dedifferentiation over time (28). As a result, many high-grade astrocytomas contain areas that appear well differentiated. Even within high-grade regions there is variable expression of critical diagnostic features. This *regional heterogeneity* is a principal cause of sampling-related errors, which are, in turn, the principal limitation of microscopic evaluation of brain biopsies. Although biopsies of a homogeneous neoplasm should result in the same diagnosis and grade, irrespective of the biopsy site, biopsies of a heterogeneous tumor may yield significantly different results. Thus, a biopsy of a GBM at different sites could yield diagnoses of LGA, AA, or GBM, or may yield only infiltrating tumor cells that defy further grading (3,29–31). Necrosis may be so extensive that biopsy yields only nondiagnostic necrotic debris. Foci of oligodendroglioma differentiation in an astrocytoma also can result in misclassification of a small biopsy. In addition to their diagnostic implications, these heterogeneity-induced grading and classification errors hobble treatment studies by producing spurious survival results.

Because representative sampling is essential for accurate diagnosis (3,29), the increasing use of stereotactic needle biopsies poses a significant problem for the pathologist. The small sample increases the chance of sampling-related errors, compared with formal open biopsy, debulking, or resection (29–31). In addition, compression artifacts may impair evaluation of cytological detail, particularly if the tissue is first used for frozen section evaluation. Despite these reservations, stereotactic biopsies are useful for diagnosis of tumors in fragile patients or from eloquent areas (32,33). We recommend that needle biopsies be taken all along an axis of the tumor so that the superficial and deep radiographic "margins" and center are all sampled (3,34). Close cooperation among surgeon, radiologist, and pathologist is essential. If the frozen section examination indicates a lower-grade tumor than the image suggests, additional tissue is needed to help resolve the discrepancy (33). Additional biopsies from the diagnostic region(s) should be processed without freezing, to permit optimum histological preparation.

We have focused on the histological expression of glioma heterogeneity. However, as the name glioblastoma multiforme indicates, heterogeneity is seen at the gross level as well and, as we shall see in the following, regional heterogeneity is seen at all levels in astrocytomas, from the gross to the molecular (20,27,35–39).

G. Current Investigations

Most grading systems are functionally three-tiered. Although it is recognized that each grade does not contain a completely homogeneous group of neoplasms, attempts at further subdivision, based on microscopic criteria alone, have not proved fruitful. Effective subclassification of AA and GBM awaits the results of ongoing molecular, immunological, and cytogenetic studies.

Among the histological features used in grading, the identification of mitotic figures most directly reflects a specific biological characteristic of malignancy. However, the mitotic count may *not* reflect the actual proliferative activity of the neoplasm, because only a small part of the proliferative cell cycle is visualized. Quantitative analysis of proliferative activity by immunohistochemical methods, including bromodeoxyuridine (BrdU) incorporation, Ki-67 and proliferating cell nuclear antigen (PCNA)-labeling indices (LI), silver-staining of nucleolar-organizing regions (AgNORs or NORs), or by flow cytometric (FCM) cell cycle analysis offer the possibility of more accurate measurement. Preliminary studies using these methods have shown good correlation with histological tumor grade and good correlation of proliferation estimates among the methods (40–52). The immunohistochemical and AgNOR methods may be particularly useful in overcoming sampling errors in small specimens, such as needle biopsies, or in biopsies from the infiltrating edge of a tumor, where the usual histological features of malignancy may be absent. In our laboratory, Ki-67 LI are reported on all gliomas. In general, labeling indices of less than 1–2% are seen in LGA, with values up to 30% seen in high-grade tumors. Caution must be exercised in evaluating proliferation measurements: systematic studies have found diagnostically significant regional heterogeneity in Ki-67 LI and FCM S-phase determinations (53,54).

Two other histological characteristics—nuclear pleomorphism and hyperchromasia—reflect abnormal, usually increased, DNA content in tumor cells (aneuploidy), but in a nonspecific, nonquantitative manner. Flow cytometry allows quantitative measurement of DNA content; however, ploidy determination by FCM has been of equivocal value in assessing astrocytomas. Most studies find a correlation between aneuploidy and aggressive tumor behavior, but others dispute this conclusion (46,55,56). Most tumors have obvious aneuploid or tetraploid populations. However, FCM currently is not sufficiently sensitive to detect differences of only one or two chromosomes. This results in many truly (albeit barely) aneuploid tumors being called diploid. Further limiting the effectiveness of ploidy studies is the observation of significant regional heterogeneity, with populations of cells of different ploidy in different regions of tumors (53).

Formal cytogenetic studies are more promising. The appearance of specific karyotypic abnormalities appears to be associated with neoplastic transformation and with malignant progression. The most common changes include loss of one chromosome 10, and trisomy of chromosome 7 (27,57–61). Numerical abnormalities of chromosomes 13, 22, and Y are less common, but also appear significant (27,57,58,60,61). Tumors may demonstrate more than one abnormal clone. The number and complexity of the chromosomal abnormalities increase with tumor grade, and the genetic instability that they indicate may have intrinsic biological and prognostic significance (27,60). In addition to these cell-to-cell differences in karyotype, regional karyotypic heterogeneity is also seen, suggesting that malignant progression may involve clonal expansion of a local mutation (27,28,36).

Structural (nonnumerical) chromosomal abnormalities also occur. Perhaps the most important is mutation of the p53 gene on chromosome 17. Most commonly, this occurs in association with loss of the p53 gene on the other chromosome 17. This loss of heterozygosity for p53 and mutation of the remaining p53 gene is associated with progression from low to high grade, and has been reported in one-third to one-half of high-grade astrocytomas (62–64).

Several growth factor and receptor pathways interact in astrocytomas. These pathways include both paracrine mechanisms, in which the stimulus to proliferate comes from an exogenous source (other tumor cells, endothelial cells), and autocrine mechanisms, by which tumor cell proliferation is self-stimulated (65–69). The platelet-derived growth factors (PDGF), transforming growth factors (TGF), and fibroblastic growth factors (FGF), all appear to have substantial roles in glioma growth (65–69). The FGF and TGF are particularly involved with tumor angiogenesis (69,70). The epidermal growth factor receptor (EGF-R) appears to play a central role in tumor proliferation. Amplification of the EGF-R gene and protein overexpression are correlated with tumor grade (71–74). Only EGF-R and PDGF have been evaluated for heterogeneity, and significant regional differences were found for both (39,75).

Recent investigations are also challenging assumptions about the lineage of glial tumors. The term *astrocytoma* suggests that these are tumors of astrocytes, and the descriptive names of the cytological subtypes reinforce this view. Current immunological data suggest that these tumors arise from more primitive astroglial progenitor cells. Type 1 astrocytes are the traditional structural and reactive fibrillary astrocytes. Type 2 (protoplasmic) astrocytes are associated with neurons and are involved with neuropil function. Type 2 astrocytes are derived from 0-2A progenitor cells, which react with the A2B5 antigen, whereas type 1 progenitor cells are negative for A2B5. The type 1 astrocyte or its precursor gives rise to traditional astrocytomas, but the type 2 astrocyte or its 0-2A progenitor cell appears to be the precursor for some astrocytomas and mixed gliomas, as well as all oligodendrogliomas (76,77). This difference in lineage and its role in tumor prognosis are discussed in the sections on oligodendroglioma and mixed glioma.

III. PILOCYTIC ASTROCYTOMAS

A. Introduction

Pilocytic astrocytomas (PAs) occur preponderantly in the first two decades, but also occur in older adults (78). The cerebellum and hypothalamus are favored locations, particularly in young persons. Hemispheric tumors are being recognized more frequently (79). Pilocytic astrocytomas appear to have a unique biology among astrocytomas. Their generally sharp circumscription makes them amenable to complete excision, particularly in the cerebellum, in which they typically occur as a cystic tumor with a mural nodule. Up to 95% of patients with cerebellar PA were disease-free 25 years after surgery (80). Similar results were obtained in a study of hemispheric tumors (79). Even subtotal resection results in long-term survival in many patients, as malignant evolution is exceptional (81,82).

B. Imaging Studies and Gross Features

Imaging studies show a mass, with well-defined borders, that is contrast-enhancing (82,83). This latter feature is important, because enhancement typically is associated with high-grade gliomas. In a well-differentiated hemispheric PA, contrast enhancement distinguishes it from a diffuse low-grade astrocytoma. However, PAs often demonstrate significant pleomorphism, and this, coupled with contrast enhancement, may result in an erroneous diagnosis of AA.

Grossly, PAs are often gray and fleshy, but a highly developed microcystic pattern may produce a more myxoid appearance. Coalescence of the microcysts into a single large cyst, with a solid mural nodule, also occurs, particularly in the cerebellum. The cystic component can be the principal cause of mass effect.

C. Microscopic Features

Two principal cell types may be found in PA (Fig. 11). The pilocyte is a well-differentiated bipolar cell with prominent, hairlike glial processes. The other cell resembles a protoplasmic astrocyte, with round nuclei and few visible processes. Areas of the latter cell type probably account for reports of apparent oligodendroglioma differentiation in PA. Microcysts that contain mucopolysaccharide material may be common, and can coalesce to form a single cyst or multiple cysts. Contrasting areas of high and low cellularity are often seen, and there may be similar variation in the density of glial fibers. Rosenthal fibers, which are densely eosinophilic rod-shaped bodies, and granular bodies, which are eosinophilic deposits of unknown origin, are seen commonly. These last two features are particularly helpful, as they are seen only in indolent neoplasms, such as PA and gangliogliomas, and not in high-grade gliomas (78). Prominent capillary networks must be distinguished from the pattern of vascular proliferation seen in high-grade astrocytomas.

Prominent cytological atypia and focal hypercellularity are not uncommon and, rarely, necrosis may be seen. An occasional mitosis may be seen in some tumors, but their usual low-

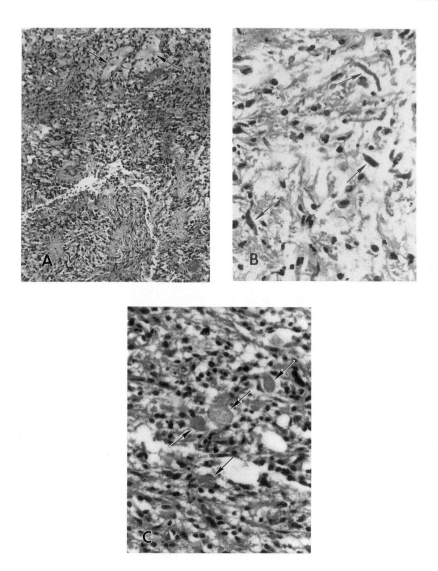

Figure 11 Pilocytic astrocytoma: (A) Tumor is characterized by pilocytes and microcysts containing mucopolysaccharide material (arrows). Note irregular distribution of tumor cells, producing nucleus- and fiber-rich regions. (B) Rosenthal fibers (arrows) may be abundant. (C) Eosinophilic granular bodies (arrows) are numerous in this example. Contrast their loose-textured appearance with the dense Rosenthal fibers seen in B (H&E; original magnification: A × 100; B, C × 400).

proliferative activity is borne out by low Ki-67 LI (84) and S-phase fraction (85). The relation of histological features to outcome is controversial. A poorer prognosis has been reported in cases with atypical features, but this conclusion is challenged by other investigators (78–80,86). Given that recurrence following total resection is rare, and can occur irrespective of histological features, we do not believe that current means of histological grading have a role in determining management.

The presence of atypical histological features in a substantial number of PAs creates the potential for their misdiagnosis as AA, especially when there is limited tumor sampling (e.g., with needle biopsies). Hemispheric tumors are of particular concern here. Furthermore, both AA and PA demonstrate diffuse contrast enhancement on MRI studies (83). Such misdiagnoses may explain many cases of very long survival in "anaplastic astrocytomas."

IV. GLIOMATOSIS CEREBRI

A. Introduction

Gliomatosis cerebri is a very rare pattern of astrocytic neoplasia. Its distinction from astrocytoma may be artificial, but traditionally it is discussed as a separate entity. It may occur at any age, but is most common in the middle-adult years (87). In the strictest linguistic sense, it may not be a "tumor" at all: there is often no mass per se; instead, neoplastic astrocytes diffusely expand large areas of the cerebral hemisphere(s) or central and infratentorial structures, or both (87–92), ultimately resulting in mass *effects*. Despite the extent of tumor, there is often a paucity of symptoms, even at diagnosis. Survival ranges from weeks to many years postdiagnosis (87,91, 92).

B. Imaging and Gross Features

Computed tomography and MRI reveal a diffuse, nondestructive process, often with slitlike ventricles, that may not be distinguishable from nonneoplastic hypodense lesions (89,92). Before the modern imaging era, the diagnosis of gliomatosis cerebri was made exclusively at autopsy, but the combination of imaging and multiple biopsies allows antemortem diagnosis (87,92).

Gross examination displays cerebral architecture that typically is expanded and distorted without a destructive mass (87–92). White matter involvement predominates, with tumor often following anatomical pathways (89), but gray matter involvement may be extensive. Sometimes, a small discrete mass may be present (87–92).

C. Microscopic Features

Microscopically, the neoplasm is often composed of spindle-shaped astrocytes that show a variable degree of fiber production. The tumor cells grow between the myelinated fibers, with little damage to the infiltrated white matter. The cellularity and cytological features are usually those of a diffuse low-grade astrocytoma, but areas with greater pleomorphism, mitotic figures, and even necrosis are sometimes observed (87–92). Low proliferative activity has been found in two cases stained for nucleolar-organizing regions (93). When present, tumor masses may demonstrate high-grade transformation.

D. Origin and Development

The origin of gliomatosis cerebri is controversial. Arguments in favor of diffuse or widespread multifocal neoplastic transformation have been made (88,90). Others, ourselves included, consider it an extreme example of diffusely infiltrating astrocytoma (94,95). The possibility that gliomatosis cerebri can be produced by both mechanisms has also been suggested (92). Low-grade astrocytomas are primarily infiltrative in the early stages of their evolution. In some high-grade astrocytomas, particularly recurrent small-cell glioblastomas, invasiveness is highly expressed. The formation of a discrete, locally destructive mass is a feature of high-grade gliomas and appears to be a property distinct from invasiveness. Gliomatosis may be the end result of low-grade tumors that never acquire the capacity to form destructive masses, or arise from high-grade tumors in which invasiveness predominates over other features.

V. PLEOMORPHIC XANTHOASTROCYTOMA

A. Introduction

The pleomorphic xanthoastrocytoma is a rare, superficial hemispheric tumor that most commonly arises in the temporal or parietal lobes (96–99). It is a tumor of children and young adults, with the diagnosis usually made in the second or third decade. However, many patients have a history of seizures with onset in childhood, which presumably are referable to the tumor (96,97,100). The increasing use of MRI to evaluate new-onset seizures may result in substantially earlier detection and treatment and this, in turn, may alter the expected course of the disease.

The tumors generally follow an indolent course, and long survival is expected (96,97). Although generally partly circumscribed, the cyst wall may have a diffusely infiltrating interface with brain, which sometimes precludes complete surgical removal (96–98). The often long interval between onset of seizures and production of symptoms of mass effect indicates that pleomorphic xanthoastrocytomas grow slowly. This was confirmed in a tumor studied by flow cytometry, that was found to have a low S-phase fraction (101). Anaplastic transformation, once considered exceptional (79), now has been reported in several cases and is associated with a rapidly fatal course (96,97,102,103).

B.   Imaging Studies and Gross Features

Grossly, the tumor is circumscribed, often sharply so. Solid areas may alternate with cystic regions, and the cysts may predominate. The solid portions of the tumor are in contact with the pia mater (96,97). Imaging studies (96,97,99,104) demonstrate uniform contrast enhancement of the solid tumor. Alternation of solid and cystic areas may produce a mottled appearance.

C.   Microscopic Features

The microscopic appearance of the pleomorphic xanthoastrocytoma reflects its name (96–99). The tumor is characterized by cellular regions composed of large, often wildly pleomorphic cells. The hyperchromatic nuclei may be multiple, and there is abundant glassy eosinophilic cytoplasm. Infrequent mitotic figures and absence of a typical vascular proliferation or necrosis belie the aggressive course suggested by the pleomorphism. The interface with brain may be sharply circumscribed, or the tumor cells may blend with the parenchyma in a manner indistinguishable from a diffuse infiltrating astrocytoma. Many of the cells tend to be lipid laden, but this feature may not be apparent. Vascular-based lymphocytic infiltrates are common, and the tumor displays a rich reticulin network.

1.   Ultrastructure

Ultrastructural studies have found abundant basement membrane material associated with the tumor cells (97,98,101,103), a feature of subpial astrocytes, but not of other astrocytic subtypes (97,98). This suggests that the pleomorphic xanthoastrocytoma may arise from the subpial astrocyte (97,98), which would be consistent with its consistently superficial location.

D.   Differential Diagnosis

The principal considerations in differential diagnosis are histiocytic tumors (in lipid-rich speci-mens), high-grade gliomas, and gangliogliomas (98,99,104). The histiocytic tumors are excluded by the consistently strong reaction for GFAP in even the lipid-filled tumor cells. As noted in the foregoing, the pleomorphic xanthoastrocytoma lacks most of the features associated with high-grade tumors. Only if the biopsy is limited to the edge of an infiltrating variant should the distinction be a challenge. Gangliogliomas may share many features with pleomorphic xanthoas-trocytomas, and differentiation may rest on finding an astrocytic, rather than neuronal, im-munohistochemical reaction pattern.

VI. ASTROBLASTOMA

A. Introduction

The astroblastoma is an exceedingly rare neoplasm of presumed astrocytic lineage. Most develop in the cerebral hemispheres in the first three decades, but have been diagnosed in older adults (105,106).

B. Pathological Features

Grossly, astroblastomas are discrete and often cystic, with the usual gray-tan cut surfaces of gliomas. Soft areas of necrosis may be a feature of high-grade tumors (106).

Most astroblastomas have a sharp interface with the surrounding brain, indicative of expansile, rather than infiltrative, growth. In its pure form, it has a striking appearance (105–108). Spindle-shaped tumor cells are oriented around blood vessels. Short, thick processes extend to the vessel. The arrangement resembles the pseudorosettes seen in ependymomas and astrocytomas. However, unlike these other tumors, few cells or cell processes are present between the perivascular clusters, producing an almost papillary appearance. Tumor cells demonstrate the expected immunoreactivity for GFAP (105,107–109), but one study suggests that the principal intermediate filament is vimentin (109). Usually, little cytological atypia and few mitoses are observed. Anaplastic features, high mitotic counts, and necrosis may be seen in pure astroblastomas. When they are accompanied by areas of typical high-grade astrocytoma, differential diagnoses between astroblastoma and anaplastic astrocytoma or glioblastoma with features of astroblastoma become problematic (105,106). The distinction may not be relevant, as these tumors behave as high-grade astrocytomas. Ependymoma is the other principal differential diagnostic consideration (105). In the absence of true rosettes or ependymal tubules, the characteristic large pseudorosettes and the intervening areas of high cellularity are still distinctive.

C. Behavior

Although the name suggests a relatively primitive tumor, the course of well-differentiated astroblastomas has been characterized as low grade, with its sharp circumscription lending a better prognosis than in diffuse low-grade astrocytomas (106,110). Anaplastic features are associated with a worse prognosis, but there is a less consistent correlation between histological features and survival than there is for astrocytomas (106,111).

VII. OLIGODENDROGLIOMA

A. Introduction

As discussed in the foregoing, the lineage of oligodendrogliomas is closely related to the astrocytoma and, as discussed in the following, their cell types often overlap. They represent from 4 to 15% of gliomas (112,113), the wide variation in estimated frequency reflecting the often subtle distinction between oligodendroglioma and astrocytoma. They occur at all ages, but are rare in childhood and adolescence (112,113). Their greatest incidence is in the fourth and fifth decade (113).

Oligodendrogliomas occur primarily in the cerebral hemispheres, particularly in the frontal and parietal lobes. They are diffusely infiltrative in a nondestructive manner, similar to low-grade astrocytomas. As a result, they can achieve great size before they produce symptoms. Like astrocytomas, the principal pattern of spread is through white matter; however, oligodendrogliomas often have a significant gray matter component, and appear to move more freely through gray matter than do most astrocytomas.

B. Imaging Studies and Gross Findings

The MRI appearance of oligodendrogliomas is typically that of a discrete, low-density lesion that shows little or no contrast enhancement. Calcification is usually apparent on CT scans. Hemorrhage and cyst formation are commonly seen (114). The MRI-defined tumor margins are often inapparent on gross examination. Instead, the white (and sometimes gray) matter may be diffusely expanded and have an abnormally firm texture (see Fig. 4). There is a gradual transition to normal dimensions. Other tumors produce discrete soft gray mass lesions (113).

C. Microscopic Features

The microscopic appearance of the classic oligodendroglioma is distinct: a uniform mosaic of cells, with clear cytoplasm, a distinct cell membrane, and centrally placed round, regular nuclei, with dispersed chromatin. A prominent network of fine, branching capillaries completes the picture (112,113). This pattern of cells, with the perinuclear halos and plexiform capillaries, has given rise to the term "fried egg cells and chicken feet vasculature," a colorfully descriptive term in the gastronomic manner favored by many pathologists.

Unfortunately, the full expression of this pattern is the exception, rather than the rule. The perinuclear halos are an artifact of autolysis and may not be well developed in promptly fixed biopsies. Similarly, the vascular pattern, which some feel is merely an exaggeration of the normal cerebral capillary network, may not be prominent.

Diagnosis often rests on recognition of the characteristic evenly spaced, bland, round nuclei, which are larger and usually paler-staining than normal oligodendroglia (112,113). Even more than LGA, oligodendrogliomas grow without destruction of the infiltrated brain and, often, do not elicit a prominent glial response. Thus, the background of the tumor contains preserved neuropil or white matter without many astrocytic fibers. The tendency to *perineuronal satellitosis*—the clustering of tumor cells around neurons in a neoplastic caricature of their normal supportive role—is not specific to oligodendrogliomas, but is characteristic and often highly expressed (112,113,115). Oligodendrogliomas may demonstrate considerable pleomorphism. In addition to variability in nuclear morphology, cells with dense eosinophilic cytoplasm, which resemble elements more typical of astrocytomas, may be present.

1. Histological Grading

Predicting the behavior of oligodendrogliomas is a challenging problem in surgical neuropathology. The relative rarity of these neoplasms compared with astrocytomas has contributed to the delayed development of a reliable histological grading system. As with astrocytomas, there is a strong correlation between age at diagnosis and outcome in oligodendrogliomas. In our studies, age at diagnosis has been a stronger predictor of survival than histological criteria.

The histological criteria and survival estimates of several commonly used grading systems are shown in Table 2. In general, oligodendrogliomas are associated with longer survival than their astrocytoma counterparts with similar histological features (112,116). Figures 12–15 illustrate typical histological patterns and are accompanied by the corresponding grades in several systems.

All of the systems effectively classify the lowest- and highest-grade tumors; however, there is considerable variability in survival among tumors in the critical middle grade(s). The four-tiered systems of Kernohan (117) and Smith et al. (118) attempt to subdivide this middle group of tumors, with mixed success. As others have reported (101), we found no significant difference in survival between Smith grades B and C, and survival varied widely within these grades. The system of Kros et al. (119) is, in fact, a reevaluation of the Smith system, which combines grades B and C and eliminates redundant criteria. The St. Anne–Mayo system is an adaptation of the system developed at the Mayo Clinic for grading astrocytomas (116,120) (see Sec. II.B).

Table 2 Comparison of Grading Systems for Oligodendrogliomas

Kernohan (117)	St. Anne–Mayo (116,120)	Smith et al. (118)	Ringertz–Burger (112)
Tumor grades are based on progressive development of hypercellularity, cellular anaplasia and mitotic activity.	Tumor grades are based on presence of specific histologic features: pleomorphism, mitoses, atypical vascular proliferation and necrosis.	Tumor grades are based on specific histologic features: pleomorphism, hypercellularity, high nuclear/cytoplasmic ratio, vascular proliferation and necrosis.	Tumor grades are based on progressive development of anaplasia.
Grade	Grade	Grade	
1	1	A	Well-differentiated
No pleomorphism. Mild hypercellularity. Neuropil persists between cells.	No features present.	No features present.	Uniform round nuclei. Mitoses rare or absent. No vascular proliferation or necrosis.
2	2	B	Anaplastic
Moderate hypercellularity with loss of neuropil between cells. Mild pleomorphism.	One feature present. (pleomorphism)	Pleomorphism and/or high cellularity and nuclear/cytoplasmic ratio.	Obvious oligodendroglioma differentiation persists.
3	3	C	Hypercellularity, pleomorphism, mitoses and vascular proliferation present. Necrosis is common.
Moderate hypercellularity and moderate pleomorphism. Mitoses present.	Two features present. (typically pleomorphism and mitoses)	Pleomorphism, high cellularity and nuclear/cytoplasmic ratio, atypical vascular proliferation.	
4	4	D	Glioblastoma Multiforme
Moderate hypercellularity with increasing pleomorphism and mitoses. Vascular proliferation and necrosis may be present.	Three or four features present. (pleomorphism, mitoses, plus vascular proliferation and/or necrosis)	All features present. (necrosis)	Focal preservation of typical oligodendroglioma indicates lineage, but tumor appears predominantly astrocytic or undifferentiated
			Typical features of GBM present: pleomorphism, mitoses, vascular proliferation and necrosis.

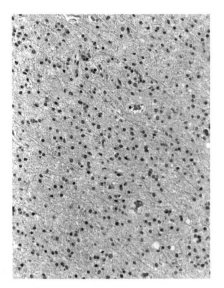

Figure 12   Oligodendroglioma: Kernohan (K): grade 1; St. Anne–Mayo (SA/M): grade 1; Smith (S): grade A; Ringertz–Burger (R/B): well differentiated. Modestly hypercellular tumor composed of cells with bland round nuclei that are larger and less densely staining compared with normal oligodendrocytes. The white matter is well preserved. There is no mitotic activity (H&E; original magnification × 100).

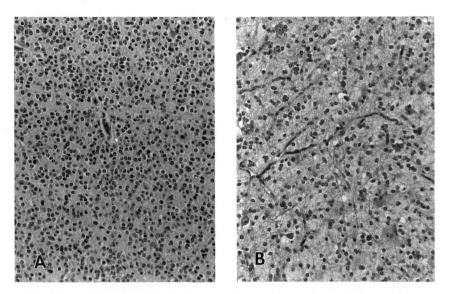

Figure 13   Oligodendroglioma: K: grade 2; SA/M: grade 2; S: grade B; R/B: well-differentiated. (A) Tumor is moderately hypercellular and almost confluent, resulting in less parenchymal preservation. The tumor cells demonstrate classic perinuclear halos. There is some pleomorphism, but nuclear contours remain round-to-oval. (B) The typical plexiform capillary network is well-seen in this region (H&E; original magnification: A, B × 200).

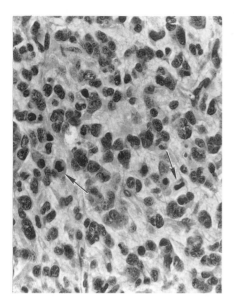

Figure 14 Oligodendroglioma: K: grade 3; SA/M: grade 3; S: grade C; R/B: anaplastic. Tumor is more hypercellular, and there is greater pleomorphism. Mitotic figures are frequently seen (arrows) (H&E; original magnification × 500).

As the comparative table reveals, the histological classification of oligodendrogliomas is less refined than for astrocytomas. For the latter, differences in grading systems relate principally to the emphasis given each of the generally accepted histological criteria. For oligodendrogliomas, there is a more fundamental disagreement about which criteria are important.

The most interesting difference among grading systems is the lack of correlation between the presence of mitoses and outcome in several systems (115,118,119). Since the capacity to proliferate and create a space-occupying mass is a major determinant of behavior in glial tumors, it is unlikely that tumor growth rate does not significantly affect survival. Besides being counterintuitive, such a conclusion also would be contrary to the literature concerning the closely related astrocytoma (120–123). The mitotic count may not accurately reflect the actual proliferative activity of a tumor. Mitotic figures represent only a small proportion of the cells undergoing proliferation, and their identification is affected by observer subjectivity and errors inherent in tumor sampling.

The distinction between an oligodendroglioma with atypical histological features, but low-grade behavior, and one with both anaplastic histology and aggressive behavior is not academic. Oligodendrogliomas are often treated using astrocytoma protocols, and the classification of a tumor as "grade 3" or "anaplastic," may subject a patient to inappropriately aggressive therapy.

D. Current Investigations

Quantitative assessment of proliferation may offer a better means of assessing this theoretically important prognostic variable. We found that proliferative activity, as measured by FCM PI, was a highly significant predictor of survival in oligodendrogliomas, and was considerably more accurate in predicting outcome than the histopathological grade (124). However, a small series evaluating the Ki-67 LI was inconclusive (125).

In contrast with the promise shown by proliferation assessment, two studies have found no correlation between aneuploidy per se, or a specific aneuploid pattern, and survival (124,126), so there appears to be no role for ploidy determination in the evaluation of oligodendrogliomas.

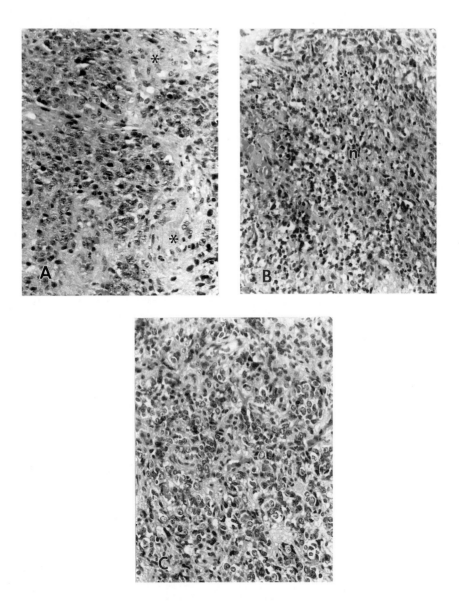

Figure 15   Oligodendroglioma: K: grade 4; SA/M: grade 4; S: grade D; R/B: glioblastoma multiforme. (A) Atypical vascular proliferation is present (*). Tumor cells are pleomorphic and poorly differentiated. (B) Karyorrhexis, indicative of early tumor necrosis is present (n). (C) In some regions, the pleomorphic tumor cells demonstrate characteristic perinuclear halos (original magnification: A–C, × 250).

Cytogenetic studies have demonstrated no consistent abnormalities. Oligodendrogliomas tend to have normal karyotypes, but simple clonal and, less commonly, complex clonal abnormalities are seen (127,128). Molecular studies found that only a small percentage of oligodendrogliomas demonstrate p53 mutations (129). Overexpression of EGF-R has been reported in 40% of oligodendrogliomas, but the significance of this observation is unknown (130).

It has been hoped that immunohistochemical markers would reliably distinguish between oligodendroglioma and astrocytoma. As alluded to earlier, oligodendrogliomas have variable expression of GFAP, so this feature cannot be used to distinguish the tumors. Mature oligodendroglia demonstrate myelin basic protein (MBP) (131), but MBP has not proved reliable in identifying oligodendrogliomas. Oligodendroglial cells arise from the 0-2A progenitor cells, which also give rise to type 2 astrocytes and express the A2B5 antigen. Cells that differentiate toward oligodendroglia express, in addition, galactocerebroside (GC), whereas those that become astrocytes express GFAP. Recent studies have found consistent expression of A2B5 and GC in oligodendrogliomas (132,133). A2B5 is also expressed in a certain proportion of astrocytomas and mixed oligoastrocytomas (132,133).

E. Heterogeneity

Although they are typically more homogeneous than astrocytomas, oligodendrogliomas also demonstrate regional heterogeneity. Diagnostically, significant regional differences have been noted in microscopic appearance, ploidy, and proliferative activity (134,135).

VIII. MIXED GLIOMA

The term *mixed glioma* is used here to describe tumors containing more than one histological pattern of glial differentiation. The principal neoplasms of mixed glial and neuronal or mesenchymal elements (i.e., ganglioglioma and gliosarcoma) are discussed separately. For practical purposes, mixed glioma means mixed astrocytoma and oligodendroglioma. This combination is sometimes called oligoastrocytoma.

The use of the diagnosis mixed glioma is highly variable among pathologists. Many pathologists prefer to name the tumor by its dominant cell type, restricting the term mixed glioma for those cases in which similar-sized, regionally distinct areas of both cell types are present (136). Others apply the term whenever a definite admixed population of a second cell type is recognizable.

Whatever the histological patterns, mixed gliomas are the result of neoplastic transformation of a single cell line that demonstrates divergent expression of astroglial differentiation, and it is likely that the behavior of the tumor will reflect the cell line that underwent neoplastic transformation. To many, the expected behavior of a mixed glioma was that predicted by its "astrocytic" component. However, a recent study found that most mixed gliomas express the A2B5 antigen, indicating origin from the 0-2A progenitor cell that gives rise to oligodendrogliomas and type 2 astrocytes (137,138). The mixed glioma cells also expressed galactocerebroside (an oligodendroglial marker) and GFAP (an astrocytic marker). Recognition of this lineage may be critical for predicting tumor behavior. Oligodendrogliomas, the best-studied tumors of this lineage, have a more favorable prognosis than astrocytomas of equivalent grade (139,140). The data suggest that a tumor with a diagnosis of mixed glioma also *may* have a better prognosis than a similar-grade astrocytoma. A correspondingly less aggressive approach to radiation therapy may be appropriate, and consideration should be paid to the new chemotherapy regimens being used to treat oligodendrogliomas (141).

IX. EPENDYMOMA

A. Introduction

The ependymoma is among the more common nonastrocytic tumors and constitutes 2–6% of all primary brain tumors (142,143). It occurs primarily in childhood and adolescence, but may occur at any age (142–145). As the name implies, ependymomas derive from neoplastic transformation of the ependyma. The normal ependyma forms an epithelial lining on the surfaces of the ventricles, and ependymomas of the brain are primarily ventricular tumors. Intrahemispheric tumors without demonstrable connection to the ventricles occur, presumably arising from rests of ependymal cells that remain following fusion of the primitive ependymal seam in embryological development. Intracranial ependymomas are often grouped into two categories, based on location. Supratentorial tumors are preponderant in adults, whereas more infratentorial tumors occur in children (142–144,146).

B. Imaging and Gross Findings

Radiologic studies of ependymomas are usually prompted by symptoms of CSF obstruction (144,145,147,148). T1-weighted MRI images disclose a hypo- to isointense contrast-enhancing mass that typically fills and expands a ventricle. They are hyperintense on T2-weighted images, and contrast enhancement may be necessary to distinguish the tumor margins from surrounding edema. Calcification may be seen by CT. A large cyst may be present. Hydrocephalus is often present (144,145,147,148).

Grossly, ependymomas are lobular, with fleshy gray-tan cut surfaces. They are exophytic, protruding into the ventricle, but have a broad-based attachment to the ventricular surface. Fourth ventricular tumors often extend through the foramena and wrap the brain stem. A sharp cleavage plane between tumor and parenchyma is usually identifiable, an important feature that allows complete surgical removal in many cases (145).

C. Microscopic Features

Ependymomas demonstrate diverse microscopic appearances (142–144,146,147,149–152). The most common growth pattern is solid and highly cellular (Fig. 16). Mucopolysaccharide deposition is relatively common and can be the dominant architectural feature, giving rise to a myxoid, often microcystic, appearance. A papillary pattern may be seen; in extreme cases, the intracerebral tumors closely resemble the myxopapillary ependymoma of the filum terminale (153). The papillary fronds have a core of glial processes that surround a central capillary. Limited invasiveness is the rule, corresponding to the gross circumscription.

Ependymomas may show both glial and epithelial features, as befits their heritage. Epithelial features include the formation of glandlike structures, which may appear as linear tubules, or as ependymal rosettes in cross-sectional profile. When present, cysts are lined by a single layer of tumor cells. The presence of these features in combination with glial regions is both striking and diagnostic; however, clear-cut epithelial differentiation is not always seen, and glial features predominate in most tumors. The most striking feature of glial differentiation is the perivascular pseudorosette. These highly fibrillary regions are essentially devoid of nuclei, in sharp contrast with the typically highly cellular surrounding tumor. The radial arrangement of cell processes extending to the blood vessel is often easily appreciated. Examination of the blood vessels often provides an explanation for the contrast enhancement on imaging studies. The vessels of ependymomas are "leaky," and pale hyaline collars often form around vessels as a result of plasma protein exudation.

Ependymomas typically have strikingly uniform, round-to-oval nuclei, with stippled chromatin. The cytoplasm may be inapparent or form an incomplete eosinophilic rim around the nucleus. Different cytological appearances also may be seen. The major variations have been given descriptive names. These cytological subtypes may be minor components of an otherwise typical ependymoma, or they may be the predominant pattern. In the latter event, the descriptive cytological term often is incorporated in the diagnosis. In the clear cell ependymoma, the bland nuclear appearance is preserved, but there is a uniform perinuclear halo, such as is seen in oligodendrogliomas (154). In the tanycytic ependymoma, cells are more spindle shaped and have more prominent fibrillary processes, resembling an astrocytoma. Tanycytic ependymomas are typically less cellular than other ependymomas, but maintain the diagnostic cellular clustering and perivascular pseudorosettes (142). Pigmented ependymomas are very rare. In these tumors, a

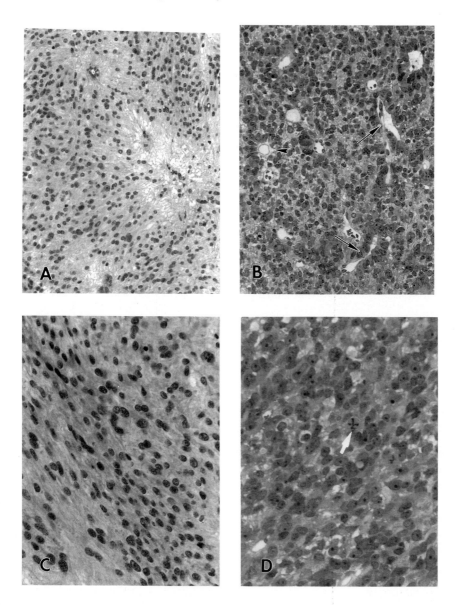

Figure 16 Ependymoma: (A) The tumor is moderately cellular. Glial fibers surround blood vessels, producing characteristic perivascular pseudorosettes. (B) True ependymal rosettes (arrowhead) and tubules (arrows) may be seen. (C) Most ependymomas have bland, round-to-oval nuclei with stippled chromatin. (D) Anaplastic ependymomas are pleomorphic, with more pronounced hypercellularity. Mitotic figures are numerous; an atypical mitosis is illustrated (arrow) (H&E; original magnification: A, B × 200; C, D × 400).

variable number of cells contain neuromelanin (155). The subtypes bear no prognostic value; their significance lies in their varied differential diagnoses.

Although their typical cellular uniformity is a helpful diagnostic feature, ependymomas demonstrate the usual spectrum of cytological and morphological atypia. Rare mitoses and moderate pleomorphism are not unusual in otherwise typical ependymomas, nor are histologically malignant tumors uncommon (145,151)

D. Immunohistochemistry

Despite the epithelial differentiation and function, the ependyma maintains GFAP as a principal intermediate filament and demonstrates limited keratin immunoreactivity. This pattern is carried over into ependymomas. Most ependymomas demonstrate diffuse staining for GFAP, vimentin, and S-100 (156,157). Although occasional keratin-positive cells may be seen, the staining pattern does not resemble the diffuse reactivity of choroid plexus tumors and metastatic carcinomas (156).

E. Growth and Behavior

Ependymomas are malignant tumors, with survival typically ranging from 2 to 20 years. Five-year survival estimates range from 50 to 76% (144,145,158). Most ependymomas grow slowly, although rapid growth is seen occasionally. As with other intracranial neoplasms, metastasis outside the CNS is not a feature of ependymomas. Dissemination and seeding through CSF pathways occurs in fewer than 10% of cases (143,145,147). Although the presence of metastatic lesions is associated with an aggressive course and less than 2-years survival, it is local recurrence at the site of the primary tumor that ultimately causes the death of the patient (143–145,147). Local radiation therapy results in longer survival and may be particularly important when residual tumor is present (143,146).

Although several factors have been associated with an aggressive course, determination of the prognosis for an individual patient is difficult. The lack of infiltrative invasiveness would seem to make ependymomas well suited to curative surgery, and most studies have found a correlation between the success of surgical extirpation and survival (144,145). The absence of residual tumor on postoperative MRI scans has been emphasized as more important than the surgical impression of "gross total removal" (GTR) (144). The age at diagnosis is an important prognostic factor: children have shorter survival, independent of tumor site (144,145,147). Shorter survival is reported in infratentorial tumors, exclusive of perioperative mortality, which is also higher than in supratentorial ependymomas (143,146,147). The meaning of this observation is uncertain because, compared with supratentorial tumors, infratentorial ependymomas have a higher frequency of subtotal resections, owing to involvement of critical structures in the wall of the fourth ventricle (146) and a higher percentage of pediatric patients. Further complicating the already confusing situation, anaplastic features may be more common in supratentorial tumors (149,158).

F. Histological Grading

With a relatively few tumors available to sort out a confusing clinicopathological spectrum, it is not surprising that the usefulness of histological grading in prognostication is controversial (143,145– 147,150,158,159). Among those who have found grading ependymomas to be useful, the usual histological features are generally accepted as being predictive of aggressive behavior: high mitotic activity, atypical vascular proliferation, and necrosis (146,149,151,159). However, these criteria seem to be difficult to apply: different series find 15–94% of ependymomas to be anaplastic (145,151). In the absence of a generally accepted grading system, the terms *anaplastic* or *poorly differentiated* ependymoma are favored to describe the tumors in which these features predominate. *Malignant* ependymoma should be avoided, since it implies a behavior that may not be forthcoming.

Current grading systems may not give proper relative emphasis to the different criteria. As noted, the extent of resection is probably a primary factor determining outcome in ependymomas and may obscure the contributions of tumor biology per se. Nevertheless, the interval to recurrence should reflect tumor growth rate. Recent studies by Schiffer et al. found that the mitotic rate was more important than the presence of necrosis or atypical vascular proliferation in determining prognosis in supratentorial ependymomas (151,160), and similar findings are reported for infratentorial tumors (161). Quantitative methods to assess proliferation would seem potentially helpful here. Single studies of FCM and BrdU were inconclusive (162,163), but a study using PCNA is promising (164).

G. Current Investigations

Molecular and cytogenetic studies in ependymomas are limited. Chromosome 17 abnormalities are most frequent, but no specific abnormality has been identified (165). A p53 mutation is not a feature of ependymomas (166). Of greatest interest, DNA sequences similar to simian virus 40 (SV40) have been found in ependymomas and choroid plexus papillomas (CPP). SV40 is closely related to the ubiquitous human papillomaviruses (BK and JC), and is tumorigenic in rats, inducing CPP (167).

H. Differential Diagnosis

The differential diagnosis of ependymomas is generally not difficult. In the lateral and third ventricles, the principal considerations are diffuse astrocytoma, oligodendroglioma, and central neurocytoma. In addition to the characteristic growth patterns, the high cellularity and minimal pleomorphism of the ependymoma are often distinctive. A similar level of cellularity in an astrocytoma is associated with anaplastic features. The tanycytic ependymoma is less cellular, and its cells closely resemble fibrillary astrocytes, but characteristic nuclear clustering and anucleate zones allow differentiation. Clear cell ependymoma may be confused with oligodendroglioma or neurocytoma. Again, identification of the characteristic morphology and immunohistochemistry allows correct diagnosis. The principal other tumors of the fourth ventricle are the medulloblastoma and pilocytic astrocytoma, which are distinguished easily from ependymoma. Papillary ependymomas in any ventricle must be distinguished from choroid plexus tumors and from metastatic carcinoma. As noted earlier, the papillary fronds in the ependymoma have gliovascular cores, in contrast with the fibrovascular cores seen in the other tumors. If necessary, the distinction can be made by immunohistochemistry: choroid plexus tumors and carcinomas demonstrate immunoreactivity for keratin, rather than GFAP.

Ependymoblastomas are supratentorial primitive neuroectodermal tumors (PNET) that occur exclusively in children (149,168). The details of their characteristic histological appearance and aggressive behavior are discussed with the pediatric tumors.

X. CHOROID PLEXUS TUMORS

A. Introduction

Choroid plexus tumors (CPT) arise from neoplastic transformation of the choroid plexus (CP) epithelium. This specialized epithelium derives from ependyma, and forms papillary protrusions into the ventricles, primarily the lateral and fourth. The choroid plexus requires a rich vascular supply to produce cerebrospinal fluid (CSF) from plasma. The vascular network creates a fibrovascular core in the papillary fronds, in contrast with the glial framework of the rest of the brain. The blood vessels are "leaky" and, as a result, CP is white on T2-weighted MRI images and demonstrates contrast enhancement.

Choroid plexus tumors account for fewer than 1% of all brain tumors (169,170); CPT are relatively more common in childhood, and account for 4% of pediatric brain tumors (171,172). Tumor location follows the distribution of normal CP. For both benign and malignant tumors, adults more commonly have fourth ventricular tumors (169,173,174), whereas in children, lateral ventricular tumors predominate (169,171,173,174). As noted earlier, a recent study has suggested a role for SV40 in the etiology of CPT (175).

B. Choroid Plexus Papilloma

1. Imaging Studies and Gross Features

Imaging studies demonstrate a diffusely enhancing, sharply circumscribed ventricular mass. Hydrocephalus is a consistent feature. Grossly, the typical choroid plexus papilloma (CPP) is a spongy red or tan mass composed of a proliferation of papillary fronds that arise from a variably broad-based stalk. Occasionally, an outgrowth of ependymal epithelium may give the appearance of encapsulation (170,171).

2. Microscopic Features

The microscopic appearance differs from normal CP, primarily in the volume and complexity of the papillary fronds (Fig. 17). A single layer of cuboidal cells with round-to-oval, bland nuclei, lines fibrovascular cores. There is little cytological atypia. Oncocytic change may be seen. Mitotic figures are not present. There is no tumor necrosis, but intratumor hemorrhage is seen frequently and may be confused with necrosis by the unwary. There is no invasion of the underlying parenchyma (170,171,176).

3. Growth and Behavior

Choroid plexus papillomas are slow-growing tumors (177,178). Their lack of invasiveness makes them amenable to curative excision. Rarely, CPP may seed locally or disseminate through CSF pathways.

C. Atypical Choroid Plexus Papilloma and Choroid Plexus Carcinoma

1. Imaging Studies and Gross Features

The imaging features are similar to CPP. Grossly, choroid plexus carcinomas (CPC) demonstrate solid areas, in addition to typical papillary regions. The attachment to the ventricular wall may be broader, and frank invasion may be appreciated. Necrosis may be seen on the cut surfaces (179,180). Implantation and subarachnoid seeding may be apparent (174).

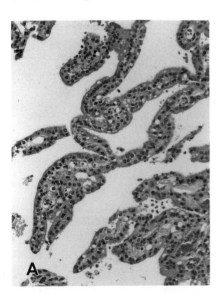 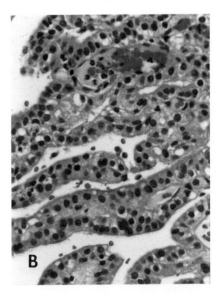

Figure 17   Choroid plexus papilloma: (A) The papillary architecture is preserved, but is more complex tnan normal choroid plexus. (B) Tumor cells demonstrate little or no atypia, with bland round nuclei (H&E; original magnification: A × 200; × 400).

2. Microscopic Features

Histological criteria for malignancy were developed in the early 1960s by Lewis (179) and Russell and Rubenstein (176) (Fig. 18). Cytological atypia, mitoses, transition to a solid growth pattern, and brain parenchymal invasion were required for a diagnosis of choroid plexus carcinoma. The last criterion often limits the usefulness of the classification system. Because the interface between stalk and ventricular surface provides an obvious landmark for excision, the underlying parenchy-

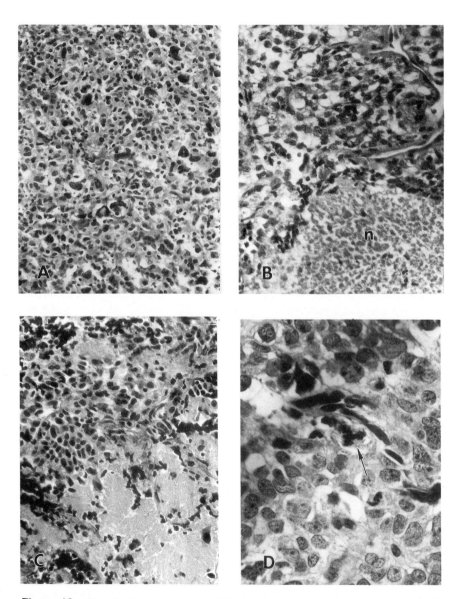

Figure 18 Choroid plexus carcinoma: (A) The papillary architecture has been replaced by a solid growth pattern. Pleomorphism may be prominent, as seen in this example. (B) A sheet of viable tumor cells abut a region of tumor necrosis (n). (C) Tumor cells infiltrate the periventricular parenchyma. (D) Atypical mitotic figures (arrow) complete the picture of malignancy. This high-power view also highlights the nuclear atypia (H&E; original magnification: A $\times$ 250; B, C $\times$ 400; D $\times$ 1000).

ma is often not sampled, and invasion cannot be evaluated. Even applying these criteria, outcome may not correlate with histological grade: typically benign-appearing CPP can behave malignantly, and choroid plexus carcinomas have been cured by simple excision. Recently, McGirr et al. have questioned the significance of the traditional criteria, including microscopic tumor invasion, and the role of histological classification of CPT in directing therapy has become unsettled (171). They describe tumors with significant cytological atypia as well as limited mitotic activity and microscopic parenchymal invasion. These "atypical" CPP have good outcomes following simple excision. The atypical CPP do not demonstrate a high mitotic rate, atypical mitoses, or tumor necrosis.

We require the presence of cytological atypia, with loss of papillary growth pattern and a high mitotic rate, including atypical mitotic figures, for a diagnosis of CPC. Tumor necrosis is also a helpful feature, but we have not seen it in the absence of the other criteria. Parenchymal invasion, if extensive, is also helpful, but sampling problems limit its usefulness as a diagnostic criterion (177).

D. Immunohistochemistry

Unlike the ependyma from which it is derived, choroid plexus and its tumors have keratin as a principal intermediate cytoskeletal protein, whereas GFAP immunoreactivity is limited or absent (170,181–183). S-100 (170,182,183) and transthyretin (183) immunoreactivity also are found consistently, whereas vimentin (182) and CEA (170,183) are less consistent.

E. Current Investigations

As is true for most glial neoplasms, limited numbers have made evaluation of new methods difficult. In the largest reported study of DNA content by flow cytometry, nine of ten tumors demonstrated at least one aneuploid peak, with five cases containing two or more aneuploid populations. However, the nearly ubiquitous presence of aneuploidy limits its usefulness in tumor classification. A strong correlation has been reported between SPF and both histological grade and tumor behavior (177). Reports of immunohistochemical assessment of proliferation in CPT are limited to isolated cases, but confirm the trend of low, but measurable, proliferation in CPP and high proliferation in CPC (176,177,184).

F. Clinical Behavior

A recent study has suggested that CPC need not follow as malignant a course as previously thought. Although early reports cite survival of 9 months for children and 3.5 years for adults, more recent studies report a 50% 5-year survival following aggressive surgery (173,177). Most studies have reported CPC to have a dismal 1-year survival rate. When longer median survival has been found, death, if it occurred, did so in the first year (173,180). Improvements in surgical and anesthesia techniques have made contributions to improved survival (173). At least as important are modern imaging techniques, which facilitate complete removal of CPC and early detection of recurrence. Early detection and intervention following recurrence may be curative.

There remains some controversy about the significance of histological features in predicting the behavior of individual CPT. However, as a group, CPC are generally assumed to behave more aggressively than CPP. It is also clear that the more rapidly a tumor grows, the earlier a recurrence will become clinically significant. The assessment of proliferation in CPT will help identify those cases that will behave like CPC, and require particularly close follow-up owing to a higher likelihood of early recurrence.

XI. GLIOSARCOMA

A. Introduction

Gliosarcomas are tumors composed of both neoplastic glial and mesenchymal cells. Although the origin and nature of the sarcomatous element remains controversial, usually, the pathogenesis is presumed to be induction of neoplasia in perivascular mesenchymal cells by a preexisting GBM (185–189). Astrocytomas produce factors that promote angiogenesis, and they may produce other important growth factors. Excessive stimulation of the blood vessels produces the atypical vascular proliferation that characterizes high-grade gliomas. Although exuberant proliferation of perivascular mesenchymal cells is common, true neoplastic transformation is rare: a sarcomatous component is found in only about 2–5% of GBM (187,190).

Occasionally, the sarcomatous component may predominate (188,191). When this happens, particularly in a superficial tumor, the term *sarcoglioma* has been used to indicate both the predominance of the sarcoma and also a reverse of the usual origin: that is, induction of the astrocytoma by a primary sarcoma. Although likely to be true in some instances, the criteria for distinction from gliosarcoma are vague and arbitrary.

Although gliosarcomas may occur at any site, an avidity for the temporal lobes has been reported (187). They may occur at any age, most commonly in older adults (185,187,192).

Gliosarcomas generally follow a grim course, paralleling that of GBM (187). Tumor behavior in response to therapy is varied. Tumor recurrence may show the same admixture of cell types seen in the primary, but may be restricted to either the glial or sarcomatous component. Systemic metastasis of the sarcomatous elements occurs at a relatively high rate compared with that for pure glial neoplasms (187,193–195). The sarcoma also readily infiltrates into the extracranial soft tissues.

B. Imaging Studies and Gross Findings

Gross examination and imaging studies demonstrate an enhancing, often superficial, partly circumscribed mass (187,188,194). The cut surfaces are typical of a high-grade glioma, but may be more firm, reflecting the sarcomatous component.

C. Microscopic Features

Microscopic examination typically shows the apparent circumscription to be illusory, with diffuse parenchymal infiltration (Fig. 19). Interestingly, the sarcoma may be circumscribed, with infiltration only by the astrocytoma. Occasionally, the glial and sarcomatous elements are present as regionally distinct masses. More commonly, fascicles and nests of both cell types interweave. The two components are usually about evenly distributed, but either element may be preponderant (185,187–189,192).

The glial tumor usually demonstrates the typical features of GBM: mitotic figures, pleomorphism, and necrosis (185,187–189,192). Tumors in which the glial component is an oligodendroglioma have been reported (196,197). Immunoreactivity for GFAP confirms the glial nature of this component of the tumors. The sarcomatous element almost always has the microscopic features of fibrosarcoma (187,188,193) or malignant fibrous histiocytoma (MFH) (192,195). The former is often well differentiated, composed of regular, moderately pleomorphic spindle cells, in orderly fascicles. Trichrome stain confirms the expected collagen production, and there is a rich reticulin network around the individual tumor cells. Immunoreactivity is limited to vimentin. More undifferentiated tumors resemble MFH, with a storiform growth pattern of cells with bizarre pleomorphism. Vimentin and antiprotease immunoreactivity has been reported in these tumors (198). Other sarcomatous patterns occasionally are present as minor components, including osteosarcoma, chondrosarcoma, and myosarcoma (190,199). Despite the appearance of angiocentric origin of gliosarcomas, angiosarcomas almost never occur, and tumor cells are consistently negative for factor VIII antigen and *Ulex europaeus* lectin reactivity, antigens that are characteristic of endothelial cells (198).

D. Differential Diagnosis

The principal differential diagnostic problem is recognition of the dual lineage; the presence of an orderly, fascicular spindle cell component should spark further evaluation for the possibility of sarcoma. All "pure" sarcomas need immunohistochemical confirmation of the absence of a *neoplastic* glial component, but care must be taken to avoid overinterpreting entrapped islands of reactive astrocytes.

XII. EMBRYONAL NEOPLASMS

A. Introduction

The embryonal neoplasms include medulloblastoma, cerebral neuroblastoma, ependymoblastoma, medulloepithelioma, and pineoblastoma. They are principally tumors of children and are more thoroughly discussed in the chapter on pediatric neoplasms (see Chap. 4). However, medulloblastomas and cerebral neuroblastomas occur with sufficient frequency in adults to merit a brief note here. Pineoblastomas also occur in adults and are discussed later in the section on pineal tumors (see Sec. XV).

B. Medulloblastoma

Medulloblastomas are tumors of the cerebellum (Fig. 20). Approximately 30% are reported to occur in adults (200). They constitute approximately 1% of all adult CNS tumors (201,202). Five-year survival estimates range from 30 to 78% (202) and are similar to those of children. Medulloblastomas grow in the fourth ventricle and invade the cerebellum. They spread along parenchymal surfaces in the subarachnoid space; before the era of radiation therapy, this created a characteristic "sugar icing" coating on the surface of the brain at autopsy. Metastases through CSF pathways are common (201–203). The soft, gray tumor mass often demonstrates areas of hemorrhage and necrosis. Medulloblastomas are characterized by small cells, with hyperchromatic nuclei that range from round to carrot shaped. Mitotic figures are numerous, and necrosis is common. A variable amount of neuropil-like stroma and several Homer–Wright rosettes are seen (200,201). A wide variety of histological patterns occur. Of particular interest, neuronal or, less commonly, glial maturation is reported in about 50% of cases (201,203,204). The tumor cells are commonly positive for neurofilament and NSE immunoreactivity, but rarely are positive for synaptophysin (201,205). Flow cytometric studies of DNA content have demonstrated a more favorable prognosis in patients with aneuploid tumors. No association has been found between proliferative activity and survival (206).

C. Cerebral Neuroblastoma

Cerebral neuroblastomas can occur at any site and are found most commonly in the frontal and parietal lobes (203,207). They are considerably less common than medulloblastomas. Survival estimates vary and are based on limited numbers, but suggest a prognosis comparable with that of medulloblastoma (203,207). Cerebral neuroblastomas are often large and well circumscribed grossly, with gray cut surfaces, marked by frequent hemorrhage and necrosis. Cysts are present in about 50% of cases (204,207). By light microscopy, the neoplastic cells are typical of PNETs. A neuropil-like network of processes and Homer–Wright rosettes may be seen (203,207–209).

Mitoses are usually readily identified (203,207–209), particularly in tumors that lack maturation. In contrast with medulloblastomas, they are reported to have consistent synaptophysin and NSE immunoreactivity, but only rarely are cells positive for neurofilament (207). Maturation along glial and neuronal lines occurs (203,207,208,210). The clinical significance of differentiation is unclear (207). In two such patients we have found low Ki-67-labeling indices and prolonged survival (Coons SW, unpublished data). Local recurrences are expected, and spread along CSF pathways is common (207,210).

D. Nomenclature

The term *primitive neuroectodermal tumor* (PNET) has been applied to the embryonal tumors, based on similar morphology, potential for divergent differentiation, behavior, and possibly cell of origin (203,204,208,210,211). Although the term is useful as a starting point for describing these often similar tumors, we agree with Rubinstein (212) that the distinctive names should be preserved. Although similar in many respects, there are morphological differences among tumors that are indicative of ontogenic or local environmental influences, irrespective of possible origin from a common progenitor cell. For example, the abundant distinctive giant ependymal rosettes and tubules that characterize ependymoblastoma suggest a fundamental difference from the other PNETs, as does the increased tendency toward divergent maturation in cerebral neuroblastomas. We should not assume that our current lack of sophistication in identifying clinically relevant differences will always be true.

XIII. GANGLION CELL TUMORS

A. Introduction

Neoplasms containing mature neuronal elements are grouped together as ganglion cell tumors. Most cases demonstrate both neoplastic neuronal, and astrocytic elements, and are classified as gangliogliomas. In the absence of an admixed neoplastic glial component, the tumors are classified as gangliocytomas (213,214) or neurocytomas (see Sec. XIV). The diagnosis of ganglion cell tumors is usually made before the age of 30 (215). The most common symptom is seizures, and patients often have a history of seizures dating back many years (215–217). As with other low-grade brain tumors, increasing use of MRI to evaluate the onset of seizures will probably result in a decrease in the typical age at diagnosis. These are rare tumors in adults, but comprise about 1–9% of pediatric tumors (216,218). They can occur at any site and rarely can be multiple, but the most common presentation is a single lesion in the temporal lobe (215,217,219,220), where they are often found in resections for intractable seizures.

B. Imaging and Gross Characteristics

Imaging studies typically show a small, well-demarcated hypodense lesion, often with prominent calcification. Signal intensity on T2-weighted images is high. Contrast enhancement is variable. Cyst formation is common, and the cyst may be the principal culprit producing mass effect (216, 221).

Grossly, the tumors are usually small, gray, and well circumscribed. When dominated by a cyst, a mural nodule is present. Calcification often produces a gritty texture to the cut surfaces and, in extreme cases, may require decalcification before sectioning (214,220,222).

C. Microscopic Characteristics

The sine qua non of ganglion cell tumors is the presence of neoplastic neurons, which are recognizable by the presence of Nissl substance in the usually abundant cytoplasm, and by the large vesicular nuclei with prominent nucleoli (Fig. 21). Silver stains disclose abnormally oriented

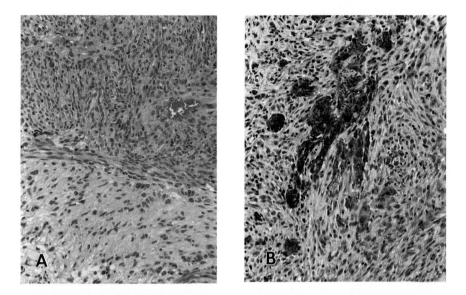

Figure 19   Gliosarcoma: (A) The pleomorphic fibrillary astrocytoma elements (A) are delineated from the more cellular fibrosarcoma (S). (B) This immunoperoxidase stain for glial fibrillary acidic protein (GFAP) reveals nests and cords of darkly staining astrocytoma cells admixed with the spindle cell sarcomatous elements (A, H&E; B, GFAP; original magnifications × 200).

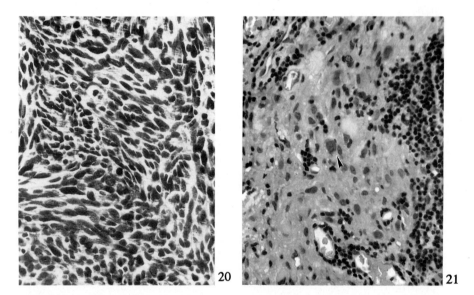

Figure 20   Medulloblastoma (PNET): The neoplasm is markedly hypercellular and lacks evidence of neuronal maturation. Typical hyperchromatic carrot-shaped nuclei are seen (H&E; original magnification × 400).

Figure 21   Ganglioglioma: Maldistributed atypical neuronal elements are seen in a background of atypical astrocytes and lymphocytic infiltrates. A binucleate neuron (arrowhead) is present; the nuclei are in different focal planes and are difficult to distinguish (H&E; original magnification × 200).

neuritic processes. Cytological features that distinguish well-differentiated tumor cells from normal neurons include the presence of binucleate and multinucleate forms, abnormal nuclear/cytoplasmic ratios, irregular distribution of Nissl substance, and abnormal neuritic processes. The neoplastic neurons are often abnormally clustered and irregularly oriented (216–218,220,222). They are associated with a finely fibrillary neuropil.

Glial elements may be inconspicuous (gangliocytoma), but most commonly there is an admixture of neoplastic neurons and astrocytes. Occasionally, the glioma component may obscure the neurons. Cellularity ranges from modest to moderate. Typically, the astrocytic component is composed of well-differentiated fibrillary astrocytes and would be classified as low-grade astrocytoma in the absence of a neuronal component. Immature neurons and cells of indeterminate origin can be identified in the more cellular tumors (216–218,220,222).

Lymphocytic and plasmocytic infiltration of fibrovascular septa is almost always seen, and may be extensive. Microcalcification is usually also present. A rich reticulin network may be seen (216–218,220,222).

Most tumors display bland cytological features, but they are capable of a striking display of atypia (217). The neuronal and glial atypia usually parallel one another. Mitoses of mature neurons have never been reported, but may be seen in the astrocytic component.

As atypia increases, distinguishing between the two cell types by routine microscopy becomes more difficult. They remain immunohistochemically distinct (217,222). The neurons demonstrate variable positivity for synaptophysin, neurofilament, vasoactive intestinal peptide, chromogranin, tyrosine hydroxylase (222), and PGP 9.5 (Johnson PC, unpublished results). The astrocytes demonstrate reactivity for GFAP.

D. Clinicopathological Correlation

Ganglion cell tumors are generally slow growing and have well-defined margins that indicate a lack of invasiveness. Their location, small size, and sharp circumscription often permit complete surgical extirpation (215). As a result, they generally follow an indolent course, with long survival or cure the norm. Even with subtotal resection, they generally have a good prognosis, and radiation therapy is indicated only for progressive disease (216,218). About 10% of gangliogliomas behave as high-grade neoplasms, with aggressive behavior and rapidly fatal course (219,220,223). The aggressive elements are always glial, by definition and by theory. The neuronal elements are considered to be locked into a maturation process that results in end-stage mature neurons that are capable of very limited further mitotic activity. Although aggressive ganglion cell tumors have the typical features of histological malignancy, studies have found that these features do not consistently predict aggressive behavior (217–220).

E. Differential Diagnosis

The differential diagnosis of ganglion cell tumors hinges on the recognition of the neurons and their neoplastic nature. A predominant astrocytic component may hinder recognition of the neurons, resulting in a diagnosis of astrocytoma being rendered. The presence of perivascular lymphocytic infiltrates is a clue that should prompt a thorough search for neoplastic neurons. At the other extreme, astrocytomas with entrapped normal neurons, or with atypical tumor cells that resemble neurons, may be misclassified as gangliogliomas. Careful evaluation of neuronal cytology and distribution and judicious use of immunohistochemistry and electron microscopy should prevent these errors. Tumors that contain a significant number of proliferative neuroblasts admixed with neurons are classified as differentiated neuroblastomas. They are felt to be biologically distinct from the ganglion cell tumors being considered here; they were discussed in previous section on embryonal neoplasms (see Sec. XII) (223).

XIV. CENTRAL NEUROCYTOMA

A. Introduction

The central neurocytoma is a rare tumor of neuronal origin, with a level of differentiation intermediate between a cerebral neuroblastoma (PNET) and a gangliocytoma or ganglioglioma (224,225). Neurocytomas have been recognized as a distinct diagnostic entity only recently, and a consensus about the name is also recent. The list of alternative names, which includes intraventricular neurocytoma, intraventricular neuroblastoma, and differentiated cerebral neuroblastoma, suggests that their neuronal origin always was recognized; however, as discussed in the following, many were originally diagnosed as oligodendroglioma or, less commonly, ependymoma.

Neurocytomas are tumors of young adults, with a few cases reported in children and older adults. They always have a prominent intraventricular component, typically in the midline, often in association with the septum pellucidum (224–233).

The rarity and relatively recent description of these tumors makes it difficult to be definitive about their behavior. Neurocytomas demonstrate a limited ability to invade, sometimes making resection difficult, and are considered low-grade malignant tumors. They are not reported to have spread through CSF pathways. They are slow growing, and in Ki-67 measurements, little proliferative activity was noted (226; Coons SW, unpublished data).

B. Imaging Studies and Gross Features

Imaging studies show them to be discrete, well-circumscribed tumors. They demonstrate diffuse contrast enhancement. Calcification is always present and tumor tissue is isodense with brain (226–229).

The gross examination is relatively uninformative: they share the same soft, gray-tan appearance of most intracerebral tumors. They may demonstrate significant calcification, but this feature also is hardly unique and is shared in particular with oligodendrogliomas (226,229).

C. Microscopic Features

Reports of the light microscopic appearance of neurocytomas are so consistent that their recent recognition is surprising (224–233) (Fig. 22). Neurocytomas are remarkable for the uniformity of constituent cells and nuclei. The cytoplasm is usually clear, giving the appearance of perinuclear halos. The cell membranes are sharply delineated. The evenly distributed nuclei are round, with lightly stippled chromatin. The sheetlike arrangement of cells lies in a variably prominent fine neuropil-like feltwork, typical of most neuronal neoplasms. When prominent, the fine capillary network creates a nested appearance. Fibrillary anucleate zones may be seen around the vessels. The formation of long columns of cells may also be seen. Mitoses are not generally present, nor is necrosis; however, otherwise classic neurocytomas may have areas with increased mitotic activity, cellularity, and a less-differentiated appearance (224,225,231). The significance of these features for tumor behavior needs further evaluation as the number of cases increases.

1. Immunohistochemistry

Neurocytomas are immunoreactive for a variety of neuronal markers, particularly NSE and synaptophysin. Neurofilament is identified less commonly. The tumor cells are negative for GFAP, but scattered entrapped astrocytes may be GFAP-reactive (224–226,228–232).

2. Ultrastructure

Electron microscopy played a major role in the confirmation of neuronal origin of neurocytomas and continues to provide useful diagnostic information (225,226,229,231,233). Neuritic cell processes containing microtubules and dense-core granules, and clear vesicles are consistent findings. Mature synapses are seen in a few cases, and intermediate filaments are found infrequently.

D. Differential Diagnosis

There are two aspects to the differential diagnosis of central neurocytoma: first, it must be recognized as a tumor of neuronal lineage and, second, the degree of differentiation must be appropriate. As we have indicated, neurocytomas may be confused with oligodendrogliomas. Both usually have remarkably uniform nuclei, prominent perivascular halos, and discrete cell boundaries. The correct diagnosis is suggested by the MRI image of a discrete intraventricular tumor that demonstrates contrast enhancement and calcium. When these features are present, it is essential for the pathologist to look for histological evidence of neuronal differentiation by immunohistochemical studies and electron microscopy. In a retrospective institutional review of five tumors originally diagnosed as intraventricular oligodendroglioma, two were identified as neurocytomas.

When the pathologist is clever, but not clever enough, the fine perivascular feltwork may be interpreted as perivascular pseudorosettes. This, coupled with the intraventricular location, will suggest a diagnosis of clear cell ependymoma. Once again, immunohistochemistry, or electron microscopy or both, will confirm the correct diagnosis.

Among the neuronal neoplasms, the absence of large ganglion cells in neurocytomas makes their distinction from gangliocytomas easy. Differentiation from the less well-differentiated neuroblastoma is more problematic. As discussed earlier, and in the chapter on pediatric neoplasms (see Chap. 4), primitive neuronal tumors may show a substantial degree of maturation. The neuronal maturation in neuroblastomas is toward large ganglion cells, which are not seen in neurocytomas. Divergent differentiation along neuronal and glial lines in neuroblastomas, with the presence of GFAP-reactive tumor cells, provides an additional point of distinction from neurocytomas (225).

The possibility that neurocytoma is part of a continuous spectrum of differentiation and behavior in neuronal neoplasms must be considered, but the consistent location, the striking appearance, and the lack of reports of similar tumors in the typical sites of other primitive neuronal tumors (cerebellum, pineal), argues for a unique origin for the neurocytoma.

XV. PINEAL PARENCHYMAL NEOPLASMS AND MISCELLANEOUS PINEAL NEOPLASMS

A. Pineal Parenchymal Neoplasms

1. Introduction

Pineal parenchymal neoplasms are rare tumors that constitute fewer than 1% of adult brain tumors (234–238). They are not even the most common tumor of the pineal, that distinction belonging to the germ cell tumors (234,239,240). They are somewhat more common in males than females (238,240,241). Pineal tumors presumably arise from neoplastic transformation of the normal or developing pineocyte (234). They range from the extremely primitive pineoblastoma to a well-differentiated tumor indistinguishable from a cerebral ganglioglioma. The pineocytoma, which uniquely resembles normal pineal tissue, is intermediate in differentiation. In general, the degree of tumor differentiation increases with the age of the patient. Pineoblastomas have their highest incidence in the first decade and are relatively rare beyond the third (234,237,238). Pineocytomas and gangliogliomas are generally tumors of the teenage years and beyond (234–238).

2. Imaging Studies and Gross Features

Radiologic studies of pineoblastomas and pineocytomas disclose diffusely contrast-enhancing posterior midline lesions. The tumors are hypodense on CT scans and have a hypointense signal on T1-weighted MRI images. Cysts may be present, producing a mottled pattern. The ventricles are often dilated owing to obstruction of CSF flow in the aqueduct (239,240,242). Calcification is often noted in pineocytomas (235,242). Examination of the whole neural axis may disclose metastatic lesions, particularly with pineoblastoma.

Grossly, pineal tumors are often well circumscribed. Their cut surfaces are gray to tan and generally firm and may demonstrate residual lobularity of the normal gland (234,238). The gross features of the tumors are not distinctive, and diagnostic differentiation occurs at the microscopic level.

3. Microscopic Features

Pineoblastoma. Pineoblastomas are densely cellular neoplasms, composed of small un-differentiated cells (Fig. 23). Typical small Homer–Wright "neural" rosettes are sometimes seen (234,237,238). This results in their categorization as primitive neuroectodermal tumors (PNETs) by some. Indeed, the histological features are often indistinguishable from medulloblastoma, and their clinical behavior is similar. Mitotic activity is typically high, and tumor necrosis is common (234,237,238). Pineoblastomas are unencapsulated and tend to be infiltrative (234,238). On silver staining, pineoblastomas have few processes, and these lack the characteristic clublike terminations of better-differentiated pineal cells (234,237). Many cells have NSE reactivity. Electron microscopy demonstrates few organelles, but microtubules may be seen. Features of more-advanced neuronal differentiation are absent (243).

Pineoblastomas also may have Flexner–Wintersteiner rosettes and fleurettes (234,237,238), which reflect a relation between pineal cells and photoreceptor cells of the retina and are indicative of retinoblastomatous differentiation. Rarely, pineoblastoma and bilateral retinoblastoma occur together, constituting a recognized genetic disorder (234).

Pineocytoma. Pineocytomas are less densely cellular than pineoblastomas. The cells and nuclei are larger, and their nuclear chromatin is less dense (Fig. 24). They may be arranged in variably sized lobules that resemble the normal or developing pineal. Mitotic figures are usually rare. The tumor cells exhibit a variable degree of neuronal differentiation. Striking, characteristic large rosettes, surrounding a fine feltwork of processes resembling neuropil, are usually present (234,235,237,238). The silver-positive processes often demonstrate the club-shaped terminations characteristic of pineal origin (234,235,237,238). Immunoreactivity for NSE is expected (235), and synaptophysin reactivity may be present. Electron microscopy demonstrates variable numbers of microtubules, clear and dense-core vesicles, and synaptic structures (238,243). Ganglionic differentiation is recognizable by the presence of typical large neurons. These often accompany the pineal rosettes or may be present exclusive of rosettes. Astrocytic differentiation may accompany the ganglion cells and can be confirmed by the presence of GFAP-reactive tumor cells. When extensive, the tumors are classified as gangliogliomas.

Tumors that have the characteristic larger cells and lobular pattern, but lack rosettes or ganglionic differentiation, have been classified as pineocytomas (234,238,242). Transition forms between pineoblastoma and pineocytoma also are described (234,238). The clinical behavior of these groups is close to that of the pineoblastoma, but with higher risk of CSF dissemination and local infiltration. Some pathologists restrict the diagnosis of pineocytoma to those tumors with neuronal differentiation (pineal rosettes or ganglion cells) that have a relatively favorable prognosis (235,237)

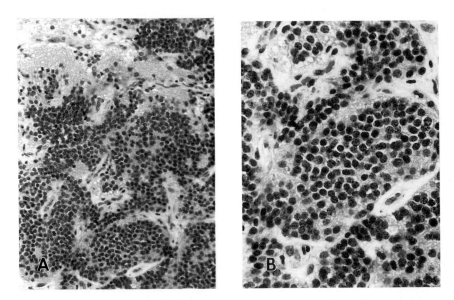

Figure 22 Neurocytoma: (A) Tumor cells grow in nests surrounded by fibrovascular septa. (B) The nuclei are round with a "salt-and-pepper" chromatin distribution. Perinuclear halos are seen in many cells and suggest oligodendroglioma, but the neuronal nuclear features are distinctive (H&E; original magnification: A × 200; B × 400).

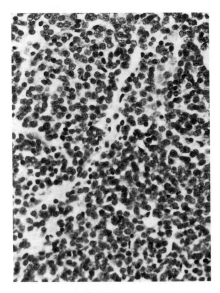

Figure 23 Pineoblastoma (PNET): Sheets of primitive tumor cells, with scant cytoplasm and round, hyperchromatic nuclei, characterize this tumor. There is no neuronal or glial maturation (H&E; original magnification × 400).

4. Clinical Considerations

Pineal tumors enlarge to compress the colliculi and the aqueduct and may invade locally (234,238). Of far greater concern for prognosis is the ability to disseminate through CSF pathways. As might be expected, the tendency toward CSF spread is inversely related to the degree of differentiation (234,235,237,238), and essentially all pineoblastomas follow this aggressive course. Craniospinal radiation typically is recommended for those tumors with the potential to disseminate. Despite this aggressive therapy, patients with pineoblastomas rarely survive 2 years (234,238). Survival with pineocytomas is variable, but has been reported for up to 29 years (234,236). Long survival is typical for adults with pineocytomas with neuronal differentiation (234–239). For these patients, aggressive surgical extirpation alone may be appropriate, with radiation therapy reserved for failure of local control or unexpected dissemination (236). Because of the nomenclature controversy, it is essential for the pathologist to specify explicitly the presence or absence of neuronal differentiation.

Historically, the high operative mortality, up to 60% in some series (240), led to the use of radiation therapy without a tissue diagnosis. Improvements in microneurosurgical techniques have resulted in significant morbidity or mortality in fewer than 2% of patients in recent series (239,240). As a result, irradiation of pineal tumors without a tissue diagnosis is no longer justifiable (236,237,239,242).

5. Differential Diagnosis

The differential diagnosis of pineal parenchymal tumors is limited. Pineoblastomas are recognized easily as primitive malignant tumors. If the characteristic rosettes are not present in the biopsy, routine hemotoxylin and eosin (H&E) staining may not allow easy distinction between a pineocytoma and the occasional anaplastic astrocytoma that occurs in the pineal region. Documentation of neuronal heritage by silver stain, immunohistochemistry, or electron microscopy should resolve the problem. Differentiation from normal pineal tissue may be more difficult, particularly for pathologists unfamiliar with the area. The pineal gland has pronounced, uniform lobularity, and the cells do not demonstrate even the mild pleomorphism of pineocytomas. This distinction is particularly critical: in our experience, small biopsies of a pineal "mass" missed the adjacent germinoma. Biopsy of pineal gland in the wall of a pineal cyst may be misdiagnosed as pineocytoma. The differentiating characteristics of the germ cell tumors are discussed in detail in the next section (see Sec. XVI)

B. Miscellaneous Neoplasms

In addition to the true pineal parenchymal tumors and midline germ cell tumors, a wide variety of other primary intracranial tumors occasionally are found in the pineal region, including astrocytomas, oligodendrogliomas, ependymomas, meningiomas, dermoids and epidermoids, paragangliomas, and hemangiopericytomas. Metastatic disease is also found (234,240). Like the germ cell tumors, these tumors do not differ significantly from those in their more common primary sites.

XVI. GERM CELL TUMORS

A. Introduction

Intracranial germ cell tumors almost always arise in the midline and are found most commonly in the pineal or suprasellar regions. Between 10 and 50% occur at two sites, usually pineal and suprasellar, or pineal and third ventricle (244–247). Their midline location parallels their presence at other extragonadal midline sites. Speculation about their origin relates to migratory pathways and disturbances of primitive streak development (244). Germ cell tumors are rare tumors that constitute fewer than 1% of all brain tumors (244,247); however they are more common than pineal parenchymal tumors in that region. They span the range of subtypes found in their other primary sites; however, the frequency of occurrence of each subtype is significantly different. Germinomas comprise 61% of all germ cell tumors and are the most common pineal region tumor of any type. Teratomas are also relatively common, with mature and immature teratomas contributing 10% and 23% to the total, respectively. Teratomas are the most common neonatal brain tumor. The remaining tumors—embryonal carcinoma, endodermal sinus tumor, and choriocarcinoma— are rare, composing no more than 3% individually and fewer than 10% in aggregate of the total germ cell tumors. As in extracranial sites, mixed tumors occur frequently (244). The germ cell tumors occur primarily in children and younger adults and, except for suprasellar germinomas, are significantly more common in males (244,245,248).

The pineal germ cell tumors are situated just above the quadrigeminal plate, and their principal symptoms relate to compression of the colliculi and cerebral aqueduct, with consequent impairment of CSF flow. Suprasellar tumors produce symptoms related to disturbances of the hypothalamus and the hypothalamic–pituitary axis.

B. Clinical Behavior

The behavior of germ cell tumors is related to cell type, and all but the teratomas are highly malignant. Dissemination through CSF pathways is common, but extracranial metastasis is rare (244,249,250). Whereas the other germ cell tumors tend to be somewhat circumscribed, germinomas tend to be infiltrative into and around adjacent brain and cranial nerves, often precluding complete resection (244). Fortunately, germinomas are highly radiosensitive, and long-term survival or cure is possible. Five-year survival is greater than 70% (251). The other high-grade tumors are less responsive to treatment, and their outlook is much less bright. Alone among the germ cell tumors, mature teratomas are often amenable to cure by complete resection (252).

C. Imaging Studies and Gross Features

On CT images, nonteratomatous germ cell tumors are iso- to hyperdense midline lesions. Magnetic resonance shows iso- to hypointense T1-weighted images. Both demonstrate homogeneous contrast enhancement (249,250,253). Blood or necrosis may produce a mottled pattern of densities and enhancement. In germinomas, imaging studies can define the presence and extent of local infiltration (248,250,253). In teratomas, cysts and mixed cellular elements also produce a variable pattern of enhancement and different tissue densities (252,254). Examination of the entire neuroaxis is indicated to evaluate the extent of disease.

Choriocarcinomas have gross hemorrhage more commonly than do other germ cell neoplasms, but only the teratoma has a distinctive gross appearance. Teratomas typically have a complex pattern of cysts and solid areas (244). A striking variant, the giant congenital teratoma, may fill and expand the cranial cavity and replace most of the brain (252).

D. Microscopic Features

The microscopic appearances of the germ cell tumor subtypes match those of their gonadal counterparts.

1. Germinoma

Germinomas are composed of cells with abundant, clear cytoplasm and large, vesicular, round-to-oval nuclei, with very prominent nucleoli (Fig. 25). The clear cytoplasm marks the presence of glycogen (which is largely washed out during tissue processing), and PAS stain typically demonstrates strong positivity that is diastase-sensitive. The noncohesive cells may be diffusely distributed or may cluster in nests outlined by fibrovascular septa. A variable infiltrate of a mixture of chronic inflammatory cells may obscure the presence of the tumor. Scattered mitoses are present (244,247,250). Increased mitotic activity and pleomorphism are sometimes seen, but the significance of these changes is unclear. Germinomas demonstrate immunoreactivity for placental alkaline phosphatase (PLAP) (245,255). Scattered cells that are reactive for markers of other germ cell tumor types, particularly human chorionic gonadotropin (hCG) (244–246,256), may be seen, but the temptation to diagnose a mixed tumor should be resisted in the absence of larger regions of the second cellular type (244). Of all the germ cell tumors, germinomas are least likely to demonstrate divergent differentiation. The interface between the tumor and brain demonstrates superficial infiltration of tumor cells, and a most striking feature is a brisk glial proliferation that can mimic astrocytoma.

By microscopy, the differential diagnosis is not generally difficult, but it is particularly dependent on an adequate biopsy. Small biopsies of reactive pineal gland may be mistaken for a parenchymal tumor. Biopsies of the interface with brain may suggest astrocytic neoplasia. The presence of a significant lymphocytic population is helpful: inflammation is not a prominent feature of other pineal neoplasms and its presence is strongly suggestive of germinoma. Inflammation that obscures the tumor cells may be confused with a primary inflammatory process.

2. Teratoma

By definition, teratomas demonstrate tissues from all germinal layers, and the presence of diverse cellular elements is diagnostic (Fig. 26). Teratomas are classified as mature if all the cellular elements demonstrate maturation and as immature if embryonal or fetal elements persist. There is uncertainly about whether or not immature teratomas are, by definition, malignant (254). Whereas some series find consistent aggressive behavior (244), others find that they may mature over time (252,254). Immature tumors may contain frankly malignant non–germ-cell elements, including carcinoma and sarcoma, and may coexist with malignant germ cell elements, most commonly embryonal carcinoma (teratocarcinoma) (244,247,249). The microscopic appearance is highly variable and has an appropriate parallel in the pattern of immunoreactivity. Diagnostically, significant markers include CEA and keratin for epithelial differentiation, and NSE for neuronal differentiation.

3. Embryonal Carcinoma

Embryonal carcinoma is characterized by sheets and anastomosing cords of poorly differentiated epithelial cells. The cells have little cytoplasm, and the pleomorphic nuclei contain irregularly distributed chromatin and prominent nucleoli. Mitoses and necrosis are frequently encountered (244). Although keratin reactivity is consistent and clearly intrinsic to embryonal carcinoma, the nature of cells reactive to other markers, most commonly alpha-fetoprotein (AFP), is unclear (244–246,256). As noted in the foregoing, embryonal carcinoma is commonly found as an element in mixed germ cell tumors and is most commonly associated with teratomas. Other neoplastic germ cell elements, including choriocarcinoma and endodermal sinus tumor, may also be present. This creates the potential for a complex pattern of immunohistochemical reactions, and it may be the cause of conflicting reports concerning the immunohistochemical reactivity of embryonal carcinoma.

4. Endodermal Sinus Tumor

Endodermal sinus tumors are characterized by the presence of Schiller–Duvall bodies, which are composed of epithelial channels containing small blood vessels lined by tumor epithelium. Other areas show lacy cords and sheets of cells. Small, apparently extracellular, amorphous eosinophilic masses are usually present. The masses stain for PAS and are diastase-resistant (244). They have been shown to be composed of AFP, and immunoreactivity for AFP is characteristic of the tumors

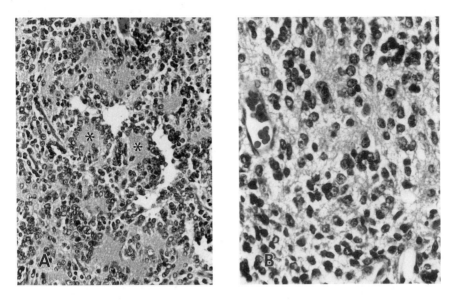

Figure 24 Pineocytoma: (A) Numerous characteristic large pineal rosettes composed of pineocytoma cells with centrally radiating neuronal processes are present (*). (B) Tumor cells have round nuclei and abundant, often thick, neuronal processes, producing a prominent neuropil-like background (H&E; original magnification: A × 200; B × 400).

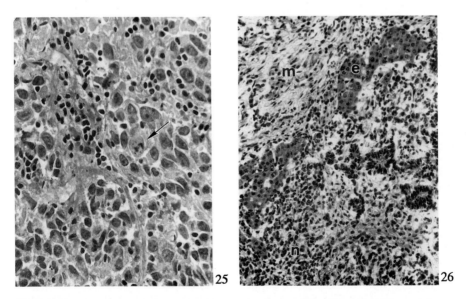

Figure 25 Germinoma: Tumor cells are poorly cohesive. They have abundant cytoplasm, and the large nuclei have a prominent nucleolus. Mitotic figures (arrow) are common. Infiltrates of small hyperchromatic lymphocytes complete the typical picture (H&E; original magnification × 400).
Figure 26 Teratoma (immature): Admixed mesenchymal (m), epithelial (e), and neuroectodermal (n) elements are present (H&E; original magnification × 200).

(244,246,249). Similar eosinophilic cytoplasmic inclusions are often seen. The appearance of endodermal sinus tumors is unique and diagnostic. As with the other germ cell tumors, endodermal sinus tumor differentiation may be seen as a minor element in another germ cell tumor, or may be the predominant feature of a mixed germ cell tumor (244).

5. Choriocarcinoma

Choriocarcinomas, similar to the other CNS germ cell tumors, are identical with their systemic counterparts. These tumors demonstrate striking pleomorphism. The diagnosis is based on the presence of syncytiotrophoblastic and cytotrophoblastic elements. The frequent presence of hemorrhage mirrors the tumor in extracranial sites (244). Immunoreactivity for hCG and human placental lactogen (hPL) are diagnostic (244,246). Because choriocarcinoma is often seen as part of a mixed germ cell tumor, other immunohistochemical markers are often positive.

E. Serum Markers

Germ cell tumors are often hormonally active, and their secretory products may be detectable in blood or in CSF. As with immunohistochemistry, the frequent occurrence of mixed germ cell tumors creates confusion over the interpretation and usefulness of immunochemical studies of serum and CSF.

Elevated serum and CSF levels of hCG are found in choriocarcinoma (244,245), whereas endodermal sinus tumors consistently have elevated AFP (244,249). Teratomas may produce a variety of compounds; CEA is among the most useful clinically (244–246). Germinomas are not associated with hormone production, but occasionally elevated levels of hCG are found, without apparent diagnostic significance (244,245).

XVII. CHORDOMA

A. Introduction

Chordomas are low-grade malignant lesions that are thought to be derived from remnants of notochord. They occur mainly at the ends of the axial skeleton, most commonly in the sacral region. We will discuss the 40% that are found at the clivus at the base of the skull (257).

B. Growth and Behavior

Chordomas occur almost exclusively in adults, primarily in the third to seventh decades (257–260). Intracranial chordomas are present at an earlier age than those in the sacrum (261). Rarely, chordomas can occur in childhood (257–259,262). Chordomas begin as *midline* tumors in the region of the clivus, an important feature in their differential diagnosis. They typically present with visual field defects and gaze disturbances and, often, headache (258–261).

In contrast to sacral chordomas, intracranial chordomas rarely metastasize. Their primary pattern of spread is by local infiltration and destruction of bone and soft tissues. Invasion of brain parenchyma is rare, but they can compress the brain stem through the dura (258–260). The infiltrative growth pattern and midline location make complete surgical removal almost impossible. Radiation therapy is employed for palliation, but is rarely curative (258–260). Chordomas grow slowly, but their progression is inexorable. Mean survival is 5–7 years (258,260,261).

C. Imaging and Gross Characteristics

Imaging studies show bony destruction involving the clivus and, sometimes, adjacent structures. Foci of calcification may be present. On MRI, the well-defined tumor mass is hypointense on T1-weighted images and hyperintense on T2-weighted images (268,269).

The gross appearance of a chordoma is of a lobulated pearl-gray mass. It is typically firm and rubbery, but a variable amount of soft mucopolysacchride material may be present. It has a pushing margin with soft tissues, where it may appear encapsulated. A similar sharp demarcation from bony surfaces is not seen (257,258,261). When abundant, the tumor has a myxoid or mucinous texture, and the diagnosis of chondrosarcoma must be considered.

D. Microscopic Features

When fully expressed, the microscopic features of chordomas are distinctive (259–261,265,266) (Fig. 27). Neoplastic cells grow in a fibrous and variably myxoid stroma. Neoplastic cells have two distinctive morphologies. Epithelioid cells with eosinophilic cytoplasm and well-defined cytoplasmic borders grow in irregular cords, small clusters or, less commonly, sheets. The morphological appearance of the second cell is that of a multiply vacuolated cell that contains mucopolysaccharide material within dilated endoplasmic reticulum; this cell is found typically in regions with a prominent myxoid stroma. This distinctive *physaliphorous* (from the Greek: bubble-bearing) cell is considered the characteristic cell of the chordoma. Transition forms between cell patterns are present, and fully developed physaliphorous cells may be rare. Nuclei are usually bland; considerable cytological atypia may be present, but is not of prognostic importance. Occasional mitotic figures may be seen. In a small series, the Ki-67 LI ranged from 0–6.3% (Coons SW, unpublished data). Chordomas share the curious immunohistochemical reactivity pattern of notochord: in addition to S-100 reactivity common to cartilage and neural connective tissues, they demonstrate keratin and epithelial membrane antigen reactivity (259, 265–270).

E. Differential Diagnosis

The clinical differential diagnosis of chordoma includes the other skull base tumors, principally craniopharyngiomas and pituitary adenomas. These tumors are distinguished easily by light microscopy. The major problematic microscopic differential considerations are metastatic adenocarcinoma and chondrosarcoma. Carcinomas are almost always pleomorphic, whereas chordomas usually demonstrate little cytological atypia. Even when atypia is present, mitotic figures are rare. In contrast, carcinomas usually display abundant mitotic figures, and the associated high growth rate also provides a clinical distinction between the tumors. The final distinction belongs to immunohistochemical analysis. Although both tumors share reactivity for epithelial markers, the additional presence of S-100 reactivity is essentially diagnostic of chordoma.

The distinction of chordoma from chondrosarcoma is less easy. The term *chondroid chordoma* traditionally has been applied to tumors described as having features of both chordoma and chondrosarcoma. The existence of this entity has been challenged by the advent of immunohistochemical analysis. Chondroid chordomas stain for S-100, but lack reactivity for the epithelial markers (266,270). These tumors should be considered low-grade chondrosarcomas, and they are discussed in more detail in the section on sarcomas.

XVIII. CRANIOPHARYNGIOMA

A. Introduction

Craniopharyngiomas are rare tumors of the skull base that arise in the region of the sella turcica. They constitute 2–3% of all brain tumors (271). Their peak incidence is in children and adolescents, but half occur in adults of any age (272,273).

Craniopharyngiomas present with symptoms typical of midline skull base tumors: disruptions of hypothalamic or pituitary function, cranial nerve disturbances (especially visual), and headache predominate (272–275).

The cell of origin of craniopharyngiomas is controversial. As the alternative name, adamantinoma, implies, the tumor bears strong resemblances to the adamantinoma of the jaw and tibia, and also to the calcifying odontogenic cyst. This has led to the suggestion that craniopharyngiomas arise from rests of enamel organ epithelium (276). Other authors dispute this origin and favor origin from squamous epithelial rests of Rathke's pouch found in the pars tuberalis of the pituitary stalk (271,275,277–282).

B. Imaging Studies and Gross Findings

Magnetic resonance imaging demonstrates variable signal intensity on T1-weighted images; high-signal intensity corresponds to the presence of cholesterol or methemoglobin from chronic hemorrhage. Signal intensity is diffusely high on T2-weighted images. Calcification is often present and is better visualized on CT scans. The tumor boundaries are best seen on MRI images (277).

Grossly, craniopharyngiomas attach to the surfaces of structures of the suprasellar region. They have irregular, lobular reddish-tan external surfaces. The sectioned surfaces demonstrate great internal complexity. Bands and nodules of fibrillary tissue separate variably sized cysts filled with cholesterol-rich ("crank-case oil") fluid. Abundant calcification is the rule, and soft necrotic debris may be found. In some cases, a single large cyst predominates (275,281).

C. Microscopic Features

The microscopic appearance of craniopharyngiomas (Fig. 28) is distinctive (271,275,281). Most are composed of nests of squamous epithelial cells that are characterized by a peripheral palisade of a basaloid layer which surrounds irregularly arranged cells that resemble the stellate reticulum cells of the epidermis. A nest may be solid, but often forms a complex trabecular network of epithelial cells and microcysts. The squamous epithelium of craniopharyngiomas demonstrates typical immunoreactivity for keratin and has no special immunohistochemical features. It usually does not undergo surface maturation with keratinization of flattened epithelial cells. This pattern may be present in the flattened epithelium of larger cysts, where it may mimic an epidermoid cyst. Microscopic nodules of keratin are often present, and the appearance of these nodules is characteristic of craniopharyngiomas. They form from the degeneration of plump squamous cells, the ghostlike outlines of which impart a distinctive appearance to the keratin debris, which is in sharp contrast to the compact, bandlike layers of keratin formed from the degeneration of flattened squamous cells at the surface of epidermoid cysts. Bands of fibrillary tissue weave between nests of epithelial cells and around cysts. The oil in the cysts is highly irritating and produces a striking fibroglial reaction, as well as a foreign body reaction to its cholesterol component. This feature alone is sufficient for a presumptive diagnosis of craniopharyngioma in a limited biopsy. The often extensive microcalcification and necrotic foci add to the complexity of the microscopic appearance. Craniopharyngiomas demonstrate diffuse immunoreactivity for keratin (279).

D. Differential Diagnosis

The differential diagnosis of craniopharyngioma is limited. The gross appearance is generally distinctive when a large enough sample is received. Microscopically, the principal consideration is epidermoid cyst, the differentiating features of which are discussed in the foregoing, and metastatic squamous carcinoma. Some authors believe that the distinction between craniopharyngioma and epidermoid cysts is artificial (271,275).

E. Growth and Behavior

Craniopharyngiomas are slow-growing, indolent tumors. Their classification as low-grade malignant tumors is more clinical than biological, and is based on the difficulty of surgical cure. The

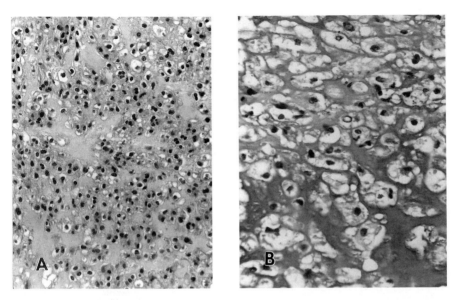

Figure 27 Chordoma: (A) Nests of epithelioid cells are present in a mucopolysaccharide-rich stroma. (B) Physaliphorous cells with their bubbly cytoplasm predominate in this tumor (H&E; original magnification: A × 250; B × 400).

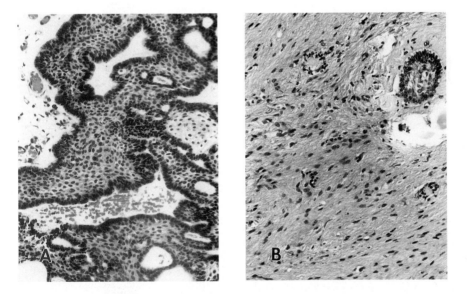

Figure 28 Craniopharyngioma: (A) Anastomosing cords of squamouslike epithelium surround cysts and loose fibrous stroma. A prominent basaloid layer surrounds the central stellate reticulumlike cells. (B) A nest of tumor cells is seen adjacent to an area of pronounced reactive gliosis. The presence of Rosenthal fibers and cytological atypia mimics pilocytic astrocytoma (H&E; original magnification: A × 200; B × 400).

tumors spread locally along intracranial surfaces and do not metastasize. As they spread, they surround and form strongly adherent fibroglial scars to any structures they encounter, including brain, cranial nerves, and critical vascular structures.

Resection is complicated further by local infiltration of brain parenchyma, which induces an exuberant gliosis, often with Rosenthal fibers, that can resemble low-grade or pilocytic astrocytoma. Bony infiltration is less common than in chordomas.

Complete surgical removal is the optimal treatment for a craniopharyngioma (272,273); however, the infiltration among the complex surfaces of the skull base usually makes complete removal impossible. Postoperative radiation therapy is employed for local control of the tumor (272–274). Repeat surgery for recurrent tumor or for cyst drainage is often necessary, and a combination of subtotal resection and radiation therapy is often preferable to debilitating radical surgery. Chemotherapy currently does not play a role in the management of craniopharyngiomas. Failure of complete initial resection and local control results in a slowly progressive course. About 50% of patients remain free of disease (272,273). Rarely, anaplastic degeneration occurs in recurrent tumors (277).

XIX. PRIMARY INTRACRANIAL SARCOMA

A. Introduction

This classification includes both the primary meningeal sarcomas and primary cerebral sarcomas. In many cases, the distinction between the two is impossible, as sarcomas involving brain parenchyma often extend to (or from) the cerebral surface (283–285) Primary sarcomas constitute fewer than 1% of all intracranial tumors (284,285). These rare neoplasms may occur at any age or site, but are most common in the first decade (283–287). As such, the principal discussion of these tumors is reserved for the chapter on childhood tumors (see Chap. 4). Malignant fibrous histiocytoma (MFH) is the exception, occurring primarily in adults (283,286).

Sarcomas arise from meningeal and perivascular mesenchyme. Intracranial involvement of skull-based osteosarcomas and chondrosarcomas also occurs, although they also may arise independently as parenchymal tumors (284,285). Rhabdomyosarcomas of children may have a distinctive origin from the primitive neuroectoderm. Neoplastic cells with rhabdomyoblastic differentiation have been identified in primitive childhood tumors, most strikingly in the medullomyoblastoma, which may be a variant of medulloblastoma (284,285). Whether these tumors are sarcomas, in the traditional sense, or are PNETs with rhabdomyoblastic differentiation is unclear.

Fibrosarcomas are the most common intracranial sarcoma, but many types occur. In addition to the tumors just noted, rhabdomyosarcomas, liposarcomas, leiomyosarcomas, and angiosarcomas have been reported (283–285,288–290).

Sarcomas are most commonly sporadic or radiation-induced, but familial cases have been reported (285,291). Sarcomas that develop following radiation therapy usually occur at least 5 years after treatment (285). In an unusual case, a postirradiation osteogenic sarcoma developed only 2 years following treatment of a familial choroid plexus carcinoma, suggesting continued influence of a familial predisposition to malignant tumor formation (Coons SW, unpublished data). Most postirradiation sarcomas are fibrosarcomas, but mixed sarcomas, which additionally include cartilaginous or osseous elements, are common (285,291,292).

B. Imaging Studies and Gross Examination

Imaging studies generally show a well-circumscribed enhancing mass (286–289). Grossly, sarcomas often appear sharply circumscribed, but some demonstrate invasiveness along meningeal pathways. The cut surfaces are fleshy and firm, except where high-grade tumors demonstrate necrosis and hemorrhage (284,285).

C. Microscopic Features

The microscopic features of intracranial sarcomas are essentially identical with their systemic counterparts, with the same range of differentiation. Lower-grade tumors are better differentiated, with moderate pleomorphism. Mitoses are present, but few. Increase in grade is accompanied by greater morphological and cytological pleomorphism, higher mitotic counts, and necrosis.

D. Differential Diagnosis

In the brain, the principal differential diagnostic consideration is high-grade astrocytoma, either alone or as an element of gliosarcoma. The absence of immunoreactivity for GFAP largely excludes a glial process. Occasionally, entrapped islands of reactive astrocytes may suggest a gliosarcoma, but the benign glial cytology does not match the expectations for a high-grade tumor (292). For meningeal-based tumors, the main distinction is from malignant meningioma. The latter characteristically demonstrates immunoreactivity for epithelial membrane antigen, and its ultrastructural features include abundant interdigitating cell processes, with numerous well-developed junctions (294,297).

E. Behavior

Despite their apparent circumscription, sarcomas generally have a very poor prognosis, which, in part, is related to tumor grade. They may spread by infiltration of adjacent brain, meninges, and bony surfaces. Subarachnoid spread and dissemination along CSF pathways also occur. Metastasis outside the nervous system occasionally occurs (284,285).

F. Chondroid Chordoma

The low-grade chondrosarcoma that arises in the region of the sella turcica merits attention. Previously called *chondroid chordoma*, this term is being replaced as evidence accumulates on its origin (294–296). Microscopically, this tumor bears superficial resemblance to those chordomas that have abundant myxoid stroma. However, vacuolated cells are not well developed, and the chondrocytes tend to be single, rather than in cords. Extensive cartilaginous differentiation is typical (294–297). The most compelling evidence comes from radiologic and immunohistochemical studies. Chordomas, by definition, are midline tumors, whereas chondroid chordomas need not be. Although both tumors demonstrate immunoreactivity for S-100, only chordomas are positive for keratin (294–297). Interestingly, this chondrosarcoma tends to be low grade, with little pleomorphism or mitotic activity. Expected survival actually far exceeds that of chordoma (284,294), partly reflecting better circumscription and surgical accessibility.

XX. PRIMARY CEREBRAL LYMPHOMA
A. Introduction

Primary cerebral lymphoma is an uncommon disease that historically constitutes approximately 1% of primary brain tumors. Although it may occur at any age, it is most common in older adults (289,290). With the advent of acquired immune deficiency syndrome (AIDS)-associated lymphomas there has been a marked increase in the number of cases, and these have occurred in younger persons (300–302). Also, for reasons that are unclear, there also has been a significant increase in lymphoma in the non–HIV-infected or otherwise immunocompromised population, especially among older patients (298). Other viral agents, particularly Epstein–Barr, as well as environmental agents, have been proposed as factors (298,299,303,304).

The initial response to therapy is almost diagnostic: marked shrinkage of the tumor is seen on imaging studies following initiation of steroid therapy (299,305), and the initial response to radiation is also gratifying (299). However, the tumors return aggressively, and in the older literature, survival beyond 2 years was unusual (301,306). Modern chemotherapy has resulted in a much-improved prognosis for sporadic lymphomas, and recent studies report median survival of about 5 years (306). In contrast, the prognosis for AIDS-associated lymphomas is abysmal. The tumors respond only transiently to therapy, and most patients die within a year of diagnosis (300,301,304,306,307). Primary cerebral lymphomas have a microscopic range that parallels their systemic counterparts, and differences in survival, based on subtypes, also parallels systemic tumors (299).

Primary lymphomas occur throughout the brain, often being periventricular. They tend to be limited to one or two sites, but may be multifocal, particularly in AIDS-associated disease.

B.   Imaging Studies and Gross Features

Imaging studies are helpful in diagnosis. The lesions tend to be dark on T1-weighted images. Peritumoral edema, as measured by the T2-weighted images, is variable, but less than that seen in metastatic carcinomas or high-grade gliomas. Lesions of sporadic disease typically show diffuse enhancement, rather than the ring-enhancing pattern of glioblastoma multiforme (305). In contrast, ring or irregular enhancement is the rule in AIDS-associated disease, reflecting a greater degree of tumor necrosis (302). The lesions may be well circumscribed, but often show vague, somewhat infiltrative margins.

The gross appearance parallels the radiologic studies (303). Circumscribed lesions may have a gray, fleshy appearance, similar to systemic lymphomas, or may be soft, mottled, and otherwise indistinguishable from a high-grade astrocytoma. The borders are often vaguely defined. Some lesions produce architectural distortion without a definite mass.

C.   Microscopic Features

The cardinal microscopic feature of primary lymphomas is their tendency to grow around blood vessels (angiocentricity) (299,307,308) (Fig. 29). Tumor cells surround and infiltrate the walls of small and medium-sized blood vessels. The lamellar arrangement of the perivascular tumor cells is highlighted by reticulin staining. The onion-skin or basket-weave appearance of rows of tumor cells within layers of reticulin is characteristic. The involvement of the blood vessels may be destructive, producing hemorrhage or infarcts. Lymphoma cells apparently infiltrate in the subarachnoid (Virchow–Robin) space between the blood vessel and brain parenchyma, the site where lymphoid cells normally reside. Perivascular tumor foci may be present at some distance from an apparently sharply defined tumor mass. Some lymphomas do not demonstrate a principal mass, but are composed of numerous angiocentric infiltrates. These lesions blur the distinction between lymphoma and lymphomatoid granulomatosis, a rare condition that can evolve into lymphoma and that characteristically involves lung and brain (308).

Most tumors form a diffuse mass of noncohesive cells that may represent a confluence of several perivascular foci. The interface with brain often appears fairly sharp, with individual tumor cells appearing to infiltrate only a short distance. Tumor necrosis, especially of single cells, and hemorrhage are common, more so in AIDS-associated disease (307). Most cerebral lymphomas, and particularly AIDS-associated tumors, are high grade (309). The microscopic correlates

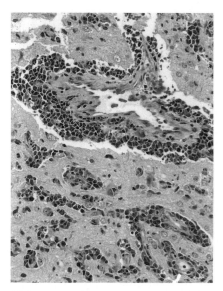

Figure 29 Lymphoma: Large pleomorphic lymphocytes demonstrate typical angiocentricity as they infiltrate gray matter (H&E; original magnification × 200).

include large cells with pleomorphic nuclei and a high mitotic rate. In addition to the typically large neoplastic cells, a polymorphous population of smaller, reactive lymphocytes is present (307).

1. Immunohistochemical Studies

Historical terms for cerebral lymphomas, such as *microglioma*, arose at a time when the nature of the tumor cells was less certain. Immunohistochemical stains have clarified the origin of primary cerebral lymphomas and also are important diagnostically (299,303,307,310). Reactivity for common leukocyte antigen (CLA) is used to confirm lymphoid origin. Interestingly, CLA reactivity often reveals much greater parenchymal infiltration by individual cells than is apparent on routine hematoxylin–eosin staining. By far, most cerebral lymphomas are B-cell neoplasms, and monoclonal reactivity for kappa or lambda light chain may be helpful diagnostically (299,303, 307,310). T-cell lymphoma occurs only rarely (299,311).

D. Differential Diagnosis

The differential diagnosis of primary cerebral lymphomas includes high-grade astrocytoma, ependymoma, PNET, metastatic systemic lymphoma, and metastatic small-cell carcinomas, all of which can be composed of "small blue cells." The characteristic vascular arrangement and lymphoid nuclear cytology usually allow easy differentiation from the nonlymphoid tumors. The immunoreactivity patterns are distinctive, and immunohistochemical analysis has become standard for confirmation. Metastatic lymphomas tend to be superficial, with a meningeal or bony base, in contrast with the deep-seated primary tumors. Nevertheless, a systemic workup may be necessary to exclude this possibility. Differentiation from inflammatory processes may be more difficult, particularly if the biopsy does not include an area of confluent tumor cells. The neoplastic lymphoid cytology may be apparent on touch or smear preparations as part of frozen section analysis, or on the permanent sections. When in doubt, monoclonality needs to be established by immunochemical methods.

ACKNOWLEDGMENT

The authors wish to thank Mrs. Dorothy R. Haskett and Mrs. Andrea Dishman for their superb support in preparation of this manuscript.

REFERENCES

1.   Burger PC, Scheithauer BW, Vogel FS. Surgical pathology of the nervous system and its coverings, 3rd ed. New York: Churchill–Livingstone, 1991:194–404.
2.   Svien HJ, Mabon RF, Kernohan JW, Adson AW. Astrocytomas. Proc Staff Meet Mayo Clin 1949; 24:54–63.
3.   Burger PC, Kleihues P. Cytologic composition of the untreated glioblastoma with implications for evaluation of needle biopsies. Cancer 1989; 63:2014–2023.
4.   Ringertz N. "Grading" of gliomas. Acta Pathol Microbiol Scand 1950; 27:51–64.
5.   Burger PC, Vogel FS, Green SB, Strike TA. Glioblastoma multiforme and anaplastic astrocytoma: pathologic criteria and prognostic implication. Cancer 1985; 56:1106–1111.
6.   Daumas-Duport C, Scheithauer B, O'Fallon J, Kelly P. Grading of astrocytomas: a simple and reproducible method. Cancer 1988; 62:2152–2165.
7.   Kim TS, Halliday AL, Hedley-Whyte ET, Convery K. Correlates of survival and the Daumas-Duport grading system for astrocytomas. J Neurosurg 1991; 74:27–37.
8.   Zulch KJ. Histologic typing of tumours of the central nervous system. International histological classification of tumours. Geneve: WHO 1979; 21:17–57.
9.   Scherer HJ. The forms of growth in gliomas and their practical significance. Brain 1940; 63:1–35.
10. Russell DS, Rubinstein LJ. Pathology of tumours of the nervous system, 5th ed. Baltimore: Williams & Wilkins, 1989:187–215, 394–420.
11. Kelly PJ, Daumas-Duport C, Scheithauer BW, Kall BA, Kispert B. Stereotactic histologic correlations of computed tomography- and magnetic resonance imaging-defined abnormalities in patients with glial neoplasms. Mayo Clin Proc 1987; 62:450–459.
12. Johnson PC, Hunt SJ, Drayer BP. Human cerebral gliomas: correlation of postmortem MR imaging and neuropathologic findings. Radiology 1989; 170:211–217.
13. Burger PC, Heinz ER, Shibata T, Kleihues P. Topographic anatomy and CT correlations in the untreated glioblastoma multiforme. J Neurosurg 1988; 68:698–704.
14. Kelly PJ, Daumas-Duport C, Kispert DB, Kall BA, Scheithauer BW, Illig JJ. Imaging-based stereotaxic serial biopsies in untreated intracranial glial neoplasms. J Neurosurg 1987; 66:865–874.
15. Barnard RO, Geddes JF. The incidence of multifocal cerebral gliomas. A histologic study of large hemisphere sections. Cancer 1987; 60:1519–1531.
16. Giangaspero F, Burger PC. Correlations between cytologic composition and biologic behavior in the glioblastoma multiforme: a postmortem study of 50 cases. Cancer 1983; 52:2320–2333.
17. Shapiro JR, Yung WA, Shapiro WR. Isolation, karyotype and clonal growth of heterogeneous subpopulations of human malignant gliomas. Cancer Res 1981; 41:2349–2359.
18. Giangaspero F, Chieco P, Lisignoli G, Burger PC. Comparison of cytologic composition with microfluorometric DNA analysis of the glioblastoma multiforme and anaplastic astrocytoma. Cancer 1987; 60:59–65.
19. Burger PC, Dubois PJ, Schold SC, Smith KR, Odom GL, Crafts DD, Giangaspero F. Computerized tomographic and pathologic studies of the untreated, quiescent, and recurrent glioblastoma multiforme. J Neurosurg 1983; 58:159–169.
20. Shapiro JR. Biology of gliomas: heterogeneity, oncogenes, growth factors. Semin Oncol 1986; 13:4–15.
21. Shapiro JR, Scheck AC, Mehta BM, Moots PL, Fiola MR. Minor subpopulation of intrinsically chemoresistant and radioresistant cells in primary gliomas become the dominant population in recurrent tumors. J Cancer Res Clin Oncol 1990; 116(suppl):1135.
22. Shapiro JR, Scheck AC. Molecular biological events in the selection of chemotherapy-resistant cells in

human malignant gliomas. In: Paoletti P, Takakura K, Walker MD, Butti, G, Pezzotta S (eds.). *Neurooncology* Amsterdam: Kluwer Academic Publishers, 1991:21–26.

23. Bronen RA, Sze G. Magnetic resonance imaging contrast agents: theory and application to the central nervous system. J Neurosurg 1990; 73:820–839.

24. Lee YY, Van Tassel P, Bruner JM, Moser RP, Share JC. Juvenile pilocytic astrocytomas: CT and MR characteristics. Am J Neuroradiol 1989; 10:363–370.

25. Wallner KE, Galicich JH, Krol G, Arbit E, Malkin MG. Patterns of failure following treatment for glioblastoma multiforme and anaplastic astrocytoma. Int J Radiat Oncol Biol Phys 1989; 16:1405–1409.

26. Shapiro JR, Shapiro WR. The subpopulations and isolated cell types of freshly resected high grade human gliomas: their influence on the tumor's evolution in vivo and behavior and therapy in vitro. Cancer Metastasis Rev 1985; 4:107–124.

27. Finlay JL, Goins SC. Brain tumors in children. Advances in diagnosis. Am J Pediatr Hematol Oncol 1987; 9:246–255.

28. McComb RD, Burger PC. Pathologic analysis of primary brain tumors. Neurol Clin 1985; 3:711–728.

29. Burger PC, Vollmer RT. Histologic factors of prognostic significance in the glioblastoma multiforme. Cancer 1980; 46:1179–1186.

30. Paulus W, Pfeiffer J. Intratumoral histologic heterogeneity of gliomas. A quantitative study. Cancer 1989; 64:442–447.

31. Glantz MJ, Burger PC, Herndon JE, Friedman AH, Cairncross JG, Vick NA, Schold SC Jr. Influence of the type of surgery on the histologic diagnosis in patients with anaplastic gliomas. Neurology 1991; 41:1741–1714.

32. Chandrasoma PT, Smith MM, Apuzzo MLJ. Stereotactic biopsy in the diagnosis of brain masses: comparison of results of biopsy and resected surgical specimen. Neurosurgery 1989; 24:160–165.

33. Dean BL, Drayer BP, Bird CR, et al. Gliomas: classification with MR imaging. Radiology 1990; 174:411–415.

34. Daumas-Duport C, Monsaingeon V, N'Guyen JP, Missir O, Szikla G. Some correlations between histological and CT aspects of cerebral gliomas contributing to the choice of significant trajectories for stereotactic biopsies. Acta Neurochir [Suppl] 1984; 33:185–194.

35. Ross GW, Rubinstein LJ. Lack of histopathological correlation of malignant ependymomas with postoperative survival. J Neurosurg 1989; 70:31–36.

36. Bigner DD. Biology of gliomas: potential clinical implications of glioma cellular heterogeneity. Neurosurgery 1981; 9:320–326.

37. Westphal M, Herrmann H-D. Growth factor biology and oncogene activation in human gliomas and their implications for specific therapeutic concepts. Neurosurgery 1989; 25:681–694.

38. Coons SW, Shapiro JR, Johnson PC. Regional heterogeneity in an astrocytoma. Comparison of flow cytometry, karyotyping, and histopathology [abstract]. J Neuropathol Exp Neurol 1991; 50:368.

39. Scheck AC, Beikman MK, Korn MC, Shapiro JR. Regional analysis of genes potentially involved in resistance to BCNU in human malignant gliomas (Abstract). Proc. Am. Assoc. Cancer Res 1991; 32:358.

40. Coons SW, Davis JR, Way DL. Correlation of DNA content and histology in prognosis of astrocytomas. Am J Clin Pathol 1988; 90:289–293.

41. Hoshino T, Prados M, Wilson CB, Cho KG, Lee K-S, Davis RL. Prognostic implications of the bromodeoxyuridine labeling index of human gliomas. J Neurosurg 1989; 71:335–341.

42. Hoshino T, Rodriguez LA, Cho KG, Lee KS, Wilson CB, Edwards MSB, Levin VA, Davis RL. Prognostic implications of the proliferative potential of low grade astrocytomas. J Neurosurg 1988; 69:839–842.

43. Zuber P, Hamou M-F, de Tribolet N. Identification of proliferating cells in human gliomas using the monoclonal antibody Ki-67. Neurosurgery 1988; 22:364–368.

44. Ostertag CB, Volk B, Shibata T, Burger P, Kleihues P. The monoclonal antibody Ki-67 as a marker for proliferating cells in stereotactic biopsies of brain tumors. Acta Neurochir 1987; 89:117–121.

45. Coons S, Johnson PC, Haskett DR. DNA content of oligodendrogliomas. Correlations with outcome, histology, and clinical variables (Abstract). Am J Neuropathol Exp Neurol 1990; 49:321.

46. Danova M, Giaretti W, Merlo F, Mazzini G, Gaetani P, Geido E, Gentile S, Butti G, Di Vinci A, Riccardi A. Prognostic significance of nuclear DNA content in human neuroepithelial tumors. Int J Cancer 1991; 48:663–667.

47. Raghavan R, Steart PV, Weller RO. Cell proliferation patterns in the diagnosis of astrocytomas, anaplastic astrocytomas and glioblastoma multiforme: a Ki-67 study. Neuropathol Appl Neurobiol 1990; 16:123–133.

48. Morimura T, Kitz K, Budka H. In situ analysis of cell kinetics in human brain tumors. A comparative immunocytochemical study of S-phase cells by a new in vitro bromodeoxyuridine-labeling technique, and of proliferating pool cells by monoclonal antibody Ki-67. Acta Neuropathol 1989; 77:276–282.

49. Plate KH, Rüschoff J, Mennel HD. Cell proliferation in intracranial tumours: selective silver staining of nucleolar organizer regions (AgNORs). Application to surgical and experimental neuro-oncology. Neuropathol Appl Neurobiol 1991; 17:121–132.

50. Nicoll JAR, Candy E. Nuclear organizer regions and postoperative survival in glioblastoma multiforme. Neuropathol Appl Neurobiol 1991; 17:17–20.

51. Hara A, Hirayama H, Sakai N, Yamada H, Tanaka T, Mori H. Nucleolar organizer region score and Ki-67 labelling index in high-grade gliomas and metastatic brain tumours. Acta Neurochir (Wien) 1991; 109:37–41.

52. Louis D, Meehan S, Ferrante R, Hedley-Whyte E. Use of the silver nucleolar organizer region (AgNOR) technique in the differential diagnosis of central nervous system neoplasia. J Neuropathol Exp Neurol 1992; 51:150–157.

53. Coons S, Johnson PC. Regional heterogeneity in flow cytometric measurements of DNA ploidy and proliferation in human gliomas (Abstract). Proc. Am. Assoc. Cancer Res 1991; 32:26.

54. Coons SW, Johnson PC. Regional heterogeneity in the Ki67 labelling indices of gliomas. J Neuropathol Exp Neurol 1992; 51:331.

55. Jiminez O, Timms A, Quirke P, McLaughlin JE. Prognosis in malignant glioma: a retrospective study of biopsy specimens by flow cytometry. Neuropathol Appl Neurobiol 1989; 15:331–338.

56. Zaprianov Z, Christov K. Histological grading, DNA content, cell proliferation and survival of patients with astroglial tumors. Cytometry 1988; 9:380–386.

57. Rasheed BK, Bigner SH. Genetic alterations in glioma and medulloblastoma. Cancer Metastasis Rev 1991; 10:289–299.

58. Jenkins RB, Kimmel DW, Moertel CA, Schultz CG, Scheithauer BW, Kelly PJ, Dewald GW. A cytogenetic study of 53 human gliomas. Cancer Genet Cytogenet 1989; 39:253–279.

59. Kimmel DW, O'Fallon JR, Scheithauer BW, Kelly PJ, Dewald GW, Jenkins RB. Prognostic value of cytogenetic analysis in human cerebral astrocytomas. Ann Neurol 1992; 31:534–542.

60. Bigner SH, Mark J, Burger PC, Mahaley MS Jr, Bullard DE, Muhlbaier LH, Bigner DD. Specific chromosomal abnormalities in malignant human gliomas. Cancer Res 1988; 88:405–411.

61. Thiel G, Losanowa T, Kintzel D, Nisch G, Martin H, Vorpahl K, Witkowski R. Karyotypes in 90 human gliomas. Cancer Genet Cytogenet 1992; 58:109–120.

62. Frankel RH, Bayona W, Koslow M, Newcomb EW. p53 mutations in human malignant gliomas: comparison of loss of heterozygosity with mutation frequency. Cancer Res 1992; 52:1427–1433.

63. Sidransky D, Mikkelsen T, Schwechheimer K, Rosenblum ML, Cavanee W, Vogelstein B. Clonal expansion of p53 mutant cells is associated with brain tumour progression. Nature 1992; 355:846–847.

64. Fults D, Brockmeyer D, Tullous MW, Pedone CA, Cawthon RM. p53 mutation and loss of heterozygosity on chromosomes 17 and 10 during human astrocytoma progression. Cancer Res 1992; 52:674–679.

65. Mauro A, Bulfone A. Oncogenes and growth factors in gliomas. J Neurosurg Sci 1990; 34:171–173.

66. Takahashi JA, Mori H, Fukumoto M, Igarashi K, Jaye M, Oda Y, Kikuchi H, Hatanaka M. Gene expression of fibroblast growth factors in human gliomas and meningiomas: demonstration of cellular source of basic fibroblast growth factor mRNA and peptide in tumor tissues. Proc Natl Acad Sci USA 1990; 87:5710–5714.

67. Akutsu Y, Aida T, Kakazawa S, Asano G. Localization of acidic and basic fibroblast growth factor mRNA in human brain tumors. Jpn J Cancer Res 1991; 82:1022–1027.

68. Maxwell M, Naber SP, Wolfe HJ, Hedley-Whyte ET, Galanopoulos T, Neville-Golden J, Antoniades

HN. Expression of angiogenic growth factor genes in primary human astrocytomas may contribute to their growth and progression. Cancer Res 1991; 51:1345–1351.

69. Maxwell M, Naber SP, Wolfe HJ, Galanopoulos T, Hedley-Whyte ET, Black PM, Antoniades HN. Coexpression of platelet-derived growth factor (PDGF) and PDGF-receptor genes by primary human astrocytomas may contribute to their development and maintenance. J Clin Invest 1990; 86: 131–140.

70. Stefanik DF, Rizkalla LR, Soi A, Goldblatt SA, Rizkalla WM. Acidic and basic fibroblast growth factors are present in glioblastoma multiforme. Cancer Res 1991; 51:5760–5765.

71. Libermann TA, Nusbaum HR, Razon N, Kris R, Lax I, Soreq H, Whittle N, Waterfield MD, Ullrich A, Schlessinger J. Amplification, enhances expression and possible rearrangement of EGF receptor gene in primary human brain tumours of glial origin. Nature 1985; 313:144–147.

72. Libermann TA, Nusbaum HR, Razon N, Kris R, Lax I, Soreq H, Whittle N, Waterfield MD, Ullrich A, Schlessinger J. Amplification and overexpression of the EGF receptor gene in primary human glioblastomas. J Cell Sci 1985; (suppl 3):161–172.

73. Agosti RM, Leuthold M, Gullick WJ, Yasargil MG, Wiestler OD. Expression of the epidermal growth factor receptor in astrocytic tumours is specifically associated with glioblastoma multiforme. Virchows Archiv [A] 1992; 420:321–325.

74. Ekstrand AJ, James CD, Cavenee WK, Seliger B, Petterson RF, Collins VP. Genes for epidermal growth factor receptor, transforming growth factor α, and epidermal growth factor and their expression in human gliomas in vivo. Cancer Res 1991; 51:2164–2172.

75. Strommer K, Hamou MF, Diggelmann H, de Tribolet N. Cellular and tumoural heterogeneity of EGFR gene amplification in human malignant gliomas. Acta Neurochir (Wien) 1990; 107:82–87.

76. Bishop M, de la Monte SM. Dual lineage of astrocytomnas. Am J Pathol 1989; 135:517–527.

77. De la Monte SM. Uniform lineage of oligodendrogliomas. Am J Pathol 1989; 135:529–540.

78. Burger PC, Scheithauer BW, Vogel FS. Surgical pathology of the nervous system and its coverings, 3rd ed. New York. Churchill–Livingstone, 1991: 234–271.

79. Palma L, Guidetti B. Cystic pilocytic astrocytomas of the cerebral hemispheres: surgical experience with 51 cases and long-term results. J Neurosurg 1985; 62:811–815.

80. Ilgen EB, Stiller CA. Cerebellar astrocytomas: therapeutic management. Acta Neurochir 1986; 81:11–26.

81. Austin EJ, Alvord JEC. Reoccurrences of cerebellar astrocytomas: a violation of Collins' law. J Neurosurg 1988; 68:41–47.

82. Ilgren EB, Stiller CA. Cerebellar astrocytomas, part II. Pathologic features indicative of malignancy. Clin Neuropathol 1987; 6:201–214.

83. Lee YY, van Tassel P, Bruner JM, Moser RP, Share JC. Juvenile pilocytic astrocytomas: CT and MR characteristics. Am J Neuroradiol 1989; 10:363–370.

84. Shibata T, Burger PC. The use of the monoclonal antibody Ki-67 in determination of the growth fraction in pediatric brain tumors. Childs Nerv Syst 1987; 3:364–367.

85. Tomlinson FH, Scheithauer BW, Hayostek CH, Parisi JE, Meyer FB, Shaw EG. Atypia and malignancy in pilocytic astrocytoma of the cerebellum: a clinicopathologic and flow cytometric study. J Neuropathol Exp Neurol 1992; 51:331.

86. Rekate HL, Rakfal SM. Controversial areas of treatment: low grade astrocytomas of childhood. In: Cohen ME, Duffner PK. Brain tumors in children. Neurol Clin 1991:9;423–440.

87. Couch JR, Weiss SA. Gliomatosis cerebri. Report of four cases and review of the literature. Neurology 1974; 24:504–511.

88. Malamud N, Wise BL, Jones OW Jr. Gliomatosis cerebri. 1952; 9:409–417.

89. Simonati A, Vio M, Iannucci AM, Toso V, Morello F, Rizzuto N. Gliomatosis cerebri diffusa. Acta Neuropathol 1981; 54:311–314.

90. Dunn J, Kernohan JW. Gliomatosis cerebri. Hum Pathol 1957; 64:82–91.

91. Schober R, Mai JK, Volk B, Wechsler W. Gliomatosis cerebri: bioptical approach and neuropathological verification. Acta Neurochir (Wien) 1991; 113:131–137.

92. Ross IB, Robitaille Y, Villemure JG, Tampieri D. Diagnosis and management of gliomatosis cerebri: recent trends. Surg Neurol 1991; 431:431–440.

93. Sakai HA, Yamada H, Tanaka T, Mori H. Assessment of proliferative potential in gliomatosis cerebri. Neurol 1991; 238:80–82.

94. Burger PC, Scheithauer BW, Vogel FS. Surgical pathology of the nervous system and its coverings, 3rd ed. New York: Churchill–Livingstone, 1991:247–250.

95. Moore MT. Diffuse cerebrospinal gliomatosis, masked by syphilis. J Neuropathol Exp Neurol 1954; 13:129–143.

96. Allegranza A, Ferraresi S, Bruzzone M, Giombini S. Cerebromeningeal pleomorphic xanthoastrocytoma. Report on four cases: clinical radiologic and pathological features (including a case with malignant evolution). Neurosurg Rev 1991; 14:43–49.

97. Kepes JJ, Rubinstein LJ, Eng LF. Pleomorphic xanthoastrocytoma: a distinctive meningocerebral glioma of young subjects with relatively favorable prognosis; a study of 12 cases. Cancer 1979; 44:1839–1852.

98. Kepes JJ, Rubinstein LJ, Ansbacher L, Schreiber DJ. Histopathological features of recurrent pleomorphic xanthoastrocytomas: further corroboration of the glial nature of this neoplasm; a study of 3 cases. Acta Neuropathol 1989; 78:585–593.

99. Kros JM, Vecht CJ, Stefanko SZ. The pleomorphic xanthoastrocytoma and its differential diagnosis; a study of five cases. Hum Pathol 1991; 22:1128–1135.

100. Hosokawa Y, Tsuchihashi Y, Okabe H, Toyama M, Namura K, Kuga M, Yonezawa T, Fujita S, Ashihara T. Pleomorphic xanthoastrocytoma; ultrastructural, immunohistochemical, and DNA cytofluorometric study of a case. Cancer 1991; 68:853–859.

101. Zorzi F, Facchetti F, Baronchelli C, Cani E. Pleomorphic xanthoastrocytoma: an immunohistochemical study of three cases. Histopathology 1992; 20:267–269.

102. Iwaki T, Fukui M, Kondo A, Matsushima T, Takeshita I. Epithelial properties of pleomorphic xanthoastrocytomas determined in ultrastructural and immunohistochemical studies. Acta Neuropathol 1987; 74:142–150.

103. Whittle IR, Gordon A, Misra BK, Shaw JF, Steers AJW. Pleomorphic xanthoastrocytoma; report of four cases. J Neurosurg 1989; 70:463–468.

104. Grant JW, Gallagher P. Pleomorphic xanthoastrocytoma. Am J Surg Pathol 1986; 10:336–341.

105. Yamashita J, Handa H, Yamagami T, Haebara H. Astroblastoma of pure type. Surg Neurol 1985; 24:218–222.

106. Bonnin JM, Rubinstein LJ. Astroblastomas: a pathological study of 23 tumors, with a postoperative follow-up in 13 patients. Neurosurgery 1989; 25:6–13.

107. Kubota T, Hirano A, Sato K, Yamamoto S. The fine structure of astroblastroma. Cancer 1985; 55:745–750.

108. Rubinstein LJ, Herman MM. The astroblastoma and its possible cytogenic relationship to the tanycyte, an electron microscopic, immunohistochemical, tissue- and organ-culture study. Acta Neuropathol 1989; 78:472–483.

109. Cabello A, Madero A, Castresana A, Diaz-Lobato R. Astroblastoma: electron microscopy and immunohistochemical findings: a case report. Surg Neurol 1991; 35:116–121.

110. Burger PC, Scheithauer BW, Vogel FS. Surgical pathology of the nervous system and its coverings, 3rd ed. New York: Churchill–Livingstone, 1991:193–437.

111. Russell DS, Rubinstein LJ. Pathology of tumours of the nervous system, 5th ed. Baltimore: Williams & Wilkins, 1989:161–168.

112. Burger PC, Vogel FS, Green SB, Strike TA. Glioblastoma multiforme and anaplastic astrocytoma: Pathologic criteria and prognostic implications. Cancer 1985; 56:1106–1111.

113. Bruner JM. Oligodendroglioma: diagnosis and prognosis. Semin Diagn Pathol 1987; 4:251–261.

114. Lee YY, Van Tassel P. Intracranial oligodendrogliomas: imaging findings in 35 untreated cases. AJR 1989; 152:361–369.

115. Mørk SJ, Halvorsen TB, Lindegaard KF, Eide GE. Oligodendroglioma: histologic evaluation and prognosis. J Neuropathol Exp Neurol 1986; 45:65–78.

116. Shaw EG, Scheithauer BW, O'Fallon JR, Tazelaar HD, Davis DH. Oligodendrogliomas: the Mayo Clinic experience. J Neurosurg 1992; 76:428–434.

117. Kernohan JW, Mabon RF, Svien HJ, Adson AW. A simplified classification of the gliomas. Proc Staff Meet Mayo Clin 1949; 24:71–75.
118. Smith MT, Ludwig CL, Godfrey AD, Armbrustmacher VW. Grading of oligodendrogliomas. Cancer 1983; 52:2107–2114.
119. Kros JM, Troost D, van Eden CG, van der Werf AJM, Uylyings HBM. Oligodendroglioma: a comparison of two grading systems. Cancer 1988; 61:2251–2259.
120. Daumas-Dupont C, Scheithauer B, O'Fallon J, Kelly P. Grading of astrocytomas. Cancer 1988; 62:2152–2165.
121. Fulling KH, Nelson JS. Cerebral astrocytic neoplasms in the adult: contribution of histologic examination to the assessment of prognosis. Semin Diagn Pathol 1984; 1:152–163.
122. Russell DS, Rubinstein LJ. Pathology of tumours of the nervous system, 5th ed. Baltimore: Williams & Wilkins, 1989.
123. Svien HJ, Mabon RF, Kernohan JW, Adson AW. Astrocytomas. Proc Staff Meet Mayo Clin 1949; 24:54–63.
124. Coons SW, Johnson PC, Haskett DR. DNA content of oligodendrogliomas: correlation with outcome, histology, and clinical variables. J Neuropathol Exp Neurol 1990; 49:321.
125. Shibata T, Burger PC, Kleihues P. Cell kinetics of oligodendroglioma and oligoastrocytoma—Ki-67 PaP study. Brain Nerve 1988; 40:779–785.
126. Kros JM, van Eden CG, Vissers CJ, Mulder AH, van der Kwast TH. Prognostic relevance of DNA flow cytometry in oligodendroglioma. Cancer 1992; 69:1791–1798.
127. Jenkins RB, Kimmel DW, Moertel CA, Schultz CG, Scheithauer BW, Jelly PJ, Dewald GW. A cytogenetic study of 53 human gliomas. Cancer Genet Cytogenet 1989; 39:253–279.
128. Di Carlo A, Mariano A, Macchia PE, Moroni MC, Behuinot L, Macchia V. Epidermal growth factor receptor in human brain tumors. J Endocrinol Invest 1992; 15:31–37.
129. Ohgaki H, Eibl RH, Wiestler OD,Yasargil MG, Newcomb EW, Kleihues P. p53 mutations in nonastrocytic human brain tumors. Cancer Res 1991; 51:6202–6205.
130. DiCarlo A, Mariano A, Macchia P, Moroni MC, Beguinot L, Macchia V. Epidermal growth factor receptor in human brain tumors. J Endocrinol Invest 1992; 15:31–37.
131. Tanaka J, Hokama Y, Nakamura H. Myelin basic protein as a possible marker for oligodendroglioma. Acta Pathol Jpn 1988; 38:1297–1303.
132. De la Monte SM. Uniform lineage of oligodendrogliomas. Am J Pathol 1989; 135:529–540.
133. Bishop M, De la Monte SM. Dual lineage of astrocytomas. Am J Pathol 1989; 135:517–527.
134. Coons S, Johnson PC. Regional heterogeneity in flow cytometric measurements of DNA ploidy and proliferation in human gliomas (Abstract). Proc Am Assoc Cancer Res 1991; 32:26.
135. Coons SW, Johnson PC. Regional heterogeneity in the Ki67 labelling indices of gliomas. J Neuropathol Exp Neurol 1992; 51:331.
136. Burger PC, Scheithauer BW, Vogel FS. Surgical pathology of the nervous system and its coverings, 3rd ed. New York: Churchill–Livingstone, 1991:202–282.
137. De la Monte SM. Uniform lineage of oligodendrogliomas. Am J Pathol 1989; 135:529–540.
138. Bishop M, De la Monte SM. Dual lineage of astrocytomas. Am J Pathol 1989; 135:517–5272.
139. Shaw EG, Scheithauer BW, O'Fallon JR, Tazelaar HD, Davis DH. Oligodendrogliomas: the Mayo Clinic experience. J Neurosurg 1992; 76:428–434.
140. Kros SM, Van Eden CG, Stefanko SZ, Waayer-Van Batenburg M, van der Kwast TH. Prognostic implications of glial fibrillary acidic protein containing cell types in oligodendrogliomas. Cancer 1990; 66:1204–1212.
141. Glass J, Hochberg FH, Gruber ML, Louis DN, Smith D, Rattner B. The treatment of oligodendrogliomas and mixed oligodendroglioma–astrocytomas with PCV chemotherapy. J Neurosurg 1992; 76:741–745.
142. Russell DS, Rubinstein LJ. Pathology of tumours of the nervous system, 5th ed. Baltimore: Williams & Wilkins, 1989:187–219.
143. Mørk SJ, Løken AC. Ependymoma. A follow-up study of 101 cases. Cancer 1977; 40:907–915.
144. Healey EA, Barnes PD, Kupsky WJ, Scott RM, Sallan SE, Black PM, Tarbell NJ. The prognostic significance of postoperative residual tumor in ependymoma. Neurosurgery 1991; 28:666–672.

145. Lyons MK, Kelly PJ. Posterior fossa ependymomas: report of 30 cases and review of the literature. Neurosurgery 1991; 28:659–665.

146. Ernestus RI, Wilcke O, Schröder R. Intracranial ependymomas: prognostic aspects. Neurosurgery 1989; 12:157–163.

147. Rawlings CE III, Giangaspero F, Burger PC, Bullard DE. Ependymomas: a clinicopathologic study. Surg Neurol 1988; 29:271–281.

148. Spoto GP, Press GA, Hesselink JR, Solomon M. Intracranial ependymoma and subependymoma: MR manifestations. Am J Neuroradiol 1990; 11:83–91.

149. Cruz-Sanchez FF, Iglesias JR, Rossi ML, Cervos-Navarro J, Figols J, Haustein J. Histologic characterization of 41 ependymomas with the help of a personal computer. Cancer 1988; 62:150–162.

150. Sutton LN, Goldwein J, Perilongo G, Lang B, Schut L, Rorke L, Packer R. Prognostic factors in childhood ependymomas. Pediatr Neurosurg 1990–91; 16:57–65.

151. Schiffer D, Chiò A, Giodana MT, Migheli A, Palma L, Pollo B, Soffietti R, Tribolo A. Histologic prognostic factors in ependymoma. Childs Nerv Syst 1991; 7:177–182.

152. Uematsu Y, Rojas-Corona RR, Llena JF, Hirano A. Distribution of epithelial membrane antigen in normal and neoplastic human ependyma. Acta Neuropathol 1989; 78:325–328.

153. Sonneland PRL, Scheithauer BW, Onofrio BM. Myxopapillary ependymoma. A clinicopathologic and immunocytochemical study of 77 cases. Cancer 1985; 56:883–893.

154. Kawano N, Yada K, Yagishita S. Clear cell ependymoma. A histological variant with diagnostic implications. Virchows Arch [A] 1989; 415:467–472.

155. McCloskey JJ, Parker JC Jr, Brooks WH, Blacker HM. Melanin as a component of cerebral gliomas. The melanotic cerebral ependymoma. Cancer 1976; 37:2373–2379.

156. Mannoji H, Becker LE. Ependymal and choroid plexus tumors. Cytokeratin and GFAP expression. Cancer 1988; 61:1377–1385.

157. Cruz-Sanchez FF, Rossi ML, Hughes JT, Cervos-Navarro J. An immunohistological study of 66 ependymomas. Histopathology 1988; 13:443–454.

158. Ross GW, Rubinstein LJ. Lack of histopathological correlation of malignant ependymomas with postoperative survival. J Neurosurg 1989; 70:31–36.

159. Shaw EG, Evans RG, Scheithauer BW, Ilstrup DM, Earle LD. Postoperative radiotherapy of intracranial ependymoma in pediatric and adult patients. Int J Radiat Oncol Biol Phys 1987; 13:1457–1462.

160. Schiffer D, Chiò A, Cravioto H, Giordana MT, Migheli A, Soffietti R, Vigliani MC. Ependymoma: internal correlations among pathological signs: the anaplastic variant. Neurosurgery 1991; 29:206–210.

161. Figarella-Branger D, Gambarelli D, Dollo C, Devictor B, Perez-Castillo AM, Genitori L, Lena G, Choux M, Pellissier JF. Infratentorial ependymomas of childhood. Correlation between histological features, immunohistological phenotype, silver nucleolar organizer region staining values and postoperative survival in 16 cases. Acta Neuropathol 1991; 82:208–216.

162. Spaar FW, Blech M, Ahyai A. DNA-flow fluorescence-cytometry of ependymomas. Report on ten surgically removed tumours. Acta Neuropathol (Berl) 1986; 69:153–160.

163. Nagashima T, Hoshino T, Cho KG, Edwards MS, Hudgins RJ, Davis RL. The proliferative potential of human ependymomas measured by in situ bromodeoxyuridine labeling. Cancer 1988; 61:2433–2438.

164. Schiffer D, Giordana MT, Mauro A, Migheli A, Pezzulo T, Vigliana MC. PCNA immunohistocytochemistry in the recognition of malignant ependymoma. J Neuropathol Exp Neurol 1992; 51:362.

165. Stratton MR, Darling J, Lantos PL, Cooper CS, Reeves BR. Cytogenetic abnormalities in human ependymomas. Int J Cancer 1989; 44:579–581.

166. Ohgaki H, Eibl RH, Wiestler OD, Yasargil MG, Newcomb EW, Kleihues P. p53 mutations in non-astrocytic human brain tumors. Cancer 1991; 51:6202–6205.

167. Bergsagel DJ, Finegold MJ, Butel JS, Kupsky WJ, Garcea RL. DNA sequences similar to those if simian virus 40 in ependymomas and choroid plexus tumors of childhood. N Engl J Med 1992; 326:988–993.

168. Rubinstein LJ. The definition of the ependymoblastoma. Arch Pathol 1970; 90:35–45.
169. Bohm E, Strang R. Choroid plexus papillomas. J Neurosurg 1961; 18:493–500.
170. Coffin CM, Wick MR, Braun JT, Dehner LP. Choroid plexus neoplasms: clinicopathologic and immunohistochemical studies. Am J Surg Pathol 1986; 10:394–404.
171. McGirr SJ, Ebersold MJ, Scheithauer BW, Quast LM, Shaw EG. Choroid plexus papillomas: long-term follow-up results in a surgically treated series. J Neurosurg 1988; 68:843–849.
172. Raimondi AJ, Gutierrez FA. Diagnosis and surgical treatment of choroid plexus papillomas. Childs Brain 1975; 1:81–115.
173. Ellenbogen RG, Winston KR, Kupsky WJ. Tumors of the choroid plexus in children. Neurosurgery 1989; 25:327–335.
174. Carpenter DB, Michelsen WJ, Hays AP. Carcinoma of the choroid plexus: case report. J Neurosurg 1982; 56:722–727.
175. Bergsagel DJ, Finegold MJ, Butel JS, Kupsky WJ, Garcea RL. DNA sequences similar to those of simian virus 40 in ependymomas and choroid plexus tumors of childhood. N Engl J Med 1992; 326:988–993.
176. Russell DS, Rubinstein LJ. Pathology of tumours of the nervous system, 5th ed. Baltimore: Williams & Wilkins, 1989:394–404.
177. Coons SW, Johnson PC, Haskett D, Rider R. Flow cytometric analysis of DNA ploidy and proliferation in choroid plexus tumors. Neurosurgery 1992; 31:850–856.
178. Coons S, Johnson PC, Dickman CA, Rekate H. Choroid plexus carcinoma in siblings: a study by light and electron microscopy with Ki-67 immunocytochemistry. J Neuropathol Exp Neurol 1989; 48:483–493.
179. Lewis P. Carcinoma of the choroid plexus. Brain 1967; 90:177–186.
180. Dohrmann GJ, Collias JC. Choroid plexus carcinoma: case report. J Neurosurg 1975; 43:225–232.
181. Miettinen M, Clark R, Virtanen I. Intermediate filament proteins in choroid plexus and ependyma and their tumors. Am J Pathol 1986; 123:231–240.
182. Doglioni C, Dell'orto P, Coggi G, Iuzzolino P, Bontempini L, Viale G. Choroid plexus tumors: an immunocytochemical study with particular reference to the coexpression of intermediate filament proteins. Am J Pathol 1987; 127:519–529.
183. Matsushima T, Inoue T, Takeshita I, Fukui M, Iwaki T, Kitamoto T. Choroid plexus papillomas: an immunohistochemical study with particular reference of the coexpression of prealbumin. Neurosurgery 1988; 23:384–389.
184. Giangaspero F, Doglioni C, Rivano MT, Pileri S, Gerdes J, Stein H. Growth fraction in human brain tumors defined by the monoclonal antibody Ki-67. Acta Neuropathol (Berl) 1987; 74:179–182.
185. Feigin IH, Gross SW. Sarcoma arising in glioblastoma of the brain. Am J Pathol 1955; 31:633–653.
186. Ho KL. Histogenesis of sarcomatous component of the gliosarcoma: an ultrastructural study. Acta Neuropathol 1990; 81:178–188.
187. Morantz RA, Feigin I, Ransohoff J. Clinical and pathological study of 24 cases of gliosarcoma. J Neurosurg 1976; 45:398–408.
188. Rubinstein LJ. The development of contiguous sarcomatous and gliomatous tissue in intracranial tumours. J Pathol Bacteriol 1956; 71:441–459.
189. Slowik F, Jellinger K, Gas ZÓ, Fischer J. Gliosarcomas: histological, immunohistochemical, ultrastructural and tissue culture studies. Acta Neuropathol 1985; 67:201–210.
190. Banerjee AK, Sharma BS, Kak VK, Ghataj NR. Gliosarcoma with cartilage formation. Cancer 1989; 63:518–523.
191. Lalitha VS, Rubinstein LJ. Reactive glioma in intracranial sarcoma: a form of mixed sarcoma and glioma ("sarcoglioma)." Cancer 1979; 43:246–257.
192. Meis JM, Martz KL, Nelson JS. Mixed glioblastoma multiforme and sarcoma. Cancer 1991; 67:2342–2349.
193. Burger PC, Scheithauer BW, Vogel FS. Surgical pathology of the nervous system, 3rd ed. New York: Churchill–Livingstone, 1991.
194. Cerame MA, Guthikonda M, Kohli CN. Extraneural metastases in gliosarcoma: a case report and review of the literature. Neurosurgery 1985; 17:413–418.

195. Smith DR, Hardman JM, Earle KM. Contiguous glioblastoma multiforme and fibrosarcoma with extracranial metastasis. Cancer 1969; 24:270–276.
196. Feigin I, Ransohoff J, Lieberman A. Sarcoma arising in oligodendroglioma of the brain. J Neuropathol Exp Neurol 1976; 35:679–684.
197. Pasquier B, Couderc P, Pasquier D, Panh MH, N'Golet A. Sarcoma arising in oligodendroglioma of the brain. Cancer 1978; 42:2753–2758.
198. Grant JW, Steart PV, Aguzzi A, Jones DB, Gallagher PJ. Gliosarcoma: an immunohistochemical study. Acta Neuropathol 1989; 79:305–309.
199. Richman AV, Balis GA, Maniscalco JE. Primary intracerebral tumor with mixed chondrosarcoma and glioblastoma–gliosarcoma or sarcoglioma? J Neuropatholol Exp Neurol 1980; 39:329–335.
200. Russell DS, Rubinstein LJ. Pathology of tumours of the nervous system, 5th ed. Baltimore: Williams & Wilkins, 1989:251–289.
201. Hubbard JL, Scheithauer BW, Kispert DB, Carpenter SM, Wick MR, Laws ED Jr. Adult cerebellar medulloblastomas: the pathological, radiographic, and clinical disease spectrum. J Neurosurg 1989; 70:536–544.
202. Farwell JR, Flannery JT. Adult occurrence of medulloblastoma. Acta Neurochir (Wien) 1987; 86:1–5.
203. Grant JW, Steart PV, Gallagher PJ. Primitive neuroectodermal tumors of the cerebrum: a histological and immunohistochemical study of 10 cases. Clin Neuropathol 1988; 7:228–233.
204. Dehner LP. Peripheral and central primitive neuroectodermal tumors. A nosologic concept seeking a consensus. Arch Pathol Lab Med 1986; 110:997–1005.
205. Kleinert R. Immunohistochemical characterization of primitive neuroectodermal tumors and their possible relationship to the stepwise ontogenetic development of the central nervous system. Acta Neuropathol 1991; 82:508–515.
206. Tomita T, Yasue M, Engelhard HH, McLone DG, Gonzalez-Crussi F, Bauer KD. Flow cytometric DNA analysis of medulloblastoma. Cancer 1988; 61:744–749.
207. Horten BC, Rubinstein LJ. Primary cerebral neuroblastoma: a clinicopathological study of 35 cases. Brain 1976; 99:735–756.
208. Mierau GW, Timmons CF, Orsini EN, Crouse VL. Intriguing case: primary cerebral neuroblastoma. Ultrastruct Pathol 1989; 13:281–289.
209. Louis DN, Swearingen B, Linggood RM, Dickersin GR, Kretschmar C, Bhan AK, Hedley-White T. Clinical study: central nervous system neurocytoma and neuroblastoma in adults—report of eight cases. J Neurooncol 1990; 9:231–238.
210. Tomita T, McLone DG, Yasue M. Cerebral primitive neuroectodermal tumors in childhood. J Neurooncol 1988; 6:233–243.
211. Rorke LB, Gilles FH, Davis RL, Becker LE. Revision of the World Health Organization classification of brain tumors for childhood brain tumors. Cancer 1985; 56:1869–1886.
212. Rubinstein LJ. Embryonal central neuroepithelial tumors and their differentiating potential. A cytogenetic view of a complex neuro-oncological problem. J Neurosurg 1985; 62:795–805.
213. Itoh Y, Yagishita S, Chiba Y. Cerebral gangliocytoma: an ultrastructural study. Acta Neuropathol 1987; 74:169–178.
214. Izukawa D, Lack B, Benoit B. Gangliocytoma of the cerebellum: ultrastructure and immunohisto-chemistry. Neurosurgery 1988; 22:576–581.
215. Silver JM, Rawlings CE, Rossitch E Jr, Zeidman SM. Ganglioglioma: a clinical study with long-term follow-up. J Surg Neurol 1991; 35:261–266.
216. Martin LD, Kaplan AM, Hernried LS, Fisher BJ. Pediatr Neurol 1986; 2:178–182.
217. Kalyan-Raman UP, Olivero WC. Ganglioglioma: a correlative clinicopathological and radiological study of ten surgically treated cases with follow-up. Neurosurgery 1987; 20:428–433.
218. Johannsson JH, Rekate HL, Roessmann U. Gangliogliomas: pathological and clinical correlation. J Neurosurg 1981; 54:58–63.
219. Russell DS, Rubinstein LJ. Pathology of tumours of the nervous system, 5th ed. Baltimore: Williams & Wilkins, 1989:289–306.
220. Burger PC, Scheithauer BW, Vogel FS. Surgical pathology of the nervous system and its coverings, 3rd ed. New York: Churchill–Livingstone, 1991:325–336.

221. Peretti-Viton P, Perez-Castillo AM, Raybaud C, Grisoli F, Bernard F, Poncet M, Salamon G. Magnetic resonance imaging in gangliogliomas and gangliocytomas of the nervous system. J Neuroradiol 1991; 18:189–199.

222. Diepholder HM, Schwechheimer K, Mohadjer M, Knoth R, Volk B. A clinicopathologic and immunomorphologic study of 13 cases of ganglioglioma. Cancer 1991; 68:2192–2201.

223. Russell DS, Rubinstein LJ. Ganglioglioma: a case with long history and malignant evolution. J Neuropathol Exp Neurol 1962; 21:185–193.

224. Louis DN, Swearingen B, Linggood RM, Dickersin GR, Kretschmar C, Bhan AK, Hedley-Whyte ET. Central nervous system neurocytoma and neuroblastoma in adults—report of eight cases. J Neurooncol 1990; 9:231–238.

225. Figarella-Branger D, Pellissier JF, Daumas-Duport C, Delisle MB, Pasquier B, Parent N, Gambarelli D, Rougan G, Hassoun J. Central neurocytomas. Am J Surg Pathol 1992; 16:97–109.

226. Barbosa MD, Balsitis M, Jaspan T, Lowe J. Intraventricular neurocytoma: a clinical and pathological study of three cases and review of the literature. Neurosurgery 1990; 26:1045–1054.

227. Bolen JW Jr, Lipper MH, Caccamo D. Intraventricular central neurocytoma: CT and MR findings. J Comput Assist Tomogr 1989; 13:495–497.

228. Nishio S, Tashima T, Takeshita I, Fukui M. Intraventricular neurocytoma: clinicopathological features of six cases. J Neurosurg 1988; 68:665–670.

229. Kim DG, Chi JG, Park SH, Chang KH, Lee SH, Jung HW, Kim HJ, Cho BK, Choi KS, Han DH. Intraventricular neurocytoma: clinicopathologic analysis of seven cases. J Neurosurg 1992; 76:759–765.

230. Von Deimling A, Kleihues P, Saremaslani P, Yasargil MG, Spoerri O, Sudhof TC, Wiestler OD. Histogenesis and differentiation potential of central neurocytomas. Lab Invest 1991; 64:585–591.

231. Von Deimling A, Janzer R, Kleihues P, Wiestler OD. Patterns of differentiation in central neurocytoma. An immunohistochemical study of elelven biopsies. Acta Neuropathol 1990; 79:473–479.

232. Wilson AJ, Leaffer DH, Kohout ND. Differentiated cerebral neuroblastoma: a tumor in need of discovery. Hum Pathol 1985; 16:647–649.

233. Pearl GS, Takei Y, Bakay RAE, Davis P. Intraventricular primary cerebral neuroblastoma in adults: report of three cases. Neurosurgery 1985; 16:847–849.

234. Burger PC, Scheithauer BW, Vogel FS. Surgical pathology of the nervous system and its coverings, 3rd ed. New York: Churchill–Livingstone, 1991:386–398.

235. Vaquero J, Ramiro J, Martinez R, Coca S, Bravo G. Clinicopathological experience with pineocytomas: report of five surgically treated cases. Neurosurgery 1990; 27:612–619.

236. Disclafani A, Hudkins RJ, Edwards MSB, Wara W, Wilson CB, Levin VA. Pineocytomas. Cancer 1989; 36:302–304.

237. Borit A, Blackwood W, Mair WGP. The separation of pineocytoma from pineoblastoma. Cancer 1980; 45:1408–1418.

238. Herrick MK, Rubinstein LJ. The cytological differentiating potential of pineal parenchymal neoplasms (true pinealomas). A clinicopathological study of 28 tumours. Brain 1979; 102:289–320.

239. Edwards MSB, Hudkins RJ, Wilson CB, Levin VA, Wara WM. Pineal region tumors in children. J Neurosurg 1988; 68:689–697.

240. Linggood RM, Chapman PH. Pineal tumors. J Neurooncol 1992; 12:85–91.

241. Müller-Forell W, Schroth G, Egan PJ. MR imaging in tumors of the pineal region. Neuroradiology 1988; 30:224–2319.

242. D'Andrea AD, Packer RJ, Rorke LB, Bilaniuk LT, Sutton LN, Bruce DA, Schut L. Pineocytomas of childhood. A reappraisal of natural history and response to therapy. Cancer 1987; 59:1353–1357.

243. Markesbery WR, Haugh RM, Young AB. Ultrastructure of pineal parenchymal neoplasms. Acta Neuropathol (Berl) 1981; 55:143–149.

244. Burger PC, Scheithauer BW, Vogel FS. Surgical pathology of the nervous system, 3rd ed. New York: Churchill–Livingstone, 1991:351–383.

245. Inoue HK, Naganuma H, Ono N. Pathobiology of intracranial germ-cell tumors: immunochemical, immunohistochemical, and electron microscopic investigations. J Neurooncol 1987; 5:105–115.

246. Yamagami T, Handa H, Yamashita J, Okumura T, Paine J, Haebara H, Furukawa F. An immunohistochemical study of intracranial germ cell tumours. Acta Neurochir 1987; 86:33–41.

247. Jellinger K. Primary intracranial germ cell tumours. Acta Neuropathol 1973; 25:291–306.

248. Linggood RM, Chapman PH. Pineal tumors. J Neurooncol 1992; 12:85–91.

249. Kirkove CS, Brown AP, Symon L. Successful treatment of a pineal endodermal sinus tumor. Case report. J Neurosurg 1991; 74:832–835.

250. Horowitz MC, Hall WA. Central nervous system germinomas. Arch Neurol 1991; 48:652–657.

251. Saitoh M, Tamaki N, Kokunai T, Matsumoto S. Clinico-biological behaviour of germ-cell tumors. J Childs Nerv Syst 1991; 7:246–250.

252. Hunt SJ, Johnson PC, Coons SW, Pittman HW. Neonatal intracranial teratomas. Surg Neurol 1990; 34:336–342.

253. Müller-Forell W, Schroth G, Egan PJ. MR imaging in tumors of the pineal region. Neuroradiology 1988; 30:224–231.

254. Drapkin AJ, Rose WS, Pellmar MB. Mature teratoma in the fourth ventricle of an adult: case report and review of the literature. Neurosurgery 1987; 21:404–410.

255. Aguzzi A, Hediger CE, Kleihues P, Yasargil MG. Intracranial mixed germ cell tumor with syncytiotrophoblastic giant cells and precocious puberty; a case report. Acta Neuropathol 1988; 75:427–431.

256. Bjornsson J, Scheithauer BW, Okazaki H, Leech RW. Intracranial germ cell tumors: pathobiological and immunohistochemical aspects of 70 cases. J Neuropathol Exp Neurol 1985; 44:32–46.

257. Burger PC, Scheithauer BW, Vogel FS. Surgical pathology of the nervous system and its coverings, 3rd ed. New York: Churchill–Livingstone, 1991:34–39.

258. Raffel C, Wright DC, Gutin PH, Wilson CB. Cranial chordomas: clinical presentation and results of operative and radiation therapy in 26 patients. Neurosurgery 1985; 17:703–710.

259. Volpe R, Mazabraud A. A clinicopathologic review of 25 cases of chordoma. Am J Surg Pathol 1983; 7:161–170.

260. Rich TA, Schiller A, Suit HD, Mankin HJ. Clinical and pathologic review of 48 cases of chordoma. Cancer 1985; 56:182–187.

261. Heffelfinger MJ, Dahlin DC, MacCarty CS, Beabout JW. Chordomas and cartilaginous tumors at the skull base. Cancer 1973; 32:410–420.

262. Kaneko Y, Sato Y, Iwaki T, Shin RW, Tateishi J, Fukui M. Chordoma in early childhood: a clinicopathological study. J Neurosurg 1991; 29:442–446.

263. Machida T, Aoki S, Sasaki Y, Iio M. Magnetic resonance imaging of clival chordomas. Acta Radiol 1986; 369:167–169.

264. Brown RV, Sage MR, Brophy BP. CT and MR findings in patients with chordomas of the petrous apex. Am J Neuroradiol 1990; 11:121–124.

265. Salisbury JR, Isaacson PG. Demonstration of cytokeratins and epithelial membrane antigen in chordomas and human fetal notochord. Am J Surg Pathol 1985; 9:791–797.

266. Brooks JJ, LiVolsi VA, Trojanoswki JQ. Does chondroid chordoma exist? Acta Neuropathol 1987; 72:229–235.

267. Abenoza P, Sibley RK. Chordoma: an immunohistochemical study. Hum Pathol 1986; 17:744–747.

268. Macdonald RL, Deck JH. Immunohistochemistry of ecchordosis physaliphora and chordoma. Can J Neurol Sci 1990; 17:420–423.

269. Miettinen M, Lehto V-P, Dahl D, Virtanen I. Differential diagnosis of chordoma, chondroid, and ependymal tumors aided by anti-intermediate filament antibodies. Am J Pathol 1983; 112:160–169.

270. Meis JM, Giraldo AA. Chordoma: an immunohistochemical study of 20 cases. Arch Pathol Lab Med 1988; 112:553–556.

271. Russell DS, Rubinstein LJ. Pathology of tumours of the nervous system, 5th ed. Baltimore: Williams & Wilkins, 1989:161–168.

272. Hoff JT, Patterson RH Jr. Craniopharyngioma in children and adults. J Neurosurg 1972; 36:299–302.

273. Baskin DS, Wilson CB. Surgical management of craniopharyngiomas. J Neurosurg 1986; 65:22–27.

274. Pollack IF, Lunsford MD, Slamovits TL, Gumerman LW, Levine G, Robinson AG. Stereotaxic intracavitary irradiation for cystic craniopharyngiomas. J Neurosurg 1988; 68:227–233.

275. Petito CK, DeGirolami U, Earle KM. Craniopharyngiomas: a clinical and pathological review. Cancer 1976; 37:1944–1952.

276. Pusey E, Kortman KE, Flannigan BD, Tsuruda J, Bradley WG. MR of craniopharyngiomas: tumor delineation and characterization. AJR 1987; 149:383–388.

277. Nelson GA, Bastian FO, Schlitt M, White RL. Malignant transformation in craniopharyngioma. Neurosurgery 1988; 22:427–429.

278. Boggan JE, Davis RL, Zorman G, Wilson CB. Intrasellar epidermoid cyst: case report. J Neurosurg 1983; 58:411–415.

279. Asa SL, Kovacs K, Bilbao JM, Penz G. Immunohistochemical localization of keratin in craniopharyngiomas and squamous cell nests of the human pituitary. Acta Neuropathol 1981; 54:257–260.

280. Banna M. Craniopharyngioma in adults. Surg Neurol 1973; 1:202–204.

281. Burger PC, Scheithauer BW, Vogel FS. Surgical pathology of the nervous system and its coverings, 3rd ed. New York: Churchill–Livingstone, 1991:193–437.

282. Goldberg GM and Eshbaugh DE. Squamous cell nests of the pituitary gland as related to the origin of craniopharyngiomas. Arch Pathol 1960; 70:293–299.

283. Paulus W, Slowik F, Jellinger K. Primary intracranial sarcomas: histopathological features of 19 cases. Histopathology 1991; 18:395–402.

284. Burger PC, Scheithauer BW, Vogel FS. Surgical pathology of the nervous system and its coverings, 3rd ed. New York: Churchill–Livingstone, 1991:112–117, 369–380.

285. Russell DS, Rubinstein LJ. Pathology of tumours of the nervous system, 5th ed. Baltimore: Williams & Wilkins, 1989:507–517.

286. Berry AD III, Reintjes SL, Kepes JJ. Intracranial malignant fibrous histiocytomas with abscess-like tumor necrosis. J Neurosurg 1988; 69:780–784.

287. Dropcho EJ, Allen JC. Primary intracranial rhabdomyosarcoma: case report and review of the literature. J Neurooncol 1987; 5:139–150.

288. Louis DN, Richardson EP JR, Dickersin GR, Petrucci DA, Rosenberg AE, Ojemann RG. Primary intracranial leiomyosarcoma. J Neurosurg 1989; 71:279–282.

289. Charman HP, Lowenstein DH, Cho KG, Dearmond SJ, Wilson CB. Primary cerebral angiosarcoma. Case report. J Neurosurg 1988; 68:806–810.

290. Mena H, Ribas JL, Enzinger FM, Parisi JE. Primary central nervous system angiosarcoma: a study of 7 cases. J Neuropathol Exp Nuerol 1990; 49:322.

291. Gainer JV, Chou SM, Chadduck WM. Familial cerebral sarcomas. Arch Neurol 1975; 32:665–668.

292. Feigin IH, Gross SW. Sarcoma arising in glioblastoma of the brain. Am J Pathol 1955; 31:633–653.

293. Ng HK, Tse CCH, Lo STH. Meningiomas and arachnoid cells: an immunohistochemical study of epithelial markers. Pathology 1987; 19:253–257.

294. Brooks JJ, LiVolsi VA, Trojanowski JQ. Does chondroid chordoma exist? Acta Neuropathol (Berl) 1987; 72:229–235.

295. Heffelfinger MJ, Dahlin DC, MacCarty CS, Beabout JW. Chordomas and cartilaginous tumors at the skull base. Cancer 1973; 32:410–420.

296. Miettinen M, Lehto V, Dahl D, Virtanen I. Differential diagnosis of chordoma, chondroid, and ependymal tumors as aided by anti-intermediate filament antibodies. Am J Pathol 1983; 112:160–169.

297. Meis JM, Giraldo AA. Chordoma. An immunohistochemical study of 20 cases. Arch Pathol Lab Med 1988; 112:553–556.

298. Eby NL, Grufferman S, Flannelly CM, Schold SC Jr, Vogel FS, Burger PC. Increasing incidence of primary brain lymphoma in the US. Cancer 1988; 62:2461–2465.

299. Hochberg FH, Miller DC. Primary central nervous system lymphoma. J Neurosurg 1988; 68:835–853.

300. Baumgartner JE, Rachlin JR, Beckstead JH, Meeker TC, Levy RM, Wara WM, Rosenblum ML. Primary central nervous system lymphomas: natural history and response to radiation therapy in 55 patients with acquired immunodeficiency syndrome. J Neurosurg 1990; 73:206–211.

301. Beral V, Peterman T, Berkelman R, Jaffe H. AIDS-associated non-Hodgkin lymphoma. Lancet 1991; 337:805–809.

302. Remick SC, Diamond C, Migliozzi JA, Solis O, Wagner H Jr, Haase RF, Ruckdeschel JC. Primary

central nervous system lymphoma in patients with and without the acquired immune deficiency syndrome. A retrospective analysis and review of the literature. J Med 1990; 69:345–360.

303. Nakhleh RE, Manivel JC, Hurd D, Sung JH. Central nervous system lymphomas. Immunohistochemical and clinicopathologic study of 26 autopsy cases. Arch Pathol Lab Med 1989; 113:1050–1055.

304. Lowenthal DA, Straus DJ, Campbell SW, Gold JWM, Clarkson BD, Koziner B. AIDS-related lymphoid neoplasia. Cancer 1988; 61:2325–2337.

305. Peretti-Viton P, Margain D, Arnaud O, Perez-Castillo AM, Graziani N. Primary and secondary lymphomas of the brain: an MRI study. J Neuroradiol 1991; 18:173–188.

306. Pollack IF, Lunsford LD, Flickinger JC, Dameshek HL. Prognostic factors in the diagnosis and treatment of primary central nervous system lymphoma. Cancer 1989; 63:939–947.

307. DeAngelis LM. Primary central nervous system lymphoma: a new clinical challenge. J Neurol 1991; 41:619–621.

308. Burger PC, Scheithauer BW, Vogel FS. Surgical pathology of the nervous system and its coverings, 3rd ed. New York: Churchill–Livingstone, 1991:359–365.

309. Sherman ME, Erozan YS, Mann RB, Kumar AA, McArthur JC, Royal W, Uematsu S, Nauta HJ. Stereotactic brain biopsy in the diagnosis of malignant lymphoma. J Clin Pathol 1991; 95:878–883.

310. Bashir R, Freedman A, Harris N, Bain K, Nadler L, Hochberg F. Immunophenotypic profile of CNS lymphoma: a review of 18 cases. J Neurooncol 1989; 7:249–254.

311. Morgello S, Maiese K, Petito CK. T-cell lymphoma in the CNS: clinical and pathologic features. J Neurol 1989; 39:1190–1196.

312. Coons SW, Johnson PC. Histopathology of astrocytomas; grading, patterns of spread and correlation with modern imaging modalities. Semin Radiat Oncol 1991; 1:2–9.

4

Pediatric Brain Tumors: Classification

Floyd H. Gilles

Children's Hospital of Los Angeles and University of Southern California School of Medicine, Los Angeles, California

I. INTRODUCTION

Tumor type, locations, and clinical outcome vary among children with brain tumors. Children and adults often have different prognoses, even with brain tumors of the same name in the same location. The bimodal age-related frequency distribution of brain tumors, with a peak in the first decade and a subsequent peak many decades later (1) suggests that the etiologies of brain tumors in children may also differ from those in adults. However, judgments about prognosis, therapy, and etiology depend on reliable, reproducible, and clinically meaningful diagnoses. Furthermore, prognoses, ideally, should reflect measured associations between the specific histological patterns within tumors and the clinical survival of children with these tumors. Unfortunately, most estimates of malignancy are based on only the naming or grading of surgical tissue samples. Finally, it is self-evident that estimates of prognosis are needed for each individual tumor category in each of the major locations in the brain. In this chapter the histological features of the most common pediatric brain tumors will be reviewed and their classification in relation to prognosis will then be considered.

II. HISTOLOGICAL FEATURES

A. Primitive Neuroectodermal Tumors

Tumors with this name (or any of its synonyms, e.g., medulloblastoma or desmoplastic medulloblastoma) are separated from their diagnostic neighbors by their high cell density and frequent content of regions of neuronal, astroglial, ependymal, or oligodendroglial elements. More rarely, they may contain regions with melanin-producing cells in fields of papillary or tubular formations or regions of striated or smooth muscle. Almost always synaptophysin-positive (2), they may contain other histological components that create dramatic patterns of streams, whorls, or islands of cells, with or without intervening streams of desmoplasia or fibrillary glial stroma. Other regions may be entirely cellular without any superimposed pattern (Fig. 1). Thus, the

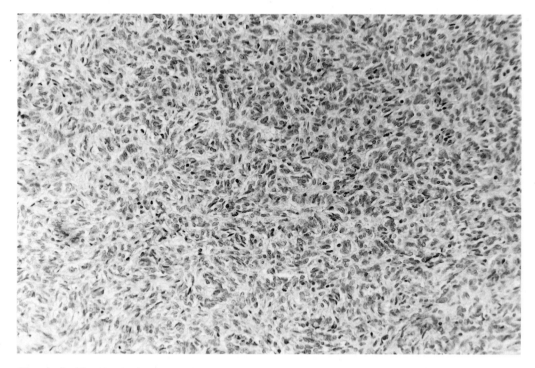

Figure 1   The histological hallmark of the primitive neuroectodermal tumor (medulloblastoma) is dense cellularity. The addition of other histological patterns may modify the diagnosis.

histological picture is inconstant and varied. These tumors are very cellular, contain relatively little stroma, and only a few blood vessels. The cells of these tumors are of moderate or variable size relative to erythrocytes, usually have a very sparse cytoplasm, are hyperchromatic, and may exhibit considerable pleomorphism. Mitotic activity is variable. Ultrastructurally, the presence of neuronal characteristics or extensive neurite production and of synaptic vesicles helps separate this neoplastic process from its diagnostic neighbor, the anaplastic astrocytoma. Although most often found in the posterior fossa, with a propensity for the cerebellum in children, a small proportion are found in several other locations in the brain.

B.   Ependymoma

The ependymomas constitute about 10% of the tumors in the Childhood Brain Tumor Consortium (CBTC) data base. These tumors usually bear some relation to a ventricular surface and either protrude into the ventricle or grow into the surrounding brain. Thus, although usually found within the cranium, some occur in the spinal cord, in relation to the buried ependymal cells of the central canal (which is usually closed by the end of gestation); in the conus medullaris, in relation to the terminal ventricle; or in the filum terminale, in relation to the ependymal deposits sometimes present in this structure. In the CBTC data base, the location of these tumors is mostly infratentorial, with smaller proportions located above the tentorium and the smallest proportion in the spinal canal. This tumor was distinguished, in 1889 by Störch, from the rest of the "gliosarcomas" on several bases. He felt that these tumors should lend themselves to surgical intervention because of their distinct margins and well-circumscribed nature. Most neuropathologists agree that the most important diagnostic feature is the presence of ependymal rosettes, even though most cases do not contain them. Ependymal rosettes are characteristic spherical structures that contain a small central lumen when cut across. Other manifestations of this variety of structure is the ependymal tubule and the ependymal surface. Störch recognized the range of these histological features as well as the feature that is, in fact, the diagnostic feature, namely, the perivascular pseudorosette (Fig. 2). These histological structures contain a central capillary or sinusoid surrounded by a relatively nucleus-free zone of fibrils and radiating processes, derived from a ring of nuclei, which form a second concentric halo around the vascular channel. Perivascular pseudorosettes may be frequent or rare in these tumors and may be separated by variable amounts of glial tissue or sheets of ependymal cells. Two subtypes may rarely be found in children—namely, the papillary and the myxopapillary ependymoma. The papillary variety is distinguished from the choroid plexus papilloma by its stroma; the papillary ependymoma has a neuroglial stroma and the choroid plexus papilloma has a fibrovascular stroma in its papillae. Anaplastic ependymomas, containing the histological features of anaplasia in addition to perivascular pseudorosettes are unfortunately all too common in children. The nonanaplastic ependymomas are often considered relatively benign (3); this, however, is not true in children (4,5).

C. Astrocytoma

Astrocytoma is a tumor of neoplastic astrocytes and, although often thought of as focal, it is likely to have an indistinct border and to grow diffusely into the surrounding neural parenchyma (Fig. 3). Sometimes it is entirely diffuse in its growth pattern. Other structures inherent in neural tissue often form foci for astrocytic growth. Intra- and perifascicular columns of neoplastic cells sometimes are found extending away from a focal nodular growth. Sometimes a diffusely infiltrating astrocytoma appears to stop at the cortical–white matter junction. In other cases, a largely intracortical astrocytoma appears to stop infiltrating at the same margin. Most astrocytomas in children, however, do not respect the cortical–white matter junction. Many cases of astrocytoma exhibit distant regions of cortical involvement consisting of only perineuronal deposits of neoplastic glial cells or only a subpial extension of the tumor in the molecular layer. Unless these tumors contain neoplastic astrocytes predominately with fibrillary or protoplasmic characteristics, they are simply labeled astrocytomas, and they may or may not be anaplastic. The decision about anaplasia rests on the histological characteristics of high cell density, hyperchromia, pleomorphism, mitotic activity, endothelial hyperplasia and hypertrophy, and necrosis. The antibody to glial fibrillary acidic protein (GFAP) will clearly stain neoplastic astrocytes, but it will also stain hypertrophic or "reactive" astrocytes in the vicinity of the tumor and, thus, it does not discriminate between the two cell populations. Occasionally, a glioblastoma multiforme will exhibit a peripheral invasion of surrounding tissue. All regions of the central nervous system are at risk for these tumors. Computed tomography (CT) and magnetic resonance imaging (MRI) scans of these tumors will clearly demonstrate the nodular aspect of astrocytoma, but will grossly underestimate the extent of the diffuse component of these tumors.

D. Fibrillary Astrocytoma

The fibrillary astrocytoma is a tumor the cells of which contain many intracytoplasmic fibrils. These fibrils may be demonstrated by special techniques (e.g., with phosphotungstic acid-hematoxylin [PTAH] or GFAP antibody).

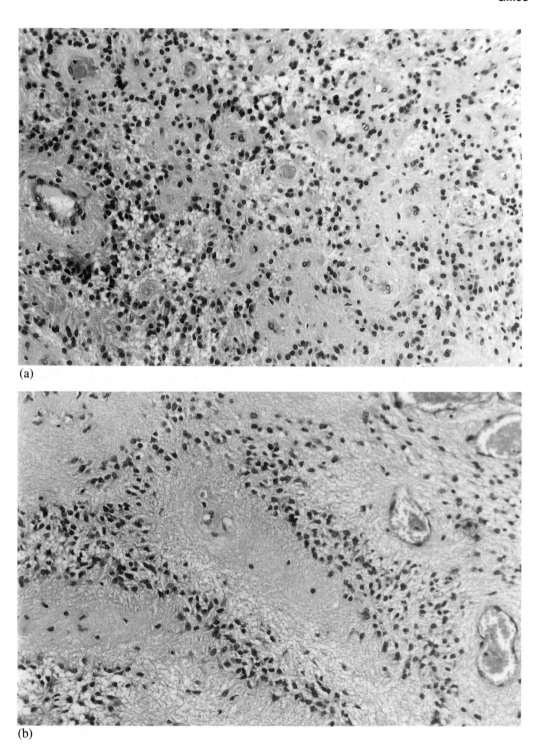

(a)

(b)

Figure 2 The perivascular pseudorosette is the primary criterion for the ependymoma. Its profile consists of a pericapillary or perivenular hypocellular zone surrounded by tumor nuclei. The perivascular zone may be narrow (a) or wide (b) and centric (a) or eccentric (b).

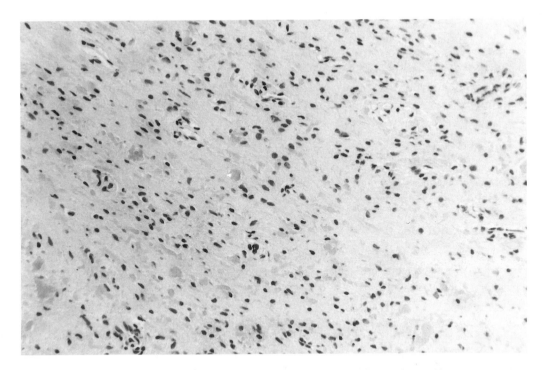

Figure 3 Some astrocytomas have no apparent margins and grow within and along white matter structures and into gray matter. The cellularity at the border gradually diminishes, but where neoplastic cells cease is difficult to determine. This example, which is readily distinguished in this photograph, merges gradually into the surrounding gray and white matter with no apparent boundary.

E. Protoplasmic Astrocytoma

The astrocytes with abundant cytoplasm in this tumor contain few or no demonstrable intracytoplasmic fibrils in PTAH stain. This tumor is easily confused with the gemistocytic astrocytoma, which is a tumor composed preponderantly of even larger, plump astrocytes, with abundant eosinophilic cytoplasm and, often, two or more nuclei. This latter tumor is rare in children [0.1% (CBTC)].

F. Xanthomatous Astrocytoma

The xanthomatous astrocytomas are largely supratentorial tumors in children and young adults (6) and, histologically, are composed of moderately cellular pleomorphic neoplastic astrocytes, many of which are very large and are lipidized. The cells contain both fat and GFAP-positive material. Lymphocytes and plasma cells are frequently found. The mitotic activity is low and the patients have a good prognosis.

G. Pilocytic Astrocytoma

The pilocytic astrocytoma was originally described as an astrocytoma composed preponderantly of fusiform cells that possess unusually long wavy fibrillary processes. A population of stellate astrocytes may also be found (see WHO definition elsewhere in this chapter). Several histological features further characterize this tumor (4). The histological appearance of proteinaceous microcavities or microcysts (Fig. 4) is almost always found, as are leptomeningeal deposits, and Rosenthal fibers. Oligodendroglial deposits may also be found. In children whose tumors have microcysts and one or more of these histological features, the outlook is very good, even with inoperable extension into the middle cerebellar peduncle. The issue of anaplastic characteristics in these tumors is always a vexing problem. Lucien Rubinstein recognized long ago that some of the astrocytes in these tumors can be very pleomorphic; focal regions of high cell density are sometimes present, and multinucleated cells often drive the pathologist into calling these tumors anaplastic. Most of the time, however, these latter features do not appear to adversely affect outcome (4,7). Having said that, however, it is clear that a small subset of pilocytic astrocytomas, containing patches of very anaplastic features, are found in those children whose tumor recurs repeatedly, sometimes becoming more anaplastic with each recurrence. (See the comments concerning the cerebellar astrocytoma elsewhere in this chapter.)

H. Mixed Gliomas

A large proportion of childhood gliomas contain mixtures of two or more cell types. Most authors do not include in this category the ependymomas and oligodendrogliomas that contain an incidental population of astrocytes. In fact, most of the latter two tumor types contain a small to moderate population of astrocytes. A surprisingly large number of childhood brain tumors, however, contain two or more cell types; the questions, then, become how to name them and how to estimate their degree of anaplasia. One practical operational method is to name them by the proportion of the

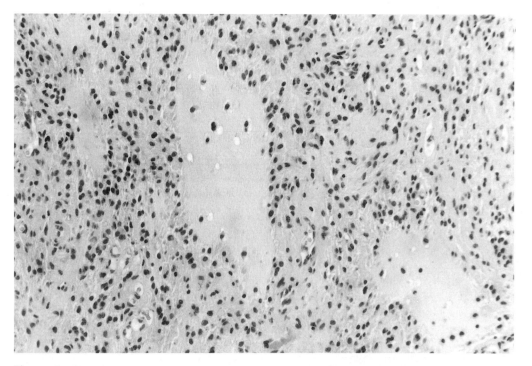

Figure 4   The microcyst or microcavity is a fairly constant component of the pilocytic astrocytoma. It is composed of a round or oval cavity, ranging in size from 20 to 200 μm or more in greatest dimension. The cavity is filled with a protein-rich fluid and may contain a few glial cells or macrophages. Often considered a degenerative phenomenon, its walls are not necrotic, nor does it contain necrotic debris. It must be distinguished from the vacuole, which is much smaller and does not apparently contain a protein-rich fluid.

section surface area occupied by each cell type. If the astrocytic component is preponderant in an ependymoma, then one would call it an astroependymoma. If anaplastic, then the anaplastic component should be in first position (e.g., anaplastic ependymoastrocytoma).

I. Ganglioglioma

There are two brain tumors in children that deserve this name; their clinical behavior is likely to be distinctly different. The *first*, a focal lesion that is commonly located in the cortex, is usually small, very firm, and well circumscribed. Often calcified, the lesions can sometimes be identified on CT scans. These tumors are often cystic and sometimes occupy a mural position in the cyst. Microscopically, the typical lesion is of low or moderate cellularity and clearly contains neurons that are either atypical for site or atypical in showing a range of neurons and astroglial cells. The neurons range in size from small to very large bizarre forms; multinucleate neurons are common. In appropriate silver preparations, the neurons have anomalous tortuous, neuritic processes that clearly differentiate them from the local nonneoplastic neuronal population. It also has another component that is glial, one of fibrillary astrocytes of low or moderate cellularity. This variety of ganglioglioma histologically contains three more features of diagnostic importance: first, and least helpful, is calcospherites of various sizes; second, is perivascular lymphocytic cuffs; and the third is an abundant network of reticulin and collagen fibrils. These tumors grow slowly, are usually small and well demarcated, and are reasonably easily recognized in neuroimages and surgically. Their outcome is usually favorable.

The *second* tumor that is also properly called a ganglioglioma is also composed of both neurons and glial cells. It is an entirely different tumor in its neuroimaging characteristics, gross appearance, and in its component histological characteristics. Grossly, it has many of the characteristics of the diffuse astrocytoma. It is ill-defined, not very firm, and is not well demarcated from the surrounding neural parenchyma in neuroimages, at gross examination, or histologically. It does not contain the ancillary histological features of calcospherites (usually), perivascular lymphocytic cuffs, or the dense network of reticulin and collagen fibrils. Its degree of anaplasia is dependent on its glial component. The tumor with these histological features is not associated with particularly good outlook, even if not anaplastic. Ganglion cell-containing tumors constitute only slightly more than 1% of the CBTC data base.

III. CLASSIFICATION OF PEDIATRIC BRAIN TUMORS AND PROGNOSIS

Diagnoses provided by pathologists are categories in classifications of brain tumors. These classifications are hypotheses about tumor biology and their natural history (8). These hypotheses need to be tested by the same rules that apply to all scientific hypotheses and theories in general (9). Brain tumor classifications are human constructs and may or may not reflect separate entities in nature. Historically, various changes in brain tumor classifications have come about in response to the perception that a new classification would be better than an old one in meeting a new or old need. In the future, brain tumor classifications may be based on etiology or on operational, agreed-upon diagnostic categories with specific histological criteria; however, this is not currently true. The designation of an individual tumor in a specific diagnostic class is often now assisted by ultrastructural examination, molecular biological tools, cytogenetics, or immunohistochemistry. Various studies have indicated that morphometry, DNA flow cytometry, lectin-binding studies, enzyme histochemistry, cell kinetic studies, as well as other techniques, may complement conventional light microscopy. Many of these studies have given us a better understanding of the biology of brain tumors, but none of these modern techniques has yet produced a better classification system than that based on regular traditional pathology.

Brain tumor classification held little interest during much of the 19th century. Most tumors were lumped together as "gliosarcomas." The lack of concern about classification may have been related to the fact that virtually all brain tumors were lethal, since neurosurgery had not yet appeared as a discipline. Surgeons, by the end of the 19th century, were making inroads into brain tumor removal. A supraorbital meningioma was removed from a child by Macewen in 1879 [reported by Anderson (10)], a cerebral glioma in 1884 (11), and a convexity meningioma in 1887 (12). At the end of the 19th century, several disparate forces (namely, improved anesthesia and the recognition that some brain tumors grow with a well-defined border) came together and changed this picture. Macewen, Keen, Horsley, and Krause continued their efforts to remove these tumors with the benefit of increased knowledge of anesthetics. Störch, in 1889, segregated a new brain tumor entity that he thought was unlike most gliomas in that it tended to grow with a sharp, distinct margin, had a distinct set of histological features (those of the ependymoma), and was resectable (13).

An association between individual histological features and brain tumor prognosis was not recognized until 1912. Tooth correlated clinical progress with specific histopathological features in gliomas and used prognosis to make therapeutic judgments (14). Tooth did not propose a new classification of brain tumors, but made two points of great importance to clinicians: namely, that the clinical courses of patients with brain tumors vary, and that a relation exists between the morphological characteristics of the tumor and the clinical course of the patient. For instance, for Tooth, astrocytomas had a slow clinical course, cavities in a brain tumor were associated with benignity, and necrosis and vascular proliferation were found in more malignant, highly cellular gliomas.

Thus, at the beginning of this century, it was established that some brain tumors appeared to be resectable, and that average survival differed for patients whose tumors had differing histological patterns. These two ideas are as important today as they were then. In 1926, Bailey and Cushing (15) proposed a new classification, based on a hypothetical histogenic analogy (16) that became the backbone of modern classification schemes. However, several years later Cushing realized that this classification still failed to provide him with the kind of prognostic information he needed to make clinical judgments (17).

Pathologists may be faced with myriad histological features or patterns, as well as with one or more cell types, when confronted with microscopic slides of a brain tumor. Each tumor varies in its own way from histologically similar tumors. Bailey recognized the variation among tumors in 1927:

> no two gliomas are alike. The gliomas do not fall into distinct groups in which all the members look alike, but consist of variant individuals with certain family resemblances. To find a typical member of each family with which the others may be recognized on comparison is about as difficult as to find a typical member of the Alpine or Dinaric races (18).

In response to the histological variability of brain tumors, four classifications or diagnostic systems evolved for evaluating brain tumors histologically, each emphasizing different aspects of tumor structure and each based on different assumptions. These classifications of brain tumors are very different conceptually. The first three diagnostic schemes or classification systems use arbitrary a priori dicta to form the backbone of the system, and the fourth uses measured associations among histological features (i.e., clusters of histological features), rather than these dicta, as well as measured associations between histological features (or clusters of histological features) and survival. These four childhood brain tumor diagnostic classification systems are based on different assumptions and different methodologies. The first is the phenetic ("look-alike") system, which employs the idea that brain tumor cells resemble cells in the normal brain (19). The second is a system that employs the idea of histogenetic analogy (15,16), namely, that the cells in brain tumors resemble the cells in certain regions and at certain stages of brain development. The third system is focused more on the need to provide a meaningful clinically relevant prognostic statement by estimating ("staging") the degree of anaplasia (20,21). The fourth uses stochastic models to identify clusters of histological features which, in turn, form the basis for a formal classification of brain tumors without the limitations of a priori dicta (4,22,23).

The phenetic system, a product of the early 19th century, antedated ideas of classification for prognostic information and appeared when pathologists dealt largely with autopsy and not surgical material. It was a product of the early 19th century. Burns, in 1800 (24), said that brain tumors resembled the brain, and Virchow, who had previously identified neuroglia, in 1864 added that brain tumor cells resemble some of the cells in the brain and coined the term glioma (19). Thus, designations of brain tumors as astrocytoma, ependymoma, and oligodendroglioma became conceptually possible, although the latter two tumors were not recognized as separate entities until much later. During this same period, Cleland (25) recognized the histological similarity between what is now called meningioma and pacchionian granulations.

The next change in brain tumor classification came early in the 20th century, with the development of the classification system based on histogenetic analogy. Ribbert, in 1918, believed that each glioma arose in neural cells that recapitualated different stages of neural development (16). The conceptual basis for the 1926 Bailey and Cushing classification of gliomas is this same histogenetic hypothesis (15) and is the backbone of many subsequent diagnostic systems, such as those of Russell and Rubinstein; Davis; and Burger and Vogel (7,26,27). Other brain tumor diagnostic systems appeared, but are not widely used.

The third classification system [developed at the Mayo Clinic and first published in the *Rocky Mountain Medical Journal* (20)] introduced the idea that brain tumor diagnosis would be simplified if each brain tumor was graded on the basis of its anaplasia; that is, its pleomorphism, density of cells, number of mitotic figures, atypical mitotic figures, level of cellular differentiation, giant cells, abnormal stromal reactions (e.g., vascular proliferation), necrosis with or without pseudo-palisades, rapidity of growth, growth by infiltration, and metastases (21). This classification system provided ease in recognizing the ends of the prognostic spectrum represented in grades I or IV, as had earlier classification systems, but failed, however, to provide exact criteria to upgrade a glioma histologically from grade I to grade II and, perhaps more importantly, from grade II to grade III. Similarly to earlier classifications, it also ignored the effect of location within the brain in the determination of prognosis. This tradition of grading has continued at the Mayo Clinic, and recently, a simplified and reproducible grading system for gliomas requiring the recognition only of the presence or absence of any of four individual histological features was introduced (28). The usefulness of this system, using nuclear atypia, mitosis, endothelial proliferation, or necrosis, has received support (29).

A generation after Kernohan introduced the Mayo Clinic method of grading, the World Health Organization (WHO) classification of tumors was developed (3,30). In the introduction to the WHO monograph on the histological typing of tumors of the central nervous system (the general preface to the entire series of WHO monographs on the histological typing of all tumors), the statement is made that WHO considers that three separate classifications of tumors are needed according to (1) anatomical site, (2) histological type, and (3) degree of malignancy. The WHO monograph, developed in 1979 for the histological typing of tumors of the central nervous system, was an attempt to satisfy the second and third foregoing criteria (3). Like all previous classifications, the 1979 WHO classification of brain tumors, and its successor in 1991 (30), is based on arbitrary, preselected microscopic characteristics. The defining histological features used in this classification, although often unclear, were borrowed from each of the three diagnostic systems mentioned earlier. Since it provided an amalgamation of the terms used in the three types of historically used brain tumor classification, it was hoped that it would increase uniformity among pathologists. The WHO brain tumor classification disregards location in the brain and may prove disappointing to clinicians who must make prognostic decisions. On the other hand, to have available a list of brain tumor diagnostic categories, agreed to by a large number of neuropathologists from many countries, represents a sizable achievement. The following perusal of the WHO definitions of a few of the common neuroepithelial tumors in children will emphasize its strengths in attempting to identify individual brain tumor entities as well as its weaknesses in failing to provide necessary and requisite histological diagnostic criteria.

A. World Health Organization Definitions of Selected Tumors of Neuroepithelial Tissue

The following section is paraphrased or quoted from the WHO manual (3) to illustrate the difference between histological descriptions that provide an overview of the wide variety of histological features that *can* be found in a group of tumors with a specific name, and the histological descriptions that provide the *necessary* and *boundary* histological criteria for admitting a tumor to each specific diagnostic tumor class. The order of the presentation of the individual tumor varieties has been rearranged somewhat from that of the original publication.

The WHO classification is based largely on the predominant cell type, although it is recognized that many neuroepithelial tumors contain mixtures of different neoplastic cells (3). For example, many astrocytomas are composed of different types of astrocytes, and many oligodendrogliomas include astrocytes that participate in the neoplastic process. Anaplastic (malignant) variants are recognized for the more differentiated of the foregoing tumor entities (i.e., in contradistinction to tumors that are classified as either poorly differentiated or embryonal, these are neoplasms of differentiated neuroepithelial cells in which variable foci of anaplasia are demonstrable).

The term *anaplasia* is here defined to include all the morphological features that are associated with a malignant biological behavior. Cellular pleomorphism may be one of these, but other features of anaplasia include increased cellularity; the presence of numerous mitotic figures, particularly atypical forms; loss or absence of cellular differentiation; the presence of mononucleate or multinucleate giant-cell formation; abnormal stromal reactions, especially vascular proliferation; and necrosis with or without pseudopalisading. Important criteria of malignant biological behavior are rapid growth, growth by infiltration, and, in some cases, metastases through the cerebrospinal pathways and even outside the central nervous system.

Medulloblastoma: A tumour composed of small poorly differentiated cells with ill-defined cytoplasmic processes and a tendency to form Homer–Wright rosettes ("pseudorosettes"). Differentiation into glial or neuronal elements has been observed in some examples. . . . Medulloblastomas correspond histologically to grade IV.

Desmoplastic Medulloblastoma: A tumour with the cellular features of a medulloblastoma, but demonstrating in addition an abundant network of reticulin fibers in its stroma. . . . Histologically it corresponds to grade III or IV.

Astrocytoma (nos): A tumour composed predominantly of astrocytes. [These are tumors that have no additional defining histological features. They are referred to as "diffuse" astrocytomas in some publications and by some laboratories].

Fibrillary astrocytoma: A tumour composed predominantly of astrocytes with many intracytoplasmic fibrils. These fibrils may be demonstrated by special techniques.

Protoplasmic astrocytoma: A tumour composed predominantly of astrocytes that contain few or no demonstrable intracytoplasmic fibrils as shown by the PTAH stain or by metallic impregnation. This cell type should not be confused with the large gemistocytic astrocyte, described below, which invariably contains intracytoplasmic fibrils largely situated at the periphery of the cell cytoplasm.

Gemistocytic astrocytoma: A tumour composed predominantly of large, plump astrocytes with abundant eosinophilic cytoplasm and one or more, usually eccentric, nuclei.

The biological behavior of these three subtypes is typically characterized by slow growth, but evolution into anaplastic forms is recognized. The gemistocytic astrocytoma is especially prone to such dedifferentiation. Astrocytomas of these three types are generally held to correspond histologically to grade II.

Anaplastic astrocytoma: An astrocytoma of one of the recognized subtypes containing areas of anaplasia. It may be difficult focally to distinguish from glioblastoma. However, the prognosis in anaplastic astrocytoma is not as invariably sinister as in the usual glioblastoma. It corresponds histologically to grade III.

Pilocytic astrocytoma: An astrocytoma composed predominantly of fusiform cells which possess unusually long wavy fibrillary processes. Stellate astrocytes are also frequently found.

The predominant cell in these tumors has been referred to as a piloid astrocyte or a "spongioblast", and is characterized by having an oval nucleus with fine chromatin and unipolar or bipolar, elongated, PTAH-positive processes. The fibrillar processes tend to form parallel bundles. Biphasic patterns consisting of pilocytic areas adjacent to loosely structured microcystic areas are commonly encountered. The microcysts show transitions to the larger cystic components which may, when situated in the posterior fossa, replace the vermis or large parts of the cerebellar hemisphere.

The stroma consists of an irregular pattern of blood vessels which may be hyalinized. Endothelial proliferation is not uncommon, especially in the walls of cysts, but this feature does not signify malignancy. Elongate eosinophilic club-shaped structures (Rosenthal fibers) and eosinophilic intracytoplasmic droplets (granular bodies) are commonly found. Calcification may also occur but is usually not conspicuous.

Included in this category are the cystic and solid cerebellar astrocytoma, the pilocytic astrocytoma of juvenile type, and the optic nerve glioma. These tumours have also been referred to as "polar spongioblastoma." Those situated in the neurohypophyseal region have sometimes been labelled "infundibuloma." When situated above the tentorium these tumours are usually midline, but large hemispheric examples are known to occur. Other types of astrocytoma can assume a typical pilocytic appearance when the shape of their component cells is influenced by their surroundings—for example, when the corpus callosum is infiltrated.

This tumour typically occurs as a slowly growing, only focally infiltrative neoplasm. Local invasion of the subarachnoid space is frequent and may be accompanied by a moderate to marked fibroblastic leptomeningeal reaction, but this phenomenon does not signify malignancy. In the cerebellum, removal often results in a cure. Evolution to an anaplastic form seldom occurs, in which case the tumour is categorized as an anaplastic astrocytoma. This tumour histologically corresponds to grade I.

Ependymoma: A tumour composed predominantly of uniform ependymal cells forming rosettes, canals, and perivascular pseudorosettes.

Ependymal rosettes are diagnostic, but perivascular rosettes are the most frequently encountered feature; the histological pattern is that of slender cell processes tapering to a point and radiating towards a central blood vessel. By light microscopy, at high powers of magnification, PTAH-positive structures called "blepharoplasts" may be demonstrated in the cytoplasm, particularly along the luminal margin of the cells forming rosettes and canals.

The tumour typically projects from an ependymal surface. The floor of the fourth ventricle, the region of the central canal of the spinal cord, the lateral and the third ventricles and, rarely, the cerebellopontine angle, are the sites of origin. The usual biological behavior is one of slow growth over a period of years, but anaplastic forms are recognized. In general, ependymomas histologically correspond to grade I, rarely II.

Anaplastic ependymoma: An ependymoma containing areas of anaplasia, or a tumour resembling a glioblastoma or medulloblastoma in which features indicative of ependymal differentiation can be recognized.

Neoplasms of this type may occur as large cystic calcified, partly papillary masses in the cerebral hemispheres of children and less commonly young adults, as well as in the fourth ventricle. They are tumours of considerable cellularity, composed of cells that may be poorly differentiated, but in which typical ependymal and perivascular rosettes are recognized. This category also includes what has been called "ependymoblastoma." Histologically the tumours of this group correspond to grades III and IV.

IV. CHILDHOOD BRAIN TUMORS

The summary observations for the following section are drawn from the data base of the Childhood Brain Tumor Consortium (CBTC) (31).

The term *primitive neuroectodermal tumor* (PNET) was introduced by Rorke to include medulloblastoma and about 18 other densely cellular ill-defined brain tumors of children (32), and it was included in a suggestion for a revision of the WHO classification of brain tumors for children (33).

The PNET and the pilocytic astrocytoma are, by far, the most frequent of childhood brain tumors (Table 1) and, together, they constitute one-half of all neural tumors of childhood (Table 2). The PNET constitutes about 20% of tumors in the CBTC (31) data base and about 94% occur infratentorially. Ependymoma and anaplastic ependymoma constitute 10% of childhood brain tumors (see Table 1). Seven percent of pediatric brain tumors are not classifiable in hematoxylin–eosin (H&E)-stained slides using criteria provided in the WHO manual (1979) or in current texts (3,7,26,27); many of these are gliomas with mixed cellular populations or are those that contain

Table 1 Frequencies of Common (>1%) Childhood Brain Tumors in the Data Base of the Childhood Brain Tumor Consortium

Name	%
Pilocytic astrocytoma	18.9
Medulloblastoma	17.2
(desmoplastic medulloblastoma 2.8%)	
Ependymoma	8.3
Unclassifiable or unknown	7.0
Craniopharyngioma	6.8
Fibrillary astrocytoma	6.5
Anaplastic astrocytoma	5.9
Astrocytoma, nos	4.7
Protoplasmic astrocytoma	2.4
Germ cell tumors (including teratoma)	2.3
Choroid plexus papilloma	1.8
Anaplastic ependymoma	1.7
Oligodendroglioma	1.2
Ganglioglioma	1.1
Less frequent tumors (<1% each)	8.7
Disagreement about diagnoses	2.7
	100.0

Table 2   Frequencies of Common (>1%) Neural Tumors in Children

Name	%
Medulloblastoma (and desmoplastic medulloblastoma)	26.3
Pilocytic astrocytoma	24.9
Ependymoma	10.9
Fibrillary astrocytoma	8.6
Anaplastic astrocytoma	7.8
Astrocytoma, nos	6.1
Protoplasmic astrocytoma	3.2
Oligodendroglioma	1.6
Ganglioglioma	1.4
Subependymal giant cell astrocytoma	1.2
Mixed oligoastrocytoma	1.2
Less frequent neural tumors (<1% each)	14.6
	100.0

anaplastic characteristics such that classification is not yet possible. Many will be classifiable in the future by using modern molecular biological, ultrastructural, cytogenetic, or immunohistochemical information.

Among supratentorial tumors, the craniopharyngioma is the most frequent tumor (Table 3). Anaplastic astrocytoma and pilocytic astrocytoma vie for second place. Unclassifiable tumors and

Table 3   Frequencies of Common (>1%) Supratentorial Childhood Brain Tumors

Name	%
Craniopharyngioma	14.9
Anaplastic astrocytoma	12.5
Pilocytic astrocytoma	12.2
Fibrillary astrocytoma	8.9
Unclassifiable or unknown	8.5
Germ cell tumors (including teratomas)	5.3
Ependymoma	5.0
Choroid plexus papilloma (including anaplastic varieties)	4.4
Astrocytoma, nos	3.7
Ganglioglioma	2.6
Subependymal giant cell astrocytoma	2.6
Oligodendroglioma	2.5
Meningioma	2.4
Anaplastic ependymoma	2.3
Mixed oligoastrocytoma	2.1
Medulloblastoma	2.0
Protoplasmic astrocytoma	1.9
Giant cell glioblastoma	1.4
Less frequent tumors (<1% each)	4.8
	100.0

fibrillary astrocytomas each constitute about 8.5%, and germ cell tumors, ependymomas, choroid plexus papillomas (all varieties), and astrocytoma (nos) are less frequent.

Three well-known supratentorial glial tumors (pilocytic astrocytoma, anaplastic astrocytoma, and ependymoma) in the CBTC data base are associated with significantly different ($p < 0.0001$) probabilities of survival in unadjusted raw estimates of survival (Fig. 5). For children with supratentorial pilocytic astrocytomas, the probability of survival is about 0.8 in the fifth postoperative year and a little less than 0.7 in the tenth postoperative year. Deaths beyond this point continue to occur, however. The ependymoma in children, whether located above or below the tentorium, is uniformly fatal (2,4), unlike the expectation provided by the WHO manual, which indicates that this tumor is grade I or II (3). The probability of survival for children with a supratentorial ependymoma is about 0.5 in the fifth postoperative year. [For the purposes of this demonstration, the supratentorial ependymomas and anaplastic ependymomas have been grouped together, as the survival associated with the latter is insignificantly different ($p = 0.811$) from the former in the CBTC data base]. The supratentorial anaplastic astrocytoma is associated with a worse outlook; the probability of survival is only 0.3 in the third postoperative year. The probability of survival of children with a supratentorial fibrillary astrocytoma is not significantly different from that of the pilocytic astrocytoma.

Among infratentorial tumors, the group of primitive neuroectodermal tumors (medulloblastoma and desmoplastic medulloblastoma) is, by far, the most frequent tumor (37.8%), followed by the pilocytic astrocytoma, ependymoma, and several other astrocytomas (Table 4). Together the primitive neuroectodermal tumors and the pilocytic astrocytoma account for two-thirds of infratentorial tumors. Other varieties of neural and nonneural tumors are far less frequent.

Children with infratentorial pilocytic astrocytoma, astrocytoma (without other distinguishing features), and anaplastic astrocytoma have significantly different survival probabilities ($p < 0.0001$) (Fig. 6). Overall, without consideration of specific location within the infratentorial compartment, children with pilocytic astrocytoma have a survival probability approaching 0.9 at 10 years after their first operation. Four years after first operation, astrocytoma, without other distinguishing histological features [astrocytoma (nos)], is associated with a much worse survival probability of 0.5. The survival probability for children with fibrillary astrocytomas lies between

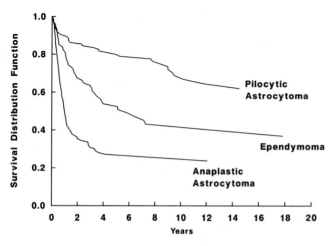

Figure 5 Comparisons of the probability of survival of children who have supratentorial pilocytic astrocytoma, ependymoma, or anaplastic astrocytoma in the CBTC data base. These are significantly ($p < 0.0001$) different. Children with a supratentorial anaplastic ependymoma have a probability of survival that is not significantly different from those with ependymoma ($p = 0.811$). Those with fibrillary astrocytoma are not significantly different from the children with pilocytic astrocytoma.

Table 4 Frequencies of Common (>1%) Infratentorial Brain Tumors

Name	%
Medulloblastoma	32.4
(desmoplastic medulloblastoma)	5.4
Pilocytic astrocytoma	28.3
Ependymoma	12.0
Fibrillary astrocytoma	3.8
Astrocytoma, nos	3.7
Protoplasmic astrocytoma	2.5
Anaplastic astrocytoma	2.4
Anaplastic ependymoma	1.7
Craniopharyngioma	1.6
Unclassifiable or unknown	1.4
Less frequent tumors (<1% each)	4.8
	100.0

that of astrocytoma (nos) and pilocytic astrocytoma, but is not significantly different from either. The few children with infratentorial protoplasmic astrocytomas have a survival distribution function that lies between those with fibrillary astrocytoma and astrocytoma (nos), but is not significantly different from any of the foregoing; however, it is significantly better than for those with anaplastic astrocytoma ($p < 0.001$). Anaplastic astrocytoma is associated with the worst probability of survival of any of the other infratentorial astrocytomas, with a survival probability of less than 0.2 at the end of the second postoperative year.

Primitive neuroectodermal tumors, ependymomas, and anaplastic ependymomas have a tendency to extend into the cervical spinal canal at the time of first presentation. Thus, for the survival distribution functions of children with tumors of the "cervicomedullary region," I have included all children with infratentorial tumors, whether or not their tumors had extended into the

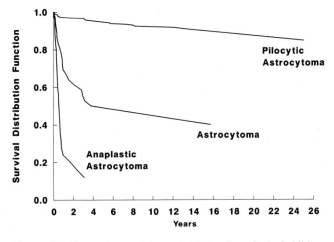

Figure 6 Comparisons of the probability of survival of children with infratentorial pilocytic astrocytoma, astrocytoma (without other distinguishing feature; nos), and anaplastic astrocytoma. These are significantly ($p < 0.001$) different and are not adjusted for location within the infratentorial compartment, age, amount of tumor removed, or decade of surgery. The probability of survival of children with an infratentorial fibrillary astrocytoma was not significantly different from those with pilocytic astrocytoma.

cervical spinal canal (Fig. 7 and Table 5). Ependymoma and PNET are not associated with significantly different survivals ($p = 0.28$). In these unadjusted estimates, the children with these tumors have survival probabilities that approach 0.5 in their third postoperative year. Anaplastic ependymoma, on the other hand, is associated with a significantly worse survival ($p = 0.02$).

V. RELIABILITY OF THE WHO CLASSIFICATION DIAGNOSIS OF CHILDHOOD BRAIN TUMORS

One of the problems faced by neurooncologists is that of comparability and reliability of the diagnostic categories in the WHO manual (or in any other diagnostic classification, for that matter). The morphological variability of the common brain tumors (18) of children has spawned a wide range of histopathological terminology [see Rorke regarding the multiple names of the densely cellular tumors of childhood (32)].

The implication of a study (34) of the reproducibility of the WHO tumor classification (Table 6) is that much misclassification of brain tumors has taken place, meaning that a high proportion of these tumors had two different diagnoses on two reviews of the same microscopic slides. Misclassification, in turn, increases the amount of variance of the survival data for a given tumor type. Furthermore, the homogeneity of groups of children with specific tumors for the clinical investigation of outcome or therapeutic response is seriously compromised. Similarly, the specificity of subsets or groups of tumor tissues to be used for basic biological investigations is seriously diminished. All three of these points are of considerable importance.

None of the commonly used classifications of brain tumors [Bailey and Cushing, Russell and Rubinstein, Kernohan, and the WHO scheme (3,7,15,21)] have been subjected to studies of the reliability of assignment of tumors to individual diagnostic categories before this study. Although our estimates of the reliability of assignment of tumors to some diagnostic categories are alarming, they are not much different from the reliability assessments for many other tumor classifications. Reliability has been assessed for three classification systems of breast carcinoma [i.e., WHO, Ackerman's, and that of the Armed Forces Institute of Pathology, all of which had low levels of reproducibility (35)]; the Dukes (36) classification of rectal carcinoma (37); and a classification

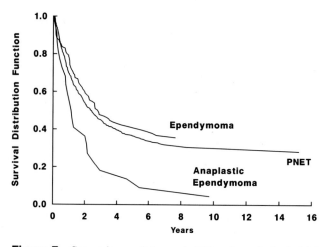

Figure 7 Comparisons of the probability of survival of children with infratentorial tumors that have a tendency to extend through the foramen magnum into the cervical canal. Children with ependymoma and PNET have similar probabilities of survival, whereas children with anaplastic ependymoma have a significantly worse outlook (p = 0.28).

Table 5 Frequencies of Common (>1%)
Spinal Canal Tumors

Name	%
Pilocytic astrocytoma	13.0
Myxopapillary ependymoma	10.0
Astrocytoma, nos	9.6
Neurilemoma	9.6
Fibrillary astrocytoma	7.8
Ependymoma	7.0
Anaplastic astrocytoma	6.1
Unclassifiable or unknown	5.2
Protoplasmic astrocytoma	4.4
Medulloblastoma	4.4
Ganglioglioma	3.5
Meningioma	3.4
Papillary ependymoma	2.6
Desmoplastic medulloblastoma	2.6
Pineoblastoma	1.7
Epidermoid	1.7
Less frequent tumors (<1% each)	7.4
	100.0

scheme for Hodgkin's disease that had levels of observer agreement too low to be scientifically useful (38). Some classifications of other tumors may also have reliability levels that seriously limit their usefulness (39–44). The recently introduced simple classification of gliomas by using four arbitrary histological features has been claimed to be reproducible (28,29).

There are two difficulties with the WHO classification of brain tumors (and all other brain tumor classifications as well) that might account for these levels of reliability. I feel that diagnoses should be based on (1) defining criteria that are *necessary* for making each specific histological diagnosis and (2) *boundary* criteria (i.e., histological features that distinguish or separate related tumor diagnoses, e.g., astrocytoma and anaplastic astrocytoma). The brain tumor classifications listed previously have in common many statements about the histological features that *may be* found in a specific tumor type. What they lack, in common, are sets of statements about the histological features that *must* be present for a tumor be placed in a specific diagnostic category. For example, to upgrade a tumor, histological features thought to indicate "anaplasia" must be found in "increased" amounts (e.g., Kernohan classification). However, at no point does this classification indicate by how much the cell density or pleomorphism must be increased to upgrade an astrocytoma to an anaplastic astrocytoma. These are boundary criteria that need to be addressed.

The WHO diagnostic categories with suboptimal reproducibility tend to have histological neighbors with which they are confused. This is not unexpected because many brain tumors share common histological features and also because features that might clearly separate one diagnostic category from the other have not yet been identified. Diagnostic neighbors become important when they differ in prognosis or expected response to therapy (e.g., pilocytic astrocytoma and anaplastic astrocytoma).

Diagnostic neighbors were identified as the substituted diagnoses in our study of observer variability (34). Pilocytic astrocytoma was a frequently substituted diagnosis within the other generally hypocellular astrocytoma categories, namely, fibrillary and protoplasmic astrocytoma and astrocytoma (nos). Each of these diagnostic categories shares some histological features with the pilocytic astrocytoma. The overall reliability of pilocytic astrocytoma was considered accept-

Table 6 P_x. The Conditional Probability of Agreement Given That One of the Reviews Resulted in the Specific Diagnosis. P_x Ranges from 0–1 with 1 Reflecting Perfect Agreement

WHO diagnosis	Number of cases[a]	P_x	95% confidence limits
Craniopharyngioma	59	0.97	(0.88–1.0)
Germinoma	12	0.92	(0.62–1.00)
Teratoma	5	0.80	(0.28–1.00)[b]
Medulloblastoma	151	0.79	(0.71–0.85)[b]
Pilocytic astrocytoma	158	0.77	(0.70–0.83)[b]
Ependymoma	87	0.77	(0.67–0.85)[b]
Subependymal giant cell astrocytoma	8	0.75	(0.35–0.97)
Choroid plexus papilloma	12	0.75	(0.43–0.95)
Neurilemoma	5	0.60	(0.15–0.95)
Desmoplastic medulloblastoma	25	0.56	(0.35–0.76)
Anaplastic astrocytoma	69	0.46	(0.34–0.59)
Giant cell glioblastoma	7	0.43	(0.10–0.82)
Unclassified tumor	44	0.39	(0.24–0.55)
Meningioma	8	0.38	(0.09–0.76)
Fibrillary astrocytoma	74	0.34	(0.23–0.46)
Ganglioglioma	14	0.29	(0.08–0.58)
Anaplastic ependymoma	22	0.23	(0.08–0.45)
Mixed oligoastrocytoma	14	0.21	(0.05–0.51)
Astrocytoma, nos	56	0.21	(0.010–0.32)[b]
Neuroblastoma	5	0.20	(0.01–0.72)
Glioblastoma	5	0.20	(0.01–0.72)
Protoplasmic astrocytoma	27	0.19	(0.06–0.38)
Pineoblastoma	10	0.10	(0.00–0.45)
Oligodendroglioma	7	0.00	(0.00–0.41)

[a]Number of cases = the total number of cases with a specific diagnosis at the first review or at the second review. The total of this column is greater than the number of cases used in the study because each case for which the diagnosis was inconsistent at the first review and the second review appears twice.

[b]P_x was significantly lower ($p < 0.05$) when this tumor was located in the supratentorial compartment. The supratentorial vs infratentorial P_x for each of these diagnoses was astrocytoma, nos, 0.10 (0.02–0.27) vs 0.33 (0.16–0.55); pilocytic astrocytoma, 0.61 (0.43–0.77) vs 0.83 (0.75–0.89); ependymoma, 0.58 (0.34–0.80) vs 0.83 (0.72–0.91); and medulloblastoma 0.27 (0.06–0.61) vs 0.83 (0.75–0.88)

Source: Ref. 43.

able, but the reliability of each of the other three diagnostic categories was relatively low. An overlap between pilocytic astrocytoma and mixed oligoastrocytoma is understandable, as pilocytic astrocytoma may contain patches of oligodendrocytes (4,45). The infrequently substituted diagnosis of anaplastic astrocytoma is more troubling because a different therapy is implied. However, the pilocytic astrocytoma may contain foci of pleomorphic astrocytes, which do not appear to influence the prognosis of pilocytic astrocytomas (4,7).

VI.   MYTHS IN PEDIATRIC NEUROONCOLOGY

Among the myths in pediatric neurooncology are three that particularly need to be addressed: (1) the unitary entity "cerebellar astrocytoma"; (2) the expected prognosis of ependymomas in children; and (3) that neuroradiologic images are representative of the extent of tumor.

A. Cerebellar Astrocytoma

The cerebellar astrocytomas were not separated as a distinct group of tumors in the classification of brain tumors proposed by Bailey and Cushing in 1926 (15). Tumors in their classification were grouped histologically by "the predominant cell type" into astrocytoma, oligodendroglioma, and so on, and the astrocytomas were further divided into fibrillary, protoplasmic, and other. In 1931, Cushing separated the cerebellar tumors from the rest of the astrocytoma group, using largely operative features, age, and high survival rates (46). He found no histological features to separate them from astrocytomas located elsewhere in the brain. He thought that the cerebellar astrocytomas were protoplasmic or fibrillary, or both. Four years later, Elvidge and associates reported 55 astrocytomas of the nervous system; 14 located in the cerebellum (47). Overall they found three varieties, namely, pilocytic, gemistocytic, and diffuse, but all of their 14 cerebellar tumors were pilocytic. Bergstrand emphasized, in 1937, that these tumors were a mixture of loose, microcystic, and dense portions; that they had a curious capillary network; that they contained characteristically shaped hyaline bodies; and that they often grew in the leptomeninges (48). Thus, he included histological features other than only the predominant cell type in his grouping of brain tumors. Bucy and Gustafson, in 1939, however, excluded all of these "degenerative" changes from a role in defining a class of tumors (49). They proposed that these tumors vary in cellularity from case to case, that the great majority of cells were stellate cells, and that these tumors were either protoplasmic or fibrillary astrocytomas. They recognized that other glial cells were present in these tumors and called them spongioblasts, astroblasts, and oligodendroglia. Bucy and Gustafson went on to say, "Cerebellar astrocytomas are, in other words, more or less fibrillary, or predominantly fibrillary or protoplasmic, as the case may be and as one prefers. . . . Fortunately all cerebellar astrocytomas are benign, slowly growing neoplasms, which are fairly well circumscribed, and complete gross enucleation apparently provides a cure in every case." Thus, the pseudoentity of a cerebellar astrocytoma with an optimistic probability of survival became ensconced: a tumor defined solely on the basis of one histological feature (e.g., any kind of astrocyte) and one clinical feature (e.g., location in the cerebellum, whether or not jointly occupying the brain stem).

Confusion about the histological definition of this tumor continued and, 1 year later, Zülch said that cerebellar astrocytomas really are composed of polar spongioblasts, with an admixture of oligodendroglia and a few mature astrocytes (50). The next advance came with the report of Ringertz and Nordenstam in 1951 (45). In their 140 cases of "cerebellar" astrocytoma, they recognized 6 in which the histological structure could not be distinguished from diffuse astrocytomas of the cerebrum. They recognized that only about one-half contained a macrocyst and that a sizable proportion (21%) simultaneously involved the brain stem [compare with the 30% of infratentorial pilocytic astrocytomas that simultaneously involved the brain stem in the CBTC database (31)]. They felt that the most characteristic structural features of these cerebellar gliomas, distinguishing them from most, but not all, cerebral gliomas, were many of the degenerative changes of earlier authors. They found common alternating loose and dense tissue, oligodendroglia (8.6% of cases), multinucleated cells, Rosenthal fibers (44% of cases), capillary proliferation (called "glomeruli" by some authors), leptomeningeal deposits (18% of cases), and calcification (18% of cases). Although their astute observations and well-written report explicitly and implicitly recognized the presence of other astroglial tumors of the cerebellum, papers summarizing the cerebellar astrocytoma have continued to be published over the succeeding four decades.

The CBTC data base gives some clarification. Clearly, the cerebellum is not unique in its ability to generate virtually all classes of gliomas. Although the pilocytic astrocytoma is by far the most frequent tumor of the cerebellum and, if not part of a tumor that occupies the middle cerebellar peduncle and brain stem, is associated with a probability of survival similar to that depicted in Figure 6. The cerebellum is also the site of other astroglial tumors, each of which is associated with its own distinctive survival probability. The astrocytoma (nos), fibrillary astrocytoma, and protoplasmic astrocytoma have indistinguishable survival probabilities that are worse than that in children with the pilocytic astrocytoma. The survival probability of the anaplastic astrocytoma in the cerebellum is much worse. All of these survival probabilities are very similar to those of the infratentorial astrocytomas as depicted in Figure 6. Some investigators still regard the cerebellar astrocytoma as a single entity (51–53). However, that anaplastic and diffuse astrocytomas also occur in the cerebellum in addition to the pilocytic astrocytoma has been widely recognized (54–59).

In 1959, Russell and Rubinstein separated juvenile from adult pilocytic astrocytomas (60). They equated the pilocytic astrocytoma of the third ventricle with a cerebellar tumor of the same name. They considered the adult variety as similar to the pilocytic areas of large hemispheric growths containing closely packed interwoven bundles of relatively broad bipolar fibrillated cells with no relation to blood vessels and little tendency to undergo microcystic degeneration. The juvenile variety is a growth in young subjects with morphologically simple tumor cells and contains regions of microcystic degeneration. The cells are not piloid but "feebly" stellate (i.e., protoplasmic astrocytes). Russell and Rubinstein make the curious statement that these account for only few cerebellar astrocytomas. Thus, they may have been describing a different tumor as "juvenile." They recognized that anaplasia is uncommon in cerebellar tumors, but that it occurs, that some cerebellar tumors are solid throughout, and that some are diffuse astrocytomas. As diagnostic criteria for the pilocytic astrocytoma, they used alternating loose and dense areas and microcysts. However, although the appellations of *juvenile* or *adult* seem ensconced in some centers, I find that they add nothing to the histological criteria that support the diagnosis of pilocytic astrocytoma.

In a study of cerebellar gliomas in children, we studied the relation of histological features to each other (clustering) and to survival in a population of 132 children with cerebellar gliomas (4). A classification system that accentuates differences in survival was derived on the bases of clustering of histological features and survival. This division was supported by the existence of differentially distributed symptoms and signs and by differences in resectability. Two of the clusters of histological features resemble current notions of the histological features of (1) pilocytic astrocytoma (glioma A) and (2) diffuse astrocytoma or astrocytoma (nos) (glioma C). Glioma A had one or more of the four cluster A histological features of microcyst, leptomeningeal deposits, Rosenthal fibers, or focus of oligodendroglia, and was associated with a 10-year survival rate of 94%. Glioma C astrocytomas had none of the cluster A features; they were simply astrocytomas without other distinguishing histological features or diffuse cerebellar astrocytomas and were associated with a 10-year survival rate of 69.2%.

In conclusion, the concept of a singular entity cerebellar astrocytoma associated with a single survival probability is not supportable historically or on the basis of the data in the data base of the Childhood Brain Tumor Consortium.

B. Survival Expectancy of Ependymomas in Children

The survival expectancy of ependymomas has been codified in the WHO manual as grade I or II (3). This may or may not be true for adults, but it is certainly *not* true for children. Shuman and colleagues found that ependymoma survival expectancy for children was very poor and rivaled that of medulloblastomas (5). In a subsequent study of cerebellar tumors in children, we showed that children whose cerebellar glioma contained perivascular pseudorosettes had a survival experience that was very poor, in that only one-fourth were alive 5 years after surgery, thereby supporting previous authors (4). In the CBTC data used in this chapter, the probability of survival of children with supratentorial or infratentorial ependymomas is between 0.4 and 0.5 at 5 years. Children with supratentorial anaplastic ependymomas had the same survival expectancy as those with ependymoma, in contrast to children with infratentorial anaplastic ependymomas in whom the probability of survival was much less (see Fig. 7).

C. Clinical Underestimation of the Extent of Gliomas by Radiologic Studies

There are many limitations of our clinical estimates of the extent of brain tumors in children. Unfortunately, neither the surgeon's estimate at the time of surgery nor the preoperative or postoperative neuroradiologic images necessarily reveal the extent of the usual glioma. The surgeon's estimate is based on his visual inspection of the tumor bed and comparison with the putative extent of the tumor in neuroradiologic images. Surgeon's estimates of 50, 91, or 95% of tumor removal are based on the assumption that the neuroradiologic images are representative of the true extent of the tumor. Unfortunately, these images indicate only disruption of cerebral anatomy, breakdown of the blood–brain barrier, or abnormal water content of tissue, and may not reveal the true extent of tumor. As an example, a 6-year-old child underwent neurosurgical exploration of a left temporal lobe lesion. There was no significant enhancement (Fig. 8), nor was there extensive T_2 hyperintense signal relative to gray matter adjacent to the lesion (Fig. 9). At operation, much of the posterior two-thirds of the temporal lobe had been replaced by an anaplastic astrocytoma. The tumor extended far afield medially toward the putamen and the thalamus, and the surgery was terminated. Postoperatively, there was no enhancement of the medial bed of the tumor (Fig. 10).

(a)　　　　　　　　　　　　　　　　(b)

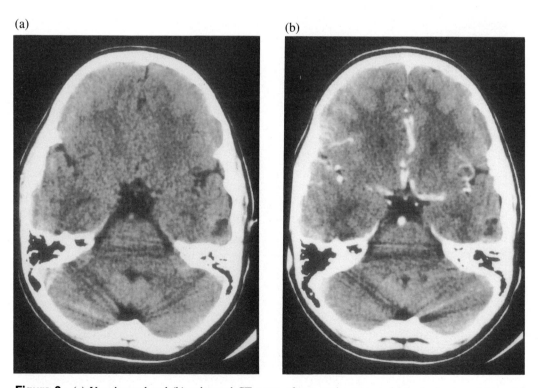

Figure 8　(a) Unenhanced and (b) enhanced CT scans of a posterior temporal lobe lesion in a 6-year-old boy. There is a small nonenhancing hypodense region that is not associated with displacement of the temporal horn of the lateral ventricle or with parahippocampal herniation.

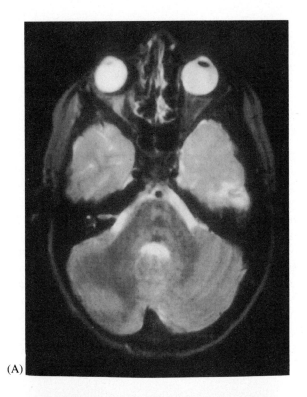

(A)

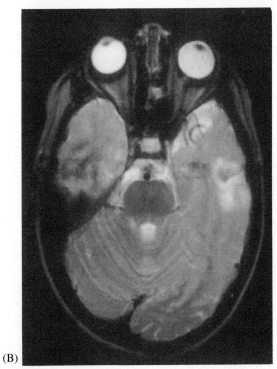

(B)

Figure 9 (A) In T2-weighted MRI images, the left temporal lesion is surrounded by a narrow hyperintense rim relative to gray matter. (B) At surgery, most of the posterior two-thirds of the left temporal lobe was occupied by an anaplastic astocytoma.

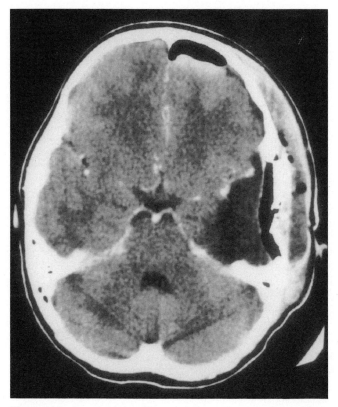

Figure 10 Postoperative CT scan fails to reveal the residual anaplastic astrocytoma that remained in the operative bed.

VII. SUMMARY

In this chapter, I have focused on the frequent brain tumors found in children, namely, on the primitive neuroectodermal tumor (PNET), pilocytic astrocytoma, the astrocytoma (nos) (i.e., without distinguishing histological characteristics or the diffuse astrocytoma), the anaplastic astrocytoma, and the ependymoma. These tumors account for almost all brain tumors in children, are associated with above-average or average intraobserver reliability (with one exception), and are associated with significantly different survivals. Poor reliability adversely influences the variance of the estimates of the probability of survival of children with these tumors and decreases the homogeneity of groups of children with "similar" tumor types for clinical trials as well as groups of tumor tissues for basic biological investigation. The less frequent glial tumors, on the other hand, are generally associated with below-average intraobserver reliability (with a few exceptions), are not well defined histologically (i.e., *defining* and *boundary* histological criteria are not widely agreed on), and may or may not be associated with specific survival expectations. Finally, I reviewed the strengths and limitations of the WHO classification of brain tumors as it applies to children, and discussed three myths currently in vogue in pediatric neurooncology, namely the pseudoentity called cerebellar astrocytoma, the notion that ependymomas are grade I or II in children, and the idea that surgical evaluation, CT or MRI images capture the true extent of tumor.

ACKNOWLEDGMENT

The data collection for this study was funded through National Cancer Institute (NCI) grant R01 CA20462. The analysis was supported in part by the Burton E. Green Foundation and NCI grant R01 CA49532.

REFERENCES

1. MacMahon B. Epidemiology of Hodgkin's disease. Cancer Res 1966; 26:1189–1200.
2. Gould VE, Jansson DS, Molenaar VM, Rorke LB, Trojanowski JQ, Lee VM, Packer RJ, Franke WW. Primitive neuroectodermal tumors of the central nervous system. Patterns of expression of neuroendocrine markers, and all classes of intermediate filament protein. Lab Invest 1990; 62:498–509.
3. Zülch K. Histological typing of tumors of the central nervous system. International histological classification of tumors, no. 21. Geneva: World Health Organization, 1979.
4. Winston K, Gilles FH, Leviton A, Fulcheiro A. Cerebellar gliomas in children. JNCI 1977; 58:833–838.
5. Shuman RM, Alvord EC Jr, Leech RW. The biology of childhood ependymomas. Arch Neurol 1975; 32:731–739.
6. Kepes JJ, Rubinstein LJ. Malignant gliomas with heavily lipidized (foamy) tumor cells: a report of three cases with immunoperoxidase study. Cancer 1981; 47:2451–2459.
7. Russell DS, Rubinstein LJ. Pathology of tumors of the nervous system, 5th ed. Baltimore: Williams & Wilkins, 1989.
8. Gilles FH. Classifications of childhood brain tumors. Cancer 1985; 56:1850–1857.
9. Popper KR. The logic of scientific discovery, 2nd ed. New York: Harper & Row, 1968.
10. Anderson JW. Tumor of the dura mater—convulsion: removal of tumor by trephining—recovery. Glasgow Med J 1879; 12:210–13 (Macewen).
11. Bennet AH, Godlee RJ. Excision of a tumor from the brain. Lancet 1884; 2:1090–1091.
12. Keen WW. Three successful cases of cerebral surgery including (1) the removal of a large intracranial fibroma, (2) exsection of damaged brain tissue and (3) exsection of the cerebral center for the left hand: with remarks on the general technique of such operations. Trans Am Surg Assoc. 1888; 6:293–347.
13. Störch H. Über die path-anat: vorgange am stützgerust des centralnervensystems. Virchows Arch 1889; 157:127–171, 197–234.
14. Tooth HH. Some observations on the growth and survival period of intracranial tumors based on the review of 500 cases, with special reference to the pathology of gliomata. Brain 1912; 35:61–108.
15. Bailey P, Cushing H. A classification of the tumors of the glioma group on a histogenetic basis with a correlated study of prognosis. Philadelphia: JB Lippincott, 1926.
16. Ribbert H. Über das spongioblastom und das gliom. Virchows Arch 1918; 225:195–213.
17. Cushing H. Tumeurs intracraniennes. Paris: Masson et Ci; 1937 (quoted by Scherer, 1940).
18. Bailey P. Histologic atlas of gliomas. Arch Pathol Lab Med 1927; 4:871–921.
19. Virchow R. Die krankhaften geschwulste. Berlin: A Hirschwald, 1864.
20. Adson AW, Svien HJ. Brain tumors: diagnosis and treatment. Rocky Mtain Med J. 1948; 45:962–968.
21. Kernohan JW, Mabon RF, Svien HJ, Adson AW. Symposium on a new and simplified concept of gliomas (a simplified classification of gliomas). Proc Mayo Clin 1949; 24:71–75.
22. Gilles FH, Winston K, Jasnow M, Leviton A, Hedley-Whyte ET. Densely cellular cerebellar tumors in children. Trans Am Neurol Assoc 1978; 103:265–268.
23. Gilles FH, Sobel EL, Tavare CJ. Childhood brain tumor classification: linnaean or traditional. Brain Tumor Pathol (Jpn) 1991; 8:155–161.
24. Burns J. Dissertation on inflammation. 1800 (quoted by Virchow, 1864).
25. Cleland J. Description of two tumors adherent to the deep surface of the dura mater. Glasgow Med J 1864; 11:148–159.
26. Davis RL. Astrocytomas. In: Minckler J, ed. Pathology of the nervous system, vol. 2. New York: McGraw-Hill, 1971:2007–2026.

27. Burger PC, Vogel FS. Surgical pathology of the nervous system and its coverings, 2nd ed. New York: John Wiley & Sons, 1982.
28. Daumas-Duport C, Scheithauer B, O'Fallon J, Kelly P. Grading of astrocytomas. A simple and reproducible method. Cancer 1988; 62:2152–2165.
29. Kim TS, Halliday AL, Hedley-Whyte ET, Convery K. Correlates of survival and the Daumas-Duport grading system for astrocytoma. J Neurosurg 1991; 74:27–37.
30. WHO working group. Histological typing of tumors of the central nervous system. A report of the second meeting in Zürich, March 28–April 1, 1990; given by John Kepes in Kyoto, Japan, 1990.
31. Childhood Brain Tumor Consortium. A study of childhood brain tumors based on surgical biopsies from ten North American institutions: sample description. J Neurooncol 1988; 6:9–23.
32. Rorke LB. The cerebellar medulloblastoma and its relationship to primitive neuroectodermal tumors. J Neuropathol Exp Neurol 1983; 42:1–15.
33. Rorke LB, Gilles FH, Davis RL, Becker LE. Revision of the World Health Organization classification of brain tumors for childhood brain tumors. Cancer 1985; 56:1869–1886.
34. Childhood Brain Tumor Consortium. Intraobserver reproducibility in assigning brain tumors to classes in the world health organization diagnostic scheme. J Neurooncol 1989; 7:211–224.
35. Stenkvist B, Bengtsson E, Eriksson O, Jarkrans T, Nordin B, Westman-Naeser S. Histopathological systems of breast cancer classification: reproducibility and clinical significance. J Clin Pathol 1983; 36:392–398.
36. Dukes CE. The classification of cancer of the rectum. J Pathol Bacteriol 1932; 35:323–332.
37. Thomas GDH, Dixon MF, Smeeton NC, Williams NS. Observer variation in the histological grading of rectal carcinoma. J Clin Pathol 1983; 36:385–391.
38. Coppleson LW, Factor RM, Strum SB, Graff PW, Rapport H. Observer disagreement in the classification and histology of Hodgkin's disease. JNCI 1970; 45:731–740.
39. Svanholm H, Starklint H, Gunderson HJG, Fabricius J, Barlebo H, Olsen S. Reproducibility of histomorphologic diagnoses with special reference to the kappa statistic. APMIS 1989; 97:689–698.
40. Pedersen L, Holck S, Schiødt T, Zedeler K, Mouridsen HT. Inter- and intraobserver variability in the histopathological diagnosis of medullary carcinoma of the breast, and its prognostic implications. Breast Cancer Res Treat 1989; 14:91–99.
41. Ismail SM, Colclough AB, Dinnen JS, Eakins D, Evans DMD, Gradwell E, O'Sullivan JP, Summerell JM, Newcombe R. Reporting cervical intra-epithelial neoplasia (CIN): intra- and interpathologist variation and factors associated with disagreement. Histopathology 1990; 16:371–376.
42. Robertson AJ, Beck JS, Burnett RA, Howatson SR, Lee FD, Lessells AM, McLaren KM, Moss SM, Simpson JG, Smith GD, Tavadia HB, Walker F. Observer variability in histopathological reporting of transitional cell carcinoma and epithelial dysplasia in bladders. J Clin Pathol 1990; 43:17–21.
43. DeVet HCW, Knipschild PG, Shouten HJA, Koudstaal J, Kwee W, Willebrand D, Sturmans F, Arends JW. Interobserver variation in histopathological grading of cervical dysplasia. J Clin Epidemiol 1990; 43:1395–1398.
44. Hastrup N, Hamilton-Dutoit S, Ralfkiaer E, Pallesen G. Peripheral T-cell lymphomas and evaluation of reproducibility of the updated Kiel classification. Histopathology 1991; 18:99–105.
45. Ringertz N, Nordenstam H. Cerebellar astrocytoma. J Neuropathol Exp Neurol 1951; 10:343–367.
46. Cushing H. Experiences with the cerebellar astrocytomas. A critical review of seventy-six cases. Surg Gynecol Obstet 1931; 52:129–204.
47. Elvidge A, Penfield W, Cone W. The gliomas of the central nervous system. Assoc Res Nerv Mental Dis Proc 1935; 16:107–181.
48. Bergstrand H. Weiteres über sog. kleinhirnastrocytome. Virchows Arch Pathol Anat 1937; 299:725–739.
49. Bucy PC, Gustafson WA. Structure, nature and classification of the cerebellar astrocytomas. Am J Cancer 1939; 35:327–353.
50. Zülch K. Hirngeschwülste im jugendalter. Zentralbl Neurochir 1940; 5/6:238–274.
51. Lapras C, Patet JD, Lapras C Jr, Mottolese C. Cerebellar astrocytomas in childhood. Childs Nerv Syst 1986; 2:55–59.

52. Austin EJ, Alvord EC Jr. Recurrences of cerebellar astrocytomas: a violation of Collin's law. J Neurosurg 1988; 68:41–47.
53. Undjian S, Marinov M, Georgiev K. Long-term follow-up after surgical treatment of cerebellar astrocytomas in 100 children. Childs Nerv Syst 1989; 5:99–101.
54. Occhiogrosso M, Spada A, Merlicco G, Vailati G, DeBenedictis G. Malignant cerebellar astrocytoma. Report of five cases. J Neurosurg Sci 1985; 29:43–50.
55. Ilgren EB, Stiller CA. Cerebellar astrocytomas. Part I. Macroscopic and microscopic features. Clin Neuropathol 1987; 6:185–200.
56. Ilgren EB, Stiller CA. Cerebellar astrocytomas. Part II. Pathologic features indicative of malignancy. Clin Neuropathol 1987; 6:201–214.
57. Bonner K, Siegel KR. Pathology, treatment and management of posterior fossa brain tumors in childhood. J Neurosci Nurs 1988; 20:84–93.
58. Itoh Y, Kowada M, Mineura K, Kojima H, Sageshima M. Primary malignant astrocytoma of the cerebellum in children. Report of a case with electron microscopic and cytofluorometric DNA evaluation. Childs Nerv Syst 1988; 4:306–309.
59. Shinoda J, Yamada H, Sakai N, Ando T, Hirata T, Hirayama H. Malignant cerebellar astrocytic tumors in children. Acta Neurochir (Wien) 1989; 98:1–8.
60. Russell DS, Rubinstein LJ. Pathology of tumors of the nervous system. London: Edward Arnold, 1959.

5

Brain Tumors: Anatomical Considerations

Ziya L. Gokaslan and Raymond E. Sawaya
**University of Texas M.D. Anderson Cancer Center,
Houston, Texas**

I. INTRODUCTION

The goal of this chapter is to present an overview of the brain anatomy, with special emphasis on material that is relevant to the clinician treating patients with brain tumors. The scope of the chapter is broad; therefore, no exhaustive efforts were made to discuss the gross or microscopic anatomical details of the central nervous system. The reader is advised to refer to the references, if he or she intends to explore a particular anatomical structure in detail. On the other hand, this chapter is designed to include pertinent neuroanatomical structures, as they might relate to function and dysfunction of the nervous system in a given patient with a brain tumor.

II. GENERAL CONSIDERATIONS

For practical purposes, the nervous system can be divided into two principal parts: (1) the central nervous system (CNS), which comprises the brain and the spinal cord; and (2) the peripheral nervous system.

The brain is the principal integrative area of the nervous system, and is divided into many separate functional parts, which will be the main topic of discussion of this chapter. The spinal cord serves two functions: a conduit for several nervous pathways to and from the brain and an integrative area for coordinating many reflex activities (1).

The peripheral nervous system consists of an extensive branching network of nerves. The nerves are made of two functional types of fibers: afferent fibers, for transmission of sensory information into the spinal cord and brain; and efferent fibers, for transmitting motor signals back from the CNS to the periphery, especially to the skeletal muscles. Some of the peripheral nerves arise directly from the brain itself, called cranial nerves, which supply mainly the head region of the body. Although the anatomy of the spinal cord and peripheral nerves is left out in this chapter because the scope of the book is limited to *brain* tumors, relevant anatomy of cranial nerves is discussed, along with the anatomy of brain, owing to their proximity and importance in clinically localizing the lesions in the brain (1).

III. GROSS ANATOMY OF THE BRAIN

The brain is the portion of the nervous system that is located in the cranial cavity. Unfortunately, several terminologies are used to describe the different portions of the brain. These are listed in Table 1 (2).

A. Cerebrum

The cerebrum is divided into right and left hemispheres by a longitudinal fissure. Each hemisphere has three surfaces, superolateral, medial, and inferior. All of these have irregular fissures or sulci demarcating convolutions or gyri. Four principal sulci are illustrated in Figure 1 (3).

Longitudinal sulcus separates the two cerebral hemispheres from each other in the midsagittal plane of the brain.

Central (rolandic) fissure extends in an approximate inferosuperior direction on the lateral side of each hemisphere and divides the cerebrum into approximately an anterior and posterior half.

Lateral (sylvian) sulcus has a short stem between the orbital surface of the frontal lobe and the temporal lobe. The Sylvian fissure extends along the lateral surface of each cerebral hemisphere for about half of its length.

Parieto-occipital sulcus originates from the side of the longitudinal fissure about one-quarter the distance between the anterior and the posterior pole of the hemisphere and then extends laterally and anteriorly for about 5 cm.

1.   The Lobes of the Cerebrum

The foregoing fissures divide the cerebrum into frontal, parietal, occipital, and temporal lobes.
     The *frontal lobe* lies in front of the central sulcus and anterosuperior to the lateral sulcus. The *parietal lobe* lies behind the central sulcus, above the posterior ramus of the lateral sulcus and in front of an imaginary line drawn between the parieto-occipital sulcus and the preoccipital notch. The *occipital lobe* lies behind the same imaginary line. The *temporal lobe* lies below the stem and posterior ramus of the lateral sulcus and is bounded behind to the lower part of the aforementioned imaginary line (3).
     Frontal Lobe.   The superolateral surface of the frontal lobe is transversed by three main sulci and thus divided into four gyri (Figs. 2 and 3). The precentral sulcus runs parallel to the central

Table 1   Various Terminologies for the Anatomical Parts of the Brain

Classical terminology	Anglized terminology	Most widely used terminology
Encephalon	Brain	Brain
Prosencephalon		
Telencephalon		Cerebrum
Diencephalon		Diencephalon (or thalamus, hypothalamus, and surroundings)
Mesencephalon	Midbrain	Mesencephalon
Rhombencephalon	Hindbrain	
Metencephalon		
Cerebellum		Cerebellum
Pons		Pons
Myelencephalon		
Medulla oblongata		Medulla (or medulla oblongata)

Source: Ref. 20.

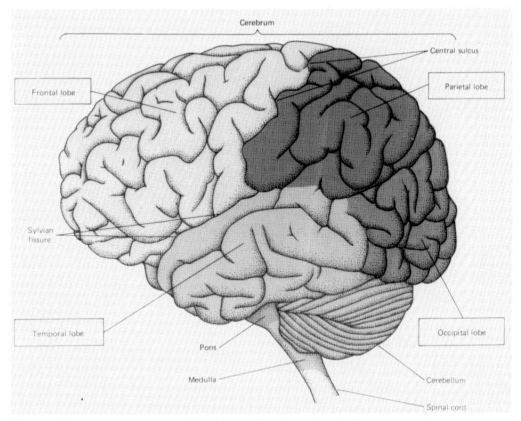

Figure 1 Superolateral surface of the brain—major lobes. (From Ref. 1)

sulcus, separated from it by the precentral gyrus, which corresponds to Brodmann's cytoarchitectonic field 4 or the great cortical somatomotor area. The precentral gyrus gives rise to most of the
corticospinal motor fibers that are responsible for the contralateral motor movement of face, arm,
leg, and trunk. The superior and inferior frontal sulci curve across the remaining part of the
surface, dividing it into superior, middle, and inferior frontal gyri. This gross anatomical division
of the superolateral surface of the frontal lobe is of limited help in determining the functionally
important areas, except for the precentral gyrus, which corresponds to area 4.

Immediately anterior to the precentral gyrus lies the premotor area (area 6), as shown in Figure
3. Area 8, frontal eye field, is located in front of the premotor area and occupies the posterior
aspect of all three frontal gyri and initiates voluntary eye movements to the opposite side. Area 44
in the dominant hemisphere is the Broca's area that is located in the posterior frontal opperculum
immediately anterior to the lower end of the motor strip (Brodmann's area 4). Broca's area in the
dominant hemisphere is the expressive center for speech. The remainder of the frontal lobe
functionally corresponds to the prefrontal area and is believed to be important for the personality
and overall motivation and initiative of a person (2,4,5).

On the medial surface of the cerebrum, the cingulate sulcus separates the cingulate gyrus from
the remainder of the frontal lobe. The cingulate sulcus curves superiorly on the medial surface of
the cerebral hemisphere and ends in the longitudinal fissure, posterior to the central sulcus. The
medial frontal lobe around the central sulcus is called the paracentral lobule and is a critical part of
the cerebrum for cortical inhibition of bladder and bowel function (2,4,5).

The orbital surface of the frontal lobe contains the olfactory sulcus in which the olfactory bulb

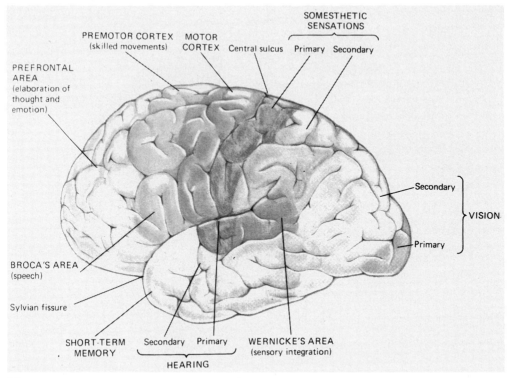

Figure 2 Superolateral surface of the brain—functionally important areas. (From Ref. 1)

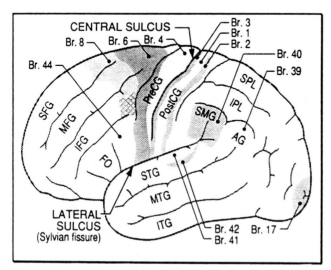

Figure 3 Superolateral surface of the brain—major sulci and gyri, cytoarchitectonic fields of clinical significance. (From Ref. 4)

and nerve are lodged. Medial to the olfactory sulcus is the straight gyrus (gyrus rectus). Laterally, the orbital gyri are separated by the orbital sulcus. This portion of the frontal lobe is functionally considered to be a part of the prefrontal area (2,5).

Frontal Lobe Function (6)

1. Precentral gyrus: motor cortex; contralateral movement—face, arm, leg, trunk
2. Broca's area: dominant hemisphere; expressive center for speech
3. Premotor (supplementary motor) cortex: contralateral head and eye movement
4. Prefrontal areas: personality, initiative
5. Paracentral lobule: cortical inhibition of bladder and bowel voiding

Tumors of the frontal lobes may manifest themselves with a constellation of symptoms, depending on what anatomically important structures are involved in the process. For instance, a high-grade glioma of the dominant frontal lobe frequently presents with contralateral hemiparesis and expressive dysphasia. A sudden hemorrhage into the tumor bed may result in deviation of the eyes to the ipsilateral side owing to involvement of the premotor cortex (frontal eye field). In contrast, however, an epileptogenic focus caused by an oligodendroglioma in the same region may cause a seizure episode, with deviation of the eyes to the contralateral side. More slowly growing tumors involving the prefrontal areas bilaterally, such as olfactory groove meningiomas, may present with signs and symptoms mimicking dementia, including loss of initiation and interest, personality changes, and loss of inhibition, along with lack of smell. Classically, a parasagittal meningioma of posterior frontal lobes causes spastic paraparesis and impairment of bowel and bladder control (6).

Parietal Lobe. The parietal lobe shows two main sulci that divide it into three gyri. The postcentral sulcus lies parallel to the central sulcus, separated from it by the postcentral gyrus, the great somatic sensory area (see Fig. 2 and 3). This part of the cortex corresponds to Brodmann's areas 1, 2, 3, and receives afferent pathways for appreciation of posture, touch, and passive movements. The remaining, larger part of the superolateral parietal surface is subdivided into superior and inferior parietal lobules (gyri) by the intraparietal sulcus, which runs backward from near the midpoint of the postcentral sulcus and usually extends into the occipital lobe, where it ends by joining the transverse occipital sulcus. The parts of the superolateral parietal cortex that lie around the Sylvian (lateral) sulcus and posterior end of the superior temporal sulcus (which extends into the parietal lobe) are named the supramarginal gyrus and angular gyrus, respectively. These regions correspond to Brodmann's field 40 and 39, and make up part of Wernicke's speech area, the receptive speech center. The dominant parietal lobe is also implicated in the skills of handling numbers and calculations. The nondominant parietal lobe, on the other hand, is important in the concept of body image and the awareness of the external environment (3,4).

Parietal Lobe Function (6)

1. Post-central gyrus: appreciation of posture, touch, and passive motion
2. Supramarginal and angular gyri: Wernicke's speech center (dominant hemisphere)
3. Nondominant parietal lobe: concept of body image, awareness of the external environment, ability to construct shapes—visual proprioceptive skills
4. Dominant parietal lobe: skills of handling numbers and calculation
5. The visual pathways: the fibers of the optic radiation (lower visual field) pass deep through the parietal lobe

Impairment of parietal lobe function can be exemplified by the tumors involving this region. Neoplastic processes affecting the sensory cortex usually cause a disturbance of sensation in the contralateral body parts. Involvement of Wernicke's area in the dominant hemisphere is associated with receptive dysphasia. Involvement of the nondominant parietal lobe, however, usually causes difficulties with concept of body image and orientation in space, resulting in anosognosia and in dressing, geographic, and constructional apraxia. Tumors of the dominant parietal lobe may be associated with Gertsmann's syndrome, which presents with finger agnosia, acalculia, agraphia, and loss of left–right discrimination. Involvement of the deep parietal white matter may cause contralateral lower homonymous quadrantanopia (6).

Temporal Lobe.   The temporal lobe is divided by superior and inferior temporal sulci into superior, middle, and inferior temporal gyri. The sulci run backward and slightly upward, in the same general direction as the posterior ramus of the lateral sulcus, which lies above them. The superior sulcus ends in the lower part of the inferior parietal lobule, and the superjacent cortex is called the angular gyrus (see Figs. 2 and 3). The superior temporal gyrus contains the primary auditory areas (transverse gyri of Heschl), which correspond to Brodmann's areas 41 and 42. The inferior surface of the temporal lobe lies on the floor of the middle cranial fossa, and it shows two anteroposterior grooves, the collateral and occipitotemporal sulci (Fig. 4). Both run almost directly forward from the occipital pole to the temporal pole. The anterior end of the collateral sulcus is called the rhinal sulcus. The parahippocampal and lingual gyri lie medial to the collateral sulcus. The dentate gyrus, a narrow fringe of cortex with transverse markings, occupies the groove between the parahippocampal gyrus and the fimbria of the hippocampus. The anterior end of the

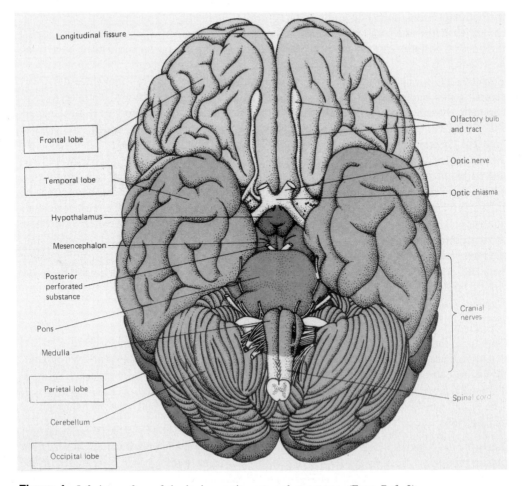

Figure 4   Inferior surface of the brain—major external structures. (From Ref. 2).

parahippocampal gyrus curves once again to form the uncus, which is partly occupied by the cortical olfactory area. The medial occipitotemporal gyrus is fusiform, and lies between the collateral and occipitotemporal sulci. The lateral occipitotemporal gyrus lies lateral to the occipitotemporal gyrus around the inferior margin of the hemisphere (3,4).

The lateral sulcus is deep and contains the "buried" temporal lobe. This buried island of cortex is referred to as the *insula* (island of Reil). Herschl's gyrus, or primary auditory cortex, lies within the insula (3).

Temporal Lobe Function (6)

1. Auditory cortex (Heschl's gyrus): dominant hemisphere—hearing of language; nondominant hemisphere—hearing of music
2. Middle and inferior temporal gyri: learning, memory
3. The limbic lobe (inferior and medial portions of the temporal lobe and hippocampus and parahippocampal gyrus): sensation of olfaction
4. Visual pathways: pass deep in the temporal lobe around the posterior horn of the lateral ventricle

Tumors of the temporal lobe may present with complex partial seizures. If the tumor involves the auditory cortex, auditory hallucinations may be the presenting symptom. Involvement of the middle and inferior temporal gyri may result in a disturbance of memory function. Tumors affecting the limbic lobe, such as medial sphenoid wing meningiomas, may be associated with olfactory hallucinations. In addition, aggressive behavior and inability to establish new memories may be seen in tumors involving this region. Dominant lobe tumors may cause receptive dysphasia. Involvement of posterior deep temporal white matter may cause contralateral upper quadrantanopia. It is usually agreed that the anterior temporal lobe can be excised up to 4.5 cm on the left side, and up to 7 cm on the right side without causing any significant neurological deficit, although variability in the location of the speech area and memory function has been well documented in the literature (6).

Occipital Lobe. The occipital lobe merges anteriorly with the parietal and temporal lobes (see Fig 1). The lateral surface of the occipital lobe shows a short transverse occipital sulcus and a lunate sulcus. On the medial surface, the calcarine sulcus extends forward and the parieto-occipital sulcus separates the occipital and parietal lobes. The visual cortex lies along the banks of the calcarine sulcus, and this area is referred to as the striate cortex. Below this lies the parastriate cortex. The striate cortex is the primary visual cortex, which corresponds to Brodman's area 17 (see Fig. 3). The parastriate cortex is known as the visual association cortex and corresponds to Brodmann's area 18. The inferior surface of the occipital lobe rests on the tentorium cerebelli and shows the posterior extension of medial and lateral occipitotemporal gyri (3,4).

Occipital Lobe Function (6)

1. The striate cortex: primary visual cortex
2. The parastriate cortex: visual association cortex

Tumors of the occipital lobe commonly present with contralateral homonymous hemianopia (6).

2. Medial Surface of the Hemispheres

The medial surfaces of the cerebral hemispheres are flat and, although separated for most of their extent by the longitudinal fissure and falx cerebri, they are connected in parts by the cerebral commissures and by the structures bounding the third ventricle (see Fig. 7).

The *corpus callosum* is the largest of the cerebral commissures and forms most of the roof of the lateral ventricle. In a median sagittal section, it appears as a flattened bridge of white fibers (see

Fig. 7). The central portion of this commissure is called the trunk. Anteriorly, the trunk is recurved to form the genu, which tapers rapidly into the rostrum. The expanded posterior end or splenium overlies the midbrain and adjacent parts of the cerebellum (7). Limited transsection of the corpus callosum, which is the means of gaining access into the third ventricle for tumors of this region during a transcallosal approach, is usually not associated with any detectable neurological deficit.

The *fornix* is the symmetric arching bundle of white fibers below the splenium and trunk of the corpus callosum. This large bundle of axons extends from the hippocampal formation to the mamillary bodies. The body of the fornix lies on the roof of the third ventricle. Anteriorly, the body separates into two columns, the columns of the fornix curving downward to the mamillary bodies. Posteriorly, it forms two symmetric arching bundles, the crura of the fornix, which end in the hippocampal formation. The fornix is part of the limbic system and is an extremely important structure for memory function (5). Damage to the fornicies bilaterally, which can occur during transcallosal excision of tumors in this region, may result in very severe memory problems and should be avoided.

The *septum pellucidum* is a thin-walled, paired structure (midplane) separating the lateral ventricles and extending between the fornix and the corpus callosum. At times, it is separated in the midline by a small cavity (cavum septum pellucidum) (8).

The *cingulate gyrus* is a crescentic convolution between the cingulate sulcus and corpus callosum. The cingulate sulcus begins below the genu of the corpus callosum and ends above the posterior part of the trunk by turning upward to cut the superior margin of the hemisphere. The cingulate sulcus separates the medial frontal and cingulate gyri. Below the genu and rostrum of the corpus callosum are small paraolfactory sulci separating the subcallosal (paraolfactory) areas and paraterminal gyrus. The cingulate gyrus is also a part of the limbic system, which contains structures important to memory (7).

The corpus callosum is the most important connecting pathway between two hemispheres. The lesions of the connecting pathways result in recognizable syndromes—the interhemispheric disconnection syndromes (6).

The lesions of the anterior corpus callosum, with interruption of the connections between the right and left association motor cortical areas, are manifested by the apraxia of left-sided limb movements. The lesion of the posterior corpus callosum and dominant occipital lobe, with interruption of connections between the visual cortex and the angular gyrus (Wernicke's area), are characterized by alexia without agraphia (6).

The limbic system contains structures important in memory. The hippocampus, a deep structure in the temporal lobe, ridges the floor of the lateral ventricle. The *fimbria* of the hippocampus consists of a loop from hippocampus → fornix → mamillary body → thalamus → cingulate gyrus → back to hippocampus. The memory process involves intermediate term memory, recent memory, and remote memory. Intermediate term memory is believed to be related to the prefrontal cortex and dorsomedial nucleus of the thalamus, and its dysfunction is well represented in Korsakoff's psychosis. Recent memory function is linked to the hippocampus, and its dysfunction is exemplified by Alzheimer's disease. Remote memory, however, is thought to be distributed throughout the entire hemisphere, but particularly in the temporal lobes. Therefore, only diffuse cerebral disorders, such as trauma or advanced Alzheimer's disease, would present with remote memory dysfunction (6).

3. Basal Ganglia

The basal ganglia are symmetric subcortical masses of gray matter that are imbedded in the lower parts of the cerebral hemispheres. Each is composed of corpus striatum, formed by the large lentiform (lenticular) and caudate nuclei, a thin sheet of gray matter termed the claustrum, and a group of small nuclei combined within the amygdaloid body or amygdala (Fig. 5) (7).

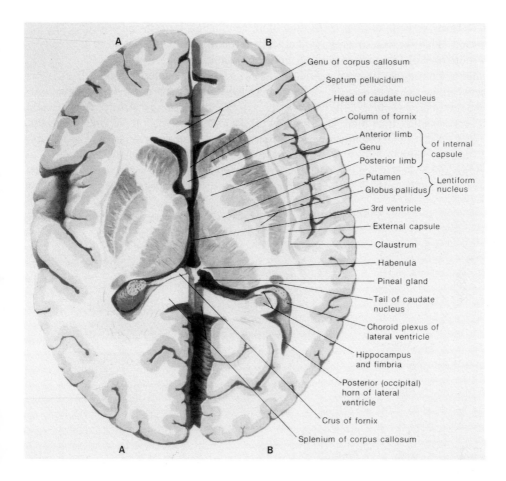

Figure 5 Axial section of the brain—basal ganglia. (From Ref. 2)

The lentiform nucleus is biconvex and is encapsulated in white matter; the laminae bounding its outer and inner surfaces are known as the external and internal capsule, respectively. The external capsule separates the lentiform nucleus from the claustrum which, in turn, is separated from the insula by a thin layer of white matter, the extreme capsule. The thicker internal capsule is angulated and conforms to the shape of the medial surface of the lentiform nucleus. The anterior part of the limb of the internal capsule is interposed between the lentiform nucleus and the head of the caudate nucleus. The posterior limb of the internal capsule separates the lentiform nucleus from the thalamus, which lies medially. The angle at the junction of the anterior and posterior limbs is termed the genu, or knee, of the internal capsule. On section, the lentiform nucleus is seen to have a darker lateral portion, the putamen, and a smaller, paler medial part, the globus pallidus (7).

The caudate nucleus resembles an elongated and curved exclamation mark. Its main part is an expanded head directly continuous with a smaller and attenuated body that merges into an elongated tail (cauda). The head bulges into the anterior horn of the lateral ventricle and forms its sloping floor. The caudate nucleus is separated from the lentiform nucleus by the anterior limb of the internal capsule (see Fig. 5), but the separation is incomplete because the head of the caudate nucleus and the putamen are connected, especially anteroinferiorly, by bands of gray matter traversing the white matter of the anterior limb. This admixture of gray and white matter produces the striated appearance that justifies the term *corpus striatum* applied to these nuclei. The head tapers into the narrower body that lies in the floor of the central part of the lateral ventricle. The tail turns downward along the outer margin of the posterior surface of the thalamus. It then curves forward into the roof of the inferior horn of the lateral ventricles (7).

The anterior limb of the internal capsule contains the frontopontine tract as well as fibers traveling between the thalamus and the various parts of the cortex (anterior thalamic radiation). The genu and the anterior portion of the posterior limb contain the most functionally critical fibers, namely, the corticobulbar tract more anteriorly and the corticospinal tract (face, shoulder, arm, hand, hip, foot, in that order, from anterior to posterior) more posteriorly (Fig. 6). The remainder of the posterior limb is mostly occupied by connecting fibers between the thalamus and cortex (superior and posterior thalamic radiation). The most posterior aspect of the posterior limb carries fibers of the auditory and optic radiations. Because of the condensation of white matter

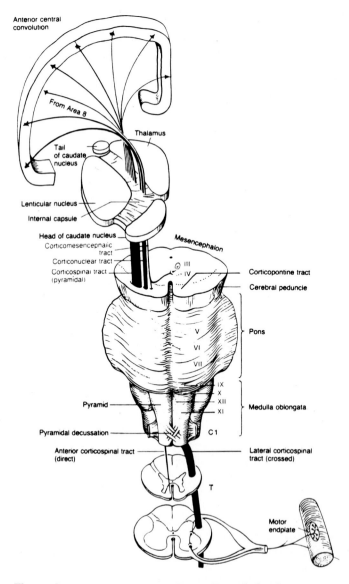

Figure 6   Major cortical motor fibers. (From Ref. 16)

tracts into a very small area, lesions involving the internal capsule may result in very dense neurological deficits involving face, arm, and leg (9).

Attempted surgical excision of the tumors in this region is usually associated with formidable neurological deficits. Therefore, this area of the brain is the preferred site for stereotaxic biopsy, if tissue is needed to establish a diagnosis.

B. Brain Stem

The brain stem is a collective term for the diencephalon, midbrain, pons, and myelencephalon (medulla oblongata). Although the cerebellum is a part of the metencephalon, the brain stem is the part of brain remaining after the cerebral hemispheres and cerebellum are removed.

1. Diencephalon

The diencephalon lies between the cerebrum and midbrain, and encloses the third ventricle. Subdivisions of the diencephalon are best depicted when viewed in a midsagittal plane (Fig. 7) (10). These subdivisions include the following:

Epithalamus.   The epithalamus is a narrow band on the roof of the diencephalon and contains the pineal gland as well as the habenular complex and posterior commissure.

Thalamus.   The thalamus is the largest division of the diencephalon. It is a large ovoid mass located above the hypothalamic sulcus and on either side of the third ventricle. It is the major relay (integrative) station interposed between many subcortical structures and the cerebral cortex. In some persons there is a small area of fusion of the dorsal thalami called the massa intermedia (interthalamic adhesion). The thalamus anatomically contains more than 30 nuclei, divided into three major groups (10).

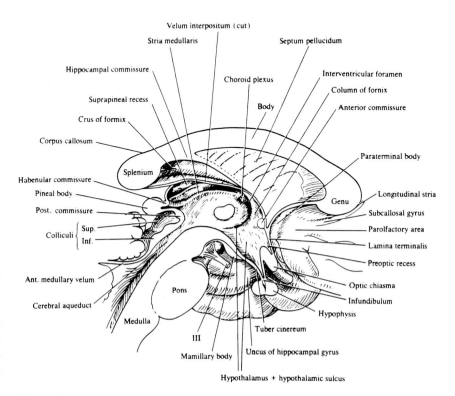

Figure 7   Midsaggital section through the brain stem. (From Ref. 5)

1. *Anterior nuclear group* contains afferent fibers from mamillary bodies (mamillothalamic tract) and efferent fibers to the cingulate gyrus (cortex). This is considered to be a part of the limbic system.
2. *Medial nuclear group* contains fibers projecting to the frontal cortex and from corpus striatum.
3. Midline nuclear group includes groups of cells lying just beneath the ependymal lining of the third ventricle and in interthalamic adhesion. These nuclei connect with nuclei in the hypothalamus and with periaqueductal gray matter.
4. *Lateral nuclear group* is the part of the thalamus that contains the pulvinar, lateral, and medial geniculate bodies, along with some other nuclei. The pulvinar connects with cortices of parietal and temporal lobes. The lateral geniculate body receives fibers from the optic tract and projects them to the visual cortex as the geniculocalcarine (optic) radiations. The medial geniculate body, on the other hand, receives fibers from the lateral lemniscus and inferior colliculus, and projects them to Herschl's gyri (temporal cortex) as the auditory radiations.

Other nuclei of functional significance in the lateral group are ventral anterior (VA) nucleus that receives input from substantia nigra and globus pallidus, and sends output to the caudate nucleus and premotor cortex (area 6) (10). The ventral lateral (VL) nucleus receives input from the globus pallidus, substantia nigra, and cerebral cortex and cerebellum (dentatorubral thalamic tract). It also has reciprocal connections with the precentral gyrus (area 4) (10). The ventral posterior (VP) nuclear complex consists of two nuclei, ventral posterior medial (VPM) and ventral posterior lateral nuclei (VPL), and receives the trigeminal pathways from the head, and the spinothalamic and medial lemniscus pathways from the trunk and limbs, respectively. These nuclei then project to the postcentral gyrus (primary somatosensory cortex) by thalamic radiation in the posterior limb of the internal capsule. Specific neurosurgical lesions in the VA thalamic nuclei interrupt connections between the basal ganglia and the premotor cortex and help relieve the rigidity and tremor in patients with Parkinson's disease. The lesions that destroy the VP nucleus of thalamus produce a contralateral hemianesthesia, with loss of sensory modalities on the face, trunk, and limbs (10).

Since attempted surgical excision of the tumors in this area is usually associated with very severe neurological deficits, including irreversible coma, stereotaxic biopsy is the preferred means of obtaining tissue to establish diagnosis for the tumors of this region.

Hypothalamus   The hypothalamus is located on the inferior aspect of the diencephalon and is bordered by the lamina terminalis anteriorly; midbrain, posteriorly; hypothalamic sulcus, dorsally; third ventricle, medially; and subthalamic nucleus laterally (see Fig. 7). The main hypothalamic structures are best depicted on a view of the ventral aspect of the diencephalon (Fig. 8). These structures include mamillary bodies, tuber cinereum, medial eminence, infundibulum, and neurohypophysis. The optic chiasm and optic tracts delineate the floor of the hypothalamus. Several visceral, limbic, and endocrine functions are controlled by the hypothalamus (10).

Supraoptic and paraventricular nuclei are associated with the release of antidiuretic hormone (ADH) and oxytocin, respectively. The hypothalamus also influences the secretory activity of the pars distalis (anterior lobe of the pituitary). The anterior hypothalamic center regulates the loss of heat, whereas the posterior hypothalamus regulates the conservation of heat. Water metabolism and drinking are influenced by the stimulation of the lateral hypothalamus. Food intake and feeding behavior are controlled in the lateral hypothalamus, whereas the satiety of feeding is controlled in the medial (ventromedial) areas. Lesions in the ventromedial area usually lead to hyperphagia and obesity, whereas lateral hypothalamic lesions cause aphagia and ultimate emaciation. Sleep is controlled by the posterior hypothalmus, and lesions in this region may result in hypersomnia. The hypothalamus also gives rise to the sympathetic pathways that descend through the brain stem to reach the intermediolateral columns of the spinal cord. Interruption of this descending sympathetic pathway causes ipsilateral Horner's syndrome (10).

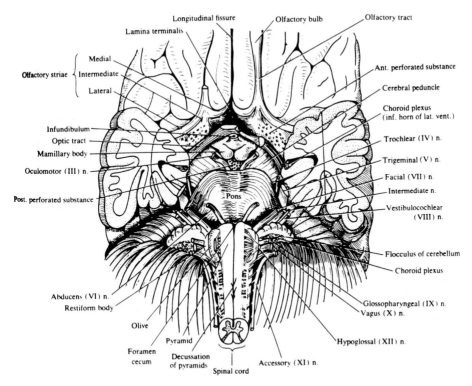

Figure 8 Basis cerebri. (From Ref. 5)

Subthalamus. The subthalamus lies ventral to thalamus and flanks the hypothalamus laterally. It has no visible or prominent external structures, but is an important subcortical center for voluntary muscle control (10).

2. Mesencephalon

The mesencephalon, or midbrain, is the smallest of the four major subdivisions of the brain stem and is positioned between the pons and diencephalon. On the ventral surface, elevations on each side are formed by the cerebral peduncles (basis pedunculi, crus cerebri) (Fig. 9). The peduncles consist almost entirely of descending fibers. The corticospinal and corticonuclear fibers occupy approximately the middle three-fifths, and the temporopontine and parietopontine fibers each occupy the lateral one-fifth (see Fig. 6). Cranial nerve III (oculomotor) emerges from the side of the fossa between the two cerebral peduncles (interpeduncular fossa). On the dorsal surface (Fig. 10), four rounded eminences, the corpora quadrigemina are arranged in pairs and called the superior and inferior colliculi. The superior colliculi are associated with the optic system. The brachium (bridgelike structure) of the superior colliculus connects with the lateral geniculate body and contains fibers from the cerebral cortex and retina to the superior colliculus. The inferior colliculi are important relay nuclei on the auditory pathway to the thalamus. The brachium of the inferior colliculus connects with the medial geniculate body. Cranial nerve IV (trochlear) emerges from the brain stem just inferior to the inferior colliculus and curves around the brain stem (3,10).

The internal gross anatomy is best demonstrated in transverse sections at the level of the superior and inferior colliculus. The section of the midbrain at the level of superior colliculi (Fig. 11(a)) shows the nucleus of cranial nerve III in the periaqueductal gray matter, and the medial

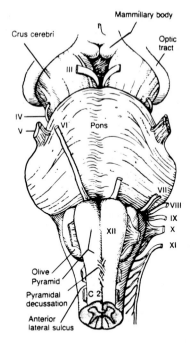

Figure 9 Brain stem structures—ventral view. (From Ref. 16)

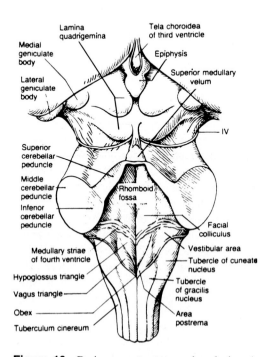

Figure 10 Brain stem structures—dorsal view (cerebellum removed). (From Ref. 16)

(a)

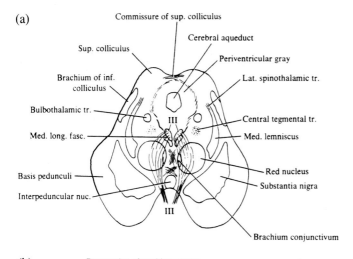

(b)

Figure 11 Midbrain—(a) section through the superior colliculi; (b) section through the inferior colliculi. (From Ref. 10)

longitudinal fasciculi (MLF) form a *V* at this level with the oculomotor nucleus cradled in the arm of the *V*. The crura on each side on the anterior portion of the midbrain are separated from the remainder of it by the substantia nigra. The red nuclei are located posteromedial to the substantia nigra, through which fibers of oculomotor nerves travel to exit from each side of the interpeduncular fossa. The cerebral aqueduct is located between the nuclei of the third nerve and the superior colliculi (10).

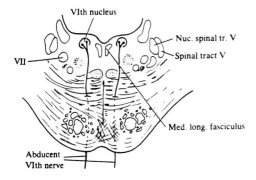

Figure 12 Lower pons (From Ref. 10)

The section through the level of the inferior colliculus (Fig. 11(b)) shows the nucleus of the fourth cranial nerve located on the ventromedial aspect of the periaqueductal gray matter. These nuclei actually invaginate the dorsal surface of the medial longitudinal fasciculi (10).

The medial lemniscus can be seen lateral to the nuclei of the third and fourth cranial nerves at the corresponding levels (10).

3. Metencephalon

The metencephalon is composed of both the pons and cerebellum in the adult. Since the latter is not defined as part of the brain stem, it will be discussed separately.

Pons.   The term *pons* means bridge, and it refers to the prominent ventral bulge of bridge between the cerebellar hemispheres (10).

The pons is located between the mesencephalon, or midbrain, and myeloencephalon, or medulla oblongata, and ventral to the cerebellum (see Fig 9) (10).

The dorsal pons is concealed by the cerebellum, whereas the ventral pons comprises a ventral bulge (see Fig. 9) that is continuous with the cerebellum through the large, paired middle cerebellar peduncles (brachium pontis) (10).

The ventral surface of the pons is closely associated with four cranial nerves (see Fig. 9): The trigeminal (V) nerve is located on its lateral aspect, and nerves VI, VII, and VIII are located in the inferior pontine sulcus, which marks the caudal boundary of the pons.

The dorsal surface of the pons (see Fig. 10) forms the rostral half of the fourth ventricle. Lateral walls of this half of the fourth ventricle comprise the three pairs of the cerebellar peduncles. Of these, the middle cerebellar peduncle serves to connect the pons with the cerebellum. In addition, the median eminence lies on the floor of the fourth ventricle, and the facial colliculus is a prominent structure located on each side of the median eminence (10).

Major internal structures of the pons include the corticospinal tract in the basilar portion, and the main sensory and motor nuclei of the trigeminal nerve more posteriorly. The other important structures are the medial lemniscus and trapezoid bodies in the dorsal pons or tegmentum.

A lower pontine section shows cranial nerve nuclei and fibers of cranial nerves VI, VII, and VIII, and will be discussed under cranial nerves (Fig. 12).

In general, most tumors of the brain stem are treated by a stereotactic biopsy and then radiation therapy. In rare instances of exophytic tumors, a more radical resection may be attempted.

Cerebellum.   The cerebellum occupies most of the posterior cranial fossa. It lies dorsal to the brain stem and is attached to the pons, medulla, and mesencephalon by three pairs of thick fiber bundles, the cerebellar peduncles (11) (see Fig. 10).

The superior cerebellar peduncle (brachium conjunctivum) is the bridge between the midbrain and the cerebellum. It carries mostly fibers projecting from the cerebellum toward the midbrain and thalamus (7). The middle cerebellar peduncle (brachium pontis) is the bridge between the cerebellum and the pons. It carries mostly fibers projecting from pons to cerebellum (12). The inferior cerebellar peduncle (restiform body) is the bridge between the medulla and cerebellum. The fibers project both to and from the cerebellum (12).

The cerebellum is composed of two large lateral masses, the cerebellar hemispheres and a midline portion known as the vermis (Fig. 13). The section of cerebellum shows a layer of gray matter that covers the surface, the cerebellar cortex, and the central gray matter, the cerebellar nuclei. In between these is the "medullary center," an internal core of white matter consisting of fibers traveling in both directions (Fig. 14) (12).

The cerebellar nuclei include the dentate nucleus (largest, most lateral), the emboliform, globose, and the fastigial nuclei (near the midline). These nuclei are present in each of the cerebellar hemispheres (see Fig. 14) (12).

The anterior lobe (paleocerebellum) consists of most of the vermis and the anterior portion of the cerebellar hemispheres. It is associated mainly with proprioceptive (spinocerebellar) input and

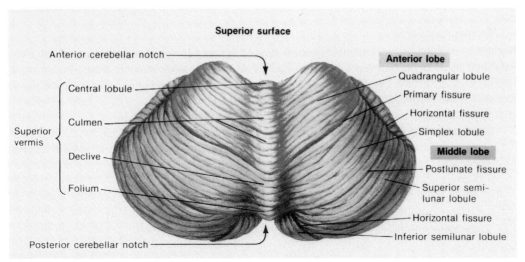

Figure 13   Cerebellum—dorsal view. (From Ref. 2)

exteroceptive input, from head and body, and plays a significant role in the regulation of muscle tone (12).

The posterior lobe (neocerebellum) consists of the bulk of the cerebellar hemisphere and part of the vermis. This part receives connections from the cerebrum and plays an essential role in the muscular coordination of phasic movements (12).

The flocculonodular lobe (archicerebellum) consists of the paired flocculi of the hemispheres (small appendages in the posterior inferior region) and unpaired nodulus, which is the inferior part of the vermis. This part is associated with the vestibular system and plays a significant role in regulating muscle tone, equilibrium, and posture through its influence on the trunk muscles (12).

In general, the cerebellar nuclei receive the axons from ipsilateral Purkinje cells that are located in the cerebellar cortex. They, in turn, provide the main output from the cerebellum, with fibers traveling mostly through the superior cerebellar peduncle to the midbrain and the thalamus (12).

Tumors affecting the cerebellar hemispheres usually cause incoordination of the ipsilateral limbs, whereas involvement of vermis results in trunkal ataxia (13).

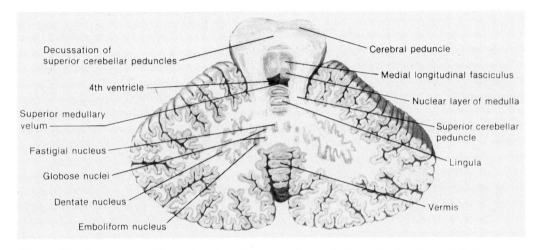

Figure 14   Cerebellar nuclei—section through the superior cerebellar peduncle. (From Ref. 7)

4. Myelencephalon

The myelencephalon, or medulla oblongata, is located between the pons and the spinal cord. The rostral half of its dorsal portion forms the caudal half of the fourth ventricle floor.

The ventral surface (see Fig. 9) of the medulla reveals the pyramids, olives, pyramidal decussation, and rootlets of cranial nerves IX, X, XI, and XII. Cranial nerves IX, X, and XI exit in the postolivary sulcus, whereas XII exists in the preolivary sulcus.

The dorsal surface of the medulla (see Fig. 10) consists of the caudal portion of the floor of the fourth ventricle. Structures found on this portion of the floor, inferior to the stria medullaris, are two prominences that are caused by underlying nuclei of hypoglossal nerves, medially, and vagus nerves, laterally (hypoglossal and vagal trigones, respectively).

The major internal anatomical structures of the myelencephalon are best depicted through a section at the level of the olive (Fig. 15). These include the fasciculus and nucleus of gracilis and of cuneatus, which form the corresponding tubercules and fasciculi externally. As shown in Figure 15, additional structures are the spinal nucleus and the tract of the fifth nerve, inferior olivary complex that causes the bulge on the surface known as olive, corticospinal tracts that comprise the pyramids at the level of the medulla, and vestibular area, medial longitudinal fasciculus (MLF), spinothalamic tract, and nuclei of the 10th and 12th nerves (10).

IV. CRANIAL NERVES

A. Olfactory Nerve (Cranial Nerve I)

The olfactory nerve is concerned with the special sense of smell (special visceral afferents). The receptors are the neuroepithelial cells of the olfactory mucosa that are distributed in the upper one-third of the nasal cavity. The axons of these cells terminate in the olfactory bulb. Second-order neurons then send their projections by the olfactory tract to the uncus and entorhinal area (anterior part of the hippocampal gyrus), to the anterior perforated substance and to the septal region (7,14).

Loss of function is manifested by anosmia (loss of smell) and may be the only sign of an olfactory groove meningioma. Therefore, sense of smell should always be tested carefully during a routine neurological examination (13).

B. Optic Nerve (Cranial Nerve II)

The primary neurons are the receptor cells of the retina: the rods and cones. The secondary neurons are the bipolar cells of the retina, and the tertiary neurons are the ganglionic cells of the retina, the axons of which form the optic nerve. The axons run over the surface of the retina and converge toward the optic papilla or disc (Fig. 16). The optic nerve then passes through the optic foramen. In

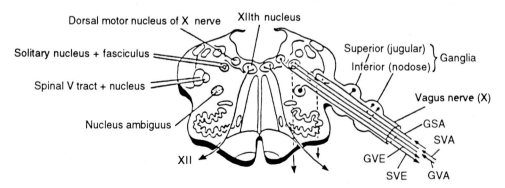

Figure 15 Medulla oblongata—section at the level of the olive. (From Ref. 10)

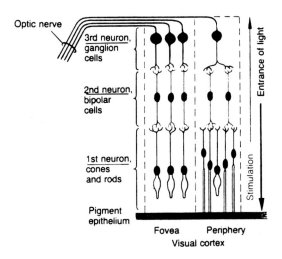

Optic nerve

3rd neuron, ganglion cells

2nd neuron, bipolar cells

1st neuron, cones and rods

Pigment epithelium

Entrance of light

Stimulation

Fovea   Periphery

Visual cortex

Figure 16   Retina. (From Ref. 16)

the cranial cavity the two nerves converge to form the optic chiasma. The fibers from the nasal retina (temporal field of vision) cross in the chiasma and join the uncrossed fibers from the temporal retina (nasal field of vision) to form the optic tracts. Optic tracts then course posteriorly and end at the lateral geniculate bodies. Most of the optic fibers terminate by forming synapses with neurons in the lateral geniculate bodies, but some bypass the bodies and course through the brachium of the superior colliculus and form synapses in the colliculus and pretectal region, thereby establishing reflex pathways. Axons of the cells in the geniculate bodies project (by optic radiations) and terminate in the visual cortex around the calcarine fissure (Fig. 17). The fibers originating from the superior colliculus and pretectal region are primarily concerned with visual reflexes. The fibers from the superior colliculus terminate in various motor nuclei of the cranial nerves and in the anterior gray column of the cervical segments of the spinal cord. Axons originating from the pretectal region, however, pass to the Edinger-Westphal nuclei (parasympathetic portion of the oculomotor nucleus) to establish a reflex (light reflex) that will constrict the pupil in response to strong light. Therefore, loss of the light reflex, without loss of vision, indicates a lesion in the pretectal region. In addition, lesions in the optic pathways cause very specific visual field defects that are most helpful in localizing the pathological processes involved. Visual pathways and corresponding visual field defects are illustrated in Figure 18 (7,14,15).

C.   Oculomotor Nerve (Cranial Nerve III)

The oculomotor nuclear complex is located in the mesencephalon at the level of the superior colliculus, near the midline, ventral to the aqueduct (Fig. 19). From these nuclei, two types of fibers emerge. General somatic efferent fibers innervate all the extraocular muscles except the lateral rectus and superior oblique. General visceral efferent fibers, on the other hand, are the parasympathetic preganglionic fibers that travel to the ciliary ganglia that, in turn, give the postganglionic fibers that terminate in sphincter pupillae and ciliary muscles. They cause the contraction of the iris sphincter muscle and relaxation of the suspensory ligament of the lens by contraction of the ciliary muscle. The origin of these fibers is in the Edinger-Westphal nucleus, which forms a part of the nuclear complex. This nucleus receives fibers from the pretectum and, thereby, participates in the pupillary light reflex. The visceral efferent components of the oculomotor nucleus also possess a convergence center that receives fibers from the visual cortex and the

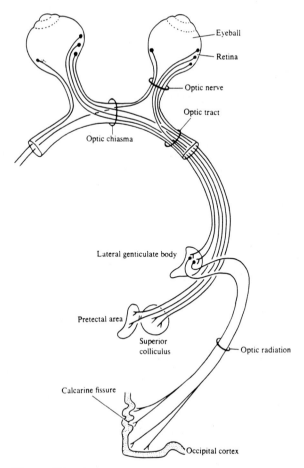

Figure 17 Visual pathways. (From Ref. 14)

frontal eye centers. The axons of the third nucleus course ventrally from the oculomotor nucleus and pass through the red nucleus to emerge in the interpeduncular fossa, medial to the basis pedunculi. After emerging from the mesencephalon, the nerve courses between the posterior cerebral and superior cerebellar arteries before piercing the dura and entering the cavernous sinus. In the sinus, the nerve lies superior to cranial nerves IV and VI, and bends down and laterally to enter the orbit through the medial aspect of the superior orbital fissure. The muscles supplied by the oculomotor nerve turn the eye upward, downward, and medially, whereas parasympathetic fibers produce constriction of pupils, participate in accommodation reflexes, and raise upper eyelids (same fiber ends in levator palpebrae superioris muscle). Total loss of function is manifested by the eye looking downward and outward, a dilated pupil and no accommodation (14).

Tumors of the cavernous sinus may cause not only the dysfunction of the 3rd nerve, but also of the 4th, 5th, and 6th cranial nerves owing to their proximity to the oculomotor nerve in their course through the sinus to the superior orbital fissure.

D.   Trochlear Nerve (Cranial Nerve IV)

The trochlear nucleus is located in the mesencephalon, at the level of the inferior colliculus, in the ventromedial portion of the central gray matter, adjacent to the medial longitudinal fasciculus

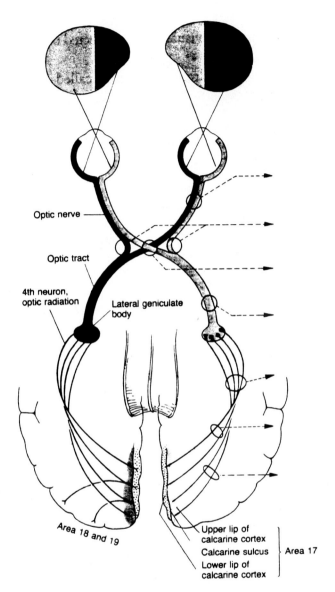

Optic nerve

Optic tract

4th neuron,
optic radiation

Lateral geniculate
body

Area 18 and 19

Upper lip of
calcarine cortex

Calcarine sulcus   Area 17

Lower lip of
calcarine cortex

Figure 18 Visual pathways and corresponding visual field defects depending on the location of the lesion. (From Ref. 16)

(Fig. 20). The somatic efferent fibers that emerge from this nucleus supply the superior oblique eye muscle that assists in turning the eye downward and outward. The trochlear nerve fibers exit from the dorsal aspect of the brain stem just below the inferior colliculus after the decussation of its fibers in the superior medullary velum. The 4th nerve swings around the lateral surface of the brain stem, passes between the posterior cerebral and superior cerebellar arteries, and pierces the dura in the anterior attaching fold of the tentorium cerebelli. The nerve then enters the cavernous sinus inferior to the third nerve and reaches the orbit through the superior orbital fissure. The loss of function is manifested by slight upward deviation of the eye and is usually difficult to detect during a routine neurological examination (14).

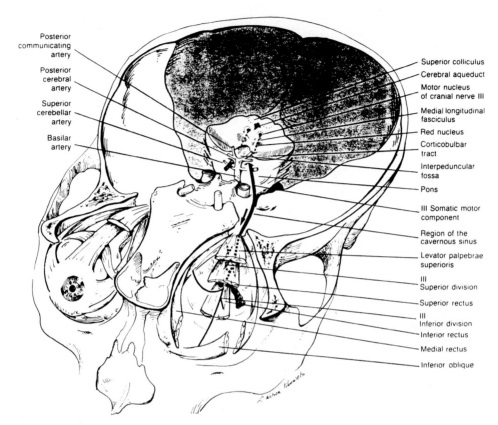

Figure 19 Oculomotor nerve. (From Ref. 15)

E. Trigeminal Nerve (Cranial Nerve V)

The trigeminal nuclear complex consists of four nuclei (three sensory and one motor).

The trigeminal motor nucleus is located in the upper part of the pons. The three sensory nuclei are the principal (pontine) sensory nucleus and the spinal nucleus of the trigeminal nerve, which receive pain, touch, and temperature fibers from the face, sinuses, teeth, and nasopharynx, and the mesencephalic nucleus, which receives proprioceptive fibers from the orbital and masticatory muscles (Fig. 21) (7,14).

Large sensory and smaller motor roots emerge through the lateral part of the pons. The sensory portion then expands over the apex of the petrous temporal bone into the trigeminal (semilunar) ganglion, which gives off ophthalmic, maxillary, and mandibular nerves. These nerves pass through the superior orbital fissure, the foramen rotundum, and the foramen ovale, respectively. The ophthalmic nerve divides into lacrimal, frontal, and nasociliary branches, which carry sensory fibers from the eye, nose, and scalp. The maxillary nerve traverses the pterygopalatine fossa, then enters the infraorbital groove, and emerges as the infraorbital nerve through the infraorbital foramen. This nerve conveys sensation from the lower eyelid, side of nose, upper lip, palate, upper jaw and teeth, part of buccal mucosae, nasal sinuses, nasopharynx, and from vessels and glands in its area of supply. The mandibular nerve has two components. The motor portion joins the nerve in the foramen ovale and gives branches supplying masticatory muscles and tensors of the soft palate and tympanic membrane. The sensory portion of the nerve conveys sensation from the lower jaw, teeth, overlying skin and mucosa, and from the auricular and part of external auditory meatus, the

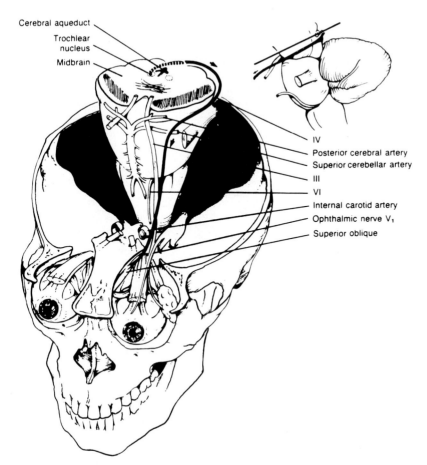

Figure 20 Trochlear nerve. (From Ref. 15)

temporal region, the temporomandibular joint and masticatory muscles, the salivary glands, the vessels in its area of supply, and the anterior two-thirds of the tongue. Loss of function is manifest by deviation of the mandible from the midline on mouth opening and lack of sensation in the corresponding areas of innervation (14).

The dysfunction of the trigeminal nerve per se is uncommon, but when it is seen, with loss of hearing or facial paralysis, it is highly suggestive of a large tumor in the cerebellopontine angle, such as an acoustic neuroma.

F. Abducens Nerve (Cranial Nerve VI)

The nucleus of the abducens nerve is located in the lateral part of the median eminence in the floor of the fourth ventricle. The fibers of the facial nerve loop (internal genu of the facial nerve) around the nucleus (Fig. 22). Of the fibers of the sixth nerve, somatic efferent fibers supply the lateral rectus muscle of eyeball. They originate from the medial side of the nucleus and travel ventrally and caudally to exit from the brain stem at the caudal border of the pons. (They pass just lateral to the corticospinal tract as they exit.) The nerve then passes forward to pierce the dura, and enters the lateral aspect of the cavernous sinus, lying inferior to the trochlear nerve. The abducens nerve enters the orbit by the superior orbital fissure (14).

The loss of function is manifested by inward deviation of the eye, and this may be the only manifestation of a clivus chordoma. In most cases, a sixth nerve palsy is a nonlocalizing sign, and may be reflective of a generalized increase in intracranial pressure.

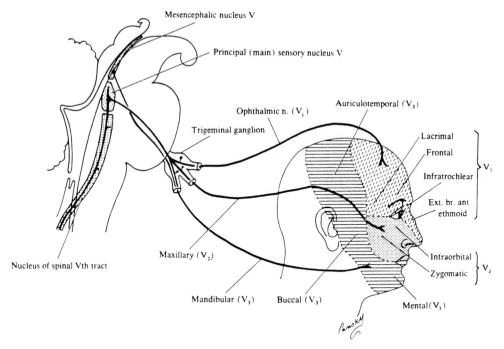

Mesencephalic nucleus V

Principal (main) sensory nucleus V

Ophthalmic n. (V₁)

Auriculotemporal (V₃)

Trigeminal ganglion

Lacrimal

Frontal

Infratrochlear

Ext. br. ant. ethmoid

} V₁

Nucleus of spinal Vth tract

Maxillary (V₂)

Infraorbital

Zygomatic

} V₂

Mandibular (V₃)   Buccal (V₃)

Mental (V₃)

Figure 21   Trigeminal nerve. (From Ref. 14)

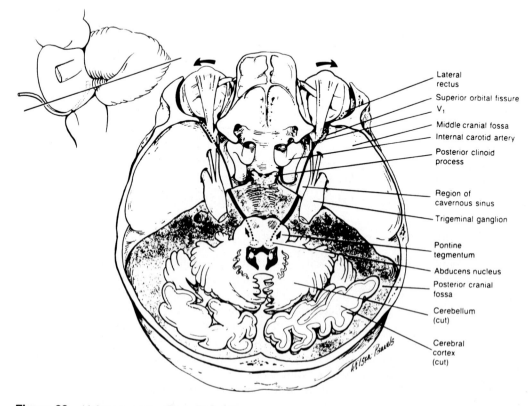

Lateral
rectus

Superior orbital fissure

V₁

Middle cranial fossa

Internal carotid artery

Posterior clinoid
process

Region of
cavernous sinus

Trigeminal ganglion

Pontine
tegmentum

Abducens nucleus

Posterior cranial
fossa

Cerebellum
(cut)

Cerebral
cortex
(cut)

Figure 22   Abducens nerve. (From Ref. 14)

G. Facial Nerve (Cranial Nerve VII)

Cranial nerve VII has three functional components: motor, secretomotor, and special sensory. Motor fibers arise in the facial nucleus in the pons and loop around the abducens nucleus; secretomotor fibers originate in the superior salivatory nucleus located near the caudal end of the motor nucleus; special sensory fibers arise from receptors in the anterior two-thirds of the tongue and soft palate, and end in a nucleus of the solitary tract (Fig. 23) (7).

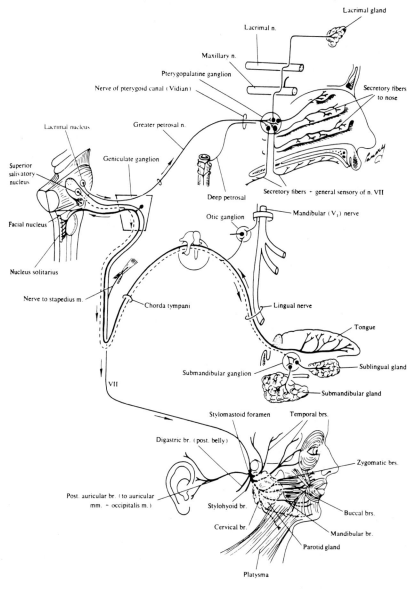

Figure 23   Facial nerve. (From Ref. 14)

The dorsal portion of the motor nucleus supplies innervation to muscles of the upper face and forehead, and receives bilateral input from the cortex, whereas the ventral portion provides innervation for the lower facial muscles and receives only unilateral cortical input through the crossed fibers (7).

The nerve emerges through the recess between the inferior cerebellar peduncles and olive as two parts: the larger motor root and the smaller nervus intermedius, containing secretomotor and special sensory fibers. Both parts enter the internal acoustic meatus alongside the vestibulocochlear nerve, run through the angulated facial canal (Fig. 24), and expand into the geniculate ganglion, which contains cell bodies of sensory fibers. The facial nerve gives off three branches, namely, the greater petrosal nerve, nerve to stapedius muscle, and the chordatympani, before it exits through the stylomastoid foramen just behind the parotid gland and spreads on the face. The greater petrosal nerve carries special sensory fibers from the soft palate, as well as preganglionic parasympathetic fibers to the pterygopalatine ganglion which, in turn, gives rise to postganglionic fibers innervating the lacrimal gland. The chordatympani nerve conveys special sensation from the anterior two-thirds of the tongue, along with preganglionic fibers to the submandibular ganglion which, in turn, gives rise to postganglionic parasympathetic fibers to the sublingual and submandibular glands. (7).

Loss of function is manifested by facial paralysis, poor secretion from glands of salivation and ageunsia (loss of taste) on the anterior two-thirds of the tongue. Some of these functions may be spared, depending on the location of injury, and help localize the lesion. Peripheral seventh nerve palsy is associated with total loss of function in all muscles of facial expression, whereas central paralysis spares the muscles of the upper face (14). A central facial paralysis may be indicative of a tumor of the opposite cerebrum, whereas a partial peripheral facial palsy is commonly seen after surgery for a large acoustic neuroma.

H. Vestibulocochlear Nerve (Cranial Nerve VIII)

The vestibulocochlear nerve has two components. The vestibular portion of the nerve conveys impulses concerned with equilibration, position, and movements of head and neck. The cochlear component is the nerve of hearing. Vestibular and cochlear nerve fibers arise from bipolar cells in vestibular and spiral cochlear ganglia, respectively. The receptor cells for the vestibular system are hair cells of the cristae and macula. The receptor cells of the cochlear component, however, are the

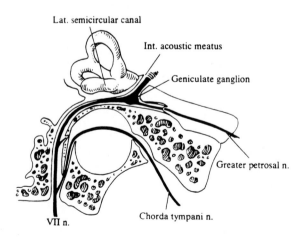

Figure 24   Facial nerve and its course through the petrous bone—major branches. (From Ref. 14)

hair cells located in the organ of Corti. Ampulla of the semicircular canals, utriculus, and sacculus are the inner ear structures related to vestibular function. Similarly, the cochlear duct of the inner ear is associated with auditory function (7).

The nerve fibers course from the internal meatus toward the pontomedullary junction and enter the groove between the pons and medulla posterolateral to the facial nerve.

Although the distal processes of bipolar cells of the vestibular ganglion end in its receptor cells, the proximal ones terminate in the vestibular nuclei located in the brain stem. There are four vestibular nuclei, and they make numerous connections (Fig. 25) (14,16).

Fibers from the superior nucleus enter the medial longitudinal fasciculus (MLF) of the same side and end in the nuclei of cranial nerves III, IV, and VI. The lateral nucleus is the origin of the vestibulospinal tract that terminates in the ventral gray column of the spinal cord. The inferior nucleus is associated with the accessory nerve and ventral gray column of the cervical cord. Fibers from the medial nucleus cross the midline and make numerous connections with the reticular formation and are associated with motor nuclei of the autonomic system (14).

These connections provide the system that helps maintain balance and the normal position of the head, and they coordinate eye movements with those of head. Their relation to autonomic motor nuclei accounts for the nausea, vomiting, and pallor, manifest with overstimulation of the

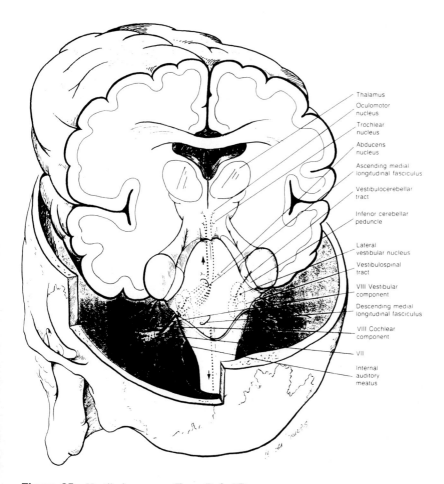

Figure 25 Vestibular nerve. (From Ref. 15)

vestibular system. There are direct and indirect connections with the cerebellar system, which are needed to exert control over the activities initiated by the stimulation of the vestibular receptors (7).

Dysfunction of the vestibular system is manifested by disturbances of equilibrium, balance, and coordination, along with vertigo and tinnitus (17).

The cochlear nerve follows a similar path (Fig. 26). The distal ends of bipolar cells end in the hair cells of the organ of Corti, whereas proximal processes travel into the brain stem and terminate in the cochlear nuclei, namely, in the dorsal and ventral cochlear nuclei. Axons of these nuclei pass rostrally to either decussate in and to form the trapezoid body, or synapse with neurons in the superior olivary nucleus. These fibers then decussate, ascend in and terminate in the inferior colliculus. The axons of these neurons then course through the brachium of the inferior colliculus to the medial geniculate body, which sends projections to the auditory area of the cerebral cortex (14).

The sensation of hearing has bilateral cortical representation and thus unilateral lesions in the CNS do not cause complete loss of hearing in either ear. However, peripheral unilateral dysfunction is associated with hearing loss in the corresponding ear (17).

Vestibulocochlear nerve dysfunction presenting with tinnitus and ipsilateral loss of hearing may be the only sign of an acoustic neuroma, which is the most common tumor of the cerebellopontine angle.

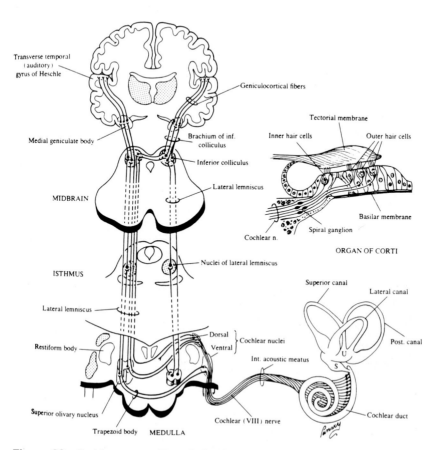

Figure 26   Cochlear nerve. (From Ref. 14)

I. Glossopharyngeal Nerve (Cranial Nerve IX)

The glossopharyngeal nerve has motor, secretomotor, special sensory, and sensory components. Motor fibers arise from cranial ends of ambiguus and dorsal vagal nuclei. Secretomotor fibers arise from the inferior salivatory nucleus. Special sensory fibers convey sensation from the posterior one-third of the tongue. Sensory fibers, in addition to those of the tongue, arise from the pharynx, fauces, tonsil, tympanic cavity, auditory tube, and mastoid cells. Visceral sensory fibers end in the combined dorsal glossopharyngeal–vagal nucleus; ordinary sensory fibers end in the spinal tract and the nucleus of the trigeminal nerve, and those concerned with special sensation, in the solitary tract nucleus (Fig. 27) (14).

The nerve emerges from the medulla above the vagus, leaves the skull through the jugular foramen, runs forward between the internal carotid artery and internal jugular vein, curves anteriorly and ends in branches to the tonsils, mucous membranes and glands, pharynx, and pharyngeal part of tongue. The motor component of the nerve supplies the stylopharyngeus muscle and helps innervate the pharyngeal muscles. A special sensory portion is the nerve of taste for the posterior one-third of the tongue. Sensory fibers convey ordinary sensation from the pharynx, pharyngeal part of the tongue, fauces, tonsils, tympanic cavity, auditory tube, and mastoid cells. It is also the chief nerve supply of the carotid body and sinus (7).

Dysfunction of the nerve is manifested with decreased gag reflex, difficulty with swallowing, and ageunsia on the posterior one-third of tongue (17).

The dysfunction of the 9th cranial nerve along with that of the 10th and 11th is suggestive of a skull base tumor, such as nasopharyngeal carcinoma involving the jugular foramen.

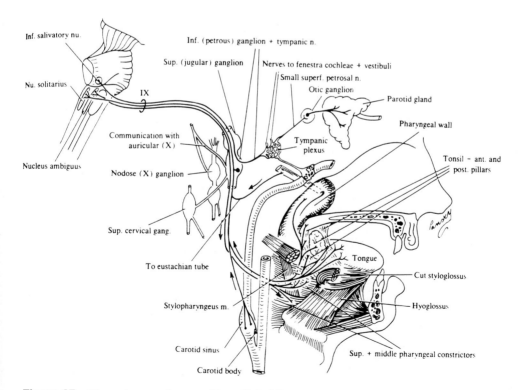

Figure 27 Glossopharyngeal nerve. (From Ref. 14)

J. Vagus Nerve (Cranial Nerve X)

The vagus nerve has three functional components: motor, sensory, and special sensory. Motor fibers for cardiac and unstriated muscles arise in the dorsal vagal nucleus, which extends throughout the length of the medulla oblongata. Motor fibers for striated muscles of the larynx and pharynx originate in the nucleus ambiguus. Afferent fibers from visceral receptors end in the mixed dorsal vagal nucleus; special sensory fibers end in the solitary tract nucleus; and somatic afferent fibers carried in auricular and meningeal branches end in the spinal tract and nucleus of the trigeminal nerve (Fig. 28) (7).

Motor fibers innervate the intrinsic laryngeal muscles and help supply pharyngeal constrictors. It also provides parasympathetic supply to the heart, respiratory system, and gastrointestinal tract. Somatic sensory fibers supply the meninges of posterior fossa and parts of auditory canal. Special sensory fibers carry some taste impulses from the epiglottis and valleculae (7).

Dysfunction to the nerve is manifest by difficulty in swallowing and speaking, loss of reflex control of circulatory system, and poor digestion owing to decreased secretion of digestive enzymes (14).

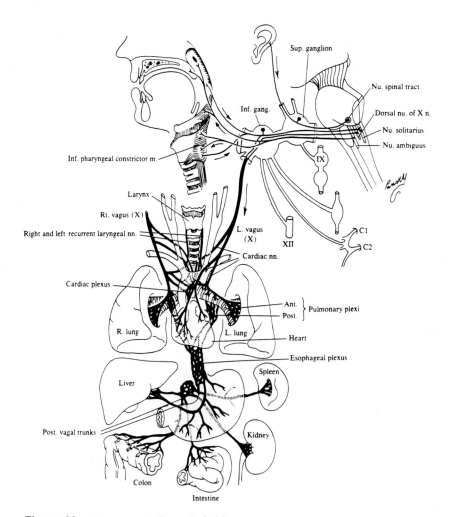

Figure 28 Vagus nerve. (From Ref. 14)

K. Accessory Nerve (Cranial Nerve XI)

The accessory nerve consists of cranial and spinal roots. The cranial root arises from the lower end of the nucleus ambiguus, whereas the spinal root originates from the spinal accessory nucleus, groups of ventral horn cells in the upper five or six cervical segments. Cranial root fibers emerge from the medulla oblongata below and in line with the glossopharyngeal and vagal nerve rootlets. Spinal rootlets originate from the lateral white column of cord, and ascend behind denticulate ligaments, uniting to form a single nerve that enters the skull through the foramen magnum behind the vertebral artery. Immediately after leaving the skull through the jugular foramen, the nerve divides into an internal and external branch. The internal branch joins the vagal nerve and provides motor fibers distributed in pharyngeal and laryngeal muscles and muscles of the soft palate (except for tensor veli palatini). The external branch carries the motor supply for the sternocleidomastoid and trapezius muscles (Fig. 29) (14).

Dysfunction of the nerve is manifested by difficulty in turning the head and possibly in swallowing (14).

L. Hypoglossal Nerve (Cranial Nerve XII)

The hypoglossal nerve has a purely motor function. It is the motor nerve of the tongue muscles. In addition it helps form the ansa cervicalis that supplies twigs to the sternohyoid, sternothyroid, and omohyoid muscles (Fig. 30) (2).

The nucleus of the nerve is located in the medulla oblongata. Nerve fibers emerge in rootlets between the pyramid and olive. They then unite to form the nerve, which passes through the

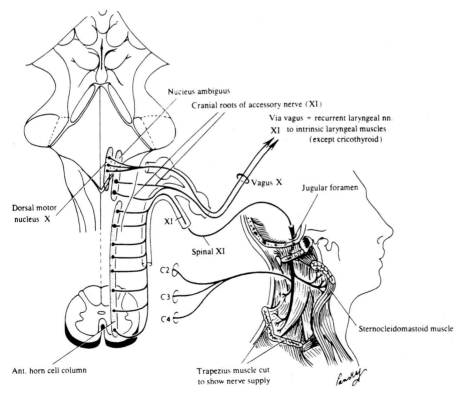

Figure 29 Accessory nerve. (From Ref. 14)

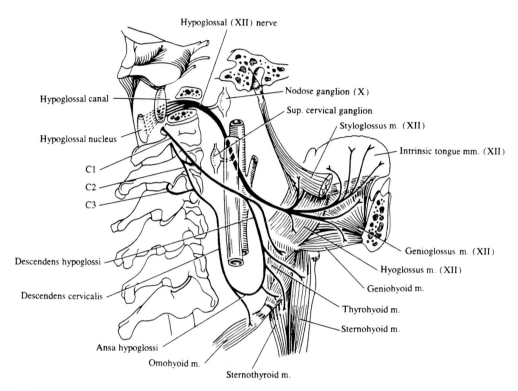

Figure 30 Hypoglossal nerve. (From Ref. 14)

hypoglossal canal of the occipital bone to leave the skull. It runs between the internal carotid artery and internal jugular vein and inclines upward into the tongue. It is joined by a filament from spinal nerve C1, which soon leaves to form the superior root (descendens hypoglossis) of ansa cervicalis (14).

Dysfunction of the nerve is manifested by paralysis of the tongue, and when seen in association with other lower cranial nerve dysfunction is highly suggestive of a skull base tumor, such as nasopharyngeal carcinoma.

V. CIRCULATION OF CEREBROSPINAL FLUID

The choroid plexus of the lateral ventricles is the largest of that found in any ventricle and produces most of the cerebrospinal fluid (CSF). The CSF flows through the interventricular foramina (of Monro) into the third ventricle, augmented by fluid formed by the choroid plexus of this ventricle, and passes through the cerebral (Sylvian) aqueduct to the fourth ventricle which also possesses a choroid plexus. The CSF from all these sources, as well as any formed in the central canal of the spinal cord escapes from the fourth ventricle into the subarachnoid space through the median aperture (of Magendie) and lateral apertures (of Luschka). The CSF then circulates through the freely communicating subarchnoid cisterns of the base of the brain. From the cisterns most of the CSF is directed upward over the cerebral hemispheres toward the superior sagittal sinus. The CSF is then absorbed into the blood through the arachnoid villi, and through the walls of capillaries of the CNS and pia mater (Fig. 31) (3).

Any impairment of CSF circulation or overproduction results in accumulation of excess CSF and hydrocephalus. Obstruction of CSF pathways results in obstructive hydrocephalus, which is

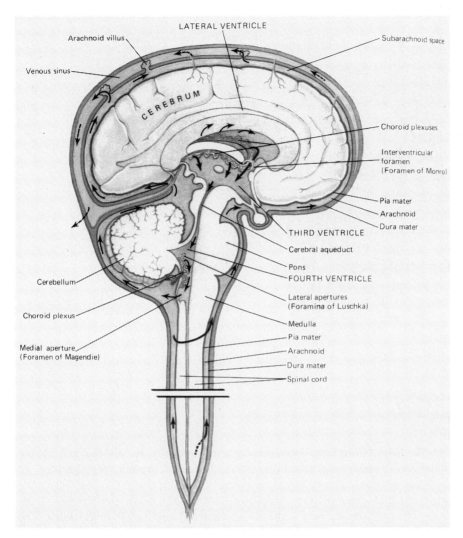

Figure 31 CSF circulation. (From Ref. 2)

the accumulation of the CSF behind the point of obstruction. However, if obstruction occurs at the absorption sites, then no compartmental dilation takes place, and the entire CSF space expands, resulting in communicating hydrocephalus. Tumors arising in the midline of the brain (such as peri-aqueductal gliomas) are likely to cause early obstructive hydrocephalus.

VI. CEREBRAL CIRCULATION

A. The Arterial Supply of the Cerebral Hemispheres

The hemispheres are supplied by the terminal branches of the carotid and basilar arteries. There are anastomoses between the various branches over the cortex, and the efficiency of these is often critical in determining the final outcome of major vessel occlusions (Fig. 32) (18).

The internal carotid artery comes off the common carotid system in the cervical region and gives off no branches extracranially. Then it enters the carotid canal, which traverses the

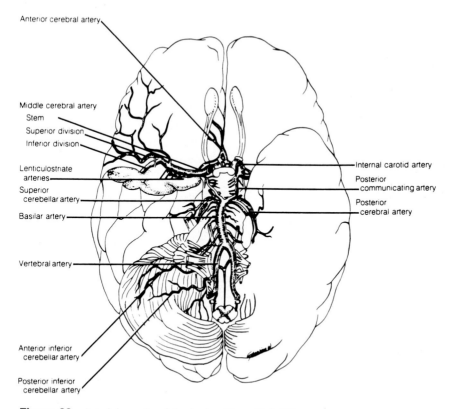

Anterior cerebral artery

Middle cerebral artery
  Stem
  Superior division
  Inferior division

Lenticulostriate
  arteries

Superior
  cerebellar artery

Basilar artery

Vertebral artery

Anterior inferior
  cerebellar artery

Posterior inferior
  cerebellar artery

Internal carotid artery

Posterior
  communicating artery

Posterior
  cerebral artery

Figure 32   Arterial supply of the brain. (From Ref. 23)

petrous temporal bone. After exiting from the carotid canal intracranially, the vessel enters into the cavernous sinus and gives several branches to the pituitary gland and to some cranial nerves. At about the level of the anterior clinoid process, it leaves the cavernous sinus, and enters the subarachnoid space and then gives off the ophthalmic, anterior choroidal, and posterior communicating arteries. The ophthalmic artery is the main source of blood supply to the retina. The anterior choroidal artery is an important vessel supplying the internal capsule, diencephalon, midbrain, and part of the medial temporal lobe. It supplies most of the choroid plexus of the lateral ventricles. The posterior communicating artery helps form the circle of Willis, and the carotid artery then bifurcates into the middle cerebral and anterior cerebral arteries (19).

The anterior cerebral artery sweeps forward and over the genu of the corpus callosum and backward as two vessels. The pericallosal and callosomarginal arteries supply the parasagittal cortex, including the entire motor and sensory cortex controlling the leg. An important branch of the anterior cerebral artery immediately after its origin is the recurrent artery of Heubner, which supplies the nerve fibers in the internal capsule destined to supply the cranial nerve nuclei and the arm on the opposite side. The anterior cerebral arteries are joined by a short anterior communicating artery, which allows collateral flow to the opposite hemisphere (18).

The middle cerebral artery enters the Sylvian fissure shortly after its origin. Here it divides into three main vessels that pass upward and backward in the fissure, giving off branches that exit along the length of the fissure to supply the surface of the hemisphere. These are the precentral, central, posterior parietal, and posterior temporal arteries. As the middle cerebral artery passes laterally, it gives off the lenticulostriate arteries that supply the basal ganglia and part of the internal capsule. Terminal branches of the main vessel reach the occipital pole and probably provide an independent blood supply to the macular cortex at the tip of the lobe (18).

The posterior cerebral arteries are formed by the bifurcation of the basilar artery. Each vessel passes around the cerebral peduncles lying between the medial surface of the temporal lobe and the upper brain stem. Along its length, it supplies the inferior and medial surfaces and the hippocampal area of the temporal lobe. The thalamogeniculate and thalamoperforating arteries are the other important vessels that supply the dorsolateral brain stem, the thalamus, posterior internal capsule, as well as the visual radiations. The main vessel terminates as the calcarine artery, supplying the visual cortex, with the exception of the macular cortex (18).

B. The Blood Supply of the Brain Stem and Cerebellum

The main blood supply is derived from the paired vertebral arteries, which join to form the basilar artery at the pontomedullary junction. The blood supply of the medulla is derived mainly from the vertebral arteries, which also give small branches to form the anterior spinal artery. Laterally, each vertebral artery gives off a variable branch, the posterior inferior cerebellar artery (PICA). It supplies a part of the medulla (see Fig. 32) (20).

The other brain stem vessels are the anterior inferior cerebellar arteries (AICA), the transverse pontine arteries, the superior cerebellar arteries (SCA), and the posterior cerebral arteries. Each gives off a long penetrating paramedian branch that supplies the central area of the brain stem, whereas the main trunk of the vessel passes around the brain stem to supply the dorsolateral quadrant of the brain stem and part of the cerebellum. The SCA supplies all the deep structures, including the nuclei. The AICA gives off the internal auditory branch that supplies the inner ear and the vestibular apparatus (20).

C. Venous Drainage of the Brain

Veins of the brain are classified as external and internal cerebral veins, and they all terminate in the dural sinuses (Fig. 33).

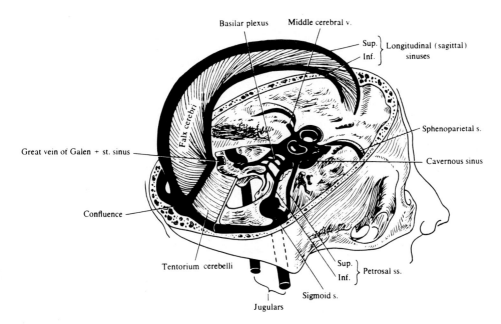

Figure 33 Cerebral venous sinuses. (From Ref. 21)

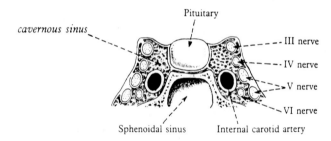

Pituitary

cavernous sinus

III nerve

IV nerve

V nerve

VI nerve

Sphenoidal sinus   Internal carotid artery

Figure 34   Cavernous sinus—coronal section at the level of the pituitary gland. (From Ref. 17)

The external cerebral veins and the middle cerebral veins drain the surface of the hemispheres, and they terminate in the superior sagittal sinus and cavernous sinus respectively (21).

The 3rd, 4th, 6th, and the first two divisions of the 5th nerve travel through the cavernous sinus. The relation of these structures to the pituitary gland in the sella tursica and the position of the cranial nerves in the cavernous sinus relative to the carotid artery is shown in Figure 34. This anatomy is clinically important in explaining the symptomatology related to tumors involving the cavernous sinus (22).

The basal veins (of Rosenthal) are formed by the veins draining the inferior surface of the brain and deep structures. They terminate in the great cerebral vein (of Galen) (21).

The internal cerebral veins are formed by a confluence of the thalamostriate vein and the anterior septal vein. They drain the adjacent periventricular structures. The internal cerebral veins are joined by the basal veins to form the great cerebral vein (of Galen) (21).

The veins of the posterior fossa are classified into superior, anterior, and posterior groups, and they drain posterior fossa structures into the vein of Galen, the superior petrosal sinus, and the sigmoid sinus, respectively (21).

REFERENCES

1. Guyton AC, Basic neuroscience, anatomy and physiology. Philadelphia: WB Saunders, 1987:2–4.
2. Guyton AC, Basic neuroscience, anatomy and physiology. Philadelphia: WB Saunders, 1987:22.
3. Netter FC, Nervous system, part I, anatomy and physiology. 1983:21–39.
4. Greenberg MS. Handbook of neurosurgery. Greenberg Graphics, 1991:91–104.
5. Pensky B, Dalmas AJ, Budd GC. Review of neuroscience, 2nd ed. New York: Macmillan Publishing, 1998:90–131.
6. Lindsay KW, Bone I, Callender R. Neurology and neurosurgery illustrated. New York: Churchill–Livingston, 1986:104–114.
7. Netter FC. Nervous system, part I, anatomy and physiology. The Ciba collection of medical illustrations. Ciba, 1983:91–110.
8. Carpenter MB. Core text of neuroanatomy. Baltimore: Williams & Wilkins, 1985:20–52.
9. Carpenter MB. Core text of neuroanatomy. Baltimore: Williams & Wilkins, 1985:221–264.
10. Pensky B, Dalmas AJ, Budd GC. Review of neuroscience, 2nd ed. New York: Macmillan Publishing, 1988:80–90.
11. Netter FC. Nervous system, part I, anatomy and physiology. The Ciba collection of medical illustrations. Ciba, 1983:198–220.
12. Pensky B, Dalmas AJ, Budd GC. Review of neuroscience, 2nd ed. New York: Macmillan Publishing, 1988:239–255.
13. Lindsay KW, Bone I, Callender R. Neurology and neurosurgery illustrated. New York: Churchill–Livingston, 1986:167–171.
14. Pensky B, Dalmas AJ, Budd GC. Review of neuroscience, 2nd ed. New York: Macmillan Publishing, 1988:133–166.

15. Wilson-Paumels L, Akesson EJ, Stewart PA. Cranial nerves, anatomy and clinical comments. Toronto: BC Decker, 1988:9–24.
16. Duus P. Topical diagnosis in neurology. Stuttgart, George Thieme Verlag, 1983:163–170.
17. Lindsay KW, Bone I, Callender R. Neurology and neurosurgery illustrated. New York: Churchill–Livingston, 1986:159–166.
18. Duus P. Topical diagnosis in neurology. Stuttgart: George Thieme Verlag, 1983:86–98.
19. Patten J. Neurological differential diagnosis. New York: Springer-Verlag, 1981:87–142.
20. Duus P. Topical diagnosis in neurology. Stuttgart: George Thieme Verlag, 1983:119–136.
21. Pensky B, Dalmas AJ, Budd GC. Review of neuroscience, 2nd ed. New York: Macmillan Publishing, 1988:120–124.
22. Duus P. Topical diagnosis in neurology. Stuttgart: George Thieme Verlag, 1983:136.
23. Simon RP, Aminoff MJ, Greenberg DA. Clinical neurology. New York: Appleton & Lange, 1989:120–148.

6

Molecular Genetic Events in Some Primary Human Brain Tumors

Henry H. Schmidek
Marion, Massachusetts

I. INTRODUCTION

Neoplasia is a multistep process, intimately linked to normal growth and differentiation, in which certain cells are altered so that they maintain the capacity to divide, which normal cells lose as they mature. The change in the cells' genetic makeup overrides the cells' normal regulatory mechanisms and results in a growth advantage that allows their continued, inappropriate proliferation. Subsequently, these cells may undergo further changes in gene expression, leading to their malignant transformation (1). The transformation of a cell may be brought about by mechanisms that involve (1) altering the expression of specific genes normally present in the susceptible cell; these genes, called protooncogenes, can be converted into transforming genes (oncogenes) by releasing them from their normal controls, augmenting their expression (gene amplification), or producing mutational changes in their DNA; or (2) as a result of losing genetic material with the loss of a tumor suppressor gene (TSG). Some of the genetic changes that have recently been implicated in the genesis of the three most common and important primary human brain tumors: the gliomas, meningiomas, and the medulloblastomas, will be examined in this chapter.

II. GLIOMAS

The gliomas constitute approximately 50% of human primary brain tumors. The most common of these tumors are astrocytic and span a spectrum of malignancy, based on clinical and neuropathological criteria, ranging from the benign, low-grade astrocytoma, such as the pilocytic astrocytoma, to an astrocytoma of an intermediate grade of malignancy, the anaplastic astrocytoma, to a neoplasm that is among the most malignant of human malignancies, the glioblastoma multiforme. A central objective of neuropathological research is to decipher the mechanisms involved in the initiation and progression of these brain tumors.

In the multistep model of carcinogenesis, tumor initiation begins with a genetic change that provides the affected cell and its descendants with a growth advantage and permits the preferential development of this clone of cells. Subsequently, these cells undergo additional genetic changes, some of which convey an additional growth advantage. A tumor that is becoming increasingly malignant characteristically reflects this evolutionary process by demonstrating increasing aneuploidy, variability of phenotype, and increasing chromosomal changes. These are the changes that have been identified as a low-grade glioma undergoes transformation to a glioblastoma. Recently, there have been some insights into some of the molecular events underlying these changes, and these involve the loss of genetic information from chromosomes 9p, 10, 13, 17p, and 22 and evidence of amplification of the epidermal growth factor receptor (EGFR) (2–5). The 17p deletions have been reported to occur in 5 of 19 low-grade gliomas, 7 of 24 anaplastic astrocytomas, and 19 of 49 glioblastomas (i.e., at about the same frequency for each grade of malignancy), suggesting that the loss of information from the short arm of chromosome 17 is an early event in the neoplastic transformation of astrocytes. The deletion of sequences from chromosomes 13, 17p, and 22 has been identified in low-grade gliomas, but at a lower frequency than of losses of 17p (3, 6–10). Loss of genetic information from chromosome 9 is a common event in intermediate- and high-grade gliomas, with this finding seen in 4 of 8 anaplastic astrocytomas, 6 to 12 glioblastomas, but none of 10 low-grade astrocytomas examined. The loss of genetic information from chromosome 10 has now been reported to occur in 59 of 84 glioblastomas, 5 of 33 anaplastic astrocytomas, and none of 32 low-grade gliomas. These findings suggest that chromosome 10 loss is a specific event associated with the evolution of a glioblastoma. Fults and associates used a large number of allelic probes and attempted to localize a region of chromosome 10 that is lost consistently among a series of anaplastic astrocytomas and glioblastomas (3). These investigators were unable to establish the location of a tumor suppressor gene on this chromosome because the losses occurred along the entire length of the chromosome, suggesting the loss of an entire chromosome may be a frequent event in these neoplasms.

A working model based on these findings suggests that the transformation of the astrocyte often involves loss of 17p and that, in the cases demonstrating a loss of heterozygosity, the p53 gene is frequently mutated and loses its growth suppressor function (11–15). The subsequent dedifferentiation of this tumor to form an anaplastic astrocytoma involves additional chromosomal loss from 9p and, among the glioblastomas, one may find evidence of these accumulated changes, as well as the loss of information from chromosome 10. In addition to this pathway, there are probably alternate routes by which, for example, a glioblastoma may arise, since a significant percentage of tumors of each grade of malignancy do not demonstrate the foregoing findings.

Glia can be stimulated to proliferate under the influence of a variety of growth factors. The binding of the epidermal growth factor (EGF) to its receptor, the epidermal growth factor receptor (EGFR), stimulates the transmembrane phosphorylation of other membrane-associated proteins, initiating a series of receptor-mediated biochemical events. The EGFR consists of 1186 amino acids, of which 557 through 1154 correspond to the protein kinase domain and autophosphorylation sites. This segment of amino acids possesses an 85% homology with the v-*erb* oncogene product, and the homology reeaches 97% for the sequences of the protein kinase domain. Two reports have identified aberrant forms of EGFR isolated from different tumors, but having similar alterations in the external domain of the receptor. Sugawa characterized six aberrant EGFR transcripts in six different glioblastoma specimens. Each tumor had a similar splicing rearrangement with an 801-bp deletion corresponding to exons 2 though 7 (16). Yamazaki observed a similar deletion in several glioma cell lines (17). These and other reports suggest that alteration of the EGFR is a relatively common event occurring in about 50% of glioblastomas and in about 15% of lower-grade gliomas. These mutations uncouple the tyrosine kinase activity of the receptor from the binding of the external ligand, and the mutated receptor stimulates cell proliferation in the absence of the appropriate environmental stimulus. The foregoing data suggest EGFR amplification as another event associated with the anaplastic transformation of the astrocyte (4, 9, 17, 18).

III. MENINGIOMAS

The meningiomas are common, usually benign, primary tumors of the nervous system, arising from the membranes covering the brain and the spinal cord. The analysis of the cytogenetic and molecular genetic properties of these tumors with current techniques has opened important vistas into trying to understand the mechanisms involved in the initiation and progression of these neoplasms (19).

For many years it has been known that chromosomal abnormalities occur in transformed cells and that such abnormalities are manifest as chromosomal translocations, rearrangements, and deletions. The cytogenetic analysis of meningioma cells in early tissue culture reveals the loss of one copy of chromosome 22 in about 65% of these tumors (monosomy 22). In addition to cases in whom a complete loss of chromosomal 22 occurs, partial loss, involving a terminal deletion of the long arm of chromosome 22, has also been reported. In hypodiploidy, the karyotype displays less than the normal diploid karyotype. Monosomy 22 is often followed by further chromosomal loss; most frequently, this involves chromosome 14 and chromosome 17. The loss of chromosome 8 is also common, occurring in almost 20% of meningiomas with monosomy 22. The tendency toward increased hypodiploidy has been positively correlated with aggressive biological behavior of the tumor, and increased hypodiploidy is seen in 75% of invasive meningiomas and 70% of recurrent tumors. In addition to a progression of hypodiploidy, meningiomatous cells in culture frequently develop structural rearrangements of other chromosomes. Meningiomas with marked hypodiploidy show a spontaneous rate of chromosomal breakage and rearrangement of 20%. Those chromosomes most frequently involved in structural rearrangements are chromosomes 1, 14, 10, and 19. Another study revealed structural rearrangements of chromosomes 1p and 11p. Frequent structural rearrangements of chromosomes 1 and 6 and of chromosomes 1 and 22 have also been reported (20–22).

Current molecular genetic techniques have permitted an improved definition of the genetic abnormalities in meningiomas that were first demonstrated by classic cytogenetic techniques. Whereas cytogenetic studies are based on the detailed analysis of a few tumor cells, molecular genetic analysis examines the DNA of millions of tumor cells, improving the resolution of analysis to a level that far exceeds that of cytogenetic techniques when sufficient probes are available.

Analysis of polymorphic DNA loci in DNA isolated from meningiomas has permitted the sublocalization of the region of chromosome 22 involved in the tumorigenesis of meningioma (19). Polymorphic DNA loci are sites at which a small mutation in the DNA alters the recognition site of a restriction endonuclease (RE), an enzyme that cleaves DNA at sequence-specific sites. These mutations are stably inherited, normal variations in DNA sequence that cause different allele fragment lengths to be produced by the RE digestion of homologous chromosomes. These fragment length variants are referred to as restriction fragment length polymorphisms (RFLPs) and are used to detect chromosomal loss or mutation in patients who are heterozygous for the DNA marker being studied. Hybridization of radiolabeled chromosome-specific DNA probes to re-digested DNA is used to compare the genetic composition of DNA isolated from a tumor specimen against normal DNA from the same patient's leukocytes. If the patient is constitutionally heterozygous for a given chromosomal marker, and if the examination of the tumor DNA reveals a loss of heterozygosity at that locus, then the loss of genetic information in the tumor is established.

Seizinger and co-workers studied 51 patients with meningiomas (22). Forty of these patients were constitutionally heterozygous for at least one chromosome 22 marker. Of those 40 informative patients, 43% demonstrated loss of heterozygosity for at least one chromosome 22 marker. All of the markers used in this study identified regions on the long arm of chromosome 22. All meningiomas that showed loss of genetic information at one chromosome 22 marker locus showed loss of genetic information at all chromosome 22 marker loci tested. This finding corresponds to karyotype data in six of these tumors, which confirmed loss of one copy of chromosome 22. Application of these techniques involving use of probes for other chromosomes (3, 6, 7, 19–21, 23–29) has revealed loss of heterozygosity in some tumors, but at a much lower frequency than is seen for chromosome 22. All tumor DNAs that demonstrated a loss of genetic material on another chromosome also showed loss of genetic information from chromosome 22, which suggests that this loss is most probably a primary etiologic event in the evolution of some meningiomas (30).

Dumanski and associates examined 22 polymorphic DNA loci on chromosome 22 in 81 cases of sporadic meningioma (20, 21). Fifty-two of these tumors showed a loss of heterozygosity at all informative loci, which is consistent with monosomy 22 in tumor DNA. Eleven percent of tumors showed loss of one constitutional allele at one or more chromosome 22 loci, but maintenance of heterozygosity at other chromosome 22 loci, which is consistent with variable terminal deletions of the long arm of chromosome 22 in the tumor DNA. This finding suggested that the meningioma locus is located within the region of 22q12.3qter.

Densitometric scanning confirms the ratio of copy number of chromosome 22 between tumor and normal DNA as approximately $1:2$, indicating that loss of alleles from one chromosome 22 is due to a simple loss of genetic material from one copy of chromosome 22 and not to mitotic recombination or to loss and reduplication of the remaining alleles.

Demonstration that about 65% of meningiomas show a loss of genetic information from the long arm of chromosome 22 supports the hypothesis that the loss of a tumor suppressor gene may be involved in the genesis of this type of tumor. This hypothesis is attractive, but does not explain the absence of a demonstrable loss of genetic information in one-third of tumors with the same neuropathological characteristics, either because the resolution of RFLP analysis does not reveal small regions of genetic loss or because a mutation in the critical locus may make the TSG nonfunctional, although without actual loss of genetic material. Alternative hypotheses are based on the speculation that other types of genetic alterations may be present in those tumors that do not have loss of chromosome 22 and that there may be alternative genetic pathways, the molecular alteration of which may result in tumors of the same neuropathological type.

Growth factors are proteins that exert a variety of important biological effects that can affect a cell's growth, development, proliferation, and survival. These agents exert their actions by specifically binding to high-affinity receptors expressed on the surface of cells and, thereby, activating intracellular signaling mechanisms. In addition, oncogenic mutations in tumor cells are often found in genes that are in growth factor-regulated pathways. The discovery that the v-*sis* oncogene encodes a molecule that is essentially identical with platelet-derived growth factor (PDGF) established the relation of oncogenes and growth factors and, since then, other oncogenes have been shown to contain growth factor-regulated genes and encode mutated forms of growth factor receptors and growth factor-regulated signal transduction molecules.

Platelet-derived growth factor is a heterodimer composed of two related polypeptide chains, A and B. PDGF-B is the cellular homologue of the v-*sis* oncogene, and the constitutive expression of PDGF proteins in cells that express PDGF receptors is associated with transformation (31–33). The human *PDGF-B* gene lies within the region of the putative meningioma gene and, therefore, is of interest in relation to this type of tumor. There is some evidence that c-*sis* maybe implicated in the tumorigenesis of meningiomas. Bolger reported a pedigree with familial meningioma in which three siblings with meningiomas carried a constitutional translocation t(14qter-on-22qter) in their peripheral leukocytes. This is a condition in which the two centrometric ends of the long arms of one chromosome 22 and one chromosome 14 are joined to form an abnormal hybrid chromosome. Two of these patients had a variant of the c-*sis* oncogene in their leukocyte DNA, revealed by RFLP analysis. The variant of the oncogene was felt to be located on the morphologically normal chromosome 22. Investigators have recently cloned, mapped, and sequenced the abnormal c-*sis* allele from one member of this family; and analyses of the structural abnormality using several different restriction enzyme digestions demonstrate DNA fragments 0.1-kb smaller than those in DNA from unaffected individuals as a result of a deletion in this gene located within an intron and an Alu sequence. The finding of an identical deletion in the familial and in a sporadic case of meningioma suggests that the c-*sis* deletion is associated with meningioma development, possibly by activating the expression of the c-*sis* gene.

The activation of c-*sis/PDGF-2* finds expression by binding to cell surface PDGF receptors. The coexpression of a potent mitogenic growth factor and its receptor in meningiomas suggests an autocrine mechanism contributing to the growth of these neoplasms. In addition to c-*sis/PDGF*, meningiomas have been screened for the amplified expression of most of the other known oncogenes. The gene for the epidermal growth factor receptor is located on the short arm of chromosome 7, and the gene encoding the receptor for insulin-like growth factor 2 is on the long arm of chromosome 7. Two cases have been reported in patients with meningiomas with specific aberrations involving chromosome 7.

Elevated levels of EGFR have been reported in some meningiomas, although amplification of the EGFR gene appears to be rare in these tumors. However, increased expression of the receptor protein has been detected, and the increased expression of this receptor in the absence of gene amplification has been reported in other tumors. Both high- and low-affinity EGF-binding sites have been detected in meningiomas. Recently, meningiomas have also been found to express both the insulin growth factor (IGF) I and insulin growth factor II in RNAs. The coexpression of these mRNAs and of c-*sis* suggests a contribution of PDGF and the IGFs to the growth of these tumors. In addition to these growth factors, significant amounts of mRNAs for basic fibroblast growth factors have been detected in meningiomas in vivo, whereas these are not detected in normal brain or meninges.

Meningioma cells probably respond to a variety of growth factors, and some of these factors may act synergistically. For example, PDGF and the insulin-like growth factors have a synergistic proliferative effect on fibroblastic cells in culture (23, 31). The synergistic effects between growth factors is commonly seen in many cell types and likely results from different receptors activating different signaling pathways. Different combinations of growth factors activate several pathways simultaneously. Recent evidence suggests that PDGF activates the expression of between 30 and 100 "competence" or "immediate early" genes (32). Several of these gene products encode transcription factors. The protooncogenes c-*fos*, c-*myc*, and c-*jun* are among these early genes activated by PDGF. These genes encode DNA-binding proteins. The c-*fos* and c-*jun* proteins combine to form a complex, AP-1, that is important in the transcriptional regulation of many genes (35). Both c-*fos* and c-*myc* have roles in cell division and cellular proliferation and may act to initiate DNA synthesis in the cell. Currently, it is unclear how oncogenes interact with the cell cycle proteins, such as cdc2 and the cyclins, and with the tumor suppressor genes, to induce cellular proliferation; however, it is probable that, in the meningiomas, both oncogenes and tumor suppressor genes have undergone losses in their regulatory domains so that there is a persistent activation of the cells' growth stimulatory apparatus, resulting in cellular proliferation and the formation of a neoplasm that usually remains benign and that exerts its effects by local pressure.

IV. MEDULLOBLASTOMA

The medulloblastoma is a member of a family of neoplasms that share many properties with the neuroblastoma, retinoblastoma, pineoblastoma, and esthesioneuroblastoma. Medulloblastomas originate in the cerebellar vermis during the first two decades of life and present as a rapidly growing brain tumor located in the posterior fossa (24, 34).

Among the discrete histological variants of the medulloblastoma are (1) the undifferentiated medulloblastoma; (2) the medulloblastoma with neuronal differentiation, with Homer–Wright rosettes, unipolar or bipolar cells with neurosecretory granules, and occasional ganglion cells; (3) medulloblastomas with glial differentiation, which includes astrocytes, oligodendrocytes, and rarely, ependymal cells. The medulloblastomas also present with a number of transitional and mixed lesions, variants that contain striated muscle (medullomyoblastoma), and melanin-producing cells (melanotic medulloblastoma).

The medulloblastoma has been hypothesized to arise following the neoplastic transformation of a hypothesized but never identified pluripotent neuroectodermal stem cell, the medulloblast (24). Malignant transformation of these stem cells could then cause them to continue to proliferate, become locally invasive, and to frequently metastasize. Until recently, the identification of the stem cells of the nervous system has been impossible; however, the tools have been developed to allow the homogeneous-appearing cells of the early nervous system to be segregated and their differentiation to be examined in an orderly manner.

Immortalization of stem cells by retroviruses incorporating an oncogene that arrests the differentiation program is one such technique. The establishment of a cell line from primary cells using retroviruses leads to the growth of such cells continuously in culture and serves as an establishment or immortalizing function which arrests the differentiation program of several cells types, including myoblasts, chondrocytes, retinal melanoblasts, and neuroretinal cells. This technique has been used by Frederiksen and colleagues to establish cell lines from the postnatally developing rat cerebellum. These investigators then used a panel of monoclonal antibodies to recognize the stages of neuronal and glial differentiation and included in this panel reagents to nestin, an intermediate filament gene, specifically expressed in central nervous system stem cells but not in differentiated cells, of the adult brain (35, 36).

A cell line, produced by the application of these techniques, which is of particular interest because it may bear a relation to identifying the putative stem cell of the medulloblastoma, has been produced by the immortalization of the postnatal rat cerebellum with a temperature-sensitive variant of the SV40 large T antigen in a retrovirus vector. This cell line, labeled ST 15, consists of a clonal population of cells that when grown at 33°C proliferate and are nestin-positive and vimentin-positive. At 39°C the large T protein is rapidly degraded, and the cells lose the nestin antigenicity and become GFAP-positive cells. The differentiation pathway adopted by the cells can be influenced by their local environment. Depending on these influences, the cells differentiate into either neurons, astrocytes, oligodendrocytes, or muscle cells. These are the properties predicted for the *medulloblast*, a stem cell the neoplastic transformation of which can produce a tumor with the potential to differentiate along neuronal, glial, oligodendroglial, myoblastic lineages, or combinations thereof. In two human medulloblastoma cell lines that I examined with the same panel of antibodies as those used on the ST 15 cell line, 282 Med and DAOY, these cell lines are composed of antivimentin- and antineurofilament-positive and anti-GFAP-negative cells. Tamura reported on the immunochemical studies of two cell lines they established of human medulloblastoma, designated ONS-76 and ONS-81 (10). Both these lines express neurofilament protein and neuron-specific enolase but do not express GFAP or S-100 protein, indicating a neuronal, but not glial, differentiation. Valtz recently reported the examination of primary cerebellar cells for evidence of muscle development (36). These primary cerebellar cells can stain with troponin T antibodies, and the troponin-positive cells have the morphological characteristics of muscle. Examination of five surgical specimens of medulloblastoma revealed nestin-positive cells in each of the tumors, although their numbers differed. The finding of the nestin-positive cells in these tumors is additional support for the concept of their derivation from a neuroectodermal stem cell.

Recent studies have shown that neoplastic transformation may result from the inactivation of tumor suppressor genes. The absence of these sequences was first demonstrated in retinoblastoma, in which the loss of both copies of the tumor suppressor gene *Rb* and its product, a DNA-binding protein, occurs in the affected cells (27, 37–39). Examination of surgical specimens of medulloblastoma has shown a loss of alleles from DNA sequences mapped to the distal part of chromosome 17 in four of nine patients (45%), and in two of these cases there was a loss of p53 sequences (25–28, 36, 40). Saylors searched for p53 mutations in 12 medulloblastoma tumor specimens, 8 xenografts, and 3 permanent cell lines and found a mutation of p53 in 1 of 3 cell lines tested, in none of the xenografts, nor in any of the primary tumors (41). Confirmatory studies of PNETs, by Raffel and associates, of 23 tumors showed a loss of genetic material from 17p in 6 of 23 tumors (42), and James and co-workers also demonstrated loss of genetic material from 17p in 5 of 11 PNETs (2). By using probes specific for 17p, the area of common loss was shown to be restricted to 17p11.2 to 17pter. Raffel sequenced p53 cDNA in eight PNETs and discovered no mutations in seven of eight tumors in exons 5–8, which contain over 90% of reported p53 mutations (42). Other reports confirm the absence of p53 mutations in PNETs (41), strongly suggesting the presence of another tumor suppressor gene besides p53, on 17p, involved in the pathogenesis of medulloblastoma. (15, 43–45).

V. CONCLUSIONS

The application of the tools of molecular genetics to problems of nervous system neoplasia has resulted in significant insights into the mechanisms related to the initiation and progression of some primary human nervous system tumors. In this chapter the current understanding of some of these events in three of the most important and common human brain tumors—the gliomas, meningiomas, and the medulloblastomas—has been examined in the context of some of the known alterations in the chromosomal, oncogene, tumor suppressor gene, and growth factor expressions of these lesions. How this information may eventually be used therapeutically is suggested by the experiment by Mercer and colleagues (13). These investigators transfected wild-type p53 into a human glioblastoma cell line and were able to arrest the proliferation of the neoplastic cells. With the identification and understanding of the genes involved in the initiation and progression of these diverse neoplasms and of the mechanisms that regulate their expression, it will be possible to tailor approaches, involving gene transfer into the neoplastic cells, that will arrest the proliferative and invasive properties of a neoplasm and possibly allow the transformed cells to undergo the normal process of cell growth and differentiation that had been derailed by their neoplastic transformation.

REFERENCES

1. Schmidek HH. The molecular genetics of nervous system tumors J Neurosurg 1987; 67:1–16.
2. James CD, Collins VP. Glial tumors. In: Levine A, Schmidek HH, eds. Molecular genetics of nervous system tumors. New York: John Wiley & Sons, 1993.
3. Fults D, Tippets RH, Thomas GA, Nakamura Y. Loss of heterozygosity for loci on chromosome 17p in human malignant astrocytoma. Cancer Res 1989; 49:6572–6577.
4. Ekstrand AJ, James CD, Cavenee WK, Seliger B. Genes for epidermal growth factor receptor, transforming growth factor alpha, and epidermal growth factor and their expression in human gliomas. Cancer Res 1991; 51:2164–2172.
5. Ruley HE, Schmidek HH. Oncogenes and nervous system tumors. In: Wilkins RH, Rengachary SS, ed. Neurosurgery update. New York: McGraw-Hill Publishing, 1990:226–232.
6. Steck PA, Saya H. Pathways of oncogenesis in primary brain tumors. Curr Opin Oncol 1991; 3:476–484.
7. Bigner SH, Mark J, Burger PC, Mahaley MS. Specific chromosomal abnormalities in malignant human gliomas. Cancer Res 1988; 48:405–411.
8. Carlbom E, Dumanski JP, Hansen M. Clonal genomic alterations in glioma malignancy stages. Cancer Res 1988; 48:5546–5551.

9. Liberman TA, Nussbaum HR, Razon N, et al. Amplification and enhanced expression and possible rearrangement of EGF receptor gene in primary human brain tumors of glial origin. Nature. 1985; 313:144–147.

10. Fults D, Pedone CA, Thomas GA, White R. Allelotype of human malignant astrocytomas. Cancer Res 1990; 50:5784–5789.

11. Finlay CA, Hinds PW, Levine AJ. The p53 proto-oncogene can act as a suppressor of transformation. Cell 1989; 57:1083–1093.

12. Hinds P, Finlay C, Levine AJ. Mutation is required to activate the p53 gene for cooperation with the *ras* oncogene and transformation. J Virol 1989; 63:739–746.

13. Mercer WE, Shields MT, Amin M, Sauve GJ. Negative growth regulation in a glioblastoma cell line that conditionally expresses human wild type p53. Proc Natl Acad Sci USA 1990; 87:6166–6170.

14. Marshall CJ. Tumor suppressor genes. Cell 1991; 64:313–326.

15. Nowell PC. Chromosomal and molecular clues to tumor progression. Semin Oncol 1989; 2:116–127.

16. Eckstrand AJ, Sugawa N, James CD, Collins VP. Amplified and rearranged epidermal growth factor receptor genes in human glioblastomas reveal deletions of sequences encoding portions of the N- and/or C-terminal tails. Proc Natl Acad Sci USA 1992; 89(10):4309–13.

17. Yamazaki H, Ohba Y, Tamaoki N, Shibuya M. A deletion mutation within the ligand binding domain is responsible for activation of epidermal growth factor receptor gene in human brain tumors. Jpn J Cancer Res 1990; 81:773–779.

18. Stromer K, Hamou MF, Diggelmann H, deTribolet N. Cellular and tumoral heterogeneity of EGFR gene amplification in human malignant gliomas. Acta Neurochir 1990; 107:82–87.

19. Atkinkson LL, Schmidek HH. Genetic aspects of meningiomas. In: Schmidek HH, ed. Meningiomas and their surgical management. Philadelphia: WB Saunders, 1991:42–47.

20. Dumanski JP, Carlbom E, Collins VP, Nordenskjold M. Deletion mapping of a locus on human chromosome 22 involved in the oncogenesis of meningioma. Proc Natl Acad Sci USA 1987; 84:9275–9279.

21. Dumanski JP, Rouleau GA, Nordensjold M. Molecular genetic analysis of chromosome 22 in 81 cases of meningioma. Cancer Res 1990; 50:5863–5867.

22. Seizinger BR, De La Monte S, Atkins L, Gusella JF. Molecular genetic approach to human meningioma: Loss of genes on chromosome 22. Proc Natl Acad Sci USA 1987; 84:5419–5423.

23. Antoniades HN, Galanopoulos T, Neville-Golden J. Expression of IGF I and IGF II genes in primary human astrocytomas and meningiomas. Int J Cancer 1992; 50:215–222.

24. Bailey P, Cushing H. Medulloblastoma cerebelli: a common type of midcerebellar tumor of childhood. Arch Neurol Psychiatry 1925; 14:192–224.

25. Bonnin JM, Perentes E. Retinal S-antigen immunoreactivity in medulloblastoma. Acta Neuropathol 1988; 76:204–207.

26. Czerwionka M, Korf HW, Hoffman O, Busch H, Schachenmayr W. Differentiation in medulloblastomas: correlation between the immunocytochemical demonstration of photoreceptor markers (S antigen, rod-opsin) and the survival rate in 66 patients. Acta Neuropathol 1989; 78:629–636.

27. Daneshvar L, Metzger AK, Edwards MS. Deletion mapping of the medulloblastoma locus on chromosome 17p. Genomics 1990; 8:279–285.

28. Tamura K, Shimizu K, Yamada M, Okamoto Y. Expression of major histocompatibility complex on human medulloblastoma cells with neuronal differentiation. Cancer Res 1989; 49:5380–5384.

29. Tohyama T, Kubo O, Katahira M, et al. Glial fibrillary acidic protein and neurofilament protein in medulloblastoma Neurol Surg 198X; 16:1243–1250.

30. Herzog R, Gottert E, Henn W, et al. Large-scale physical mapping within the region 22q12.3–13.1 in meningioma. Genomics 1991; 19:1041–1046.

31. Wagner BJ, Cochran BH. Growth factors—the PDGF paradigm. In: Levine AJ, Schmidek HH, eds. Molecular genetics of nervous system tumors. John Wiley & Sons, 1993.

32. Cochran BH. The molecular action of platelet-derived growth factor. Adv Cancer Res 1985; 45:183–216.

33. Curran T, Franza BR Jr. *fos* and *jun*: The AP-1 connection. Cell 1988; 55:393–397.

34. Lopes BS, VandenBerg SR, Scheithauer BW. World Health Organization classification of nervous

system tumors. In: Levine AJ, Schmidek HH, eds. Molecular genetics of nervous system tumors. New York: John Wiley & Sons, 1993.

35. Frederiksen K, Jat JS, Valtz N, Levy D, McKay R. Immortalization of precursor cells from mammalian CNS. Neuron 1988; 1:439–448.

36. Valtz NL, Hayes TE, Norregard T, Liu S, McKay RD. An embryonic origin for medulloblastoma. New Biol 1991; 3:364–371.

37. Malkin D, Li FP, Strong LC, Fraumeni JF. Germ line p53 mutations in a familial syndrome of breast cancer, sarcomas, and other neoplasms. Science 1990; 250:1233–1238.

38. Friend SH, Bernards R, Rogelj S, et al. A human DNA segment with properties of the gene that predisposes to retinoblastoma and osteosarcoma. Nature 1986; 323:643–646.

39. Biegel JA, Rorke LB, Packer RJ, et al. Isochromosome 17q is the most common structural abnormality in CNS primitive neuroectodermal tumors. Pediatr Neurosci 1989; 14:153.

40. Cogen PH, Daneshvar L, Metzger AK, Edwards MS. Deletion mapping of the medulloblastoma locus on chromosome 17p. Genomics 1990; 8:279–285.

41. Saylors RL, Sidransky D, Friedman HS, Bigner SH, Bigner DD, Vogelstein B, Brodeur GM. Infrequent p53 gene mutations in medulloblastomas. Cancer Res 1991; 51(17):4721–4723.

42. Karnes PS, Raffel C. Pediatric brain tumors. In: Levine A, Schmidek HH, eds. Molecular genetics of nervous system tumors. New York: John Wiley & Sons, 1993.

43. Mashiyama S, Murakami Y, Yoshimoto T, Sekiya T. Detection of p53 mutations in human brain tumors by single-stranded conformation polymorphism analysis of polymerase chain reaction products. Oncogene 1991; 6:1313–1318.

44. Metzger AK, Sheffield VC, Duyk G, Daneshvar L. Identification of a germ-line mutation in the p53 gene in a patient with an intracranial ependymoma. Proc Natl Acad Sci USA 1991; 88:7825–7829.

45. Levine AJ, Momand J, Finlay CA. The p53 tumor suppressor gene. Nature 1991; 351:453–456.

Clinical Presentation of the Brain Tumor Patient

Diana L. Kraemer

Yale University School of Medicine, New Haven, Connecticut

Dennis E. Bullard

Rex Hospital and Raleigh Neurosurgical Clinic, Raleigh, North Carolina

I. INTRODUCTION

The clinical presentation of brain tumors is often stereotyped by textbooks, educators, and clinicans when, in fact, the variety of manifestations of these multifaceted tumors is almost unlimited. Practicality, however, forces us to deal with generalities, and so it will be with this chapter. Fred Plum (1) has outlined two major approaches to the diagnosis of neurological diseases: pattern recognition and logic and probability. With the first, the clinician recognizes the signs and symptoms as a clinical syndrome, based upon his or her prior experience. This form of diagnosis is used by all of us in both our clinical practices and daily life to deal with situations for which there is a basis of underlying knowledge and experience. A zebra is seen because a zebra has been seen before. The second is the process of attempting to define the signs and symptoms, based on known physiological and anatomical principles. It is used more often in the situation for which a clinical problem does not fit with previously seen or known syndromes. It is also used by inexperienced clinicians who are attempting to correlate their basic medical knowledge with early clinical experience. We see a zebra because it looks like a donkey, but it has black and white stripes. All physicans use both approaches separately or in combination at different times in their careers and as means of verifying their thinking before committing a patient to a series of expensive diagnostic tests or potentially dangerous treatment regimens. Accordingly, both approaches will be covered to some degree in this chapter. First, symptomatology, according to location of a mass lesion, will be discussed. This will allow the clinician to review neurological localization in a classic, generalized sense. Following this introduction, symptoms according to tumor type will be presented. We hope this will allow the clinician to gain an understanding of the "personality" of different tumor types as they present clinically, and will reinforce the more traditional understanding of the nervous system. To expand upon the metaphor used earlier in this chapter, a zebra may be easier to spot if one knows where it hides in the jungle.

In today's litigious and financially limited world, the clinician is often placed in the difficult situation of having to decide how far to pursue a patient's complaints. As always, an extensive and carefully taken history, followed by a meticulous clinical examination, will provide the solution in most cases. Unfortunately, the diseases that beset the nervous system are often subtle in their manifestation; the patient may be aware of the disease process long before clinical manifestations occur in the neurological examination. The patient may recognize a change in his or her perception of the world, or the ability to function in it, long before the disease process will have overcome the plasticity and redundancy present within the central nervous system. Conversely, an underlying disease can affect the ability of the patient either to be aware of the changes occurring or to prevent the accurate reporting of them. Therefore, one caveat should always prevail for even the most experienced examiners: when an appropriate patient or his or her family is significantly concerned about a neurological or potentially neurological complaint, the physician should never hesitate nor be faulted for seeking neurological consultation or further testing. Cost-effectiveness is a term that can be used by politicians and planners with impunity, but it has only limited application to the individual clinician on the firing line. The clinician is the patient's advocate against both human disease and the bureaucratic process, an often unenviable, but necessary, role.

II. CLINICAL EXAMINATION

As with the general medical history, the neurological history will usually provide the clinician with a differential diagnosis that can be appropriately narrowed by the performance of a detailed neurological examination. In many instances, the unique aspects of the nervous system and the diseases that are affected will allow the specificity of symptoms to delineate the disease process more clearly and precisely. At other times, the disease process will affect the ability of the patient to provide an adequate history. When this occurs, it becomes crucial that family and friends be interviewed to provide an accurate and complete history. The neurological examination in the hands of a master clinician can provide a wealth of information. Its intricacies, however, often make a detailed examination impractical for routine office screening. The neurological history, therefore, can allow the clinician to focus the examination on those areas that are most likely to provide diagnostic information while doing a simplified examination of other systems (Table 1).

The neurological examination is outlined in Table 1. Mental status testing, cranial nerve examination, motor testing, sensation evaluation, and deep tendon reflex evaluation are further categorized in Tables 2–9. In addition, the neurovascular structures should be evaluated, and mechanical signs of both nerve root irritation and supporting structures should be tested. The tests are arranged as they are usually performed so that coordination may be tested last. In this way, the examiner has identified gross motor deficits and can better evaluate the combination of faculties required to truly test coordination. With practice, a thorough neurological examination can be done in a reasonable amount of time.

The neurological examination always begins with the mental status evaluation (see Table 2). A large part of this test can be performed while obtaining the neurological history. The faculties to be assessed by the clinician include level of consciousness, orientation, immediate short-term and remote memory capabilities, and language capacity. In this last category, speech and writing can

Table 1 The Neurological Examination

Mental status
Cranial nerves
Motor examination
Sensation
Deep tendon reflexes
Neurovascular examination
Mechanical signs
Coordination

Table 2 Mental Status Examination

Level of Consciousness
  Alert
  Lethargic
  Obtunded
  Stuperous
  Comatose
Orientation
  Person
  Place
  Time
Memory
  Immediate memory
    Digit repetition: forward and backward
  Short-term memory
    Delayed object recall
  Long-term memory
    Place of birth, mother's maiden name, reasonable graphic and historical events
  Language testing
    Spontaneous speech
  Comprehension
    Three-step command
  Repetition
    Single words expanding to short sentences
  Object identification
  Reading capability
  Writing
    Simple letters expanding to sentences
Higher Cortical Functioning
  Abstract thinking
  Calculation

Table 3 Cranial Nerves

    I: Smell
   II: Visual acuity, fields, and fundoscopic evaluation
III, IV, and VI: Extraocular movements and pupillary response
    V: Facial sensation, corneal reflex and massiter bulk and power
  VII: Facial movements: spontaneous and volitional
 VIII: Hearing and Rinne and Weber's tests
IX and X: Gag
   XI: Neck movement: active and passive
  XII: Tongue movement and mass

Table 4 Motor Examination

Muscle mass
Tone
Individual motor strength

Table 5   Deep Tendon Reflexes

Brachioradialis
Biceps
Triceps
Knees
Ankles
All to be done with and without recruitment

Table 6   Sensation

Pinprick
Light touch
Temperature
Vibration
Position sense

Table 7   Mechanical Signs

Cervical range of motion
   Nuchal rigidity
Spurling's sign: foraminal compression test
Lumbar Evaluation
   Straight-leg raising
   Reverse straight-leg raising
   Head bending
   Range of motion at the hip

Table 8   Neurovascular Examination

Blood pressure and pulse while lying, sitting, and standing
Cardiac examination for bruits, irregular beats or murmurs
Evaluation for bruits over the neck and great vessels
Pulse Obliteration
   Adson's maneuver
   Military maneuver

Table 9   Coordination

Finger-to-nose test
Rapid alternating movements
Heal-to-shin test
Gait Examination
   Normal gait, heel-and-toe walking
   Tandem gait
   Romberg's test

be broken down into both expressive, repetitive, and receptive components. Lastly, the higher cortical functions, which include the fund of information, abstract thinking, and the ability to calculate, should be tested. Many of these elements can be evaluated during the course of the history by providing a sympathetic ear, asking simple questions to guide the conversation, and most importantly, listening carefully.

Pursuing any speech deficit found reassures the patient that the clinician is interested in his or her problems (the patient is usually aware of an acquired speech deficit) and makes the patient feel more at ease. Moreover, the patient who cannot comprehend simple one-step commands or attend for more than several seconds will be unable to comply with further neurological testing. The goals and limitations of the neurological examination may be defined while taking the patient's history, thereby making the process more enjoyable for all.

When examining the cranial nerves, it is usually most simple and expedient to test them in serial order (see Table 3). As Sir William Osler pointed out in *A Way of Life*, "Life is a habit, a succession of actions that become more or less automatic" (2). This does not mean that every patient needs to differentiate cinnamon from cloves during testing of olfactory nerve function or that minor changes on red–green perception be tested if they have no visual symptoms. However, by repetitively and serially testing visual acuity, general fields of vision, extraocular movement, facial movement and sensation, bilateral hearing, swallowing and tongue movements, the examiner will become adept at picking up subtle abnormalities in this portion of the neurological examination and will be able to focus more attention on the pertinent areas under suspicion.

The same general principles are true for motor testing (see Table 4). The muscle bulk and general condition of the patient are first noted so that strength testing can be done in an appropriate context. Individual muscle groups should be isolated and tested so that associative and secondary muscles cannot be used to mask true weakness. If the specific movement caused pain, note this clearly so that future testing can be compared impartially and accurately. Testing of tone and deep tendon reflexes (DTR) can be done synchronously. When moving the limbs into appropriate positions for DTR testing, it is necessary to ensure that the tone and tension between the two sides is symmetric. If it is not, then the reason for it must be established as being a real difference in tone or merely poor positioning.

The neurovascular examination is largely self-explanatory and designed to exclude significant vascular compression as the cause for a given complaint (see Table 8).

Gait and coordination are tested last. To evaluate these functions, the component parts must be assessed first. If a person has a weak deltoid, then finger-to-nose testing must compensate for that factor. In the same way that mental status testing can be assessed while taking the history and mechanical testing can be done during the motor evaluation, coordination can be assessed and rechecked repetitively during the preinterview walk to the examination room. Fine motor coordination and spontaneous movement can be assessed, in large part, during the general examination, and fine details can be confirmed as a formal portion of the neurological examination.

Many detailed and complex topics have just been covered all too lightly. We would refer the clinician to one of the several excellent texts devoted to the neurological examination and to suggest that they expand their knowledge and experience by using these tests frequently and lovingly (3–7).

III. CLINICAL PRESENTATIONS BY SYMPTOMS AND SIGNS

A. Localizing Value of Common General Symptoms

Neurological symptoms are as manifest as the imagination allows; obvious examples of aberrant perception in art are the works of Van Gogh and Lewis Carroll. Although the senior author does have one fascinating patient who draws superb watercolors to show how she perceives her dysfunction, for the sake of expediency and because most of us will not routinely be presented with these types of problems, we have chosen to deal with the most common of the complaints that have significant neurological potential: headaches, dizziness, and alterations in consciousness. Each of these is an extensive topic by itself, and each has had compendiums written about it. We will deal with each by itself in the belief that they can be addressed in a truncated, but reasonable, fashion.

1. Headache

Tumors cause headaches through several mechanisms: the brain parenchyma itself has no pain fibers; therefore, pain afferents arising on intracranial vessels and meninges that cause this symptom may arise from local pressure, direct invasion of the meninges, diffuse intracranial pressure, or irritative phenomena such as hemorrhage. In general, these headaches will progressively worsen. Occasionally, changes in cerebrospinal fluid (CSF) dynamics can make these features less pronounced, allowing for waxing and waning of symptoms until the later stages of the disease. Slowly growing tumors, such as meningiomas, can be massive in size with little subjective or objective findings because of the brain's amazing ability to compensate over time for displacement and deformation. In contrast, a small hemorrhage within a long-standing asymptomatic tumor can result in the new onset of headaches or changes in neurological functioning if the adjacent brain is incapable of accommodating the sudden change in pressure or volume.

Virtually every individual will have a headache at some time in his or her life. Many will have frequent headaches, and a substantical number will have headaches of sufficient clinical frequency or intensity to require medical attention. The multitude of books and articles on this topic attest to the overall frequency and importance of this general problem. When to proceed with costly and potentially invasive testing is a question frequently posed to the primary physician (Table 10).

When obtaining the history of headaches, it is crucial to take a meticulous history that will allow the symptom or symptoms to be placed in an appropriate context. Several factors should alert the clinician to the potential for a serious underlying neurological problem. These include the recent onset of severe headaches in a individual with no previous history of similar problems; headaches associated with severe pain, nausea, or vomiting; the association of visual dysfunction, weakness, speech problems, vertigo, or a change in level of consciousness. Of significant concern is a prolonged, subacute duration of symptoms, in terms of weeks or months, unlike the less significant history of headaches dating back years. When the patient or family can present clear indication of additional changes, then the course is clear and studies should be performed. Less sophisticated families often express changes in function in simple, but difficult to understand, terms. "Mama just isn't right" may include symptoms ranging from an altered level of consciousness to changes in bowel habits. In days past, physicians often knew their patients well enough on a

Table 10 Significant Factors Associated with Headaches

Symptoms
    New onset in previously asymptomatic patient
    Severity in a stoical patient
    Associated nausea or projectile vomiting
    Associated neurological dysfunction
        Memory changes
        Alterations in speech
        Blurred or double vision
        Motor, sensory, or coordination changes

professional and often personal basis to allow them to decipher the nature and seriousness of the complaints and to judge when a problem required further evaluation. Today, that is often not true, and physicians have to make a judgment based on a single meeting or a limited number of prior visits. A general rule of thumb is that with any of the foregoing features or with a patient who is appropriately concerned, a computed tomography (CT) or magnetic resonance imaging (MRI) scan should be performed. Frequently, an unenhanced CT will exclude hydrocephalus or significant mass effect. Unfortunately, some tumors are isodense with brain unless contrast is given, thereby adding the associated risks of a reaction to the dye. We tend to prefer an MRI as a single definitive test when the clinician is truly concerned about an intracranial lesion. An MRI permits better visualization of soft tissue, will define subtle lesions such as those seen with infiltrating gliomas or smaller metastatic tumors, and gives better visualization of the posterior fossa.

A multitude of clinical adages concerning headache have an underlying basis in reality: nocturnal headaches or early morning headaches are frequently associated with increased intracranial pressure; pulsatile headaches are associated with vascular dilation, as seen with migraine or migraine variants; and tension headaches occur toward the end of the day and are nuchal in location. It is equally true that many common beliefs are unfounded: eating does not always relieve headaches associated with hypoglycemia, aspirin will almost never stop the pain of a migraine headache or a tumor-related headache in an adult, but will sometimes be remarkably effective with children. Furthermore, headache associated with a subarachnoid hemorrhage does not necessarily have to be the worst one an individual has ever suffered. For practical purposes, only headaches associated with classic migraine and with a recognizable prodrome can be considered clearly diagnostic by history alone. However, even this fairly obvious guideline is prone to exception; the rare occipital tumor may present with an aura that is virtually indistinguishable from migraine. Therefore, the lesson to be gleaned is that pattern recognition is a useful screening approach to many signs and symptoms, but logic and probability must always be involved as a fail-safe mechanism.

Certain factors can strongly suggest a serious underlying cause for headache, but in the early stages of tumor growth, very few presenting symptoms or signs are clearly diagnostic unless sufficient tumor obstructive hydrocephalus has developed.

2. Vertigo and Dizziness

Vertigo represents the sensation of either the individual or the environment moving and represents a syndrome that is easily described, but can be multifactorial. A discrepancy between sensory inputs and spatial orientation must exist before vertigo can occur. The great degree of overlap among the systems subserving these functions creates the multiple causes involved. Patients will also use various words or phrases to describe their problem: lightheadedness, dizziness, unsteadiness, or "spinning around." Most of the time the problem will be nonneurological. When the patients describe the sensation of either the room or they themselves spinning or moving back and forth, or that they are being forced forward or backward, then a more serious implication of vestibular or cerebellar dysfunction exists. Although the temporal lobe may conceivably be involved, the more likely area of involvement will be the vestibular apparatus or the posterior fossa. In both instances, careful examination of the cranial nerves is crucial. If any abnormalities are found or an adequate nonneurological explanation cannot be confirmed with symptom resolution, an MRI should be performed to exclude a posterior fossa lesion. Because hearing is difficult to test adequately in the office, when in doubt, audiometric testing should be performed. A sensorineural hearing loss requires an MRI to exclude a cerebellopontine angle (CPA) tumor.

Even though vertigo is relatively easy to describe, categorizing it and differentiating it from dizziness or imbalance is somewhat more difficult. Numerous authors have attempted to subdivide these symptoms. The schema employed by Brandt appears to be a very satisfactory way of approaching the problem (8). He has broken these complaints down into four major types: rotational, sustained rotational, positional, and dizziness with postural imbalance. Attacks of rotational or positional vertigo are seldom associated with tumors in children or adults. Sustained rotational vertigo, however, can occasionally be seen with acoustic neuromas, other cerebellopontine angle mass lesions, or brain stem lesions. Dizziness and postural imbalance are associated with mass lesions within the brainstem or cerebellum, or by lesions that cause compression in these areas.

The physical examination is particularly important with these symptoms because of the difficulty in consistently obtaining a totally accurate history and because of the frequency with which the symptom is seen and is associated with no clearly identifiable or treatable problem. This last feature is the one that makes it all too easy for the busy clinician to lose focus on the fine details of the examination and to hear instead the often loud background noise of functional findings.

The patient must be clinically tested to exclude extracranial vascular disease, and there must be a careful evaluation of cranial nerves and coordination. When facial weakness, change in facial or oral sensation, or findings suggestive of increased intracranial pressure or cerebellar dysfunction are noted; the presence of a posterior fossa or brain stem lesion must be entertained, and a neuroimaging procedure should be performed. It is usually better to proceed first with an MRI because of its superiority in visualizing lesions of the posterior fossa. As previously mentioned, all patients with a unilateral sensorineural hearing loss or unilateral unexplained tinnitus must also be further evaluated to exclude a small acoustic neuroma or other cerebellopontine angle mass. Patients with normal general examinations and laboratory values are a more difficult problem. When an extensive general examination has been completed and is unremarkable, the yield on intracranial studies is so low that time, rather than immediate imaging, may be the better alternative. Frequent follow-up visits and careful explanation of the potential problems and alternatives should be both medically and legally appropriate.

3. Alterations in Consciousness

Alterations in consciousness include both the level of consciousness and quality of consciousness. The former is characterized by a range of changes from mild transient lethargy to a complete loss of consciousness, such as a syncopal episode or complex generalized seizure. *Syncope* is sudden transient loss of consciousness that generally is not associated with a focal aura, but will have generalized presyncopal warning signs, such as dizziness or blurred vision, and is followed by a nonfocal neurological examination (9,10). Most causes of syncope are cardiological, although autonomic impairment or metabolic causes occur in approximately 30% of episodes. Syncope is statistically more common than seizures, although up to 5% of the population may have a seizure at some point in their life. Seizure activity results from abnormal synchronous neuronal discharge. The clinical manifestation of such a neuronal discharge depends on the site of origin and subsequent area of brain to which the seizure spreads. Generally, seizures will be more likely to have a focal warning aura, be more acute in onset, be lacking in a predisposing cardiac history or change in position, and have a more delayed and often focally abnormal postictal state. Tonic–clonic phenomena and incontinence are more often seen with seizures. Broadly, seizures can be grouped as either focal, when involving only limited motor or sensory manifestations, or complex partial or generalized, if a transient alteration or loss of consciousness occurs.

The history will often provide the clinician with enough evidence to pursue a focused evaluation. Most first episodes, however, should have baseline metabolic, cardiac, and neurological studies performed, including blood chemistry and hematology profiles, electrocardiogram (ECG), and CT or MRI scans.

Alterations in quality of consciousness are more complex phenomena to categorize and diagnose. The inner workings of the brain provide the individual with perception of the world and allow the person to interface with it. To define when a change in behavior or level of consciousness is significant is difficult at best. More so than even the evaluation of headache complaints, the diagnosis of changes in level or quality of consciousness require precision and completeness in history-taking. Two specific personal examples clearly stand out. The senior author had a very pleasant talk with a history professor while examining him for the ostensible complaint of forgetfulness and headaches. The general impression after the visit was that the professor was substantially smarter than the neurosurgeon and that his neurological examination was normal. Later the patient's wife called to outline a clear history of progressive change in behavior and early-morning headaches. The CT scan then demonstrated a bifrontal meningioma only slightly smaller than a pineapple. The second example is of a farmer from a rather isolated part of a nearby state, who presented with rather generalized complaints including right body weakness. At the end of the examination, the author was convinced that the patient had not only a right hemiparesis, but also a clear expressive dysphasia. After talking to the wife of the patient, their son, and the family physician over the telephone and obtaining an MRI scan of the head, which was normal, and of the spine, which was not, it became obvious that a regional dialect, a spinal cord tumor, and an inattentive physician were the dominant factors at play.

The first thing to be done in this setting is to determine that a change has occurred. The individual history, supplemented necessarily and obligatorily by the observations of family and friends, should allow this question to be answered. The nature of the change then becomes the next problem to solve. Is it a focal or diffuse process? What is its temporal course? Is it worsening, improving, or remaining stable? Are there obvious external factors: drugs, systemic illness, or social changes? These are obvious when reading the text in the office or hearing a lecture in school; in the reality of the emergency or examining room, the discipline to thoroughly explore the situation before acting is difficult to maintain but crucial to a satisfactory conclusion.

B. Localizing Value of Specific Neurological Signs

1. Supratentorial Lesions

The Mental Status Examination. The cerebral cortex constitutes the bulk of the mass within the human brain. Relatively small proportions of the cortex subserve the primary modalities of motor function and sensation. Most of the cerebral cortex provides associative neural networks for integration of input received through the primary sensory modalities, leading to human understanding and learning, which represent the higher cortical functions. The mental status examination is designed to test the functioning of these integrated neural networks. Formal mental status testing through neuropsychological testing batteries can help delineate specific deficits of higher cognitive function, but is outside the scope of the bedside or office clinical examination. However, a modified examination may be performed in the office to screen the functioning of large areas of the cerebral cortex in a succinct manner. When used appropriately, the mental status examination provides objective evidence of the presence or absence of cortical disease. A topographical display of the localizing value of particular aspects of the mental status examination is provided in Figure 1. Details of the mental status examination will be discussed further in the following paragraphs. The reader is referred to the excellent text by Strub and Black for an enjoyable and comprehensive discussion of the fine details of the mental status examination (11).

Frontal Lobe Lesions. Frontal lobe lesions are responsible for initiation of action and interpretation of emotion. Tumors within the frontal lobes produce changes in personality that vary from patient to patient. Symptoms are most prominent when both frontal lobes are involved, but can occur with unilateral lesions. Orbitofrontal tumors often cause disinhibition of behavior, manifest as social inappropriateness, quick irritability, profanity, lack of concern, and jocularity. Dorsal midline lesions often cause abulia with poor initiation of thought and motion. Lesions over

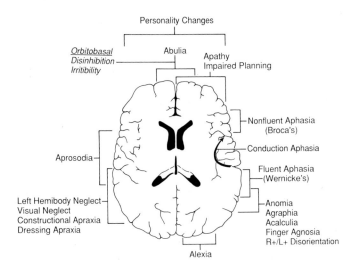

Figure 1   Cerebral localization: the mental status examination (see text for details).

the dorsolateral convexities tend to cause apathy, reduced drive, depressed mentation, and impaired planning.

Tumors within the premotor areas have subtle effects upon the neurological examination. Spasticity, contralateral ataxia, and frontal release signs occur. Destruction of the frontal eye fields by tumor may lead to a transient loss of voluntary gaze to the contralateral side and conjugate eye deviation toward the side of the lesion. Unilateral or bilateral midline lesions may lead to urinary incontinence or retention.

Aphasias are best characterized by defining specific deficits in fluency, comprehension, and repetition. A rapid screen aphasia battery, which tests naming, repetition, and comprehension, can be added to the basic neurological examination when the clinician notices reduced fluency, frequent word-finding pauses, or circumlocutory speech during the initial interview. Broca's aphasia is characterized by a nonfluent, motor aphasia with poor spontaneity of speech and dysarthria. Various degrees of such an "expressive" aphasia occur with lesions within the frontal lobes within or adjacent to Broca's area. Despite the clinician's natural tendency to forgive the minor error in speech, it is in the patient's best interest to pursue such findings until the examiner is comfortable that they are appropriate for the patient's level of education. Most aphasias are paralleled by similar defects in writing function.

Motor function is compromised when tumors arise from or compress the precentral sulcus. Spastic paralysis of the contralateral side of the face, arm or leg, or both, are seen. Changes may be subtle; the earliest finding may be the presence of a pronator drift or an inability to hop on one foot, and the clinician may rely on these findings to justify decisions when considering further diagnostic tests.

Seizures are frequently seen with frontal tumors. Focal motor seizures involving an arm or a leg may occur with tumors abutting the primary motor cortex. Partial complex seizures with predominant complex motor automatism or bicycling motion may occur with prefrontal or parasagittal lesions. Generalized seizures may also arise from the frontal lobes without a preceding aura.

Temporal Lobe Lesions.   The clinical presentation of tumors within the temporal lobes depends on the location and physiology of the particular lesion. Tumors within the anterior temporal lobe may remain clinically silent until quite large if their presence is not heralded by seizure activity. Motor deficits may occur by compression of frontal cortex along the Sylvian fissure in such tumors. In contrast, medial lesions may cause only a subtle loss of verbal memory on the dominant side, or visual spatial memory on the nondominant side, which may be quantified only by formal neuropsychological testing. Severe short-term memory loss caused by bilateral hippocampal tumor involvement is rarely seen, but may occur. Likewise, bilateral lesions of the primary auditory cortex are required before cortical deafness will occur. Such a lesion is more likely to occur from occlusive vascular disease.

Aphasia is seen with tumors within the posterior temporal lobe, near the temporal–parietal–occipital junction. Such lesions are characterized by deficits in comprehension, word-finding ability, and naming without affecting fluency. Fluent, nonsensical speech, with frequent paraphasic errors, is characteristic of the classic Wernicke's aphasia. On rare occasion, such a patient will be treated for psychosis before the true nature of the lesion is identified. The clinician is always justified in obtaining an imaging study in the confused or nonsensical patient who has previously behaved normally.

Parietal Lobe Lesions. Parietal lobe lesions may affect primary sensory cortex or adjacent association cortex. Lesions within the primary sensory cortex rarely lead to complete sensory loss, but they will lead to an inability to identify more subtle and complex sensory input, such as the ability to identify objects placed within the hand (stereognosis) or symbols written within the hand (graphesthesia).

Parietal association cortex is responsible for the integration of auditory and visual inputs; therefore, parietal lobe lesions lead to a combination of deficits in word comprehension and multimodality integration that can present as various clinical syndromes. Deficits in language comprehension and naming can arise from tumors near the temporoparietal junction. More posteriorly, tumors arising near the angular gyrus may cause all or part of the symptoms collectively described as Gerstman's syndrome in which agraphia, acalculia, finger agnosia, and right/left disorientation occur. Lesions at the parieto-occipital border will lead to alexia. Involvement of the white matter tract connecting the parietal and frontal lobes will lead to a conduction aphasia, in which language comprehension and fluency are unaffected, but the patient is unable to repeat phrases and may show deficits in naming. A similar hierarchy of the nonverbal comprehension of speech exists in the nondominant hemisphere. Deficits in the ability to express appropriate emotionally labile syntax or comprehend nonverbal cues, such as inflection and intonation in speech, have been classified as aprosodias. The antomical localization of these functions within the nondominant hemisphere correlates roughly with similar deficits in motor or comprehension abilities in the dominant hemisphere.

Neglect syndromes can arise with parietal lesions in either hemisphere; however, they are seen more frequently with nondominant hemispheric lesions. Neglect syndromes may be subtle, with the only finding on examination being extinction on one-half of the body to bilaterally presented simultaneous tactile stimuli, or they can be manifest as a complete inattention to one-half of the environment, including the patient's own body. *Apraxia*, the inability to formulate and perform complex motor behaviors, may be seen with lesions of either hemisphere. However, the clinical syndrome of left hemibody and visual spatial neglect in the presence of a constructional apraxia and dressing apraxia strongly suggests a lesion of the nondominant posterior parietal region.

Occipital Lobe Lesions. Occipital lobe lesions lead to visual field deficits in most patients. Homologous deficits of all or one part of the one-half of the visual field will occur with unilateral occipital lobe lesions. Disorders of eye movement, including the loss of smooth pursuit movements and failure of visual fixation can occur. Positive symptomatology, such as flashing lights or colored objects, may occur. Alexia may occur if the dominant occipital lobe and commissural fibers traveling through the posterior corpus callosum are interrupted. Associated deficits, such as agraphia and the inability to recognize colors and faces, may occur with encroachment upon the parietal occipital junction.

Infratentorial Lesions. Infratentorial lesions cause symptoms by compressing or invading brain stem structures, or by causing hydrocephalus. Brain stem nuclei are located in close proximity to one another, allowing involvement by tumors of multiple cranial nerves or ascending or descending pathways. Localization is aided by the findings of associated cranial nerve deficits. Lesions within the midbrain often show ocular disturbances; those within the midpons will involve the 5th, 6th, and 7th cranial nerves; and those tumors encroaching on the medulla will be associated with difficulties with balance and glutition. Although the brain stem syndromes associated with ischemic stroke may involve only millimeters of a specific region, most brain stem findings will be more diffuse and possibly more subtle, as compressive lesions may only partially interfere with normal function.

Lesions involving the midbrain tectum often lead to disorders of gaze, which are collectively referred to as the dorsal midbrain syndromes, of which Parinaud's syndrome is most commonly known. Defects in vertical gaze, conversion, and lid retraction, pupillary abnormalities with disturbances of accommodation, station and light-near dissociation, and rotational nystagmus are seen with dorsal midbrain compression. The lesions most commonly responsible for such compression are the posterior third ventricular tumors, of which pineal region tumors are most common. However, metastatic or infiltrating astrocytomas may provoke all or part of the defects discussed. In children and infants with hydrocephalus, bilateral lid retraction and paralysis of upward gaze, known as the "sunset sign," may occur.

Third nerve palsies, with or without associated long-tract findings, may occur with tumors involving the posterior fossa. Intrinsic lesions, such as astrocytomas, may cause an ipsilateral third nerve palsy and contralateral ataxia (Benedikt's syndrome), or hemiplegia (Weber's syndrome). In addition, extrinsic mass lesions within the interpeduncular fossa may cause Weber's syndrome by compressing the cerebral peduncle and exiting third nerve roots. Compression of the third nerve alone within the subarachnoid space is most commonly seen with posterior communicating artery aneurysms. Likewise, an isolated, complete third nerve palsy with pupillary sparing suggests an ischemic neuropathy, as is seen in diabetics, rather than a compressive neuropathy from tumor. This can be explained physiologically by the fact that pupillary innervation is most peripheral within the third nerve, making it susceptible to compression, but relatively resistant to ischemia, as it receives blood supply from vessels within the nerve and also externally from the vasa nervorum. Rarely, chordomas, clival meningiomas, or pituitary tumors with lateral, rather than superior, invasion may cause isolated fourth nerve findings (12).

IV. CLINICAL PRESENTATION BY TUMOR TYPE

Significant localizing information may be derived from the general neurological examination, which has been discussed in the previous pages. In addition, general classifications of brain tumors exist that help describe the most common presenting scenarios and that help guide the diagnostic workup before biopsy. An understanding of the "personality" of these different tumors should be helpful for the clinician who is presented with a patient complaining of new neurological symptoms. The focus of the second half of this chapter will be to aid the clinician in understanding the relative incidence, location, and predominant signs and symptoms of over 90% of adult brain tumors. The most common locations of primary brain tumors are presented diagrammatically in Figure 2. The relative incidence of occurrence and average postoperative survivals are presented as well to provide a sense of the likelihood that a patient may harbor a particular tumor type (Fig. 3).

The clinical presentation of any intracranial mass lesion is dependent on the histological appearance, rate of growth, location, fate of adjacent tissue, and age of the patient. Tumors intrinsic to the brain parenchyma may either displace surrounding tissue or destroy it. If such a tumor resides in eloquent brain, then focal symptoms may develop early in the disease; for

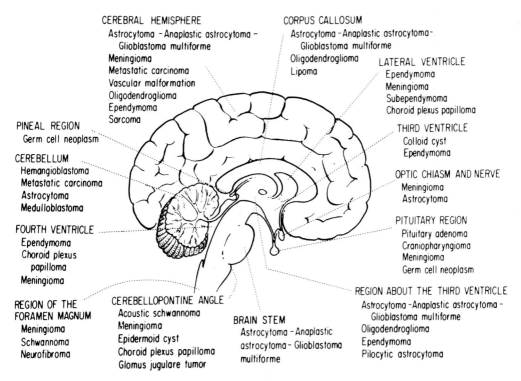

Figure 2 Topographic distribution of intracranial tumors during adulthood. (From Ref. 13)

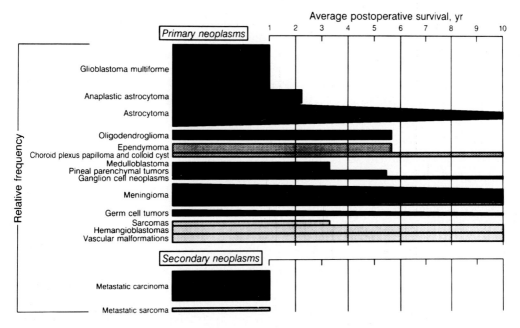

Figure 3 Central nervous system tumors: incidence and survival rates. Primary and metastatic tumefactions of the brain are represented here. Their relative incidences and average postoperative survivals are indicated, respectively, by the width and length of the individual arms. (From Ref. 13)

example, the patient with a low-grade astrocytoma in the motor cortex may present with subtle hand clumsiness that limits the ability to perform work duties. However, many areas of the brain are relatively silent clinically and may allow substantial tumor growth to occur before subtle neurological symptoms arise, as in the elderly patient, brought in by family members who can no longer tolerate the person's "forgetfulness," in whom a right temporal lobe malignant astrocytoma is found. Extrinsic lesions show the same dependence on location for clinical presentation; a parasellar meningioma may compress the optic nerve and become clinically manifest by visual disturbances when it is smaller than the size of a pea, whereas the same tumor originating only centimeters away, within the olfactory groove, may grow to the size of a lemon before personality changes become manifest and lead to diagnosis. Tumors may cause symptoms based on irritative phenomenon (i.e., seizures, aseptic meningitis) or on ablative phenomenon, such as visual defects or hemiparesis. Confusion and lethargy may be due to direct tumor involvement, to increased intracranial pressure, or to hydrocephalus. Cranial nerve palsies may be due to compression or to invasion of cranial nerves in the subarachnoid space, stretch from hydrocephalus, or direct invasion of the nucleus of origin by an infiltrating tumor within the brain stem.

Clearly, the various clinical manifestations of brain tumors defy strict classification. A general understanding of the most common symptoms and signs of tumors should be within the reach of most clinicians. The following text is designed to provide a succinct introduction to the most common primary brain tumors for general use. In addition, sufficient detail has been included to make this section a quick reference source for those clinicians who wish to update their knowledge base when confronted with a particular clinical situation.

A. Glial Tumors

Glial tumors account for approximately half of all intracranial tumors. They are derived from astrocytes, oligodendroglia, and ependymal cells. Most gliomas in adults are derived from astrocytes and can be classified into five subtypes: fibrillary, gemistocytic, protoplasmic, pilocytic, and subependymal giant-cell tumors. Almost all adult gliomas are fibrillary astrocytomas. Fibrillary astrocytomas display a wide range of growth characteristics from low-grade, indolent lesions, to high-grade, malignant glioblastomas. The gemistocytic and protoplasmic astrocytomas follow a clinical course similar to the intermediate-grade tumor known as anaplastic astrocytoma (13) and will not be discussed separately. Pilocytic astrocytomas and subependymal giant cell astrocytomas represent distinct biological and clinical subtypes that warrant separate discussion, despite their relatively uncommon occurrence.

1. Fibrillary Astrocytomas

The classification of fibrillary astrocytomas remains controversial and confusing despite several formal attempts at reclassification in the past decade. Pathologically, these tumors form a continuum ranging from the low-grade, well-differentiated lesion that is barely distinguishable from normal brain, to the intermediate, moderately dedifferentiated tumor commonly known as the anaplastic astrocytomas, to the highly anaplastic, bizarre-appearing, malignant neoplasm know as glioblastoma multiforme. It is likely that these neoplasms represent a pathological continuum not only in different patients, but also chronologically in the individual patient. In patients who receive serial biopsies over time, the evolution from well-differentiated, to anaplastic astrocytoma, to glioblastoma multiforme can be followed (14). The difficulty in developing a universally accepted classification system stems from the semantic limitations in defining the diffuse melding of one tumor type into another. Regardless of the classification system used, it is crucial for the primary care physician to have a working understanding of the natural history of these primary astrocytic tumors, as the clinical presentation differs among them.

Low-Grade Astrocytomas. Low-grade, or well-differentiated, astrocytomas, represent the most indolent form of the fibrillary astrocytomas. They represent 10–30% of all astrocytomas. The mean age of presentation is 35 years of age, with a male preponderance of 1.3:1. Computed tomography most often shows a focal, nonenhancing mass lesion in the frontal or temporal lobes. The MRI scan reveals a nonenhancing lesion with increased signal changes on T1- and T2-weighted imaging. Often, these signal changes are accompanied by little to no mass effect, making MRI the superior diagnostic modality. Consequently, as more subtle changes are appreciated on imaging studies, the mean age of diagnosis has fallen, and the presenting clinical scenario has changed (15). In a study including patients diagnosed within the CT era, 90% presented with seizures, and 78% had a normal neurological examination (16).

The signs and symptoms of this particular group of patients are particularly subtle and require and increased awareness on the part of the physician to pursue diagnostic evaluation. The hallmark of these tumors is seizures, which may be of some localizing value. Tumors in the frontal lobes may cause complex partial seizures with prominent arm posturing, such as a fencing stance or a bicycling motion of the legs. Temporal lobe tumors often begin with an aura, followed by loss of contact and oral or manual automatism. Periolandic lesions may cause focal motor seizures. Occipital tumors may cause positive visual symptoms, such as flashing white or colored spots or lines. Such symptoms in an adult, particularly one with no previous history of migraine, provide sufficient ground to justify a diagnostic-imaging study, even in the presence of a normal neurological examination. The duration of seizures may precede the diagnosis by many years, with up to 40% of patients having seizures for more than 5 years before diagnosis (16).

Anaplastic Astrocytomas. The anaplastic fibrillary astrocytoma follows a biological and clinical course more aggressive than the low-grade astrocytoma but does not share all of the malignant features seen on pathological examination, nor does it follow the same rapidly fatal clinical course as the glioblastoma multiforme. Patients with these tumors represent a clinical cohort who appear to have a different clinical presentation and prognosis than either the more benign or the more malignant astrocytomas; however, it is important for the clinician to understand that an individual patient's presentation and fate are dependent on the relative degree of anaplasia present in that particular tumor.

Anaplastic astrocytomas occur at a mean age of 45 years, which is roughly a decade later than low-grade astrocytomas and a decade before the presentation of gliobastoma. They occur in relative proportion to the amount of white matter seen in the brain; over 90% occur in the white matter of the cerebral hemispheres, with a relative distribution proportional to the volume of each lobe (Fig. 4). Symptoms are present for an average of 6–24 months before diagnosis of the tumor, reflecting a more rapid growth rate than seen in low-grade astrocytomas. Headache and alteration in mentation are seen in 50–70% of patients. On neurological examination, 50% will show signs of altered mentation; 60% will show signs of hemiparesis. Roughly half will have either a failure of vision, hemianopsia, or papilledema (17). The reader should keep in mind that the incidence for these symptoms is derived from a study that, in part, was performed before the CT era. It is likely that more sophisticated, noninvasive imaging will lead to earlier diagnosis in the face of more subtle neurological symptoms and may help stabilize the progression of the disease (15,18).

Astrocytomas can occur within the diencephalon, optic pathways, or brain stem, and occur in adults with a frequency that is roughly one-tenth that seen in the pediatric population. In the adult, anaplastic astrocytomas or glioblastoma multiforme will occur more frequently than the low-grade lesion associated with childhood. Signs of a rapidly growing mass lesion within critical brain stem parenchyma and symptoms of increased intracranial pressure are the most common presentations. Hydrocephalus caused by obstruction of CSF pathways is common. Radiation therapy can slow progression, but median survival remains no better than 1–3 years (19).

Glioblastoma Multiforme. Glioblastoma multiforme accounts for one-half of all astrocytic tumors, and approximately one-quarter of all primary brain tumors seen in adult patients. The

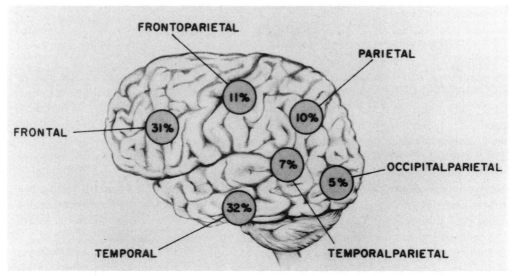

Figure 4   Distribution of malignant gliomas within the adult brain. (From Ref. 54)

mean age of presentation is 62. The incidence of glioblastomas increases with each decade of life, and shows a greater male preponderance in each passing decade. Overall, the male/female ratio is 1.5:1 (13,20,21). Glioblastomas are highly anaplastic, infiltrating tumors that invade and destroy surrounding brain tissue. Necrosis is a pathological hallmark of the lesion. This is represented on CT studies as a central area of decreased tissue density, surrounded by an outer ring of abnormally enhancing tissue, which represents breakdown of the blood–brain barrier within the advancing margins of the tumor. These tumors may present as a malignant transformation of a known preexisting anaplastic astrocytoma, or may present de novo in a patient with no known previous disease. If left untreated, survival is usually measured in weeks to months.

Symptom duration at the time of presentation is fewer than 6 months in two-thirds of patients. Symptoms lasting significantly longer than this suggest dedifferentiation of a preexisting astrocytoma. Patients present with symptoms of a rapidly growing intracranial mass with signs of increased intracranial pressure and focal neurological deficits. Headache, with associated papilledema is present in over 60% of patients. Vomiting, presumably from increased intracranial pressure, is present in one-third of patients. Mental status changes are present in two-thirds, and one-third will show a decreased level of consciousness. Hemiparesis is present in 70%; over one-third will have a hemianopia and one-third will have aphasia. Seizures are the presenting symptom in only 20% of patients (17).

2.   Oligodendrogliomas

Oligodendrogliomas are low-grade neoplastic tumors derived from oligodendrocytes. They occur as tumors composed solely of oligodendroglia, or can be found as a component in a mixed tumor in which both oligodendroglial and astrocytic cell lines are represented. Oligodendrogliomas account for 5–10% of all glial tumors, and mixed oligoastrocytomas represent another 3% of glial tumors (3,19). They show a similar heterogeneity of tissue type from the more well-differentiated, clinically indolent tumor to the poorly differentiated, malignant tumor. Likewise, they show the same propensity to dedifferentiate with time to a more biologically aggressive tumor (22).

The clinical presentation of both tumor types is similar to that seen in low-grade astrocytomas, with few minor exceptions. Oligodendrogliomas present with a similarly high incidence of seizures, being present in up to 88% of patients, and show the same long interval between symptom onset and tumor recognition (23). Mean age of presentation is 44 years of age, with a male/female ration of 2:1 (24). They occur slightly more often in the frontal lobes and have a tendency to show calcification on CT imaging. Surgical resection is usually the initial treatment; however, tumor recurrence can eventually be expected. Survival rates are better than those seen for astrocytomas of similar grades (15,23,24).

3. Pilocytic Astrocytomas

Pilocytic astrocytomas are a distinct subgroup of astrocytomas that differ biologically from the more common fibrillary astrocytoma. They are relatively benign, slowly growing lesions that show less tendency to invade surrounding brain parenchyma and have minimal tendency toward malignant dedifferentiation. Pilocytic astrocytomas may arise from the optic nerves, chiasm, or tract, hypothalamus, brain stem, cerebellum, or cerebral hemispheres. These lesions usually occur during childhood and are discussed more in Chapter 4.

Pilocytic astrocytomas that arise from the cerebral hemispheres may present in young adults. Tumors that arise in the cerebral hemispheres are usually associated with large cystic components that produce significant mass effect. Symptoms of focal neurological deficits referable to the site of origin will occur in two-thirds of the patients. Headache and papilledema from increased intracranial pressure will present in two-thirds of patients. In addition, two of three patients will have seizures. The goal of treatment is gross total resection. Long-term survival and seizure control are common with complete excision (19,25,26).

4. Giant Cell Subependymal Tumors

Subependymal giant cell astrocytomas are glial tumors that arise in the subependymal layer of the lateral ventricle. They are slow-growing, relatively benign lesions, with the pathologically characteristic giant astrocyte from which the tumor derives its name. These tumors are seen frequently with tuberous sclerosis but can occur independently. Subependymal giant cell astrocytomas may be found during neuroimaging procedures in a patient with tuberous sclerosis who is being evaluated for mental retardation and seizures. These rare tumors have a tendency to originate in the region of the foramen of Monro. In this position, they can easily grow into the lateral ventricles and cause obstruction of CSF outflow through the foramen of Monro, leading to symptoms of hydrocephalus (19).

5. Choroid Plexus Papillomas

Choroid plexus papillomas are benign glial tumors that arise from ependymal cells present in normal choroid plexus. They are rare tumors, representing fewer than 1% of glial tumors. They are far more common in children, in whom they tend to occur in the lateral ventricle or third ventricle and present clinically at a mean age of 1 year with hydrocephalus, macrocephaly, and bilateral sixth nerve palsies caused by the hydrocephalus. In adults, these lesions are more common in the posterior fossa. They occur in the fourth ventricle, where they cause hydrocephalus, or in the cerebellopontine angle, where they arise from choroid plexus exiting at the foramen of Lushka. In this latter position, they cause symptoms by compression of the cerebellar hemisphere or focal cranial nerve deficits through the same mechanism. Hydrocephalus appears more likely to be caused by obstruction of CSF flow or destruction of absorptive mechanisms by a high CSF protein content than by an overproduction of CSF; however, investigation to support both hypotheses is still required (27,28). When technically possible, complete resection should be performed and leads to long-term cure.

6. Ependymomas

Ependymomas are highly malignant primary brain tumors that arise from the wall of the ventricles, or arise from fetal rests of ependymal cells in extraventricular sites. Approximately two-thirds of ependymomas occur in the posterior fossa, where they usually arise from the floor of the fourth ventricle. Obstruction of the fourth ventricle can lead to hydrocephalus, papilledema, compression of the cerebellum, leading to ataxia and displacement of the cerebellar tonsils into the foramen magnum, which may in turn lead to neck pain and stiffness. Ependymomas occur in the supratentorial space in approximately one-third of the patients. Supratentorial lesions are found in young adults. Those tumors that arise from the ventricular walls will produce signs of ventricular obstruction, hydrocephalus, and increased intracranial pressure. Ependymomas arising in the cerebral hemispheres will cause focal signs referable to the site of origin, and are associated with seizure activity in 30% of patients (19,29).

B. Neuronal Neoplasms

1. Gangliogliomas

Gangliogliomas are mixed tumors that are composed of neoplastic glial and neuronal cell types. The incidence of occurrence ranges from 0.4–7.6%, with the higher percentages being seen in pediatric series. Tumors are usually recognized in teens or young adults. Seventy-five to one-hundred percent present with seizures, often during the teenage years. Seizures often occur for years before the detection of the tumor (30,31).

Tumors occur within the temporal and frontal lobes in most cases, but can occur anywhere, including the deep central gray matter, hypothalamus, and cerebellum. They are slowly growing, indolent lesions that may not recur if completely resected. Therefore, temporal tumors that present with seizures carry the best prognosis. If undetected, tumors may grow to an excessive size before recognition. In such cases, patients may present with signs of intracranial mass lesions, with headache, nausea and vomiting, and occasionally focal neurological signs that localize to the site of origin. The clinical course after partial resection is variable. Long-term survival is common. Recurrence and progression of symptoms may occur in some, but not all, patients, giving the disease a far more favorable prognosis than is seen with glial tumors (30).

2. Neurocytomas

Central neurocytomas are rare intracranial lesions that have received increased attention within the neurosurgical literature. They are presented here for completeness. Histopathologically, this tumor is characterized by a uniform neoplastic cell population, with features of neuronal differentiation. They occur most often in young adults. Tumors are intraventricular in location, and usually present with symptoms and signs of hydrocephalus, with headache, nausea, visual impairment, papilledema, and disturbances of mentation. A highly variable interval of preoperative symptoms can be observed, with an average period of 11 months. Surgical resection is the treatment of choice, and can lead to long-term cure; however, recurrences, with or without malignant histological cytology, have been reported recently, suggesting that the biological behavior of these lesions may not be as favorable as previously assumed (10).

C. Meningiomas

Meningiomas account for 20% of intracranial tumors. They occur intracranially twice as often in women as in men, beginning after puberty and occurring with increasing incidence until the eighth decade of life, with a peak annual incidence of 7.2:100,000 (21). There is a marked increase in symptomatic occurrence between 40 and 60 years of age. Multiple meningiomas may be present in 1–2% of symptomatic patients. Incidental meningiomas may be found in up to 2–3% of autopsy series (21), which suggests that a large percentage of meningiomas remain asymptomatic throughout life. Approximately 2% of meningiomas occur in children. When present, they are likely to be large and are often more malignant than those seen in adults (32).

Several risk factors have been identified in association with meningioma. Cranial irradiation increases the incidence of meningioma. Meningiomas occur more frequently in patients with both central and von Recklinghausen's neurofibromatosis (32). Rare familial association has been documented. Head injury, particularly with depressed skull fracture, may affect the development of some meningiomas, but this is not a major etiologic factor (33).

Meningiomas are seen more frequently in patients with breast cancer. Interestingly, 41% of patients who have both a meningioma and either breast cancer or a female reproductive tract malignancy will harbor a third primary malignancy (33). Therefore, hypervigilance in this small group of patients is of paramount importance.

Many clinicians have had the uncomfortable experience of treating a patient who becomes symptomatic from a meningioma during pregnancy. Despite this clinical observation, a recent study has not confirmed an increased incidence (33). Those tumors that do become symptomatic during pregnancy tend to do so in the second and third trimesters. Proposed causal factors for symptoms include increased tumor mass due to hydroscopic swelling and vacuolation, engorgement of tumor vessels, or sodium retention, with increased fluid volume and parenchymal edema of the surrounding brain. Symptoms have been reported to regress after completion of pregnancy (21,33).

Various pathological classifications have been proposed for meningiomas. More than 80% of benign tumors belong to the meningotheliomatous, transitional, or fibroblastic varieties (21). A recurrence rate of 10–15% has been cited for benign lesions that were thought to be totally excised (13), but recurrence varies widely, depending on location of tumor and degree of resection. Fewer than 10% of meningiomas are malignant. Clinical criteria for malignancy include rapid recurrence, distant metastasis, and direct brain invasion. Pathological criteria include high cellularity, necrosis, mitosis, and abnormal sheeting of cells. Hemangiopericytomas are historically a subclassification of angioblastic meningiomas, which are currently the subject of renewed clinical interest (13). These dural-based lesions show no male/female bias, occur earlier in life, with a peak incidence in the fourth through sixth decades, and show a high tendency to recur and metastasize. Clinical symptoms may be referable to the organ bearing the metastasis, of which the most common are lung and bone. Ten-year survival is no better than 40% (13,15).

Meningiomas may arise from any surface of the cranium, and are most common along the cerebral convexities. They may occur near suture lines or along reflections of the dura, such as the falx, sphenoid wing, tuberculum sellae, or tentorium. Meningiomas arise from arachnoidal cells, without necessarily having an attachment to the adjacent dura mater, leading to their presence within the ventricles, or rarely, from deep within the Sylvian fissure. A pictorial display of the most common sites of occurrence is provided in Figure 5 to aid in understanding the relative sites of occurrence within the brain.

Meningiomas are extrinsic brain lesions that produce symptoms from compression of adjacent brain or cranial nerves. Mass effect may result from tumor volume, adjacent brain edema, or obstruction of CSF pathways. Meningiomas irritate adjacent brain parenchyma, leading to seizures in 40% of patients. Hyperostosis occurs frequently in bone adjacent to or infiltrated by meningioma, and can lead to stenosis of cranial nerve exit foramen or facial deformity. Symptoms vary according to the location of the tumor and the reaction of structures adjacent to it, and will be discussed according to specific sites. In general, headache is the most common symptom, being present in 36% of patients in one study, followed by confusion, focal weakness, and seizures. Paresis was the most frequently found sign, occurring in 30% of patients. Only 26% of patients had a normal neurological examination (21).

The many potential sites for meningioma attachment leads to a vast array of possible clinical presentations. Each is relatively uncommon; however, many are fairly stereotypic for mass lesions in particular locations and may be of great localizing help to the clinician confronted with a particular complaint. Many of the localizing signs and symptoms of a meningioma can be extrapolated to other brain tumors that present in similar locations.

1. Convexity Meningiomas

Meningiomas occurring over the convexities of the cerebral hemispheres are most common, accounting for one-third of all tumors. Symptoms vary according to location. Frontal tumors may be silent for long periods and may be quite large by the time of detection. These frontal tumors do not generally show the same symptoms of dementia, personality change, and incontinence that are associated with the more medial parasagittal or olfactory groove meningiomas; rather, symptoms of increased intracranial pressure, with visual blurring, diplopia, and papilledema occur. An expressive aphasia may be present caused by compression of Broca's area. Eventual motor involvement of the arm and face may occur with enlarging tumor size, but the leg remains relatively spared with convexity lesions. Tumors located more posteriorly, adjacent to primary motor or sensory cortex, are usually much smaller at the time of diagnosis, as symptoms occur

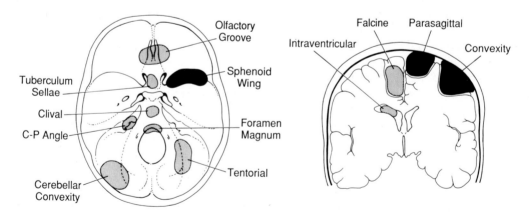

Figure 5 Meningiomas: sites of origin and relative incidence of occurrence. Solid regions represent the most common sites of origin. Stippled regions indicate uncommon sites of origin. No inference about the size of the tumor should be construed from this diagram.

early. Specifically, focal motor seizures of the face or hand are the most common presenting symptoms of perirolandic convexity meningiomas. Parietal meningiomas may cause sensory seizures, or a receptive aphasia, if located over the dominant hemisphere. Tumors over the temporal or occipital convexities are uncommon (34).

2. Parasagittal Meningiomas

Parasagittal and falcine meningiomas represent one-fourth of meningiomas. Anterior tumors are more likely to cause dementia because of bifrontal involvement. Posterior tumors show focal motor signs with either seizures or weakness of one or both legs. Occipital lesions present with headache and partial or complete hemianopia. Epilepsy arising from the occipital cortex, with associated positive visual phenomenon, is uncommon. Occlusion of the sagittal sinus by tumor occurs slowly and usually allows the development of collateral venous drainage. Therefore, sagittal sinus obstruction is usually asymptomatic unless venous stasis within the stenotic sinus leads to acute thrombosis (34).

3. Skull Base Meningiomas

Meningiomas may arise from the skull base. Most anteriorly they may originate from the olfactory groove or orbital roof. Posteriorly they may arise near the anterior clinoid and parasellar region, cavernous sinus, or sphenoid wing. Clinical presentation is highly variable and dependent on the neural structures adjacent to the tumor.

Meningiomas along the sphenoid wing are "en plaque" meningiomas, meaning that they have a diffuse dural attachment, are flatter, and are more likely to invade adjoining bone or dural structures. Dural invasion along the medial sphenoid wing can lead to cavernous sinus involvement, with multiple cranial neuropathies, involving the 3rd, 4th, 6th, and first two divisions of the 5th cranial nerves. Medial extension can lead to involvement of the paranasal sinuses. Stenosis of the optic foramen by hyperostosis or direct tumor expansion can lead to a compressive optic neuropathy. Hyperostosis along the sphenoid wing can lead to exophthalmos or rarely, facial deformity, if the malar eminence is involved. Intracranial extension along the lateral sphenoid wing leads to signs of increased intracranial pressure or signs of a frontal or temporal mass lesion, depending on the direction of tumor extension. Rarely, tumors may arise solely within Meckel's cave. Such tumors will present with trigeminal nerve dysfunction and pain. Medial extension may lead to cavernous sinus involvement, and posterior extension will lead to symptoms of a cerebellopontine angle tumor.

Olfactory groove meningiomas often become quite large before detection. Patients may present for evaluation of dementia, failing vision, headache, or seizures. More than 90% have anosmia on examination, but most will not voice this as a spontaneous complaint (35). The rare clinical triad of the Foster–Kennedy syndrome with anosmia, ipsilateral compressive optic neuropathy, and papilledema in the opposite fundus from increased intracranial pressure from the large tumor mass, classically occur in these patients. Tuberculum sellae, or parasellar tumors occur just posterior to the olfactory groove meningiomas but present quite differently. They lie adjacent to the optic nerves and usually cause symptoms of asymmetric visual loss owing to compression of the chiasm or optic nerve and are often quite small on presentation because of this early clinical manifestation.

4. Intraventricular Meningiomas

Most intraventricular meningiomas occur in the lateral ventricles and are large by the time of diagnosis. The most common presenting symptoms are headache, personality changes, and disturbances of vision. Seventy-two percent show a homonymous visual field defect, 62% showed contralateral weakness, and aphasia was seen in 50% of patients when the lesion occurred in the dominant hemisphere (15).

5. *Posterior Fossa Meningiomas*

Posterior fossa meningiomas account for 6–12% of all meningiomas (15,21). They occur most commonly along the tentorium, cerebellar hemispheres, and cerebellopontine angle, but they can also be found along the clivus and the anterior margin of the foramen magnum. Clinical syndromes are specific to location.

Meningiomas of the cerebellar pontine angle are the most common posterior fossa meningiomas. Their presentation is similar, but not identical with that seen with acoustic neuromas, and they are presented for discussion under that heading.

Tumors of the tentorium may expand both above and below the tentorium. Extension into the occipital lobes may cause visual field defects or seizures. Inferior expansion can lead to brain stem and cerebellar compression, gait disturbance, and ataxia. Long-standing progressive facial numbness and eighth nerve dysfunction can occur. Some patients have obstructive hydrocephalus and increased intracranial pressure (15,34). Tumors over cerebellar hemispheres lead to appendicular signs or, when larger, cause obstructive hydrocephalus.

Foramen magnum meningiomas, while uncommon, are frequently included in the differential diagnosis of posterior fossa syndromes and cervical spondylosis and, therefore, warrant discussion. They are difficult tumors to diagnose, as the general symptoms are common with many other diseases, and truly localizing signs are minimal. Half of patients present with suboccipital or posterior neck pain that worsens with neck movements. Dysesthesias is one or both upper extremities is the most common presenting symptom. A cartwheeling motor involvement of the extremities often follows, in which weakness of one arm will be followed by weakness in the ipsilateral leg, then the contralateral leg, then the arm. Paresis of the spinal accessory nerve occurs in 25%, and hypalgesia in the C-2 dermatome, when present, is a reliable localizing sign (15,34). The foramen magnum is routinely included on most diagnostic studies of the brain stem or cervical spine to avoid missing this lesion. Clival meningiomas are less common, and symptoms are often long-standing before detection. In general, patients show a progression of cranial nerve palsies, cerebellar signs, pyramidal tract deficits, and hydrocephalus (15).

D. Schwannomas

Schwannomas are benign neoplasms of Schwann cell origin. Schwann cells supply myelin to peripheral nerves and, therefore, schwannomas must originate from distal portions of the cranial nerves once the oligodendroglia, which myelinate the proximal several millimeters of nerves exiting the brain stem, are replaced by Schwann cells. Schwannomas tend to arise from sensory nerves. The vestibular portion of the eighth cranial nerve is most commonly involved, giving rise to the vestibular schwannoma, which is more commonly referred to as the acoustic neuroma or acoustic neurinoma. Rarely, schwannomas may arise from the fifth cranial nerve and account for fewer than 1% of intracranial tumors (36). Schwannomas occur most often in the fifth and sixth decades of life and show a relatively equal male/female ratio (35).

1. *Acoustic Neuroma (Schwannoma)*

The hallmark clinical presentation of the acoustic neurinoma is unilateral sensory neural hearing loss, with loss of high-tone frequencies and speech discrimination predominating (34). The patient may complain of losing the ability to understand talk on the telephone with one ear. Tinnitus and dizziness are common, but true vertigo is rare. As the tumor expands out of the internal auditory canal into the cerebellopontine angle, it will stretch and compress adjacent nerves. The facial nerve (cranial nerve VII) is remarkably resistant to stretch and is rarely involved until late in the disease, when the tumor is quite large. However, the fifth nerve is susceptible to compression, primarily in tumors larger than 3 cm in diameter. Progressive diminution of the corneal reflex, followed by facial numbness will occur as the tumor enlarges. Ticlike pain is uncommon. Therefore, a patient with unilateral hearing loss and facial numbness, or a diminished corneal reflex, should be considered to have an acoustic neuroma until proved otherwise by neuroimaging procedures; gadolinium-enhanced MRI is the most sensitive diagnostic test available today (38).

With further tumor enlargement, compression of the cerebellum and brain stem will occur, with associated ataxia and long tract findings. Lower cranial nerve findings can occur with downward growth of large lesions, with difficulty in swallowing and in aspiration, and with vocal cord paresis and hoarseness developing from 9th, 10th, and 11th cranial nerve palsies. Rarely, hydrocephalus and papilledema will occur from obstruction of CSF outflow pathways.

The differential diagnosis of cerebellopontine angle lesions include many uncommon neuropathological entities. Of these, the meningioma is most likely to occur and is of interest clinically as the presentation is slightly different. The fifth nerve and seventh nerve are involved before hearing function is impaired. Facial pain is more common than is seen with acoustic neurinomas and may mimic the lancinating pain of tic douloureux (38).

Other rare tumors may invade the cerebellopontine angle. They include epidermoid or dermoid cysts, arachnoid cysts, exophytic pontine gliomas, cerebellar hemangioblastomas, choroid plexus papillomas, and skull base lesions. Any such tumor will usually present with a combination of one or multiple cranial nerve palsies, involving the 5th through 12th nerves as they exit the brain stem, and may have associated cerebellar signs or long tract findings caused by cerebellar or brain stem compression.

2. *Trigeminal Schwannomas*

Trigeminal schwannomas represent fewer than 1% of intracranial tumors. They are often discovered incidentally and may not present a clinical problem. When symptomatic, however, they most commonly present with trigeminal dysfunction. Diminished facial sensation with diminished corneal reflex is the most common finding. Facial pain is common, but true trigeminal neuralgia is uncommon.

Posterior fossa extension can occur; therefore, multiple cranial neuropathies primarily involving the 6th, 7th, and 8th cranial nerves are common. Cerebellar signs and long-tract findings are seen in up to one-fourth of patients, owing to posterior fossa compression. In fact, fewer than one-fourth of patients will have symptoms referable to the trigeminal nerve alone (36). Therefore, the possibility of a trigeminal nerve tumor may be suspected in the patient who presents with facial pain, trigeminal dysfunction and associated cranial nerve palsies, and long-tract findings.

E. Pituitary Adenomas (see also Chap. 11)

Pituitary adenomas are benign, slowly expanding lesions that arise from the anterior body of the pituitary. They represent 10–20% of all primary intracranial tumors and are almost twice as likely to occur in women as in men (20,21). Traditionally, pituitary adenomas were classified into chromophobic, basophilic, or acidophilic adenomas in an attempt to relate hormonal activity with histology. This system has proved inadequate as modern technology has permitted classification based on immunocytochemistry and electron microscopy. Tumors are now classified according to their hormonal activity and size on presentation. Microadenomas are tumors that measure less than 10 mm. They are usually hormonally active, which leads to their discovery. Macroadenomas measure more than 10 mm. Most macroadenomas do not secrete physiologically active hormones. Those tumors that do produce biologically active hormones will most commonly secrete prolactin. Tumors that secrete growth hormone or corticotropin (ACTH) will cause acromegaly or Cushing's disease, respectively. Tumors that produce gonadotropic hormones or thyroid-stimulating hormone are extremely rare. Occasionally, more than one hormone may be produced by an adenoma; however, usually these subunits are immunoreactive but not biologically active.

The clinical hallmark of the pituitary macroadenoma is a bitemporal hemianopia caused by compression of the optic chiasm. Symmetric involvement of the chiasm is the most usual presenting sign seen with pituitary adenomas. Asymmetric involvement of the optic nerves and chiasm may occur, depending on the size of the lesion and direction in which the tumor extends. Bedside screening tests will exclude many large adenomas. The presence of an afferent pupillary defect, also known as the Marcus–Gunns sign, suggests a prechiasmal optic neuropathy. Any reproducible deficit found on visual field examination by confrontation may be produced by chiasmal or retrochiasmal tumors. Such signs, particularly in a patient with a history suggesting hormonal dysfunction, warrant a specific diagnostic neuroimaging examination. Magnetic resonance imaging has supplanted CT in sensitivity in discerning sellar and parasellar abnormalities.

Varying degrees of hypopituitarism may result by direct involvement of the pituitary gland or compression on the pituitary stalk by an adenoma. Vague symptoms, including lethargy, malaise, cold intolerance, alterations in skin and hair texture, and gonadal dysfunction may develop. Headache may be seen owing to mass effect on the sella or other local pain-sensitive structures. If the tumor reaches massive proportions, obstructive hydrocephalus may occur. Medial extension, with invasion of the cavernous sinus, may lead to multiple cranial neuropathies. Lateral extension may lead to parenchymal involvement of the frontal or middle temporal fossae. Seizures are uncommon.

Hypersecretory pituitary adenomas produce specific signs that may be useful in diagnosis. Prolactinoma will cause galactorrhea and amenorrhea in women but less striking symptoms in men. Galactorrhea is much less common. Men with prolactinomas may present with decreased libido, impotence, and oligospermia.

Hypersecretion of growth hormones results in enlargement of the distal extremities, face, and various soft tissues, producing acromegaly. Excess growth hormone lead to systemic disturbances including hypertension, diabetes, organomegaly, and arteriosclerotic vascular disease, which can lead to a decrease in life expectancy. Microadenomas may secrete excess ACTH, leading to hypercortisolemia. Cushing's disease refers to the specific syndrome of hypercortisolemia occurring as a pituitary tumor. Cushing's syndrome refers to the less specific diagnosis of hypercortisolemia resulting from pituitary, adrenal, or ectopic cortisol production when the etiologic agent has not been defined. Clinical features of hypercortisolemia include centripetal obesity, muscle atrophy and proximal weakness, hirsutism, and purple striae. Metabolic disturbances including hypertension, impaired glucose tolerance, gonadal endocrine abnormalities, and compromise of the immune system may occur (39).

F. Craniopharyngiomas

Craniopharyngiomas are epithelial tumors that are postulated to arise from embryonic squamous cell rests of an incompletely involuted hypophyseal–pharyngeal duct. They occur in the midline, along the nasopharynx, sellar region, suprasellar region, and they may extend or arise into the third ventricle. Tumors enlarge by progressive desquamation of epithelial cells into the center of the encapsulated tumor. Craniopharyngiomas represent between 2.5 and 4% of all brain tumors (21,40). They are considered a disease of childhood; however, roughly one-half of all craniopharyngiomas arise in adults and may be found in any decade of life.

Craniopharyngiomas produce symptoms and signs of visual impairment in approximately 80% of adult patients, with symptoms referable to parasellar mass lesions. Endocrine dysfunction is common and most often presents with sexual or menstrual dysfunction in over 80% of adult patients. Almost half of patients present with headache. Large tumors in adults may cause mental status changes, with memory loss, apathy, and hypersomnia. Hydrocephalus can be seen with large tumors (40).

G. Primary Central Nervous System Lymphomas (see also Chap. 17)

Primary central nervous system (CNS) lymphomas have accounted for approximately 1% of CNS tumors and fewer than 1% of all lymphomas in large, retrospective series (41,42). Primary CNS lymphomas have been increasing in prevalence in several populations, namely the elderly and in patients with either congenital immunodeficiency or acquired immune deficiency syndrome (AIDS). Primary CNS lymphomas occur clinically in 2% (43) of AIDS patients and have been found in 7% of AIDS patients at autopsy. As these populations increase, the frequency of occurrence of primary CNS lymphoma has been projected to exceed that of pituitary adenoma by the early 1990s (42,44).

Primary CNS lymphomas are B-cell, non-Hodgkin tumors that show cytology similar to that seen in large-cell immunoblastic or small, noncleaved cell lymphomas. Nodular lymphomas are not seen (13,43). There is a male preponderance in the disease, exclusive of the male bias seen in the AIDS population. The age at presentation in the AIDS population is 37.0 years; in the non-AIDS population, it occurs most commonly in the seventh decade (20,43).

Almost all primary CNS lymphomas occur in the brain parenchyma; rarely, meningeal disease occurs. The diagnosis of primary intracranial lymphoma by definition excludes the presence of diffuse systemic disease, with exception of concomitant ocular disease (45,46). In contrast, approximately 10% of patients with systemic lymphoma develop secondary seeding of the CNS, most of which occurs in the meninges (41). The site of presentation of the lymphoma is clinically useful but not pathognomonic for directing further diagnostic evaluation.

Clinical presentation of the primary CNS lymphoma depends on the location of these deep-seated, multifocal mass lesions. Patients may present clinically with a rapidly growing mass lesion, with focal neurological deficits, with or without signs of increased intracranial pressure. Sixty percent present with signs of confusion, lethargy, memory loss, or altered consciousness. Approximately 40–60% will have a focal deficit, such as a hemiparesis or aphasia, with or without an associated decrease in cognition. Headache in association with other neurological symptoms is rare. Papilledema occurs in 14%. Seizures occur in 15–30% of patients. Cranial nerve palsies can occur and suggest posterior fossa involvement or meningeal disease and are, therefore, probably secondary lymphomatous seeding from systemic disease (41,43,45).

H. Pineal Region Tumors

Pineal region tumors represent fewer than 1% of all primary intracranial neoplasms (21). The pathological presentation of lesions that may appear within the region of the pineal gland is vast and ranges from the benign arachnoid cyst or meningioma to the highly malignant undifferentiated teratoma. Most pineal region tumors present in children or young adults. The reader is referred to Chapter 4 for more detailed discussion of pathology and treatment of these tumors. Occasionally, pineal region tumors may occur in the adult and are of interest because of the specific clinical syndromes that may result from these lesions.

The symptomatology of pineal region tumors depends largely on the size of the lesion and its ability to compress or invade surrounding brain parenchyma. Compression of the quadrigeminal plate may cause ocular findings. Paralysis of upward gaze, pupillary abnormalities, and nystagmus and abnormalities of convergence of the eyes may occur. Distinct oculomotor paresis may occur with direct invasion of the membrane. Compression of the cerebral aqueduct or tumor enlargement into the posterior third ventricle may lead to hydrocephalus, with associated headache, mental status changes, and papilledema. Posterior extension can cause compression or invasion of the cerebellum, resulting in dysmetria, hypotonia, and intention tremor (47).

I. Colloid Cysts

Colloid cysts are rare, benign tumors filled with mucin that are found in the anterior third ventricle at the level of the foramen of Monro. Symptoms arise from intermittent or chronic obstruction of CSF flow from the lateral ventricles, leading to hydrocephalus. They constitute fewer than 1% of primary CNS tumors but have achieved notoriety owing to their dramatic ability to cause precipitous neurological decline because of acute hydrocephalus caused by impaction of the tumor at the foramen of Monro, leading to coma and death. In the era before CT, these lesions were characterized by the aforementioned sudden-death syndrome, often preceded by the history of positional headaches and an intermittent dementia. Additional presentations include the occurrence of "drop attacks" caused by sudden bilateral leg weakness, which is thought to be due to rapid stretch upon the corticospinal nerve fibers over the convexities of the cerebral hemispheres brought on by acute hydrocephalus. These attacks could be separated by periods of days or years, depending on the frequency of obstruction of CSF outflow (48).

A recent review has helped define the clinical presentation of patients diagnosed since the CT era. Not surprisingly, the scenarios are not as dramatic as with those tumors that were previously diagnosed by pneumoencephalography. Seventeen patients were reviewed: 15 complained of frontal or occipital headache, but a positional headache was noted in only 4. Nausea, vomiting, and papilledema were present in only half of the patients. Seven patients complained of visual symptoms, including scintillating scotomata in 2 and blurred vision in 5. Weakness, most often in both legs, was reported by 6 patients. Transient loss of consciousness was described by 4 patients. One presented in coma, and 1 developed a grand mal seizure. Clinical examination suggested elevated intracranial pressure without localizing signs in 15; 7 patients had bilateral papilledema and 5 had decreased visual acuity. Palsy of upward gaze was documented in 3 cases, and 3 patients had gait ataxia. Four patients had signs of an organic mental disorder and 1 had been diagnosed erroneously as having normal-pressure hydrocephalus before CT scanning. Six patients had entirely normal neurological examinations (49). Mean age at presentation was 30 years of age, with a range from 19 to 62 years. The clinical presentation in this recent series of patients is of clinical interest for several reasons. Although this disease is rare, it is prototypical for any mass lesion that can lead to intermittent obstructive hydrocephalus. It demonstrates the valuable effect neuroimaging has had on the early detection of tumors, leading to decreasing morbidity. It allows critical evaluation of a disease that has caused fear in clinicians for decades and has redefined the classic presentation of the disease. In addition, it points out that papilledema is not found universally in these patients, who are at extremely high risk for herniation caused by lumbar puncture.

J. Dermoid and Epidermoid Tumors

Dermoids and epidermoids are rare lesions that together represent fewer than 2% of brain tumors (50). They are thought to arise from developmental inclusion cysts which may occur within the scalp, calvarium, or brain. Epidermoid cysts enlarge by progressive desquamation of stratified squamous epithelium into the interior of the encapsulated tumor, whereas dermoids are composed of more complex dermal elements, which may include hair and sebaceous glands. Dermoids tend to occur in pediatric patients and are most likely to be found in the midline. The most common example of this lesion is the soft, fluctuant, midline nasal dermoid seen in infants. Epidermoids present in patients between the ages of 20 and 40, and are more likely to occur off the midline.

Intracranial cysts enlarge slowly over years. As they do so, their pliable capsules may surround, displace, or compress adjacent neural and vascular structures. Rupture of the cyst wall may allow keratin to spill into the subarachnoid space, leading to irritative phenomenon, such as aseptic meningitis. The most common locations of these cysts can be divided into four categories:

suprasellar–chiasmatic, parasellar–Sylvian fissure, retrosellar–cerebellopontine angle, and basilar–posterior fossa (50). Suprasellar cysts most commonly produce symptoms of visual impairment, with or without endocrine dysfunction. Parasellar cysts may extend into the anterior, middle, or posterior fossae, where they may cause mass effect and symptoms referable to the site of compression. Parasellar–Sylvian fissure lesions may present with symptoms referable to either frontal lobe or temporal lobe compression, including motor deficits and trigeminal nerve deficits. Cysts that arise in the retrosellar–cerebellopontine angle tend to envelop the upper cranial nerves of the posterior fossa. Early symptoms are irritative rather than dysfunctional; therefore, trigeminal neuralgia is common. As the cyst enlarges, multiple deficits of cranial nerves V, VII, and VIII will occur, which are often accompanied by nystagmus, cerebellar ataxia, and hemiparesis. Cysts at the base of the posterior fossa will surround the lower cranial nerves, leading to dysarthria and dysphasia. Cerebellar deficits and long-tract findings are attributed to brain stem compression.

Intraventricular tumors are rare but can occur. When seen, they are most frequent within the fourth ventricle. Their slow growth and pliable nature can allow a great variety of symptoms, which can wax and wane over years. As with most intraventricular tumors, symptoms include headache and alteration in mentation. With tumors of the fourth ventricle, local compressive events, with cranial nerve palsies, ataxia, and hemiparesis, may also occur.

Lesions within the skull usually present as painless, slowly enlarging mass lesions that can cause significant bony deformity. Neurological symptoms will arise if adjacent neural foramena become compromised.

The neuroimaging study of choice for diagnosis of dermoid and epidermoid tumors is MRI. The CT imaging of the posterior fossa and skull base is less detailed than the MRI, and may miss lesions that are isodense with CSF.

K. Medulloblastomas

Medulloblastomas are malignant neoplasms that are found most commonly in the posterior fossa in children. Rarely, similar-appearing tumors may be found in the cerebral convexities and may occasionally occur in adults. The reader is referred to the Chapter 4 for discussion of presenting symptoms of these lesions in children.

Medulloblastomas may occasionally arise in adults. Mean age of presentation in one recent series was 26 years. The most common presenting symptoms were headache, ataxia, weakness, and nausea. Most common neurological findings at the time of diagnosis were gait ataxia, limb dysmetria, paresis, nystagmus, and papilledema. Hydrocephalus was present in most patients. In adults, medulloblastomas occur more frequently in the cerebellar hemisphere than within the fourth ventricle, in contrast with children. Prognosis is similar to those lesions found in children (19,51).

REFERENCES

1. Plum F. Approach to the patient, including general management. In: Wingaarden JB, Smith LA, Jr, eds. Cecil textbook of medicine. Philadelphia: WB Saunders, 1985:1965–1966.
2. Osler W. A way of life. New York: Paul B Hober, 1937.
3. DeJong RN. The neurological examination, 4th ed. Hagerstown Md: Harper & Row, 1979.
4. Massey EW, Pleet AB, Scherokman BJ. Diagnostic tests in neurology: a photographic guide to bedside techniques. Chicago: Yearbook Medical Publishers, 1985.
5. Mayo Clinic and Foundation. Clinical examinations in neurology. Philadelphia: WB Saunders, 1981.
6. Rengachary SS. Cranial nerve examination. In: Wilkins RH, Rengachary SS, eds. Neurosurgery, vol 1. New York: McGraw-Hill, 1985:50–70.
7. Rosenberg M. Neuro-ophthalmology. In: Wilkins RH, Rengachary SS, eds. Neurosurgery, vol 1. New York: McGraw-Hill, 1985:71–101.

8. Brandt T. Vertigo and dizziness in diseases of the nervous system. In: Asbury AK, McKhann GM, McDonald WI, eds. Clinical neuro-biology. Philadelphia: WB Saunders, 1986:561–576.

9. Wayne HH. Syncope-physiologic considerations and an analysis of the clinical characteristics in 510 patients. Am J Med 1961: 30;418.

10. Yasargil MG, Von Ammon K. Von Deimling A, Valavanis A, Whichmann W, Wiestler OD. Central neurocytomas: histopathologic variants therapeutic approaches. J Neurosurg 1992; 76:32–37.

11. Strub RL, Black FW. The mental status examination in neurology, 2nd ed. Philadelphia: FA Davis, 1985.

12. Talbert OR. General methods of clinical examination. In: Youmans JR, ed. Neurological surgery, vol 1, 3rd ed. Philadelphia: WB Saunders, 1990:3–36.

13. Burger PC, Scheithauer BW, Vogel FS. Surgical pathology of the nervous system and its coverings, 3rd ed. New York: Churchill-Livingstone, 1991.

14. Muller W, Afra D, Schroder R. Supratentorial recurrence of gliomas. Morphological studies in relation to time intervals with astrocytoma. Acta Neurochir 1977; 39:75–91.

15. Guthrie BL, Laws ER. Supratentorial low-grade gliomas. In: Rosenblum ML, ed. The role of surgery in brain tumor management. Philadelphia: WB Saunders, 1990:1–18.

16. Piepmeier JM. Observations on the current treatment of low-grade astrocytic tumors of the cerebral hemispheres. J Neurosurg 1987; 67;177–181.

17. McKeran RO, Thomas DGT. The clinical study of gliomas. In: Thomas DGT, Graham DI, eds. Brain tumors: scientific basis, clinical investigation and current therapy. Boston: Butterworth, 1980:194–230.

18. Garcia DM, Fulling KH, Marks JE. The value of radiation therapy in addition to surgery for astrocytomas of the adult cerebrum. Cancer 1985; 55:9919–9927.

19. Harsh GR, Wilson CB. Neuroepithelial tumors of the adult brain. In: Youmans JR, ed. Neurological surgery. Philadelphia: WB Saunders, 1990:3040–3136.

20. Berens ME, Rutka JT, Rosenblum ML. Brain tumor epidemiology, growth and invasion. In: Rosenblum MD, ed. The role of surgery in brain tumor management. Neurosurg Clin North Am 1990; 1:1–18.

21. Sutherland GR, Florell R, Louw D, Choi NW, Sima AAF. Epidemiology of primary intracranial neoplasms in Manitoba, Canada. Can J Neurol Sci 1987; 14:586–592.

22. Muller W, Afra D, Schroder R. Supratentorial recurrence of gliomas: morphological studies in relation to time intervals with oligodendrogliomas. Acta Neurochir 1977; 39:15–25.

23. Bullard DE, Rawlings CE, Phillips B, Cox EB, Schold SC, Burger PC, Halperin EC. Oligodendroglioma. Cancer 1987; 60:2179–2188.

24. Shaw EG, Daumas-Duport C, Scheithauer BW, et al. Radiation therapy in the management of low-grade supratentorial astrocytomas. J Neurosurg 1989; 70:853–861.

25. Clark GB, Henry JM, McKeever PE. Cerebral pilocytic astrocytoma. Cancer 1985; 56:1128–1133.

26. Palma L, Guidetti B. Cystic pilocytic astrocytomas of the cerebral hemispheres. J Neurosurg 1985; 62:811–815.

27. Boyd MC, Steinbok P. Choroid plexus tumors: problems in diagnosis and management. J Neurosurg 1987; 66:800–805.

28. Laurence KM. The biology of choroid plexus papilloma in infancy and childhood. Acta Neurochir 1979; 50:79–90.

29. Dohrmann GJ. Ependymomas. In: Wilkins RH, Rengachary SS, eds. Neurosurgery. New York: McGraw-Hill, 1985:767–771.

30. Silver JM, Rawlings CE, Rossitch ER, Zeidman SM, Friedman AH. Gangliomas: a clinical study with long-term follow-up. Surg Neurol 1991; 35:261–266.

31. Sutton LN, Packer RJ, Schut L. Gangliolimas. In: Wilkins RH, Rengachary SS, eds. Neurosurgery update I. New York: McGraw-Hill, 1990:461–464.

32. Choux S. In: Schmidek HH, ed. Meningiomas and their surgical management. Philadelphia: WB Saunders, 1991.

33. McCormick PW, Coccia C. Coagulopathy, cerebrovascular disease and other conditions associated with meningioma. In: Schmidek HH, ed. Meningiomas and their surgical management. Philadelphia: WB Saunders, 1991.

34. Maxwell R. Posterior fossa meningiomas. In: Schmidek HH, ed. Meningiomas and their surgical management. Philadelphia: WB Saunders, 1991.

35. Ojemann RG, Martuza. Acoustic neuroma. In: Youmans JR, ed. Neurological surgery, 3rd ed, vol. 5. Philadelphia: WB Saunders, 1990:3316–3350.
36. Post KD, McCormick PFC. Trigeminal neurinoma. In: Wilkins RH, Rengachary SS, eds. Neurosurgery update I. New York: McGraw-Hill, 1991:346–353.
37. Kenan PD. In: Wilkins RH, Rengachary SS, eds. Neurosurgery, vol 1. New York: McGraw-Hill, 1985:698–705.
38. Bucheit WA, Delgado TE. In: Wilkins RH, Rengachary SS, eds. Neurosurgery New York: McGraw-Hill, 1985:720–729.
39. Tindall GT, Barrow DL. Tumors of the sellar and parasellar area in adults. In: Youmans JR, ed. Neurological surgery. Philadelphia: WB Saunders, 1990:3447–3498.
40. Carmel PW. Brain tumors of disordered embryogenesis. In: Youmans JR, ed. Neurological surgery. Philadelphia: WB Saunders, 1990:3223–3249.
41. Neuwelt EA, Gumerlock MK, Dahlborg SA. Lymphomas of the brain in adults. In: Youmans JR, ed. Neurological surgery. Philadelphia: WB Saunders, 1990:3137–3151.
42. Rosenblum JL, Levy RM, Bredesen DE. Neurosurgical implications of the acquired immunodeficiency syndrome (AIDS). Clin Neurosurg 1988; 34:419–445.
43. So YT. Primary central nervous system lymphoma in acquired immune deficiency syndrome: a clinical and pathological study. Ann Neurol 1986; 20:566–672.
44. Levy RM, Bredesen DE. In: Rosenblum ML, Levy M, Bredesen ML, eds. AIDS and the nervous system. New York: Raven Press, 1988.
45. Pepose JS, Holland GN, Nestor MS, Cochran AJ, Foos RY. Acquired immunodeficiency syndrome: ophthalmic manifestations in ambulatory patients. Ophthalmology 1983; 90:874–878.
46. Rockwood EJ, Azkov ZN, Bay JW. Combined malignant lymphoma of the eye and CNS. J Neurosurg 1984; 61:369–374.
47. Schmidek HH, Waters A. Pineal masses: clinical features and management. In: Wilkins RH, Rengachary SS, eds. Neurosurgery. New York: McGraw-Hill, 1985:688–693.
48. Kelly R. Colloid cysts of the third ventricle: analysis of twenty-nine cases. Brain 1951; 74:23–65.
49. Hall WA, Lunsford LD. Changing concepts of the treatment of colloid cysts. J. Neurosurg 1987; 66:186–191.
50. Conley FK. Epidermoid and dermoid tumors: clinical features and surgical management. In: Wilkins RH, Renchachary SS, eds. Neurosurgery. New York: McGraw-Hill, 1985:668–673.
51. Osenbach RK, Robertson S, Traynelis V. Medulloblastoma in adults: A review of 91 cases [Abstract]. Presented at the American Association of Neurological Surgeons, San Francisco, 1991.
52. Burger PC. Classification and biology of brain tumors. In: Youmans JR, ed. Neurological surgery. Philadelphia: WB Saunders, 1990:2967–2999.
53. Kelly PJ. Volumetric stereotactic surgical resection of intra-axial brain mass lesions. Mayo Clin Proc 1988; 63:1186–1198.
54. Salcman M, Kaplan RS. Intracranial tumors in adults. In: Moosa AR, Bobson MC, Schimpff SC, eds. Comprehensive textbook of oncology. Baltimore: Williams & Wilkins, 1986.

8

The Radiology of Brain Tumors: General Considerations and Neoplasms of the Posterior Fossa

Solomon Batnitzky and Donald A. Eckard
University of Kansas Medical Center, Kansas City, Kansas

I. INTRODUCTION

The diagnosis, localization, and management of intracranial neoplasms demand precise and accurate neuroradiologic evaluation. The radiologic examination of the skull and its contents uses many specialized-imaging techniques that permit remarkable accuracy both in pathological and anatomical diagnosis.

These imaging techniques include:

1. Plain films of the skull
2. Radionuclide brain scanning
3. Ultrasound
4. Angiography
5. Computed tomography
6. Magnetic resonance imaging

Before the introduction of computed tomography (CT) and, more recently, magnetic resonance imaging (MRI), the diagnosis of an intracranial space-occupying lesion was made using invasive techniques such as pneumography and cerebral angiography. These techniques rely on indirect radiographic findings of a mass lesion, such as displacement, deformity, and distortion of the ventricular system, subarachnoid spaces, and cerebral vasculature. In some cases, however, the angioarchitecture can suggest the correct histological diagnosis.

The introduction of CT in the early 1970s and MRI in the late 1980s revolutionized the practice of neuroradiology. Both CT and MRI permit direct visualization of the central nervous system (CNS). Both of these imaging techniques provide exquisite images of both normal and pathological intracranial anatomy.

Owing to the general availability of CT and MRI, patients suspected of having an intracranial neoplasm are now spared the risk and discomfort of invasive procedures, such as pneumoencephalography, ventriculography, and cerebral angiography. Pneumoencephalography and ventriculography have been rendered obsolete by CT and MRI. Cerebral angiography is no longer performed routinely as in the past, although it continues to be of value in certain clinical situations. The role and indications for cerebral angiography in the evaluation of patients with suspected intracranial tumors will be discussed later in this chapter.

This chapter provides an overview of the neuroradiologic approach to the diagnosis of intracranial tumors, with the emphasis on the CT and MRI findings.

II. RADIOIMAGING TECHNIQUES

A. Plain Films of the Skull

In the past, plain film examination of the skull was the initial and one of the main diagnostic tools in the evaluation of patients with suspected intracranial disease. Plain roentgenograms of the skull can provide important and useful information. They can demonstrate the presence of intracranial calcifications (Figs. 1 and 2), evidence of raised intracranial pressure, midline shift of a calcified pineal gland, erosion of adjacent bone by an intracranial neoplasm (Fig. 3), the presence or absence of bony metastatic deposits (Fig. 4), and areas of reactive bone formation, such as hyperostosis of the cranium secondary to a meningioma (Fig. 5). All of these radiographic findings are, for the most part, nonspecific. The incidence of positive findings, even in a selected series of patients with a proven intracranial tumor, is very low (1). The importance and use of plain skull films has declined markedly secondary to the widespread use of CT and MRI. Plain skull films are only occasionally obtained today and are reserved for secondary evaluation to answer specific questions raised by either the CT or MRI examination.

B. Radionuclide Brain Scanning

In the past, the radionuclide brain scan was a helpful diagnostic tool in the evaluation of patients with suspected intracranial tumors. With the introduction of CT and MRI, the indications for its use are less clear, and radionuclide brain scanning has been effectively replaced by CT and MRI.

A potentially very useful role of radionuclide agents is the development of so-called tumor-seeking radiopharmaceuticals, such as thallium-201 (2), which can be very helpful in the evaluation of the brain following radiation treatment for an intracranial neoplasm. Differentiation of radionecrosis from recurrent tumor is a very difficult clinical and imaging problem. Tumor-seeking radiopharmaceuticals, such as thallium-201, may help in differentiating recurrent tumor from radiation necrosis and postoperative changes (Fig. 6). The use of single-photon emission CT (SPECT) further improves and enhances the reliability of thallium-201.

Figure 1 Calcified convexity meningioma: Lateral skull radiograph demonstrates large well-defined, homogeneous calcification in the frontoparietal convexity region. On the posterior aspect of the tumor, an enlarged vascular groove is seen entering the tumor. This enlarged vascular groove was secondary to a hypertrophied posterior branch of the middle meningeal artery that supplied the tumor.

Figure 2 Calcified oligodendroglioma: Lateral skull radiograph demonstrates a large area of dense nodular calcification in the occipital lobe.

Figure 3 Meningioma with osseous destruction: Lateral skull radiograph demonstrates erosion and destruction of the frontal bone secondary to underlying frontal meningioma. The patient presented with a 5-year history of a progressively enlarging left forehead mass.

Figure 4 Multiple myeloma: Lateral skull radiograph demonstrates multiple, discrete "punched-out" lesions with well-defined and nonsclerotic margins. The relatively uniform size and round shape are important features in differentiating myelomatosis from malignant metastases.

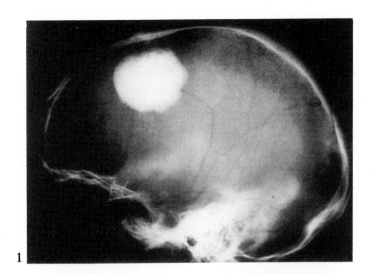

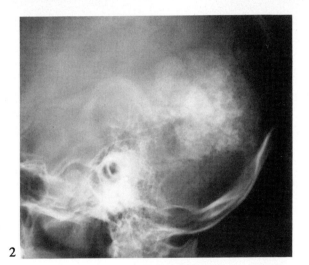

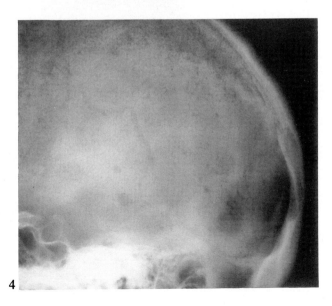

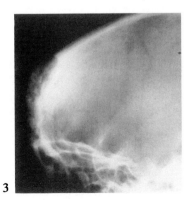

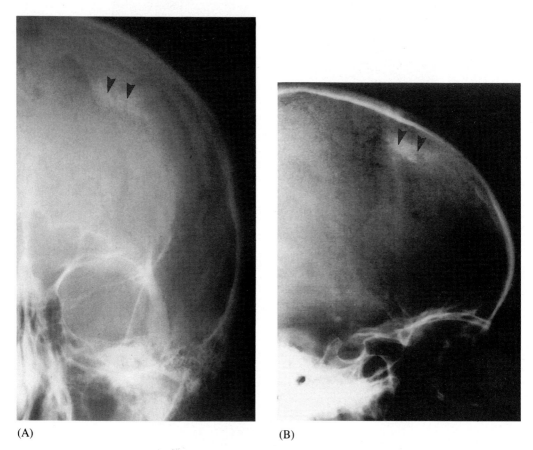

(A)   (B)

Figure 5 Hyperostosis of the cranium secondary to meningioma: (A) Frontal and (B) lateral skull radiographs demonstrate hyperostosis (arrowheads) in the left frontal bone secondary to underlying meningioma.

C. Ultrasound

The routine use of ultrasound in the evaluation of the brain is limited because of the inability of this technique to penetrate bone. The major use of ultrasound is in the evaluation of neonates who have patent fontanelles and as an intraoperative procedure after craniotomy for the localization and characterization of intracranial mass lesions.

D. Cerebral Angiography

In the era of CT and MRI, the emphasis of angiography has changed from diagnosis to more accurate evaluation of known intracranial processes. Angiography can provide important pre-operative information to the neurosurgeon by demonstrating the vascular supply to a tumor and the position and relation of the major intracerebral vessels, both arterial and venous, to the tumor mass. In many instances the angioarchitecture of the tumor may suggest the correct pathological diagnosis (Figs. 7 and 8). However, caution should be exercised when attempting to establish a histological diagnosis based on the cerebral angiogram alone. Angiography can also rule out or demonstrate an intracranial aneurysm that can mimic an intracranial tumor (Fig. 9). Occasionally, angiography is useful for the diagnosis of meningioma or other vascular tumors, such as paragang-liomas and hemangioblastomas. Angiography may be helpful to differentiate an infarct from a

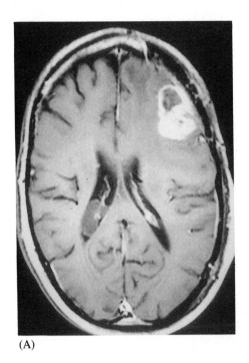

(A)

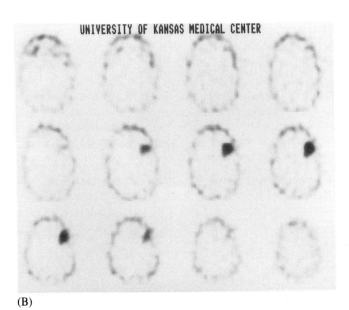

(B)

Figure 6 Recurrent glioblastoma multiforme; role of thallium brain scan: A 52-year-old man, status postresection of left frontal glioblastoma multiforme: (A) post-gadolinium axial T1-weighted MRI; (B) thallium-201 radionuclide brain scan. The post-gadolinium MRI (A) demonstrates an inhomogeneous enhancing mass, with a large necrotic component in the left frontal lobe. The thallium radionuclide brain scan (B) demonstrates increased uptake of thallium in the region of the left frontal lobe, consistent with tumor recurrence. Thallium-201, being a potassium analogue localizes to living tissue. In situations of radiation necrosis thallium-201 would not localize to this area, as the cells in this region are no longer viable.

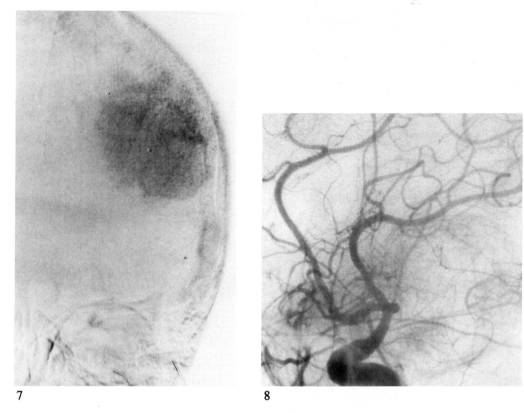

7   8

Figure 7 Vascular stain secondary to meningioma: Selective left carotid angiography demonstrates uniform homogeneous stain characteristic of a meningioma.
Figure 8 Angioarchitecture of glioblastoma multiforme: Arterial phase of left carotid angiogram demonstrates left temporal lobe mass as evidenced by elevation of middle cerebral artery group. Numerous small tumor vessels are seen within the mass as well as areas of avascularity. This angiographic picture is consistent with a glioblastoma multiforme, but is nonspecific and may also be seen with a metastasis.

glioma. Angiography remains essential in the preliminary evaluation of potential therapeutic interventional neuroradiologic procedures.

E. Computed Tomography

The introduction of CT for clinical use in the early 1970s profoundly affected the practice of neurosurgery, neurology, and other medical specialties. It revolutionized the approach to the diagnosis of intracranial disease. It became apparent soon after its introduction that CT was the only examination necessary for most problems.

A differential x-ray absorption of 5% or more is generally required to distinguish different soft tissues on plain radiographs. Computed tomography is able to differentiate between many soft tissues in which the differential absorption may be as little as 0.5%. With its remarkable ability to detect and display minute differences in tissue densities, CT opened new vistas of radiologic diagnosis. The overall accuracy, especially when performed without and with intravenous iodinated contrast material, approaches 98% for the diagnosis of a lesion versus no lesion (3).

The advent of MRI has challenged the supreme role that CT had established for itself in the

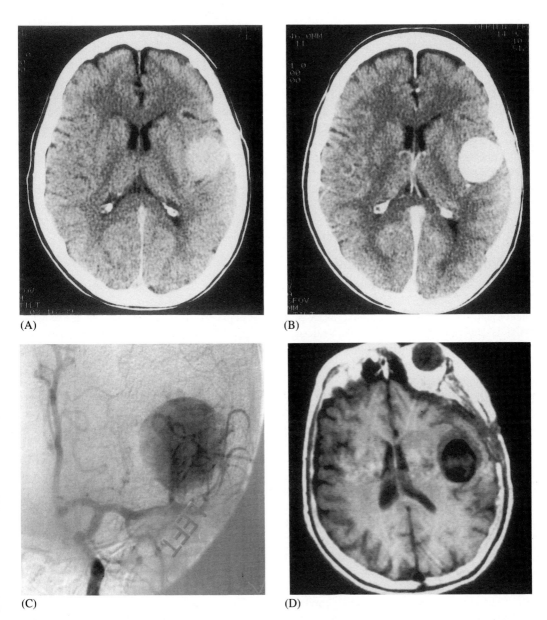

(A)

(B)

(C)

(D)

Figure 9 Giant middle cerebral artery aneurysm mimicking meningioma: (A) precontrast axial CT scan; (B) postcontrast axial CT scan; (C) frontal view of left carotid angiogram; (D) axial T1-weighted MRI. Precontrast CT scan (A) demonstrates round hyperdense mass in the left parietal region. This mass demonstrates marked uniform homogeneous enhancement following the administration of intravenous contrast material (B). Left carotid angiography (C) demonstrates a giant middle cerebral artery aneurysm. The T1-weighted MRI (D) demonstrates the characteristic signal void caused by flowing blood within the aneurysm. Within the central portion of the aneurysm, there is an area of increased signal intensity probably representing sluggish flow or clot. Perianeurysmal edema is noted anterior to the aneurysm.

past. Computed tomography is superior to MRI in several clinical situations. It is superior to MRI in the evaluation of bony structures and calcification. Acute intracranial hemorrhage is more reliably and easily evaluated with CT than with MRI. If a rapid study is desired, CT is a better modality than MRI. Critically ill patients with life-support systems are difficult to examine by MRI because the MRI examination takes much longer and requires more patient cooperation than a CT examination. In addition, many of the life-support systems are ferromagnetic and cannot be used with MRI. However, new nonferromagnetic life-support systems are now available, which helps overcome this problem to some degree.

Although MRI is superior to CT for the evaluation of most disease processes of the central nervous system as will be discussed in the following section, one should not underestimate the role of CT in the diagnosis of intracranial tumors. Computed tomography is still an outstanding and very accurate imaging modality. In addition, the cost of a CT examination is less than an MRI examination. Computed tomography is more universally and more readily available than is MRI. As a result, probably more intracranial tumors are evaluated with CT than with MRI.

F. Magnetic Resonance Imaging

The recent addition of MRI to our diagnostic armamentarium has been the major innovation in medical imaging of the 1980s. Like CT, MRI is a computer-based imaging modality that depicts anatomical sections in tomographic slices of varying thickness. It is universally recognized that MRI is superior to CT as the diagnostic-imaging modality for the evaluation of a suspected intracranial tumor (4–7) (Figs. 10 and 11). The increased sensitivity of MRI over CT applies to metastatic disease as well (8,9).

Although anatomically, MRI scans are similar to CT scans, the MRI information is fundamentally different from CT information. In CT and conventional radiography, the gray–scale-ordering never changes. Bones always appear as the whitest issue on images, followed by muscle and fat, and air always appears black. Unlike CT and conventional radiography, the gray–scale-ordering in MRI is highly variable and potentially confusing. It is beyond the scope of this chapter to discuss the physics of MRI. The reader is referred to standard texts for this purpose (6,7, 10–12). With MRI, a knowledge of the effects of and interrelations among scanning parameters on image quality is important for accurate image interpretation. To understand how an MRI image is created and can be manipulated to answer clinical questions, some fundamental principles of MRI will be briefly discussed in the following. It should be emphasized that this description is very basic and simplifies the very complex physics of MRI.

The MRI technique is based on the effects that a large magnetic field and radiofrequency pulses have on the nuclei of hydrogen atoms present in body tissue. Hydrogen is ideally suited for MRI because it is the most sensitive of the stable nuclei to a nuclear magnetic resonance effect and the hydrogen atom is also the most abundant nucleus in the body.

Multiple parameters can affect tissue signal intensity and contrast in an MR image. These can be divided into extrinsic (equipment) parameters and intrinsic (tissue) parameters.

Figure 10 Fibrillary astrocytoma; superiority of MRI over CT: (A) postcontrast axial CT scan; (B) axial T2-weighted MRI. Postcontrast CT scan (A) demonstrates an ill-defined area of enhancement in the left basal ganglia region with ill-defined surrounding lucency. The T2-weighted MRI (B) demonstrates an obvious well-defined area of abnormal increased signal intensity in the same area as (A).

Figure 11 Fibrillary astrocytoma; superiority of MRI over CT: (A) double-dose postcontrast axial CT scans; (B) axial T2-weighted MRI: (C) coronal T2-weighted MRI. Double-dose postcontrast axial CT scans (A) demonstrates no abnormality. The patient had three normal CT scans without and with intravenous contrast material over a period of 12 months. The T2-weighted MRI (B,C) demonstrate an obvious area of abnormal increased signal intensity in the left parietal convexity region.

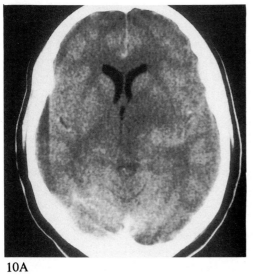

10A

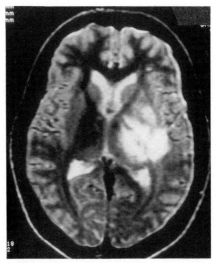

10B

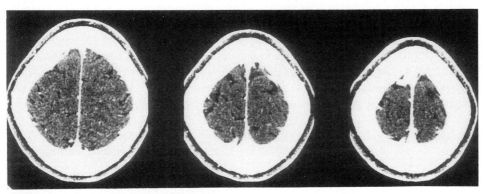

11A

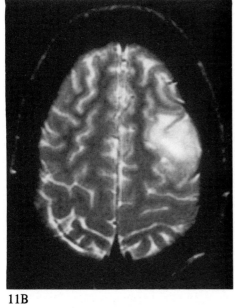

11B

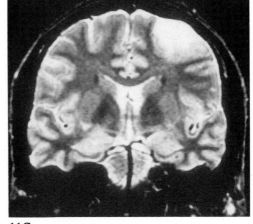

11C

Major extrinsic parameters include the pulse-timing intervals (TR,TE), variation in magnetic field strength from one unit to another, field of view, matric size, section thickness, and so on. The reader is again referred to standard texts for description and details of these parameters.

The principal intrinsic parameters are the T1 relaxation time, T2 relaxation time, and proton density of the imaged tissues.

Relaxation is the process that occurs in tissues after cessation of the radiofrequency pulse, in which the physical changes that were caused by the radiofrequency pulse returns to the state they were in before application of the pulse. The time it takes for the voltage to decay or for relaxation to occur is expressed by two time constants: the T1 and T2 relaxation times. These two components of relaxation proceed at different rates, depending on the nature of the tissue. Each tissue has its own T1 and T2 relaxation times; different tissues have different T1 and T2 relaxation times.

Images can be created to emphasize either the T1 or T2 characteristics of a tissue by altering the pulse sequences. T1-weighted images have a short TR and a short TE. The TR (repetition time) and TE (echo time) refer to equipment parameters. T2-weighted images have long TR and long TE. Proton-density (spin-density, balanced image, intermediate image) has long TR and short TE.

The degree of whiteness or blackness of a tissue or organ depends on its T1 and T2 relaxation times, on the hydrogen concentration in the tissue, and also on whether the pulse sequence is chosen to emphasize the T1 or T2 characteristics of the tissue. These have been called T1- and T2-weighted images. For the purposes of simplicity the terms T1-weighted and T2-weighted will be used in this chapter. Although it is useful to use the terms T1- and T2-weighted images, it should be noted that these terms cannot be rigidly defined. There is a smooth spectrum from T1- to T2-weighted images. All images have some degree of T1 and T2 weighting within them. A proton density image gives a relative balance to the T1 and T2 components, with neither being especially emphasized.

Tissues with long T1 relaxation times yield a much weaker signal than tissues with short T1 relaxation times. On the other hand, tissues with long T2 relaxation times produce a strong signal and appear white.

Fat has short T1 and intermediate T2 relaxation times and, therefore, appears white on T1-weighted images and intermediate intensity on T2-weighted images. It parallels the intensity of subcutaneous fat. Air has a low hydrogen concentration and always appears black. Flowing blood usually appears black because the excited hydrogen atoms flow away from the plane of interest before they have had time to return a signal. Cerebrospinal fluid (CSF) has a very long T1; therefore, it appears black on T1-weighted images. It has a long T2 relaxation time; therefore, it appears white on T2-weighted images.

Because of marked T1 differences between white and gray matter, these areas are sharply distinguished on T1-weighted images. T1-weighted images produce excellent anatomical details. T1-weighted images demonstrate exquisitely the anatomical distortion produced by a tumor. White and gray matter have similar T2 relaxation times; therefore, they are poorly differentiated on T2-weighted images, which appear anatomically less esthetic than T1-weighted images. However, many disease processes, including neoplasia, have T2 relaxation times far longer than gray or white matter and, therefore, are sharply highlighted on T2-weighted images.

MRI has several advantages over other imaging modalities:

1. There are no known adverse biological effects.
2. MRI does not use ionizing radiation. Although the amount of radiation used by CT is relatively low, it is obviously preferable not to use any ionizing radiation.
3. MRI exhibits substantially greater tissue contrast resolution than has been achieved by any other imaging modality. MRI has been reported to supply additional information not available on CT in as many as 50% of patients evaluated by both techniques (13). Because of

MRI's ability to detect small changes in the water content of tissues, it may define an abnormality or the extent of an abnormality much more readily than CT.

4. MRI provides significantly more information about intrinsic tissue characterization than does CT.

5. The increased sensitivity of MRI over CT applies to metastatic disease, especially when intravenous contrast is used with MRI.

6. Beam-hardening artifacts seen with CT do not occur with MRI. These artifacts on CT make diagnosis difficult, if not impossible, in some patients. In the posterior fossa, middle cranial fossa, craniocervical junction, and in evaluating for meningeal lesions MRI is far superior to CT.

7. With MRI, multiple projections can be obtained with ease. With CT, direct coronal images require that the patient must hyperextend his or her neck. This can be difficult, cumbersome, and painful and, many times, this is not possible. In most cases, direct sagittal images on CT are not possible. The multiplanar capability of MRI allows clearer and more accurate definition of a tumor. In addition, the multiplanar capability of MRI is very helpful in making the distinction between an intra- and extra-axial lesion. The determination of a tumor's extra-axial origin, as opposed to an intra-axial origin, has significant clinical importance. The location of a mass affects treatment planning and is predictive of prognosis. For example, extra-axial masses are most frequently benign.

8. MRI has the ability to define subacute and chronic collections of blood much better than does CT.

9. MRI is superior in the evaluation of the contents of a cystic lesion.

10. Patients with allergies to iodinated contrast material can easily be evaluated with MRI.

Contraindications for magnetic resonance imaging:

1. Cardiac pacemaker
2. Ferromagnetic cerebral aneurysm clips
3. Metallic foreign body near the eye
4. Cochlear implants.

G. Tumor Enhancement

The use of contrast agents is a familiar method of enhancing diagnostic images generated by x-rays and radionuclide-imaging techniques. The most common contrast enhancement agents in use in diagnostic radiology are iodine, used in conventional x-rays and CT examinations, and technetium, employed in radionuclide imaging. Both of these agents are directly detected by the image-detecting devices. Iodine absorbs x-rays and thus appears as a white area on the x-ray image. Technetium is a radioactive substance the presence of which is detected by scintillation probes or cameras and appears as a group of dots on the scan. The first MRI contrast agent to be released for clinical use was gadolinium diethylemetriamine pentaacetic acid (GdDPTA). Gadolinium-containing agents, such as GdDPTA, unlike iodinated contrast agents, are not directly detected. Instead, GdDPTA is a paramagnetic agent that alters the magnetic environment of the imaged tissues so that the resulting image is enhanced.

Paramagnetic materials themselves do not produce any signals. However, the effect is solely due to a change in the signal of hydrogen nuclei contained in the tissue in which the agent resides. Paramagnetic agents shorten the T1 and T2 relaxation times of neighboring hydrogen nuclei. A decrease in T1 induces a net increase in signal intensity; that is, enhancement of the image. A decrease in T2 produces a net decrease in signal intensity. Thus, in the clinical setting, when using gadolinium-containing agents, only T1-weighted sequences are obtained.

Unlike iodinated contrast agents used in CT, no direct relation exists between the concentration of gadolinium-containing agents and the observed signal intensity. With CT, the amount of iodine injected is critical to ensure an adequate load of contrast material; at least 40 g of iodine is necessary in an adult.

Endothelial cells of cerebral capillaries have fused membranes, called tight junctions, which are probably the most important feature in regulating capillary permeability in the brain (14). This is known as the *blood–brain barrier* (BBB). The capillaries of the normal brain are impermeable to intravascular-injected contrast agents. Capillaries of tissues outside the nervous system are fenestrated with discontinuities in their basement membranes, with wide intercellular gaps permitting the free passage of protein molecules from the lumen of the capillary into the extravascular space. The blood–brain barrier interfaces are not found in some regions of the brain (15). These areas include the choroid plexus, pituitary gland, cavernous sinus, pineal gland, and dura. Capillaries in these areas are fenestrated and normally allow the diffusion of contrast material into the extracellular space and exhibit normal enhancement following the intravenous injection of contrast agents.

In a variety of pathological conditions, including tumors, infections, and demyelinating disease, disruption of the blood–brain barrier occurs, with resulting enhancement both on CT and MRI following the injection of intravenous contrast material.

Tumors have a tendency to provoke the formation of capillaries in their tissue. Tumor capillaries in gliomas may have near-normal features with a functioning blood–brain barrier. These areas of tumor tissue will not enhance following the injection of intravenous contrast material. In other, more malignant, gliomas, there is stimulation of capillaries the endothelia of which are fenestrated and, therefore, have no blood–brain barrier (5,15). These tumors enhance following the injection of intravenous contrast material.

Metastatic lesions possess non-CNS capillaries that are similar to their tissue of origin. Thus, brain metastases almost always enhance. Extra-axial tumors, such as meningiomas, arise from tissues the capillaries of which do not possess a blood–brain barrier. Therefore, these tumors enhance following the injection of intravenous contrast material. There is no correlation between CT and MRI enhancement and angiographic findings of hypervascularity. The formation of tumor capillaries that do not possess a blood–brain barrier is presumed to be the explanation for tumor enhancement on CT and MRI, rather than active destruction of the barrier by the tumor.

It is important to stress that the lack of enhancement following the injection of intravenous contrast material both on CT and MRI does not necessarily signify absence of a tumor (5).

Early experience with CT determined that postcontrast CT scans were essential (unless contraindicated) in the evaluation of intracranial tumors. The postinfusion CT scan enhances areas of abnormality that may not be seen, or be well-defined before contrast injection.

Even though the mechanism of enhancement is identical for both CT and MRI (5,15,16), MRI is generally more sensitive for contrast enhancement than CT. Tumor enhancement on MRI following intravenous injection of gadolinium-containing agents is more sensitive than tumor enhancement on CT using iodinated contrast material (5,7).

Indications and advantages of gadolinium-containing contrast agents:

1. It improves the delineation of intracranial lesions.
2. It distinguishes nonspecific high-intensity foci in the deep white matter from metastases or lymphoma.
3. It provides additional radiologic information about and characterization of tumor location, size, and configuration.
4. It greatly enhances comparative intensity between surrounding tissue and the mass.

5. Regions of edema are visualized more often and with greater delineation in postcontrast studies than in preinjection scans.
6. It substantially improves the ability of MRI to detect multiple lesions.
7. It is the best-imaging technique to visualize leptomeningeal spread and involvement.
8. It has a more acceptable safety profile than traditional iodinated contrast agents.
9. Because it does not contain iodine, it may be used in patients who have an allergy to iodine.

III. GENERAL CHARACTERISTICS OF BRAIN TUMORS

The specificity of both CT and MRI lags behind the exquisite sensitivity of these imaging modalities. Furthermore, the distinction between benign and malignant brain tumors is not as clear as it is for other organ system tumors.

There are many CT and MRI characteristics of brain tumors that help in distinguishing one type of brain tumor from another. In fact, in many cases, the specific tumor type itself can be diagnosed with a high degree of certainty, depending on the characteristics of the brain tumor.

The general characteristics of brain tumors are discussed in general terms. They will be described in more detail in the discussion on each tumor type.

Location. Certain tumors are found in specific locations. It is important to determine whether a tumor is extradural or intradural. Features of an extradural location include:

1. Demonstration of brain displacement by the mass from adjacent bone and dura
2. Widening of the cisternal subarachnoid space adjacent to the tumor
3. Broad surface of the tumor abutting a dural or osseous surface
4. Bone erosion or hyperostosis

As discussed previously, most extra-axial masses are benign. The location of a mass is predictive of prognosis and affects treatment planning.

Multiplicity. Although multiple primary gliomas and multiple meningiomas occur, tumor multiplicity usually indicates metastatic disease.

Calcification. Tumor calcification is better evaluated by CT than by MRI (18). The presence and character of tumor calcification is important to the diagnosis. Benign tumors tend to calcify more frequently than malignant ones. Calcification in malignant tumors is uncommon unless malignant degeneration of the benign tumor has occurred. Tumors such as craniopharyngioma, oliogodendroglioma, and meningioma commonly calcify.

Hemorrhage. Certain primary intracranial tumors, such as glioblastoma multiforme (Fig. 12), ependymoma, oligodendroglioma, and metastatic tumors, such as melanoma, lung carcinoma, renal cell carcinoma, and choriocarcinoma, tend to bleed. The identification of intratumoral hemorrhage can be most helpful in diagnosis.

Although CT is superior to MRI in the evaluation of acute hemorrhage, subacute and chronic hemorrhage is far better evaluated with MRI. On MRI, intratumoral hemorrhage, as opposed to benign intracerebral hemorrhage, tends to be heterogeneous, with mixed stages of blood present owing to continual, repeated, or intermittent bleeding (19).

A. Necrosis

The presence of necrosis within a tumor suggests a malignant or more aggressive lesion. The biochemical changes related to necrosis escape detection on CT unless the necrosis is cystic.

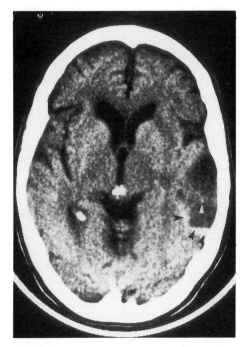

Figure 12 Hemorrhage in glioblastoma multiformé. Noncontrast CT scan demonstrates a left temporoparietal mass with areas of acute hemorrhage (arrowheads) within the tumor.

It will then appear as an area of decreased attenuation similar to CSF. The MRI features of necrosis are complex. Necrosis can be either low- or high-signal intensity on T1- and T2-weighted images. The presence of hemorrhage or several naturally occurring paramagnetic cations and free radicals shorten relaxation times, whereas areas of cystic necrosis prolong relaxation times (5,20). The intensity of cystic necrosis parallels the intensity of CSF on T1- and T2-weighted images, although occasionally, tumor cysts have a slightly higher-signal intensity than pure CSF on T1- and T2-weighted images. This is due to proteinaceous debris or dilute concentrations of paramagnetic substance, which can shorten T1 enough to alter the intensity of these images (21).

B. Margination

Smooth, sharply defined margins favor the diagnosis of a benign lesion, whereas irregular, poorly defined margins favor the diagnosis of a malignant neoplasm.

C. Intensity

Most intracranial tumors exhibit low-signal intensity on T1-weighted images and high-signal intensity on T2-weighted images. In some tumors, such as meningiomas, the degree of relaxation appears shorter, and this can be an important distinguishing feature. Thus, meningiomas tend to be iso- or hypointense on T1-weighted images and iso- to mildly hyperintense on T2-weighted images.

Fat-containing neoplasms (teratoma, dermoid, and lipoma) characteristically are bright on T1-weighted images and have an intermediate intensity on T2-weighted images. Fat parallels the intensity of subcutaneous fat.

D. Contrast Enhancement

Homogeneous contrast enhancement favors a benign process, whereas inhomogeneous contrast enhancement favors the diagnosis of a more aggressive or malignant lesion.

E. Hypervascularity

Large vessels indicative of hypervascularity may be seen in some tumors, such as hemangioblastoma and glioblastoma, on T1- and T2-weighted images. These vessels appear as linear or serpentine regions of signal void within the tumor mass.

The salient CT and MRI differential diagnostic features of the five most common types of intracranial tumors seen in the adult (6) are listed in Table 1.

IV. POSTERIOR FOSSA TUMORS

Posterior fossa tumors represent about 20% of intracranial tumors in adults; however, in the pediatric-age group (22,23), the posterior fossa is the most common site of primary intracranial tumors. Intracranial neoplasms constitute the second most common location of tumors in childhood. In children, posterior fossa neoplasms are more frequent than supratentorial neoplasms when all pediatric ages are grouped together. However, supratentorial tumors are more common in the first year of life (5,24). Infratentorial lesions are preponderant from 4 to 11 years of age, and both locations are equally frequent through the rest of the pediatric period. Excluding the first year of life and adolescence, 60–70% of brain tumors in the pediatric-age group appear in the posterior fossa.

It is useful to classify posterior fossa mass lesions according to their location into the following broad categories:

1. Anterior compartment of the posterior fossa
2. Posterior compartment of the posterior fossa

The fourth ventricle is the reference point. Lesions anterior to the fourth ventricle are part of the anterior compartment, and lesions involving the fourth ventricle and posterior to the fourth ventricle are in the posterior compartment.

Tumors of the posterior compartment of the posterior fossa include mainly intra-axial tumors involving the cerebellar hemisphere, vermis, and fourth ventricle. However, extra-axial tumors, such as meningioma or arachnoid cyst may also occur in this compartment.

The anterior compartment of the posterior fossa can be divided into intra-axial tumors and extra-axial tumors. Intra-axial tumors of the anterior compartment of the posterior fossa are essentially brain stem tumors.

Extra-axial masses of the posterior compartment involve mainly the cerebellopontine angle (CPA), but also the clivus, the dura, and vertebrobasilar system.

Although this classification is somewhat arbitrary and has some overlap, it is useful and simple.

A. Posterior Compartment of the Posterior Fossa

Most lesions found in this compartment are intra-axial tumors of the fourth ventricle and cerebellum. Seventy-five percent of pediatric brain tumors involve the cerebellum. In adults, the most common neoplasm in the cerebellum is a metastasis. Hemangioblastoma is the most common primary adult intra-axial posterior fossa tumor found, but it is less common than a metastasis.

Table 1 Differential Diagnostic Features of Cerebral Neoplasms

Characteristic	Supratentorial astrocytoma	Malignant astrocytoma/glioblastoma	Meningioma	Hematogenous metastasis	Lymphoma (primary and secondary)/leukemia
Preinfusion CT density	Decreased to isodense, mixed	Variable: decreased to increased, mixed	Isodense to increased homogeneous[a]	Variable: decreased to increased	Isodense to hyperdense
MR intensity T1-weighted image	Hypo- to isointense	Hypo- to isointense rim; hypointense center	Isointense	Hypo- to hyperintense (melanoma, bleed) nodule, hypointense periphery (edema)	Lymphoma: slightly hypointense to gray matter. Leukemia: isointense to white matter
T2-weighted image	Hyperintense	Hyperintense	Isointense to mildly hyperintense[a]	Hyperintense	Lymphoma: isointense to slightly hyperintense to gray matter[a]. Leukemia: isointense to white matter
Calcification	Common	Uncommon, unless malignant degeneration of benign astrocytoma	Frequent	Uncommon	Unknown
Hemorrhage	Rare	Common	Rare	Common in certain metastases	Rare
Degree of enhancement	None to moderate[a]	Moderate to marked, occasionally minimal	Marked	Moderate to marked	Moderate to marked
Homogeneity of enhancement	Unusually patchy	Ring, solid	Homogeneous	Homogeneous or ring	Homogeneous
Tumor margins after contrast	Irregular, poorly defined	Mixed: sharp, irregular	Sharp	Sharp	Irregular
Edema	Minimal	Abundant	Minimal to mild	Abundant	Minimal
Mass effect	Variable: none to moderate	Moderate to marked	Variable: slight to moderate	Frequently marked	Slight

[a]Denotes significant differential characteristic.
Source: After Ref. 6.

1. Cerebellar Astrocytoma

Cerebellar astrocytoma is the most common posterior fossa tumor in the child (5,22). This tumor exhibits peak incidence in the middle of the first decade of life and is encountered infrequently in adult life. Posterior fossa astrocytoma can occur anywhere in the cerebellum, either in the midline (vermis) or hemisphere.

Cerebellar astrocytomas comprise two pathological subgroups (5,23):

1. Juvenile pilocytic astrocytoma, which accounts for 85% of cerebellar astrocytomas
2. Fibrillary variety (15%), which is similar to the cerebral astrocytoma of the adult

The pilocytic astrocytoma is well circumscribed, partially cystic, and often has a mural nodule of vascular solid tissue. The fibrillary type tends to be more infiltrative and is more frequently anaplastic.

On MRI, pilocytic cerebellar astrocytoma appears as a well-demarcated mass that may be solid, mixed cystic and solid (Fig. 13), or cystic, with a mural nodule often located in the wall of the cyst. Fifty percent of cerebellar astrocytomas are cystic, and an additional 20% are partially so (22).

On T1-weighted images, the solid portion of the tumor is hypointense to the normal brain (Fig. 14). The cystic portion is either isointense to CSF or may be hyperintense both on T1- and T2-weighted images, probably because of its proteinaceous contents. Following the intravenous administration of gadolinium-containing agents, the solid portion of the tumor enhances (see Fig. 14). In the cystic variety, the mural nodule exhibits marked enhancement. The cyst wall may or may not enhance.

Cerebellar astrocytomas may resemble hemangioblastomas. However, the latter tumor is rare in the pediatric-age group. The CT pattern is variable. In up to 20% of cases calcification may be

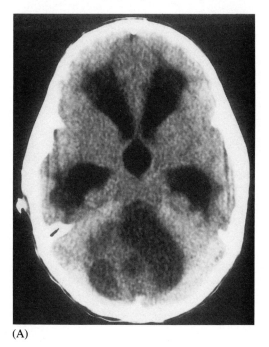 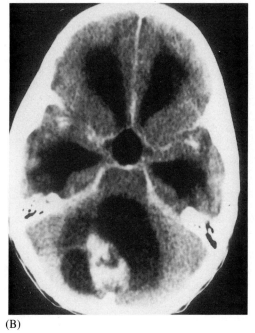

(A)   (B)

Figure 13 Cerebellar astrocytoma: (A) pre- and (B) postcontrast axial CT scans demonstrate marked hydrocephalus of the lateral and third ventricles. A large midline posterior fossa mass is noted that shows dense enhancement in its midportion following the administration of intravenous contrast material (B).

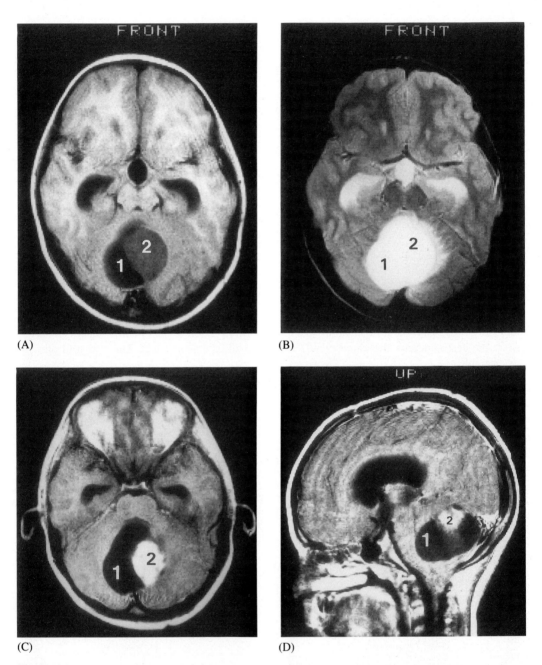

(A)   (B)

(C)   (D)

Figure 14   Pilocytic astrocytoma, cerebellum: (A) axial T1-weighted MRI; (B) axial T2-weighted MRI; (C, D) axial and sagittal T1-weighted MR images following the administration of contrast material. Axial images (A–C) and sagittal MRI (D) show a large midline mass that is partly cystic (1) with a mural nodule of solid tumor (2). On the T2-weighted MRI (B) both the cystic and solid portions of the tumor exhibit increased signal intensity. Enhancement is noted in the solid portion of the tumor (C,D).

demonstrated (22). This is more readily detected on CT. However, the presence or absence of calcification has little value in the differential diagnosis of this tumor. These tumors tend to be hypodense. The cystic variety appears as a fairly well-defined circular lucency with a mural nodule. Following the intravenous administration of iodinated contrast, there may be a ringlike pattern enhancement, as well as enhancement of the mural nodule (Fig. 15).

The solid type on precontrast scans may have a slightly increased density, decreased density, or may be isodense with the surrounding brain. Following the intravenous administration of contrast material, 40% of tumors will enhance in a homogeneous pattern.

2. Medulloblastoma

Medulloblastoma is a highly malignant brain tumor. It is the second most common brain tumor in children (5,23), although, in some series, it is rated as the most common posterior fossa neoplasm of childhood (22,25–27).

Pathologically, medulloblastoma is often included in the primitive neuroectodermal tumor group (PNET). These tumors are thought to originate from primitive or undifferentiated neuroepithelial cells, which display considerable histopathological heterogeneity. The prototype of these tumors is the cerebellar medulloblastoma. The term PNET is somewhat controversial and, for the purposes of this chapter, the term medulloblastoma will be used.

Although they occur at any age, the peak incidence is 1–10 years of age (22). These tumors have a second peak at 20–24 years of age (23,28). Medulloblastomas occur most commonly in the midline. They develop in the vermis of the cerebellum and roof of the fourth ventricle (Fig. 16). Approximately two-thirds of the patients show extension into the cerebellar hemispheres or brain stem (Fig. 17).

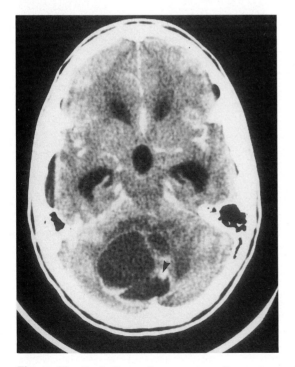

Figure 15 Cerebellar cystic astrocytoma: Postcontrast axial CT scan demonstrates enhancement around the wall of the cystic tumor. Enhancement is noted in the mural nodule of the solid portion of the tumor (arrowhead).

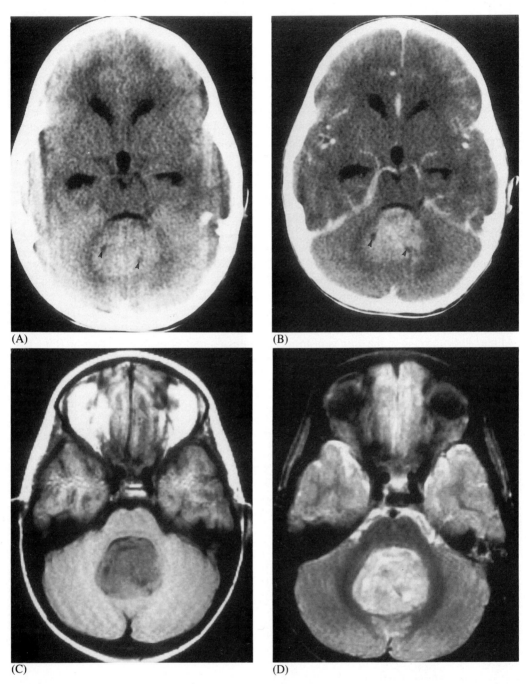

(A)   (B)

(C)   (D)

Figure 16   Medulloblastoma of fourth ventricle: (A, B) pre- and postcontrast axial CT scans; (C, D) axial T1- and T2-weighted MR images; (E) axial T1-weighted MRI following the intravenous administration of gadolinium. Pre- and postcontrast (A,B) demonstrate a large hyperdense mass that fills and displaces the fourth ventricle anteriorly. Mild inhomogeneous contrast enhancement is noted (B). Small intratumoral areas of cystic necrosis are noted. Obstructive hydrocephalus is also present. The mass is of low-signal intensity on the T1-weighted image (C) and exhibits increased signal intensity on the T2-weighted image (D). The small intratumoral areas of cystic necrosis seen on the CT scan are also seen on the MR images. The tumor exhibits marked enhancement on the postcontrast scan (E).

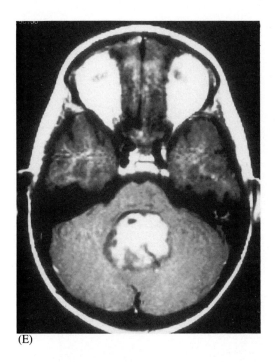

(E)

Certain intracranial neoplasms may exhibit frequent and widespread tumor dissemination throughout the subarachnoid space. Medulloblastoma, perhaps more than any other tumor, is known for its tendency to seed the subarachnoid space both intracranially and within the spinal canal (Fig. 18). To a lesser extent, ependymoma, astrocytoma, dysgerminoma, and choroid plexus carcinoma seed the subarachnoid space. Deutsch and Reigel (29) reported an incidence of 36.4% of clinically unsuspected lesions in the spinal canal, as demonstrated by myelography, in newly diagnosed medulloblastoma patients. These findings mandate evaluation of the spinal canal, even in those patients for whom there is no clinical suspicion of spinal disease. This may be accomplished by either myelography or, more commonly, by gadolinium-enhanced MRI of the spine. North et al. (30) reported subarachnoid spread in 30% of medulloblastomas seen on the initial cranial CT study.

Medulloblastoma exhibits T1 and T2 lengthening. It is hypointense on T1-weighted images and hyperintense on T2-weighted images. Compared with other brain tumors, medulloblastoma often exhibits a relative low-signal intensity on T2-weighted images and may appear nearly isointense to brain parenchyma. The marked hypercellularity of the tumor, with scant cytoplasm and a high nucleus/cytoplasm ratio, is thought to be responsible for this phenomenon.

Following the intravenous administration of contrast, medulloblastoma exhibits marked homogeneous enhancement (see Fig. 16). Intravenous contrast is also important to demonstrate leptomeningeal spread, both in the head and in the spine (see Fig. 18).

Medulloblastomas exhibit increased density, compared with the surrounding brain, on preinfusion CT scans (22) (see Fig. 16). This is often very helpful in differentiating these tumors from ependymoma or astrocytoma. Following the intravenous administration of iodinated contrast material, the tumor enhances homogeneously. However, about 10% of these tumors fail to enhance after the intravenous administration of contrast (Fig. 19).

A lateral hemispheric location may be seen in some patients, especially in older ones. These laterally situated medulloblastomas develop secondary to tumor extension through the foramen of Luschka into the CPA (Fig. 20). Other atypical features of medulloblastoma include areas of cystic formation or necrosis (27). Calcification occurs in about 10% of patients.

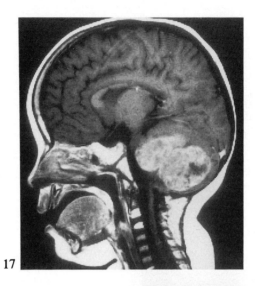

17

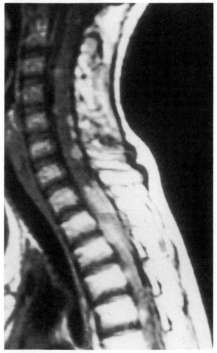

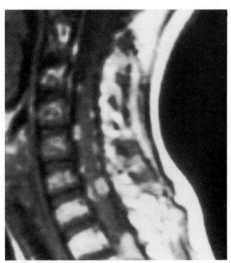

18A   18B

Figure 17 Extension of medulloblastoma into brain stem and cerebellar hemisphere. Sagittal T1-weighted MRI after the administration of gadolinium demonstrates a large inhomogeneously enhancing mass that extends into the brain stem and cerebellar hemisphere. Multiple small intratumoral areas of cystic necrosis are noted.

Figure 18 Seeding into spine of medulloblastoma (drop metastases): (A,B) sagittal T1-weighted MR images of (A) cervical and (B) thoracic spine following the intravenous administration of gadolinium demonstrates multiple enhancing masses of various size in the cervical and thoracic spinal canal.

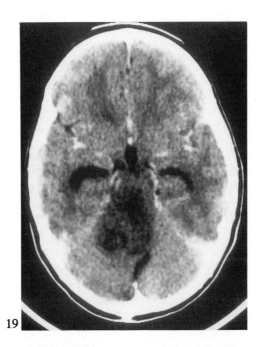

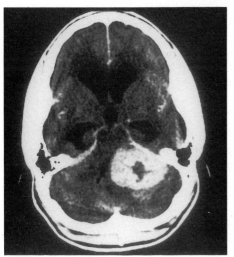

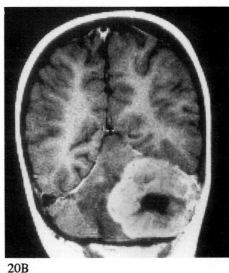

20A   20B

Figure 19   Medulloblastoma with no enhancement: Postcontrast axial CT scan demonstrates a large mass that fills the fourth ventricle and that exhibits no enhancement after the intravenous administration of iodinated contrast material.

Figure 20   Laterally situated medulloblastoma: (A) axial and (B) sagittal T1-weighted MR images following the intravenous administration of gadolinium, demonstrate a lateral hemispheric location of the tumor. A fairly large central cystic component of the tumor is noted.

3. Ependymoma

Ependymoma is a neoplasm composed of, and usually derived from, differentiated ependymal cells. In childhood, intracranial ependymoma is more commonly infratentorial (70%) than supratentorial (30%) (22). In children younger than 2 years of age, 92% are infratentorial. Posterior fossa ependymoma arises from the ependymal surface of the floor of the fourth ventricle and is primarily a tumor of the fourth ventricle. Most posterior fossa ependymomas present within the first decade of life. The mean age at diagnosis is approximately 1–5 years (22). Posterior fossa ependymoma has a second peak at the age of 34 years (22).

Ependymoma often invades the cerebellar hemispheres and brain stem. The tumor may extend through the foramen of Luschka of the fourth ventricle into the CPA cisterns. It can also extend through the foramen of Magendie through the vallecula into the cisterna magna. In about 10% of cases the tumor may extend through the foramen magnum into the dorsal aspect of the cervical spinal canal (31). This has been termed "plastic ependymoma," and this appearance is highly suggestive of the diagnosis (32).

Multiplanar imaging is particularly helpful in identifying the intraventricular location of the tumor. However, as the tumor grows, it often invades surrounding parenchyma. It then may be difficult to distinguish this tumor from tumors arising in the cerebellum. The signal intensity changes are generally characterized by T1 and T2 lengthening (Fig. 21). Cystic or necrotic changes may exhibit increased T1 and T2 relaxation times. Subacute to chronic hemorrhage may be seen.

Ependymomas are associated with small amounts of bleeding over a long period, leading to hemosiderin deposition on the pial surface. Ependymomas are the most common cause of superficial siderosis, which appears as a thin line of hypointensity surrounding the exposed surfaces of the brain. It is more prominent on T2-weighted images and is better demonstrated with higher field strength units.

On CT, the features of ependymoma are variable. The tumor may exhibit increased density, decreased density, and isodensity on noncontrast scans (27). Calcification is seen in about 50% of ependymomas (Fig. 22). In about 10% of medulloblastomas calcification is also seen. Thus, calcification is not pathognomonic of ependymomas. Central necrosis and cyst formation are common with ependymomas.

Following the intravenous administration of iodinated contrast material, most tumors show patchy enhancement (27). Some tumors will enhance uniformly. A small percentage will not enhance at all following the administration of contrast.

4. Subependymoma

Subependymoma is considered a variant of ependymoma (33). These tumors are often an incidental finding at autopsy, even when large enough to fill the fourth ventricle. They are characterized by a very benign course and are slow-growing tumors. They are usually seen in men

---

Figure 21 Fourth ventricular ependymoma: (A) sagittal T1-weighted MRI; (B) axial T2-weighted MRI. Sagittal T1-weighted MRI (A) demonstrates a large iso- to slightly hypointense inhomogeneous mass filling the fourth ventricle and compressing the pons and medulla. Herniation of the cerebellar tonsil is noted (arrowhead) as well as obstructive hydrocephalus. The T2-weighted MRI (B) in the same patient demonstrates a large midline mass in the posterior fossa that exhibits inhomogeneous increased signal intensity. Areas of intratumoral cystic necrosis are noted.

Figure 22 Fourth ventricular ependymoma: (A) precontrast axial CT scan; (B) postcontrast axial CT scan. Precontrast CT scan (A) demonstrates a midline isodense mass. Areas of calcification are noted in the left side of the mass (arrowheads). The fourth ventricle is effaced and displaced anteriorly. Marked obstructive hydrocephalus is noted. The postcontrast CT scan (B) demonstrates intense inhomogeneous enhancement of the tumor.

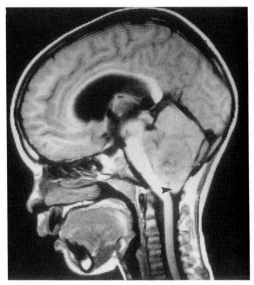

21A

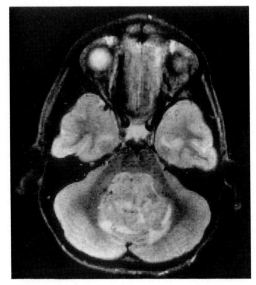

21B

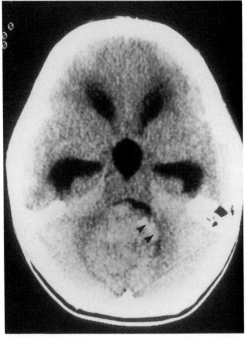

22A

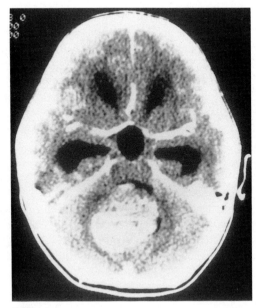

22B

with a mean age of 60 years at the time of presentation. Occasionally, these tumors grow large enough to cause symptoms by causing obstructive hydrocephalus.

Subependymomas tend to calcify, and they are solid and relatively homogeneous. The fourth ventricle is the most common site (75%) for subependymoma (34). These tumors can also occur in the lateral ventricle and aqueduct of Sylvius.

5. Hemangioblastoma

Hemangioblastoma is a histologically benign tumor occurring exclusively within the neuroaxis, most commonly in the posterior fossa (35). Hemangioblastoma is the most common primary adult intra-axial posterior fossa tumor. It can also occur in the medulla and spinal cord. Supratentorial involvement is distinctly uncommon (35).

Hemangioblastoma may be part of the von Hippel–Lindau complex (VHL complex), or it may occur sporadically. The VHL complex is an autosomal dominant disorder characterized by retinal angiomas; cerebellar, medullary, and spinal hemangioblastomas; renal cell carcinoma; cysts; and angiomatous tumors of several visceral organs (see Chap. 18). Fewer than 20% of patients with hemangioblastoma have the VHL complex (36).

The peak incidence is in the fifth and sixth decades of life for the nonfamilial or sporadic hemangioblastoma. Hemangioblastomas that are part of the VHL complex present in younger adults, with a peak incidence in the third decade of life and the second peak in the fifth decade (35). In familial cases, hemangioblastomas tend to be multiple (35). In the nonfamilial or sporadic variety multiplicity is rare.

Hemangioblastomas demonstrate several morphological patterns:

1. Cyst with mural nodule
2. Solid tumor
3. Solid tumor with intratumoral cyst

Seventy percent of cerebellar hemangioblastomas tend to be cystic, with a highly vascularized solid mural nodule situated in the wall of the cyst (35,36). Characteristically, the mural nodule is superficial and abuts pia mater. Entirely solid hemangioblastomas occur in about 30% of patients. Some solid tumors may contain intratumoral cysts.

Magentic resonance imaging is more sensitive and specific than CT for the diagnosis of cerebellar hemangioblastoma (36) (Fig. 23).

One of the goals of preoperative imaging is to locate the mural nodule. This is important, not only to make a specific diagnosis, but also because the cyst is bound to recur unless the mural nodule is removed at the time of surgery. If CT or MRI does not demonstrate the mural nodule, it may be necessary to perform angiography to demonstrate this nodule or additional smaller lesions (Figs. 24 and 25).

Vertebral angiography is highly sensitive to detect the mural nodule and additional smaller hemangioblastomas. Hemangioblastomas are very vascular, with an intense tumor stain appearing in the arterial phase and persisting well into the venous phase. Although a hypertrophied artery supplying the tumor may be demonstrated, no obvious draining veins are seen. It has not yet been

---

Figure 23 Cerebellar hemangioblastoma: (A,B) axial T1- and T2-weighted MR images; (C) axial T1-weighted MRI following the intravenous administration of gadolinium. A large cyst occupies the right cerebellar hemisphere. On the periphery of the cyst, a solid mural nodule (arrow) is noted. The mural nodule is iso- to hypointense on the T1-weighted MRI (A). On the T2-weighted MRI (B) both the cyst and mural nodule exhibit increased signal intensity, with the cyst exhibiting greater T2 lengthening than the mural nodule. Following the intravenous administration of gadolinium, the mural nodule exhibits marked enhancement (C).

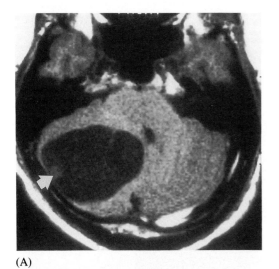

(A)

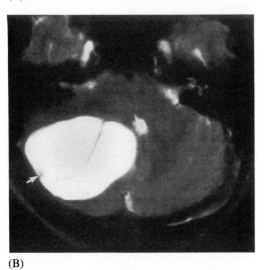

(B)

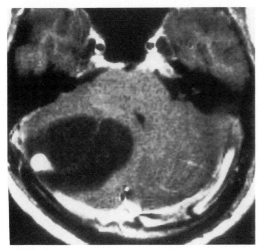

(C)

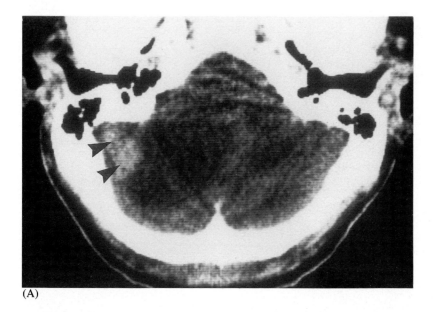

(A)

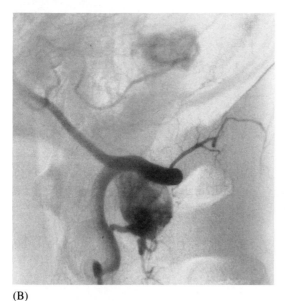

(B)

Figure 24 Multiple hemangioblastomas: (A) postcontrast axial CT scan; (B) lateral projection of left vertebral angiogram. Postcontrast CT scan (A) demonstrates enhancing mural nodule (arrowheads) associated with a large right cerebellar cyst. The arterial phase of the left vertebral angiogram (B) demonstrates two densely enhancing masses. In addition to the mural nodule seen on the CT scan (A), a second hemangioblastoma is demonstrated in the upper cervical spinal canal. This area was not imaged on the CT scan of the head.

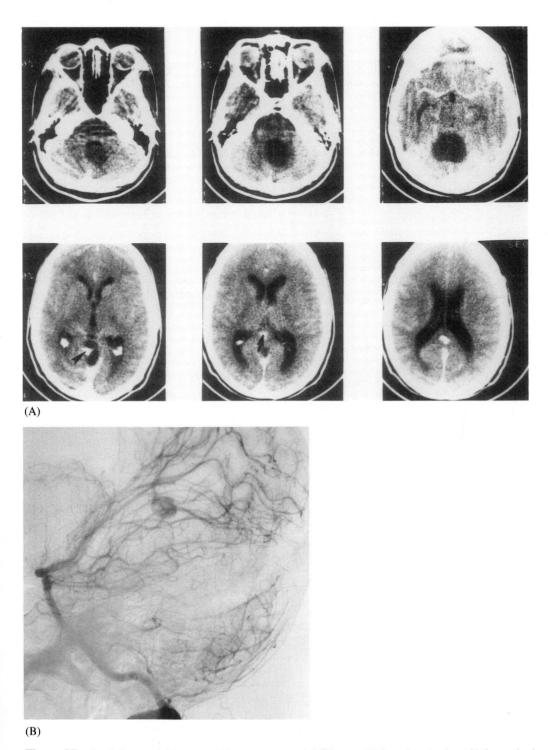

(A)

(B)

Figure 25 Cystic hemangioblastoma: (A) postcontrast axial CT scan; (B) lateral projection of left vertebral angiogram. Postcontrast axial CT scan (A) demonstrates a midline cystic mass. The arrowhead points to the enhancing mural nodule on the upper aspect of the cyst. The arrow points to the normal-enhancing pineal gland. Left vertebral angiography (B) confirms the diagnosis of the mural nodule by demonstrating the characteristic intense stain of the mural nodule in the arterial phase of the angiogram.

established whether high resolution contrast-enhanced MRI is as sensitive as angiography for detecting smaller lesions.

Some specific almost pathognomonic features of hemangioblastoma on MRI include:

1. Cystic nature of mass
2. Peripheral pial-based mural nodule of solid tissue that enhances markedly following the intravenous injection of contrast material

Large vessels may be seen in the periphery of the tumor or within the tumor mass, which appear as serpentine or linear regions of signal void both on T1- and T2-weighted images.

The signal intensity of the cyst is variable. It may be isointense to CSF on T1- and T2-weighted images. However, if the cyst contains paramagnetic cations secondary to hemorrhage or nonparamagnetic protein concentrates, the cyst intensity can be slightly high relative to CSF on T1- and T2-weighted images. The mural nodule is hypointense on T1-weighted images and hyperintense on T2-weighted images (see Fig. 24). The mural nodule enhances markedly following the intravenous administration of contrast material (see Fig. 23).

On precontrast CT, the tumor appears as an area of decreased attenuation. Following the intravenous administration of iodinated contrast material the mural nodule is seen as an area of enhancement in the wall of the cyst (see Figs. 24 and 25). Solid hemangioblastomas enhance homogeneously following intravenous contrast material administration.

6. Lymphoma

Primary CNS lymphoma constitutes fewer than 1.5% of all CNS neoplasms (37). However, its incidence is increasing and has tripled over the past decade (5). Parenchymal intracranial lymphoma is almost exclusively non-Hodgkin's in type.

Lymphoma can be focal or multiple, most commonly presenting in the deep gray matter structures (basal ganglia and thalamus), periventricular regions, cerebellum (Fig. 26), and brain stem. The reader is referred to the discussion of lymphoma in Chapter 17 for more details.

7. Metastases

Metastatic deposits are the most common intra-axial posterior fossa tumors in adults. Although they may have a variety of appearances, most metastases are round and well demarcated. Edema often surrounds cerebellar metastases, but it is less prominent than that observed with cerebral metastases. Multiplicity is an important diagnostic feature, but this is not always true. A single metastasis may occur in 49% of patients (38). The most common sites of origin are lung, breast (Figs. 27 and 28), skin (melanoma), gastrointestinal tract, and genitourinary tract.

Signal intensity patterns of metastases on MRI are nonspecific, in that most tumors exhibit prolonged relaxation times on T1- and T2-weighted images (i.e., they have low-signal intensity on T1-weighted images and high-signal intensity on T2-weighted images).

An MRI scan can be more specific in many cases. Metastases from melanoma, choriocarcinoma, and renal cell carcinoma have a particular tendency to bleed, and this is well demonstrated on MRI. Nonhemorrhagic melanoma metastases can be hyperintense on T1-weighted images and isointense on T2-weighted images. This relaxation enhancement pattern has been ascribed to the free-radical content of melanin (5). Areas of nonhemorrhagic cystic necrosis within a metastasis can be seen as an area of signal intensity that parallels CSF. Necrosis may also shorten relaxation times, appear bright on T1-weighted images and have a decreased signal on T2-weighted images. This is due to the release of intracellular, naturally occurring paramagnetic agents (Fe, Cu) with free-radical peroxidation (5).

Although the inherent sensitivity of conventional MRI (T1 and T2) to detect metastases is

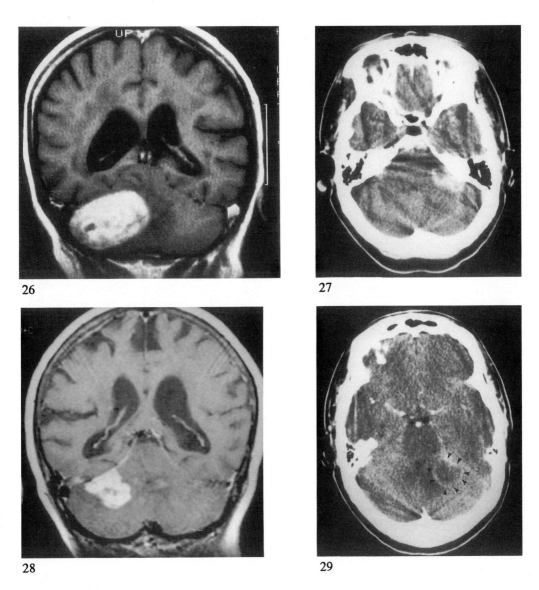

26 27

28 29

Figure 26 Non-Hodgkin's lymphoma, cerebellar hemisphere: Postcontrast T1-weighted MRI demonstrates a large inhomogeneously enhancing mass in the right cerebellar hemisphere. Areas of cystic necrosis are also seen.

Figure 27 Metastatic breast carcinoma: Postcontrast axial CT scan demonstrates an enhancing mass in the left CPA.

Figure 28 Metastatic breast carcinoma: Coronal T1-weighted MRI, following the intravenous administration of gadolinium, demonstrates a right-sided, intensely, but inhomogeneously, enhancing dural-based mass with irregular margins. The tentorium to which the mass is attached also enhances, suggesting tumor extension along the tentorium.

Figure 29 Metastatic lung carcinoma: Postcontrast axial CT scan demonstrates peripheral ring enhancement (arrowheads) around a necrotic mass above the left CPA. Peritumoral edema is also noted.

high, the intravenous administration of contrast increases the sensitivity of detection of intracranial metastases (8,9). Contrast MRI detects many lesions that otherwise may go undetected.

The pattern of enhancement varies. Solid (see Fig. 28), nodular, and ringlike enhancement may be seen. Contrast with MRI is also an excellent modality to detect leptomeningeal involvement. Although not as sensitive as MRI, postcontrast CT is also an excellent modality to detect metastases. On CT, most metastases demonstrate homogeneous or ringlike enhancement (see Figs. 28 and 29). Cystic areas may also be seen on CT.

B. Intra-axial Tumors of the Anterior Compartment of the Posterior Fossa

1. Brain Stem Gliomas

Glioma is the most common neoplasm involving the brain stem. The peak incidence for brain stem glioma is aged 4–13 years. The term *brain stem glioma* designates a group of glial tumors intrinsic to the brain stem. About 70% of brain stem gliomas are anaplastic astrocytomas or glioblastoma multiforme. Approximately 20% resemble the more benign juvenile pilocytic astrocytoma (23). Gangliomas, ependymomas, and hemangioblastomas also occur within the brain stem.

Brain stem glioma most often involves the pons (Fig. 30), followed by the midbrain. The tumor exhibits rostrocaudal spread into the thalamus or the medulla, respectively. Primary brain stem gliomas of the medulla are uncommon (Fig. 31), but frequently tend to be malignant. The tumor may also spread through the cerebellar peduncles into the cerebellum. Brain stem glioma can be exophytic and present as a CPA tumor.

Before the advent of MRI, the diagnosis of brain stem glioma was difficult even with CT. The diagnosis was often based solely on indirect signs of subtle enlargement or distortion of the pons on CT (see Fig. 30). Magnetic resonance imaging has dramatically advanced the diagnosis of these neoplasms by providing superb anatomical detail, combined with ability to differentiate the tissue characteristics of the tumor on T1- and T2-weighted images (39).

The MRI features of brain stem glioma are variable. Intratumoral heterogeneity is present on T1- and T2-weighted images (see Fig. 30). On T1-weighted images, brain stem gliomas may exhibit a hypointense or isointense signal intensity. They may appear as poorly defined areas of increased signal on T2-weighted images. Hemorrhage may often be present. Cysts or areas of necrosis are not uncommon. The MRI scan will also demonstrate the enlargement and distortion of the pons. Hydrocephalus is a late concomitant finding and occurs less frequently and later than with other posterior fossa tumors. Effacement of the prepontine cistern and encasement of the basilar artery will be demonstrated by MRI.

Contrast enhancement occurs in about 50% of cases (31) (see Figs. 30 and 31); it may be focal and irregular, and large portions of the tumor may not enhance. There is no relation between enhancement and histological malignancy. Some low-grade astrocytomas show striking enhancement, whereas some glioblastomas do not enhance at all.

Calcification is rare in untreated gliomas. Calcification may develop within brain stem gliomas following radiation therapy. Recent and old hemorrhage is a common finding.

C. Extra-axial Tumors of the Anterior Compartment of the Posterior Fossa

Eighty percent of extra-axial lesions of the posterior fossa are found in the cerebellopontine angle cistern.

Magnetic resonance imaging is considered the primary and often the definitive imaging examination for the detection of CPA lesions.

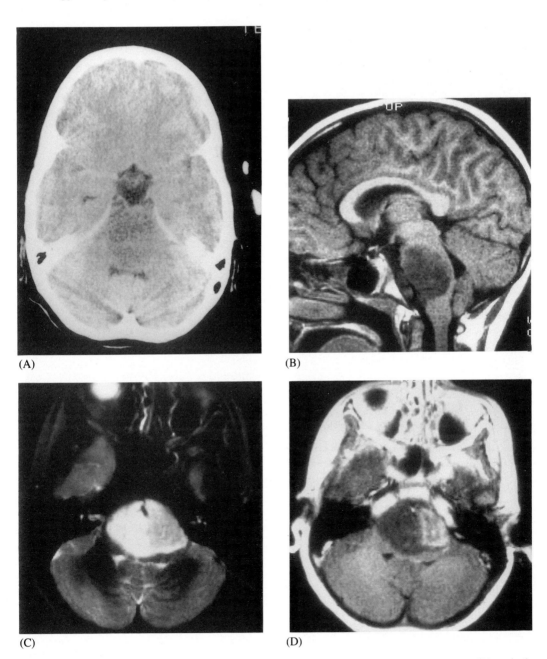

Figure 30 Brain stem glioma; superiority of MRI over CT: (A) postcontrast axial CT scan; (B) sagittal T1-weighted MRI; (C) axial T2-weighted MRI; (D) axial T1-weighted MRI after the intravenous administration of gadolinium. Postcontrast axial CT scan (A) demonstrates subtle findings of a brain stem mass. An ill-defined area of decreased attenuation is seen in the brain stem. The fourth ventricle is displaced posteriorly and its shape is distorted and effaced by the mass. Sagittal T1-weighted MRI (B) demonstrates a large, well-defined mass in the pons and medulla that displaces the fourth ventricle and aqueduct posteriorly. This mass exhibits inhomogeneous decreased signal intensity. Axial T2-weighted MRI (C) shows that the mass exhibits inhomogeneous increased signal intensity, with the left side showing less increase in signal intensity than the right side. Following the intravenous administration of gadolinium, the T1-weighted MRI (D) reveals an area of inhomogeneous enhancement in the left side of the tumor.

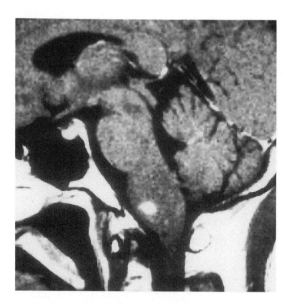

Figure 31 Glioma of medulla: Post-gadolinium sagittal T1-weighted MRI demonstrates a nodular area of enhancement that exhibits hypo- to isointense signal in the swollen and enlarged medulla. The tumor extends into the upper cervical area.

Intra-axial neoplasms from the brain stem, vermis, cerebellar hemisphere, or fourth ventricle may extend into the CPA. However, most CPA neoplasms are extradural in origin, arising from the meninges, nerve roots, or vascular structures. Cerebellopontine angle mass lesions include:

1. Acoustic schwannoma
2. Meningioma
3. Epidermoid and dermoid cysts
4. Schwannomas of other cranial nerves
5. Arachnoid cyst
6. Cholesterol granuloma
7. Ependymoma
8. Choroid plexus papilloma
9. Glomus tumor
10. Lipoma
11. Chordoma
12. Metastases
13. Lymphoma

1. Acoustic Schwannoma

Acoustic schwannoma is the most common neoplasm of the CPA and internal auditory canal (IAC) accounting for 85–90% of all CPA and IAC tumors (40,41). It constitutes approximately 7–8% of all primary intracranial tumors (42).

Acoustic nerve schwannoma (neuroma, neurinoma, neurilemoma), like a schwannoma elsewhere in the body, arises from the neural sheath of the nerve. Acoustic schwannoma can arise anywhere along the entire course of the eighth cranial nerve, and almost all of them arise from the vestibular portion of the eighth cranial nerve. Tumors arising from the cochlear division are less common. The peak incidence of presentation usually occurs between 40 and 60 years of age.

These tumors generally involve the intracanalicular portion of the nerve and, in most instances, also demonstrate a mass in the cerebellopontine angle. Frequently, these neoplasms are seen in association with neurofibromatosis 2 (NF2) in which they are typically bilateral. Bilateral tumors may also occur in a familial form not associated with neurofibromatosis (43).

On precontrast CT scans, acoustic schwannomas are isointense with gray matter. The tumor is centered on the internal auditory meatus. Cisternal widening and canal enlargement are noted in about 90% of the cases. Following the intravenous administration of iodinated contrast material, there is pronounced homogeneous enhancement of the tumor.

Enhanced CT scans cannot exclude the presence of a small intracanalicular acoustic schwannoma. Lesions smaller than 0.5 cm and completely intracanalicular previously required gas cisternography CT to demonstrate these tumors (44). High-resolution multiplanar MRI is the examination of choice for demonstration of these lesions.

Acoustic schwannomas are well demarcated, with smooth margins. They are mildly hypointense on T1-weighted images, exhibiting a heterogeneous pattern (Figs. 32 and 33). On T2-weighted images these tumors exhibit heterogeneous hyperintensity (see Fig. 32). The heterogeneous pattern, consisting of ill-defined regions of mild hypointensity and isointensity on T1-weighted images and hyperintense and isointense on T2-weighted images, probably represent areas of different cell types. Well-defined oval regions within the tumor of hypointensity on T1-weighted images and hyperintensity on T2-weighted images similar to that of CSF probably represent cystic change within the tumor. Tumors with marked vascularity or focal nodular calcifications will reveal areas of hypointensity on T1- and T2-weighted images.

Large CPA tumors have a broad-based surface along the petrous ridge. In acoustic schwannoma there is usually an intracanalicular portion of the tumor associated with a cisternal mass. Widening of the IAC will usually be appreciated best on axial MRI scans. Coronal images usually do not demonstrate the entire length of the canal in a single slice (45). About 20% of acoustic schwannomas, however, have no intracanalicular component or only a very small knuckle of tumor extending into the canal (42). Lesions without intracanalicular extension can be difficult to differentiate from a CPA meningioma.

Acoustic schwannoma, unlike meningioma, tends to be rounded, rather than sessile, in configuration, exhibiting acute angles between the lesion and petrous bone. They tend to be centered in or near the porus acousticus. Only rarely do acoustic schwannomas extend into the middle fossa, in contradistinction to meningomas, which frequently extend into the middle fossa.

Following the intravenous administration of gadolinium-containing agents, acoustic schwannomas enhance markedly (Fig. 33). Contrast enhancement may be homogeneous, but is frequently inhomogeneous. Usually tumor within the internal auditory canal can be demonstrated on noncontrast MRI; however, contrast enhancement will demonstrate smaller intracanalicular tumors that may not be seen on the noncontrast examination (see Fig. 33). Contrast enhancement may also show extension of the tumor into the canal in the absence of canal expansion. With the use of intravenous gadolinium, tumors as small as 2–3 mm in diameter can be clearly demonstrated (46).

2. Meningioma

The posterior fossa, including the foramen magnum, is the site for 10–12% of all intracranial meningiomas (43). Most meningiomas arise in the CPA and are the second most common neoplasm to occur in this location (Figs. 34 and 35). However, the incidence of CPA acoustic schwannoma is three to four times that of a CPA meningioma. Other locations in the posterior fossa at which meningiomas occur include the cerebellar convexities, lateral sinus, clivus, and foramen magnum (Fig. 36).

Findings on CT and MRI differ little from the findings of meningiomas in the supratentorial compartment. The CPA meningiomas are broad based and smoothly marginated. They have a

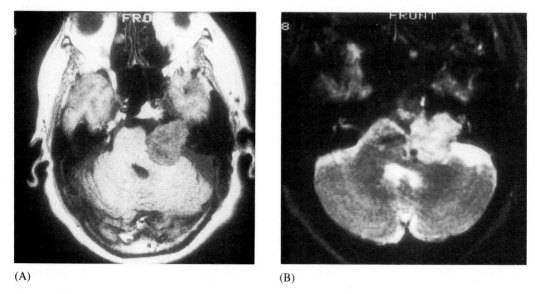

(A)   (B)

Figure 32   Acoustic schwannoma: (A) axial T1-weighted MRI; (B) axial T2-weighted MRI. Axial T1- and T2-weighted MRI images (A,B) demonstrate a large left CPA tumor that is heterogeneous and is associated with brain stem compression. The tumor is hypointense on T1-weighting (A) and hyperintense on T2-weighting (B):

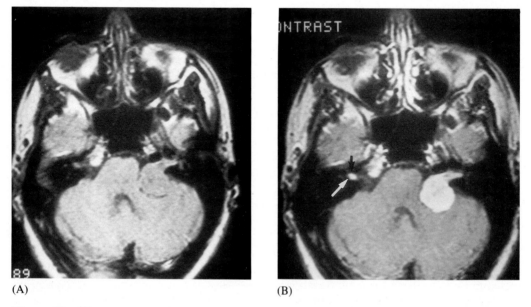

(A)   (B)

Figure 33   Bilateral acoustic schwannomas: (A) axial T1-weighted MRI; (B) post-gadolinium axial T1-weighted MRI. Precontrast T1-weighted MRI (A) shows a large left CPA mass. Following the intravenous administration of gadolinium, the T1-weighted MRI (B) shows enhancement of the left-sided acoustic schwannoma as well as enhancement in a right intracanalicular tumor (arrow).

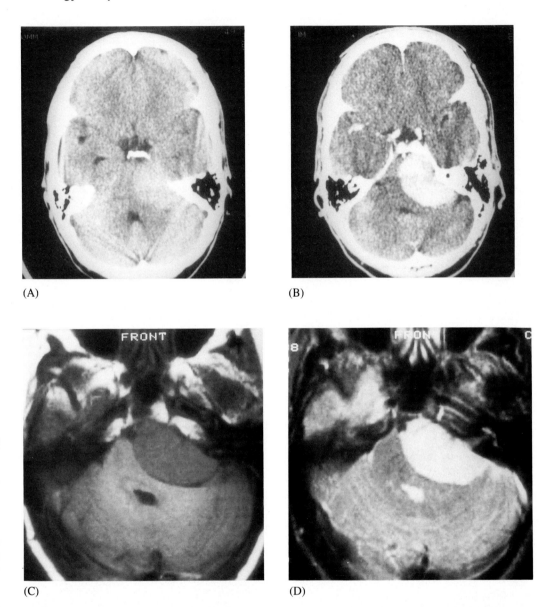

Figure 34 Cerebropontine angle meningioma: (A) precontrast axial CT scan; (B) postcontrast axial CT scan; (C) axial T1-weighted MRI; (D) axial T2-weighted MRI. Precontrast CT scan (A) demonstrates a large hyperdense CPA mass that enhances homogeneously after the intravenous administration of iodinated contrast material (B). The mass has a dural-based attachment to the petrous bone. The T1-weighted MRI (C) shows a large hypointense mass with a more hypointense rim. This latter finding represents a CSF cleft. The broad-based dural attachment and the identification of a CSF cleft are findings confirming the extradural location of the tumor. The tumor exhibits increased signal intensity on T2-weighted MRI (D). Hyperintense meningiomas on T2-weighted images are associated with syncytial or angioblastic elements (see Chap. 9).

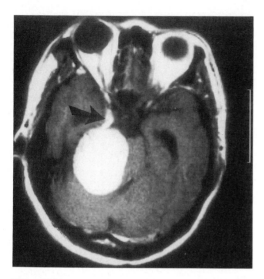

Figure 35 Cerebropontine angle meningioma with supratentorial extension: Post-gadolinium axial T1-weighted MRI demonstrates a large right-sided enhancing CPA mass. Right paracavernous extension of the mass is indicated by the arrow.

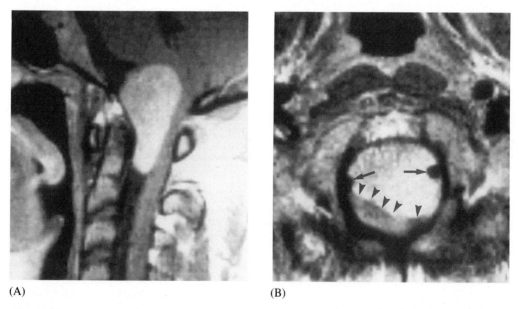

(A)   (B)

Figure 36 Foramen magnum meningioma: (A) post-gadolinium sagittal T1-weighted MRI; (B) post-gadolinium axial T1-weighted MRI. Post-gadolinium sagittal (A) and axial (B) T1-weighted MR images demonstrate a large pear-shaped homogeneously enhancing mass occupying the anterior three-fourths of the foramen magnum. The medulla and upper cervical spinal cord are compressed by the mass. The anterior edge of the medulla is indicated by the arrowheads on the axial scan (B), which also demonstrates both vertebral arteries (arrows). The left vertebral artery is encased by the tumor.

homogeneous hyperdense appearance on noncontrast CT (see Fig. 34). In some instances, they may be isodense. Calcification is very common and ranges from diffuse calcification to areas of punctate calcification. Following the intravenous administration of iodinated contrast material, these tumors enhance homogeneously (see Fig. 34). If a tumor is densely calcified, the enhancement is difficult to appreciate.

On MRI, meningiomas tend to be isointense to gray matter, exhibiting a heterogeneous texture both on T1- and T2-weighted images. On T1-weighted images, some meningiomas may be hypointense (see Fig. 34); on T2-weighted images, meningioma is often less hyperintense relative to the gray matter when compared with other tumors. Occasionally, meningioma exhibit increased signal on T2-weighted images. Acoustic schwannomas usually show increased T1 and T2 relaxation features when compared with meningiomas; however, the overlap between both tumors precludes a safe differentiation based on tissue parameters alone. Peritumoral hyperintense edema occurs in 75% of cases, and this is best appreciated on the T2-weighted images. Signal inhomogeneity or microcyst or cyst formation is common and occurs in about 20% of patients. However, frank cyst formation is rare, occurring in fewer than 2% of cases. Marked homogeneous enhancement is noted following the intravenous injection of gadolinium (see Fig. 35).

Meningiomas may extend upward and anteriorly into the parasellar region. This produces the characteristic comma sign of a meningioma (see Fig. 35). The CPA acoustic schwannomas, in contradistinction, tend to grow in a posterior direction into the ambient cistern.

The lack of intracanalicular signal alteration or lack of intracanalicular contour abnormality produced by meningioma is a helpful finding in differentiating meningiomas from acoustic schwannomas. Although most meningiomas do not involve the internal auditory canal, occasionally extension into and enlargement of the IAC is seen with meningiomas (46) (Fig. 37).

Marked punctate or confluent foci of decreased signal on T2-weighted images usually indicates calcification. This occurs in 25% of cases (47). Calcification is unusual with schwannomas, occurring in 5% of cases. Hyperostosis in the temporal bone, secondary to meningioma, occurs less commonly than with meningiomas located in other parts of the cranium.

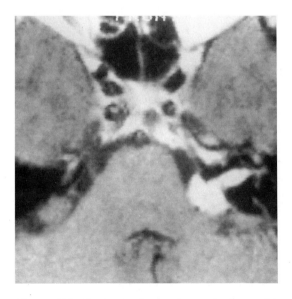

Figure 37 Cerebropontine angle meningioma with extension into the internal auditory canal: Post-gadolinium axial T1-weighted MRI demonstrates an enhancing left CPA mass with a fingerlike extension into the internal auditory canal.

3. Epidermoid Cyst

Epidermoid cyst (epidermoidoma and cholesteatoma) is an uncommon lesion accounting for approximately 1% of all intracranial tumors. These lesions arise from ectodermal elements that become sequestered at the time of closure of the neural groove during the third to fifth weeks of embryonic life. Histologically, epidermoid cysts are composed of epidermis and associated connective tissue. This lesion represents an embryonic malformation, rather than a true neoplasm, but it is regarded as a tumor because of its expanding nature. Because of their characteristic glistening white capsule with a "mother-of-pearl" sheath, these lesions have been termed *tumeurs perlees* or pearly tumors (48). Although these lesions are congenital and can present at any age, they do not usually present until the fourth or fifth decade of life (49).

Cranial epidermoids may be either intradural (90%) or extradural (10%) (50). Intradurally, the preferred location is the basal surface of the brain (subarachnoid cisterns), with 40% of these lesions being found in the CPA. They can also occur in the fourth ventricle as well as supratentorially.

Epidermoids of the CPA are the third most common tumor in this region after acoustic schwannoma and meningioma. These lesions grow by progressive desquamation of epithelial cells with their conversion to keratin and cholesterin. Cholesterin is a lipid and is a breakdown product of keratin. Because the breakdown products are soft and because the pliable capsule wall continues to grow slowly, these tumors can literally grow into any available space, conforming to the shape of the adjacent brain and cerebrospinal fluid spaces in which they are growing. They usually reach a very large size before symptoms develop. The tumor grows slowly, is soft, and is very pliable.

On CT scan, an epidermoid cyst typically presents as a mass with low attenuation values (50) (Figs. 38 and 39). However, lesions of relatively high density can also occur. This range of values reflects the varying amounts of low-density lipid and high-density keratin in the desquamative debris of the tumor.

Discrete foci of calcification may be noted in the tumor capsule of an epidermoid, but calcification is uncommon. Generally, epidermoid tumors do not enhance after the intravenous injection of iodinated contrast material. This reflects the avascular nature of their contents and the thin avascular walls. On occasion, some enhancement at the margin of the lesion is seen, and this is attributed to reactive changes.

It can be difficult at times to differentiate an epidermoid from an arachnoid cyst on the density characteristics. The lobulated configuration of epidermoids, compared with the smooth surface of an arachnoid cyst, helps to differentiate these lesions.

The use of intrathecal water-soluble nonionic contrast agents in conjunction with CT can often demonstrate the characteristic filigree, frondlike, or cauliflower appearance of these lesions by opacifying the interstices of the tumor (50) (see Fig. 39). This is pathognomonic for epidermoid.

On T1-weighted MR images epidermoids exhibit mild hypointensity (between CSF and brain parenchyma) (see Fig. 38). The signal characteristics of T2-weighted images are similar to or greater than CSF (see Fig. 38), usually with significant heterogeneity of the signal intensity. On spin-density sequences, epidermoids are almost never isointense with CSF. This helps differentiate epidermoids from arachnoid cysts. The signal characteristic of most epidermoids may be related to the manner in which lipid cholesterin moieties are arranged. Intercalation of these moieties about the bound hydrogen of adjacent water, may account for the unexpected "waterlike" signal characteristics of epidermoids.

Cases of T1-weighted hyperintense epidermoids may occur rarely (51,52). These correspond to the hyperdense epidermoids that may be seen on CT (53).

The eccentric anatomical location, absence of T2-weighted hyperintense edema, signal inhomogeneity, scalloped or serpiginous margins, help differentiate these lesions from arachnoid cysts.

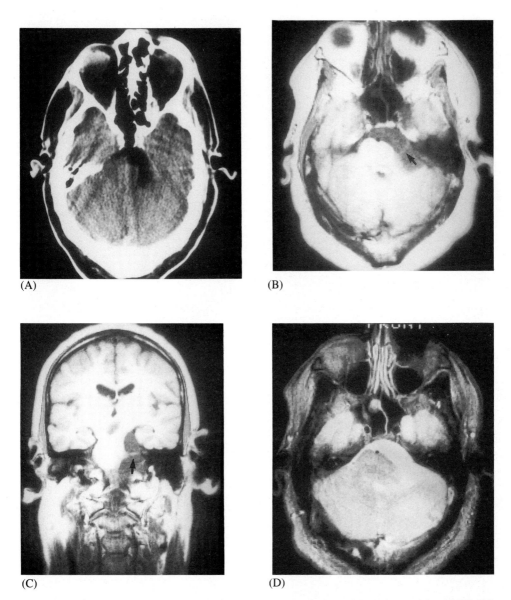

Figure 38 Peripontine epidermoid: (A) precontrast axial CT scan; (B) axial T1-weighted MRI; (C) coronal T1-weighted MRI; (D) axial T2-weighted MRI. The CT scan (A) demonstrates a left CPA mass with decreased attenuation extending medially to involve the prepontine cistern. Postcontrast CT scan (not shown) did not demonstrate any enhancement. Axial (B) and coronal (C) T1-weighted images demonstrate decreased signal intensity that is slightly greater than the decreased signal intensity of CSF. Stretching of the left trigeminal nerve (arrow) is noted (B,C). Insinuation of epidermoid tumors around nerves is a characteristic feature of these lesions. T2-weighted MRI (D) shows the tumor to be hyperintense.

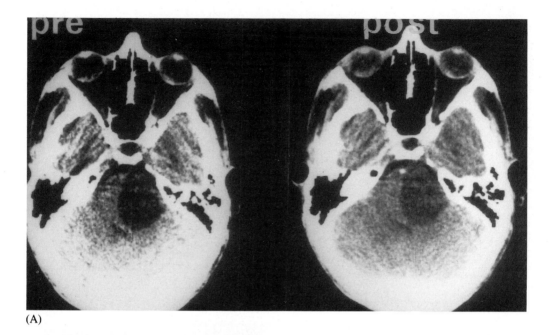

(A)

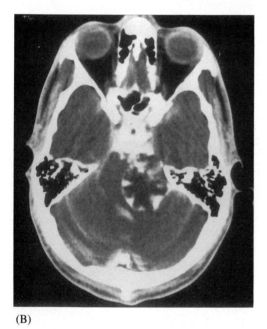

(B)

Figure 39 Epidermoid cyst: (A) pre- and postcontrast axial CT scans; (B) axial CT scan following the injection of intrathecal, nonionic water-soluble contrast material. Pre- and postcontrast CT scans (A) demonstrate a large area of decreased attenuation in the left CPA. No enhancement is seen on the postcontrast scan. Following the intrathecal administration of nonionic water-soluble contrast material, the CT scan (B) demonstrates the characteristic and almost pathognomonic picture of an epidermoid. Contrast material is seen opacifying the interstices of the tumor, producing the characteristic filigree, frondlike or cauliflower appearance.

4. Dermoid Cysts

Intracranially dermoid cysts are rarer tumors than epidermoid cysts (23). Dermoid cysts arise from the inclusion of ectodermal elements in the neural tube at its time of closure. Histologically, dermoid cysts contain dermal appendages, such as hair follicles, sweat glands, and sebaceous glands, in addition to epidermis. They enlarge by secretion of these glands. Clinically, they usually present in the third decade and are most commonly located in the posterior fossa in the midline, but they may occur in the cisterns about the sella and elsewhere. They may also have an intraventricular location.

Dermoid cysts typically demonstrate marked hyperintensity on T1-weighted images owing to their fatty content, which consists of triglycerides and unsaturated fatty acids (54) (Figs. 40 and 41). On T2-weighted images, the cysts usually exhibit hypointensity. These cysts may rupture into the subarachnoid space or the ventricle, in the case of intraventricular dermoids. Subarachnoid or intraventricular rupture will demonstrate droplets and streaks of high-signal intensity within the CSF on T1-weighted images. Within the ventricles, a fat–fluid level may be seen. On T1-weighted images a high-signal intensity fluid level will be present anterior to the hypointensity of CSF, whereas on T2-weighted sequences, an intermediate and low-signal fluid collection will be observed anterior to the high-signal intensity of CSF. A markedly hypointense band on the posterior margin of the ruptured dermoid contents, which represents a chemical shift artifact, may be seen. This confirms the fatty nature of these lesions.

The CT attenuation of dermoid cysts approximates fat (see Fig. 41). The major differences between epidermoids and dermoids are shown in Table 2.

5. Schwannomas Involving Other Cranial Nerves

Schwannomas may occur on other cranial nerves apart from the eighth nerve. The MRI appearance of schwannomas of other cranial nerves that involve the CPA are similar to acoustic schwannomas.

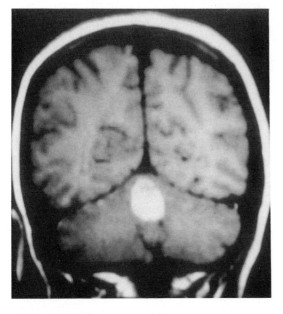

Figure 40 Posterior fossa dermoid: Coronal T1-weighted MRI demonstrates a midline oval mass of increased signal intensity. The T2-weighted MRI (not shown) reveals that the mass exhibited decreased signal intensity.

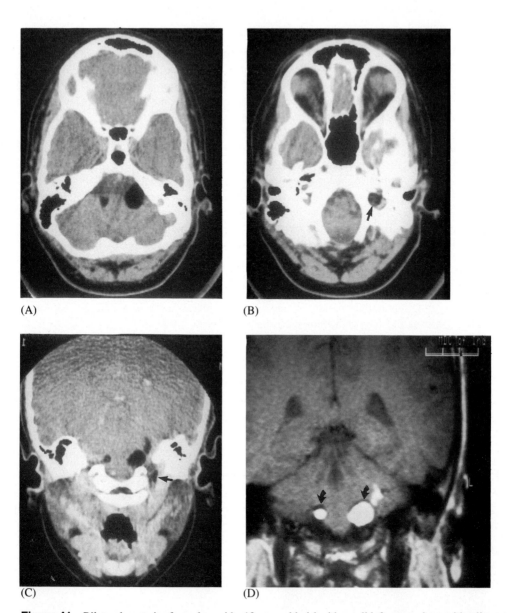

Figure 41 Bilateral posterior fossa dermoids; 12-year-old girl with small left external ear with adjacent skin tag: (A,B) noncontrast axial CT scans; (C) noncontrast coronal CT scan; (D) coronal T1-weighted MRI. The axial and coronal CT scans (A–C) demonstrate bilateral fat density masses, the left side greater than the right. The left-sided mass can be seen to enter the left jugular foramen (B,C) (straight arrows). Coronal T1-weighted MRI (D) demonstrates that these masses exhibit hyperintense signals. The hypointense rim surrounding the superior aspect of these masses (curved arrows) is due to chemical shift artifact observed adjacent to fatty structures. The T2-weighted MRI (not shown) demonstrated iso- to hypointense signal within the lesions.

Location of the central portion of the tumor within or near the nerve of origin helps localize the nerve from which it arises.

   Schwannoma of the trigeminal nerve (Figs. 42 and 43) is next in frequency to eighth nerve tumors. Schwannoma of the trigeminal nerve may occur along the course of the fifth nerve, involving its pontine cisternal segment or extension into Meckel's cave at the petrous apex and the cavernous sinus. The signal characteristics of these tumors approximate acoustic schwannomas.

Table 2 Major Differences Between Epidermoid and Dermoid Cysts

Characteristic	Epidermoid	Dermoid
Histology	Epidermal elements and connective tissue	In addition, dermal appendages (hair follicles, sweat and sebaceous glands)
Frequency	Ten times more frequent than dermoids	
Age of clinical onset	Peak onset: 5th decade	Younger patients: 1st and 2nd decades
Sex distribution	Male preponderance	Growth is slightly more rapid than epidermoids; enlarges by glandular secretions as well as by desquamation; tends to rupture more commonly than epidermoid
Sites of preference	Often in lateral location: diploe of skull, pons, cerebellopontine angle, ventricular system, optic chiasm, parapituitary area, and collicular plate	May also occur in same locations, but there is avidity for the midline (cerebellum), upper and outer quadrant of the orbit, scalp, and paranasal regions
Associated anomalies	No definite association.	Associated developmental anomalies of skeleton, dermal sinuses; tufts of external hair, focal skin pigmentation are often present.
Calcification	Uncommon	Common

Location and symptomatology provide the key to diagnosis. Location anterior to the CPA near the petrous tip or extension into the Meckel's cave and the middle fossa are suggestive of the trigeminal schwannoma.

Schwannomas of other cranial nerves will demonstrate intensity characteristics similar to those of acoustic schwannoma.

6. Arachnoid Cyst

Arachnoid cyst is a developmental lesion representing 1% of all intracranial masses. One-half to two-thirds occur in the middle cranial fossa (55). Arachnoid cysts may also be found in the posterior fossa in the CPA and foramen magnum region. The CPA is the second most common site for arachnoid cysts in the posterior fossa. The midline or lateral retrocerebellar location is the most common infratentorial location. Arachnoid cysts do not calcify and do not enhance following the intravenous administration of contrast.

These lesions have smooth round margins. The signal intensity on MRI will usually follow that of CSF. They are of low-signal intensity on T1-weighted images and high-signal intensity on T2-weighted images. The signal intensity is homogeneous, which helps differentiate it from epidermoids. On CT, arachnoid cysts are hypodense (matching CSF).

7. Cholesterol Granuloma

Cholesterol granuloma (cholesterol cyst, giant cholesterol cyst) is an expansile lesion of the petrous apex that thins and erodes bone. These lesions may be confused with epidermoids. It occurs in extensively pneumatized temporal bones. Obstruction of airflow from pneumatized air cells causes repetitive cycles of hemorrhage and granulomatous reaction (56). An inflammatory reaction to the

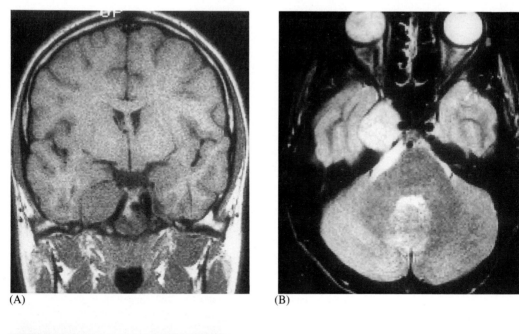

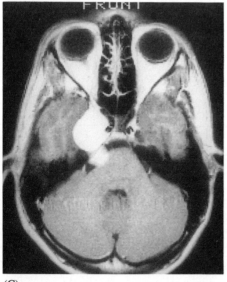

(C)

Figure 42 Trigeminal schwannoma: (A) coronal T1-weighted MRI; (B) axial T2-weighted MRI; (C) post-gadolinium axial T1-weighted MRI. Coronal T1-weighted MRI (A) demonstrates a large right-sided isointense mass centered in Meckel's cave. The hypointense rim around the lateral aspect of the mass represents a CSF cleft, indicating the extradural location of the mass. Axial T2-weighted MRI (B) demonstrates increased signal intensity in the mass. Axial T1-weighted MRI following the intravenous administration of gadolinium (C) demonstrates marked homogeneous enhancement of the mass and also demonstrates involvement of the pontine cisternal segment of the trigeminal nerve.

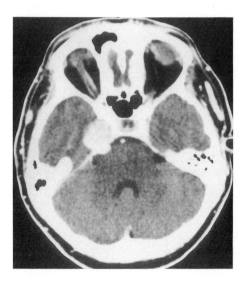

Figure 43 Trigeminal schwannoma: Postcontrast axial CT scan demonstrates a homogeneously enhancing mass centered in the right Meckel's cave and also involving the pontine cisternal segment of the trigeminal nerve.

cholesterol crystals from the breakdown products of blood leads to extensive bone erosion. Although these lesions are rare, they are much more common than previously realized (57, 58). They are probably the most common primary petrous apex lesion. Cholesterol granuloma may also involve the middle ear and mastoid.

These lesions are hyperintense on T1- and T2-weighted images (Fig. 44), thereby differentiating this mass from an epidermoid tumor (59,60). It does not enhance following intravenous gadolinium administration.

The CT scan demonstrates a sharply and smoothly marginated expansile mass of the petrous apex (57,58,61). It is isodense, does not contain calcium, and demonstrates no enhancement following the intravenous administration of contrast material.

8. *Choroid Plexus Papilloma*

Choroid plexus papillomas are uncommon histologically benign neoplasms that arise from epithelial cells of the choroid plexus. They represent about 3% of all intracranial neoplasms in children and about 0.5% of those in adults (62). In the course of neoplastic transformation, some of these epithelial cells may express glial characteristics that are consistent with the ontogeny of the parent organ (23). In addition, the tumors share with normal choroid plexus the physiological property of CSF production (23). The oversecretion by these neoplasms is a well-recognized phenomenon. Although they occur at any age, 40–50% present in the first decade of life. About 20% are identified in children younger than 1 year of age. In children, the left atrial trigone is the classic location for these neoplasms (23,62,63). Multiple papillomas exist in 3–7% of cases (23,63). In adults, choroid plexus papilloma occurs in the midline in the fourth ventricle or in its lateral recess (Figs. 45 and 46).

Involvement of the CPA occurs, in about 9% of these cases, from direct extension of a fourth ventricular papilloma, from distant CSF seeding, or as a primary CPA lesion arising from the small choroidal tuft that normally protrudes from the foramen of Luschka (64) (see Fig. 45). Normally, a small tuft of choroidal plexus accompanies the lateral medullary velum as it exits the foramen of Luschka and extends into the CPA (65,66). This has been termed Bochdalek's flower basket

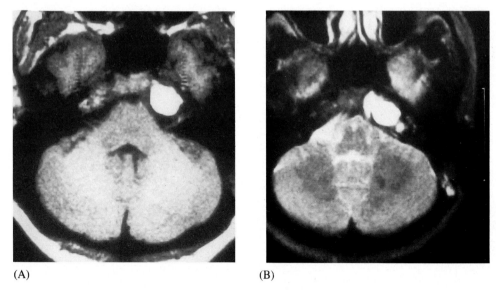

(A)   (B)

Figure 44 Cholesterol cyst: (A) axial T1-weighted MRI; (B) axial T2-weighted MRI. (A) T1- and (B) T2-weighted MR images demonstrate a well-defined petrous apex mass on the left side. This mass is hyperintense on both T1- and T2-weighted MR images.

(Bochdaleksches Blumenkorbchen). This is a site from which choroid plexus papilloma can arise and is totally extra-axial and extraventricular in location. Extra-axial and extraventricular ependymoma can arise in the same location from the lateral medullary velum (67,68).

Choroid plexus papilloma has a lobulated margin and is iso- to slightly hypointense on T1-weighted images (see Fig. 45). On T2-weighted images the tumor exhibits heterogeneous hyperintensity (see Fig. 45). Following the intravenous administration of gadolinium, the tumor enhances markedly (see Figs. 45 and 46). Hydrocephalus secondary to obstruction of the ventricular outlets or from the presence of hemorrhage and its associated adhesions is present in most, but not all, cases. Hydrocephalus may also be secondary to increased CSF production by these tumors.

On CT, choroid plexus papilloma is iso- to slightly hyperdense on preinfusion scan. Postcontrast scans demonstrate marked enhancement.

About 10–20% of choroid plexus papillomas are malignant (62,69). These have been referred to as choroid plexus carcinomas. These tumors show a marked propensity to metastasize through the CSF pathways. Tumor extension outside the ventricular system into the adjacent parenchyma suggests malignancy (62). Choroid plexus carcinoma tends to present at a slightly older age, but usually within the first 5 years of life (70).

9. *Ependymoma of the fourth ventricle and its lateral recesses not infrequently extends into the CPA as an exophytic mass. These exophytic tumors often have an irregular lobulated surface.*

In some instances, an ependymoma may involve the CPA and be totally extra-axial, without any involvement of the fourth ventricle (Figs. 47 and 48). These ependymomas arise in the CPA from the lateral medullary velum (67,68). The lateral medullary velum is a thin plate of glial tissue and is analogous to the anterior and posterior medullary velum of the fourth ventricle. The lateral medullary velum is lined by ependymal cells and extends through the foramen of Luschka into the CPA.

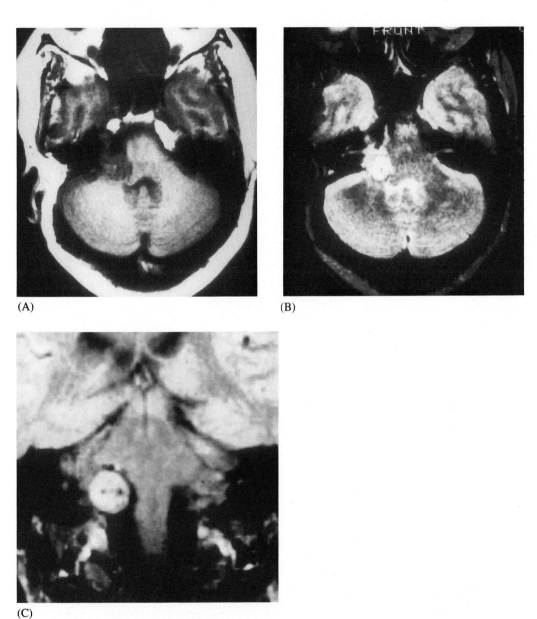

(A)

(B)

(C)

Figure 45 Extra-axial CPA choroid plexus papilloma: (A) axial T1-weighted MRI; (B) axial T2-weighted MRI; (C) post-gadolinium coronal T1-weighted MRI. The T1-weighted MRI (A) reveals a hypointense right-sided CPA mass that is hyperintense on the T2-weighted MRI (B). Coronal T1-weighted MRI following the intravenous administration of gadolinium (C) demonstrates an enhancing right-sided CPA mass. Internal hypointense structures that represent internal vascular structures are noted within the tumor.

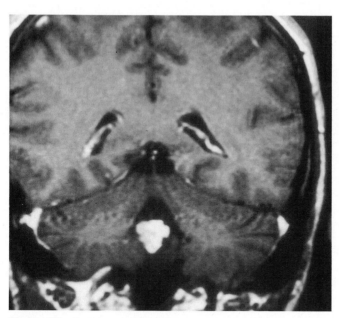

Figure 46 Fourth ventricular choroid plexus papilloma: Post-gadolinium coronal T1-weighted MRI demonstrates an enhancing mass within the fourth ventricle. This mass has the characteristic lobulated appearance of a choroid plexus papilloma.

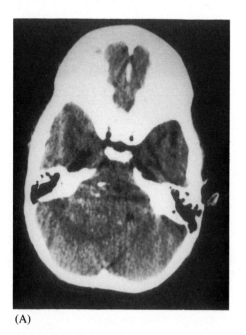
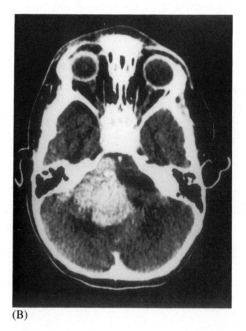

(A)   (B)

Figure 47 Extra-axial CPA ependymoma: (A) noncontrast axial CT scan; (B) postcontrast axial CT scan; (C) axial T1-weighted MRI; (D) coronal T1-weighted MRI; (E) axial T2-weighted MRI. Precontrast CT scanning (A) demonstrates a large right CPA mass with punctate calcification. The mass enhances markedly following the intravenous administration of contrast material (B). MRI demonstrated the tumor to be heterogeneous. The tumor is hypointense on T1-weighting (C,D) and hyperintense on T2-weighting (E). On the coronal image (D) note the mass affect on the brain stem.

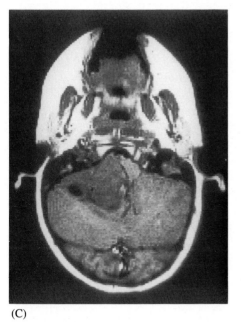

(C)

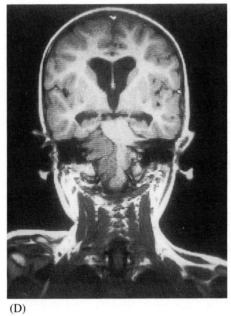

(D)

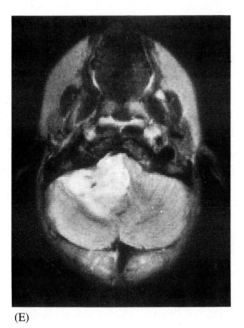

(E)

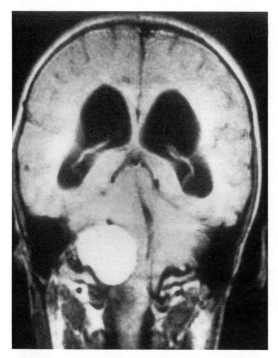

Figure 48 Extra-axial ependymoma: Post-gadolinium coronal T1-weighted MRI demonstrates a large right-sided extra-axial CPA enhancing mass, which effaces and displaces the medulla and pons across the midline. Note there is no connection between the mass and the fourth ventricle.

10. Glomus Tumor

Glomus tumor (paraganglioma, chemodectoma) is the second most common temporal bone tumor and the most common tumor involving the middle ear. Glomus tumor is a highly vascular, benign tumor that arises from the paraganglionic cells of the sympathetic nervous system. It occurs in adults over the age of 30 with an average age of 50 years, and is two to three times more common in women than in men (71).

Glomus tumors are classified according to their location. In decreasing order of frequency, they arise in the jugular foramen (glomus jugulare), middle ear (glomus tympanicum), and in the oropharyngeal–nasopharyngeal carotid space (glomus vagale). Tumors from these locations may extend into the CPA (72).

On T1-weighted images, glomus tumors exhibit mixed hypointense and isointense signal (Fig. 49). The hypointensity reflects flowing blood in the vascular structures. The isointense portion reflects the solid portion of the tumor. On T2-weighted images, glomus tumors exhibit increased signal in the solid portion of the tumor (see Fig. 49) and persistent flow void in the vascular portion. The MRI appearance of signal void caused by the high flow of the serpentine tumor vessels has been termed salt-and-pepper pattern. Following the injection of intravenous gadolinium, heterogeneous enhancement occurs in almost all cases.

An MRI scan will also demonstrate the superior extension of the tumor into the middle ear, involvement of the petrous carotid canal, and extension of the tumor into the jugular vein; however, CT is superior to MRI in demonstrating adjacent bone destruction (see Fig. 49).

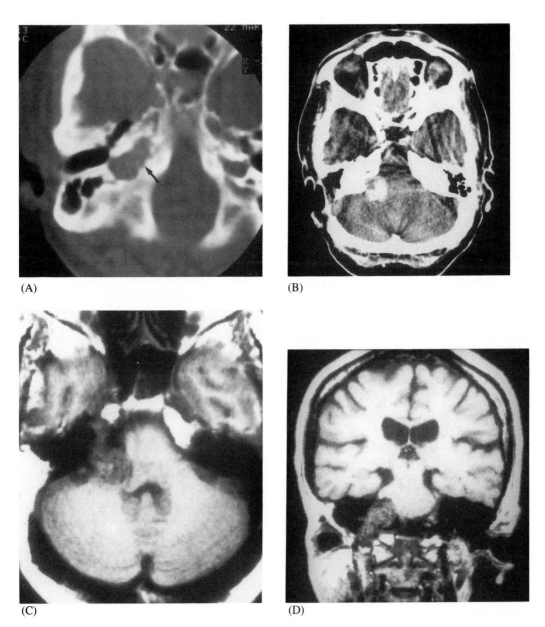

(A)   (B)

(C)   (D)

Figure 49 Glomus jugulare: (A) axial CT scan (bone windows); (B) postcontrast axial CT scan; (C) axial T1-weighted MRI; (D) coronal T1-weighted MRI; (E) axial T2-weighted MRI; (F) Left external carotid angiogram. Axial CT (bone windows) (A) demonstrates enlargement and erosion of the right jugular foramen (arrow). There is enhancement of a right CPA mass (B) axial and coronal (C,D). T1-weighted MR images demonstrate a well-defined hypointense mass in the right CPA. The coronal image (D) reveals jugular invasion by the tumor. The tumor is hyperintense on T2-weighting (E). External carotid angiography (F) shows a hypervascular mass with a dense blush. The primary supply to the tumor was the ascending pharyngeal artery.

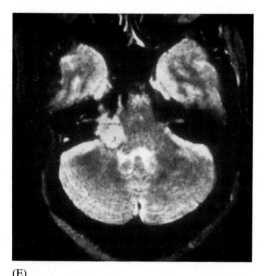

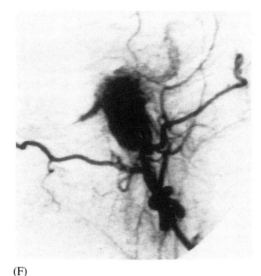

(E)   (F)

Figure 49 Continued

11. Lipoma

Lipomas produce a pathognomonic MRI appearance. On T1-weighted images, they appear as hyperintense lesions (Fig. 50). On T2-weighted images they exhibit intermediate signal that approximates the signal of subgaleal fat.

The quadrageminal plate and the CPA are the most frequent posterior fossa locations of lipomas.

Most posterior fossa lipomas are asymptomatic. Cerebellar vermian agenesis is rarely associated with posterior fossa lipomas.

12. Chordoma

Chordoma is a slow-growing tumor that arises from notocord remnants in the spheno-occipital synchondrosis or clival region. Chordomas present clinically in the third or fourth decades of life (43).

On CT, these lesions appear as iso- or hyperdense masses. In 30–50% of cases calcification can be observed. Following the intravenous administration of iodinated contrast material, variable contrast enhancement may be noted. A CT scan will also demonstrate bone destruction of the clivus, foramen magnum, petrous bone (Fig. 51), and sella turcica.

Chordomas often have a frondlike or cauliflowerlike appearance. Usually chordomas are hypointense on T1-weighted images and hyperintense on T2-weighted images (see Fig. 51). T1-weighted images will also demonstrate destruction or replacement of the hyperintense T1-weighted clival marrow signal by one of intermediate intensity. Although both CT and MRI are sensitive techniques in detecting chordomas, MRI is superior in delineating the full extent of the tumor (73).

Occasionally, especially with calcified lesions, intermediate and inhomogeneous T2-weighted signal characteristics occur. Following the intravenous administration of gadolinium, minimal heterogeneous enhancement may be noted.

13. Lymphoma

Diagnosis of an extra-axial lymphoma in the CPA is extremely rare (40,74,75). The imaging features are similar to lymphomas found elsewhere in the CNS.

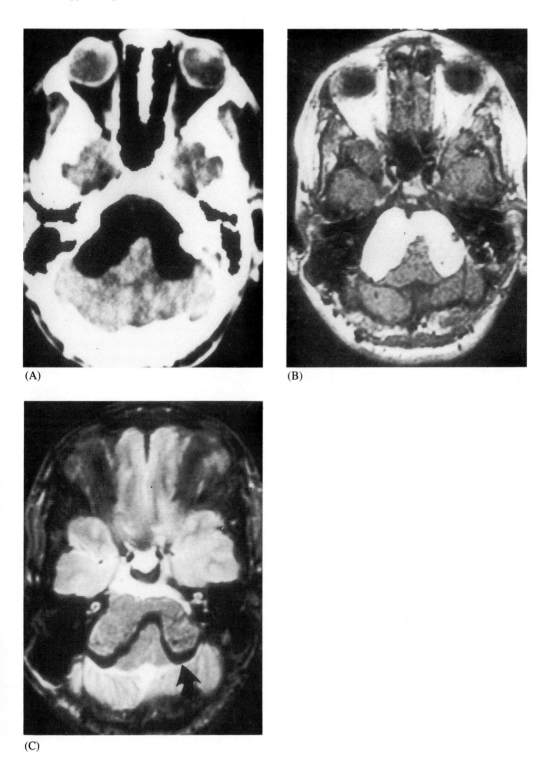

Figure 50 Lipoma: (A) noncontrast axial CT scan; (B) axial T1-weighted MRI; (C) axial T2-weighted MRI. The CT scan (A) demonstrates a low-density anterior compartment posterior fossa mass. This mass is hyperintense on T1-weighting (B) and hypointense on T2-weighting (C). The signal characteristics of the mass mimics that of fat. A chemical shift artifact (arrow) typical for fat is noted.

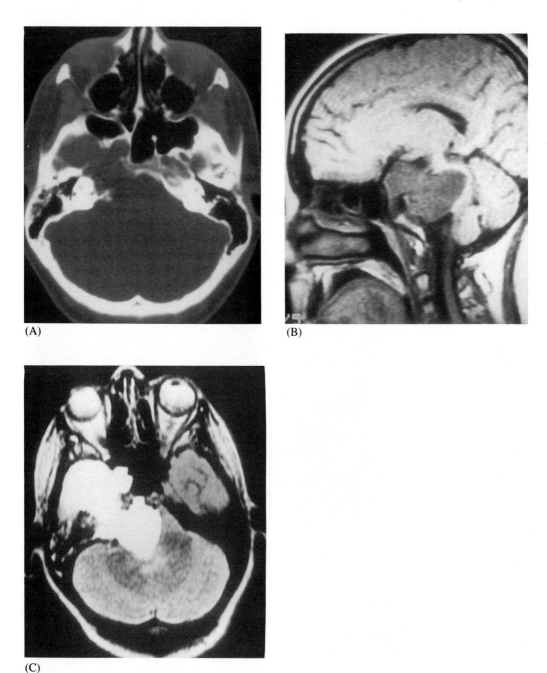

(A)

(B)

(C)

Figure 51 Chordoma: (A) axial CT scan (bone windows); (B) sagittal T1-weighted MRI; (C) axial T2-weighted MRI. The CT scan (A) demonstrates an area of bone destruction involving the clivus, right petrous apex, and middle cranial fossa. Sagittal T1-weighted MRI (B) demonstrates a large mass with decreased signal intensity. This mass extends into the posterior fossa and middle cranial fossa. The mass exhibits increased signal intensity on T2-weighting (C). In addition to the posterior extension of the tumor into the posterior fossa, the tumor occupies virtually the entire middle cranial fossa on the right side.

References

1. Stenhouse D. Plain radiography of the skull in the diagnosis of intracranial tumors. Br J Radiol 1948; 21:287–300.
2. Hisada K, Tonami N, Miyamae T, Hiraki Y, Yanazaki T, Maeda T, Nakajo M. Clinical evaluation of tumor imaging with ^{201}Tl chloride. Radiology 1978; 129:497–500.
3. Baker HI, Houser OW, Campbell JR. National Cancer Institute study: evaluation of CT in the diagnosis of intracranial neoplasms. Radiology 1980; 136:91–96.
4. Lee BCP, Kneeland JB, Cahill PT, Deck MDF. MR recognition of supratentorial tumors. AJNR 1985; 6:871–878.
5. Atlas SW. Intraaxial brain tumors. In: Atlas SW, ed. Magnetic resonance imaging of the brain and spine. New York: Raven Press, 1991:223–326.
6. Latchaw RE, MR and CT imaging of the head, neck and spine, 2nd ed. St Louis: Mosby Year Book, 1991.
7. Stark DD, Bradley WG. Magnetic resonance imaging. St Louis: Mosby Year Book, 1992:3–554.
8. Healy ME, Hesselink JR, Press GA, Middleton MS. Increased detection of intracranial metastases with intravenous Gd-DTPA, Radiology 1987; 165:619–624.
9. Russel EJ, Geremia GK, Johnson CE, Huckman MS, Ramsey RG, Washburn-Bleck J, Turner DA, Norusis M. Multiple cerebral metastases: detectability with Gd-DTPA-enhanced MR imaging. Radiology 1987; 165:609–617.
10. Horowitz AL. MRI physics for radiologists. A visual approach, 2nd ed. New York: Springer-Verlag, 1989.
11. Edelman RR, Hesselink JR. Clinical magnetic resonance. Philadelphia: WB Saunders, 1990:3–376.
12. Atlas SW. Magnetic resonance imaging of the brain and spine. New York: Raven Press, 1991:1–128.
13. Packer RJ, Batnitzky S, Cohen ME. Magnetic resonance imaging in the evaluation of intracranial tumors of childhood. Cancer 1985; 56:1767–1772.
14. Reese TS, Karnovsky MJ. Fine structural localization of blood–brain barrier to exogenous peroxidase. J Cell Biol 1967; 34:207–217.
15. Sage MR. Blood–brain barrier: phenomenon of increasing importance to the imaging clinician. AJR 1982; 138:887–898.
16. Weinman HJ, Brasch RC, Press WR, Wesbey GE. Characteristics of gadolinium-DTPA complex: a potential NMR contrast agent. AJR 1984; 142:619–624.
17. Graif M, Bydder GM, Steiner RE, Niendorf P, Thomas DGT, Young IR. Contrast-enhanced MR imaging of malignant brain tumors. AJNR 1985; 6:855–862.
18. Oot RF, New PFJ, Pile-Spellman J. The detection of intracranial calcifications by MR. AJNR 1986; 7:801–809.
19. Atlas SW, Grossman RI, Gomori JM, Hackney DB, Goldberg HI, Zimmerman RA, Bilaniuk LT. Hemorrhagic intracranial malignant neoplasms: spin-echo MR imaging. RAdiology 1987; 164:71–77.
20. Kovalikova Z, Hoehn-Berlage MH, Gersonde K, Porschen R, Mittermayer C, Franke RP. Age-dependent variation of T1 and T2 relaxation times of adenocarcinoma in mice. Radiology 1987; 164:543–548.
21. Hackney DB, Grossman RI, Zimmerman RA, Joseph PM, Goldberg HI, Bilaniuk, LT, Spagnoli MV. Low sensitivity of clinical MR imaging of small changes in the concentration of nonparamagnetic protein. AJNR 1987; 8:1003–1008.
22. Naidich TP, Zimmerman RA. Primary brain tumors in children. Semin Roentgenol 1984; 19:100–114.
23. Russel DS, Rubinstein LJ. Pathology of tumors of the nervous system, 5th ed. Baltimore: Williams & Wilkins, 1989.
24. Farwell JR, Dohrmann GJ, Flannery JT. Central nervous system tumors in children. Cancer 1977; 40:3123.
25. Segall HD, Zee CS, Naidich TP, Ahmadi J, Becker TS. Computed tomography in neoplasms of the posterior fossa in children. Radiol Clin North Am 1982; 20:237–253.
26. Chin HW, Maruyama Y, Young AB, Medulloblastoma: recent advances and directions in diagnosis and management: part 1. Curr Probl Cancer 1984; 8:1–54.

27. Segall HD, Batnitzky S, Zee CS, Ahmadi J, Bird CR, Cohen ME. Computed tomography in the diagnosis of intracranial neoplasms in children. Cancer 1985; 56:1748–1755.
28. Hubbard JL, Scheithauer BW, Kispert DB, Carpenter SM, Wick MR, Laws ER. Adult cerebellar medulloblastomas. The pathological, radiographic and clinical disease spectrum. J Neurosurg 1989; 70:536–544.
29. Deutch M, Reigel DH. Myelography and cytology in the treatment of medulloblastoma. Int J Radiat Oncol Biol Phys 1981; 7:721–725.
30. North C, Segall HD, Stanley P, Zee CS, Ahmadi J, McComb JG, Early CT detection of intracranial seeding from medulloblastoma. AJNR 1985; 6:11–13.
31. Fitz CR, Rao KCVG. Primary tumors in children. In: Lee SH, Rao KCVG, eds. Cranial computed tomography and MRI. New York: McGraw-Hill, 1987:365–412.
32. Courville CB, Broussalian SL. Plastic ependymomas of the lateral recess. Report of eight verified cases. J Neurosurg 1961; 18:792–799.
33. Rorke LB, Gilles FH, DAvis RL, Becker LE. Revision of the World Health Organization classification of brain tumors for childhood brain tumors. Cancer 1985; 56:1869–1886.
34. Scheithauer BW. Symptomatic subependymoma. Report of 21 cases with review of the literature. J Neurosurg 1978; 49:689–696.
35. Rengachary SS. Hemangioblastomas. In: Wilkins RH, Rengachary SS, eds. Neurosurgery. New York: McGraw-Hill, 1985:772–782.
36. Lee SR, Sanches J, Mark AS, Dillon WP, Norman D, Newton TH. Posterior fossa hemangioblastomas: MR imaging. Radiology 1989; 171:463–468.
37. Schwaighofer BW, Hesselink JR, Press GA, Wolf RL, Healy ME, Bertholy DP. Primary intracranial CNS lymphoma: MR manifestations. AJNR 1989; 10:725–729.
38. Delattre JY, Krol G, Thaler HT, Posner JB. Distribution of brain metastases. Arch Neurol 1988; 45:741–744.
39. Lee BCP, Kneeland JB, Walker RW, Posner JB, Cahill PT, Deck MDF. MR imaging of brainstem tumors. AJNR 1985; 6:159–163.
40. Morrison AW, King TT. Space-occupying lesions of the internal auditory meatus and crebellopontine angle. Adv Otorhinolaryngol 1984; 34:121–142.
41. Hasso AN, Smith DS. The cerebellopontine angle. Semin Ultrasound CT MR 1989; 10:280–301.
42. Goldberg HI. Extraaxial brain tumors. In: Atlas SW, ed. Magnetic resonance imaging of the brain and spine. New York: Raven Press 1991:327–278.
43. Pomerantz SJ. Posterior fossa, skull base, craniocervical junction. In: Pomerantz SJ, ed. Craniospinal magnetic resonance imaging. Philadelphia: WB Saunders, 1989:248–274.
44. Pinto RS, Kricheff II, Bergeron RT, Cohen N. Small acoustic neuromas: detection by high resolution gas CT cisternography. AJR 1982; 139:129–132.
45. Goldberg HI, Spagnoli MV, Grossman RI, Hackney DM, Zimmerman RA, Bilaniuk LT. High field MRI evaluation of acoustic neuroma. Acta Radiol [Suppl] 1986; 369:173–175.
46. Hasso AN, Moody E. Imaging of the cerebellopontine angle. In: Huckman MS, ed. ARRS categorical course syllabus. Neuroradiology. Reston: American Roentgen Ray Society, 1992:177–185.
47. Pomeranz SJ. MR of supratentorial neoplasm. In: Pomeranz SJ, ed. Craniospinal magnetic resonance imaging. Philadelphia: WB Saunders, 1989:208–247.
48. Cruveilhier C. Anatomie pathologique du corps humain, vol 1, book 2. Paris: Bailliere, 1829.
49. Tampieri D, Melanson D, Ethier R. MR imaging of epidermoid cysts. AJNR 1989; 10:351–356.
50. Gao P, Osborn AG, Smirniotopoulos JG, Harris CP. Epidermoid tumor of the cerebellopontine angle. AJNR 1992; 13:863–872.
51. Houston LW, Hinke ML. Neuroradiology case of the day. AJR 1986:637.
52. Tekkok IH, Cataltepe O, Saglan S. Dense epidermoid cyst of the cerebellopontine angle. Neuroradiology 1991; 33:255–257.
53. Braum IF, Naidich TP, Leeds NE, Koslow M, Zimmerman HM, Chase NE. Dense intracranial epidermoid tumors. Computed tomographic observations. Radiology 1977; 122:717–719.
54. Newton DR, Larson TC III, Dillon WP, Newton TH. Magnetic resonance characteristics of cranial epidermoid and teratomatous tumors. AJNR 1987; 8:945.

55. Galassi E, Piazza G, Gaist G, Frank F. Arachnoid cysts of the middle cranial fossa: a clinical and radiological study of 25 cases treated surgically. Surg Neurol 1980; 14:211–219.

56. Nager GT, Vanderveen TS. Cholesterol granuloma involving the temporal bone. Ann Otol 1976; 85:204–209.

57. Graham MD, Kemink JL, Latack JT, Kartush JM. The giant cholesterol cyst of the petrus apex: a distinct clinical entity. Laryngoscope 1985; 95:1401–1406.

58. Lattack JT, Malcolm DG, Kemink JL, Knake JE. Giant cholesterol cysts of the petrous apex: radiologic features. AJNR 1985; 6:409–413.

59. Griffin C, De La Paz R, Enzmann D. MR and CT correlation of cholesterol cysts of the petrous bone. AJNR 1987; 8:825–829.

60. Greenberg JL, Oot RF, Wismer GL, DAvis KR, Goodman ML, Weber AE, Montgomery WW. Cholesterol granuloma of the petrous apex: MR and CT evaluation. AJNR 1988; 9:1205–1214.

61. Lo WWM, Solti-Bohman LG, Brackmann DE, Gruskin P. Cholesterol granuloma of the petrous apex. CT diagnosis. Radiology 1984; 153:705–711.

62. Batnitzky S. Intraventricular meningioma. In: Weinberg PE, Batnitzky S, Bentson JR, Bryan RN, Naidich TP, Sackett JF, Zimmerman RA, eds. Neuroradiology text and syllabus. Reston: American College of Radiology 1990:714–744.

63. Radkowski MR, Naidich TP, Tomita T, Byrd SE, McLone DG. Neonatal brain tumors: CT and MR findings. J Comput Assist Tomogr 1988; 12:10–20.

64. Ken JG, Sobel DF, Copeland B, Davis J III, Kortman KE. Choroid plexus papillomas of the foramen of Luschka: MR appearance. AJNR 1991; 12:1201–1203.

65. Bochdalek VA. Anleitung zur praktischen zergliederung des menschlichen gehirnes, nebst einer anatomischen beschreibung desselben; mit besonderer rüchsicht auf das kleine gehirn. Prague: G Haase Söhne, 1983.

66. Hälfte E. Topographische and stratigraphische anatomie des kopfes. In: Pernkopf E, ed. Topographische anatomie des menschen IV. München: Urban & Schwarzenberg, 1957:47.

67. Kernohan JW, Woltman HW, Adson AW. Gliomas of the cerebellopontine angle. J Neuropathol Exp Neurol 1948; 7:349–367.

68. Kernohan JW, Sayre GP. Tumors of the central nervous system. In: Atlas of tumor pathology. Washington DC: Armed Forces Institute of Pathology, 1952:F35–48.

69. Carpenter DB, Michelsen WJ, Hays AP. Carcinoma of the choroid plexus. Case report. J Neurosurg 1982; 56:722–729.

70. Barkovich AJ, Edwards MSB. Brain tumors of childhood. In: Barkovich AJ, ed. Pediatric neuroimaging. New York: Raven Press, 1990:149–203.

71. Hasso AN, Hinshaw DB Jr, Kief-Garcia ML. Neoplasms of the cranial nerves and skull base. In: Stark DB, Bradley WG Jr, eds. Magnetic resonance imaging. St Louis: Mosby Year Book, 1992:851–889.

72. Remley KB, Coit WE, Harnsberger HR, Smoker WRK, Jacobs JM, McIff EB. Pulsatile tinnitus and the vascular tympanic membrane: CT, MR and angiographic findings. Radiology 1990; 174:383–389.

73. Sze G, Uichanco LS III, Brant-Zawadzki MN, Davis RL, Gutin PH, Wilson CB, Norman D, Newton TH. Chordomas: MR imaging. Radiology 1988; 166:187–191.

74. Yang PJ, Seeger JF, Carmody RF, Mehta BA. Cerebellopontine angle lymphoma. AJNR 1987; 8:368–369.

75. Nakada T, St John JN, Knight RT. Solitary metastasis of systemic malignant lymphoma to the cerebellopontine angle. Neuroradiology 1983; 24:225–228.

9

The Radiology of Brain Tumors: Supratentorial Neoplasms

Solomon Batnitzky and Donald A. Eckard
University of Kansas Medical Center, Kansas City, Kansas

I. GLIAL TUMORS

Primary cerebral gliomas represent the largest single group of intracranial tumors, and constitute 40–45% of all such tumors (1).

There are three classes of neuroglial cells: astrocytes, oligodendroglia, and ependymal cells (2). Each of these neuroglial elements may undergo neoplastic transformation. The following gliomas will be considered:

Glioblastoma multiforme (highly anaplastic astrocytoma)
Fibrillary astrocytoma
Gliomatosis cerebri
Juvenile pilocytic astrocytoma
Subependymal giant cell astrocytoma
Oligodendroglioma
Ependymoma
Ganglioglioma
Choroid plexus papilloma

The vast majority of adult gliomas are supratentorial, whereas in childhood, 70–80% of these tumors are infratentorial (1).

The degree of malignancy ranges from the most benign end of the spectrum—the pilocytic astrocytoma, which is usually found in the pediatric age group—to the most malignant end of the spectrum, consisting of glioblastoma multiforme.

Although computed tomography (CT) performed without and with intravenous contrast has provided a high degree of sensitivity and consistency in the diagnosis of intracranial gliomas (3–5), magnetic resonance imaging (MRI) is more sensitive than CT in the diagnosis of these lesions, both in terms of tumor detection and more completeness in delineation of the lesion (6). However, the preoperative neuroradiologic evaluation with either MRI or CT is often inconclusive for the histological grade of the glioma (6–9). Furthermore, it is well known that prolongation of T2 in most gliomas is not even specific for a neoplasm. Increased signal on T2-weighted images is a nonspecific finding and can be seen in ischemic and inflammatory lesions of the brain, as well as in neoplastic lesions (8–10).

The specificity of both CT and MRI lags far behind the exquisite sensitivity of these imaging modalities.

A. Glioblastoma Multiforme

Glioblastomas represent the most malignant end of the spectrum of neuroglial tumors, representing approximately 15–20% of all intracranial tumors and nearly half of cerebral gliomas (1).

Glioblastoma is the most common primary supratentorial neoplasm in adults. The peak age of diagnosis is between 45 and 55 years of age. As with gliomas, in general, these lesions show a male preponderance. Although glioblastomas can involve any lobe and may frequently involve more than one lobe, the frontal lobe is the most commonly involved site, followed by the temporal lobe. Bihemispheric involvement through the corpus callosum—the so-called butterfly glioma—is not uncommon (Fig. 1). Multicentric glioblastomas are rare, occurring in approximately 5% of cases (1). Superficially located lesions tend to invade the leptomeninges and dura, with subsequent dissemination through the subarachnoid spaces.

On MRI, glioblastoma exhibits marked heterogeneity both on T1- and T2-weighted images. However, this is most marked on the T2-weighted images (Figs. 2 and 3). Central necrosis and hemorrhages of varying ages may also be demonstrated (see Fig. 2). Glioblastoma, similar to certain other intracranial neoplasms (ependymoma, metastases), has a characteristic tendency to bleed. Demonstration of hemorrhage within the tumor can be an important clue in the diagnosis of

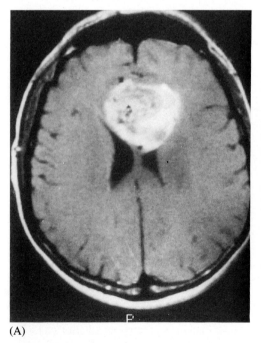
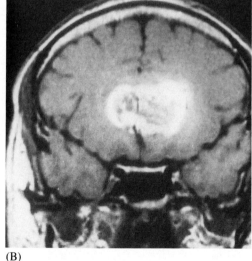

(A)   (B)

Figure 1   Butterfly glioblastoma multiforme: Post-gadolinium (A) axial and (B) coronal T1-weighted MR images. Post-gadolinium MRI (A,B) demonstrate a large heterogeneously enhancing, partially solid and necrotic midline mass involving the corpus callosum and both cerebral hemispheres.

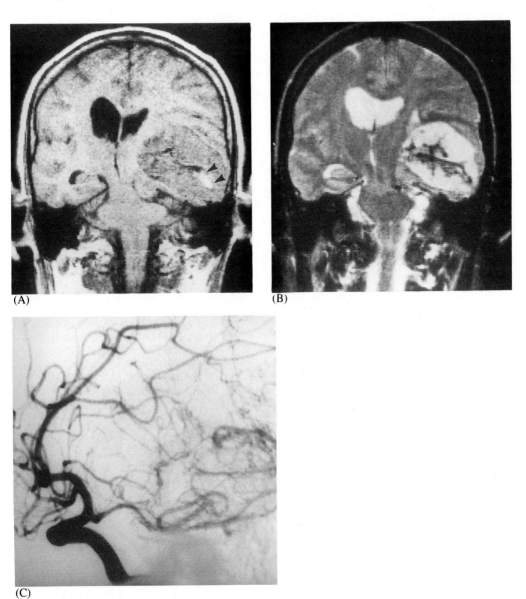

Figure 2 Glioblastoma multiforme: (A) coronal T1-weighted MRI; (B) coronal T2-weighted MRI; (C) lateral projection of early arterial phase of left carotid angiogram; (D) lateral projection of late arterial and early capillary phase of left carotid angiogram. Coronal T1-weighted MRI (A) demonstrates a heterogeneous hypointense mass in the left temporal lobe. An area of increased signal intensity owing to methemoglobin (arrowheads) representing subacute–chronic hemorrhage is noted within this mass. Linear areas of signal void reflecting the hypervascular nature of the glioblastoma are also noted within the tumor. There is left-to-right shift of the ventricular system. The T2-weighted MRI (B) shows heterogeneous increased signal intensity within the tumor. The linear or serpentine regions of signal void seen in (A) are again noted. Left carotid angiography (C) demonstrates a left temporal lobe mass as evidenced by elevation of the middle cerebral artery. Marked neovascularity with AV shunting and early-draining veins is noted. In the late arterial–early capillary phase (D) a marked tumor stain is seen, with early opacification of the lateral and sigmoid sinuses.

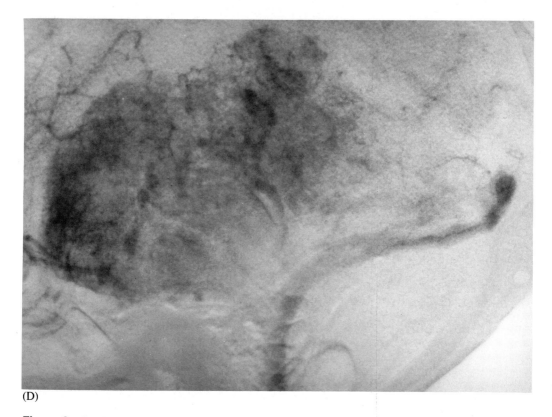

(D)

Figure 2 Continued

these tumors. The CT scan is very sensitive in demonstrating the presence of acute hemorrhage (see Fig. 12, Chap. 8). Because of the paramagnetic properties of many of the blood breakdown products, hemorrhage is uniquely depicted by MRI (see Fig. 2).

Linear or serpentine regions of signal void reflecting hypervascular nature of glioblastomas are commonly seen. Calcification is rare in glioblastomas. Glioblastomas exhibit extensive mass effect mainly caused by peritumoral edema, which is usually moderate to severe.

A characteristic feature of glioblastoma is that the tumor margins are blurred, indicating the infiltrating nature of the neoplasm (9). There is no clear margin microscopically at which tumor cells stop and edema or normal brain begin (1). On MRI and CT one cannot define the margins of the tumor. The radiologist and neurosurgeon should be aware that neoplastic tissue extends beyond the recognizable regions of the abnormality, as demonstrated by MRI and CT (9–11).

Although the mechanism of enhancement is identical for both CT and MRI, it appears that tumor enhancement on MRI with gadolinium-containing agents is more sensitive than tumor enhancement on CT with iodinated contrast material (9,12). Enhancement following the intravenous administration of gadolinium-containing contrast agents is variable. Enhancement is usually heterogeneous. It may be thick, irregular, and ringlike around areas of necrosis, or it may be dense, nodular, or linear in character (see Figs. 1–4). Enhancement is helpful in determining the site of stereotactic surgical biopsy, as areas of enhancement correlate with the areas of tumor tissue on pathologic examination (11,13); however, these areas do not correlate with the degree of hypervascularity, as demonstrated on angiography.

The CT and MRI features of glioblastoma are identical with those seen in metastases and radiation necrosis (9). On noncontrast CT, glioblastomas appear as zones of high and low density.

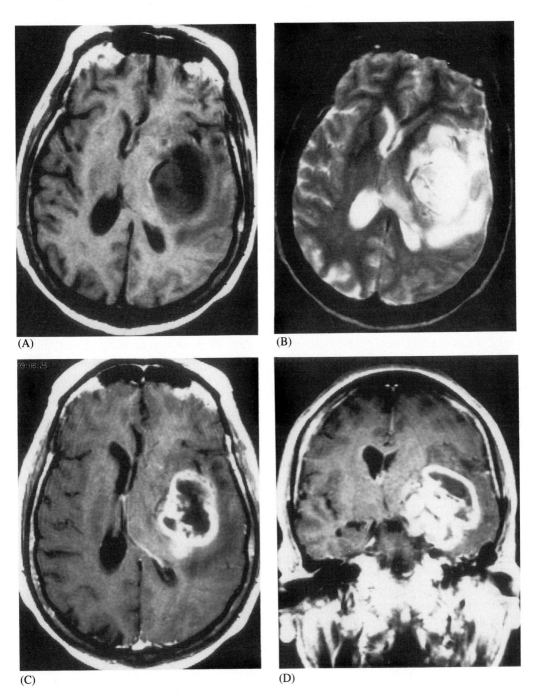

(A)

(B)

(C)

(D)

Figure 3 Glioblastoma multiforme: (A,B) axial T1- and T2-weighted MR images; (C) post-gadolinium axial T1-weighted MRI; (D) post-gadolinium coronal T1-weighted MRI. Axial T1- and T2-weighted MR images demonstrate a large left-sided heterogeneous mass that exhibits decreased signal intensity on T1-weighting (A) and increased signal intensity on T2-weighting (B). Pronounced peritumoral edema is seen, which appears as decreased signal on T1-weighting and increased signal on T2-weighting. The mass produces a left-to-right shift of the ventricular system. A thick, irregular ring of enhancement, highly suggestive of malignant neoplasm, is seen on the post-gadolinium MR images (C,D). Necrotic areas that do not enhance are seen throughout the tumor.

The tumor margins are blurred. The tumor exhibits moderate to marked edema. Following the intravenous administration of contrast material, inhomogeneous contrast enhancement is nearly always present. Thick, irregular ringlike enhancement around areas of necrosis is frequently demonstrated (Figs. 5 and 6).

1. Angiography

Many glioblastomas are highly vascular lesions that exhibit neovascularity and arteriovenous shunting. The neovascularity consists of abnormal vessels in the interstices of the tumor, which appear tortuous and irregular in caliber, with areas of localized dilatation and constriction. Puddling and vascular staining, representing contrast accumulation in the proliferating capillaries or sinusoids, are often seen. Few if any normal arteries are seen within the tumor parenchyma itself. Tumor vessels surrounding an area of necrosis, which appears as an avascular area, produce the so-called ring sign.

Arteriovenous shunting with early venous opacification is commonly seen in glioblastomas. This is nonspecific and can also be seen in metastases, infarcts, arteriovenous malformations (AVM), inflammatory lesions, and toxic processes. It may sometimes be difficult to distinguish between a very vascular glioblastoma and an AVM. The large feeding arteries and draining veins are usually more evident in an AVM.

The tumor blush of a glioblastoma is seen during the arterial phase of the angiogram (see Fig. 8, Chap 8; and Fig. 2 in this chapter). Because of the vascularity of the mass and arteriovenous shunts, the tumor may have emptied completely during the venous phase of the angiogram.

Glioblastomas may be avascular angiographically. It is important to note that absence of neovascularity does not preclude the possibility of a highly malignant lesion. Angiographically, a metastatic deposit may be indistinguishable from a glioblastoma.

B. Fibrillary Astrocytoma

Astrocytomas constitute 25–30% of hemispheric gliomas in adults (1). The peak incidence of supratentorial astrocytomas is between 20 and 50 years of age. Fibrillary astrocytomas can be divided into two types: diffuse and circumscribed (1). The diffuse forms of fibrillary astrocytomas are most often encountered in the cerebral hemispheres of adults and in the brain stem in children and adolescents. In the cerebellum, diffuse fibrillary astrocytomas are more commonly seen in aged and middle-aged adults. The circumscribed form of fibrillary astrocytomas is characteristically found in the cerebellum and in the diencephalic region of young patients, with only occasional involvement of one of the cerebral lobes.

Gemistocytic astrocytomas are restricted to the cerebral hemispheres and, as a pure form, are extremely rare (1). Foci of gemistocytic astrocytomas comprise considerable areas within diffuse fibrillary cerebral astrocytomas (1).

Infiltrating astrocytomas may arise in any part of the hemisphere, with a relative sparing of the occipital lobes (15). They constitute a widely heterogeneous group of tumors that behave differently biologically, pathologically, and clinically.

Low-grade astrocytomas generally have a better prognosis than higher-grade lesions. However, it is recognized that over the years a substantial portion of low-grade lesions dedifferentiate into more malignant grades (9). The pathologically diffuse, infiltrative form of fibrillary astrocytomas make up about 75% of hemispheric astrocytomas in adults (1,9). These tend to be solid tumors and calcification is present in many. Dural and leptomeningeal invasion, subarachnoid and subependymal seeding are rare unless malignant degeneration has occurred.

On MRI, these tumors are relatively homogeneous, although heterogeneity is occasionally seen. Focal cystic areas can sometimes be seen.

These tumors are iso- to hypointense on T1- and hyperintense on T2-weighted images (see

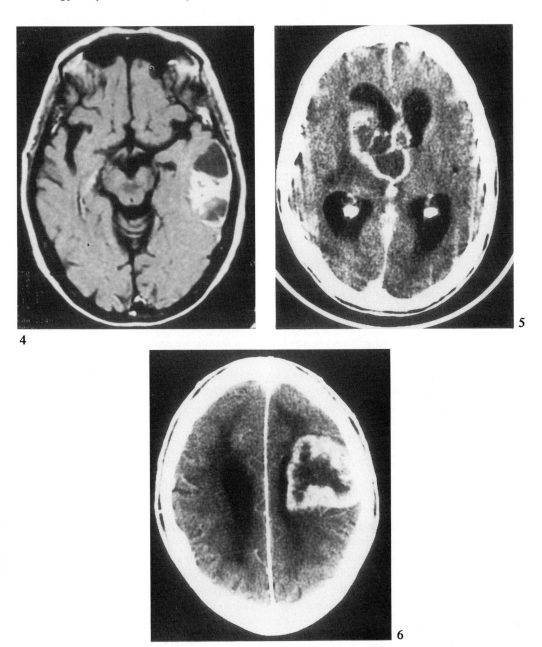

Figure 4 Glioblastoma multiforme: Post-gadolinium axial T1-weighted MRI demonstrates marked heterogeneous enhancement of a left parietal mass. Cystic and necrotic areas are seen in the anterior and posterior portions of the tumor.

Figure 5 Glioblastoma multiforme: Postcontrast axial CT scan demonstrates irregular peripheral ringlike enhancement around a necrotic mass in the right basal ganglia region. The mass crosses the midline to involve the left hemisphere.

Figure 6 Glioblastoma multiforme: Postcontrast axial CT scan demonstrates thick irregular ring enhancement in a left frontoparietal convexity mass.

Figs. 10 and 11, Chap. 8). On CT, these tumors are hypo- to isodense with the surrounding brain. These tumors are not usually associated with peritumoral edema. On MRI, because of its superior contrast resolution, these tumors can be clearly demonstrated as abnormal areas of increased signal intensity (see Figs. 10 and 11, Chap. 8). Calcification on CT is demonstrated in about 20% of tumors (16). Calcification is not as well appreciated on MRI as it is on CT. As with glioblastomas, the radiologist and neurosurgeon should be cognizant that tumor tissue may extend beyond the margins of abnormal signal intensity (9,11).

Contrast enhancement is variable. Contrast enhancement may be homogeneous; it may be focal, nodular or ringlike. Low-grade astrocytomas often do not enhance, whereas the higher-grade tumors do; however, there is a considerable degree of overlap.

The differential diagnosis includes metastasis, lymphoma, cerebritis or abscess, and cerebral infarction.

C. Gliomatosis Cerebri

Gliomatosis cerebri is a rare, diffusely infiltrative glial neoplasm that may involve nearly the entire brain substance. The posterior fossa, brain stem, and spinal cord may also be involved. Gliomatosis cerebri represents the most extreme end of the spectrum of diffuse astrocytoma (1). The peak incidence is in the second to fourth decades of life (17).

On MRI, ill-defined regions of increased signal intensity on T2-weighted images, associated with sulcal and ventricular effacement, are the prominent features of this tumor. Contrast enhancement is usually not a common feature.

The diffuse nature of this condition may be confused with an extensive demyelinating or dysmyelinating disease. The diagnosis of gliomatosis cerebri is made by biopsy of the tumor, although MRI and clinical features may suggest the diagnosis.

D. Juvenile Pilocytic Astrocytoma

The most common form of astrocytoma in the pediatric age group is juvenile pilocytic astrocytoma (JPA). This tumor represents the most benign form of glial astrocytoma (1). These tumors are often, but not always, associated with neurofibromatosis. The cerebellar hemisphere is the most common location of JPA. Supratentorially, it may be found in the cerebral hemispheres and in the diencephalon (chiasm hypothalamus, floor of third ventricle) (18) (Figs. 7 and 8). The peak incidence is in the first two decades of life (9).

The JPA is a well-circumscribed mass, often associated with a vascular tumor nodule in the wall of the cyst. More than two-thirds of cases show cyst formation (18).

On MRI, the solid portion of the tumor is slightly hypointense on T1-weighted images and hyperintense on T2-weighted images (see Figs. 7 and 8). The cystic portion of the tumor is isointense to cerebrospinal fluid (CSF) on T1- and T2-weighted images. It may be hyperintense both on T1- and T2-weighted images in some cases, probably owing to its proteinaceous contents. Following the intravenous administration of gadolinium-containing contrast material, the solid portion of the tumor enhances. The mural nodule in the cystic variety of the tumor exhibits marked enhancement following intravenous contrast injection. Absence of accompanying peritumoral edema is a characteristic feature of this tumor.

Chiasmal or hypothalamic JPA are less commonly associated with macrocysts, although microcysts may be present (9) (see Figs. 7 and 8).

E. Subependymal Giant Cell Astrocytoma

Subependymal giant cell astrocytoma is a rare form of astrocytoma, characteristically, but not always, associated with tuberous sclerosis. It is found in 3–14% of patients with tuberous sclerosis

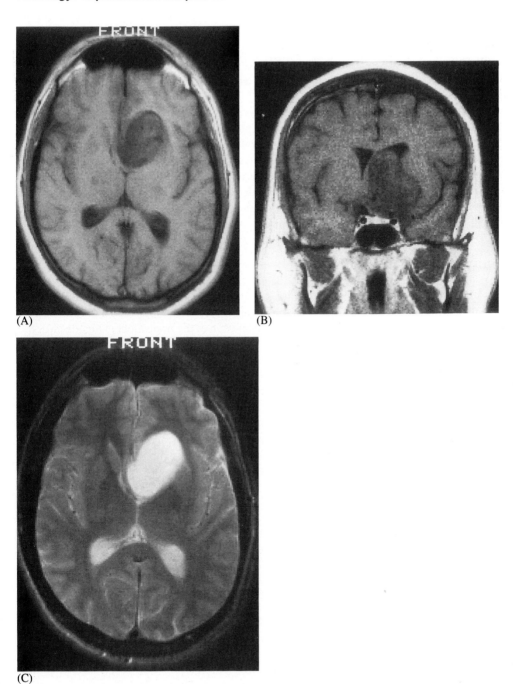

Figure 7 Chiasmal–hypothalamic pilocytic astrocytoma: (A) axial T1-weighted MRI; (B) coronal T1-weighted MRI; (C) Axial T2-weighted MRI. T1- and T2-weighted MR images (A,B) demonstrate a well-circumscribed heterogeneous left-sided suprasellar mass that extends superiorly into the left frontal horn. This mass is hypointense on T1-weighted images (A,B) and hyperintense on the T2-weighted MRI (C).

(19–21). The peak age of incidence is 5–10 years. The tumor is almost exclusively located along the wall of the ventricle nearer the foramen of Monro and presents as an intraventricular mass that frequently obstructs this foramen, causing hydrocephalus (20). The diagnosis is established by the characteristic location of the tumor and by the presence of other features of tuberous sclerosis (cortical tubers, heterotopic gray matter).

On MRI, these lesions are iso- or hypointense on T1-weighted images (Fig. 9). On T2-weighted images, these tumors are hyperintense and are heterogeneous. In contradistinction, benign tubers exhibit little signal increase on T2-weighted images. Calcification seen as signal void areas may be seen in the giant cell tumors. Most giant cell astrocytomas enhance following the intravenous administration of gadolinium-containing agents (22,23) (see Fig. 9).

On CT, the lesion is a well-circumscribed isodense or hyperdense mass and demonstrates intense homogeneous contrast enhancement. The tumor may contain some calcification. Subependymal tubers of tuberous sclerosis are typically nearly totally calcified and do not enhance following the intravenous administration of iodinated contrast material (24).

F. Oligodendroglioma

Oligodendroglioma is a slow-growing glial neoplasm. It is relatively uncommon, representing 5–7% of all intracranial neoplasms (25). The peak incidence is in the fourth to fifth decades of life.

Most oligodendrogliomas involve the centrum semiovale of the frontal lobe. Oligodendrogliomas are rarely found in the cerebellum. They are solid infiltrating tumors, with poorly defined borders. Focal cystic necrosis and intratumoral hemorrhage is common. Calcification is extremely common (see Fig. 2, Chap. 8).

On MRI, the tumors exhibit mixed intensity patterns. Up to 90% are calcified on CT (26). Conventional spin-echo MRI is not sensitive to calcification. However, gradient-echo imaging improves the sensitivity of MRI to detect calcification (27).

Edema is present in only 50% of cases (28). Contrast enhancement occurs in about half of the cases (29). The differential diagnosis is usually between an astrocytoma and an oligodendroglioma. Astrocytomas usually are more homogeneous, are not calcified, and are often located deeper in the hemisphere.

It should be stressed again that potentially all areas of contiguous abnormality around an oligodendroglioma, including edema, may represent microscopically infiltrating tumor.

A CT scan demonstrates a calcified, irregularly-marginated, deep mixed-density tumor. Low-grade oligodendrogliomas do not enhance. High-grade tumors usually show enhancement following the intravenous administration of contrast material.

G. Ependymoma

Ependymomas are slow-growing glial neoplasms. An infratentorial location predominates in 75% of pediatric patients (see discussion under posterior fossa in Chap. 8). In the older age group, however, supratentorial ependymomas tend to occur more frequently than the infratentorial tumor (30).

Supratentorial ependymoma is usually a single large tumor that arises in the cerebral white matter, most frequently the frontal or parietal lobes, areas remote from the ventricular wall, presumably from fetal rests of ependymal cells (31,32). It may also involve the atrium of the lateral ventricle, the foramen of Monro, or the third ventricle (Fig. 10).

Ependymomas demonstrate varying degrees of malignancy. The higher-grade tumors have less distinct margins. On MRI, they exhibit prolonged T1 and T2 features. They are poorly circumscribed with variable edema. Contrast enhancement occurs in most cases (see Fig. 10). On noncontrast CT, the tumors are iso- to slightly hypodense. A dense ependymoma usually suggests

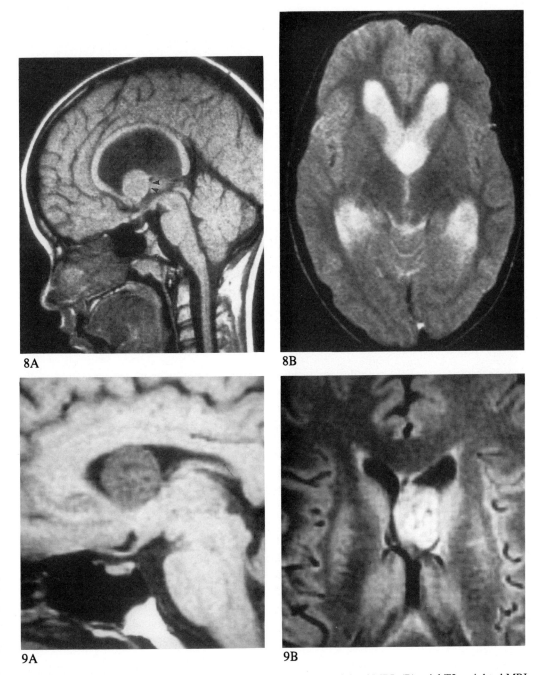

Figure 8 Hypothalamic pilocytic astrocytoma: (A) sagittal T1-weighted MRI; (B) axial T2-weighted MRI. Sagittal T1-weighted MRI (A) demonstrates a well-circumscribed isointense mass anterior to the foramen of Monro (arrowheads) extending up into the floor of the frontal horns of the lateral ventricles. This mass exhibits increased signal intensity on T2-weighted MRI (B). It mimics a colloid cyst; however, a colloid cyst arises in the roof of the third ventricle posterior to the foramen of Monro.

Figure 9 Subependymal giant cell astrocytoma in a patient with tuberous sclerosis: (A) sagittal T1-weighted MRI; (B) axial spin-density MRI. Sagittal and axial MR images demonstrate a well-circumscribed left-sided mass, anterior to the foramen of Monro, which occupies the left frontal horn of the lateral ventricle. This mass is heterogeneous and is hypointense on the T1-weighted MRI (A) and hyperintense on the spin density MRI (B).

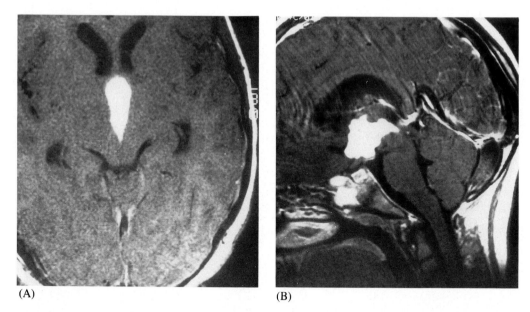

(A)   (B)

Figure 10 Third ventricular ependymoma: post-gadolinium (A) axial and (B) sagittal MR images show an intensely enhancing intra-third ventricular mass.

a hemorrhagic event. Following the intravenous administration of contrast, these tumors usually enhance. Enhancement may be either homogeneous or inhomogeneous. Calcification is seen in 50% of cases on CT (33,34). Calcification tends to be multiple and punctate in nature.

Cystic tumors are more common in the supratentorial variety of ependymomas than in the infratentorial type (33,34). In fact, 70% of supratentorial ependymomas will show cystic change.

Ependymoblastoma is an aggressive and undifferentiated variant of ependymoma. It often follows resection of a lower grade lesion and frequently seeds the subarachnoid spaces of the brain or spine. Whereas 66% of ependymomas are found infratentorially, 81% of ependymoblastomas occur supratentorially (32).

H. Ganglioglioma

Ganglioglioma is a slow-growing tumor that affects children and young adults. Ganglioglioma is a tumor in which differentiated ganglion cells and mature neuroglia show cytological features of neoplasia (35,36). Ganglioglioma constitutes about 3% of brain tumors in children (31). These tumors can arise supra- and infratentorially as well as in the spinal cord. The temporal lobe is the most frequent site (Fig. 11), followed by the occipital, frontal, and parietal lobes, in decreasing order of frequency (35–40). Ganglioglioma is regarded as a low-grade malignancy, with a slow clinical course (35).

Gangliogliomas are well-circumscribed tumors that may be either cystic or solid (39,40).

Figure 11 Solid ganglioglioma: (A) sagittal T1-weighted MRI; (B) axial spin-density MRI; (C) Axial T2-weighted MRI. Sagittal T1-weighted MRI (A) demonstrates a large well-demarcated mass occupying the temporal lobe. This mass is hypointense, but not to the same extent as CSF on the T1-weighted MRI. The mass exhibits increased signal intensity on T2-weighted MRI (C), mimicking the signal characteristics of CSF. Peritumoral edema, shown by increased signal intensity, is also noted. Although the signal characteristics of the mass are similar to CSF on T2-weighting, the spin-density image (B) clearly demonstrates that the mass exhibits increased signal on spin density, whereas the CSF is hypointense. The T1-weighted MRI (A) also shows a clear difference in signal characteristics between the tumor and the CSF.

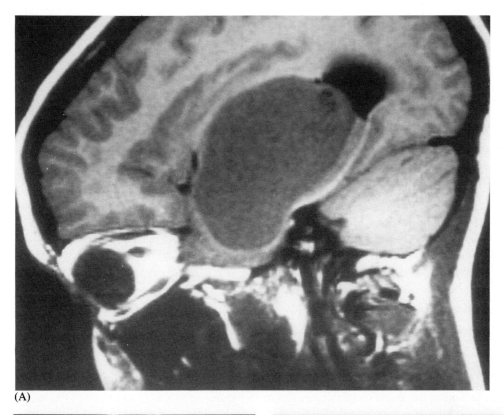

(A)

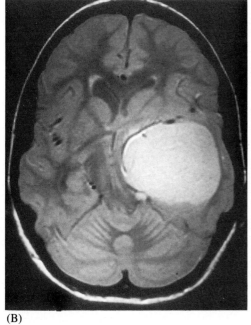

(B)

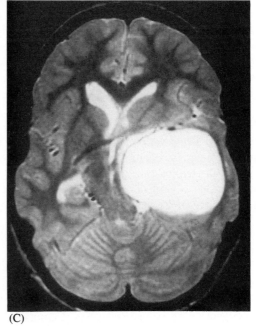

(C)

Cystic tumors occur in 38% of cases (39,40). Calcification is seen in about one-third of these. The MRI features of ganglioglioma are nonspecific. These tumors may be iso- or hypointense on T1-weighted images. On T2-weighted images, increased signal intensity is noted, which is inhomogeneous in character (see Fig. 11). In the cystic variety, markedly prolonged T2 relaxation may be seen. The solid nodule exhibits intermediate signal intensity. Most gangliogliomas exhibit contrast enhancement following the administration of intravenous gadolinium-containing agents.

On noncontrast CT, these lesions appear as isodense or low-density lesions, with little or no shift of the adjacent structures. Following the intravenous administration of iodinated contrast material, moderately intense homogeneous enhancement is seen in about 30% of cases.

I. Choroid Plexus Papilloma

Choroid plexus papilloma is derived from epithelial cells of the choroid plexus and represents about 3% of all intracranial neoplasms in children and about 0.5% of those in adults (32). Supratentorial choroid plexus papillomas involve the trigone of the lateral ventricle, particularly on the left side, and less commonly, the third ventricle (Figs. 12 and 13) (see discussion under posterior fossa tumors in Chap. 8).

II. LYMPHOMA

Primary CNS lymphoma constitutes approximately 1.5% of all CNS neoplasms (41). Although it has been relatively rare, it is increasing in prevalence, largely because patients with immunodeficiency states, such as acquired immune deficiency syndrome (AIDS), patients undergoing long-term immunosuppression therapy, patients with congenital immunodeficiency syndromes, and organ transplant recipients, are susceptible to development of these tumors. Excluding lymphoma in immunocompromised patients, there has also been an increase in the prevalence of primary CNS lymphoma worldwide. Some estimates predict it will be the most common primary brain neoplasm in the 1990s (9). Parenchymal intracranial lymphoma is almost exclusively of the non-Hodgkin's type. Controversy has surrounded the origin of primary intracranial lymphoma, which has also been referred to in the past as reticulum cell sarcoma, microglioma, periepithelial sarcoma, adventitial sarcoma, plasmacytic myeloma, round cell sarcoma, and reticulohistiocytic granulomatous encephalitis (41).

The prognosis is poor. Untreated patients survive an average of only 1.5 months after diagnosis. Treated patients, with solitary parenchymal lesions, have a median survival of 45 months, patients with multiple lesions have a median survival of 9 months, and those with meningeal involvement or subependymal involvement at diagnosis survive 7.5 months (9). Treatment with steroids can have a dramatic effect on the appearance of lymphoma, as seen with imaging studies, with complete regression of brain lesions reported as early as 8 h after administration of intravenous steroids (9).

Lymphoma can be focal or multiple, most commonly presenting in the deep gray matter structures (basal ganglia and thalamus), periventricular regions, cerebellum and brain stem. Up to 30% of patients demonstrate leptomeningeal involvement (28).

On MRI, lymphoma is most often slightly hypointense on T1-weighted images and slightly hyperintense on proton-density and T2-weighted images relative to gray matter (41). However, this is not always true, and lymphoma can be very hyperintense on the T2-weighted images or have heterogeneous signal characteristics. Homogeneous enhancement following intravenous gadolinium is generally observed (Fig. 14). A feature seen on both MRI and CT is the paucity of mass

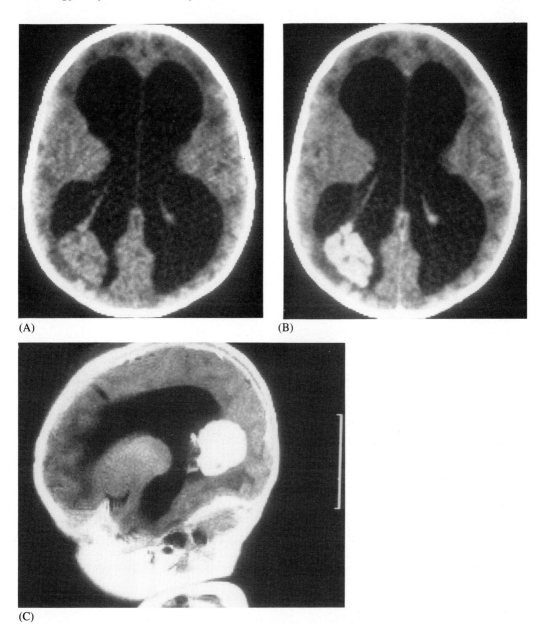

(A)

(B)

(C)

Figure 12 Choroid plexus papilloma of the trigone of the lateral ventricle in 6-week-old boy: (A) precontrast axial CT scan; (B) postcontrast axial CT scan; (C) post-gadolinium sagittal T1-weighted MRI. Precontrast CT scan (A) demonstrates a large isodense filling defect in the right trigone of the lateral ventricle. Marked hydrocephalus is present. Following the intravenous administration of contrast material (B) this mass enhances markedly. The enhanced mass has a nodular or cauliflower appearance. The post-gadolinium sagittal MRI (C) clearly demonstrates the enhancing tumor in the region of the trigone of the lateral ventricle.

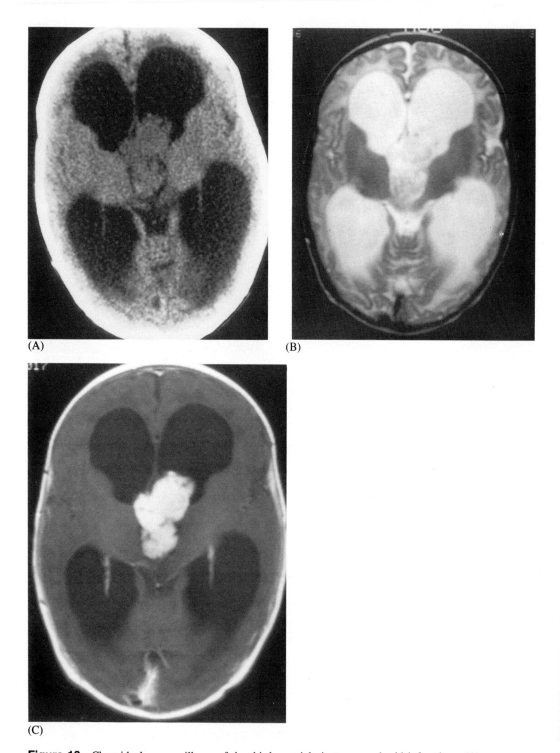

Figure 13 Choroid plexus papilloma of the third ventricle in two-month-old infant boy: (A) precontrast axial CT scan; (B) axial T2-weighted MRI; (C) post-gadolinium axial T1-weighted MRI. Precontrast CT scan (A) reveals a large isodense mass in the third ventricle that extends through the foramen of Monro into the left frontal horn of the lateral ventricle. Marked hydrocephalus is present. The T2-weighted MRI (B) shows that this mass is hyperintense, but less than that of CSF. The post-gadolinium MRI (C) reveals marked enhancement of the mass, which has a nodular character.

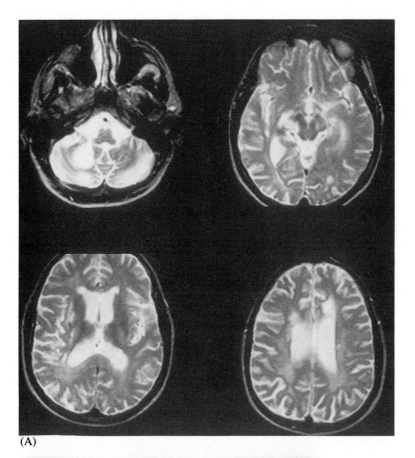

(A)

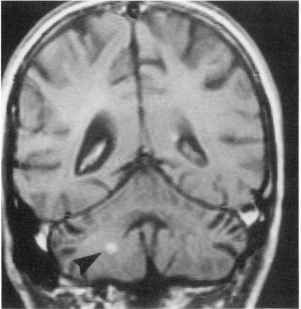

(B)

Figure 14 (See next page for legend.)

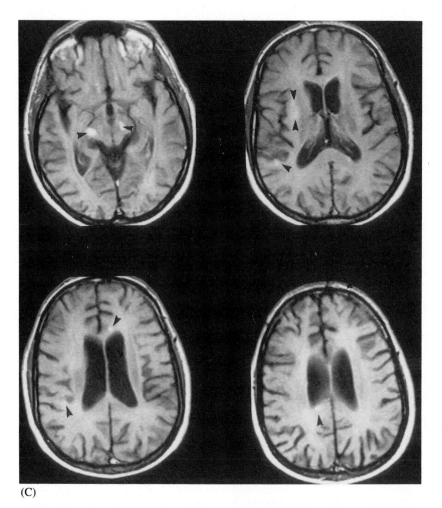

(C)

Figure 14 Primary CNS lymphoma: (A) axial T2-weighted MR images; (B) post-gadolinium coronal T1-weighted MRI; (C) post-gadolinium axial T1-weighted MR images. Axial T2-weighted MR images (A) demonstrate abnormal areas of increased signal intensity in the right cerebellar hemisphere, brain stem bilaterally, basal ganglia and periventricular regions, and subcortical areas. The post-gadolinium images (B,C) demonstrate enhancement (arrowheads) of many of the abnormal areas seen in (A).

effect and edema, given the size of the mass. This is a helpful feature in distinguishing these masses from primary glial tumors and metastases. Lymphomatous masses do not calcify, and hemorrhage is uncommon.

The most common CT appearance of intracranial lymphoma is of an isodense or hyperdense mass, relative to gray matter on unenhanced scans, which shows homogeneous enhancement after contrast administration (see Fig. 14).

Although lymphoma in patients with AIDS can have the appearance just described, it can also have an atypical appearance, with ring enhancement. In patients with AIDS, it can be very difficult to distinguish lymphoma from toxoplasmosis or other less common inflammatory lesions. This difficulty is in part related to the fact that opportunistic infections in immunocompromised patients will present with less edema owing to a diminished inflammatory response (42). Dina has reported that the most reliable features in distinguishing between primary CNS lymphoma and toxoplasmosis are that patients with lymphoma more commonly show subependymal spread, associated with a focal mass, and more commonly show increased density on CT (43).

Intracranial metastases from systemic lymphoma initially involve the leptomeninges or, less commonly, the dura (Fig. 15). Spread along the Virchow–Robin spaces can occur and produce a parenchymal mass. It is very unusual to see a parenchymal mass from systemic lymphoma without leptomeningeal involvement. Other than the fact that parenchymal involvement is more common in primary lymphoma, secondary lymphoma is indistinguishable from primary lymphoma on imaging studies (44).

III. LEUKEMIA

Leukemic involvement, similar to secondary lymphoma, initially involves the leptomeninges, with occasional spread into the Virchow–Robin spaces, producing a parenchymal leukemic mass ("chloroma").

Imaging studies are notoriously poor for detecting leptomeningeal seeding. MRI with intravenous contrast, however, is superior to CT. A subtle clue to the presence of leptomeningeal tumor may be the presence of slight ventricular enlargement, believed to be due to a slowing of the CSF circulation over the convexities by the leptomeningeal tumor (45,46).

Parenchymal leukemic deposits, if present, are better visualized on imaging studies. These lesions are generally isointense to white matter on T1-weighted images and isointense or of increased signal intensity on T2-weighted images (47,48). Enhancement following intravenous gadolinium is generally seen (Fig. 16). Leukemic deposits are generally isodense or slightly increased in density on nonenhanced CT and enhance homogeneously after intravenous contrast. The borders of the lesions may be sharp, but are commonly ill-defined, secondary to infiltration into surrounding parenchyma.

IV. NEUROFIBROMATOSIS

Neurofibromatosis (NF) is no longer considered a single disease, but is now recognized as a heterogeneous group of diseases. The two most common subtypes that account for over 99% of cases of NF have been designated NF-1 and NF-2. In 1988, an NIH Consensus Conference recommended the adoption of uniform clinical criteria to define the two most common subtypes, NF-1 and NF-2 (49) (see criteria Table 1). Neurofibromatosis-1, also known previously as von Recklinghausen's disease or peripheral neurofibromatosis, has been linked with an abnormality of chromosome 17. It is an autosomal dominant disorder affecting approximately 1:4000 individuals. Roughly, one-half the cases are inherited, with nearly 100% penetrance, and the other one-half of cases are believed to be due to spontaneous mutation (50). Neurofibromatosis-2, also known as bilateral acoustic neurofibromatosis or central neurofibromatosis, has been linked to an abnormality of chromosome 22. It is an autosomal dominant disorder occurring in about 1:50,000 persons.

Neurofibromatosis-1 is characterized by multiple cutaneous skin lesions (cafe au lait spots and neurofibromas), mesodermal dysplasias, and nervous system tumors. The intracranial lesion most commonly encountered in NF-1 is the optic glioma, which has been estimated to occur in 5–15% of patients. Conversely, approximately 25–50% of patients with an optic chiasm glioma have NF-1 (51,52). Astrocytomas, glioblastomas, and ependymomas are other glial tumors that can occur in patients with NF-1. Since the advent of MRI, it has also been discovered that many NF-1 patients have abnormal focal areas of increased signal intensity on T2-weighted images, most commonly in the cerebellar peduncles, basal ganglia, brain stem, and optic radiations (53–55). There is generally no mass effect, edema, or contrast enhancement of these lesions. If the basal ganglia are

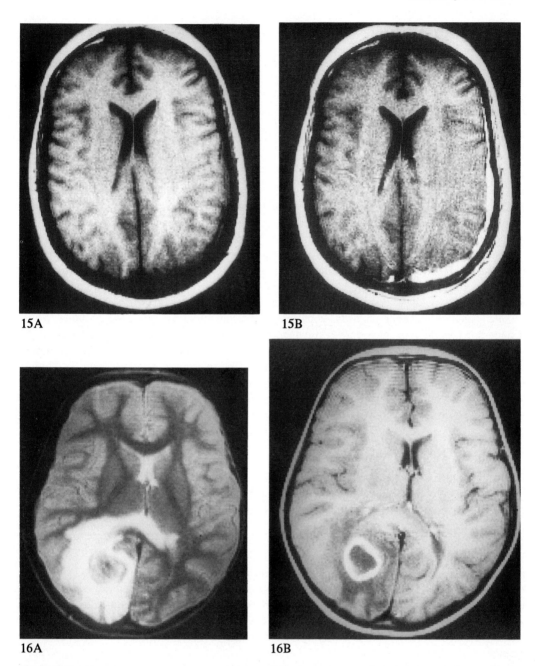

15A   15B

16A   16B

Figure 15 Systemic lymphoma, with dural involvement: (A) axial T1-weighted MRI; (B) post-gadolinium axial T1-weighted MRI. No definite abnormality can be seen on the T1-weighted MRI (A). The post-gadolinium MRI (B) reveals left-sided dural enhancement secondary to lymphoma.

Figure 16 CNS leukemia: (A) axial T2-weighted MRI; (B) post-gadolinium axial T1-weighted MRI. The T2-weighted MRI (A) demonstrates a heterogeneous mass of decreased signal intensity in the right occipital lobe. This mass is surrounded by marked peritumoral edema, which appears as increased signal intensity. Following the intravenous administration of gadolinium (B) ringlike enhancement is demonstrated.

involved, the lesions may also appear as areas of increased intensity on T1-weighted images. They are generally not seen on CT scanning. Autopsy studies have suggested that these lesions may represent hamartomas, heterotopias, glial dysplasias, or infarcts, although the true nature of many of these lesions is unknown (56). The lesions are most commonly seen in childhood and regress with advancing age. It is recommended that patients with these lesions be followed yearly to be sure they are not actually slowly growing gliomas.

Patients with NF-1 also develop plexiform neurofibromas, which are usually locally aggressive tumors coursing along the entire nerve of origin. These tumors may occur around the eyelid and orbit, frequently causing proptosis, and extending in retrograde fashion into the ipsilateral cavernous sinus (52). Sphenoid wing dysplasia is often an associated finding, producing a harlequin eye appearance on plain skull radiographs. It is felt, however, that the empty orbit appearance is caused by a mesodermal dysplasia of the sphenoid bone and is not secondary to erosion from an associated tumor (1,57). These patients may also have absence of portions of the squamous occiput along the lambdoid suture.

Patients with NF-1 may also develop arterial occlusive disease, with involvement of the aorta, celiac, mesenteric, renal, and intracranial blood vessels (58).

Intracranial lesions most commonly encountered in NF-2 include schwannomas (most commonly acoustic neuromas) and meningiomas (Fig. 17). The tumors are often multiple, with bilateral acoustic schwannomas being the hallmark of the disease. Whereas the tumors encountered in NF-1 arise primarily from the glial elements, the tumors encountered in NF-2 arise primarily from the coverings of the central nervous system.

The NIH Consensus Conference recommended that in NF-1, imaging tests to detect these intracranial problems should be reserved for patients with clinical symptoms. However, in patients with a family history of NF-2, it was recommended that all patients should have an MRI at puberty even if asymptomatic to detect occult neoplasms. It was felt that surgery or possibly stereotactic radiosurgery should be considered in patients with acoustic neuromas, even if the tumors are small and asymptomatic, since the possibility of preserving hearing is improved if the lesions are treated when small (49).

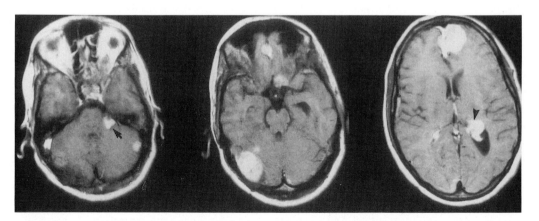

Figure 17 Neurofibromatosis 2: Post-gadolinium axial MR images demonstrate multiple, bilateral homogeneously enhancing masses representing multiple meningiomas, including an intraventricular meningioma in the left trigone of the lateral ventricle (arrowhead). A left-sided acoustic schwannoma (arrow) is also seen.

Table I.   Diagnostic Criteria for Neurofibromatosis-1 and Neurofibromatosis-2

(From the NIH Consensus Development Conference) (49)

1. *Neurofibromatosis-1*

The criterion for NF-1 includes two or more of the following:

1. Six or more cafe au lait spots over 5 mm in greatest diameter (prepubertal) and over 15 mm in greatest diameter (postpubertal)
2. Two or more neurofibromas of any type or one plexiform neurofibroma
3. Freckling in the axillary or inguinal regions
4. Optic glioma
5. Two or more Lisch nodules (iris hamartomas)
6. A distinctive osseous lesion, such as sphenoid dysplasia or thinning long bone cortex, with or without pseudoarthrosis
7. A first-degree relative (parent, sibling, or offspring) with NF-1 by the foregoing criteria.

2. *Neurofibromatosis-2*

The criterion for NF-2 includes one of the following:

1. Bilateral eighth nerve masses seen with appropriate imaging techniques (e.g., CT or MRI).
2. NF-2 in a first-degree relative, and either a unilateral eighth nerve mass or two of the following: neurofibroma, meningioma, glioma, schwannoma, or juvenile posterior subcapsular lenticular opacity.

V.   BRAIN TUMORS IN THE FIRST YEAR OF LIFE

Intracranial tumors presenting in the first year of life are an interesting group of lesions. These tumors account for approximately 10% of all pediatric brain tumors. The most common tumors found in this age group include teratomas, hamartomas, choroid plexus neoplasms (see Figs. 12 and 13), primitive neuroectodermal tumors (Fig. 18), and astrocytomas (Fig. 19).

Supratentorial tumors are more common than posterior fossa tumors in the first year of life. Almost half of the supratentorial tumors are astrocytomas of diencephalic origin. Suprasellar tumors are seen more commonly during the first year of life than during the rest of the pediatric age period.

Many of these tumors are huge at the time of presentation. This has been attributed to the elasticity of the infant skull and the capacity for functional adaptation of the immature nervous system.

VI.   MENINGIOMA

Meningiomas constitute 15–18% of all intracranial neoplasms (47,59). Meningiomas are the most common benign intracranial neoplasms and represent the largest group of operable intracranial tumors with a favorable outcome (60). Of all primary intracranial tumors, meningiomas are second in frequency only to gliomas. Meningiomas arise from arachnoid cells embedded in the dura and can be found wherever there is dura. The term *meningioma* was coined by Harvey Cushing in 1922 for tumors arising from the meninges (61).

Meningiomas are tumors of adults, with the age of incidence ranging between 20 and 60 years (59). The peak incidence is near the age of 40. A definite female preponderance is seen (59).

Meningiomas are distinctly rare in childhood, with fewer than 2% of meningiomas occurring in the pediatric age group (59). The female preponderance does not exist in the pediatric age group, where there is also a frequent association of neurofibromatosis (59).

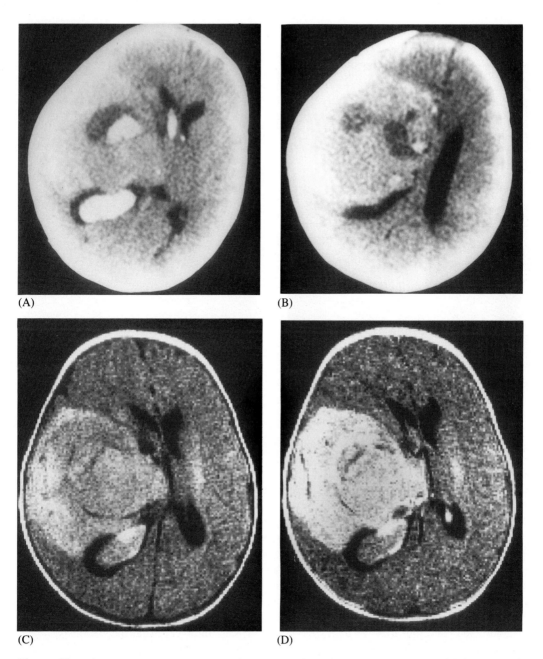

Figure 18 Primary CNS neuroblastoma in 6-week-old infant girl: (A,B) precontrast axial CT scans; (C) axial T1-weighted MRI; (D) post-gadolinium axial T1-weighted MRI; (E) post-gadolinium coronal T1-weighted MRI. Precontrast axial CT scans (A,B) demonstrate a large right-sided heterogeneous mass that displaces the ventricular system across the midline. Areas of acute hemorrhage are noted within the mass, and hemorrhage is also seen in the right frontal horn and in the trigone region, extending into the occipital horn. Areas of mottled calcification are noted throughout the mass, especially anteriorly near the anterior margin of the mass (B). In addition, areas of decreased attenuation are noted within the mass. These areas represent chronic hemorrhage or cystic or necrotic changes within the mass. This tumor is seen as a heterogeneous hyperintense mass on the T1-weighted MRI (C). Linear areas of signal void are noted within the mass. The areas of acute hemorrhage in the frontal horn and trigone region seen in (A) and (B) are seen as hyperintense regions within the lateral ventricle (C). Following the intravenous administration of gadolinium (D,E), the mass exhibits inhomogeneous enhancement.

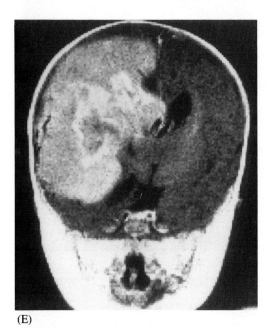

(E)

Figure 18   Continued

Most meningiomas are solitary, but multiple meningiomas can occur alone or in association with neurofibromatosis. Most meningiomas are well demarcated, round or oval, frequently lobulated tumors attached to the dura.

There appears to be a close relation between the distribution of arachnoid granulations and the favorite sites for development of meningioma (59). The most common locations are the convexity or parasagittal areas (30–40%) (62). Approximately 50% of convexity meningiomas are parasagittal or attached to the sagittal sinus. Most of these are found in the middle third of the dural sinus, with the anterior third being the next most common location. The sphenoid wing, particularly the medial third, is the next most common site (15–20%). The olfactory groove, planum sphenoidale, and diaphragma sellae account for approximately 10% of intracranial meningiomas.

Other favorite sites for development of meningiomas are in the posterior fossa (5–10%). Meningiomas in the posterior fossa involve the cerebellopontine angle (CPA), clivus, foramen magnum, and tentorium, both its upper and lower surfaces. Intraventricular meningiomas, pineal meningiomas, and meningiomas involving the orbits are less common sites.

The histopathological classification of meningiomas in widest use today is that proposed by Courville (63) and later modified by Russel and Rubinstein (1). Meningiomas are divided into four basic subtypes: fibroblastic, transitional, syncytial, and angioblastic. Mixed types also occur.

Fibroblastic meningiomas are characterized by elongated cells, with sparse cytoplasm embedded in a dense collagenous matrix. The distinctive feature of transitional meningiomas is the presence of whorl formation (tumor cells arranged in an onion-skin fashion). When these calcify, they are known as psammoma bodies. Marked psammomatous calcifications may be a dominant feature of these tumors. Syncytial meningiomas (meningoepithelial, endotheliomas) are characterized by moderate cellularity, consisting of polygonal cells, often poorly defined and arranged in lobules. Coexistent microcystic changes are relatively common in this subtype. The distinctive features of angioblastic meningiomas are their high cellularity and vascularity.

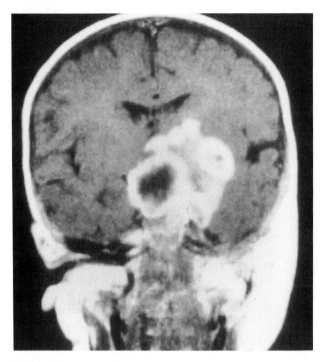

Figure 19 Hypothalamic chiasmal glioma in 6-month-old boy: Postcontrast coronal CT scan demonstrates a very large inhomogeneously enhancing suprasellar mass that contains cystic and solid components. The mass extends into the left cerebral hemisphere.

A. Plain Skull Film Findings

Approximately 30–60% of meningiomas show some type of bony abnormality or calcification on plain skull films (14,64) (see Fig. 1, Chap. 8). The abnormal findings include the following:

1. Reactive hyperostosis, which is typical of a meningioma (see Fig. 5, Chap. 8). It may assume the form of diffuse bony thickening or spicule formation. The degree of reactive bone does not necessarily correspond to the size of the tumor. In some cases, the tumor may extend through the diploe and project into the scalp, producing a palpable mass. Meningiomas of the tuberculum sellae and planum sphenoidale result in a reactive hyperostosis, causing an appearance of a "blister" of the bone. This is due to upward herniation of the posterior ethmoid air cells or sphenoid sinus. It is probable that this herniation is due to localized bony weakness.
2. Rarely, meningiomas may cause only bony destruction (see Fig. 3, Chap. 8).
3. Increase in number, size, and tortuosity of the vascular grooves on the inner table of the skull is caused by hypertrophied feeding meningeal arteries (Fig. 20).
4. Unilateral abnormal enlargement of the foramen spinosum because of a hypertrophied middle meningeal artery (see Fig. 20) is best seen on the submentovertex view. The diagnostic value of a unilateral enlarged foramen spinosum is limited and should be evaluated with caution.
5. Calcification: Approximately 10% of meningiomas will demonstrate calcification on plain skull films (14,64). Calcification may be dense and homogeneous, with well-defined margins, which many times represent the true size of the tumor (see Fig. 1, Chap. 8). In other cases, calcification may be curvilinear, speckled, granular, or cloudlike in character.

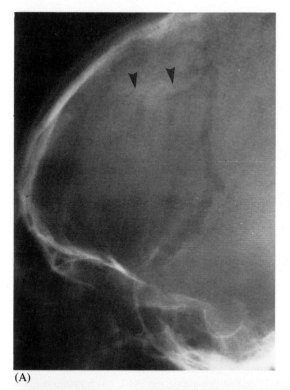

(A)

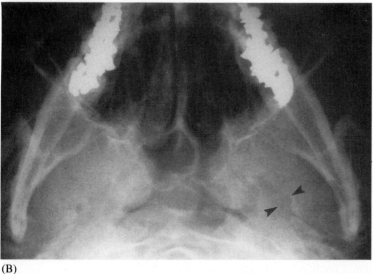

(B)

Figure 20 Meningioma: (A) lateral skull radiograph; (B) submentovertex view of skull; (C) lateral view of left selective external carotid angiogram (arterial phase); (D) lateral view of capillary phase of left selective external carotid angiogram; (E) lateral view of venous phase of left selective internal carotid angiogram. Lateral skull radiograph (A) demonstrates a very prominent enlarged tortuous vascular groove caused by an enlarged hypertrophied anterior branch of the middle meningeal artery, which is demonstrated in (C). Hyperostosis of the cranium (arrowheads) is also noted. The submentovertex view (B) demonstrates an enlarged foramen spinosum (arrowheads) caused by the hypertrophied middle meningeal artery on the left side. Left selective external carotid angiography (C) demonstrates the enlarged hypertrophied anterior branch

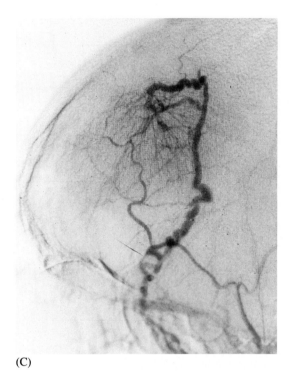

(C)

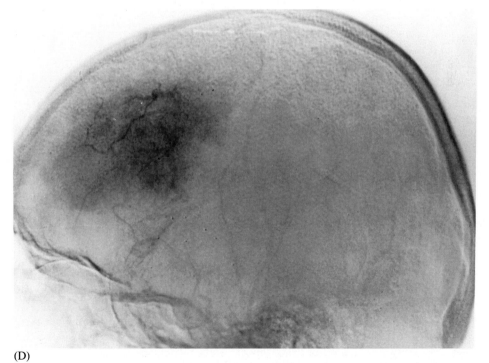

(D)

of the middle meningeal artery supplying the tumor. A sunburst or radial appearance of the arteries at the hilus of the tumor is well seen. The capillary phase of the external carotid angiogram (D) demonstrates the characteristic uniform homogeneous stain of a meningioma. The venous phase of the internal carotid angiogram demonstrates an avascular mass, indicating that the entire blood supply to the tumor is derived from the external carotid circulation.

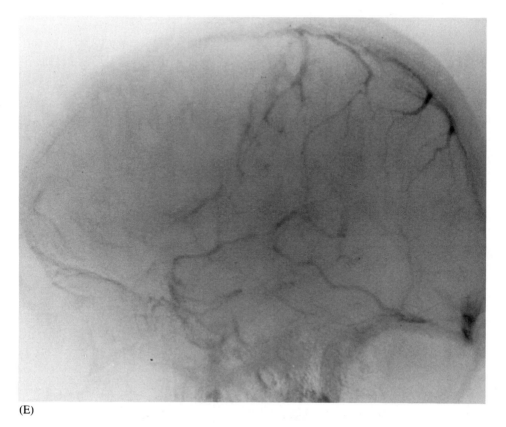

(E)

Figure 20   Continued

B.   Magnetic Resonance Imaging and Computed Tomography Findings

On T1-weighted images, most meningiomas are isointense to slightly hypointense to gray matter (65) (Fig. 21). On T2-weighted images, the MRI appearance of meningiomas is varied. Most meningiomas are isointense to mildly hyperintense (65). It may be difficult to distinguish a meningioma from contiguous brain parenchyma, particularly if the mass is small and there is little or no mass effect (Fig. 22). Some meningiomas, however, may exhibit hypo- or marked hyperintensity on T2-weighted images. Elster has shown that the varied MRI appearance of meningiomas has a clear histological basis and that a crude prediction of pathological subtypes is possible in over 75% of cases (65).

Meningiomas that are markedly hypointense to cortex on T2-weighted images are those meningiomas with preponderantly fibroblastic or transitional elements. Hyperintense meningiomas on T2-weighted images are associated with syncytial or angioblastic elements.

The intensity pattern is heterogeneous in most meningiomas (66,67). This is most evident on T2-weighted images. This heterogeneous intensity pattern is due to the presence of one or more factors: tumor vascularity, cystic foci, or calcifications. Tumor vascularity is seen as low-signal punctate or curvilinear areas on both T1- and T2-weighted images. Cystic foci appear as smooth, rounded low-signal intensities on T1-weighted images. On T2-weighted images these foci are hyperintense. Calcifications appear as coarse irregular, nodular, punctate, or curvilinear areas of signal void within the tumor on both T1- and T2-weighted images.

Secondary features such as the degree of edema, cyst formation, and the presence of

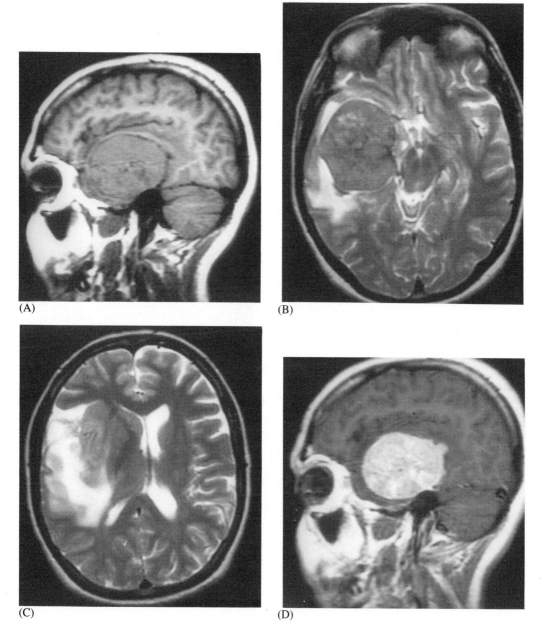

Figure 21 Sphenoid wing meningioma: (A) sagittal T1-weighted MRI; (B,C) Axial T2-weighted MR image; (D) post-gadolinium sagittal T1-weighted MRI; (E) lateral radiograph of early arterial phase of right selective internal carotid angiogram; (F) lateral radiograph of late arterial phase of selective internal carotid angiogram. Sagittal T1-weighted MRI (A) demonstrates a large well-defined heterogeneous iso- to slightly hypointense mass. This mass is isointense on T2-weighted MR images (B,C). Peritumoral edema, which appears as increased signal intensity, is seen on the T2-weighted MR images (B,C). Cystic foci, which appear as small, round hyperintense areas within the tumor, are also seen (B). A CSF interface, which appears as a low-intensity cleft on the T1-weighted MR images and exhibits high-signal intensity on T2-weighted images, can clearly be seen on the T1- and T2-weighted MR images (A,B). The identification of CSF cleft between the tumor surface and the brain surface indicates that the mass is extra-axial in location. Following the intravenous administration of gadolinium, marked homogeneous enhancement of the tumor is seen (D). Right selective internal carotid angiography demonstrates that the tumor is supplied by a hypertrophied branch of the meningohypophyseal trunk—the so-called artery of Bernasconi and Casinari (arrowheads) (E). In the late arterial phase (F) a uniform homogeneous stain is seen.

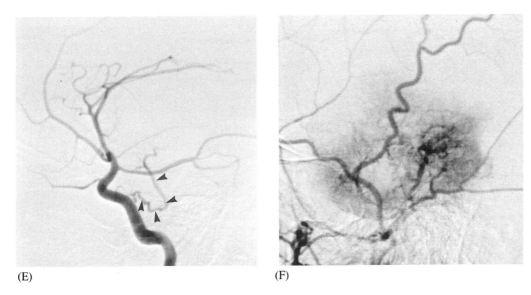

(E)   (F)

Figure 21 Continued

calcification can lead to a more accurate histological prediction in over half the remaining isointense meningiomas (65).

Central necrosis or cyst formation is more common in syncytial and angioblastic meningiomas. Coexistent microcystic changes, which are relatively common in syncytial meningiomas, also contribute to the prolonged T2 values in these histological subtypes.

Approximately 50% of meningiomas are associated with vasogenic edema (67–69) (see Fig. 21). The presence and degree of peritumoral edema is variable and is independent of the location and size of the meningioma. It is not at all unusual for small meningiomas to be associated with marked edema, whereas large meningiomas often incite little or no edema. Posterior fossa meningiomas are rarely associated with edema. Although varying amounts of edema can be seen with any histological type of meningioma, fibroblastic and transitional tumors usually tend to be associated with mild or moderate degrees of edema. Severe edema tends to be associated with syncytial or angioblastic meningiomas (65). Meningioma associated with a well-defined cystic mass may also occur (Fig. 23).

A CT scan is superior to MRI in detecting calcification. The presence of visible calcium on MRI, which may appear as rimlike, nodular, or punctate areas of low-signal intensity in an otherwise isointense tumor, suggests a transitional or fibroblastic cell type. However, calcification may not always be seen on MRI, even when the meningioma is densely calcified on a CT examination (47). This phenomenon can be explained by the fact that the signal from tumor tissue matrix obscures the signal void caused by the presence of calcification. By using gradient-echo imaging, the sensitivity for the detection of calcification on MRI is markedly improved (9).

The diagnosis of a meningioma necessitates that the mass must be extra-axial. Usually, the extra-axial location of a meningioma is obvious; however, there are times when this is not always true. Criteria that are helpful in establishing the extra-axial location of a meningioma include a broad-based dural or bony margin, bony hyperostosis, or any invasion. Hyperostosis is present in up to 27% of cases of meningiomas (47,66). However, hyperostosis may be difficult to appreciate on MRI.

Goldberg has shown that the identification of various anatomical interfaces interposed between the tumor surface and the brain surface is highly specific for extra-axial localization (67). Three

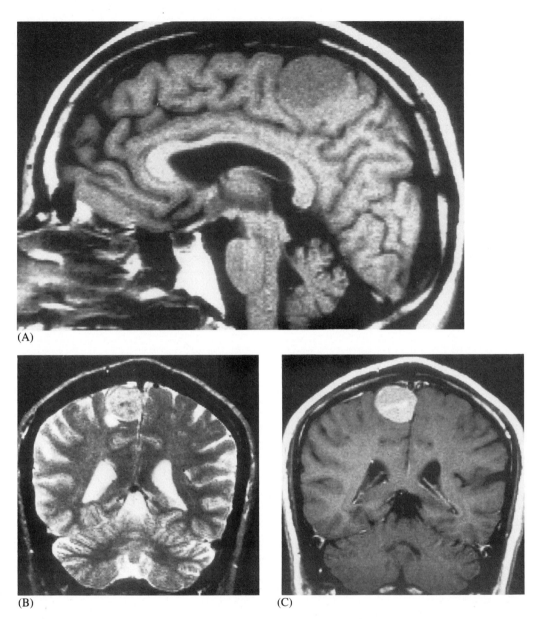

Figure 22 Parafalcine meningioma; pre- and postembolization: (A) sagittal T1-weighted MRI; (B) coronal T2-weighted MRI; (C) post-gadolinium coronal T1-weighted MRI; (D) lateral projection of right selective external carotid angiogram; (E) frontal projection of left selective external carotid angiogram; (F) lateral projection of right selective external carotid angiogram following embolization of the tumor. Sagittal T1-weighted MRI (A) demonstrates an isointense mass that exhibits increased signal intensity on the T2-weighted MRI (B). The parafalcine location is well seen on the coronal T2-weighted MRI (B) as well as on the post-gadolinium coronal T1-weighted MRI (C), which demonstrates uniform homogeneous enhancement of the tumor. The right selective external carotid angiogram (D) demonstrates that the tumor is supplied by a hypertrophied anterior branch of the middle meningeal artery. Left selective external carotid angiography (E) reveals that the tumor is also supplied by the contralateral external carotid artery. Following embolization of the tumor, right selective external carotid angiography reveals that the vascularity and blood supply to the tumor has been substantially reduced (F).

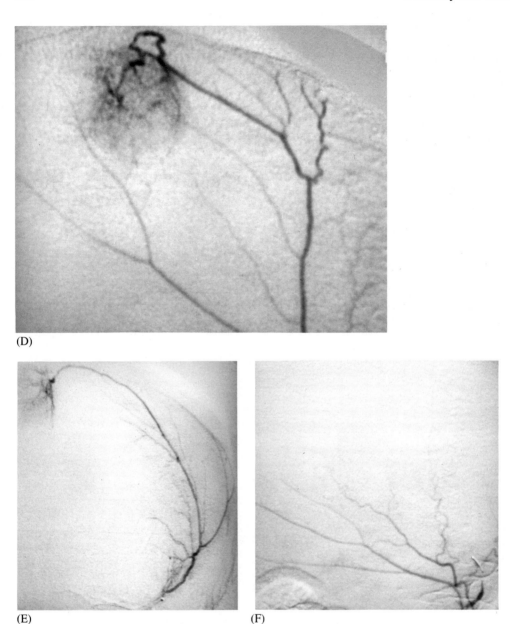

(D)

(E)   (F)

Figure 22 Continued

different anatomical interfaces may be identified on MRI. These consist of pial vascular structures, CSF clefts, and dural margins. One or more of these interfaces can usually be identified with almost all meningiomas, although the interfaces may not be found along the full tumor–brain interface (66,67). Pial blood vessel interfaces appear as punctate and curvilinear areas of signal void on T1- and T2-weighted images or along one or more of the tumor–brain margins (see Figs. 21 and 22). The CSF interfaces appear as low-intensity clefts on T1-weighted images and exhibit high-signal intensity on T2-weighted images (see Fig. 21). These CSF clefts appear isointense on proton-density images. A thin isointense rim, representing the proton cerebral cortex, separates the CSF clefts from edema. Vascular rims may be seen within the CSF clefts. The dural margin

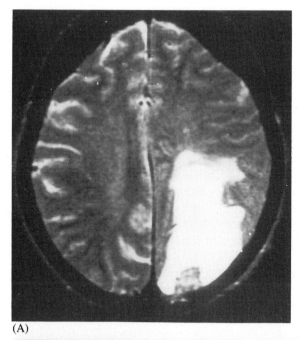

(A)

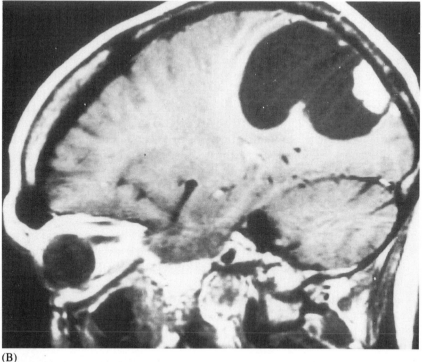

(B)

Figure 23 Meningioma associated with well-defined cystic mass: (A) axial T2-weighted MRI; (B) post-gadolinium sagittal T1-weighted MRI. Axial T2-weighted MRI (A) demonstrates a dural-based slightly hypointense mass in the occipital region. This mass is surrounded by a well-defined mass of increased signal intensity. The post-gadolinium sagittal T1-weighted MRI (B) demonstrates uniform homogeneous enhancement of the solid portion of the tumor. The cystic portion is clearly seen as a well-marginated area of decreased signal intensity.

interface is seen as a low-intensity rim on all imaging sequences and is seen primarily in meningiomas of the cavernous sinus (67).

An MRI scan is superior to CT (with and without contrast) in demonstrating these interfaces (67). In patients in whom the interfaces are identified on MRI, CT with and without contrast can identify them in fewer than 50% of the tumors (66,67).

An intra-axial mass (glioma or metastasis) in the corticomedullary junction may simulate a meningioma, especially if there is a large amount of surrounding cerebral edema. An extra-axial mass, such as a meningioma, displaces the cortex from the inner table of the skull, buckling the underlying white matter, but leaving the junction intact—white matter buckling (70). An intra-axial mass will destroy the gray–white matter junction. In addition, extra-axial masses compress the adjacent portions of the brain together, producing arcuate bowing and compression of adjacent cortical convolutions in an onion-skinlike configuration, beginning at the margin of the tumor (67). Large intracerebral masses located near the surface of the brain tend to spread the parenchymal areas apart and do not produce this accordionlike compression.

The use of intravenous gadolinium is very important in evaluation of meningiomas (71–74). As stated previously, in many instances it may be difficult to distinguish a meningioma from contiguous brain parenchyma, particularly if the meningioma is isointense and if there is little or no mass effect. Following the intravenous administration of gadolinium, marked homogeneous enhancement of the tumor is noted (see Figs. 21–25). This is because the capillaries of the meningioma have no blood–brain barrier.

An MRI scan demonstrates the relation of the vascular structures to the tumor. In parasellar meningiomas, MRI, particularly when used with gadolinium, will demonstrate whether the internal carotid arteries are encased by the tumor (75) (Fig. 24).

Venous sinus invasion is demonstrated on MRI by the partial or complete obliteration of the sinus flow void with a soft-tissue mass (Fig. 26). The intensity of tissue within the venous sinus is usually similar to that of the adjacent tumor mass (see Fig. 26) and will show marked enhancement following the intravenous administration of gadolinium.

Contrast will also demonstrate infiltration of adjacent dural surfaces, which may not be apparent on noncontrast scans (see Fig. 25). This may be of import in surgical planning. However, it may be difficult to differentiate dural infiltration from reactive dural thickening and enhancement, without tumor infiltration (67,76). The latter may also be seen in meningiomas. Dural thickening and enhancement in continuity with margins of an intracranial tumor adds another MRI feature of extraaxial-based tumors.

Intraventricular meningiomas arise from arachnoid cells of the tela choroidea or from cell rests within the stroma of the choroid plexus. Intraventricular meningiomas account for a small fraction of all intracranial meningiomas (fewer than 0.5%) (32). Although intracranial meningiomas are much more rare in children than in adults, the percentage of meningiomas located within the ventricular system is much higher in children (15–17%) than in adults (0.5–1%) (32). Clinically evident intraventricular meningiomas have been reported in patients ranging in age from 3.5 to 72 years. The peak incidence is during the third and fourth decades of life.

Most intraventricular meningiomas arise in the region of the trigone of the lateral ventricle (Fig. 27). The left lateral ventricle is affected more often than the right. About 12% of these tumors are located more anteriorly in the lateral ventricle, near the foramen of Monro. Those meningiomas located in the lateral ventricles do not produce symptoms until they have attained considerable size. Meningiomas of the third and fourth ventricles may produce symptoms earlier because of the earlier development of associated hydrocephalus. Meningiomas of the third ventricle are extremely rare, but when they occur, they tend to arise in the posterior portion of the third ventricle and may present with symptoms mimicking those of a pineal region tumor (32). Intraventricular meningiomas consistently show a high frequency of calcification compared to meningiomas located

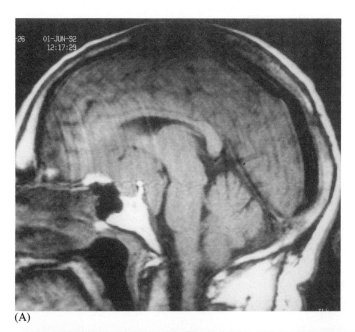

(A)

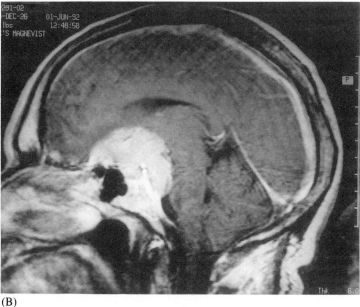

(B)

Figure 24 Large parasellar and suprasellar meningioma with vascular encasement: (A) sagittal T1-weighted MRI; (B) post-gadolinium sagittal T1-weighted MRI; (C) post-gadolinium coronal T1-weighted MRI. Sagittal T1-weighted MRI (A) demonstrates a large isointense suprasellar mass that extends behind the clivus, displacing and effacing the midbrain and pons. The extra-axial location of the mass is confirmed by the CSF cleft seen on the superior aspect of the mass. Following intravenous administration of gadolinium, the mass enhances uniformly (B,C). The coronal scan (C) demonstrates encasement of the middle and anterior cerebral arteries as well as the supraclinoid internal carotid artery. The tumor elevates and stretches the middle and anterior cerebral arteries.

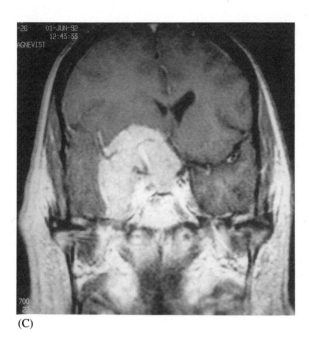

(C)

Figure 24 Continued

elsewhere intracranially (32). The CT and MRI characteristics of intraventricular meningiomas are similar to meningiomas in other locations.

On nonenhanced CT, meningiomas appear as homogeneous masses that are isodense or slightly hyperdense (Fig. 28). Calcification is present in approximately 18% of cases. The appearance of calcification is variable and may appear as nodular, very fine, or punctate (psammomatous). In some instances, the entire tumor may be calcified. Following the intravenous administration of iodinated contrast material, intense enhancement of a homogeneous nature occurs (see Figs. 25 and 28). When an entire meningioma is densely calcified, no enhancement is visible following the intravenous administration of contrast.

On CT it may be difficult, if not impossible, to distinguish between a meningioma, schwannoma, and aneurysm (47). Angiography is the definitive imaging test for the diagnosis of an aneurysm. However, if the aneurysm is thrombosed, the diagnosis may be difficult on CT.

Magnetic resonance imaging is an excellent technique to differentiate meningiomas and schwannomas from an aneurysm (see Fig. 9, Chap. 8). If the aneurysm is patent, MRI will demonstrate a signal void caused by rapidly moving blood. If the aneurysm is partially thrombosed, MRI will demonstrate a mixture of hypo- and hyperintense signals, as well as hemosiderin deposition.

C. Angiography

Meningiomas have angiographic characteristics that are recognizable in over half the cases. Most meningiomas receive their blood supply from the external carotid circulation (see Figs. 20 and 22). As the tumor increases in size, with involvement of the leptomeninges, the meningioma may acquire a dual blood supply by parasitizing adjacent cerebral vessels. The central portion or core of the tumor is supplied by the external carotid artery, and the peripheral portion of the tumor is supplied by branches of the internal carotid artery (Fig. 29).

It is often helpful to perform selective external and internal carotid angiography to achieve a

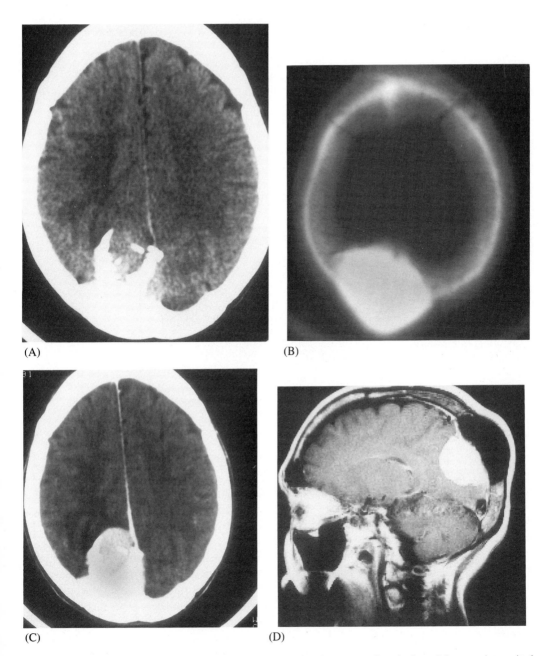

(A)

(B)

(C)

(D)

Figure 25 Occipital meningioma, with marked osseous involvement and occlusion of the superior sagittal sinus: (A) axial precontrast CT scan; (B) axial precontrast CT scan (bone windows); (C) postcontrast axial CT scan; (D) post-gadolinium sagittal T1-weighted MRI; (E) Lateral projection of right internal carotid angiogram (venous phase). Precontrast CT scan (A) demonstrates a densely calcified mass in the right occipital region. On a higher axial image (B) photographed at bone window settings, a dense ossified component of the tumor, which protrudes posteriorly beyond the cranium, is seen. The soft-tissue component of the tumor enhances following the intravenous administration of contrast material (C). The sagittal post-gadolinium MRI (D) demonstrates homogeneous enhancement of the tumor as well as enhancement of the dura anterior and posterior to the tumor. The osseous component of the tumor expands the cranium and exhibits decreased signal intensity. In the lateral projection of the venous phase of the carotid angiogram (E) there is no opacification of the posterior half of the superior sagittal sinus, indicating that it is occluded by the tumor. The posterior half of the superior sagittal sinus also did not opacify on the left carotid and vertebral angiograms. (For orientation the arrowhead points to the torcular.)

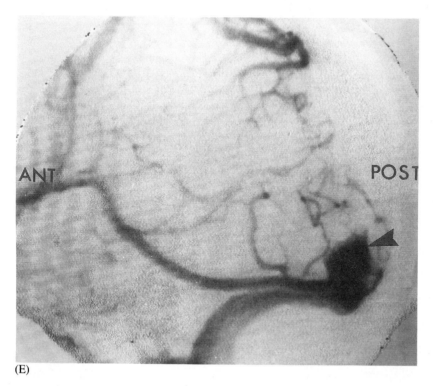

(E)

Figure 25 Continued

better definition and more accurate evaluation of the tumor. Furthermore, in some patients the meningioma may receive additional blood supply from the contralateral external carotid artery (see Figs. 22 and 30). Therefore, it may be necessary to perform bilateral carotid angiography to demonstrate the full blood supply to the meningioma.

In the arterial phase, angiography may demonstrate dilated tortuous feeding vessels, usually from the external carotid artery. In approximately two-thirds of cases, meningiomas reveal a characteristic and almost pathognomonic angioarchitecture, consisting of a homogeneous tumor stain that appears in the late capillary phase and persists through the late venous phase (32) (see Fig. 21; and Fig. 7, Chap. 8). Angiography may also demonstrate a sunburst appearance of the arteries at the hilus or attachment of the meningioma to the dura (see Figs. 20 and 29). Upon reaching the tumor, the feeding artery branches into a myriad of very tiny vessels that appear to begin at a central point and then branch out in a sunburst or radial pattern.

Some meningiomas are associated with early draining veins.

Some meningiomas, particularly at the skull base and CPA do not demonstrate the characteristic tumor blush.

The objectives of angiography are:

1. To serve as a road map for surgery
2. To confirm encasement of carotid or vertebral arteries and their branches
3. To consider and plan preoperative embolization as an adjunct to surgery
4. To confirm or exclude patency of major dural sinuses (see Fig. 25)
5. To confirm the diagnosis of meningioma, if the diagnosis is in doubt following CT and MRI

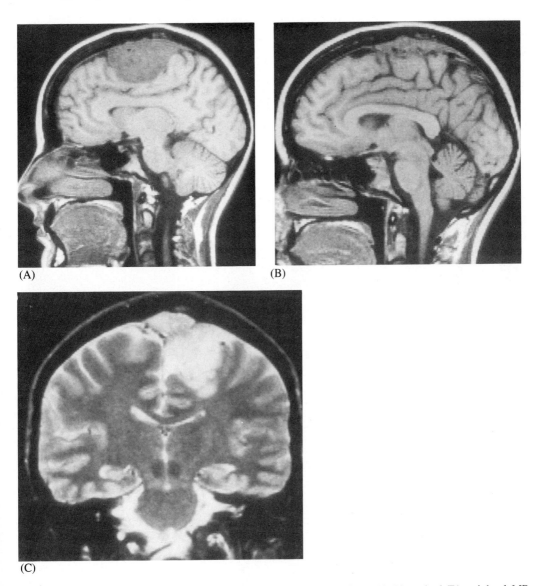

Figure 26 Falx meningioma, with invasion of superior sagittal sinus: (A,B) sagittal T1-weighted MR images; (C) coronal T2-weighted MRI. Sagittal T1-weighted MRI images (A,B) demonstrate a hypointense extra-axial mass, with superior sagittal sinus invasion. On the coronal T2-weighted MRI (C) the mass exhibits increased signal intensity. The tumor in the superior sagittal sinus exhibits increased signal intensity similar to that of the tumor.

VII. COLLOID CYSTS OF THE THIRD VENTRICLE

Colloid cysts of the third ventricle (paraphyseal or neuroepithelial cysts) are rare lesions representing approximately 0.5% of all brain tumors (77). Colloid cyst of the third ventricle is a developmental anomaly that arises in the anterosuperior part of the third ventricle immediately posterior to the foramen of Monro. The cyst usually projects downward into the third ventricle and, to a variable extent, upward and forward. The cyst is well circumscribed, smooth, and spherical, with diverse sizes from 0.3 to 3–4 cm in diameter (77). It may have a narrow pedicle or broad

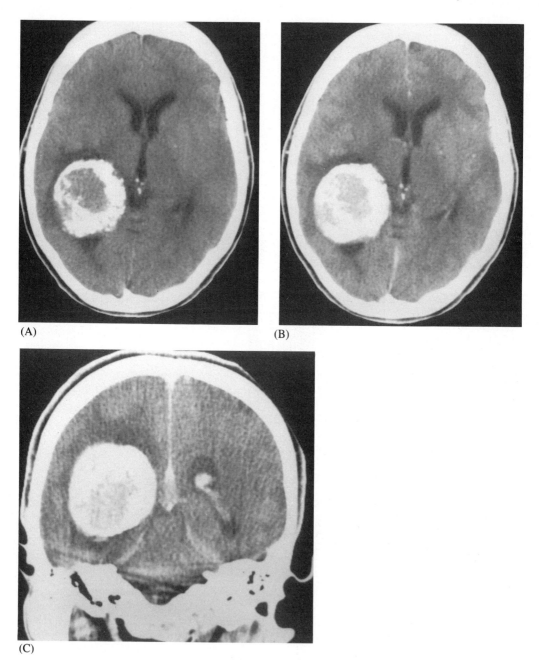

(A)

(B)

(C)

Figure 27 Intraventricular meningioma: (A,B) pre- and postcontrast axial CT scans; (C) postcontrast coronal CT scan. The precontrast CT scan (A) reveals peripheral calcification in a large mass in the region of the right trigone of the lateral ventricle. Some peritumoral edema is also evident. There is only a slight shift of the ventricular system from right to left. Postcontrast axial and coronal CT scans (B,C) show homogeneous enhancement of the mass. Both the axial and coronal images confirm the intraventricular localization of the tumor. (From Ref. 33.)

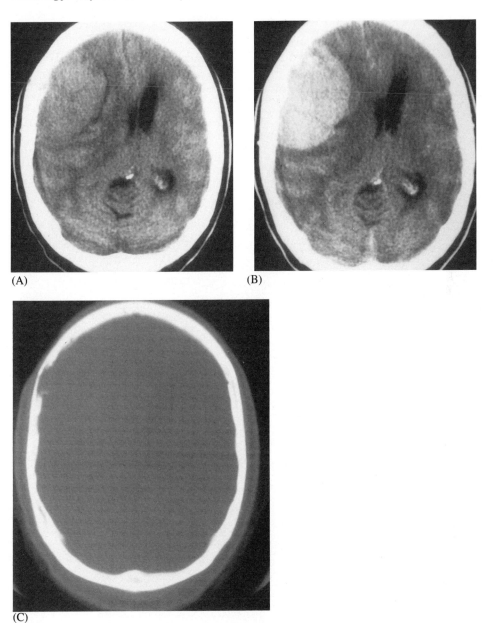

(A) (B)

(C)

Figure 28 Convexity meningioma; CT features and bone erosion of inner table of skull: (A) precontrast axial CT scan; (B) postcontrast axial CT scan; (C) axial CT scan (bone windows). Precontrast CT scan (A) demonstrates a hyperdense mass in the right frontal convexity area. The ventricular system is displaced across the midline. The extra-axial location of the mass is confirmed by the CSF cleft seen on the medial aspect of the tumor. Following the intravenous administration of contrast material (B), the mass enhances uniformly and homogeneously. Erosion of the inner table of the skull is demonstrated on the axial CT scan photographed at bone window settings (C).

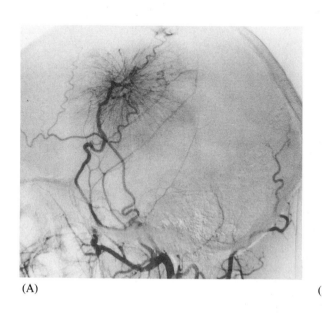

(A)

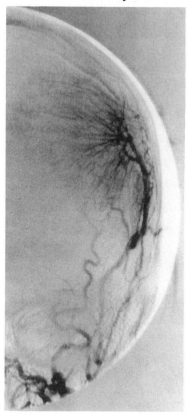

(B)

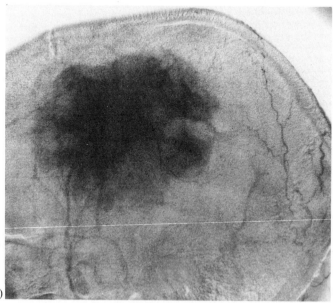

(C)

Figure 29 Convexity meningioma: (A) lateral projection of arterial phase of left selective external carotid angiogram; (B) frontal projection of arterial phase of left selective external carotid angiogram; (C) lateral projection of the late capillary–early venous phase of left selective external carotid angiogram; (D) lateral projection of venous phase of left selective internal carotid angiogram. Arterial phase of the left selective external carotid angiogram (A,B) shows a hypertrophied anterior branch of the middle meningeal artery

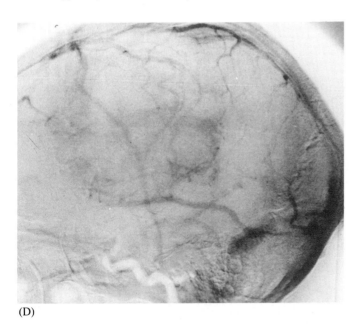

(D)

supplying the convexity meningioma. A sunburst appearance of the arteries at the hilus of the meningioma is noted. The late capillary–early venous phase of the selective external carotid angiogram (C) demonstrates a uniform homogeneous stain. Note that multiple areas on the periphery of the tumor do not stain on the external carotid examination. These areas, however, are supplied by the internal carotid artery (D) and exhibit a uniform homogeneous stain on the selective internal carotid examination.

sessile base. It is attached to the choroid plexus of the roof of the third ventricle to a rather variable extent. The cyst is filled with a homogeneous viscus material containing cellular debris; hence, the term *colloid cyst.*

Histologically, a colloid cyst is benign, but by virtue of its position, a colloid cyst may produce marked dilatation of the lateral ventricles by intermittently or persistently obstructing one or both foramina of Monro (77).

The MRI findings of colloid cysts are inconsistent, ranging from hypo- to iso- to hyperintensity on all pulse sequences (47) (Fig. 31). The signal character may be homogeneous or heterogeneous.

Approximately 60% of colloid cysts are lined by ciliated epithelium secreting mucinous material (28). These colloid cysts exhibit short T1 relaxation times and irregular shortening of T2 relaxation (28). This MRI appearance may be partially related to the heavy protein or mucoid content of the cyst (28). More than one-half of cysts exhibiting bright signal on T1-weighted images exhibit centrally shortened T2 relaxation, with a circumferentially hyperintense T2-weighted image capsule (78). This central paramagnetic effect may be related to spectroscopically confirmed cyst contents, such as magnesium, copper, or iron (79). In other cases, generalized decreased signal intensity may be seen on T2-weighted images (see Fig. 31).

Some colloid cysts may be lined by cuboidal epithelial cells that secrete a serous fluid which mimics CSF. These colloid cysts exhibit long T1 and T2 relaxation characteristics.

Following intravenous administration of gadolinium-containing agents, colloid cysts may demonstrate mild enhancement in the periphery of the cyst (see Fig. 31). In many cases, no enhancement is identified.

On noncontrast CT, colloid cysts are isodense or hyperdense (80,81) (see Fig. 31). Rarely,

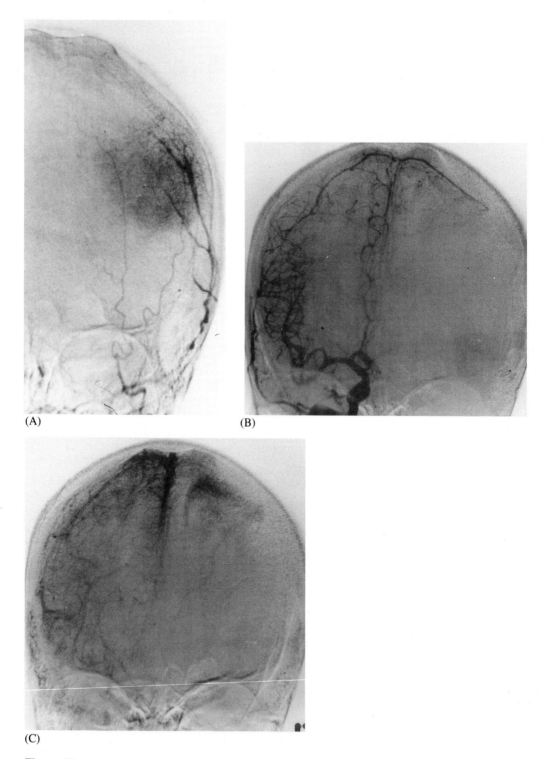

(A)

(B)

(C)

Figure 30 Convexity meningioma supplied by contralateral external carotid artery: (A) frontal projection of left selective external carotid angiogram; (B) frontal view of right common carotid angiogram (arterial phase); (C) frontal view of right common carotid angiogram (venous phase). The selective left external carotid angiogram (A) demonstrates a uniform homogeneous stain characteristic of meningioma in the parietal convexity region. The right common carotid angiograms (B,C) reveal that the superior and part of the lateral and medial aspects of the tumor are supplied by a hypertrophied meningeal artery that is the continuation of the right posterior branch of the middle meningeal artery, which crosses the midline to supply the tumor.

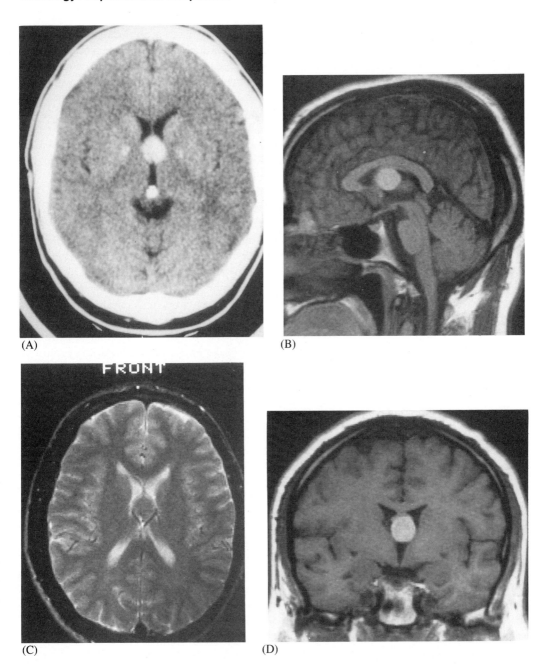

(A) (B)

(C) (D)

Figure 31 Colloid cyst of the third ventricle: (A) precontrast axial CT scan; (B) sagittal T1-weighted MRI; (C) axial T2-weighted MRI; (D) post-gadolinium coronal T1-weighted MRI. The precontrast CT scan (A) demonstrates a hyperdense, round midline mass in the region of the foramen of Monro. Incidental note is also made of bilateral basal ganglia calcification, which was not of any clinical significance. Postcontrast CT scan (not shown) did not demonstrate enhancement. The T1-weighted MRI (B) demonstrates a hyperintense mass arising in the roof of the third ventricle behind the foramen of Monro and extends into the floor of the lateral ventricle. This mass is hypointense on the T2-weighted MRI (C). Note that the internal cerebral veins are splayed laterally by this mass. The postcontrast coronal MRI (D) reveals mild peripheral enhancement of the mass.

hypodense lesions on CT can be seen (82). Following the intravenous administration of iodinated contrast material, colloid cysts enhance to a mild degree in most cases (80). The enhancement may be secondary to blood vessels in the wall of the cyst or to leakage of contrast into the cyst cavity. Occasionally, no enhancement can be appreciated following intravenous contrast administration.

VIII. SELLAR AND PARASELLAR LESIONS

The sella turcica is a saddle-shaped depression in the floor of the sphenoid bone, which contains the pituitary gland and the inferior infundibulum. The sella is bordered anteriorly, inferiorly, and posteriorly by the sphenoid bone, superiorly by the diaphragma sella, and laterally by the cavernous sinuses. Above the diaphragma sella is the CSF-filled suprasellar cistern through which courses the superior infundibulum, the optic chiasm, the supraclinoid carotid arteries, and the circle of Willis. Laterally, the dura-lined cavernous sinuses contain the carotid arteries and the oculomotor (III), trochlear (IV), first and second divisions of the trigeminal (V1 and V2) and the abducens (VI) nerves. Lesions that present in the sellar and parasellar region can arise from these structures, from adjacent brain structures such as the hypothalamus, or from distant sites.

The pituitary gland is divided into three lobes: the adenohypophysis, the pars intermedia, and the neurohypophysis. The anterior adenohypophysis develops from the upward migration of Rathke's pouch, which is an ectoderm-lined diverticulum from the embryonic mouth. The adenohypophysis is responsible for the synthesis of prolactin, corticotropin (adrenocorticotropic hormone; ACTH), and growth hormone (GH). Release of these hormones is under the control of the hypothalamus.

The posteriorly located neurohypophysis, infundibulum, and supraoptic and paraventricular nuclei of the hypothalamus derive from a down growth of the neuroectoderm of the diencephalon. Antidiuretic hormone and oxytocin are synthesized in the hypothalamus and stored in the neurohypophysis until their release is dictated by the hypothalamus.

Between the adenohypophysis and the neurohypophysis is the pars intermedia, which is an embryonic vestige and normally not of any significance. It may contain occasional glandlike spaces representing remnants of the Rathke cleft.

The pituitary gland normally measures 3–8 mm in height, with a flat or slightly concave upper surface (83,84). In young adult women, the gland may be slightly larger, measuring up to 12 mm in height, with a bulging or convex upper margin (85).

The pituitary gland is best imaged using MRI, largely because the dense bone at the base of the skull does not cause significant artifact on MRI. An MRI scan also has substantially greater soft-tissue contrast and has multiplanar capability. Evaluation of possible pituitary lesions is best performed with T1-weighted images and, therefore, T2-weighted images are usually not performed. Thin-section coronal and sagittal images both before and after contrast are most helpful. The anterior pituitary gland shows homogeneous, intermediate signal intensity on both T1-weighted and T2-weighted images, roughly paralleling the signal intensity of normal cerebral white matter. The posterior pituitary shows increased signal intensity on T1-weighted images, probably owing to T1 shortening caused by lipoproteins that serve in transport of neurophysins from the hypothalamus (86). It exhibits decreased signal intensity on T2-weighted images. Following the administration of intravenous contrast, the pituitary gland shows homogeneous enhancement.

Not only is the pituitary gland optimally imaged on MRI, but so are the other structures in the parasellar region. The infundibulum, originating from the median eminence of the hypothalamus and inserting on the superior pituitary gland, is well seen on sagittal and coronal images. The optic nerves, optic chiasm, and optic tracts are visualized and generally parallel the signal intensity of cerebral white matter. The cavernous sinuses forming the lateral border of the sella are seen, but the thin medial dural reflection and the individual cranial nerves are not generally visualized as distinct structures. Because the medial wall is not visualized, it is often very difficult to accurately determine cavernous sinus invasion by a pituitary mass. The carotid arteries can be seen as areas of flow void within the cavernous sinuses.

A. Pituitary Adenoma

The most common lesion to involve the pituitary gland region is the pituitary adenoma, which arises from the adenohypophysis and accounts for about 10–15% of all intracranial neoplasms (87,88). Adenomas are classified by size into macroadenomas, which are larger than 10 mm, and microadenomas, which are smaller than 10 mm. They can further be classified into nonfunctioning and functioning types. The functioning or secreting types of adenomas can further be divided into types based on the hormone they secrete. Prolactin-secreting adenomas are most common, with GH- and ACTH-secreting types being less common.

Clinical signs and symptoms depend on the tumor's functional status, size, and degree and direction of extrasellar extension. Not surprisingly, nonfunctional tumors tend to be large at the time of diagnosis and usually present secondary to their compressive effects on adjacent structures, such as the optic chiasm. The size of functional adenomas at presentation is variable. Forty percent of prolactin-secreting adenomas and 85% of ACTH-secreting adenomas are smaller than 10 mm at diagnosis (88). On the other hand 95% of growth hormone-secreting adenomas are larger than 10 mm at the time of diagnosis because radiologic evaluation is usually delayed in these patients (88).

Microadenomas typically appear as an area of decreased signal intensity within the otherwise homogeneous anterior pituitary gland (Fig. 32). Gadolinium-enhanced images are very helpful in patients with equivocal or negative noncontrast studies. Following the administration of intravenous contrast, the adenoma will appear as an area of decreased signal intensity within the dense, homogeneous enhancing pituitary gland (Fig. 32). If delayed scans are performed, the adenoma may become isointense or even increased in signal intensity, compared with the normal pituitary gland, as it absorbs contrast more slowly than the normal gland. Secondary signs of a microadenoma include asymmetric bulging along the superior or inferior surface of the gland or lateral deviation of the infundibulum. However, patients with normal pituitary glands may also show infundibular tilt secondary to ectopic positioning of the pituitary gland or ectopic insertion of the infundibulum.

Microadenomas can also be visualized in many patients with CT scanning. Contrast-enhanced coronal images are generally necessary and show the adenoma as an area of decreased density in the otherwise densely enhancing pituitary gland. Asymmetric bulging of the gland and infundibular tilt may also be helpful signs. However, MRI should be used as the initial screening study unless there is a contraindication.

Macroadenomas are generally isointense to gray matter on T1-weighted images (Fig. 33). The T2-weighted appearance is variable. Most macroadenomas enhance after the administration of intravenous gadolinium in either a homogeneous or nonhomogeneous pattern. Most, but not all, macroadenomas are centered in the sella turcica. They often extend superiorly into the suprasellar cistern and abut or compress the optic chiasm (see Fig. 33). They may extend inferiorly into the sphenoid sinus or even postero-inferiorly to the clivus. Invasion of the cavernous sinus is also often present, but is difficult to evaluate on imaging studies as discussed in the foregoing. The sensitivity of MRI to cavernous sinus invasion is approximately 55% (89). Carotid artery encasement is the most specific sign of cavernous sinus invasion (see Fig. 33). Carotid artery displacement, however, does not mean there is cavernous sinus invasion (89).

Hemorrhage accompanying pituitary adenoma is seen in approximately 18% of macroadeno-

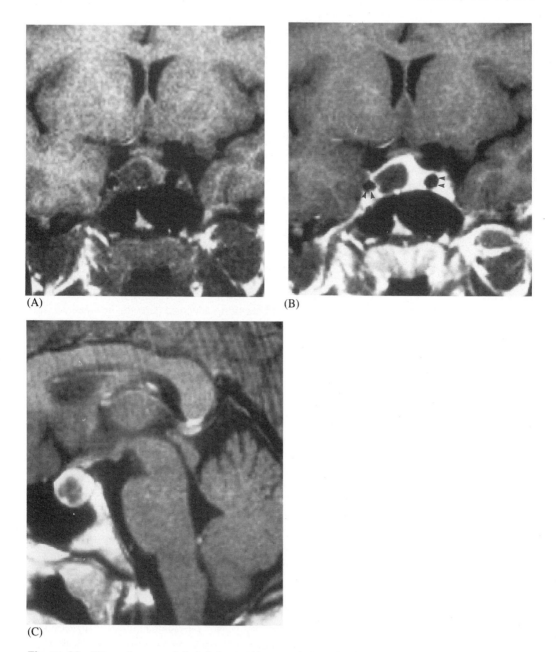

(A)   (B)

(C)

Figure 32 Microadenoma of the pituitary: (A) coronal T1-weighted MRI; (B) post-gadolinium coronal T1-weighted MRI; (C) post-gadolinium sagittal T1-weighted MRI. The T1-weighted MRI (A) demonstrates a right-sided hypointense mass in the pituitary that produces an upward convex margin to the pituitary gland. Following the administration of gadolinium (B,C), the adenoma appears as an area of decreased signal intensity within the dense homogeneous enhancing pituitary gland. This mass measured less than 10 mm. The arrowheads point to the signal void of the internal carotid arteries within the cavernous sinus.

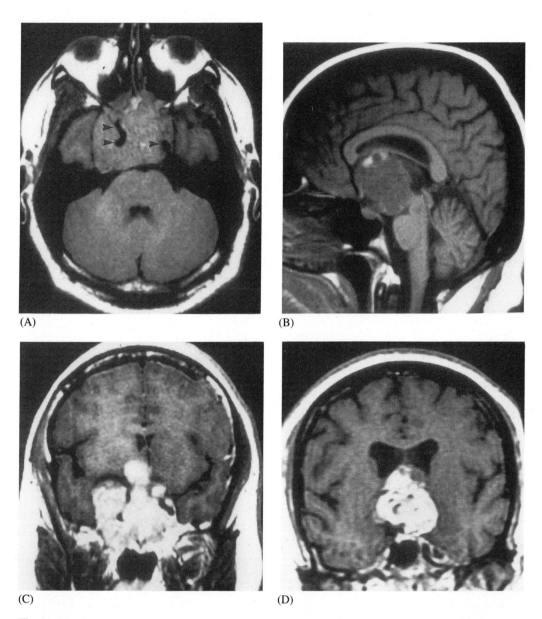

(A)

(B)

(C)

(D)

Figure 33 Large pituitary adenoma: (A) axial T1-weighted MRI; (B) sagittal T1-weighted MRI; (C,D) post-gadolinium coronal T1-weighted MR images. The T1-weighted MR images (A,B) demonstrate a large isointense mass with anterior, lateral, and superior extension. The mass encases the cavernous carotid arteries (arrowheads). Areas of increased signal intensity within the mass, representing areas of hemorrhage, are noted. The post-gadolinium coronal MR images (C,D) demonstrate uniform homogeneous enhancement. Encasement of the cavernous and supraclinoid carotid arteries are also seen (C,D).

mas (see Fig. 33) and approximately 5% of microadenomas (87). Hemorrhage on MRI in a pituitary tumor is most often seen as an area of increased signal intensity on T1-weighted images. Despite the presence of hemorrhage seen on MRI, most patients do not present with acute symptoms (apoplexy) (90). Focal areas of necrosis also can occur, presenting with the appearance of cysts within the adenoma.

Computed tomography imaging of macroadenomas is less sensitive than MRI for the reasons previously discussed. However, CT may occasionally be helpful if evaluation for bony erosion is deemed necessary.

Occasionally, a plain lateral skull film obtained for another reason will show serendipitous enlargement of the sella turcica. In these patients, macroadenoma should be excluded with MRI.

B. Meningioma

Meningiomas are the second most common tumor to arise in the pituitary region (87). Suprasellar meningiomas commonly arise from the diaphragma sellae or tuberculum sellae (Fig. 34). Meningiomas in this region also commonly arise from the dural wall of the cavernous sinus and the greater wing of the sphenoid. Their imaging characteristics may be similar to adenomas. However, they are generally not centered in the sella. Schwannomas should also be included in the differential diagnosis. Imaging features of meningiomas and schwannomas are discussed elsewhere in this chapter.

C. Craniopharyngioma

Craniopharyngiomas are epithelial neoplasms that arise from squamous epithelial rests along the involuted hypophyseal–Rathke's duct (91). They constitute 3–5% of all intracranial neoplasms. Chronic headache is the most common presenting complaint in adults, but they can also present

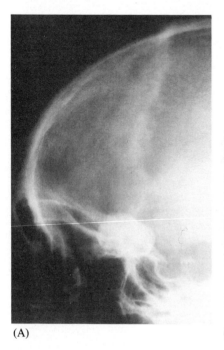
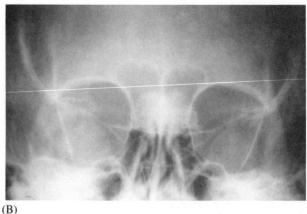

(A)   (B)

Figure 34 Calcified tuberculum sellae meningioma: (A) lateral and (B) frontal skull radiographs demonstrate densely calcified midline oval mass in region of tuberculum sellae.

with visual field disturbances, hydrocephalus or hypothalamic–hypophyseal axis dysfunction secondary to their mass effect. Children may present clinically secondary to growth failure. Craniopharyngiomas are benign, slow-growing neoplasms that most frequently present in children or young adults.

These tumors may be cystic, solid, or mixed solid and cystic. The cystic portions of the tumor often contain cholesterol crystals or, occasionally, hemorrhagic breakdown products. If this is the case, the cystic portions of the tumor often show high-signal intensity on T1-weighted images and low-signal intensity on T2-weighted images. If instead, the cyst contains proteinaceous fluid, it may be isointense to adjacent brain or of decreased signal intensity on T1-weighted images and increased in signal intensity on T2-weighted images (Fig. 35). The solid components of the tumor generally show moderate-signal intensity on T1-weighted images and high-signal intensity on T2-weighted images. These portions generally enhance following the administration of intravenous gadolinium-containing products, as does the wall of the cystic component. Calcification is commonly present in the solid portions of the tumor or in the walls of the cystic components (see Figs. 35 and 36). This is poorly imaged with MRI. If the tumor is completely calcified, it may show decreased signal intensity on T2-weighted images and frequently on T1-weighted images as well. The location of these tumors is usually suprasellar, but they can also be intrasellar. If large, they may also extend into the subfrontal regions, the temporal regions, or the posterior fossa, making their site of origin difficult to discern.

As with all lesions in the parasellar region, CT now plays a secondary role compared with MRI. However, if the diagnosis is uncertain after MRI imaging, CT may be very helpful in that it will demonstrate the tumoral calcification, which may permit a more specific diagnosis (see Figs. 35 and 36). Suprasellar calcification as evident on plain skull films is present in about 75–80% of craniopharyngiomas in children and in 40% of these tumors in adults (14). Calcification may be granular, linear, patchy, or dense. On CT, 92–95% of cases will demonstrate calcification (14). On CT, both the cystic and solid portions are usually low density, but higher density than CSF. Rarely, they are of high density on CT. Contrast enhancement in the solid portions and within the cyst walls is usually seen.

D. Rathke's Cleft Cyst

Rathke's cleft cysts are also known as pars intermedia cysts, intrasellar colloid cysts, and Rathke's pouch cysts. These cysts are believed to form from epithelial remnants of Rathke's cleft, which is a remnant of Rathke's pouch. Rathke's pouch is an ectodermal extension of the embryonic oral cavity, from which the anterior and intermediate lobes of the pituitary gland arise.

The wall of a Rathke's cyst is composed of a single layer of squamous, cuboidal, or columnar epithelial cells, intermixed with a random number of secretory goblet cells. The contents of the cyst can be serous or mucinous (88).

Most of these cysts remain small (<3 mm) and asymptomatic. Rarely, they become large, producing visual disturbances, headache, diabetes insipidus, or hypopituitarism. They are predominantly intrasellar, often closely related to the pars intermedia. They can also be found in the suprasellar region or in both the intrasellar and suprasellar regions.

On both CT and MRI, these lesions are discrete and well circumscribed. When seen on CT, they appear low density and occasionally exhibit an enhancing rim. On MRI, they may have high- or low-signal intensity of both T1- and T2-weighted images, depending on the contents of the cyst, which can range from CSF-like fluid, to hemorrhagic, to mucinous, to a thick fibrous type material (Fig. 37). Calcification is not a feature of these lesions, which may be helpful in differentiating them from a cystic craniopharyngioma. These lesions can be very difficult to differentiate from a microadenoma when small and intrasellar.

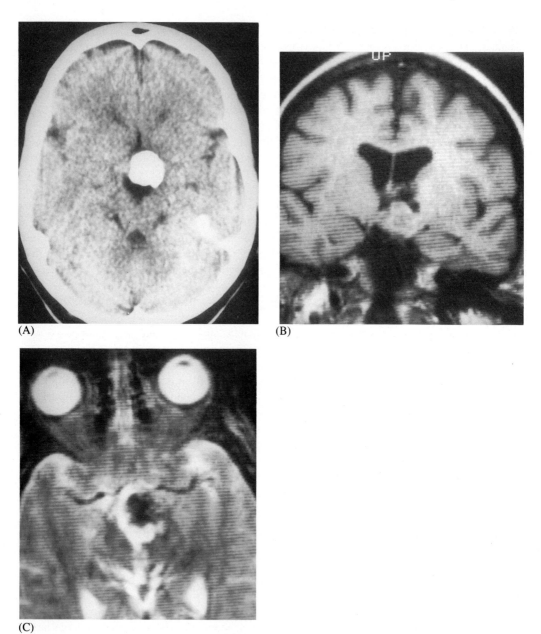

(A)   (B)

(C)

Figure 35 Craniopharyngioma: (A) precontrast axial CT scan; (B) coronal T1-weighted MRI; (C) axial T2-weighted MRI. Precontrast CT scan (A) demonstrates a dense, round area of suprasellar calcification anterior to a lucent area of CSF density. The coronal T1-weighted MRI (B) demonstrates the suprasellar mass, which exhibits areas of increased and decreased signal intensity. The calcification is not appreciated on the T1-weighted MRI. However, on the T2-weighted MRI (C), the area of calcification is seen as a large signal void area surrounded by the cystic component of tumor, which exhibits increased signal intensity.

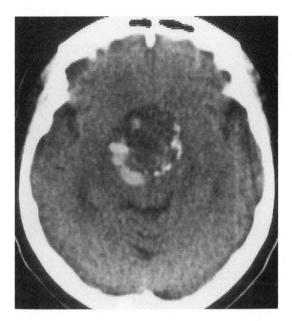

Figure 36 Craniopharyngioma: Noncontrast axial CT scan demonstrates dense irregular peripheral calcification in a suprasellar mass. On the postcontrast study (not shown) heterogeneous enhancement in the central portion of the tumor was demonstrated.

E. Optic Gliomas

Optic nerve gliomas can affect the optic nerve, optic chiasm, or both. When the area of the chiasm is involved, it is often difficult to determine the exact site of origin (optic chiasm versus hypothalamus). Gliomas of the optic chiasm and hypothalamus constitute 10–15% of supratentorial tumors in children (51). The usual age of presentation is 2–4 years. In contradistinction, gliomas of the optic nerve present at a slightly older age (6 years) (51).

Twenty to fifty percent of patients with gliomas of the optic chiasm and hypothalamus have NF-1 (51,52). In NF-1 patients, the tumor usually begins in the intraorbital segment of the optic nerve and extends toward the eye or the brain in a fusiform fashion.

Tumors originating within the optic nerve grow extremely slowly and are histologically similar to juvenile pilocytic astrocytoma (51). Tumors originating from the optic chiasm and hypothalamus behave differently. They are often invasive (92) and, on histological examination, are identical to gliomas located in the cerebral hemispheres (93).

An MRI scan is the procedure of choice in the evaluation of optic gliomas. On T1-weighted images these tumors are hypointense, and on T2-weighted images, they exhibit hyperintensity (Fig. 38). Following the administration of intravenous contrast, inhomogeneous enhancement is usually demonstrated (see Fig. 38).

Extension of chiasmatic lesions along the optic tracts is often noted. This is particularly true when associated with neurofibromatosis.

F. Other Parasellar Lesions

Other tumors that can occur in this region include germinomas (Fig. 39), epidermoids, schwannomas, chordomas, chondrosarcomas, arachnoid cysts, hypothalamic hamartomas, and metastases (Fig. 40). Most of these tumors are discussed elsewhere in this chapter and in Chapter 8.

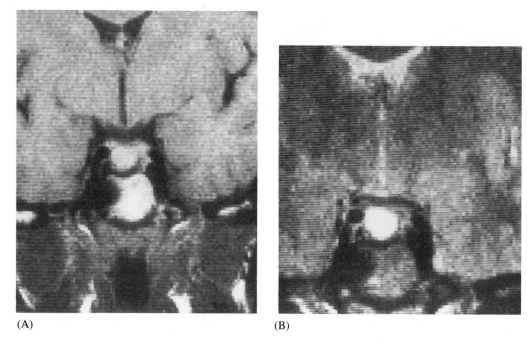

(A)   (B)

Figure 37   Rathke's cleft cyst: (A) coronal T1-weighted MRI; (B) coronal T2-weighted MRI. Coronal T1- and T2-weighted MR images (A,B) demonstrate a discrete, well-circumscribed intrasellar mass that exhibits increased signal intensity on both T1- and T2-weighted images.

When the patient presents with a lesion in the pituitary region, other conditions besides tumors also need to be considered. Perhaps most important of these is an aneurysm of the cavernous or supraclinoid internal carotid artery. Aberrant position of the carotid artery is another important, but rare, condition to avoid confusing with a tumor. Usually these lesions can easily be distinguished from tumor by MRI. Inflammatory and granulomatous conditions, such as adenohypophysitis, meningitis, sarcoidosis, and histiocytosis X, also need to be considered.

IX. PINEAL REGION TUMORS

Pineal region tumors can be broadly divided into five different groups: germ cell tumors; pineal parenchymal cell tumors; pineal cysts; tumors of adjacent structures invading the pineal region, such as glioma, meningioma, ganglioglioma, and ganglioneuroma; and metastatic disease. The first three groups will be discussed in this section. Clinically, these patients may present with one or more of the following problems: (1) hydrocephalus secondary to aqueductal compression; (2) Parinaud's syndrome caused by tectal compression, which consists of paralysis of upward gaze, failure of convergence, and dissociation of the light reflex and accommodation; and (3) endocrinological abnormalities, such as precocious puberty in male patients with germ cell tumors.

A. Germ Cell Tumors

Tumors of germ cell origin account for approximately 70% of all pineal region neoplasms (28). They include germinoma, mature teratoma, teratocarcinoma, embryonal carcinoma, yolk sac tumor (endodermal sinus tumor), choriocarcinoma, and mixed germ cell tumors. Germ cell tumors in the CNS tend to occur in midline locations, such as in the pineal region, in the suprasellar area

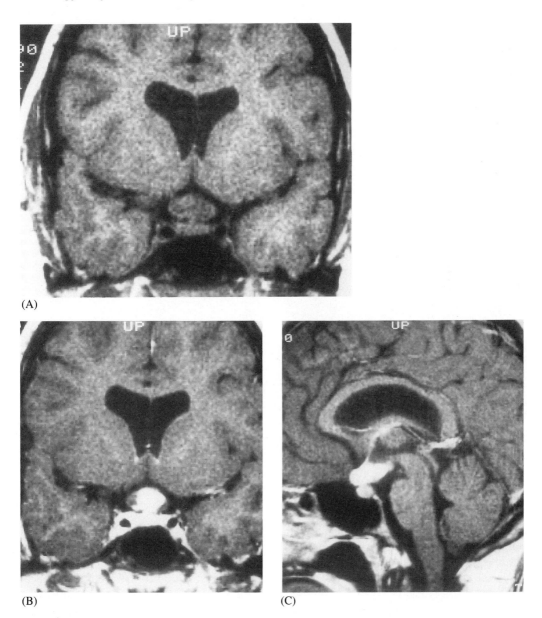

(A)

(B)   (C)

Figure 38 Optic nerve glioma: (A) coronal T1-weighted MRI; (B) post-gadolinium coronal T1-weighted MRI; (C) post-gadolinium sagittal T1-weighted MRI. Coronal T1-weighted MRI (A) demonstrates a markedly enlarged optic chiasm, which is isointense. Following the intravenous administration of gadolinium (B,C), this mass enhances homogeneously except for a small area situated laterally on each side. The pituitary and cavernous sinuses enhance normally.

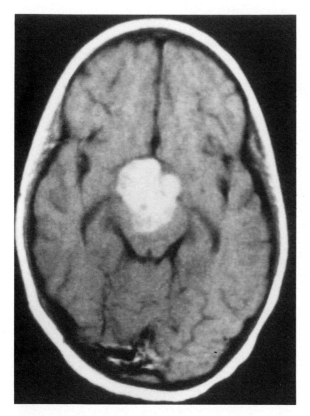

Figure 39 Suprasellar germinoma: Post-gadolinium axial T1-weighted MRI demonstrates a large enhancing suprasellar mass that shows posterior extension. No pineal involvement was demonstrated in this patient, who was a female.

(where they have been called ectopic pinealomas), and in the fourth ventricle. Basal ganglia germ cell tumors also occur, but are less common. Germinomas are the most common neoplasm in the pineal region, accounting for approximately 50% of all pineal neoplasms (28). Histologically, they are identical with seminoma of the testes and ovarian dysgerminoma (28). Recently, it has been suggested that elevated levels of serum or CSF placental alkaline phosphatase may be a specific tumor marker for germinoma (94,95). Pineal region germinomas occur primarily in patients in the first three decades of life and almost exclusively in males. In spite of the fact that germinomas are likely to invade adjacent brain structures and seed the subarachnoid space, patients with these tumors have a good survival rate because they are very radiosensitive.

Suprasellar germinomas are a group of tumors that are histologically identical to the pineal germinomas (32). These tumors arise in or beneath the anterior part of the third ventricle. Although many suprasellar germinomas represent anterior extension of a pineal germinoma, suprasellar germinomas have existed free of any pineal involvement (32) (Fig. 39). Unlike pineal germinomas, which occur almost exclusively in young males, suprasellar germinomas occur preponderantly in women (32).

Teratoma is the second most common germ cell tumor in the pineal region. These lesions are derived from all three germinal layers and thus can contain hair, teeth, bone, fat, and different soft-tissue elements. These tumors show a great deal of variation in their histological maturity and,

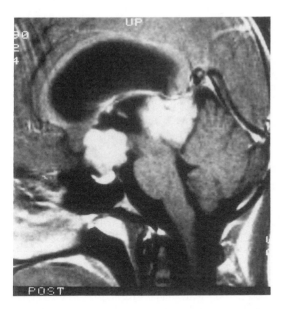

Figure 40 Dysgerminoma with pineal and suprasellar involvement: Post-gadolinium sagittal T1-weighted MRI demonstrates intense enhancement in a large pineal region mass as well as similar enhancement in a large suprasellar mass.

thus, demonstrate a great deal of variability in their biological behavior and clinical course. They are usually partially cystic and often contain evidence of hemorrhage. Embryonal carcinoma, yolk sac tumor, and choriocarcinoma are less common. Yolk sac tumors produce alpha-fetoprotein (AFP) (96–98) and choriocarcinomas produce human chorionic gonadotropin (hCG) (96–98). Embryonal carcinomas that contain multiple differentiated extraembryonic structures produce both AFP and hCG. Embryonal carcinoma has the potential to differentiate into mature or immature teratoma, choriocarcinoma, or yok sac tumor (99).

On MRI, germinomas are usually isointense to white matter on T1-weighted images and isointense to slightly hyperintense relative to white matter on T2-weighted images (100). Following the intravenous administration of gadolinium-containing compounds, intense homogeneous enhancement is seen in most cases (Fig. 40). It is not unusual to see evidence of metastatic spread to adjacent brain structures, to the surrounding subarachnoid spaces, or to the ventricles (Fig. 41).

On imaging, pineal germinomas generally appear as well-circumscribed, homogeneous masses that are inseparable from the pineal gland. Pineal germinomas generally do not calcify or contain cysts, although the pineal gland itself, which is surrounded by the tumor, is usually calcified (101). In fact, calcification of the pineal gland seen on CT in a child younger than 6 years old should suggest the possibility of a pineal region tumor (102). On CT, most germinomas are of increased density, and they generally show intense homogeneous enhancement (101).

Teratomas, on the other hand, generally have a very heterogeneous appearance on both CT and MRI, secondary to the presence of fat, calcium, hemorrhage, and soft-tissue elements. Enhancement is variable (9). Pineal choriocarcinomas and yolk sac tumors are similar in appearance to germinomas on imaging studies (101).

B. Pineal Cell Tumors

Pineocytoma and pineoblastoma are tumors that arise from the neuroepithelial cells of the pineal gland itself. They are each less common tumors than either germinomas or teratomas, together accounting for fewer than 20% of all pineal region tumors (47). There is no striking sex predisposition (9). Pineocytoma is more commonly a tumor of adults and generally has a well-defined margin (9). Pineoblastomas, on the other hand, are more common in children and tend to disseminate early into the subarachnoid spaces, generally having a poor prognosis. This tumor appears histopathologically identical to other primitive undifferentiated neoplasms, such as medulloblastoma, and is considered one of the primitive neuroectodermal tumors. In reality, elements of pineocytoma and pineoblastoma often coexist within the same neoplasm or exist in a transitional form, making categorization into one or the other type difficult at histopathological examination and on imaging studies (9).

Triretinoblastoma is a rare condition that consists of pineoblastoma in association with retinoblastoma, which is usually bilateral. It is most often inherited.

Imaging studies generally show lobulated, solid masses, which enhance with contrast, involving the pineal gland (Figs. 42 and 43). Pineoblastoma is generally larger than pineocytoma and often shows evidence of invasion of surrounding structures. These tumors show calcification more frequently than do germinomas, especially pineocytoma. On MRI, pineoblastomas are generally isointense or hypointense relative to gray matter on T1-weighted images and isointense to slightly hyperintense on T2-weighted images. This is probably related to the low water content of this tumor, which is a highly cellular undifferentiated tumor with scant cytoplasm. Lower-grade pineocytomas, however, are less cellular and contain more cytoplasm, thus appearing brighter on T2-weighted images. Pineal gland tumors on CT are generally isodense or of increased density on unenhanced scans, often show calcification, and enhance densely (101).

C. Pineal Cysts

Pineal cysts are very common lesions at autopsy (9). Computed tomography generally does not recognize these lesions, but MRI, which is a much more sensitive test, shows many of these cysts, sometimes causing confusion and occasional misdiagnosis. These cysts rarely cause symptoms, even if large.

The diagnosis of a pineal cyst can be made if a round, well-defined, homogeneous lesion is identified in the pineal region. The signal intensity of the cysts is somewhat variable, possibly related to the protein content of the cystic fluid, previous hemorrhage in some of the lesions, or isolation of the cystic fluid from the pulsatile flow of the CSF. They are generally decreased in signal intensity on T1-weighted images and isointense to CSF or increased in signal intensity on proton-density and T2-weighted images. The pineal cyst itself does not enhance after contrast, but the surrounding pineal gland or adjacent veins may give the appearance of an enhancing rim to the cyst.

In summary, a variety of lesions occur in the pineal region. Computed tomography and especially MRI studies are very sensitive in detecting lesions in this region, but are not generally specific. The multiple-imaging planes that can be obtained easily with MRI are excellent at delineating the relation of the mass to adjacent structures. Helpful clues to the correct diagnosis of tumors in this region include determining the exact site of origin of the tumor (e.g., pineal gland, tectum, tentorial incisura), CT and MRI features (Table 2), the age and sex of the patient, and the identification of serum of CSF tumor markers. However, biopsy of the lesion is often necessary to obtain a precise diagnosis.

X. METASTASES

Involvement of the brain by metastases may occur by hematogenous spread and from direct extension of the tumor (e.g., pituitary tumor, glomus jugulare, nasopharyngeal carcinoma, and

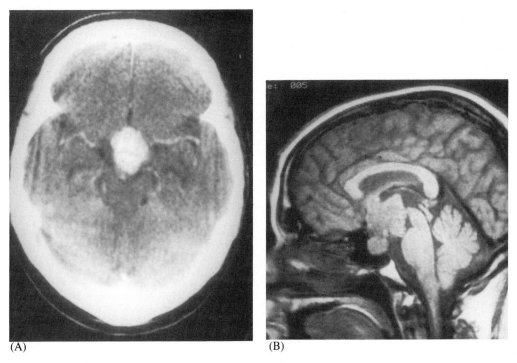

(A) (B)

Figure 41 Metastatic disease from bronchogenic carcinoma to sellar and suprasellar regions: (A) postcontrast axial CT scan; (B) sagittal T1-weighted MRI. Postcontrast CT scan (A) demonstrates an enhancing suprasellar mass. The sagittal T1-weighted MRI (B) demonstrates an isointense mass in the sella with superior extension into the suprasellar region and third ventricle.

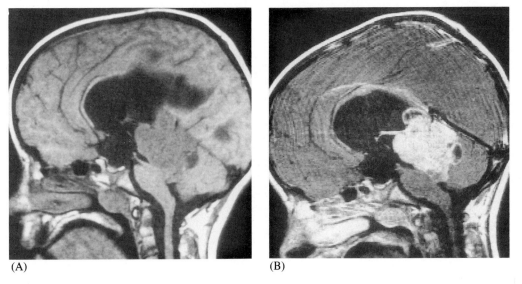

(A) (B)

Figure 42 Pineocytoma: (A) sagittal T1-weighted MRI; (B) post-gadolinium T1-weighted MRI. Sagittal T1-weighted MRI (A) shows a large hypointense mass arising in the pineal region and compressing and displacing the third ventricle and aqueduct. Obstructive hydrocephalus is present. Following the intravenous administration of gadolinium (B), marked enhancement is seen in the tumor. Areas of cystic and necrotic changes are present within the tumor.

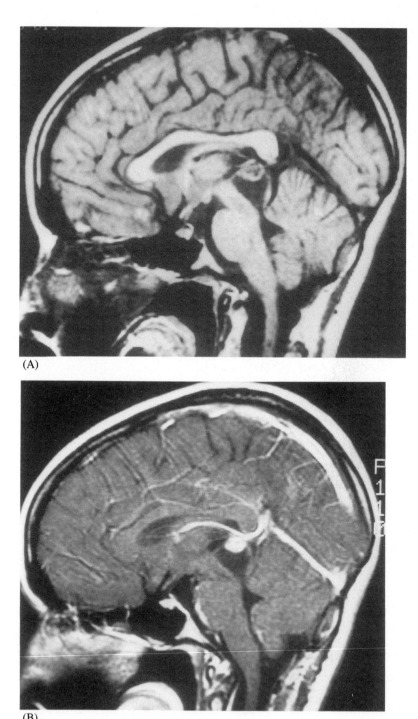

(A)

(B)

Figure 43 Pineocytoma: (A) sagittal T1-weighted MRI; (B) post-gadolinium sagittal T1-weighted MRI; (C,D) post-gadolinium axial T1-weighted MR images. Sagittal T1-weighted MRI (A) demonstrates a well-defined isointense mass in the pineal region. The central portion of the mass shows areas of signal void. This mass has an inferior cystic component that is hypointense. Following the intravenous administration of gadolinium (B,C), the solid portion of the mass enhances uniformly. The cystic component of the mass is seen inferior to the enhancing solid component of the sagittal image (B) and is also seen on axial image (C).

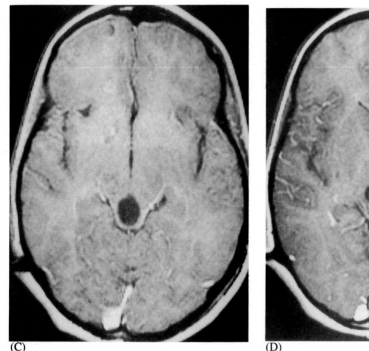
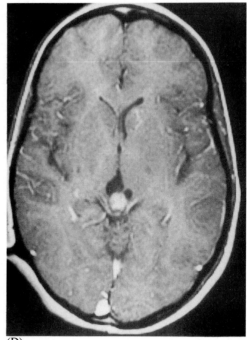

(C)   (D)

from neoplasms involving the paranasal sinuses and orbit). Metastatic deposits by nematogenous spread account for more than 50% of all intracranial neoplasms (14). Lung and breast carcinoma are the most common metastatic lesions. Other primary sites that can metastasize to the brain include kidney, pancreas, prostate, stomach, and testes. Although melanomas and choriocarcinomas are relatively uncommon lesions, they show a great predisposition to metastasize to the brain. In addition, these lesions show an increased tendency to present as hemorrhagic metastases (103) (Fig. 44). Carcinoma of the lung, thyroid, and kidney may also present with hemorrhage (103–105). Metastases are commonly multiple (Fig. 45). However, a single metastasis may occur in 49% of patients. Meningeal carcinomatosis may occur in about 10–15% of cases (14). Meningeal involvement may be present with or without parenchymal involvement. In 5–15% of surgically proved cases, no primary cancer can be clinically identified (14).

Generally speaking, brain metastasis exhibits isointense to hypointense signal relative to gray matter on T1-weighted images. Metastases are isointense or hyperintense on T2-weighted images.

Magnetic resonance imaging following the intravenous administration of gadolinium-containing agents is superior to contrast-enhanced CT in the evaluation of metastatic disease (47,106–109). Most metastases enhance to a moderate or marked degree following intravenous administration of gadolinium-containing agents.

Peritumoral edema in metastatic disease is variable, but generally moderate to marked edema is present (110).

Certain primary tumors have a propensity to metastasize to the meninges (Fig. 46). Adenocarcinoma of the lung, breast, stomach, and colon, and lymphoma and leukemia fall into this category. An MRI scan following the intravenous administration of gadolinium-containing agents is superior to CT in demonstrating meningeal involvement.

The findings on noncontrast CT are variable. Metastatic tumors may be hypo- or isodense on noncontrast CT, with or without surrounding edema. Metastases from carcinoma of the lung,

Table 1 Pineal Region Tumors

Characteristic	Germinoma	Teratoma	Pineocytoma	Pineoblastoma	Glioma	Meningioma
Age	Child	Child	Adult	Child	Child	Adult
Sex	Male	Male	Male and female	Male and female	Male and female	Male and female
Margin	Well-defined	Variable	Well-defined	Ill-defined	Ill-defined	Well-defined
Calcification	Rare	Typical	Common	Common	Uncommon	Common
Hemorrhage	Common	Typical	Common	Common	Uncommon	Common
MRI T1-weighted image	Isointense	Hypo- and hyperintense	Iso- or hypointense	Iso- or hyperintense	Iso- or hyperintense	Iso- or hyperintense
MRI T2-weighted image	Iso- or hyperintense	Hypo- and hyperintense	Hyperintense	Iso- or hyperintense	Hyperintense	Iso- or hyperintense
Homogeneity	Homogeneous	Heterogeneous	Heterogeneous	Homogeneous	Homogeneous or heterogeneous	Homogeneous or heterogeneous
Spread	Common	Variable	Uncommon	Common	Common	Rare
Metastases	Yes	Variable	No	Yes	Variable	Very rare
Enhancement	Dense	Variable	Dense	Dense	Variable	Dense
Nonenhanced CT	Slightly hyperdense	Ca, fat, soft-tissue elements	Hyperintense	Hyperdense	Hypointense	Iso- or hyperdense
Prognoses	Excellent	Variable	Variable	Poor	Variable	Excellent
Serum markers	Placental alkaline phosphatase					

Source: Adapted from Ref. 9.

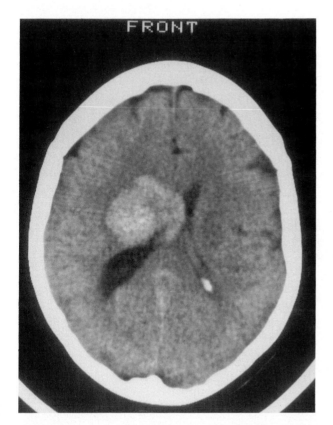

Figure 44 Hemorrhagic metastasis, carcinoma of the lung: Noncontrast axial CT scan demonstrates a large, right-sided, dense mass, representing acute hemorrhage within the mass. This mass extends into the body of the right lateral ventricle. Flecks of calcification are also noted within this mass. Right-to-left midline shift is noted. On the postcontrast CT scan (not shown), additional enhancing masses were demonstrated.

kidney, colon; melanoma; choriocarcinoma, and various sarcomas, all may exhibit hyperdensity on noncontrast CT. Following the intravenous administration of contrast, most metastases enhance to a moderate or marked degree (Fig. 47). Some authorities have advocated performing high-dose contrast CT whenever there is a question of metastatic disease (111,112). In such cases, multiple lesions not otherwise detected with a single dose of contrast and lesions difficult to define may become evident. High-dose contrast CT may also provide greater diagnostic information in the evaluation of primary neoplasms. However, MRI with gadolinium is superior to CT, even when used following the administration of high-dose iodinated contrast material in the evaluation of metastatic disease.

Recent studies have shown that high-dose gadolinium MRI provides greater diagnostic information than routine doses of gadolinium in the evaluation of metastatic disease, by providing increased lesion conspicuity and increased lesion detection (113,114).

Certain metastases, particularly osteogenic sarcoma and mucinous carcinoma of the colon, are dense on CT owing to the presence of calcification and ossification (115).

The calvarium is the site of approximately 5% of brain metastases. Bone destruction with either well-defined or diffuse leptomeningeal involvement occurs in 15% of patients with calvarial metastases. Bone window settings on CT are important to evaluate accurately the calvarium for metastatic involvement.

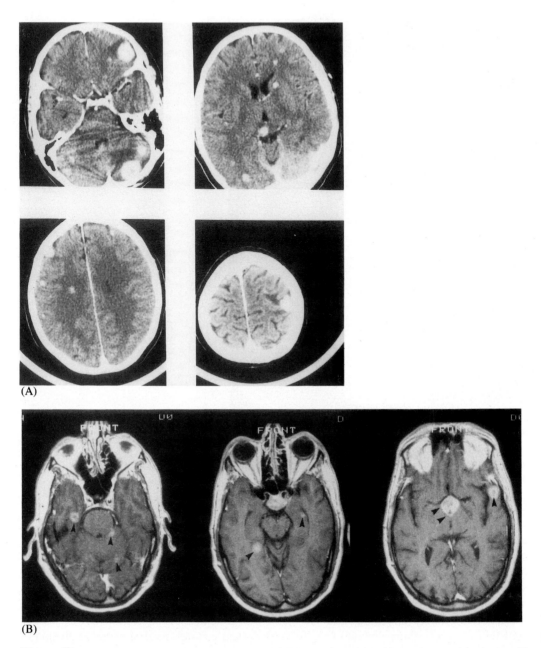

(A)

(B)

Figure 45   Multiple metastases: (A) postcontrast axial CT scans in patient with carcinoma of the breast; (B) post-gadolinium axial T1-weighted MR images in another patient with bronchogenic carcinoma. Postcontrast axial CT scans (A) demonstrate multiple enhancing masses of various sizes in both the supra- and infratentorial compartments. Post-gadolinium T1-weighted MR images (B) reveal bilateral multiple enhancing masses (arrowheads) of varying size, some exhibiting ringlike enhancement and others solid enhancement. The sella and suprasellar areas also reveal metastatic involvement.

A. Angiography

Approximately 50% of intracranial metastases are hypervascular (116). Metastases are usually round, well-circumscribed masses that exhibit neovascularity and arteriovenous shunting (Fig. 48). The spectrum of vascularity ranges from intense staining, to zones of avascularity.

The most common vascular metastases are from lung carcinoma, breast carcinoma, and hypernephroma. The presence of multiple, small round vascular lesions favor metastatic disease. A solitary metastatic deposit sometimes is indistinguishable from a glioblastoma or a meningioma.

XI. TUMOR EMBOLIZATION

Tumor embolization is a procedure usually used preoperatively to reduce the vascularity of a tumor and thereby facilitate a more complete and safe removal, with less blood loss and damage to adjacent tissues. It is also possible that embolization makes tumor recurrence less likely by producing necrosis at the site of dural attachment (117). The most common indications for tumor embolization include meningiomas (see Fig. 22), glomus tympanicum tumors, glomus jugulare tumors, glomus vagale tumors, juvenile angiofibromas, vascular schwannomas and, less commonly, sarcomas, metastatic tumors, and hemangioblastomas. Most of these tumors are supplied by external carotid artery branches or dural branches.

Before embolization, it is important to obtain appropriate imaging studies, such as CT or MRI, or both, to map the location and extent of the tumor and surrounding vital structures such as adjacent nerves, brain tissue, major vascular structures, and osseous and soft-tissue structures. It is also important to obtain a high-quality selective arteriogram to evaluate the extent of tumor vascularity, evaluate for potential dangerous collateral vessels, and evaluate for possible eloquent vessels supplying cranial nerves or brain tissue. Tumor embolization may be performed at the same time as the diagnostic arteriogram, or at a later date. If the embolization is extensive and complex, it may even be performed over several sessions.

The goal of embolization is to destroy the intratumoral vascular bed. Merely blocking the larger supplying vessels is not nearly as effective as blocking the small intratumoral vessels and in fact can make surgery more difficult if collateral arterial supply develops, especially if from unusual or surgically inaccessible sites. After embolization of the intratumoral vascular bed, secondary embolization of the larger extratumoral arteries may augment the process of intratumoral thrombosis and further aid the surgeon.

In order not to damage surrounding normal tissue, it is important to use microcatheters that allow distal superselective catheterization. These soft microcatheters also are less prone to cause spasm in the sensitive branches of the external carotid artery. Usually, microparticles such as Avitene, polyvinyl alcohol particles, or Gelfoam powder are used as embolic agents. It is important to use particles small enough to penetrate to the intratumoral vascular bed, as discussed earlier. Surgery should ideally be performed within several days of tumor embolization to achieve best results. This is especially true if using Avitene or Gelfoam for the embolization, as these are not permanent embolic agents. Fluid agents such as the cyanoacrylates or absolute ethanol may be desirable under certain circumstances. Absolute ethanol has been effective in destroying meningiomas without surgery on short-term follow-up (Ferguson RDG, personal communication). Whether these tumors are completely destroyed will require further follow-up. It is a technique, however, that can occasionally be used in nonsurgical candidates.

Patients usually tolerate embolization quite well. In most institutions, the procedure is performed with the patient awake with intravenous sedation. The embolization procedure is usually only slightly more painful than the diagnostic arteriogram. Following the embolization, some

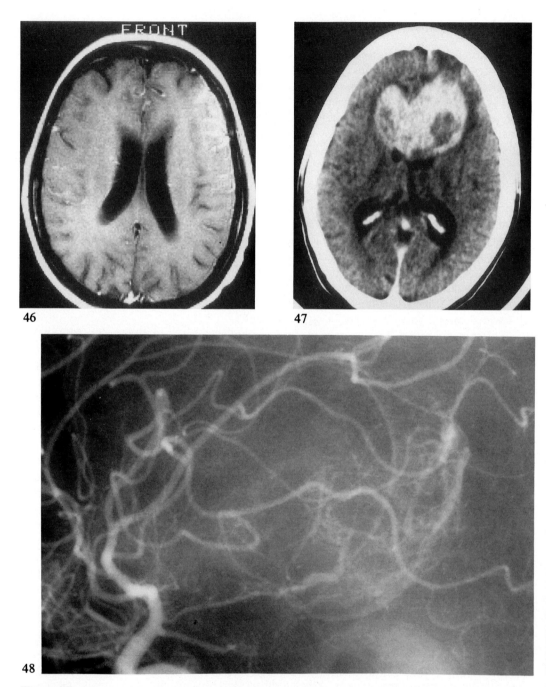

Figure 46 Meningeal carcinomatosis, carcinoma of the breast: Post-gadolinium axial T1-weighted MRI demonstrates bilateral meningeal enhancement secondary to meningeal carcinomatosis.

Figure 47 Metastatic disease from carcinoma of the lung mimicking butterfly glioma: Postcontrast axial CT scan demonstrates marked enhancement of a large mass that involves both frontal lobes and corpus callosum. The frontal horns are effaced and displaced posteriorly. Within the mass areas of necrosis are present.

Figure 48 Metastatic lung carcinoma: Lateral projection of the arterial phase of the left carotid angiogram demonstrates a left temporal lobe mass. Neovascularity and AV shunting is noted within this mass. The angiographic appearance is indistinguishable from a glioblastoma.

patients develop a headache or pain, which readily responds to oral or intravenous narcotics and is usually of short duration. Occasionally, patients develop fever following embolization, which is also of short duration. The main dangers of embolization include stroke, cranial nerve damage, skin necrosis, and poor postoperative wound healing. These complications are all quite rare in experienced hands.

In some skull base and neck tumors with an intimate relation to the internal carotid artery, internal carotid artery invasion, or with extensive vascular supply from the internal carotid artery, embolizations may be helpful. If sacrifice of the carotid artery is possible at surgery, but not certain, preoperative temporary balloon occlusion testing of the internal carotid artery can be performed to evaluate tolerance to carotid artery occlusion.

Finally, selective intra-arterial chemotherapy may be delivered into the tumor bed. Whether this is helpful in the long-term has yet to be established.

REFERENCES

1. Russel DS, Rubinstein LJ. Pathology of tumors of the nervous system, 5th ed. Baltimore: Williams & Wilkens, 1989.
2. Kernohan JW, Mabon RF, Svien HG, Adson AW. A simplified classification of the gliomas. Mayo Clin Proc 1949; 24:71–75.
3. Steinhoff H, Lanksch W, Kazner E, Grumme T, Meese W, Lange S, Aulich A, Schindler E, Wende S. Computed tomography in the diagnosis and differential diagnosis of glioblastomas. Neuroradiology 1977; 14:193–200.
4. Kendall BE, Jakubowski J, Pullicino P, Symon L. Difficulties in diagnosis of supratentorial gliomas by CAT scan. J Neurol Neurosurg Psychiatry 1979; 42:485–492.
5. Baker HI, Houser OW, Campbell JR. National Cancer Institute study: evaluation of CT in the diagnosis of intracranial neoplasms. Radiology 1980; 136:91–96.
6. Lee BCP, Kneeland JB, Cahill PT, Deck MDF. MR recognition of supratentorial tumors. AJNR 1985; 6:871–878.
7. Lilja A, Bergstrom K, Spannare B, Olsson Y. Reliability of computed tomography in assessing histopathological features of malignant supratentorial gliomas. J Comput Assist Tomogr 1981; 5:625–636.
8. Smith AS, Weinstein MA, Modic MT, Pavlicek W, Rogers LR, Budd LR, Bukowski RM, Purvis JD, Weick JK, Duchesneau PM. Magnetic resonance with marked T2-weighted images: improved demonstration of brain lesions, tumor and edema. AJNR 1985; 6:691–697.
9. Atlas SW. Intraaxial brain tumors. In: Atlas SW, ed. Magnetic resonance imaging of the brain and spine. New York: Raven Press, 1991:223–326.
10. Darwin RH, Drayer BP, Riederer SJ, Wang HZ, MacFall JR. T2 estimates in healthy and diseased brain tissue: a comparison using various MR pulse sequences. Radiology 1986; 160:375–381.
11. Earnest F IV, Kelly PJ, Scheithauer BW, Kall BA, Cascino TL, Ehman RL, Forbes GS, Axley PL. Cerebral astrocytomas: histopathologic correlation of MR and CT contrast enhancement with stereotactic biopsy. Radiology 1988; 166:823–827.
12. Graif M, Bydder GM, Steiner RE, Niendorf P, Thomas DGT, Young IR. Contrast-enhanced MR imaging of malignant brain tumors. AJNR 1985; 6:855–862.
13. Burger PC, Vogel S, Green SB, Strike TA. Glioblastoma multiforme and anaplastic astrocytoma. Cancer 1985; 56:1106–1111.
14. Azar Kia B. Intracranial neoplasms. In: Sarwar M, Azar Kia B, Batnitzky S, eds. Basic neuroradiology. St. Louis: Warren H Green, 1983:535–637.
15. McKeran RO, Thomas T. The clinical study of gliomas. In: Thomas DGT, Graham DI, eds. Brain tumors. Scientific basis, clinical investigation and current therapy. London: Butterworths 1980:194.
16. Holland BA, Kucharcyzk W, Brant Zawadzki M, Norman D, Haas DK, Harper PS. MR imaging of calcified intracranial lesions. Radiology 1985; 157:353–356.
17. Couch J, Weiss S. Gliomatosis cerebri. Neurology 1974; 24:504–511.

18. Lee Y, Van Tassel P, Bruner JM, Moser RP, Share JC, Juvenile pilocytic astrocytomas: CT and MR characteristics. AJNR 1989; 10:363–370.

19. De Recondo J, Haguenau M. Neuropathologic survey of the phakomatoses and allied disorders. In: Vinker PJ, Bruyn GW, eds. Handbook of clinical neurology: the phakomatoses. Amsterdam: North-Holland, 1972:19–71.

20. Sima AAF, Robertson DM. Subependymal giant-cell astrocytoma: case report with ultrastructural study. J Neurosurg 1979; 50:240–245.

21. Frerebeau P, Benezech J, Harbi H. Intraventricular tumors in tuberous sclerosis. Childs Nerv Syst 1985; 1:45–48.

22. McLaurin RL, Towbin RB. Tuberous sclerosis: diagnostic and surgical considerations. Pediatr Neurosci 1985; 12:43–48.

23. Tsuchida T, Kanata K, Kawanata M. Brain tumors in tuberous sclerosis. Childs Brain 1984; 8:271–283.

24. Lee BCP, Gawler J. Tuberous sclerosis: comparison of computed tomography and conventional neuroradiology. Radiology 1978; 127:403–407.

25. Rubinstein LJ. Tumors of neuroglial cells. In: Firminger HI, ed. Atlas of tumor pathology, tumors of the cerebral nervous system, fasicle 6. Washington DC: Armed Forces Institute of Pathology, 1972:257–263.

26. Williams AL. Tumors. In: Williams AL, Haughton VM, eds. Cranial computed tomography. St Louis: CV Mosby, 1985:148–239.

27. Atlas SW, Grossman RI, Hackney DB, Gomori JM, Campagna N, Goldberg HI, Bilaniuk LT, Zimmerman RA. Calcified intracranial lesions: detection with gradient-echo-acquisition rapid MR imaging. AJNR 1988; 9:253–259.

28. Pomerantz SJ. MR of supratentorial neoplasm. In: Pomerantz SJ, ed. Craniospinal magnetic resonance imaging. Philadelphia: WB Saunders, 1989:208–247.

29. Lee Y, Tassel PV. Intracranial oligodendrogliomas: imaging findings in 35 untreated cases. AJNR 1989; 10:119–127.

30. Fitz CR. Neoplastic diseases. In: Gonzalez CF, Grossman CB, Masdeu JC, eds. Head and spine imaging. New York: John Wiley & Sons, 1985:483–521.

31. Naidich TP, Zimmerman RA. Primary brain tumors in children. Semin Roentgenol 1984; 19:100–114.

32. Batnitzky S. Intraventricular meningioma. In: Weinberg PE, Batnitzky S, Bentsen JR, Bryan RN, Naidich TP, Sackett JF, Zimmerman RA, eds. Neuroradiology test and syllabus. Reston: American College of Radiology, 1990:714–744.

33. Swartz JD, Zimmerman RA, Bilaniuk LT. Computed tomography of intracranial ependymomas. Radiology 1982; 143:97–101.

34. Coulon RA, Till K. Intracranial ependymomas in children: a review of 43 cases. Childs Brain 1977; 3:154–168.

35. Johansson JH, Rekate HL, Roessmann U. Gangliogliomas: pathological and clinical correlation. J Neurosurg 1981; 54:58–63.

36. Sutton LN, Packer RJ, Rorke LB, Bruce DA, Schut L. Cerebral gangliomas during childhood. Neurosurgery 1983; 13:124–128.

37. Zimmerman RA, Bilaniuk LT. Computed tomography of intracerebral gangliogliomas. J Comput Assist Tomogr 1979; 3:24–30.

38. Denierre B, Stinchnoth FA, Hori A, Spoerri O. Intracerebral gangliomas. J Neurosurg 1986; 65:177–182.

39. Dorne HL, O'Gorman MN, Melanson D. Computed tomography of intracranial gangliogliomas. AJNR 1986; 7:281–285.

40. Castillo M, Davis PC, Takei Y, Hoffman JC Jr. Intracranial ganglioglioma: MR, CT and clinical findings in 18 patients. AJNR 1990; 11:109–114.

41. Schwaighofer BW, Hesselink JR, Press GA, Wolfe RL, Healy ME, Bertholy DP. Primary intracranial CNS lymphoma: MR manifestations. AJNR 1989; 10:725–729.

42. Levy RM, Bredesen DE, Rosenblum ML. Neurological manifestations of the acquired immu-

nodeficiency syndrome (AIDS): experience at UCSF and a review of the literature. Neurosurgery 1985; 62:475–495.

43. Dina TS. Primary central nervous system lymphoma versus toxoplasmosis in AIDS. Radiology 1991; 179:823–828.
44. Brant-Zawadzki M, Enzmann DR. Computed tomographic brain scanning in patients with lymphoma. Radiology 1978; 129:67–71.
45. Lee YY, Glass JP, Geoffray A, Wallace S. Cranial computed tomographic abnormalities in leptomeningeal metastasis. AJNR 1984; 5:559–563.
46. Pederson H, Clausen N. The development of cerebral CT changes during treatment of acute lymphocytic leukemia in childhood. Neuroradiology 1981; 22:79–84.
47. Latchaw RE. MR and CT Imaging of the head, neck and spine, 2nd ed. St Louis: Mosby Year Book, 1991.
48. Leonard KJ, Mammourian AC. MR appearance of intracranial chloromas. AJNR 1989; 10(suppl):67–68.
49. National Institutes of Health consensus development. Neurofibromatosis. Arch Neurol 1988; 45:575–578.
50. Rubenstein AE. Neurofibromatosis: a review of the clinical problem. Ann NY Acad Sci 1986; 486:1–13.
51. Barkovich AJ, Edwards MSB. Brain tumors of childhood. In: Barkovich AJ, ed. Pediatric neuroimaging. New York: Raven Press, 1990:149–203.
52. Pont MS, Elster AD. Lesions of skin and brain: modern imaging of the neurocutaneous syndromes. AJR 1992; 158:1193–1203.
53. Brown EW, Riccardi VM, Mawad M, Handel S, Goldman H, Bryan RN. MR imaging of optic pathways in patients with neurofibromatosis. AJNR 1987; 8:1031–1036.
54. Hurst RW, Newman SA, Cail WS. Multifocal intracranial MR abnormalities in neurofibromatosis. AJNR 1988; 9:293–296.
55. Bognanno JR, Edwards MK, Lee TA, Dunn DW, Roos KL, Klatte EC. Cranial MR imaging in neurofibromatosis. AJR 1988; 151:381–388.
56. Duffner PK, Cohen ME, Seidel FG, Shucard DW. The significance of MRI abnormalities in children with neurofibromatosis. Neurology 1989; 39:373–378.
57. Rubinstein LJ. Tumors of the central nervous system. Washington DC: Armed Forces Institute of Pathology, 1972:300–313.
58. Tomsick TA, Lukin RR, Chambers A, Benton C. Neurofibromatosis and intracranial arterial occlusive disease. Neuroradiology 1976; 11:229–234.
59. Kepes JJ. Meningiomas: biology, pathology, and differential diagnosis. New York: Masson, 1982.
60. Rosenbaum AE, Rosenbloom SB. Meningiomas revisited. Semin Roentgenol 1984; 29:8–26.
61. Cushing H. The meningimas (dural endotheliomas). Their source and favored seats of origin [Cavendish Lecture]. Brain 1922; 45:282–316.
62. Osborne AG. Handbook of neuroradiology. St Louis: CV Mosby, 1991:303.
63. Courville CB. Pathology of central nervous system, 3rd ed. Mountain View, CA: Pacific, 1950:383–397.
64. Ozonoff MB, Burrow EH. Intracranial calcification. In: Newton TH, Potts DG. Radiology of the skull and brain. The skull. St Louis: CV Mosby, 1971:855–858.
65. Elster AD, Challa VR, Gilbert TH, Richardson DN, Contento JC. Meningiomas: MR and histopathologic features. Radiology 1989; 170:857–862.
66. Spagnoli MV, Goldberg HI, Grossman RI, Bilaniuk LT, Gomori JM, Hackney DB, Zimmerman RA. Intracranial meningiomas: high-field MR imaging. Radiology 1986; 161:369–375.
67. Goldberg HI. Extraaxial brain tumors. In: Atlas SW, ed. Magnetic resonance imaging of the brain and spine. New York: Raven Press, 1991:327–378.
68. New PFJ, Aronow S, Hesselink JR. National Cancer Institute study: evaluation of computed tomography in the diagnosis of intracranial neoplasms IV. Meningiomas. Radiology 1980; 136:665–675.
69. Smith HP, Challa VR, Moody DM, Kelly DL Jr. Biological features of meningiomas that determine the production of cerebral edema. Neurosurgery 1981; 8:428–433.

70. George AE, Russel EJ, Kricheff II. White matter buckling: CT scan of extra-axial intracranial mass. AJNR 1980; 1:425–430.

71. Bydder GM, Kingsley DPE, Braun J, Niendorf HP, Young IR. MR imaging of meningiomas including studies with and without gadolinium-DTPA. J Comput Tomogr 1985; 9:690–697.

72. Berry I, Brant-Zawadzki M, Osaki L, Brasch R, Murovic J, Newton TH. Gd-DTPA in clinical MR of the brain: 2 extraaxial lesions and normal structures AJNR 1986; 7:789–793.

73. Haughton VM, Rimm AA, Czervionke LF, Breger RK, Fisher ME, Papke RA, Hendrix LE, Strother CM, Turski PA, Williams AL, Daniels DL. Sensitivity of Gd-DTPA-enhanced MR imaging of benign extraaxial tumors. Radiology 1988; 166:829–833.

74. Watabe T, Azuma T. T1 and T2 measurements of meningiomas and neuromas before and after Gd DTPA. AJNR 1989; 10:463–470.

75. Zimmerman RD, Flemming CA, Saint-Louis LA, Lee BCP, Manning JJ, Deck MDF. Magnetic resonance imaging of meningiomas. AJNR 1985; 6:149–157.

76. Tokumaru A, O'uchi T, Eguchi T, Kawamoto S, Kokubo T, Suzuki M, Kameda T. Prominent meningeal enhancement adjacent to meningioma on Gd DTPA-enhanced MR images: histopathologic correlation. Radiology 1990; 175:431–433.

77. Batnitzky S, Sarwar M, Leeds NE, Schechter MM, Azar Kia B. Colloid cysts of the third ventricle. Radiology 1974; 112:327–341.

78. Scotti G, Scialfa N, Colombo N, Landon L. MR in the diagnosis of colloid cysts of the third ventricle. AJNR 1987; 8:370–372.

79. Donaldson JO, Simon RH. Radiodense ions within a third ventricular colloid cyst. Arch Neurol 1980; 37:246.

80. Ganti SR, Antunes JL, Louis KM, Hilal SK. Computed tomography in the diagnosis of colloid cysts of the third ventricle. Radiology 1981; 138:385–391.

81. Powell MP, Torrens MJ, Thomson JLE, Horgan JG. Isodense colloid cysts of the third ventricle: a diagnostic and therapeutic problem resolved by ventriculoscopy. Neurosurgery 1983; 13:234–237.

82. Michels LD, Rutz D. Colloid cysts of the third ventricle. Arch Neurol 1982; 39:640–643.

83. Gonzalez JG, Elizondo G, Saldivar D, Nanez H, Todd LE, Villareal JZ. Pituitary gland growth during normal pregnancy: an in vivo study using magnetic resonance imaging. Am J Med 1988; 85:217–220.

84. Wiener SN, Rzesotarski MS, Droege RT, Pearlstein AE, Shafron M. Measurement of pituitary gland height with MR imaging. AJNR 1985; 6:717–722.

85. Swartz JD, Russell KB, Basile BA, O'Donnell PC, Popky GL. High resolution CT appearance of the intrasellar contents in women of childbearing age. Radiology 1983; 147:115–117.

86. Fullerton GD. Physiologic power of magnetic relaxation. In Stark DD, Bradley WG, eds. Magnetic resonance imaging. St Louis: CV Mosby 1988:36–55.

87. Johnsen DE, Woodruff WW, Allen IS. MR imaging of the sellar and juxtasellar regions. Radiographics 1991; 11:727–758.

88. Norman D. Sellar and parasellar lesions. In: Categorical course. Neoplasms of the central nervous system. Chicago: American Society of Neuroradiology 1990:65–71.

89. Scotti G, Yu CY, Dillon WP. MR imaging of cavernous sinus involvement by pituitary adenomas. AJNR 1988; 9:657–664.

90. Ostrov SG, Quencer RM, Hoffman JG. Hemorrhage within pituitary adenomas: how often associated with pituitary apoplexy syndrome? AJNR 1989; 10:503–510.

91. Zimmerman RA. Imaging of intrasellar, suprasellar and parasellar tumors. Semin Roentgenol 1990; 25:174–197.

92. Alvord EC, Lufton S. Gliomas of the optic nerve or chiasm: outcome by patient's age, tumor site and treatment. J Neurosurg 1988; 68:85–98.

93. Amador LV. Brain tumors in the young. Springfield: Charles C Thomas, 1983:1–453.

94. Shinoda J, Miwa Y, Sakai N. Immunohistochemical study of placental alkaline phosphatase in primary intracranial germ cell tumors. J Neurosurg 1985; 63:733–739.

95. Shinoda J, Yamada H, Norboru S. Placental alkaline phosphatase as a tumor marker for primary intracranial germinoma. J Neurosurg 1988; 68:710–720.

96. Perlin E, Engeler JE, Edson M. The value of serial measurement of both human chorionic gonadotropin and alpha-fetoprotein for monitoring germinal cell tumors. Cancer 1976; 37:215–219.

97. Allen JC, Nisselbaum J, Epstein F. alpha-Fetoprotein and human chorionic gonadotropin determination in cerebrospinal fluid. J Neurosurg 1979; 51:368–374.

98. Sun MJ, Qang YC, Liu MY. alpha-Fetoprotein, human chorionic gonadotropin and carcinoembryonic antigen in pineal region tumors. Chin Med J (Engl) 1986; 38:272–279.

99. Yoshida K, Toya S, Ohtani M. Extraneural metastasis of choriocarcinomatous element in pineal germ cell tumor. J Neurosurg 1985; 63:463–466.

100. Tien RD, Barkovich AJ, Edwards MSB. MR of pineal tumors. AJNR 1990; 11:557–565.

101. Chang T, Teng MMH, Guo WY, Sheng WC. CT of pineal tumors and intracranial germ cell tumors. AJNR 1989; 10:1039–1044.

102. Zimmerman RA, Bilaniuk LT. Age-related incidence of pineal calcification detected by computed tomography. Radiology 1982; 142:659–662.

103. Mandifour TI. Intracranial hemorrhage caused by metastatic tumors. Neurology 1977; 27:650–655.

104. Gildersleeve N Jr, Kao AH, McDonald CJ. Metastatic tumor presenting as intracerebral hemorrhage. Radiology 1977; 124:109–112.

105. Ginoldi A, Wallace S, Shalen P, Luna M, Handel S. Cranial computed tomography of malignant melanoma. AJNR 1980; 1:531–535.

106. Claussen C, Laniado M, Schorner W, Niendorf HP, Weinmann HJ, Fiegler W, Felix R. Gadolinium-DTPA in MR imaging of glioblastomas and intracranial metastases. AJNR 1985; 6:669–674.

107. Felix R, Schorner W, Laniado M, Niendorf HP, Claussen C, Fiegler W, Speck U. Brain tumors: MR imaging with gadolinium DTPA. Radiology 1985; 156:681–688.

108. Healy ME, Hesselink JR, Press GA, Middleton MS. Increased detection of intracranial metastases with intravenous Gd-DTPA. Radiology 1987; 165:619–624.

109. Russel EJ, Gerenia GK, Johnson CE, Huckman MS, Ramsey RG, Washburn-Bleck J, Turner DA, Norusis M. Multiple cerebral metastases: detectability with Gd-DTPA-enhanced MR imaging. Radiology 1987; 167:609–617.

110. Potts DG, Albott GF, von Sneidern JV. National Cancer Institute study: evaluation of computed tomography in the diagnosis of intracranial neoplasms. III. Metastatic tumors. Radiology 1980; 136:657–664.

111. Hayman LA, Evans RA, Hinck V. Delayed high iodine dose contrast computed tomography: cranial neoplasms. Radiology 1980; 136:677–684.

112. Shalen PR, Hayman LA, Wallace S, Handel SF. Protocol for delayed contrast enhancement in computed tomography of cerebral neoplasms. Radiology 1981; 139:397–402.

113. Yuh WTC, Engelken JD, Huhonen MG, Mayr NA, Fisher DJ, Ehrhardt JC. Experience with high-dose gadolinium MR imaging in the evaluation of brain metastases. AJNR 1992; 13:335–345.

114. Runge VM, Kirsch JE, Burke VJ, Price AC, Nelson KL, Thomas GS, Dean BL, Lee C. High-dose (Gadoteridol in MR imaging of intracranial neoplasms. J Magn Reson Imaging 1992; 2:9–18.

115. Ruelle A, Macchia G, Gambini C, Andrioli. Unusual appearance of brain metastasis from adenocarcinoma of colon. Neuroradiology 1986; 28:375.

116. Osborn AG. Introduction to cerebral angiography. Hagerstown: Harper & Row, 1980:273.

117. Berenstein A, Kricheff II. Microembolization technique of vascular occlusion: radiologic pathologic and clinical correlation. AJNR 1981; 2:261–267.

10

The Preoperative and Postoperative Management of the Brain Tumor Patient

Roberta P. Glick
University of Illinois Medical Center and
Cook County Hospital, Chicago, Illinois

Don Penny
University of Illinois Medical Center, Chicago, Illinois

Avery Hart
Cook County Hospital, Chicago, Illinois

I. NEURO-ONCOLOGY TEAM APPROACH

The diagnosis and management of the patients with brain tumors is always a grave and difficult situation, with profound implications for the patients and their families. The effect of surgery on a patient's survival and quality of life, the treatment of the tumor and its recurrence, and the advances in diagnosis and therapy, all must be considered. In addition, the recent scientific knowledge in the field of molecular biology has led to a rapid accumulation of new information. Thus, the treatment rendered to brain tumor patients varies widely, and it is often difficult for the general neurosurgeon to keep abreast of all the new developments in neuro-oncological diagnosis, therapy, and research.

To meet these challenges, subspecialization has emerged within the field of neurosurgery, with neuro-oncology recognized as a legitimate field of subspecialization. At our institution, we have developed a multidisciplinary neuro-oncology team that includes members from neurosurgery, neurology, neuropsychiatry, medical and pediatric oncology, neuro-ophthalmology, endocrinology, neuropathology, neuroradiology, radiation therapy, social work, nursing, and basic science. This team approach can be used for both preoperative and postoperative treatment planning, as a forum for discussion of controversial therapeutic issues, for the development of clinical treatment protocols, and for educational programs for residents.

On a regular basis, the neuro-oncology team can review clinical cases and make recommendations concerning the type of surgery and adjunctive therapy most appropriate for each tumor type, based upon multifactorial patient considerations (see later), the current status of knowledge, and the available treatment options. Once a treatment plan has been formulated, this information is presented to the patient and family at a family meeting. We usually have such a family conference at least three times: once in the office, once in the hospital before surgery, and again postoperatively. It must be remembered, however, as Vick once said, "It is the attending physician who is at the core of what is meant by the total care of the patient and his or her role in the outcome of therapy for patients can be literally quite vital" (1).

A. Support Group

The diagnosis of a brain tumor creates a unique stress to patients and to their families. A support group can be helpful in providing practical information concerning brain tumors and their various treatments, as well as psychological and social support (see Chap. 33).

It is now recognized that by providing information and education, along with emotional support, health professionals can help reduce anxiety, enhance and strengthen the patient's coping skills, and encourage positive thinking and improved self-image. In addition, many support groups offer legal and financial help and resources to alleviate the difficult social situation that may be created by a prolonged illness or disability. It is recommended that such interaction with a support group begin soon after the diagnosis is made, as this may facilitate coping with the changes that occur for patients and families from the time of their acute inpatient treatment, to their outpatient therapy and throughout their illness. The support group is usually led by health professionals and may include physicians, psychologists, nurses, social workers, and even clergy. Another important service offered by support groups involves genetic counseling for certain types of tumors, mainly the phakomatoses (e.g., neurofibromatosis). The National Brian Tumor Foundation and the Joint Section of Tumors of the AANS/CNS has recently published a list of brain tumor support groups in North America (2).

II. GENERAL CONSIDERATIONS

A. Preoperative Diagnostic Evaluation

The initial management of any intracranial lesion first depends upon a prompt and accurate diagnosis. Although computed tomography (CT) scanning has been used extensively in the past, magnetic resonance imaging (MRI), because of its sensitivity, anatomical detail, and its ability to image the brain in three dimensions, has become the most valuable tool for neuro-oncological diagnosis as well as operative planning. Gadolinium enhancement is considered essential in the diagnosis of most brain tumors. Often patients are referred from an outside center or have been seen by several physicians before treatment, and the outside studies are several weeks old. We recommend that the patient have recent imaging studies done within 2 weeks of surgery or other therapy to evaluate whether the tumor characteristics have changed (i.e., size, invasion, extent of edema, shift, or multiplicity of lesions). Thus, MRI or CT studies may need to be repeated preoperatively. In addition, in patients harboring metastatic tumors and in primary central nervous system (CNS) tumors with the propensity to metastasize or seed the CNS, preoperative staging, with cranial and spinal gadolinium-enhanced MRI is recommended.

Angiography is not routinely used for diagnostic purposes, but is performed preoperatively in specific tumors; for example, when it is necessary to identify tumor vascularity and feeding vessels, to determine the patency of major vessels or sinuses, for the embolization of meningiomas or other vascular tumors, and for operative planning.

Lumbar puncture is also not considered a routine diagnostic procedure and may even be dangerous in some situations. However, if it can be accomplished safely, it may be helpful in certain situations. For example, the evaluation of biochemical markers (i.e., alpha-fetoprotein, human chorionic gonadotropin, carcinoembryonic antigen, and placental alkaline phosphatase) in both cerebrospinal fluid (CSF) and blood can provide diagnostic clues to identifying specific types of tumors. These markers are especially useful for the germ cell tumors (choriocarcinoma, germinoma, teratoma, yolk sac tumor, embryonal carcinoma) and certain metastatic tumors. The CSF cytological studies can occasionally be diagnostic in such cases. Pre- or postoperative CSF cytological assessment with cytospin is part of the staging of certain metastatic tumors or primary

CNS tumors that may spread through CSF pathways (e.g., ependymoma, medulloblastoma). The CSF may be obtained directly from the ventricular system in those patients with ventricular access devices (e.g., shunt, Ommaya reservoir) or by lumbar puncture, if deemed safe. It should be emphasized here again that lumbar puncture can be extremely dangerous in the presence of raised intracranial or intraspinal pressure caused by mass lesions, precipitating the onset of herniation of neural structures.

Radionuclide brain scanning is no longer used to diagnose brain tumors. Recently, however, the use of single-photon emission computed tomography (SPECT) and xenon cerebral blood flow studies has created a new role for nuclear medicine in the understanding of brain tumor biology, especially permeability and blood flow dynamics.

Perhaps the most significant development in the understanding of brain tumor metabolism is the advent of 18-fluoro-2-deoxyglucose positron emission tomography (PET) scanning to study glucose metabolism. It has been shown in meningiomas and gliomas that the more malignant or aggressive the tumor, the higher the rate of glucose metabolism (3). Thus, PET scanning can be used as a preoperative diagnostic tool, but because of its limited availability and expense it is still considered experimental.

B. Preoperative Planning

Once the diagnosis of an intracranial tumor is confirmed, surgical planning depends on several factors, which are both tumor-related and patient-related (4).

The type of surgery (biopsy, open craniotomy, radical versus limited) and even the decision to operate, may be affected by a variety of factors directly related to the tumor. Tumor factors include the location (deep versus superficial; eloquent versus silent brain area), size, vascularity, composition (solid versus cystic), and multiplicity. Previous surgical intervention, radiotherapy, and adjunctive therapies should also be considered in surgical planning.

Important preoperative consideration must be given to those factors primarily related to the patient. Neurological status, as assessed by the Karnofsky score (Table 1), and age appear to be powerful predictors of clinical outcome. In patients with gliomas, a Karnofsky score over 70 (indicating independent care) and age younger than 40 are associated with a better prognosis (5).

Table 1 Karnofsky Performance Scale

Score	Characteristic
100	Normal; no complaints; no evidence of disease
90	Able to carry on normal activity; minor symptoms
80	Normal activity with effort; some symptoms
70	Cares for self; unable to carry on normal activity
60	Requires occasional assistance; cares for most needs
50	Requires considerable assistance and frequent medical care
40	Disabled; requires special assistance and care
30	Severely disabled; hospitalized, death not imminent
20	Very sick; active supportive treatment needed
10	Moribund; fatal processes are rapidly progressing

It is extremely important to evaluate any medical condition of the patient that may increase the risk of surgery and to correct abnormalities preoperatively. We will elaborate on some of the major medical factors in the following sections.

Finally, one must consider the patients' and their families' desires which are usually, but not always, to prolong survival and preserve the quality of life. It is here that family conferences with the attending physician and support group referral can be most helpful.

III. THE MEDICAL "TUNE-UP"

A. Nutrition

Nutritional status has recently been recognized as an important pre- and postoperative factor in patient outcome. The most valuable index for assessing nutritional status is weight loss. In studies for gastrectomy, a 30% weight loss preoperatively resulted in a tenfold increase in operative mortality (6). Weight loss of 10–15% is usually not of great consequence, whereas a 20% loss increases one's susceptibility to stress, and a 30% loss increases morbidity and mortality (7). In nutritional management, the term *nitrogen* is often used interchangeably with protein. An unreplaced nitrogen loss of 20 g for 2 weeks can result in 20–30% weight loss. Most patients are in negative nitrogen balance after elective craniotomy owing to an increased nitrogen excretion associated with neurological injury, but this is usually transient, mild, and not attributable to steroid administration (8).

Although most nutritional studies have examined patients with head injury, subarachnoid hemorrhage, or intracerebral hematoma, we need to consider this factor in brain tumor patients as well. In addition to caloric intake and nitrogen excretion, attention must be paid to vitamin and mineral deficiencies that can be associated with chronic disease states or alcoholism, or prolonged postoperative parenteral alimentation. Vitamin deficiency may develop in normal individuals within 1–2 weeks. An increased need for zinc and ascorbic acid has been identified in trauma patients. Parenteral alimentation-induced deficiencies may include those of copper, zinc, chromium, selenium, and trace minerals. Such vitamins and minerals are necessary not only for normal metabolic processes, but are an essential part of the wound-healing process.

Neurological recovery from brain damage can also be influenced by environmental factors, such as nutritional status (9).

Most patients can begin oral alimentation within 1–3 days after surgery. The most desirable route of alimentation is always enteral.

In patients unable to protect their airway because of a decreased gag or obtundation, or are unable to eat for any other reasons, we usually insert a Doboff tube for feedings because it is safer than a nasogastric tube in preventing aspiration. If prolonged tube-feeding is required, a percutaneous jejunostomy tube can be placed. In patients who lack alimentary tract function, parenteral hyperalimentation should be considered early in the postoperative course. It is usually administered through a separate central venous line. Standard solutions are now available commercially and include glucose, electrolytes, amino acids, fat, multivitamins, and trace elements. Electrolyte levels, liver function tests, and glucose levels must be monitored, and solutions must be adjusted to treat abnormalities appropriately.

In addition to its role in the pre- and postoperative period to enhance wound healing, proper nutrition is thought to be an important epidemiological factor in carcinogenesis and cancer prevention, and it may be an important part of cancer treatment. In fact, a recent international conference sponsored by the American Cancer Society, Centers for Disease Control, and National Cancer Institute was convened to discuss the role of nutrition in cancer treatment (10).

B. Cardiac Status

Preexisting cardiac disease can contribute to an increased risk at surgery. This can occur intraoperatively, related to the cardiotoxic effect of certain anesthetics, as well as postoperatively. In the preoperative assessment, a history of previous myocardial infarct or symptoms of chest pain, dyspnea on exertion, or peripheral edema may indicate myocardial ischemia or ventricular dysfunction. In addition to the routine 12-lead electrocardiogram (ECG) and chest x-ray, stress testing, a dipyridamole (Persantine), thallium radionuclide multiple gated image acquisition (MUGA) scan (for patients unable to perform the treadmill), or echocardiogram are performed to evaluate myocardial kinetics. Coronary angiography occasionally may be necessary. We recommend preoperative medical consultation for evaluation of most of our neurosurgical patients and, in specific cases, further cardiac evaluation. In patients with cardiovascular disease, intraoperative and postoperative monitoring includes placement of a Swan–Ganz pulmonary artery catheter for pulmonary wedge pressure and cardiac output as well as a routine arterial line for arterial blood gas determinations and blood pressure monitoring.

In the postoperative period, we routinely check chest x-ray films, ECG, arterial blood gas values, and electrolyte levels. These tests are as important for the postoperative neurosurgical patient, as for any patient with a sudden change in mentation, loss of consciousness, or obtundation, as occasionally a cardiac cause may be found (e.g., atrial fibrillation, causing emboli and stroke).

C. Pulmonary Status

Patients with pulmonary dysfunction are also at increased risk for perioperative complications. When the patient gives a history of chronic cough, productive sputum, or smoking, routine chest x-ray studies, pulmonary function tests, and arterial blood gas assessments are needed. In addition, preoperative medical or anesthesia consultation can help assess the patient's pulmonary operative risks and recommend preoperative treatments that may improve pulmonary status (e.g., bronchodilators, chest physiotherapy, antibiotics, or oxygen therapy). We also recommend that all patients discontinue smoking at least 1 week before surgery.

In the postoperative period, we routinely check chest x-ray films, arterial blood gas levels, and ECG. We usually keep the head of the bed elevated at least 45°–90° postoperatively to improve intracranial pressure and also to help with bronchial toilet. Early mobilization is usual, and we often order incentive spirometers for our patients to help improve respiratory function postoperatively.

One of the most common infections encountered postoperatively is that involving the lower respiratory tract. In a recent study, lower respiratory tract infections occurred in 32% of patients undergoing surgery for brain tumors, with a 21% incidence of pneumonia (11). Several factors have been identified that increased the risk of developing respiratory infection. These included tumor type (meningiomas had the highest incidence), age older than 60 years, cardiac failure, preoperative disturbances of consciousness, and the use of preoperative corticosteroids. In this study, the incidence was reduced by keeping those patients at risk intubated postoperatively for 3 days, although this is not the usual practice. Other factors associated with increased risk for developing postoperative respiratory infections are diabetes mellitus, smoking, alcoholism, the presence of malignant disease, an increased preoperative hospital stay, and care in the intensive care unit.

D. Coagulation Assessment

The coagulation and hematological status of the patient is routinely screened preoperatively by obtaining a complete blood count and coagulation profile. Other helpful tests include bleeding times, platelet aggregation studies, and a liver function profile. Abnormalities, such as severe anemia, which may be associated with chronic disease states or alcoholism, may need to be corrected preoperatively. Patients with coagulation abnormalities with a history of hemophilia or of medications associated with coagulopathy, including chemotherapy, need further evaluation and preoperative correction of coagulation defects. Hematological consultation can be helpful when transfusion therapy is needed, especially in guiding the use of pre- and postoperative vitamin K, coagulation factors (fresh-frozen plasma, factor VIII, platelets, cryoprecipitate, factor IX), blood and serum products, or supplemental iron therapy.

In addition, if a patient has been anticoagulated with aspirin or warfarin (Coumadin) preoperatively, these need to be discontinued or switched to heparin in the hospital until the time of surgery, at which time heparin reversal with protamine sulfate may be indicated when reversal does not occur rapidly enough. The safety of anticoagulation in the immediate postoperative period is controversial. Although some authors suggest that anticoagulation may be safe several days after craniotomy (12), many physicians routinely wait 2–3 weeks. One must weigh the need for anticoagulation (e.g., mechanical heart valve) versus the risk of bleeding into the operative site postoperatively. Anticoagulation therapy is further discussed in the next section on deep vein thrombosis (DVT).

E. Deep Vein Thrombosis

One of the major, and fortunately preventable, causes of postoperative morbidity and mortality is deep vein thrombosis (DVT). It occurs in 30–40% of neurosurgical patients (13). Its sequella, pulmonary embolism (PE), is fatal in 1–2% of patients (13). Because of this high incidence of DVT, and the risk of hemorrhage associated with anticoagulation for the treatment of DVT, it is important to focus on its *prevention* in brain tumor patients.

In general, the risk factors for developing DVT and PE include age, prolonged immobilization, malignancy, congestive heart failure, oral contraceptives, pregnancy, superficial phlebitis, and certain disease states. In neurosurgical patients, the length of the operation is an additional factor. Thus, preventive measures include the avoidance of prolonged immobilization. We advocate the continued mobilization of patients both pre- and postoperatively. If the patient is immobilized, then mechanical intermittent pneumatic compression of the calf is the best method of preventing DVT, both pre- and postoperatively. However, its effect on PE is unknown. In addition, we recommend intraoperative mechanical compression for operations lasting over 3 h.

The suspicion of DVT must be taken seriously, and patients who complain of calf or chest pain, leg edema, swelling, shortness of breath, or hemoptysis, need an expedient and thorough evaluation to confirm or eliminate the diagnosis of DVT or PE. Routine laboratory tests, such as chest x-ray studies and ECG may be suggestive for the diagnosis of PE, but are nonspecific. The diagnosis of DVT can usually be made by noninvasive techniques, such as the ^{125}I-fibrinogen uptake test and Doppler ultrasound. The radionuclide ventilation–perfusion lung scan, showing the characteristic pattern of normal ventilation in an area of underperfusion is considered more specific. Occasionally, pulmonary angiography may be necessary to confirm the diagnosis.

Prophylactic anticoagulation has been used in neurosurgical patients in both the pre- and postoperative period. So-called low-dose heparin (5000 IU) given subcutaneously twice daily can effectively reduce the risk of DVT and is used in some centers both pre- and postoperatively, usually until the patient is ambulatory. However, it is associated with an increase in postoperative wound hematomas (14). Several centers are now testing the effectiveness of an ultra-low-dose regimen, in which the heparin is given less frequently, in lower doses, and for a shorter time. Currently, under study is the use of the synthetic heparin analogue, dihydroergotamine, and dextran.

The treatment of DVT and PE usually requires anticoagulation therapy (e.g., heparin and warfarin, streptokinase, or urokinase). In neurosurgical patients, anticoagulation in the immediate postoperative period carries the risk of hemorrhage into the operative site. Although some authors assert the safety of anticoagulation several days after craniotomy (12), most physicians feel uncomfortable before 2–3 weeks postoperatively. For the use of streptokinase and urokinase, NIH guidelines recommend waiting 2 months after a neurosurgical procedure (15). Therefore, for the treatment of pre- or postoperative PE, we recommend vena caval interruption either by ligation or the placement of a Greenfield filter.

F. Metabolic Disturbances and Fluid and Electrolytes

In the preoperative assessment of patients with brain tumors, screening electrolyte profiles and liver function or enzyme tests are routinely performed. These are used to screen for liver failure, uremia, or other systemic diseases. The most common metabolic problems encountered in brain tumor patients involve abnormalities of glucose metabolism and fluid and electrolyte disorders [e.g., the syndrome of inappropriate antidiuretic hormone (SIADH)].

G. Diabetes

Because of its high prevalence in the general population (approximately 5% in the United States), diabetes is a common metabolic problem that needs special consideration in the brain tumor patient. Patients are routinely screened for diabetes with the preoperative electrolyte profile. Those with a history of familial diabetes, or who complain of symptoms suggestive of diabetes, such as thirst, polyuria, polyphagia, and weight loss, should also have fasting blood sugar levels performed. If the baseline fasting blood sugar value is above 150 mg/dl, further endocrinological evaluation, including a glucose tolerance test is mandatory.

In the initial diagnosis of a brain tumor, CT scanning with contrast is frequently utilized. One must be cautious in administering contrast agents to diabetic patients because of the associated risk of renal damage. Therefore, we recommend the use of MRI when possible. If CT is necessary, the patient must be kept well hydrated before and after the procedure, preferably with intravenous normal saline, to prevent such a complication.

Once the diagnosis of brain tumor is confirmed, patients are usually treated with corticosteroids both pre- and postoperatively. In the known diabetic patient, whether insulin-dependent or not, the administration of corticosteroids, in addition to the stress of the surgery itself, may exacerbate their hyperglycemia. It is advisable in these patients to use a lower dose of steroids when possible, and to closely monitor their blood and urine carefully for evidence of hyperglycemia, glucosuria, or hyperosmolarity. Abnormalities in glucose metabolism must be corrected. On rare occasions, an insulin drip may be required. For most diabetic patients, endocrinology consultation is recommended to help with medication dosage and metabolic monitoring.

In the diabetic patient dehydrating agents such as mannitol must also be used with caution, since they may cause hyperosmolar states. Hypovolemia in diabetic patients can have serious systemic consequences (e.g., renal failure). We recommend that normovolemia should be maintained by the use of normal saline when intravenous fluids are required. In the postoperative period, we try to rapidly taper steroids, and we continue to closely monitor blood and urine electrolyte levels and osmolarity.

One must remember that diabetes is a systemic disorder and these patients are at risk for various types of vascular diseases, including stroke and myocardial infarction. In addition, probably related to small-vessel disease, diabetic patients are at an increased risk for infections, including wound infections. Meticulous attention must be given to surgical techniques that preserve tissue blood supply. Good nutrition and oxygenation may also help reduce this risk.

H. Syndrome of Inappropriate Secretion of Antidiuretic Hormone

Although several types of electrolyte disorders can occur, patients with brain tumors most often develop hyponatremia caused by SIADH, either in the preoperative or more commonly in the postoperative period. The syndrome is defined by the patient having a less than adequately dilute urine relative to their serum in the presence of normal kidney and heart function and normo-volemia. This syndrome implies a relative water intoxication. Confirmative laboratory diagnostic tests include urine and serum electrolyte and osmolarity assessments. This condition usually indicates the presence of elevated intracranial pressure or pathology. The initial treatment of SIADH is fluid restriction. We usually start with a restriction to a total of 1500 ml/day, but have restricted fluids to 500 ml/day when necessary. In addition, we recommend that when intravenous fluids are necessary, they should be in the form of normal saline, and that intravenous medication should also be given in minimal volume using normal saline, not 5% dextrose in water. If the hyponatremia does not correct, further volume reduction can be obtained with intravenous furosi-mide (Lasix) given judiciously. If the degree of hyponatremia is very severe, or the drop in serum sodium concentration is quite precipitous, seizures can occur, and can be life-threatening. In such situations, intravenous infusion of 3% saline may become necessary. We usually give 1 L in a 24-h period as a continuous infusion. In most cases, however, the syndrome is self-limiting. In persistent or chronic cases of SIADH or when further fluid restriction is not possible, the antibiotic demeclocycline has been used.

I. Infections and Antibiotics

Neurosurgical procedures encompass operations with widely disparate risks for infection, depend-ing on whether they are clean, (i.e., craniotomy), clean-contaminated (transphenoidal hypophysec-tomy), or dirty-contaminated (excision of brain abscess). Infection in brain tumor patients can occur either preoperatively or postoperatively, and can occur either intracranially or extracranial-ly.

The risk of postoperative infections can often be reduced by preoperative preventive measures. Aside from wound infections, most postoperative infections involve the respiratory or urinary tract. We routinely screen patients preoperatively with urinalysis, chest x-ray, and complete blood count (looking for leukocytosis). In addition, open sores or draining skin wounds, sinus infections, and even dental abscesses, can be sources of infection and should be evaluated and treated preoperatively.

Infections of the genitourinary and respiratory tracts are potentially preventable, as they are often related to instrumentation, such as urethral and other forms of in-dwelling catheters and lines. Prolonged use of in-dwelling catheters and lines either pre- or postoperatively should be avoided when possible. When they are necessary, meticulous attention must be given to regularly checking them for early signs of phlebitis or infection. Intravenous lines are changed every 48–72 h. If a patient develops a fever of unknown origin, all lines should be removed and changed.

The risk of wound infection can be reduced by attention to those factors that affect the process of wound healing, both in the pre- and postoperative period (16). In brief, there are three major phases of wound healing: the inflammatory phase, involving cellular migration; the proliferative or connective tissue phase; and the reorganization or remodeling phase.

Important systemic factors that affect wound healing include the patient's age and nutritional status, hypoxia, anemia, uremia, malignant disease, and infections. The administration of certain drugs, either cytotoxic (e.g., chemotherapy) or anti-inflammatory (e.g., corticosteroids), and x-ray irradiation, can all adversely affect the various phases of wound healing. Although cortisone inhibits the inflammatory response that occurs in the initial stages of wound healing, steroid administration is not a major determinant of wound infection after clean craniotomy (17).

Adequate nutritional support is vital for wound healing and infection prevention, and is important in both the preoperative and postoperative periods, as discussed previously on nutrition. Deficiencies in proteins, amino acids, vitamins, or trace minerals can adversely affect fibroblast activity and collagen formation, which are essential parts of wound healing.

Local factors that affect wound healing include blood supply, mechanical stress, surgical technique, and suturing technique. Other general factors that may increase the chance of postoperative wound infections include a prolonged operative time, reoperations, surgery on previously irradiated wounds, multiple personnel changes in the operating room, breaks in sterile technique, and the use of postoperative drains. Technical measures that can be employed by the neurosurgeon to reduce the wound infection rate include scalp shampooing with antiseptic solution, careful intraoperative attention to designing the skin flap to preserve an adequate blood supply, gentle tissue handling, meticulous hemostasis, and frequent wound irrigation.

In one study, Mollman and Haines found that CSF leak, concomitant extracranial infections, and whether or not perioperative antibiotics were used were the major risk factors for developing neurosurgical wound infections (18).

The reported incidence of infections after clean craniotomy in most neurosurgical centers is less than 5% (19). Clean surgery is considered a procedure in which there is no break in sterile technique and there is no entry into the respiratory, gastrointestinal, or genitourinary tract. The true incidence of postoperative infections is difficult to ascertain, as hospitals vary from one to another on the definition of infection, the method of diagnosing infections (i.e., clinical or laboratory), and whether the calculation of the infection rate includes extracranial infections, such as urinary tract infections and pneumonia.

Although postoperative intracranial infections can be the result of hematogenous or direct contiguous spread from extracranial sources, most neurosurgical infections involving the surgical wound, the bone flap, the dura, the brain itself, and the CSF–ventricular system are more often the result of perioperative contamination, as suggested by the types of microorganisms cultured. The microorganisms most commonly found are the gram-positive *Staphylococcus aureus* and *S. epidermidis,* accounting for approximately 87% of postoperative wound infections. Gram-negative organisms account for approximately 8% of infections, whereas mixed cultures of gram-positive and gram-negative organisms are found in 8% of infections (19).

The types of infection vary from a superficial wound infection, to more complicated infections, such as empyema and brain abscess. Because any form of infection can be potentially disastrous for neurosurgical patients, prophylactic antibiotics are usually recommended, even in clean neurosurgical procedures such as craniotomy and ventricular shunting operations. The use of parenteral prophylactic antibiotics has been demonstrated to reduce the incidence of postoperative infections (20–28). Antibiotics are not usually administered prophylactically beyond the perioperative period unless a foreign body, such as a shunt, has been used during surgery (29).

A variety of prophylactic antibiotic regimens have been used by neurosurgeons to reduce postoperative infection. Until recently, the choice of antibiotic was often based on previous training and habits. The most popular antibiotic protocol currently in use is the Malis regimen (24). By using a combination of preoperative intramuscular aminoglycoside, intravenous vancomycin, and intraoperative streptomycin irrigating solutions, he achieved a zero incidence of intraoperative infection in 1730 cases. This impressive result has been confirmed at several other institutions using similar combinations of antibiotics. Some of the antibiotic regimens that have been reported to be effective in reducing the incidence of postoperative neurosurgical wound infections are shown in Table 2 (20,21,24,26,28). Although reports differ in the overall postoperative infection rate, most studies support the use of prophylactic antibiotics. For a more extensive review, we recommend the excellent papers by Dempsey et al. (19) and Haines and Goodman (23).

Wound infections in brain tumor patients are treated in the same manner as infections in any neurosurgical patient. Stitch abscesses are opened, drained, and the suture removed. Subgaleal purulent accumulations require drainage in the operating room, with the removal of the bone flap and any other foreign bodies (e.g., acrylic or mesh). Those patients with abscesses or empyema are treated with surgical drainage. Multiple culture samples are always obtained at the time of surgery, and broad-spectrum antibiotics are initially started until culture sensitivities are available, at which time antibiotics are changed to the most appropriate ones. We usually begin with nafcillin or vancomycin, plus an aminoglycoside, and metronidazole (Flagyl). Patients with subdural empyema and brain abscesses after craniotomy for tumor have a higher morbidity and mortality rate than patients in whom these complications do not occur. Infectious disease consultation can be very helpful in guiding antibiotic therapy in these patients.

J. Anticonvulsants and Seizures

Supratentorial cerebral tumors are commonly associated with seizures, either pre- or postoperatively. Although tumors themselves do not cause seizures, their presence and the effect they have on the surrounding adjacent cortex induce electrophysiological instability and as a result, seizures. Numerous theories have been proposed to account for the pathophysiological mechanisms causing seizures. These include ischemic and metabolic changes, as well as mechanical factors, such as compression or traction.

Patients with brain tumors may present clinically with seizures. This incidence is as high as 35% in some reported series (30). Neurosurgical procedures are associated with a 17% risk of developing postoperative seizures (31). Those patients with a preoperative history of seizures have an even further increased risk of developing postoperative seizures.

The location of the tumor influences the risk of seizures. Those tumors located near the motor or sensory cortex, as well as the temporal lobes, are known to be the most epileptogenic. Patients undergoing operative procedures in the more epileptogenic areas, such as the mesial temporal lobe or the pre- and postcentral regions are particularly predisposed to postoperative convulsions.

The tumor histological type also correlates with the frequency of seizures, with benign lesions

Table 2 Protocols for Antibiotic Prophylaxis

Protocol	Ref.
1. Gentamicin 80 mg im	24
Vancomycin 1 g iv	
Streptomycin 50 mg/L (irrigating fluid)	
2. Vancomycin 1 g iv	20
3. Oxacillin 200 mg/kg/24 h iv and q4h × 24 h	21
4. Cefazolin 1 g iv	28
Gentamicin 80 mg iv (1 h before incision then q6h)	
5. Cephalothin 2 g iv	26
Bacitracin 50,000 U/50 ml (irrigating fluid)	

(e.g., low-grade gliomas and meningiomas) having a higher incidence than the more malignant tumors, such as glioblastoma (32,33).

The occurrence of seizures in an already-compromised brain causes further neurological morbidity because of associated metabolic changes (e.g., lactic acidosis), ischemia, and edema; resulting in severe neurological deficit, coma, or even death. Thus, antiepileptic prophylaxis is recommended for most patients with supratentorial brain tumors, both pre- and postoperatively (34). Anticonvulsants are usually continued for up to 6–12 months postoperatively. When discontinuing anticonvulsants, we recommend an initial electroencephalogram (EEG), and if free of seizures or spikes, we slowly taper medications, decreasing the dose on a weekly basis, and checking frequent interval EEGs.

Several pharmacological regimens currently exist for seizure prophylaxis. Since the introduction of phenytoin in 1938, it has become the mainstay of most prophylactic protocols, although phenobarbital and carbamazepine (Tegretol) are effective alternatives. In the past, some centers have recommended two anticonvulsants preoperatively, usually phenytoin and phenobarbital (34), but this has not been the more recent procedure. We recommend the use of single agents at therapeutic levels. Therapeutic serum drug levels should be achieved preoperatively and maintained postoperatively to minimize seizure activity. Before prescribing anticonvulsants, one should become familiar with the most commonly prescribed drugs, namely phenytoin, phenobarbital, and carbamazepine, and the pharmacological properties of the drugs, methods of administration, absorption, distribution, metabolism, elimination, efficacy, dosage, and side affects. Certain anticonvulsants are available only in oral form and would be unsuitable for those patients who are not able to have oral intake. Whether or not a patient has a known allergic reaction (e.g., Stevens–Johnson syndrome) or side effects to particular drugs should be considered before commencing anticonvulsant medication. Some patients with coexistent systemic diseases or metabolic tumors may not be eligible for certain drugs because of impaired absorption, metabolism, or elimination, as a result of their disease. We will briefly review the pharmacological properties of the two most widely used anticonvulsants in neurosurgical patients: phenytoin and phenobarbital (35,36).

Phenytoin is the most commonly prescribed anticonvulsant and is known to be the least sedating and the most effective anticonvulsant existing today. This low incidence of sedation is particularly advantageous when caring for brain tumor patients, as the level of consciousness is an important clinical monitor that often reflects changes in intracranial pressure. Anticonvulsant-induced somnolence could confuse the clinical picture and is preferably avoided. Phenytoin's mechanism of action in the prevention of seizures is believed to be through the stabilization of excitable neuronal membranes. In 1955, Woodbury demonstrated that phenytoin activates the sodium pump of neuronal membranes, reducing the level of intracellular sodium (37). It is poorly absorbed from the gastrointestinal tract and most of it binds to plasma proteins once in circulation. The half-life of phenytoin ranges from 7 to 42 h. The form of seizures most effectively treated by phenytoin includes grand mal seizures, partial seizures, including those that secondarily generalize, and focal seizures. Phenytoin is ineffective in psychomotor seizures and absence seizures, and when treating these forms of epilepsy, other anticonvulsants should be considered. The average adult dosage for phenytoin is usually 300–400 mg/day, and therapeutic serum concentrations in the range of 10–20 mg/dl should be achieved. The axiom that CNS toxicity cannot occur in serum levels of less than 20 μg/L is no longer true, as it has been shown that CNS toxicity can occur at levels below 10 μg/L. Rapid loading with phenytoin is sometimes indicated, and this can be accomplished by either the intravenous or the oral route of administration, or a combination of both. The initial intravenous dose is usually 15–20 mg/kg, in both adults and children. However, the infusion rate should not exceed 50 mg/min, as it can induce cardiac arrhythmias, hypotension, or cardiac arrest. An oral loading dose of 1000 mg, in divided doses, can usually be given without undue side effects. Serum concentrations of phenytoin reflect protein-bound drug, which is approximately 90% of the phenytoin. Free phenytoin (i.e., not protein-bound) accounts for approximately 10% of the serum concentration. This ratio can change with abnormal metabolic conditions (e.g., liver failure) and may account for toxicity in patients with previous therapeutic levels. Central nervous system toxicity is manifest clinically by nystagmus, ataxia, dizziness, or mental status changes, or a combination thereof. However, phenytoin-induced changes in sensorium usually reflect an advanced toxic condition.

Phenobarbital, one of the longer-acting barbituates used to treat seizures, was introduced in 1912 by Hauptmann (38). The CNS effects of phenobarbital include both anticonvulsant and sleep-inducing effects. The seizure types most responsive to phenobarbital are the generalized tonic–clonic (grand mal) and simple partial (focal motor and sensory) seizures. Absence seizures (petit mal) are complex partial seizures and are not controlled with phenobarbital. The gastrointestinal absorption, metabolism, and elimination of this agent is slow. In fact, it has the longest half-life of any of the antoconvulsants, ranging from 53 to 140 h in adults. The oral dose of phenobarbital is 1–3 mg/kg per day. The usual adult dose is approximately 90–100 mg/day. Therapeutic serum concentrations range from 10 to 40 mg/L. The mechanism of action of the barbiturates on seizures involves their ability to affect multiple, but nonselective, aspects of synaptic transmission.

K. Intracranial Pressure

A variety of pathological lesions can cause elevated intracranial pressure, including intracranial hematomas, abscesses, generalized edema, and tumors. As the cranium in the adult is a rigid, bony structure that contains neurons, glia, CSF, and blood, it is both protective and restrictive; thus it cannot expand to accommodate a space-occupying lesion without a concomitant rise in the intracranial pressure (ICP) (39). Any significant or rapid rise in ICP can cause a reduction in the cerebral perfusion pressure and cerebral blood flow, leading to brain ischemia and subsequent infarction. The presence of a brain tumor in the supratentorial compartment usually causes a slow increase in brain volume from tumor growth. Several deleterious effects occur on the surrounding brain as the brain tries to compensate for changes in intracranial pressure. Compensatory mechanisms are accomplished by changes in the brain substance, CSF, and the blood volume. As the tumor grows, the gyri become flattened, the sulci are narrowed, and the CSF is displaced from the intracranial subarachnoid space into the spinal subarachnoid space. With continued tumor growth, the ventricle on the side of the lesion becomes effaced and, subsequently, there will be a midline shift as compensatory measures are exhausted. Further compensation can be achieved only by reduction in cerebral blood volume and compression of the major intracranial venous sinuses. With progressive increase in the size of the tumor, major intracranial shifts occur, with subsequent frank herniation. The major herniation syndromes include subfalcine, tentorial, central diencephalic, and tonsillar herniation.

Clinically, brain tumor patients may present with signs and symptoms of raised intracranial pressure. These include headache, nausea and vomiting, lethargy, drowsiness, and papilledema. Chronically raised intracranial pressure can cause erosion of the skull, and especially of the clinoid processes, the lesser wing of the sphenoid, and the orbital plates. In addition, brain tumors induce edema of the surrounding brain, perhaps caused by the release of certain vascular permeability factors, which contribute to the overall space-occupying effect and cause further elevation in the intracranial pressure. Without treatment, significantly increased intracranial pressure leads to neurological deterioration and eventually death. Thus, it is essential to treat raised intracranial pressure in all neurosurgical patients.

Occasionally, a patient with a brain tumor may present precipitously because of a rapid rise in intracranial pressure as a result of an acute hemorrhage or an associated seizure. Treatment in such cases becomes emergent.

Preoperatively, most patients are treated with corticosteroids for the brain edema that causes the raised intracranial pressure commonly associated with brain tumors (36,40). We usually prescribe 4–6 mg of dexamethasone (Decadron) every 6 h, beginning several days before elective surgery in the stable patient, and increase the dose to 10 mg on the day before surgery. Occasionally, higher doses are required and are used. Postoperatively, we continue the same dose of steroids for 3 days, considered to be the time of maximal postoperative brain swelling, after which time we taper steroids as rapidly as tolerated by the patient (usually over the course of 1 week). Some patients, especially those with malignant tumors or those who have been receiving steroids for a prolonged time preoperatively, may not tolerate the tapering of steroids and may require them for a longer period. We routinely prescribe concomitant antacids with corticosteroids.

In preoperative patients who are neurologically unstable as a result of their increased intracranial pressure, further therapy is required. In these patients, osmotic diuretics, such as intravenous mannitol (34), are given in preparation for urgent surgery. We usually use bolus infusions of mannitol, prepared as a 20% solution and given in doses of 50–150 ml every 4–6 h, depending on the weight of the patient (0.25–1 mg/kg per day), as needed to control the ICP. Osmolarity should be regularly monitored and maintained below 320 mOsm/L. In the obtunded or comatose patient, intubation for hyperventilation and barbiturate-induced coma (41,42) may be required to reduce intracranial pressure in preparation for emergent surgery. In such patients, we will place an intracranial pressure monitor to guide therapy.

Surgery for resection of the tumor or for decompression effectively reduces intracranial pressure and provides tissue for diagnosis. In patients with hydrocephalus, ventriculostomy or ventriculoperitoneal shunting will help alleviate raised intracranial pressure and can facilitate surgery.

Postoperatively, fluid restriction, including the use of diuretics such as furosimide, may well minimize cerebral edema (41,42).

L. Premedication and Neuroanesthesia

We do not usually premedicate neurosurgical patients with brain tumors until they are in the operating room. Before entering the operating suite, the patient may be given midazolam for sedation, as it induces amnesia without causing significant respiratory depression. We avoid the use of narcotics because they cause respiratory depression and hypoventilation, leading to hypercarbia, which further increases intracranial pressure.

Postoperatively, similar precautions exist concerning respiratory depression and hypoventilation in the presence of raised intracranial pressure. Most craniotomy patients do not have severe amounts of pain, and we usually use either ibuprophen or acetaminophen (Tylenol) for pain relief. Narcotics are generally avoided. In patients who do require stronger analgesia, low doses of codeine, 15–30 mg every 4–6 h, can be used when needed.

III. THE DIAGNOSIS AND MANAGEMENT OF BRAIN TUMORS DURING PREGNANCY

The diagnosis and management of the patient with a brain tumor becomes even more problematic when the patient is also pregnant. The implications for the diagnosis and treatment of the brain tumor, as well as the management of the pregnancy and the effects of treatment on the fetus, raise many medical questions as well as several significant controversial ethical issues.

Recently, there has been an increased interest in the treatment of brain tumors occurring during pregnancy, as a result of recent advances in our understanding of the mechanisms of tumor biology that link tumor growth and development to certain hormonal influences that may be present during pregnancy.

In addition, with the advent of noninvasive diagnostic testing (e.g., MRI), we now have a relatively safe and sensitive means of diagnosing neurological problems. Thus, we will briefly discuss some of the pre- and postoperative considerations in the case of the pregnant woman who has a brain tumor.

A.   Epidemiology

It has been estimated that each year in the United States, 89 pregnant women will have a primary brain tumor diagnosed (i.e., 1 : 44,000 pregnancies) (43). Although the incidence of primary brain tumors occurring in pregnancy is no higher than that in nonpregnant women, there have been numerous reports of alterations in the growth rate of certain tumors during pregnancy (44). In addition, while tumors in some patients become symptomatic during pregnancy, other patients experience resolution of their symptoms postpartum, and a few tumors present only in the postpartum period (44). These data again suggest the importance of hormonal influences in certain tumors.

Of the more than 30 known primary intracranial tumors that can occur during pregnancy, meningiomas, gliomas, acoustic neuromas, and pituitary tumors account for over 85% of brain tumors diagnosed during pregnancy. Other tumors that may occur, although with less frequency, are hemangioblastoma, neurofibromas, and spinal tumors. Although there are no specific extracranial tumors that are more likely to metastasize to the brain as a result of pregnancy, choriocarcinoma has a high propensity for brain metastasis, although it invariably presents in the postpartum period or later (45).

B.   Clinical Presentation

Generalized symptoms of raised intracranial pressure are headache, nausea, and vomiting. The headache is often worse in the morning, upon awakening. Because these very symptoms might be confused with the common symptoms of morning sickness in the pregnant patient, there is often a delay in making the diagnosis of an intracranial tumor during pregnancy. Other nonspecific symptoms related to increased intracranial pressure or mass effect caused by the brain tumor include lethargy and changes in mental status.

Pituitary tumors usually present with signs and symptoms of endocrinopathy (e.g., amenorrhea–galactorrhea, Cushing's syndrome, acromegaly). During pregnancy, hormonal influences are thought to cause the rapid growth of certain pituitary tumors such as prolactinomas. Patients with such tumors may present with signs of increased intracranial pressure or more commonly, neurological compression (i.e., progressive visual loss). Rarely, pituitary apoplexy can occur.

C.   Diagnostic Evaluation

Magnetic resonance imaging is rapidly becoming the procedure of choice for imaging most lesions of the central nervous system. Benefits of MRI include superior brain and spinal cord detail, which can be obtained in a single study in the axial, sagittal, and the coronal planes without exposure to ionizing radiation.

Because it does not expose the patient to ionizing radiation, MRI provides an especially attractive alternative to CT in pregnant patients. Although there is no evidence that MRI affects the fetus, MRI does expose it to intense magnetic and electromagnetic fields. In certain epidemiological studies, chronic exposure to electromagnetic fields has been associated with an increased incidence of brain tumors in adults (46). There is no evidence that such exposures harm the fetus, based on experience to date which includes direct imaging of the gravid uterus and the fetal brain, as well as the maternal brain, with MRI scanners of less than 2 Tesla strength (47,48). However, MRI is presently not FDA-approved for use during pregnancy. Given this fact, it is prudent to avoid MRI during the first trimester and to obtain written informed consent for the procedure at any stage of pregnancy when the test is deemed necessary (49).

Gadolinium–DTPA is an intravenous ferromagnetic material used for contrast enhancement in MRI and is particularly sensitive for demonstrating brain tumors. Currently, there is also very little evidence concerning the safety of this agent for the fetus. Fortunately, for most MRI examinations, the administration of contrast material may not be required. Since gadolinium is not yet FDA-approved for use during pregnancy, it requires the signing of specific consent and release forms.

Computed tomography (CT) of the brain becomes the alternate procedure of choice in the diagnosis of a CNS tumor during pregnancy, when MRI is not available or when the patient is unable to undergo MRI scanning.

In the special instance of a rapidly deteriorating patient, CT scanning may be the procedure of choice over MRI because of its ready availability and quick-scanning capability. However, CT does have an associated radiation risk to the conceptus. At fetal exposures of less than 10 rad, no adverse effects have been identified statistically, compared to the background rate of spontaneous abnormalities, that occur in roughly 3% of livebirths, and spontaneous abortions that occur in roughly 30% of all pregnancies (50). Medically indicated exposures of up to 5 rad are considered acceptable in pregnancy when unavoidable. The patient routinely receives between 2.5 and 3 rad to the head from a standard head CT (compared with 1–1.5 rad from plain skull x-rays). The fetal exposure from a standard skull series is under 10 rad (51). For CT scanning, fetal dosage is about 1 mrad or less per slice (52). This dose can be further reduced by shielding the uterus with lead aprons placed both above and below the patient. The upper limit for cerebral angiography is estimated at 100 mrad; actual exposures may approach this figure, depending on technical factors (53).

In the diagnosis of brain tumors, it may be necessary to obtain two separate CT scans of the brain: a noncontrast and a contrast-enhanced scan (i.e., after the infusion of intravenous iodinated contrast material). Postinfusion scans more accurately detect the presence and delineate the location of a lesion. They also give more information on the vascularity and size of a lesion. In many instances, the tumor is apparent only after the administration of contrast material and, therefore, contrast improves the diagnostic yield of CT scanning.

The risk of administering iodinated contrast material to the fetus as well as the additional radiation exposure of a second CT scan must be weighed against the immediate need for the test. Experience with iodinated contrast agents in pregnancy is limited. They have been used for intravenous injection in the diagnosis of deep vein thrombosis, and for intra-amniotic injection in the diagnosis of various obstetrical conditions. One infant exposed to intravenous contrast within the first trimester was born with undescended testes (54). The relation to exposure is unknown, and more serious malformations have not yet been reported. Some infants exposed to intra-amniotic contrast later in pregnancy have developed neonatal hypothyroidism caused by suppression of the fetal thyroid by iodine (55). The risk of this problem after maternal intravenous administration is probably quite low. As with other drugs of uncertain safety, use of contrast in the first trimester should be avoided.

When a lesion is not considered to be life-threatening, or occurs late in pregnancy, scanning is sometimes deferred until after delivery.

As with enhanced CT, angiography requires the administration of iodinated contrast material and carries the same concomitant risks to the fetus as discussed under CT scanning with contrast infusion. However, MRI can usually provide adequate information on the involvement of the normal intracranial vasculature and can differentiate vascular abnormalities (e.g., giant aneurysm) from tumor. When MRI is available, it can supplant cerebral angiography in the pregnant patient in most instances.

D. Glucocorticoids (Dexamethasone) and Osmotic Agents (Mannitol)

Management of brain edema and increased intracranial pressure associated with intracranial tumor may necessitate therapy with dexamethasone. Experience with dexamethasone in pregnancy in this circumstance is limited, but glucocorticoids have been used extensively for other conditions associated with gestation.

Dexamethasone and bethamethasone given briefly antepartum have found wide acceptance for prevention of neonatal respiratory distress syndrome in premature birth (56). In the largest study to date, mothers at gestational ages between 26 and 37 weeks received parenteral dexamethasone, 5 mg every 12 h to a maximum of 20 mg. Among subjects receiving the full course of steroids, dexamethasone plasma levels in infants delivered within 12 h after the last maternal dose averaged 12% of maternal levels. No adverse effects occurred on short-term or long-term follow-up (57,58). Fetal dexamethasone levels may reach higher levels, approaching maternal concentrations, in pregnancies at term (59).

Systematic data concerning more chronic administration of dexamethasone in pregnancy are unavailable. The data for corticosteroids in general do not suggest any teratogenic effect in humans, although they do cause congenital abnormalities in some laboratory animals (60). One study found that prednisone causes some retardation of intrauterine growth when given at a dose of 10 mg daily throughout pregnancy (61).

Suppression of the fetal adrenal gland by maternal administration of corticosteroids is rare, perhaps because regimens are either short-term or low-dose for most indications. However, regimens likely to be used in neurosurgical settings may indeed cause fetal adrenal suppression, requiring replacement of neonatal hydrocortisone at birth (62). Labor and delivery are physiologically stressful, so that neurosurgical patients who have received long-term high-dose therapy with glucocorticoids during any period of pregnancy should receive supplemental steroids in the peripartum period (63).

Acute management of increased intracranial pressure may also require the administration of mannitol. Mannitol crosses the placenta and is excreted by the fetal kidney into amniotic fluid (64,65). Osmotic shifts may theoretically result in some change in toxicity, but no adverse effects have been demonstrated.

E. Radiation Therapy

Radiation exposure in utero carries a risk of several adverse fetal outcomes, including spontaneous abortion, anatomical malformations (notably microcephaly), growth retardation, mental retardation, and possibly childhood cancer (50,66). The risk is concentrated in first-trimester exposure; exposure later in pregnancy carries less risk. However, risks are low at low exposures. As discussed earlier, for exposures of under 10 rad, no adverse effects can be identified statistically against the background rate of spontaneous abnormality of roughly 3% of live births and spontaneous abortions in roughly 30% of all pregnancies (50).

Radiation therapy in pregnancy inevitably exposes the fetus to more radiation than does diagnostic imaging. Fortunately, conceptus dose from scatter is relatively low when conventional radiation therapy is delivered to parts distant from the uterus.

Because radiotherapy does confer benefit for malignant brain tumors, but does pose a risk to the fetus, reduction in fetal dosage is desirable. One solution would be to hold all or part of the radiation dose until the postpartum period if delivery is imminent.

An examination of recurrence patterns and the incidence of radiation necrosis following radiotherapy has led to the proposal of using focal, rather than whole-brain irradiation for malignant glioma in most cases (67). The exposure rate for scattered radiation is proportional to field size (68). Therefore, the use of limited fields is especially important in the pregnant patient. Substitution of heavy-charged particles for photons in external beam irradiation also reduces scatter. Several clinical trials in nonpregnant patients have used a variety of heavy-particle beams with good results, but none of these studies were with malignant tumors (69).

Newer experimental forms of radiotherapy include the use of interstitial brachytherapy, with low-energy radioisotopes implanted intratumorally. This type of therapy minimizes radiation dose to tissues remote from the tumor. Geometric attenuation follows the inverse square law. Moreover, absorption and scattering by intervening tissue results in rapid exponential decline in exposure levels. For iodine-125 (energy 35 keV), this physical attenuation halves the dose for every 2 cm of tissue traversed (70,71). This treatment has not yet been studied in pregnant patients.

F.   Chemotherapy

The administration of antineoplastic drugs to the pregnant cancer patient is fraught with hazard. Many are teratogenic in the first trimester of pregnancy; after the first trimester, ongoing risks continue, including spontaneous abortion, premature birth, intrauterine growth retardation, and other fetal toxicity (72). Unfortunately, the same properties that improve permeability of the chemotherapeutic agent across the blood–brain barrier also promote transport across the placenta. Thus, the principal chemotherapeutic agents most active against malignant gliomas, namely the nitrosoureas, would also be efficiently delivered to the fetus. Furthermore, some nitrosoureas are not only teratogens, but are also transplacental carcinogens when tested in animals (73).

Thus, chemotherapy of malignant brain tumors in pregnancy is inadvisable. No such treated cases have yet been reported. Only one patient has been reported who received a nitrosourea during pregnancy for malignancy. In this unusual case, a pregnant woman with refractory diffuse large-cell lymphoma was treated with carmustine (BCNU) plus procarbazine, followed by streptozocin. She elected this course "despite explanation of the likely teratogenic and carcinogenic effects on the fetus" and, nonetheless, bore a genotypically and phenotypically normal fetus at 35 weeks of gestation (74).

G.   Pituitary Tumors

There appears to be some controversy over the treatment of pituitary tumors (and especially prolactinomas) during pregnancy. In one study, it was reported that of those patients entering pregnancy with a known pituitary tumor, 25% developed visual problems, of which one-half required surgery or radiation during their pregnancy (75). In another study, Kelly found only 15% of patients with known prolactinomas treated with bromocriptine, developed visual symptoms when bromocriptine was discontinued during pregnancy (76). Because bromocriptine is not tumoricidal, when it is discontinued the tumor may increase in size or it may infarct (43,77,78). In some cases, bromocriptine has been restarted during pregnancy, if patients become symptomatic upon its discontinuance (79).

Many pregnant women with pituitary tumors who required transphenoidal surgery for the relief of visual symptoms have not shown an increase in fetal abnormalities (43,79–81).

H. Perioperative Management

When intracranial tumor necessitates emergent or urgent neurosurgical intervention in pregnancy, knowledge of gestational alterations in physiology and anatomy must guide perioperative management. Beyond the first trimester, gravid patients should not be positioned in the supine position, to avoid compromising vena caval blood return and uteroplacental blood supply. Patients should be positioned in a partial left lateral decubitus position, when possible, with the right hip tipped upward at about 15° (82).

Despite restrictive lung mechanics caused by the gravid uterus, pregnant women exhibit physiological hyperventilation. Baseline PCO_2 is usually about 30 mm Hg, with an associated respiratory alkalosis, which is partially compensated by the kidneys. Perioperative ventilator management should maintain this state of hyperventilation, even if intracranial pressure is not elevated. Maternal acidosis and hypoxia are detrimental to fetal welfare and should be assiduously avoided (82).

Lower esophageal sphincter tone and gastric motility are decreased in pregnancy. This phenomenon increases the risk of gastric aspiration, particularly with altered mental status. Perioperative antacids should be considered for this purpose, as well as for prophylaxis of stress ulceration. The safety of cimetidine in pregnancy, however, has not been established (82).

Glomerular filtration increases in pregnancy, and normal serum creatine levels fall below 1.0 mg/dl (typically to the range of 0.5 mg/dl). The risk of urinary tract infection increases in pregnancy, with an attendant risk of premature labor. Therefore, urinary catheterization should be avoided or minimized (82).

Pregnant women manifest a hypercoagulable state, which is compounded by neurosurgical intervention and consequent immobilization. Therefore, consideration must be given to the prevention of deep vein thrombosis and subsequent pulmonary emboli. Heparin is safe in pregnancy, but generally contraindicated before and after intracranial operation. Intermittent pneumatic calf compression devices should be used instead (83).

If antibiotic prophylaxis is desired for a neurosurgical procedure, fetal considerations impose some constraints: Penicillins and cephalosporins are safe, but may not cover the organisms of concern (i.e., methicillin-resistant staphylococci (84).

In clinical experience, trimethoprim–sulfamethoxazole has not been associated with adverse fetal outcomes. However, theoretical objections have been raised because trimethoprim is a folate antagonist and, therefore, might be teratogenic in humans. In addition, the sulfonamide component can cause neonatal kernicterus, and thus this combination should not be used in the third trimester. Clindamycin appears to be safe in pregnancy, as does gentamicin; dosage of the latter must be adjusted owing to increased renal clearance (84). Vancomycin should be avoided because of potential fetal ototoxicity (84).

I.   Cesarean Section

An important management consideration for the pregnant patient harboring a brain tumor is the need for cesarean section during delivery. Essential to this question is the presence and severity of raised intracranial pressure (ICP) in the mother. Although uterine contractions do not necessarily increase the ICP of the mother, abdominal pressure during the second stage of labor does cause a significant increase in ICP (43). Thus, in the presence of raised ICP, cesarean section is often recommended, but the decision depends on the judgment of the physician concerning what is an acceptable level of ICP. In patients in whom the level of ICP is not thought to be dangerous, vaginal delivery may be considered. A multiparous woman will be more likely to tolerate vaginal delivery without severe increases in ICP (43).

Santoul, in 1971 (85), recommended that cesarean section be considered under the following conditions: when a malignant tumor is diagnosed, but not yet treated; when a moribund maternal state might ensue; if neurosurgical intervention is required in the last 2 months; in cases of abnormal fetal presentation; or when forceps delivery under general anesthesia is required. For most other patients, Santoul recommended natural delivery.

Recently, Simon offered a different view given that very few mothers actually develop complications from ICP during delivery (43). He recommended that cesarean section be done solely for obstetrical reasons and to avoid the second stage of labor. When there is concern over ICP, forceps delivery should be performed.

In our own experience, the recommendation for cesarean section has been based on both maternal and fetal considerations: the nature and location of the tumor (i.e., malignancy, size, necessary treatments), the severity of the raised intracranial pressure, the neurological condition of the mother, and the fetal health, size, and position. This calls for the joint involvement of both the obstetrician and neurosurgeon, working together as a team to assess the medical situation accurately and to make a clinical judgment concerning appropriate recommendations for management of the pregnancy.

REFERENCES

1. Vick NA, Wilson CB. Total care of the patient with a brain tumor. Neurol Clin 1985; 3:705–710.
2. Support groups for brain tumor patients and families in North America. San Francisco: National Brain Tumor Foundation, 1991.
3. DiChiro T, Hatazawa JL. Glucose utilization by intracranial meningiomas as an index of tumor aggressivity and probability of recurrence: a PET study. Radiology 1987; 164:512.
4. Rosenblum M. General surgical principles, alternatives, limitations. Neurosurg Clin North Am 1990; 1:19–36.
5. Byar DP, Green SP, Strike TA. Prognostic factors for malignant glioma. In: Walker MD, ed. Oncology of the nervous system. Boston: Martinus Nijhoff, 1983:379.
6. Studley HO. Percentage of weight loss: a basic indicator of surgical risk in patients with peptic ulcer disease. JAMA 1936; 106:458–460.
7. Clifton GL, Turner H. Nutrition and parenteral therapy. In: Wilkins RH, Rengachary SS, eds. Neurosurgery update. New York: McGraw-Hill, 1990:209.
8. Young B, Ott L, Norton J, et al. Metabolic and nutritional sequelae in the non-steroid treated head injury patient. Neurosurgery 1985; 17:784–791.
9. Finger S, Stein DG. Brain damage and recovery. New York: Academic Press, 1982.
10. Nutrition and cancer, proceedings of international conference. Cancer Res 1992; 52 (suppl):2019S–2126S.
11. Dauch WA, Landau G, Krez D. Prognostic factors for lower respiratory tract infections after brain tumor surgery. J Neurosurg 1989; 70:862–868.
12. Allen, MB, Johnston DW. Preoperative evaluation: complications, their prevention and treatment. In: Youmans J, ed. Neurological surgery. vol 2. Philadelphia: WB Saunders, 1990:875.
13. Powers SK, Edwards MB. Prophylaxis of thromboembolism in neurosurgical patients. Neurosurgery 1982; 10:509–513.
14. Barnett HG, Clifford JE, Llewllyn RC. Safety of mini-dose heparin administration for neurosurgical patients. J Neurosurg 1977; 47:27–30.
15. National Institutes of Health. Thrombolytic therapy in thrombosis. Stroke 1981; 12:17–21.
16. Wilkin RH. Principles of neurosurgical operative technique. In: Wilkins RH, ed. Neurosurgery. New York: McGraw-Hill, 1935:427–433.
17. Wright RL. Postoperative craniotomy infections. Springfield: Charles C Thomas, 1966.

18. Molman HO, Haines SJ. Risk factors for postoperative neurosurgical wound infection: a case control study. J Neurosurg 1986; 64:902–906.
19. Dempsey R, Rapp R, Young B, et al. Prophylactic antibiotics in clean neurosurgical procedures: a review. J Neurosurg 1988; 69:52–57.
20. Blomstedt G, Kytta J. Results of a randomized trial of vancomycin prophylaxis in craniotomy. J Neurosurg 1988; 69:216–220.
21. Djingian M, Lepresle E, Homs JB. Antibiotic prophylaxis during prolonged clean neurosurgery. J Neurosurg 1990; 73:383–386.
22. Geraghty J, Feely M. Antibiotic prophylaxis in neurosurgery. J Neurosurg 1984; 60:724–728.
23. Haines S, Goodman M. Antibiotic prophylaxis of postoperative neurosurgical wound infection. J Neurosurg 1982; 56:103–105.
24. Malis L. Prevention of neurosurgical infection by intraoperative antibiotics. Neurosurgery 1979; 5:339–343.
25. Quartey G, Polyzoidis K. Intraoperative antibiotic prophylaxis in neurosurgery: a clinical study. Neurosurgery 1981; 8:669–671.
26. Savitz M, Katz S. Rational for prophylactic antibiotics in neurosurgery. Neurosurgery 1981; 9:142–144.
27. Sharpiro M, et al. Randomized clinical trial of intramicrobial operative antibiotic prophylaxis of infection after neurosurgical procedures. J Hosp Infect 1986; 8:283–295.
28. Young R, Lawner P. Perioperative antibiotic prophylaxis for prevention of postoperative neurosurgical infections. J Neurosurg 1987; 66:701–705.
29. Schmidt K, Gjerris F, Osgaard O, et al. Antibiotic proplyaxis in cerebrospinal fluid shunting: a prospective randomized trial in 152 hydrocephalic patients. Neurosurgery 1985; 17:1–5.
30. Rasmussen T. Surgery of epilepsy associated with brain tumors. Adv Neurol 1975; 8:227–239.
31. Foy PM. Copeland G, Shaw M. The incidence of postoperative seizures: Acta Neurochir 1981; 55:253–264.
32. Boarini D, Beck D, Van Guilder J. Postoperative prophylactic anticonvulsant therapy in cerebral gliomas. Neurosurgery 1985; 16:1690–292.
33. North JB. Anticonvulsant prophylaxis in neurosurgery. Br J Neurosurg 1989; 3:425–428.
34. Rovit R, et al. Management of patients following brain tumor surgery—part II: preoperative preparation, general and postoperative considerations. Contemp Neurosurg 1986; 8:1–6.
35. Niedermeyer E. The epilepsies—diagnosis and management. Philadelphia: Urbansi Schwarzenberg, 1990.
36. North JB, Penhall R, Hanieh A, et al. Phenytoin and postoperative epilepsy. a double blind study. J Neurosurg 1983; 58:672–677.
37. Woodbury D. Mechanisms of action of anticonvulsants. In: Jasper HH, Ward AA, Pope A, eds. Basic mechanisms of the epilepsies. Boston: Little, Brown & Co, 1969:41–75.
38. Hauptmann A. Luminal bei epilepsie. Munchen Med Wochenschr 1912; 59:1907–1918.
39. Rogers M, Traystman R. An overview of the intracranial vault: physiology and philosophy. Critical Care Clin North Am 1985; 1:1–15.
40. Shapiro H. Intracranial hypertension. Anesthesiology 1975; 43:445–471.
41. Haun J. Cerebral edema and neurointensive care. Pediatr Clin North Am 1980; 3:587–631.
42. Miller D, Becker D, Ward J, et al. Significance of intracranial hypertension in severe head injury. J Neurosurg 1977; 47:503–516.
43. Simon RH. Brain tumors in pregnancy. Semin Neurol 1988; 8:214–221.
44. Roelvink CA, Kamphorst W, VanAlphen HAM, Rao BR. Pregnancy-related primary brain and spinal tumors. Arch Neurol 1987; 44:209–215.
45. Ishizuka T, Tomoda Y, Kaseki S, et al. Intracranial metastasis of choriocarcinoma. Cancer 1983; 52:896–903.
46. Preston-Martin S, Mack W, Henderson BE. Risk factors for gliomas and meningiomas in males in Los Angeles county. Cancer Res 1989; 49:6137–6143.
47. Weinreb J. Obstetrics. In: Stark DD, Bradley WG Jr, eds. Magnetic resonance imaging. St Louis: CV Mosby, 1988:1297–1322.

48. Pavlicek W. Safety considerations. In: Stark DD, Bradley WG Jr, eds. Magnetic resonance imaging. St Louis: CV Mosby, 1988:244–257.

49. National Radiological Protection Board, U.K. Revised guidelines on acceptable limits of exposure during nuclear magnetic resonance clinical imaging. Br J Radiol 1983; 56:974–977.

50. Mole RH. Radiation effects on pre-natal development and their radiological significance. Br J Radiol 1979; 52:89–101.

51. National Council on Radiation Protection and Measurements. Medical radiation exposure of pregnant and potentially pregnant women. NCRP Report No. 54, 1977.

52. McCullough EC, Payne JT. Patient dosage in computed tomography. Radiology 1978; 129:457–463.

53. Wagner LK, Lester RG, Saldana LR. Exposure of the pregnant patient to diagnostic radiation: a guide to medical management. Philadelphia: JB Lippincott, 1985.

54. Kiekegaard A. Incidence and diagnosis of deep vein thrombosis associated with pregnancy. Acta Obstet Gynecol Scand 1983; 62:239–243.

55. Rodesch F, Camos M, Ermans, AM, Dodion J, Delange F. Adverse effect of amniofetography on fetal thyroid function. Am J Obstet Gynecol 1976; 126:723–726.

56. Thomas RL. Corticosteroid therapy in the prevention of respiratory distress syndrome. In: Niebyl JR, ed. Drug use in pregnancy, 2nd ed. Philadelphia: Lea & Febiger, 1988:117–126.

57. Collaborative group on antenatal steroid therapy. Effect of antenatal dexamethasone administration on the prevention of respiratory distress syndrome. Am J Obstet Gynecol 1981; 141:276–287.

58. Collaborative group on antenatal steroid therapy. Effect of antenatal dexamethasone administration on the infant: long term follow-up. J Pediatr 1984; 104:259–267.

59. Osathanondh A, Tulchinsky D, Kamali H, Fencl M deM, Taeusch HW. Dexamethasone levels in treated pregnant women and newborn infants. J Pediatr 1977; 90:617–620.

60. Sidhu RK, Hawkins DR. Corticosteroids. Clin Obstet Gynaecol 1981; 8:383–404.

61. Reinisch JM, Simon NG, Karow WG, Gandelman R. Prenatal exposure to prednisone in humans and animals retards intrauterine growth. Science 1978; 202:436–438.

62. Evans MI, Chrousos GP, Mann DW, et al. Pharmacologic suppression of the fetal adrenal gland in utero. JAMA 1985; 253:1015–1020.

63. Byyny RL. Withdrawal from glucocorticoid therapy. N Engl J Med 1976; 195:30–32.

64. Basso A, Fernandez A, Althabe O, Sabini G, Piriz H, Belitsky R. Passage of mannitol from mother to amniotic fluid and fetus. Obstet Gynecol 1977; 49:628–631.

65. Bain MD, Copas KD, Landon MJ, Stacey TE. In vivo permeability of the human placenta to insulin and mannitol. J Physiol 1988; 399:313–319.

66. Brent RL. The effects of embryonic and fetal exposure to x-rays, microwaves, and ultrasound. Clin Perinatol 1986; 13:615–648.

67. Hochberg FH, Pruitt A. Assumptions in the radiotherapy of glioblastoma. Neurology 1980; 30:907–911.

68. National Council on Radiation Protection and Measurements. Structural shielding design and evaluation for medical use of x-rays and gamma rays of energies up to 10 MeV. NCRP Report No. 49, 1976.

69. Nelson DF, Urtasun RC, Saunders WM, Gutin PH, Sheline GE. Recent and current investigations of radiation therapy of malignant gliomas. Semin Oncol 1986; 13:46–55.

70. Krishnaswamy V. Dose distribution around an I-125 seed source in tissue. Radiology 1978; 126:489–491.

71. Shalek RJ, Stovall M. Dosimetry in implant therapy. In: Attix FH, Tochilin E, eds. Radiation dosimetry, 2nd ed. New York: Academic Press, 1969:743–807.

72. Doll DC, Ringenberg QS, Yarbro JW. Management of cancer during pregnancy. Arch Intern Med 1988; 148:2058–2064.

73. Transplacental carcinogenesis. Lancet 1976; 1:506.

74. Schapira DV, Chudley AE. Successful pregnancy following continuous chemotherapy before conception and throughout pregnancy. Cancer 1984; 54:800–803.

75. Magyar DM, Marshall JR. Pituitary tumors and pregnancy. Am J Obstet Gynecol 1978; 132:739–751.

76. Kelly WF, Doyle FH, Mashiter K, et al. Pregnancies in women with hyperprolactinemia: clinical course and obstetric complications of 41 pregnancies in 27 women. Br J Obstet Gynaecol 1979; 86:698–705.

77. Dommerhold HBR, Assies J, Van der Werf AJM. Growth of a prolactinoma during pregnancy. Br J Obstet Gynaecol 1981; 88:62–70.

78. O'Donovan PA, O'Donovan RJ, Ritchie EH, et al. Apoplexy into a prolactin secreting macroadenoma during early pregnancy with successful outcome. A case report. Br J Obstet Gynaecol 1986; 93:389–391.

79. Wilson CB. A decade of pituitary microsurgery: the Herbert Olivecrona lecture. J Neurosurg 1984; 61:814–833.

80. Samaan NA, Schultz PN, Leavens TA, et al. Pregnancy after treatment in patients with prolactinoma: operations versus bromocriptine. Am J Obstet Gynecol 1986; 155:1300–1305.

81. Hammon CH, Haney AF, Land MR, et al. The outcome of pregnancy in patients with treated and untreated prolactin secreting pituitary tumors. Am J Obstet Gynecol 1983; 147:148–157.

82. Barron WM. The pregnant surgical patient: medical evaluation and management. Ann Intern Med 1984; 101:683–691.

83. Turpie AGG, Gallus AS, Beattie WS, Hirsh J. Prevention of venous thrombosis in patients with intracranial disease by intermittent pneumatic compression of the calf. Neurology 1977; 27:435–438.

84. Hamod KA, Khouzani VA. Antibiotics in pregnancy. In: Niebyl JR, ed. Drug use in pregnancy, 2nd ed. Philadelphia: Lea & Febiger, 1988:29–36.

85. Soutoul JH, Gouase A, Gallier J, Santini JJ. Neurochirurgie et grossesse. Rev Fr Gynecol 1971; 66:603–618.

11

Tumors of the Pituitary Gland

Daniel L. Barrow and George T. Tindall
Emory University School of Medicine,
Atlanta, Georgia

I. INTRODUCTION

Neoplastic disorders of the pituitary gland may present in a variety of ways owing to the gland's major role in endocrine homeostasis and its anatomical location. The region of the pituitary gland and sella turcica has an intimate relation with several tissue types, including neural, endocrine, vascular, meningeal, and skeletal. Therefore, a myriad of pathological possibilities may arise from this small anatomical area. However, the majority of neoplastic processes arising from the region of the pituitary gland are pituitary adenomas. Therefore, this chapter will concentrate primarily on these lesions. Pituitary adenomas are readily treatable entities, often curable, and generally carry an excellent prognosis if recognized and managed appropriately.

II. CLINICAL FEATURES

Pituitary adenomas usually come to clinical attention in one of three ways. First, in the current era of modern imaging techniques, such as computed tomography (CT) and magnetic resonance imaging (MRI), it is not uncommon for an asymptomatic pituitary adenoma to be discovered incidentally on a neuroimaging study being performed for unrelated reasons, such as following a head injury or evaluation of headache or other nonspecific neurological symptoms. Second, symptomatic lesions generally come to medical attention as a result of an endocrinopathy related to excessive production of one or more pituitary hormones. Third, pituitary adenomas may come to attention as a result of mass and pressure effects of the enlarging adenoma on surrounding intracranial structures.

A. Endocrinopathy

The pituitary gland is divided into two lobes: the anterior lobe (adenohypophysis), and the posterior lobe (neurohypophysis). The anterior lobe is the primary source of the anterior pituitary hormones: thyrotropin (thyroid-stimulating hormone; TSH), corticotropin (adrenocorticotropin; ACTH), growth hormone (somatotropin; GH), prolactin (luteotropin hormone; PRL), melanocyte-stimulating hormone (MSH), luteinizing hormone (LH), and follicle-stimulating hormone (FSH). Pituitary adenomas may present through excessive secretion of any of these hormones. The three most commonly encountered clinical syndromes that result from a hormone-secreting pituitary adenoma, in order of frequency, are (1) the amenorrhea–galactorrhea syndrome (hyperprolactinemia), (2) acromegaly (excess GH), and (3) Cushing's disease (excess ACTH with hypercortisolism). Pituitary adenomas secreting excessive amounts of TSH, LH, or FSH have been described, but are rare.

A pituitary adenoma secreting excessive amounts of prolactin, the prolactinoma, is most common in women. The clinical presentation usually consists of infertility, amenorrhea or irregular menstrual periods, and galactorrhea (1). The discharge from the nipples is usually a thin, milky white fluid that may appear spontaneously or in response to nipple manipulation. Galactorrhea is less common in men with prolactinomas. Hyperprolactinemia in men may cause impotence and hypogonadism. Because of the relative paucity of clinical symptoms in males, prolactinomas are usually significantly larger at presentation than in women, with the latter often presenting with symptomatic tumors smaller than 1 cm in diameter. It has been postulated that hyperprolactinemia may be a predisposing factor in osteoporosis (2).

Patients with acromegaly have a distinctive appearance that includes overgrowth of the head and extremities. The fingers and toes are noticeably widened, and patients often report a progressive increase in shoe and ring size. Additionally, patients with acromegaly have a reduced life expectancy owing to a combination of impaired glucose tolerance, cardiomyopathy, and hypertension (3,4).

The clinical characteristics of patients with Cushing's disease are identical to those of any patient with hypercortisolism and are easily recognized by an experienced clinician. In the early stages of the disease, however, the diagnosis may be overlooked. The features of Cushing's disease include centripetal obesity with "moon" facies, "buffalo hump," abdominal striae, hirsutism, acne, glucose intolerance, hypertension, and psychiatric disturbances. As with acromegaly, patients with Cushing's disease have a reduced life expectancy (5).

The typical clinical features of various hypersecreting pituitary tumors are summarized in Table 1.

Table 1 Clinical Features of Endocrinopathies

Syndrome	Hormonal Excess	Clinical Features
Acromegaly	GH	Enlargement of hands and feet, distortion of facial features, peripheral nerve entrapment syndromes, gigantism (when prepubertal)
Cushing's disease	ACTH	Centripetal obesity, purple striae, ecchymoses, hirsutism, psychiatric disturbances, hypertension, glucose intolerance
Nelson's syndrome	ACTH	Hyperpigmentation
Amenorrhea–galactorrhea syndrome	PRL	Amenorrhea or oligomenorrhea, variable galactorrhea
Thyroid-stimulating (TSH)-secreting adenoma (rare)	TSH	Features of hyperthyroidism
Luteinizing hormone (LH)- or follicle-stimulating hormone (FSH)-secreting adenoma (rare)	LH, FSH	No known specific clinical features

Source: Ref. 75.

B. Mass Effects of Pituitary Tumors

Any pituitary tumor may reach a size at which it produces symptoms by impinging on one or more surrounding anatomical structures, usually the optic chiasm and the adjacent pituitary gland. Presentation by mass effect is most common for nonfunctional or nonsecretory adenomas, although secretory tumors may present in this manner. Other sellar and parasellar lesions, both neoplastic and nonneoplastic, may produce mass effect symptoms similar to or identical with those caused by a pituitary adenoma. Clinical findings caused by distortion or compression of surrounding structures by a pituitary tumor include headache, visual impairment, hypopituitarism, extraocular palsies, facial pain, seizures, and those related to hydrocephalus or pituitary apoplexy.

Sellar and parasellar lesions, including nonfunctional pituitary adenomas other than a prolactinoma, may cause modest elevations of serum prolactin (30–100 ng/ml). The elevated prolactin levels in these instances result from a mechanism referred to as the *stalk effect*. The stalk effect is characterized by an elevation of serum prolactin caused by the impaired delivery of the prolactin-inhibiting factor (PIF), dopamine, to the pituitary (6,7). The PIF normally passes down the stalk from the hypothalamus in the hypophyseal portal system and inhibits the release of prolactin from the normal adenohypophyseal lactotrophs (8). Any structural lesion that compresses the stalk will interfere with the delivery of PIF to the lactotrophs, which respond by secreting an unrestrained, elevated level of prolactin, usually in the range of 30–100 ng/ml. Lesions causing hyperprolactinemia by this mechanism have been referred to as *pseudoprolactinomas*.

A pituitary tumor that produces and secretes an abnormally high level of prolactin is referred to as a *prolactinoma*. Here, the mechanism of hyperprolactinemia is due to direct tumor secretion, not stalk effect, and in these cases, serum prolactin levels are usually higher than 150 ng/ml.

The characteristic visual field defect caused by a pituitary adenoma is a bitemporal hemianopia caused by compression of the optic chiasm. Decreased visual acuity, with optic pallor or optic atrophy, may also occur. Pituitary adenomas cause headache by stretching or distorting the pain-sensitive diaphragm sella or adjacent dura. Compression of the normal pituitary gland will result in progressive pituitary dysfunction and, ultimately, panhypopituitarism. Invasion of the adjacent cavernous sinus by pituitary tumors may cause compressive cranial neuropathies of the cranial nerves enclosed in the wall or interior of the cavernous sinus. Clinically, this will result in diplopia, ptosis, and facial numbness or pain.

If the suprasellar portion of a pituitary tumor obstructs the foramina of Monro of the third ventricle, the patient will develop obstructive hydrocephalus. This may cause headache, papilledema, lethargy, and if untreated, may lead to coma or death. On rare occasions, a very large pituitary tumor will irritate or compress the medial temporal lobe and result in seizures.

Pituitary apoplexy refers to the acute onset of neurological signs and symptoms resulting from the rapid enlargement of a pituitary adenoma caused by hemorrhage or infarction, with resultant sudden swelling (9,10,11). Patients may present with a constellation of symptoms that mimic a spontaneous subarachnoid hemorrhage, including sudden onset of severe headache, nausea, vomiting, photophobia, nuchal rigidity, and alteration in the level of consciousness. Additionally, they may exhibit a sudden decrease of vision, diplopia, and the clinical findings of acute adrenal insufficiency. Such patients should be diagnosed and treated expeditiously.

III. CLINICAL EVALUATION

A. Endocrinological Testing

Endocrinological evaluation of patients suspected of harboring a pituitary tumor includes an assessment of pituitary hormone reserve to detect hypopituitarism and special tests to evaluate for excessive secretion of pituitary hormones by functional pituitary adenomas.

1. Assessment of Pituitary Hormone Reserve

Determination of the status of anterior pituitary function includes assessment of the thyroidal, adrenal, and gonadal axes. Posterior pituitary function is assessed by determining if there is adequate antidiuretic hormone (ADH). It is not necessary to routinely test adult patients for deficiencies of PRL or GH, as these situations are not clinically significant.

Thyroidal Axis   Determination of serum thyroxine (total or free T_4) is an appropriate screening test for the hypothalamic–pituitary–thyroid axis. If the T_4 level is normal, one can reasonably assume that this axis is intact. If the serum T_4 is low, if hypothyroidism is clinically suspected, or if more precise testing is indicated, a thyrotropin-releasing hormone (TRH) stimulation test can be performed. Following the intravenous administration of 500 μg of TRH, there normally should be a twofold increase in the peak serum TSH value at 30 min. An impaired TSH response to TRH in a patient with a low serum T_4 level indicates a pituitary abnormality.

Adrenal Axis.   A normal morning serum or plasma cortisol level is a strong indicator of an intact hypothalamic–pituitary–adrenal axis. A simple stimulation test using cosyntropin (a potent preparation of ACTH) will add to the reliability of this determination. This is performed by obtaining a baseline blood sample for cortisol, giving 250 μg of cosyntropin intramuscularly or intravenously, and repeating cortisol samples at 30 or 60 min, or both. A normal response is a plasma cortisol rise of more than 7 $\mu g/dl$ and a peak value of over 20 $\mu g/dl$.

A variety of more sensitive tests of adrenal insufficiency may be performed and include an insulin tolerance test, the metyrapone test, and the measurement of ACTH levels after the administration of corticotropin-releasing factor (CRF).

Gonadal Axis.   In addition to a careful history and physical examination, integrity of the hypothalamic–pituitary–gonadal axis is verified by serum gonadotropins (LH and FSH) and sex steroid (estradiol in women, testosterone in men) assessment.

Prolactin.   Serum PRL levels should be measured in all patients with suspected hormonally silent or nonsecretory pituitary tumors. Levels ranging from more than 25 to less than 150 ng/ml may be due to pressure of the tumor on the hypothalamus or pituitary stalk. Levels over 150 ng/ml are usually due to a prolactinoma.

Posterior Pituitary.   Patients with a deficiency of antidiuretic hormone (ADH) will usually provide a history of nocturia, urinary frequency, and polydipsia. If there is clinical suspicion of diabetes insipidus, a 24-h urine collection should be performed to determine volume, with further tests of ADH done if volume is excessive. A more detailed evaluation of ADH requires a water deprivation test to demonstrate normal urinary concentration or a hypertonic saline infusion test to measure the ADH response to an osmotic stimulus.

2. Special Endocrine Testing

Additional endocrine tests that are obtained in certain endocrinopathies include the following: *acromegaly*: GH levels, somatomedin-C levels, glucose suppression, TRH test, growth hormone releasing factor (GHRF) levels; *Cushing's syndrome (disease)*: urinary free cortisol, low- or high-dose dexamethasone suppression, metyrapone test, ACTH levels; *prolactinoma*: serum PRL levels × 2; chlorpromazine (CPZ) test, TRH test.

In these situations testing is useful in making a positive diagnosis of the specific endocrinopathy, in identifying the source of the disorder (i.e., the pituitary in Cushing's syndrome), and in evaluating the effectiveness of a given therapy. Recommended tests for each of the endocrinopathies follow.

Acromegaly.   In addition to the baseline endocrine studies just cited, patients with suspected or proved acromegaly should undergo special studies including basal levels of GH, GH–glucose suppression test, determination of somatomedin-C levels, TRH stimulation test, and GHRF levels.

Basal levels of GH are elevated (i.e., over 10 ng/ml) in about 90–95% of patients with acromegaly. When 100 g of glucose is orally administered to a normal individual, serum GH levels fall to less than 5 ng/ml when measured 2 h later. In patients with acromegaly, the elevated levels of GH will not suppress to the 5 ng/ml level during the 2 h following a glucose load. In some cases of acromegaly, a paradoxical rise in the GH levels occurs.

Clemmons et al. found that somatomedin-C levels, determined by radioimmunoassay, appeared to provide a reliable means of confirming the diagnosis of acromegaly (12). In their study, the mean fasting serum somatomedin-C concentration was 6.8 U/ml (range, 2.6–21.7) for acromegalic subjects as compared with 0.67 U/ml (range, 0.31–1.4) for normal subjects (12). The determination of somatomedin-C levels is useful in patients who are suspected of having acromegaly, but who do not have significantly elevated basal GH levels. Somatomedin-C levels may also be an indicator of response to treatment.

Thyrotropin-releasing hormone test. Although the TRH test is not essential in establishing the laboratory diagnosis of acromegaly, it has potential value in assessing the effectiveness of treatment. A significant rise in serum GH follows the administration of TRH in acromegalic patients, as opposed to no significant change in GH in normal subjects. This laboratory finding may have predictive value for long-term cure following surgery. Patients who appear to be cured immediately after surgery, but who show an abnormal GH response to TRH, seem to be at greater risk for recurrence than patients who show normal responses following an operation.

Growth hormone-releasing factor levels. Circulating GHRF levels in acromegaly are generally below the sensitivity of present radioimmunoassays, but are measurable by bioassays. This is also true of levels in normal patients. As the assays become more sensitive, there may be other indications for this test, but the only current indication is to diagnose acromegaly caused by tumors producing ectopic GHRF (13).

Cushing's Syndrome (Disease). There are two important phases in the special endocrine evaluation of patients with Cushing's syndrome. These include establishing the diagnosis of hypercortisolism and identifying the source of the disease.

Establishing diagnosis of hypercortisolism (Cushing's syndrome). Measurement of free cortisol in a 24-h urine sample, urinary free cortisol (UFC), in the unstressed patient is an excellent assessment of cortisol production. An elevation of UFC, especially greater than twice the upper limit of normal, is strongly suggestive of Cushing's syndrome. For most patients, a 24-h urine sample can be accurately collected on an outpatient basis.

Another useful screening test for Cushing's syndrome is the overnight dexamethasone suppression test. A dose of 1 mg of dexamethasone is administered at bedtime and plasma cortisol determined the following morning. If plasma cortisol does not fall to less than 5 ng/dl, the diagnosis of Cushing's syndrome is very likely. *Normal* suppression nearly excludes Cushing's syndrome. The determination of UFC in a 24-h urine sample coupled with the overnight dexamethasone suppression test forms a very powerful screening study that can be done on outpatients to establish the presence of hypercortisolism.

Plasma cortisol levels in normal subjects follow the circadian rhythm of ACTH secretion. The values are relatively high early in the waking day, become low as time for sleep approaches, and reach a nadir during the middle of sleep. Patients with Cushing's syndrome tend to lose the normal circadian rhythm and have relatively high values at all hours. In Cushing's syndrome, plasma cortisol concentrations usually range from 15 to 25 ng/dl, regardless of time of day, whereas in normal subjects morning values range from 12 to 25 ng/dl, and late-evening values from 1 to 8 ng/dl. There is considerably more overlap in morning values between normal subjects and patients with Cushing's syndrome than with late-evening values, which are more diagnostic.

Identifying the source of the disease. Once the diagnosis of hypercortisolism (Cushing's syndrome) is suggested, more specialized tests are used to determine the cause. The most common cause is a partially autonomous, ACTH-secreting pituitary adenoma (Cushing's disease), which accounts for about 60% of cases (14). A primary adrenal disease, either an adrenal adenoma or adrenal carcinoma, accounts for about 25% of cases. An ectopic source of ACTH is found in about 15% of cases, usually from one of the following neoplasms: small-cell carcinoma of the lung, bronchial or intestinal carcinoid, thymoma, pancreatic islet cell tumor, medullary carcinoma of the thyroid, or pheochromocytoma. These three major causes of Cushing's syndrome—pituitary, adrenal, or ectopic ACTH—can be distinguished on the basis of biochemical and morphological studies. However, the etiological diagnosis of Cushing's syndrome remains one of the most difficult in neuroendocrinology.

Currently, the major tests used in the differential diagnosis of Cushing's syndrome are (1) dexamethasone suppression test; (2) inferior petrosal sinus blood sampling for ACTH levels before and during administration of CRF; (3) radiologic studies (e.g., MRI or CT of sella, adrenal glands). A summary of typical laboratory findings in various types of Cushing's syndrome/disease is shown in Table 2.

Standard dexamethasone suppression test. Originally developed by Liddle, this test consists of evaluating the response of urinary excretion of 17-hydroxycorticosteroids (17-OHCS) to step-wise increases in dexamethasone (15). Serial 24-h urine collections are done for 6 days. The first 2 days are basal collections. The next 2 days the patient takes 0.5 mg dexamethasone (low-dose) every 6 h for 48 h, and the final 2 days the patient takes 2 mg dexamethasone (high-dose) every 6 h for 48 h. All collections are corrected to creatinine excretion and expressed as mg 17-OHCS per gram creatinine per 24 h. Basal values greater than 7 mg/g creatinine per 24 h are elevated. Normal individuals suppress on low-dose dexamethasone to less than 50% of basal or less than 4 mg/g creatinine per 24 h on the second day of collection. Patients with Cushing's disease fail to suppress on low-dose dexamethasone but suppress to less than 50% of basal levels on high-dose dexamethasone (see Table 2). Patients with primary adrenal disease or ectopic ACTH production fail to

Table 2 Typical Laboratory Findings in Types of Cushing's Syndrome

Tests	Normal subjects	Cushing's disease pituitary origin	Ectopic ACTH syndrome	Adrenal tumor
Plasma cortisol	10–25 μg/dl	High	High	High
	Rhythmic	Nonrhythmic	Nonrhythmic	Nonrhythmic
UFC	Normal	Increased	Increased	Increased
Response to low-dose dexamethasone				
Urinary 17-0HCS	Decreased	No change	No change	No change
Plasma cortisol	Decreased	No change	No change	No change
Response to high-dose dexamethasone				
Urinary 17-0HCS	Decreased	Decreased	No change	No change
Plasma cortisol	Decreased	Decreased	No change	No change
Response to metyrapone				
Urinary 17-0HCS	Increased	Increased	No change	No change (rarely increased)

Source: Ref. 76.

suppress to either low- or high-dose dexamethasone. This test is very sensitive and specific when done in the standard fashion. Major factors can confuse interpretation, especially alterations in dexamethasone metabolism and periodic hormonogenesis, which can be found with all three causes of Cushing's syndrome.

3. Prolactinomas

In patients with suspected or proven prolactinomas, the baseline studies, as outlined previously, are obtained. In addition, we believe that at least two separate determinations of fasting morning serum PRL values should be obtained. For practical purposes, serum PRL levels over 150 ng/ml are diagnostic of a PRL-secreting pituitary tumor (prolactinoma). Values under 150 ng/ml and, certainly, values between 20 and 100 ng/ml can be caused by several other conditions, including hypothyroidism and ingestion of certain drugs. Pituitary or suprasellar lesions (including nonfunctional pituitary tumors) that interfere with the normal delivery of PIF to the adenohypophysis can cause hyperprolactinemia. Usually, the serum PRL values are less than 100 ng/ml in this situation.

B. Neuro-ophthalmological Evaluation

Because of the proximity of the pituitary gland to the optic nerves and chiasm, patients with sellar and parasellar neoplasms frequently develop abnormalities of visual acuity and fields. Consequently, we recommend a formal neuro-ophthalmological evaluation preoperatively in all patients with lesions potentially compromising the optic apparatus. This includes quantitative visual field testing using a Goldman perimeter (an assessment of visual acuity), and ophthalmoscopic assessment of the optic discs. These studies are also important in the postoperative evaluation to determine the effectiveness of therapy and in following patients who are being managed nonoperatively.

In the situations in which a formal neuro-ophthalmological evaluation cannot be obtained, some bedside methods are useful in evaluating the integrity of the visual system. In addition to testing visual fields by confrontation, the examiner may also place two similarly colored objects in different visual fields (temporal and nasal) of the same eye. The patient is instructed to maintain fixation on the examiner's nose, and each eye is tested separately. The object seen in the intact hemifield will appear brighter or richer in hue than the other.

Testing for an afferent pupillary defect or Marcus–Gunn pupil is a sensitive method for detecting an optic neuropathy. The test is performed by first shining a bright light in one eye, observing the speed and extent of pupillary contraction, and then quickly moving the light to the other eye and making the same observations. In a normal patient, the initial reaction of the pupil to illumination is constriction, and this response should be bilaterally symmetric. On the side of a lesion of the prechiasmal portion of the optic nerve, there will be initial dilatation, as opposed to normal constriction, of the pupil, indicating a relative afferent pupillary defect.

C. Neuroradiological Evaluation

The field of medical imaging has undergone a technological revolution over the past two decades. This dramatic change in imaging has been particularly evident in neuroimaging. In imaging lesions in the sellar and parasellar areas, a number of indirect and relatively inaccurate procedures have given way to the refined and graphic images of CT and MRI (see Chaps. 8 and 9). Most of the studies previously used need only be mentioned for historic purposes, as CT and MRI alone, or in combination, provide excellent images of most lesions in this anatomical area. Previously used neurodiagnostic-imaging modalities include plain skull films, sellar polytomography, pneumoencephalography, metrizamide cisternography, and cerebral angiography. Plain skull films are still useful in assessing the contour and pneumatization of the sphenoid sinus for the surgeon planning transsphenoidal operations, and cerebral angiography is necessary to provide accurate detail of the intracranial vasculature in planning surgical approaches to intracranial aneurysms or vascular malformations in the parasellar area. However, CT or MRI, or both, provide images that permit one to make a well-defined differential diagnosis and to plan an appropriate surgical approach. An MRI study will also demonstrate a flow void created by flowing blood, to rule out the presence of an intracranial aneurysm mimicking a pituitary adenoma.

1.   Pituitary Microadenomas

Pituitary microadenomas are arbitrarily defined as adenomas that are equal to or less than 10 mm in diameter. Both CT and MRI are useful in demonstrating pituitary microadenomas, although MRI is a superior technique where accuracy approaches 70% (16). The administration of an iodinated contrast medium will improve the CT detection rate. Following the infusion of contrast, the normal pituitary will enhance immediately, whereas the adenoma will not enhance for 30 min or more. Typically, a pituitary microadenoma will appear as a low-density area, located laterally in the gland. The diaphragm sella may be slightly elevated and the pituitary stalk may be shifted.

The T1-weighted coronal MRI is the most useful sequence for visualizing the pituitary gland, adenoma, carotid arteries, infundibulum, and optic chiasm. Pituitary microadenomas will appear as areas of decreased signal intensity on T1-weighted images. With the use of the paramagnetic contrast agent, gadolinium-DTPA, the normal pituitary gland, infundibulum, and cavernous sinus will enhance, whereas the microadenoma will not immediately enhance (Fig. 1).

2.   Pituitary Macroadenomas

Pituitary macroadenomas are arbitrarily defined as adenomas that are equal to or larger than 10 mm in diameter. These larger pituitary tumors are readily detected by both CT and MRI. On CT, pituitary macroadenomas appear as a well-delineated mass that enhances homogeneously after the administration of intravenous contrast (Fig. 2).

The MRI study has some advantages over CT in imaging pituitary macroadenomas. It will image the lesion in multiple planes, better demonstrate the relation of the tumor to the optic chiasm, and will also rule out the presence of an intra- or parasellar aneurysm. The T1-weighted image provides the best anatomical detail. Pituitary adenomas are isointense with brain, but enhance following the administration of contrast (Fig. 3). Magnetic resonance imaging is helpful in determining whether a large adenoma has invaded the cavernous sinus (Fig. 4). Areas of cyst formation and hemorrhage are well delineated by both CT and MRI, although hemorrhage is visualized to better advantage on MRI. Acute hemorrhage within a tumor will show up as an area of high signal on T1-weighted images and as either high or low signal on T2-weighted images.

IV.   TREATMENT

A variety of treatment options and combinations of treatments are available for pituitary tumors. These options include periodic follow-up with no specific treatment, surgery, medical therapy, and radiation therapy.

A.   Natural History

The natural history of pituitary adenomas is not completely known. Small incidental adenomas are a relatively common finding at both autopsy or on imaging studies. Furthermore, an unknown number of pituitary microadenomas will remain dormant, and some have actually been shown to decrease in size and disappear on imaging studies (17). Therefore, the mere presence of a pituitary microadenoma does not necessitate treatment. For asymptomatic or relatively asymptomatic

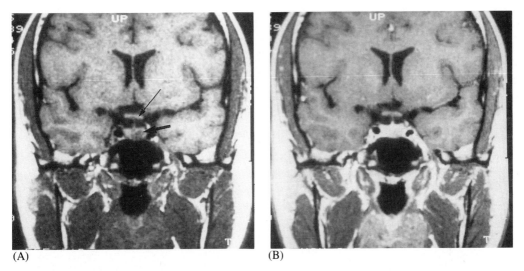

(A)   (B)

Figure 1 (A) Coronal MRI demonstrates a low-intensity microadenoma on the left side of the pituitary gland (short arrow). The optic chiasm is well visualized (long arrow). (B) Following the administration of gadolinium, there is enhancement of the normal gland, but not of the microadenoma.

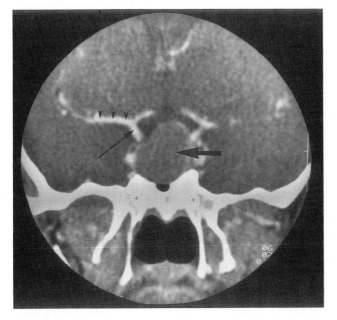

Figure 2 Coronal contrast-enhanced CT shows a large pituitary tumor with suprasellar extension (short arrow). Note enhancement of the internal carotid (long arrow) and middle cerebral arteries (arrowheads).

patients, periodic endocrinological, neuro-ophthalmological, and radiologic follow-up may be an appropriate method for management.

Macroadenomas, on the other hand, have shown their growth potential and, in our opinion, usually require some form of treatment. This is particularly true for lesions associated with visual loss. Likewise, Cushing's disease and acromegaly are entities that can impair health and may significantly reduce life expectancy (3–5); thus, these patients require some form of definitive

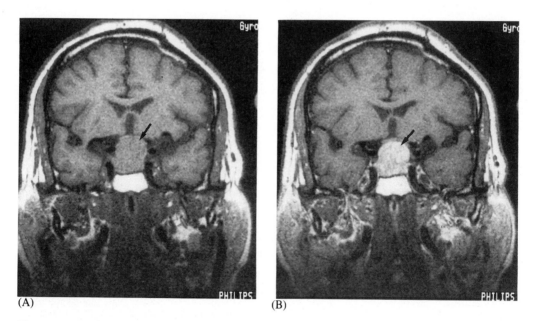

Figure 3 Coronal MRI (A) before and (B) after gadolinium reveals an enhancing sellar mass, with suprasellar extension (arrow).

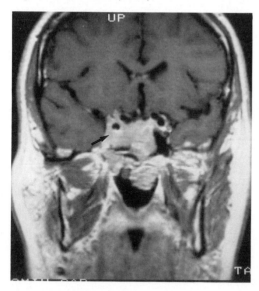

Figure 4 Coronal MRI demonstrates a large pituitary adenoma invading the right cavernous sinus (arrow).

treatment. Hyperprolactinemia may be associated with an accelerated form of osteopenia which, in turn, may set the stage for later osteoporosis (2). This potential complication is the only known health consequence of this endocrine state.

B. Medical Treatment

Medical options for managing pituitary adenomas depend largely on the type of tumor. Specific tumor types have reasonable medical options for treatment, whereas other tumors have either no or poor medical options.

1. Prolactinomas

Prolactin-secreting pituitary adenomas have the most widely used and studied medical option in the form of the dopamine agonist, bromocriptine. Bromocriptine is a potent inhibitor of the synthesis and release of PRL by the pituitary gland and is effective in reducing hyperprolactinemia, regardless of its etiology. Unfortunately, this drug has no tumoricidal activity. It reduces the size of tumors by reducing cytoplasmic volume (18–27). Consequently, when the drug is withdrawn, the tumor will usually reexpand, the symptoms will recur, and the hyperprolactinemia will return in most patients with these tumors (28,29).

Bromocriptine is well tolerated by most patients. Postural hypotension is a common side effect, but may be managed by initially administering small doses of the drug in the evening and gradually increasing to a full dose.

Although there does not appear to be any increased incidence of fetal abnormalities or multiple births with the use of bromocriptine during pregnancy, most United States physicians recommend discontinuation of the drug during pregnancy (30). Occasionally, this can result in rapid enlargement of the tumor and may require urgent surgical treatment. This potential threat occurs only in larger tumors.

The short-term use of bromocriptine for 6–8 weeks before surgical treatment has been advocated as a means of reducing the size of prolactinomas preoperatively (28,29). It is believed that this reduction would enhance the cure rate with subsequent transphenoidal surgery. Although some authors have reported that this may be true, it has been our experience that preoperative bromocriptine therapy for 6 weeks does not favorably enhance the surgical results.

The long-term use (1 year or more) of bromocriptine, however, is associated with a significant reduction in the expected surgical cure rate when compared with patients not taking the drug (31,32). This appears to be due to an increase in fibrosis of the tumor, making clean, complete surgical removal less likely (31,32).

Another potential complication of bromocriptine treatment, especially with large tumors, is the development of a cerebrospinal fluid (CSF) leak during treatment. This is due to exposure of a defect in the sellar floor and dura after a responsive tumor shrinks as a result of bromocriptine therapy (33–36).

Bromocriptine is a good option in the management of many patients with prolactinomas. Especially in patients with excessive levels of serum PRL (e.g., over 750 ng/ml), the chance of surgical cure is low, and bromocriptine will usually control tumor size and PRL levels. (37)

2. Growth Hormone-Secreting Tumors

The medical options for GH-secreting tumors are not as practical or effective as for PRL-secreting tumors. Some GH-secreting tumors will respond to bromocriptine, but generally require larger doses of the drug and frequently do not result in normalization of GH levels, if they respond at all.

The other medical option is a somatostatin analogue, octreotide. This drug has been shown to decrease GH levels and tumor size in a significant number of patients (38–40). Unfortunately, the drug must be given subcutaneously in three divided doses daily and is expensive. As with bromocriptine, the agent is not tumoricidal and must be taken indefinitely.

3. Corticotropin-Secreting Tumors

Again, there are no good, practical, long-term medical options for Cushing's disease. Many drugs have been used, including adrenal toxins, serotonin antagonists, and dopamine agonists, with variable results. The most commonly used medical treatment currently is ketoconazole, an antifungal agent that inhibits adrenal steroidogenesis (41,42).

Medical therapy is generally reserved for patients who are medically unsuitable for surgery, for surgical and radiation therapy failures and, occasionally, for preparation of a patient for surgery.

4. Nonfunctional Pituitary Tumors

Occasional nonfunctional tumors have been reported to respond to bromocriptine, but for practical purposes, there is no specific medical therapy available for this group of tumors.

C. Surgical Treatment

Most pituitary tumors are best-managed by surgical removal. This is particularly true of those tumors for which there is no good medical option. Although the surgical approach is dictated by anatomy of the tumor, almost all pituitary adenomas are most safely and effectively managed by transphenoidal microsurgery. The advantages of the transphenoidal operation include a more rapid and direct approach to the pituitary gland; better differentiation of tumor from gland; less probability of injury to the optic chiasm, nerves, and olfactory tract; and less trauma to the patient. The shape and direction of tumor growth are more important factors in choosing the surgical approach than the actual tumor size and volume. One should consider using a transcranial approach when a pituitary adenoma has an intracranial extension to the subfrontal, retrochiasmatic, or middle fossa regions. A transcranial approach is also indicated when the suprasellar portion of a tumor is separated from the intrasellar portion by a tight bottleneck constriction, which is a relatively rare situation.

Surgery is the treatment of choice for pituitary tumors associated with acromegaly and Cushing's disease. Availability of the medical option of bromocriptine for PRL-secreting pituitary adenomas makes decision-making for patients with these lesions more difficult. We generally recommend surgery for patients with symptomatic tumors associated with a serum PRL level lower than 750 ng/ml. The surgical cure rate for patients with PRL levels over 1000 ng/ml is poor and, in these patients, bromocriptine is a more attractive therapeutic alternative.

The role of surgery for microprolactinomas is more controversial. Certainly, for the young woman desiring pregnancy, surgery is a good option. In some patients it is appropriate to recommend no therapy, but rather to follow the patient closely with periodic MRI studies and PRL determinations. For example, a woman with a microprolactinoma, with modest elevation of PRL, who does not desire pregnancy may choose this option, and we believe this is a reasonable choice. The literature as well as our personal experience shows that a number of cases of microprolactinomas do not enlarge over an extended period, despite no formal therapy (17). After considering the pros and cons, the use of bromocriptine is also an appropriate choice.

D. Radiation Therapy

Radiation therapy of pituitary tumors has a history nearly as long as that for transphenoidal surgery. Gramegna first used radiation therapy to treat a pituitary adenoma in 1907, 1 year after Schloffer pioneered the transphenoidal operative approach to the pituitary gland (43). Before the rekindling of interest in transphenoidal surgery in the late 1960s, radiation therapy played a major role in the primary treatment of many pituitary adenomas. Currently, radiation therapy remains a therapeutic option for many pituitary and parasellar tumors. Its role, however, has been largely supplanted by medical and surgical options that have been previously described. The current role of radiation therapy is primarily in the management of recurrent lesions, incompletely excised neoplasms, and in the unusual patient who is unable to tolerate either transphenoidal surgery or medical therapy.

In discussing the role of radiation therapy for pituitary tumors, one must distinguish between electromagnetic and focused-beam radiation. Conventional megavoltage radiotherapy is the most widely used form of radiation. This refers to the use of photon irradiation (x-rays or gamma rays) with a beam energy of at least 1.2 million electron volts. Sources for this type of radiation include cobalt-60 units and linear accelerators. Pituitary radiation is usually given as a single course in four or five fractions per week for 4½–5 weeks. A total tumor dose of 45–50 Gy in 1.8 Gy/day fractions is recommended, although the total may be increased to 50–55 Gy for large and invasive tumors or for craniopharyngiomas. With conventional radiation, it is impossible to protect the normal pituitary gland. The optic chiasm and the hypothalamus are also exposed, especially with larger tumors.

Focused-beam radiation refers to the delivery of beams of high-energy particles, such as electrons, protons, alpha-particles, neutrons, negative pi-mesons, and heavy-charged particles. Although there has been a renewed recent interest in the field of stereotactic radiosurgery, using primarily the gamma knife, stereotactic linear accelerators, and proton beam radiation, these techniques have been used in the management of pituitary tumors since 1946, and a large experience with these techniques accumulated during the 1960s and 1970s.

Our attitude on the use of radiation therapy for pituitary tumors is relatively conservative. In general, we recommend the use of radiation therapy for documented recurrence of certain pituitary tumors following surgical excision. The advent of modern transsphenoidal surgery and imaging modalities, such as CT and MRI, has raised the question of whether radiation therapy should be administered in the immediate postoperative period or after tumor recurrence is documented by appropriate imaging studies. Although data to answer this question are presently unavailable, our approach has been to reserve radiation therapy for documented recurrence.

1. Prolactinomas

Given the excellent results obtained with transphenoidal surgery and medical therapy with bromocriptine, there is a minimal role for radiation therapy in the management of prolactinomas.

2. Acromegaly

Radiation therapy appears to be useful in treating acromegaly that persists after surgery. Many of the studies addressing the role of radiation therapy as the primary modality of treatment for acromegaly were performed before the availability of GH assays. Results were evaluated on the basis of improvement in endocrine activity and mass effect of the tumor. Eastman et al. reported beneficial therapeutic results in 47 acromegalic patients treated with 40–50 Gy of conventional supervoltage therapy followed for a period of 10 years after treatment (44). In the majority, GH levels progressively fell over the 10-year interval and were less than 10 ng/ml in 81% and less than 5 ng/ml in 69% of the patients. The subjective physical manifestations and metabolic effects of GH excess improved significantly over time and paralleled the fall of GH levels. On the other hand, the prevalence of hypopituitarism, which was low before treatment, increased progressively during the follow-up period and was documented in 9 of 19 patients 10 years after treatment. Although these results indicate that conventional radiation therapy is an effective mode of treatment for acromegaly, these results are not as impressive as modern surgical series. Until the role of medical therapy for acromegaly improves, radiation therapy will continue to play a role only in the recurrent and invasive tumors causing acromegaly.

The experiences of Kjellberg and Kliman and Lawrence et al. indicate that acromegaly can be well controlled using heavy-particle radiation therapy, with relatively few side effects (45,46). Kjellberg reported the results of 431 acromegalic patients treated with proton beam radiosurgery and obtained a "remission" rate of 80% (e.g., GH less than 10 ng/ml 4 years after therapy was administered) (45). His series reported a failure rate of 10% and approximately 10% of his patients developed hypopituitarism, requiring replacement of thyroid or steroid medication. Lawrence et al. obtained levels of GH lower than 10 ng/ml in 90% of 258 acromegalic patients within 5 years of heavy-particle therapy (46).

3. Cushing's Disease

Overall, conventional radiation therapy is effective in controlling Cushing's disease in 50–80% of patients. The interval between therapy and clinical or biochemical remission varies from months to a year, but is shorter than that required to control GH levels in acromegalic patients undergoing irradiation.

Of 124 patients treated by Kjellberg and Kliman with proton beam radiation, approximately 65% underwent complete remission with restoration of normal clinical and laboratory findings (47–50). Another 20% were improved to the point that no further therapy was felt to be necessary. The 15% who were failures were treated by adrenalectomy or open hypophysectomy. Thirteen of their patients required replacement hormonal therapy and 1–4% of patients developed temporary oculomotor disturbances, with one patient developing a visual field defect.

The excellent results obtained with transphenoidal surgery in both adults and children makes it the therapy of choice in our opinion. As with acromegaly, radiation therapy is reserved for patients with Cushing's disease who have documented recurrence of an invasive tumor that is believed to be surgically incurable. However, even in these cases, preliminary surgical debulking by a transphenoidal procedure may be a reasonable option and may enhance the effectiveness of subsequent radiation therapy.

4. Nonfunctional Adenomas

Much of the literature on radiation therapy for nonfunctional adenomas was published before the use or availability of laboratory and histological techniques allowing a modern classification of pituitary adenomas. Many of the adenomas included in these older series undoubtedly contained PRL-secreting tumors and possibly other hyperfunctional tumors of various types. Many of the larger series were collected when craniotomy, rather than transphenoidal surgery, was the surgical procedure of choice. It is apparent from the literature that the control rate for nonfunctional adenomas is about equal between radiation alone and surgery plus radiation, both of which are superior to the control rates obtained with surgery alone (51–61). It is our opinion that surgery provides a definitive diagnosis and debulking of the tumor for rapid decompression. If a complete resection cannot be accomplished, radiation therapy will usually increase the recurrence-free survival rate. As stated earlier, whether the radiation should be given immediately after surgery or when there is documented recurrence on imaging studies remains controversial.

V. OTHER SELLAR AND PARASELLAR LESIONS

A variety of neoplastic and nonneoplastic masses may arise in the vicinity of the sella turcica, causing hypothalamic or pituitary dysfunction and may mimic a pituitary adenoma. Table 3 lists most neoplastic and nonneoplastic lesions that may occur in proximity to the pituitary gland. The most commonly encountered lesions that affect pituitary function and mimic pituitary tumors are craniopharyngiomas, meningiomas, and intracranial aneurysms. The management of intracranial aneurysms is beyond the scope of this chapter as it does not represent a neoplastic disorder.

A. Craniopharyngiomas

Craniopharyngiomas constitute approximately 2.5% of all brain tumors (62). These tumors exhibit a bimodal age incidence, with one peak in the first decade of life and the second peak in the fifth to seventh decades (63). Approximately 50% occur in patients younger than 20 years of age and represent the most common nonglial tumors in children, constituting approximately one-half of sellar/chiasmal tumors in this age group. Males and females are equally affected. Craniopharyngiomas are believed to arise from squamous epithelial rests persisting from Rathke's pouch, a

Table 3 Lesions of the Sella and Parasellar Region

Neoplastic disorders
  Pituitary adenohypophyseal origin
    Pituitary adenomas
    Carcinomas
  Pituitary nonadenohypophyseal origin
    Sarcomas
    Granular cell tumors
    Craniopharyngiomas
  Nonpituitary origin
    Meningiomas
    Hypothalamic and optic gliomas
    Chordomas
    Dermoid and epidermoid cysts
    Teratomas and teratoid tumors, including germinomas
    Lipomas
    Melanomas
    Paragangliomas
    Gangliocytomas
    Chondromas
    Hemangioblastomas
    Olfactory neuroblastomas
    Lymphoproliferative disorders
    Tumors of skeletal origin
    Metastases
Nonneoplastic disorders
  Nonneoplastic cysts
    Rathke's pouch cyst
    Mucoceles
    Arachnoid cysts
  Aneurysms and other vascular malformations
  Inflammatory disorders
    Abscesses
    Sarcoidosis
    Histiocytosis X
    Lymphocytic hypophysitis

Source: Ref. 75.

diverticulum arising from the stomodeum during embryogenesis. Craniopharyngiomas may present with a variety of clinical features, including (1) visual disturbances, resulting from the involvement of the optic nerves, chiasm, or tract; (2) endocrine dysfunction, resulting from compression of the pituitary gland, stalk, or the ventral basal hypothalamus; (3) increased intracranial pressure from obstruction of the CSF pathways at the foramen of Monro or aqueduct of Sylvius; and (4) symptoms, such as somnolence, autonomic seizures, and chronic hyponatremia, that indicate intrinsic hypothalamic involvement.

Craniopharyngiomas are readily identified on CT or MRI, although MRI has replaced CT as the primary-imaging modality for these tumors. The appearance of craniopharyngiomas on MRI is somewhat variable, depending on the presence of cholesterol crystals, calcification, and hemorrhage (Fig. 5).

Most neurosurgeons agree that complete removal of craniopharyngiomas is the most desirable

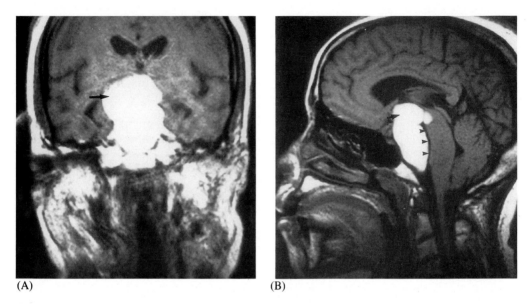

Figure 5 (A) Coronal and (B) sagittal MRI demonstrates a large cystic craniopharyngioma with suprasellar extension (arrow) and impingement upon the front of the brain stem (arrowheads).

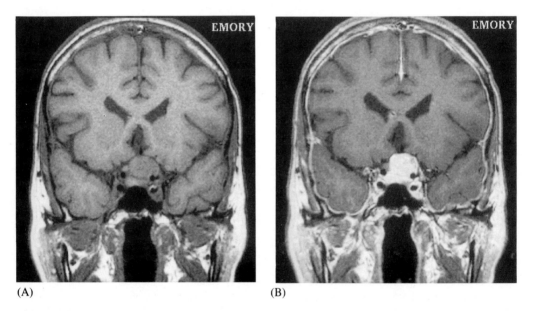

Figure 6 Coronal MRI (A) before and (B) after the administration of gadolinium illustrates a meningioma arising from the planum sphenoidale.

treatment and offers the best chance of long-term cure of the disease (64–66). A number of series report excellent results with attempted radical removal, including some series with no mortality and very low risk (66–70). Unfortunately, some craniopharyngiomas cannot be removed completely without exposing the patient to unacceptable risk. The surgeon must determine individually whether a given tumor is able to be completely removed and temper a desire for complete removal with the realization that this may not be possible.

Radiation therapy is an option for incompletely excised craniopharyngiomas. Survival rates for patients treated with surgery and radiation are better than those for patients treated with radiation alone (68,71–74). However, one must not overlook the hazards of radiation therapy, including radiation necrosis, endocrine deficiency, optic neuritis, dementia, and decreased capacity for intellectual performance in children (67). As with pituitary adenomas, if subtotal excision of the tumor is performed, radiation therapy may be withheld until there is documented recurrence of the tumor. At that time, the decision for reoperation or institution of radiation therapy must be individualized.

B. Meningiomas

Meningiomas are extra-axial tumors arising from the meningothelial cells occurring primarily in the arachnoid villae. Meningiomas that occur in the region of the pituitary gland may take their dural origin from the tuberculum sella, medial sphenoid wing, olfactory groove, optic nerve sheath, anterior clinoid process, or anterior fossa over the roof of the orbit. These lesions may compress the pituitary gland and hypothalamus or infundibulum.

Meningiomas are readily imaged on CT or MRI. With either of these imaging modalities, the use of intravenous contrast is helpful in outlining the entire extent of the neoplasm (Fig. 6). Angiography is often helpful in determining the vascular supply to meningiomas, both for diagnostic purposes and for preoperative embolization to decrease blood flow in preparation for surgery. Meningiomas are usually histologically benign tumors that may be cured by surgery alone if they are completely excised. If residual tumor is left behind, this may be followed accurately with postoperative MRI or CT, and recurrences may be treated with reoperation. Radiation therapy is beneficial in those patients in whom recurrent tumor is surgically inaccessible or in patients who cannot tolerate surgery for medical reasons.

REFERENCES

1. Forbes AP, Henneman PH, Griswold GC, et al. Syndrome characterized by galactorrhea, amenorrhea and low urinary FSH: comparison with acromegaly and normal lactation. J Clin Endocrinol Metab 1954; 14:265.
2. Klibanski A, Neer RM, Beitins IZ, Ridgway EC, Zervas, NT, McArthur JW. Decreased bone density in hyperprolactinemic women. N Engl J Med 1980; 303:1511–1514.
3. Evans HM, Briggs JH, Dixon JS. The physiology and chemistry of growth hormone. In: Harris GW, Donovan BT, eds. The pituitary gland, vol 1. Berkeley: University of California press, 1966.
4. Wright AD, Hill DM, Lowy C, Fraser TR. Mortality in acromegaly. Q J Med 1970; 39:1–16.
5. Plotz CM, Knowlton AI, Ragan C. The natural history of Cushing's syndrome. Am J Med 1952; 13:597–614.
6. Ezrin C, Horvath E, Kovacs K. Anatomy and cytology of the normal and abnormal pituitary gland. In: De Groot LJ, Cahill GF Jr, Odell WD, Martini L, Potts JT Jr, Nelson DH, Steinberger E, Winegrad AI, eds. Endocrinology, vol 1. New York: Grune & Stratton, 1979: 103–122.
7. Foncin JF, Billet R, Le Beau J. A propos des tumeurs hypophysaires extensives a secretion corticotrope (etude ultrastructurale). Ann Endocrinol 1972; 33:449–454.
8. MacLeod RM. Regulation of prolactin secretion. In: Ganong WF, Martini L, eds. Frontiers in neuroendocrinology, vol 4. New York: Raven Press, 1976: 169–194.
9. Earle KM, Dillard SH Jr. Pathology of adenomas of the pituitary gland. In: Kohler PO, Ross GT, eds. Diagnosis and treatment of pituitary tumors. Amsterdam: Excerpta Medica, 1973: 3–16.
10. Mohanty S, Tandon PN, Banerji AK, et al. Haemorrhage into pituitary adenomas. J Neurol Neurosurg Psychiatry 1977; 40:987.
11. Wakai S, Fukushima T, Teramoto A, Sano K. Pituitary apoplexy: its incidence and clinical significance. J Neurosurg 1981; 55: 187–193.

12. Clemmons DR, Van Wyk JJ, Ridgway EC, Kliman B, Kjellberg RN, Underwood LE. Evaluation of acromegaly by radioimmunoassay of somatomedin-C. N Engl J Med 1979; 301:1138–1142.
13. Thorner MO, Perryman RL, Cronin JM, Rogol AD, Draznin M, Johanson A, Vale W, Horvath E, Kovacs K. Somatotroph hyperplasia: successful treatment of acromegaly by removal of a pancratic islet tumor secreting a growth hormone-releasing factor. J Clin Invest 1982; 70:965–977.
14. Cassar J, Doyle FH, Lewis PD, Mashiter K, Van Noorden S, Joplin GF. Treatment of Nelson's syndrome by pituitary implantation of yttrium-90 or gold-198. Br Med J 1976; 2:269–272.
15. Liddle GW. Tests of pituitary–adrenal suppressibility in the diagnosis of Cushing's syndrome. J Clin Endocrinol Metab 1960; 20:1539–1560.
16. Newton DR, Dillon, WP, Norman D, Newton TH, Wilson, CB. Gd-DTPA-enhanced MR imaging of pituitary adenomas. AJNR 1989; 10:949–954.
17. Weiss MH, Teal J, Gott P, Wycoff R, Yadley R, Apuzzo MLJ, Giannotta SL, Kletzky O, March C. Natural history of microprolactinomas: six-year follow-up. Neurosurgery 1983; 12: 180–183.
18. Aronoff SL, Daughaday WH, Laws ER Jr. Bromocriptine treatment of prolactinomas [letter]. N Engl J Med 1979; 300:1391.
19. Besser GM, Thorner MO. Bromocriptine in the treatment of the hyperprolactinaemia–hypogonadism syndromes. Postgrad Med J 1976; 52(suppl 1): 64–70.
20. Chiodini P, Liuzzi A, Cozzi R, Verde G, Oppizzi G, Dallabonzana D, Spelta B, Silvestrini F, Borghi G, Luccarelli G, Rainer E, Horowski R. Size reduction of macroprolactinomas by bromocriptine or lisuride treatment. J Clin Endocrinol Metab 1981; 53:737–743.
21. Corenblum B, Webster BR, Mortimer CB, Ezrin C. Possible anti-tumour effect of 2-bromo-ergocryptine (CB-154, Sandoz) in two patients with large prolactin-secreting pituitary adenomas [abstract]. Clin Res 1975; 23:614A.
22. McGregor AM, Scanlon MF, Hall K, Cook DB, Hall R. Reduction in size of a pituitary tumor by bromocriptine therapy. N Engl J Med 1979; 300:291–293.
23. Parkes D. Drug therapy—bromocriptine. N Engl J Med 1979; 301:873–878.
24. Thorner MO, Evans WS, MacLeod RM, et al. Hyperprolactinemia: current concepts of management, including medical therapy with bromocriptine. In: Goldstein M, et al, eds. Ergot compounds and brain function: neuroendocrine and neuropsychiatric aspects, vol 23. New York: Raven Press, 1980.
25. Thorner MO, Martin WH, Rogol AD Jr, Morris JL, Perryman RL, Conway BP, Howards SS, Wolfman MG, MacLeod RM. Rapid regression of pituitary prolactinomas during bromocriptine treatment. J Clin Endocrinol Metab 1980; 51:438–445.
26. Thorner MO, Perryman RL, Rogol AD, Conway BP, MacLeod RM, Login IS, Morris JL. Rapid changes of prolactinoma volume after withdrawal and reinstitution of bromocriptine. J Clin Endocrinol Metab 1981; 53:480–483.
27. Wass JAH, Moult PJA, Thorner MO, Dacie JE, Charlesworth M, Jones AE, Besser GM. Reduction of pituitary-tumour size in patients with prolactinomas and acromegaly treated with bromocriptine with or without radiotherapy. Lancet 1979; 2:66–69.
28. Barrow DL, Tindall GT, Kovacs K, Thorner MO, Horvath E, Hoffman JC Jr. Clinical and pathological effects of bromocriptine on prolactin-secreting and other pituitary tumors. J Neurosurg 1984; 60:1–7.
29. Tindall GT, Kovacs K, Horvath E, Thorner MO. Human prolactin-producing adenomas and bromocriptine: a histological, immunocytochemical, ultrastructural, and morphometric study. J Clin Endocrinol Metab 1982; 55:1178–1183.
30. Turkalj I, Braun P, Krupp P. Surveillance of bromocriptine in pregnancy. JAMA 1982; 247:1589–1591.
31. Landolt AM, Keller PJ, Froesch ER, et al. Bromocriptine: does it jeopardise the result of later surgery for prolactinomas? Lancet 1982; 2:657.
32. Landolt AM, Osterwalder V. Perivascular fibrosis in prolactinomas: is it increased by bromocriptine? J Clin Endocrinol Metab 1984; 58:1179–1183.
33. Baskin DS, Wilson CB. CSF rhinorrhea after bromocriptine for prolactinoma [letter]. N Engl J Med 1982; 306:178.
34. Cole IE, Keene M. Cerebrospinal fluid rhinorrhoea in pituitary tumors. J R Soc Med 1980; 73:244–254.
35. Landolt AM. Cerebrospinal fluid rhinorrhea: a complication of therapy for invasive prolactinomas. Neurosurgery 1982; 11:395–401.

36. Wilson JD, Newcombe RLG, Long FL. Cerebrospinal fluid rhinorrhoea during treatment of pituitary tumours with bromocriptine. Acta Endocrinol 1983; 103:457–460.

37. Barrow DL, Mizuno J, Tindall GT. Management of prolactinomas associated with very high serum prolactin levels. J Neurosurg 1988; 68:554–558.

38. Pereira JL, Rodriguez-Paras MJ, Leal-Cerro A, et al. Acromegalic cardiopathy improves after treatment with increasing doses of octreotide. J Endocrinol Invest 1991; 14:17.

39. Vance ML, Harris AG. Long-term treatment of 189 acromegalic patients with the somatostatin analog octreotide. Results of the International Multicenter Acromegaly Study Group. Arch Intern Med 1991; 151:1573–1578.

40. Lund E, Jørgensen J, Christensen SE, Weeke J, Ørskov H, Harris AG. Reduction in sella turcica volume. An effect of long-term treatment with the somatostatin analogue, SMS 201–995, in acromegalic patients. Neuroradiology 1991;33:162–164.

41. Khanderia U. Use of ketoconazole in the treatment of Cushing's syndrome. Clin Pharm 1991; 10:12–13.

42. Tabarin A, Navarranne A, Guerin J, Corcuff J-B, Parneix M, Roger P. Use of ketoconazole in the treatment of Cushing's disease and ectopic ACTH syndrome. Clin Endocrinol 1991; 34:63–69.

43. Gramegna A. Un cas d'acromegalie traite par la radiotherapie. Rev Neurol 1909; 17:15–17.

44. Eastman RC, Gorden P, Roth J. Conventional supervoltage irradiation is an effective treatment for acromegaly. J Clin Endocrinol Metab 1979; 48:931–940.

45. Kjellberg RN, Kliman B. Proton radiosurgery for functioning pituitary adenomas In: Tindall GT, Collins WF, eds. Clinical management of pituitary disorders. New York: Raven Press, 1979:315–334.

46. Lawrence JH, Born JL, Linfoot JA, Chong CY. Heavy particle radiation treatment of pituitary tumors. JAMA 1970; 214:2061.

47. Dohan FC, Raventos A, Boucot N, et al. Roentgen therapy in Cushing's syndrome without adrenocortical tumor. J Clin Endocrinol Metab 1957; 17:8.

48. Edmonds MW, Simpson WJK, Meakin JW. External irradiation of the hypophysis for Cushing's disease. Can Med Assoc J 1972; 107:860–862.

49. Heuschele R, Lampe I. Pituitary irradiation for Cushing's syndrome. Radiol Clin Biol 1967; 36:27–31.

50. Orth DN, Liddle GW. Results of treatment in 108 patients with Cushing's syndrome. N Engl J Med 1971; 285:243–247.

51. Bloom HJG. Radiotherapy of pituitary tumors. In: Jenkins JS, ed. Pituitary tumors. New York: Appleton-Century-Crofts, 1973.

52. Correa JN, Lampe I. The radiation treatment of pituitary adenomas. J Neurosurg 1962; 19:626–631.

53. Emmanuel IG. Symposium on pituitary tumours: historical aspects of radiotherapy, present treatment technique and results. Clin Radiol 1966; 17:154–160.

54. Bouchard J. Radiation therapy of tumors and diseases of the nervous system. Philadelphia: Lea & Febiger, 1966.

55. Hayes TP, Davis RA, Raventos A. The treatment of pituitary chromophobe adenomas. Radiology 1971; 98:149–153.

56. Horrax G, Smedal MI, Trump JG, et al. Present-day treatment of pituitary adenomas: surgery versus x-ray therapy. N Engl J Med 1955; 252:524.

57. Kramer, S. Treatment of pituitary tumors by radiation therapy. In: Seydel HG, ed. Tumors of the nervous system. New York, John Wiley & Sons, 1975:91–115.

58. Pistenma DA, Goffinet DR, Bagshaw MA, Hanbery JW, Eltringham JR. Treatment of chromophobe adenomas with megavoltage irradiation. Cancer 1975; 35:1574–1582.

59. Urdaneta N, Chessin H, Fischer JJ. Pituitary adenomas and craniopharyngiomas: analysis of 99 cases treated with radiation therapy. Int J Radiat Oncol Biol Phys 1976; 1:895–902.

60. Sheline GE. Conventional radiation therapy in the treatment of pituitary tumors. In: Tindall GT, Collins WF, eds. Clinical management of pituitary disorders. New York: Raven Press, 1979:287–314.

61. Salmi J, Grahne B, Valtonen S, Pelkonen R. Recurrence of chromophobe pituitary adenomas after operation and postoperative radiotherapy. Acta Neurol Scand 1982; 66:681–689.

62. Olivecrona H. The surgical treatment of intracranial tumors. In: Olivecrona H, Tonnis W, eds. Handbuch der neurochirurgie, vol 4. Berlin: Springer-Verlag, 1967.

63. McLone DG, Raimondi AJ, Naidich TP. Craniopharyngiomas. Childs Brain 1982; 9:188–200.

64. Amacher AL. Craniopharyngiomas: The controversy regarding radiotherapy. Childs Brain 1980; 6:57–64.

65. Carmel PW. Craniopharyngiomas. In: Wilkins RR, Rengachary SA, eds. Neurosurgery, vol 1. New York: McGraw-Hill, 1985:905–916.

66. Hoffman HJ, Hendrick EB, Humphreys RP, Buncic JR, Armstrong DL, Jenkin RDT. Management of craniopharyngioma in children. J Neurosurg 1977; 47:218–227.

67. Hoff JT, Patterson RH Jr. Craniopharyngiomas in children and adults. J Neurosurg 1972; 36:299–302.

68. Carmel PW, Atunes JL, Chang CH. Craniopharyngiomas in children. Neurosurgery 1982; 11:382–389.

69. Matson DD, Crigler JF Jr. Management of craniopharyngioma in childhood. J Neurosurg 1969; 30:377–390.

70. Sweet WH. Recurrent craniopharyngiomas. Therapeutic alternatives. Clin Neurosurg 1980; 27:206–229.

71. Kramer S. Craniopharyngioma. The best treatment is conservative surgery and postoperative radiation therapy. In: Morley TP, ed. Current controversies in neurosurgery. Philadelphia: WB Saunders, 1976:336–343.

72. Kramer S, McKissock W, Concannon JP. Craniopharyngiomas: treatment by combined surgery and radiation therapy. J Neurosurg 1961; 18:217–226.

73. Richmond IL, Wara WM, Wilson CB. Role of radiation therapy in the management of craniopharyngiomas in children. Neurosurgery 1980; 6:513–517.

74. Sung DI, Chang CH, Harisiadis L, Carmel PW. Treatment results of craniopharyngiomas. Cancer 1981; 47:847–852.

75. Tindall GT, Barrow DB, eds. Disorders of the pituitary. St. Louis: CV Mosby, 1986: 71, 130.

76. Liddle GW. Pathogenesis of glucocorticoid disorders. Am J Med 1972; 53:638.

12

The Management of the Patient with a Low-Grade Cerebral Astrocytoma

Robert A. Morantz
University of Kansas School of Medicine,
Kansas City, Kansas and University of Missouri,
Kansas City, Missouri

I. INTRODUCTION

Advances in neurodiagnostic technology have caused a resurgence of interest in the optimal management of cerebral astrocytomas. When pneumoencephalography and then cerebral angiography were the only methods of brain tumor detection, most patients presented with large high-grade lesions, since they were diagnosed late in the course of their disease. The treatment of such malignant gliomas has thus far been disappointing. With the advent of computerized tomography (CT) and magnetic resonance imaging (MRI), however, we are now able to detect smaller, less malignant lesions in younger patients. The widespread use of stereotactic biopsy has allowed us to obtain pathological confirmation of tumor foci in many more cases than was previously possible. When the histological diagnosis indicates that a low-grade astrocytoma is present, we seek the therapy that offers the longest survival, best quality of life, and lowest risk of side effects. The issue of side effects is especially important, since these tumors affect patients who are relatively young; thus, they can be expected to have a fairly long postoperative survival. After reviewing what is known about the behavior of low-grade astrocytomas, we will then formulate rational guidelines for their management.

II. NOMENCLATURE

Low-grade astrocytomas arise from the supporting cells of the central nervous system (CNS). These tumors have been called *astrocytomas* in the three-tiered World Health Organization (WHO) classification. They correspond to the grade I and II astrocytomas as classified by Kernohan et al. (1) or to what have been called *low-grade astrocytomas* in the past. Most of these tumors would fall into the grade II class in the newly proposed Daumas-Duport grading system, although the number of patients who would fall into their class III category is not yet clear (2,3). Low-grade astrocytomas include lesions that previously were classified as fibrillary or protoplasmic. Some types of astrocytomas appear to have a prognosis that is unique: specifically, the gemistocytic astrocytoma seems to have a high incidence of conversion into a more malignant form and therefore has a worse prognosis than other low-grade astrocytomas (4). For this reason, it will not be included in this discussion. Tumors with a pathological diagnosis of malignant glioma, anaplastic astrocytoma, astrocytoma grade III or IV, and glioblastoma multiforme are also not covered. Although many of our findings will also apply to low-grade oligodendrogliomas and mixed oligodendroglioma–astrocytoma, there is little agreement about how such lesions should be graded and few studies in the literature that address their optimal treatment. Consequently, this chapter will focus specifically on low-grade astrocytomas, rather than on all low-grade glial tumors.

III. CASE STUDIES

To illustrate the wide variety of clinical courses that may be followed by these patients, and the concomitant difficulties in management that are presented, we present the following eight case studies:

Case 1. A 36-year-old man presented who had sought medical attention 14 years previously when he had experienced a generalized seizure. An EEG, lumbar puncture, and cerebral angiogram were negative. He was placed on a regimen of anticonvulsants and did well for 4 years, when he again began to have generalized seizures. A CT scan revealed a minimal area of decreased density in the left frontal lobe (Fig. 1a), which was interpreted as an area of infarction. A biopsy of the lesion was recommended, but the patient refused. He then underwent yearly follow-up CT scans, which were interpreted as showing no change in the lesion. He remained neurologically stable (experiencing one or two seizures each year) for 3½ more years, when he began to have speech difficulty. A CT scan revealed a large enhancing left frontal lesion (see Fig. 1b), which at the time of surgery was found to be a malignant glioma. Postoperatively he received radiation therapy, but subsequently died 18 years after his initial seizure.

Case 2. At the age of 35 a man presented with an epileptic seizure characterized by tonic–clonic movements of his left upper extremity. At that time he had a workup that included a lumbar puncture, electroencephalogram (EEG), and CT scan, all of which were reported as being normal. Four years later the patient was taken to the emergency room after experiencing another seizure. At this point, a CT scan was carried out that revealed a nonenhancing hypodense area in the left medial temporal lobe (Fig. 2a). The patient was taken to surgery during which a subtotal resection of what was shown to be a grade II astrocytoma was carried out. Postoperatively the patient was treated with 60 Gy of localized radiation therapy to the tumor and a 2-cm margin. The patient returned to work as an executive and has continued to be perfectly normal at the time of his last follow-up examination, which is 9 years after the onset of his symptoms. His MRI scans do not reveal tumor recurrence (see Fig. 2b).

Case 3. A 35-year-old man presented with a grand mal seizure and hesitancy of speech. A CT scan (Fig. 3a) revealed a lucent lesion in the left frontotemporal region. At surgery, a firm, nonvascular grade II atrocytoma could not be easily demarcated from the surrounding brain and consequently a subtotal resection was accomplished. Postoperatively the patient was given 40 Gy of whole-brain radiation, with a 20-Gy boost to the tumor bed. He returned to full employment and had no symptoms for 6½ years. He then developed speech difficulty and confusion. A CT scan revealed tumor recurrence (see Fig. 3b). He was operated on and found to have an anaplastic astrocytoma. He died 2 months after surgery.

Case 4. A 48-year-old man presented with a 9-month history of temporal lobe seizures. A CT scan with contrast was thought to be normal; MRI showed a nonenhancing, circumscribed left anterior temporal lobe lesion (Fig. 4a,b). At surgery a gross total resection of a grade II astrocytoma was carried out. The patient refused radiation therapy and was doing well with no evidence of tumor recurrence on MRI scan 3 months after surgery (see Fig. 4c,d). Four months

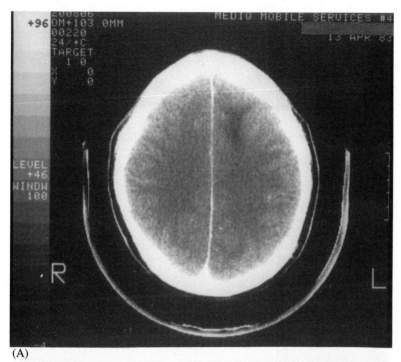

(A)

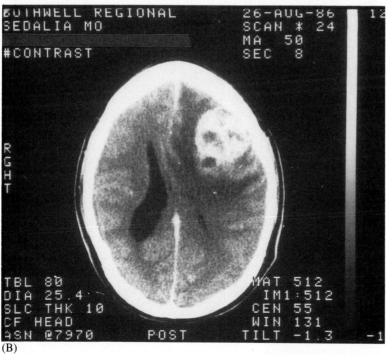

(B)

Figure 1 Case 1: (A) enhanced CT scan showing an area of decreased density in the left frontal lobe. (B) CT scan 3½ years later showing an enhancing lesion in the left frontal lobe.

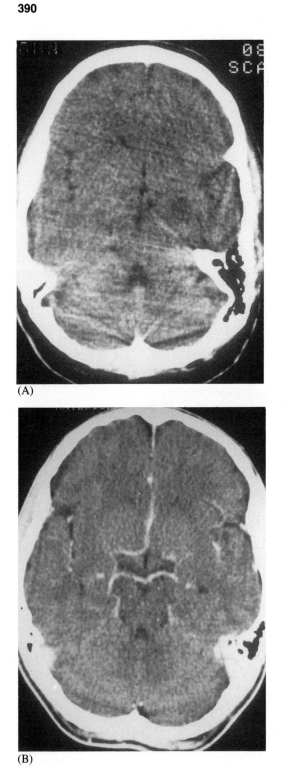

(A)

(B)

Figure 2 Case 2: (A) Enhanced CT scan showing a small lucent lesion in the left temporal lobe. (B) Enhanced CT scan 5 years later showing no evidence of tumor recurrence.

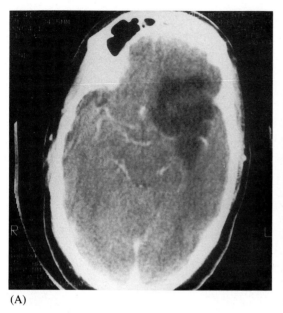

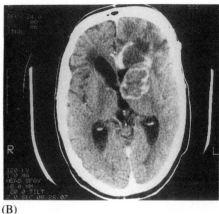

(A)   (B)

Figure 3   Case 3: (A) Enhanced CT scan showing a lucent area in the left frontotemporal region. (B) Enhanced CT scan 6½ years later showing evidence of tumor recurrence that is now an anaplastic astrocytoma.

later (7 months postoperatively) he presented with headaches and speech difficulty. The CT and MRI scans now revealed an enhancing lesion with surrounding edema (see Fig. 4e–g). At the second operation a malignant glial tumor was found. In spite of receiving postoperative radiation therapy and chemotherapy, the patient died 14 months later.

Case 5.   A 44-year-old man began to have generalized seizures in September 1984. A CT scan revealed a nonenhancing low-density lesion in the left occipital region (Fig. 5a). The patient refused biopsy. A follow-up CT scan 3 months later again revealed a low-density area in the same region, which was confirmed by MRI scanning (see Fig. 5b). A stereotactic biopsy revealed a grade II astrocytoma. Postoperatively he did well and received a course of radiation therapy—45 Gy to the tumor plus a 3-cm margin, with a 10-Gy boost to the tumor bed. He did well until 11 months later, when he began to complain of headache. A repeat CT scan (see Fig. 5c) showed medial extension of the tumor to the corpus callosum. Repeat stereotactic biopsy now revealed an anaplastic astrocytoma. In spite of carmustine (BCNU) chemotherapy he died 8 months later.

Case 6.   A 14-year-old boy presented with a 1-year history of headache and decreased visual acuity. A CT scan (Fig. 6a) revealed a contrast enhancing lesion along the orbital surface of the frontal lobe and in the parasellar area. At surgery, a grade II astrocytoma was found in the subfrontal region, and a biopsy was performed. Eighteen months later he was given radiation therapy (40 Gy to the whole brain with a 20-Gy boost to the tumor). Recent CT scans (see Fig. 6b,c) have revealed no growth of the tumor. He is presently doing well and is gainfully employed 9 years after diagnosis and 7 years after radiation therapy.

Case 7.   A 31-year-old woman presented with the chief complaint of visual hallucinations consisting of a "circle of light." A CT scan was performed (Fig. 7a), which revealed a focal enhancing lesion in the left parietal occipital area. This was confirmed on MRI (see Fig. 7b). At surgery a soft, grayish, well-circumscribed lesion was encountered, and gross total surgical excision was accomplished. Pathological review indicated a pilocytic astrocytoma. Localized radiation therapy (40 Gy to a 3-cm margin, with a 14-Gy boost to the tumor bed) was given. The

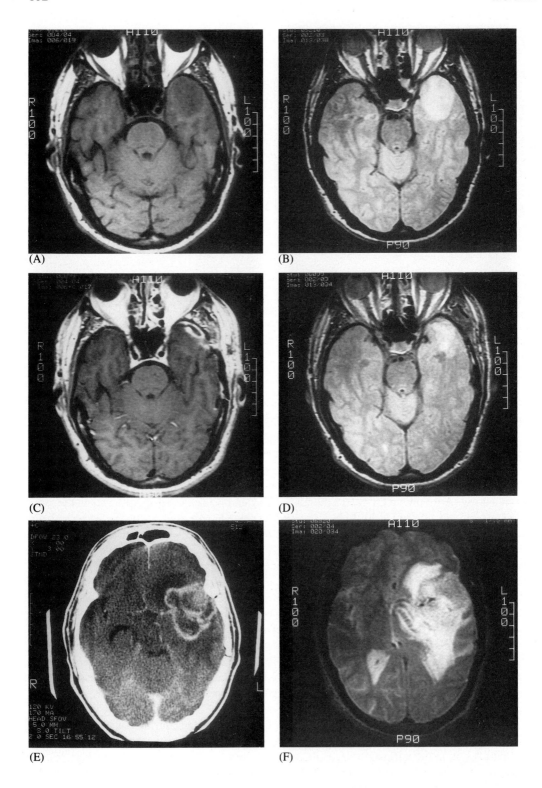

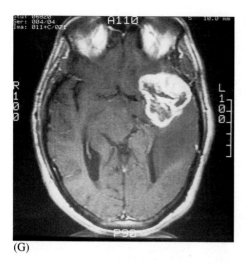

(G)

Figure 4 Case 4: (A) MRI scan (T1 image) revealing a circumscribed left anterior temporal lobe lesion. (B) MRI scan (T2 image) of the same area. (C) MRI scan 3 months later (T2 image) was interpreted as showing postoperative changes. (D) Enchanced MRI scan (after gadolinium) reveals no definite evidence of tumor recurrence. (E) Enhanced CT scan 4 months later revealing recurrence of a malignant tumor. (F) MRI scan (T2 image) revealing recurrent tumor with surrounding edema. (G) Enhanced MRI scan (after gadolinium) revealing recurrence of a malignant tumor.

patient is asymptomatic and has returned to work. There is no evidence of tumor recurrence on repeat MRI (see Fig. 7c,d) performed 5½ years after surgery.

Case 8. A 29-year-old man presented with a 6-month history of intermittent numbness of the left side of the body. His neurological examination at that time was within normal limits. A CT scan showed a 5-cm low-density lesion in the right temporal area (Fig. 8a). At surgery, a subtotal resection of a grade II astrocytoma was accomplished. Postoperatively the patient received 40 Gy to a 9 × 9-cm area and a 20-Gy boost to a smaller 7 × 7-cm area surrounding the tumor. The patient did well for the next 5 years, during which time his annual MRI scans were interpreted as showing no evidence of tumor growth. He then began to have gait difficulty and left-sided apraxia. A repeat MRI scan showed an enhancing area within the left cerebellum (see Fig. 8c). A stereotactically guided suboccipital craniectomy was then carried out, which revealed a glioblastoma multiforme of the left *cerebellar* hemisphere. The patient received radiosurgery to this area, but in spite of this, he died 6 months later, or 5½ years after his initial presentation. An autopsy confirmed recurrence of the low-grade astrocytoma of the right temporal lobe (Fig. 8d), as well as a new glioblastoma multiforme of the left *cerebellar* hemisphere (see Fig. 8e). There was no anatomical connection between the two areas, and the intervening brain was tumor-free on microscopic examination.

IV. EPIDEMIOLOGY, CLINICAL PRESENTATION, AND DIAGNOSTIC WORKUP

Astrocytomas of the cerebrum account for 10–15% of all brain tumors and constitute between 25 and 40% of all gliomas (5). They occur preponderantly in young and middle-aged patients, with a peak incidence in those between 35 and 45 years of age. Some, but not all, studies indicate that there may be an increased incidence in males. Astrocytomas arise primarily in the convexity of the brain, roughly in proportion to the relative mass of the different lobes; therefore, the frontal lobes

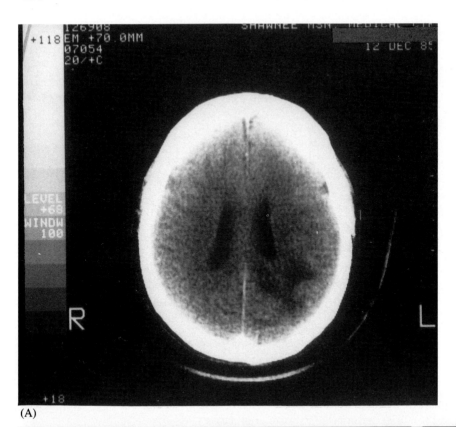

(A)

(B)

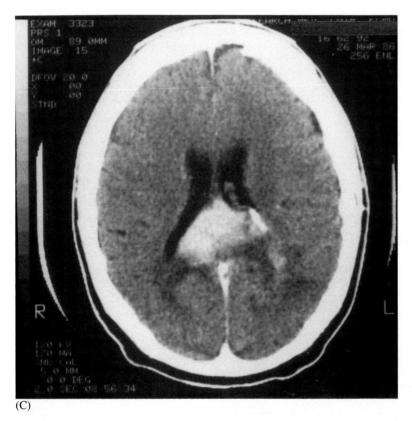

(C)

Figure 5 Case 5: (A) Enhanced CT scan demonstrating a lucent area in the left occipital region. A repeat enhanced CT scan 3 months later still revealed a lucent area with no enhancement. (B) MRI scan (T2 image) confirms a lesion in the left occipital area. (C) Repeat enhanced CT scan 1 year after the first study now reveals an enhancing lesion in the area of the splenium of the corpus callosum.

are their most common location. On gross examination they are often firm, whitish, tumors. When growth is deep within the brain, degeneration into small and large cysts may occur.

As in all brain tumors, low-grade astrocytomas may produce signs and symptoms in one of several ways: (1) by the destruction of local neurons subserving a specific function, (2) by compression of neighboring tissue, or (3) by producing increased intracranial pressure. The most common presenting symptom of a low-grade astrocytoma is an epileptic seizure. This is due to the irritation of cortical neurons by surrounding tumor infiltration. Headache and personality changes may be due to increased intracranial pressure. Whether or not the patient presents with a focal neurological deficit, such as speech difficulty, will depend on the precise location of the tumor.

In the past, the neuroradiologic procedures used to diagnose this lesion included isotope brain scanning and cerebral angiography. The isotope brain scan, in many cases, would not demonstrate the lesion, whereas the angiogram would usually show a mass lesion (without evidence of abnormal vascularity) if the tumor was large enough. In recent years the diagnostic procedures of choice have become CT scanning or MRI, or both. On CT scanning, the tumor may or may not enhance; whether such enhancement of the lesion correlates with a poorer prognosis is controversial. Silverman and Marks (6) reported that contrast enhancement had no prognostic value in patients with these tumors, whereas Piepmeier (7), in a larger series, concluded that those patients whose tumors enhanced on CT scanning had a poorer prognosis than those whose lesions did not

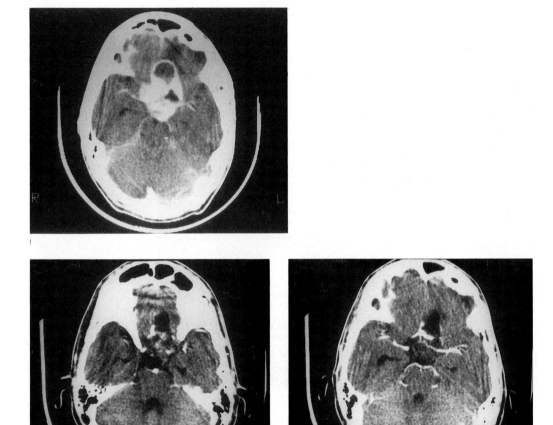

(B)   (C)

Figure 6   Case 6: (A) Enhanced CT scan demonstrating an enhancing lesion along the orbital surfaces of the frontal lobes and in the parasella area. (B,C) Repeat CT scans 5 years later reveal lucency, but less enhancement, in the same area.

enhance. This later finding was even more strongly supported by a recent study of McCormack et al., who found that contrast enhancement on the CT scan was associated with almost seven times the risk of tumor recurrence relative to those tumors not showing such enhancement (8).

The CT scan findings then, in a typical case, will usually reveal a nonenhancing or minimally enhancing lesion the density of which is lower than that of the surrounding brain. If the tumor is large enough, mass effect on the surrounding (ventricular) structures will be seen. When enhancement does occur, it is generally faint and homogeneous. The CT scan appearance may be unchanged over a period of many years.

Most clinicians now believe that MRI scanning is the procedure of choice to diagnose this tumor. The MRI scan may be abnormal, even when the CT scan is completely normal (9). On MRI, a low-grade astrocytoma typically presents a low-intensity area on T1-weighted images, whereas there is almost always an increase in signal intensity, corresponding to an increase in relaxation time, on T2-weighted images. The area of increased signal intensity is usually homogeneous and well-circumscribed, with no evidence of hemorrhage or necrosis. In many patients, it is quite difficult to differentiate the tumor from surrounding areas of edema on

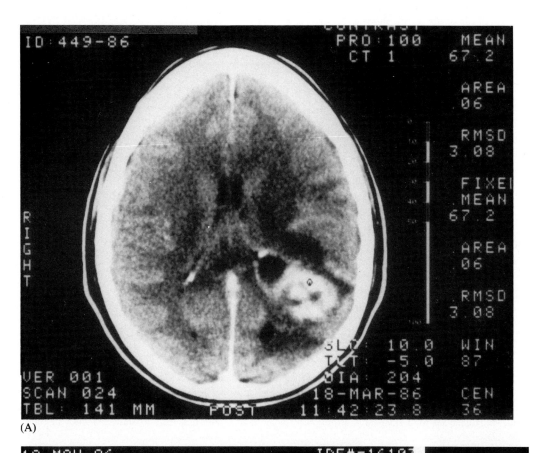

(A)

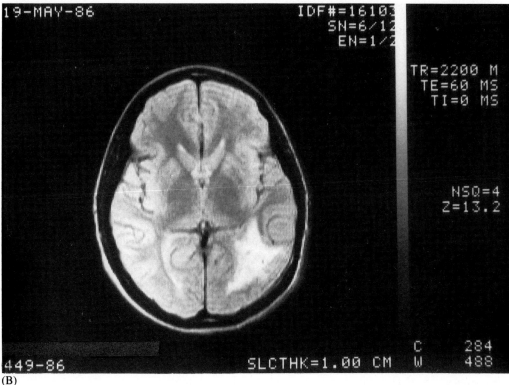

(B)

Figure 7 (See next page for legend.)

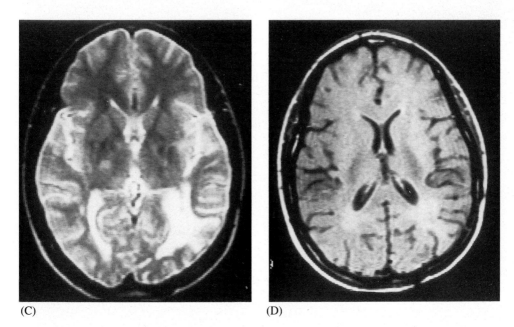

(C)   (D)

Figure 7   Case 7: (A) Enhanced CT scan reveals a focal enhancing lesion in the left occipital area. (B) MRI scan (T2 image) confirms the lesion, although differentiation between the tumor and surrounding edema cannot be made. (C) MRI scan (T2 image) 3 years later still reveals evidence of edema of the left occipital lobe. (D) Enhanced MRI scan (after gadolinium) done at the same time fails to show evidence of tumor recurrence.

MRI. Although the data are still not definitive, it does not appear that the use of an MRI contrast agent such as gadolinium will appreciably improve the ability to detect small lesions. Recent studies employing serial stereotactic biopsies of various abnormal regions detected by CT and MRI scans in patients with low-grade gliomas have indicated that there is infiltration of tumor cells into areas that were previously thought to contain only edematous white matter (10).

There also would appear to be a role for postitron emission tomography (PET) scanning in the diagnosis and treatment of these patients. A low-grade astrocytoma will be hypometabolic and, therefore, "cold" on PET scanning (11). However, when dedifferentiation to a more malignant state occurs within a low-grade astrocytoma, this area will be hypermetabolic and, consequently, will appear as a "hot spot" on PET scanning. This information may be extremely valuable in determining a site for stereotactic biopsy or for determining whether the patient should be treated with postoperative radiation therapy (12).

V.   BASIC BIOLOGY

The cell cycle can be divided into four stages, based on the nuclear DNA content. In the DNA synthesis (S) phase the cells duplicate DNA. The proportion of cells in this S-phase can be identified by flash-labeling the tissue in vitro or in vivo by briefly exposing the cells to a labeled DNA precursor, such as radioactive thymidine. The proportion of S-phase cells labeled in this manner is called the *labeling index*, and gives a rough approximation of the proliferative activity of the tissue being studied. One of the characteristics differentiating a low-grade astrocytoma from its more malignant counterparts is that low-grade tumors typically have a labeling index of less than 1%, compared with the values of 5–15% for glioblastoma (13).

The *growth fraction* is an index of the proportion of proliferating cells in relation to the total tumor cell population. Yoshii and associates estimated the growth fraction of low-grade astrocyto-

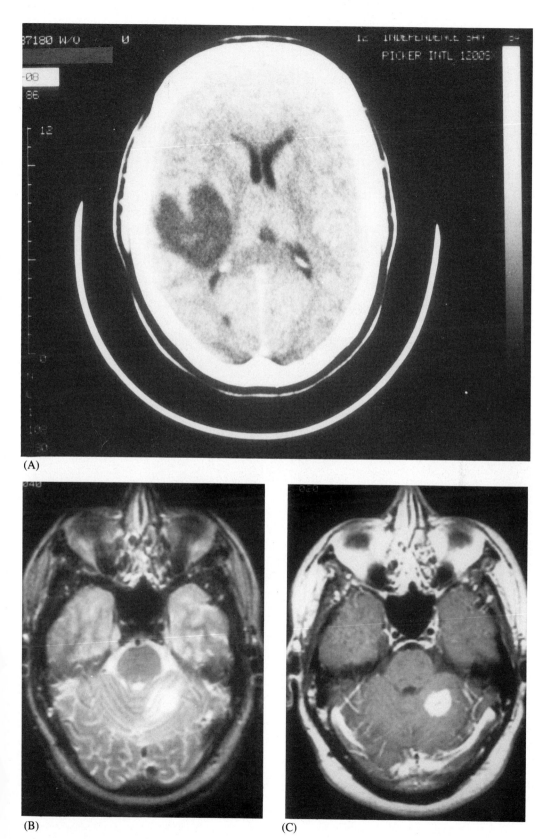

Figure 8 (See next page for legend.)

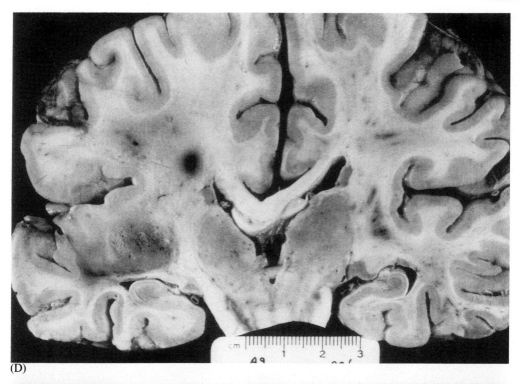

(D)

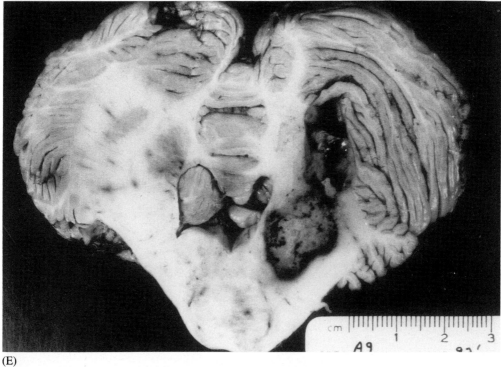

(E)

Figure 8 Case 8: (A) Enhanced CT scan reveals a 5-cm low-density lesion of the right temporal lobe. (B) MRI scan (T2 image) showing tumor and edema in the left cerebellar hemisphere. (C) MRI scan (T1 image with contrast) showing enhancing tumor of left cerebellar hemisphere. (D) Autopsy specimen of right temporal lobe revealing low-grade astrocytoma. (E) Autopsy specimen of left cerebellum revealing glioblastoma multiforme.

mas to be 2–7%, compared with 9–46% in malignant gliomas (14). Thus, most cells within a low-grade astrocytoma are relatively quiescent, rather than actively engaged in producing nucleic acids and undergoing cell division. In 1984, Hoshino postulated two mechanisms that might be responsible for the inherent slowness of growth of low-grade gliomas (15). The first concerns the mode of proliferation. Evidence from kinetic studies, outlined earlier, suggest that well-differentiated low-grade gliomas proliferate conservatively; only one of two daughter cells retains mitotic activity, and the other stops dividing. The second mechanism concerns the possible lack of traffic between the noncycling and cycling pool. If the cycling population does not increase and only sterile noncycling cells are added as the tumor grows, the growth fraction will decrease steadily. The determination of the proliferative potential may be of more than academic importance. Hoshino and associates measured the bromodeoxyuridine (BRDU)-labeling indexes in 47 patients, all of whom histologically were said to have low-grade astrocytomas. They found that 60% of the patients had labeling indexes of less than 1%, whereas 40% of the patients had labeling indexes of 1% or more. The patients were then followed for evidence of recurrence for a period up to 3½ years. In those patients with labeling indexes of less than 1%, only three died of recurrent tumor, whereas 60% of those with labeling in excess of 1% experienced a recurrence during the same follow-up time (16).

If these results are confirmed in other studies, they may have important therapeutic implications. It is well-known that in spite of histologic similarity, all low-grade astrocytomas do not behave in a biologically similar manner. Thus, it may be reasonable to treat patients whose low-grade astrocytomas have a relatively high-labeling index more aggressively (i.e., with postoperative radiation therapy) than those whose tumors have a lower-labeling index (and thus could be treated with observation alone).

VI. PROGNOSTIC FACTORS

In defining significant factors affecting prognosis, we must first separate out from other low-grade astrocytomas the pilocytic variant, which appears to have an excellent prognosis, no matter how radical the surgical resection and regardless of whether postoperative adjuvant radiation therapy is given (17,18). Next, almost all studies have found that patients having either a Kernohan or Daumas-Duport grade I designation have a better prognosis that those whose histological classification is that of grade II. As mentioned previously, it is generally agreed that the prognosis is worse for those having a gemistocytic astrocytoma (4).

Relative to other significant factors affecting prognosis, most recent studies indicate that a young age at the time of diagnosis is the most important factor associated with a prolonged survival. Laws et al found that other factors correlating with a prolonged survival were gross total surgical removal, lack of major preoperative neurological deficit, long duration of symptoms before surgery, seizures as a presenting symptom, lack of major postoperative neurological deficit, and having had surgery performed within recent decades (19). More recent papers have not been in agreement, however, on the positive prognostic import of all of these factors. For instance, Sofietti et al. (20) agreed that gross total removal was associated with a higher 5-year survival rate than subtotal removal, whereas Weir and Grace (21), Piepmeier (7) and Vertosick (22) did not find that extensive surgery was significantly correlated with the length of survival. However, most previous studies indicated that patients who received only a biopsy had a poorer prognosis than those who received gross total resection. Nevertheless, it must be said that the issue of whether or not there is an advantage to gross total removal, compared with smaller resections, has not yet been definitively answered. In spite of this, most would agree that lobectomy has no place in the routine treatment of these tumors, and that a gross total resection should be attempted, it it can be accomplished without a significant risk of producing neurological deficit.

Some authors have reported that the presence of tumor cysts within the lesion improves the prognosis (9,19), whereas others have found that the presence of such cysts is not significantly related to the patient's survival (7,23).

VII. SAMPLING AND DEDIFFERENTIATION

Scherer (24) was one of the first to emphasize that careful examination of all areas of an astrocytoma was required to determine the presence or absence of small anaplastic foci. In his classic study he made careful sections of the cerebral hemispheres of 18 patients with astrocytomas and determined foci of anaplasia in 13. In a similar manner Russell and Rubinstein (25) examined 55 autopsy specimens of patients whose clinical diagnosis was astrocytoma. In over 50% of these cases areas of anaplastic change were found. From another prospective, Russell and Rubenstein analyzed a series of 129 autopsy cases of glioblastoma and concluded that approximately 28% could be considered to have arisen from a preexisting astrocytoma. In addition, a recent paper found that the presence of areas of low-grade astrocytoma within a more malignant tumor was associated with a better prognosis, compared with those patients whose tumors on histological examination had no such areas of low-grade tumor present (26).

The issue of dedifferentiation is extremely important and has been studied by several authors. Muller and co-workers (27) examined 72 patients whose pathological diagnosis at the time of initial surgery was astrocytoma. At the time of recurrence, 14% had tumors that were pathologically unchanged, 55% were reclassified as having anaplastic astrocytoma, and 30% were reclassified as having glioblastoma multiforme. The time interval between the initial pathological diagnosis and the second operation averaged 31 months. They concluded that, in approximately two-thirds of all astrocytomas (i.e., including both astrocytomas and anaplastic astrocytomas), one can expect an increase in malignancy (i.e., dedifferentiation). In 79 patients with recurrent tumor documented at either subsequent surgery or autopsy, Laws et al. found that a change to astrocytoma grade III or IV had occurred in approximately 50% (19). Soffietti et al. reported that 79% of their astrocytoma patients who had recurrent tumor had anaplastic areas at either reoperation or autopsy (20). More recently, Vertosick and associates, in their series of 25 patients with well-differentiated astrocytomas, found that none of the 8 deaths were due to the progressive growth of the low-grade astrocytoma. Rather, 7 of the 8 deaths occurred in patients whose tumors had dedifferentiated into an anaplastic astrocytoma or a glioblastoma (22). McCormack et al. also found that dedifferentiation occurred in six of seven patients with recurrent tumor (8). They did, however, have several patients with deep-seated lesions who died of progressive spread of their low-grade tumor, rather than as a consequence of dedifferentiation to a higher degree of malignancy.

The literature is not unanimous, however, in the high incidence of dedifferentiation that occurs in these tumors, since Piepmeier found that malignant transformation was seen in only 13% of patients at the time of second operation or autopsy (7). This number is almost certainly low, however, because the patient population reviewed in this study had a median follow up of only 5 years, and such malignant dedifferentiation will undoubtedly occur in more patients as the follow-up time increases.

Although this is still the subject of some debate, and no definite answer can be provided, it is fair to suggest that the presence of anaplastic areas at the time of a second resection or biopsy in a patient with a previously diagnosed low-grade astrocytoma is not necessarily the result of an initial sampling error. Rather, in as many as one-half of the cases, dedifferentiation of a low-grade astrocytoma to a more malignant form occurs.

Recent research may offer clues to the molecular genetic basis of the process of dedifferentiation. In cancer of the colon, the progression from the more benign polyp to the overt cancer is reflected in an increasing number of genetic abnormalities within the genome of the cell. In a recent experimental study that has looked at this question relative to intrinsic brain tumors, the number of genetic abnormalities increased when one compared low-grade astrocytomas with anaplastic astrocytomas and glioblastomas (28). Thus, a reasonable hypothesis would be that a glial cell experiences a small number of "genetic hits" to change it into a low-grade astrocytoma. If these same cells then experience further alterations in their genetic makeup (e.g., by activation of protooncogenes or elimination of tumor suppressor genes), they will then undergo dedifferentiation to a more malignant phenotype.

The crucial clinical issue, however, remains that of whether radiation therapy, or any other form of adjuvant therapy, can retard the change of low-grade astrocytoma cells to a more malignant state or, alternatively, whether radiation therapy can destroy small anaplastic foci already present within the astrocytoma, as has been suggested in one pathological study (29).

VIII. SURGICAL TREATMENT

A. Timing of Operation

It is a general rule of surgical oncology that surgery should be carried out as early in the course of malignancy as possible. However, it has never been proved that earlier treatment of a low-grade astrocytoma produces an increase in life span, as measured from the time of diagnosis. Furthermore, since tumors are being detected in more and more patients while they are neurologically intact and since operative intervention in some locations carries a significant risk of postoperative morbidity, some prefer to delay surgery when the lesion has not shown a change in appearance on sequential radiologic studies (30). Unfortunately, since it is almost impossible to make a precise pathological diagnosis by neuroradiologic procedures alone, this consideration would appear to be outweighed, in most instances, by the necessity of obtaining pathological confirmation of the nature of the lesion.

B. Type of Surgery

Most, but not all, of the retrospective studies have indicated that patients who underwent gross total removal of their lesions experienced a longer survival than those who did not. We must be careful in evaluating such data, however, since it is likely that the patients in these two groups are not comparable. More specifically, in those patients whose tumors were widely infiltrating into vital areas, surgical judgment ruled out gross total removal. In spite of this, however, given the general oncological principle that one should try to obtain the maximum reduction of tumor burden possible, and the known propensity of residual cells to undergo malignant dedifferentiation, it would appear prudent to attempt gross total removal of those lesions in which this can be done without producing a postoperative neurological deficit (31).

C. Technical Aspects

If a standard craniotomy is carried out, in many instances, the Cavitron ultrasonic aspirator (CUSA) will be helpful. As in surgery for other intrinsic brain tumors, the tumor should be entered as close to the center as possible and then progressively removed toward the periphery. In many instances, it is quite difficult to be certain of the interface between frank tumor tissue and normal surrounding brain. As indicated previously, studies by Kelly and others have shown that in low-grade astrocytomas there may be no such clear interface (10). Consequently, the surgeon should err on the conservative side when potentially important areas of brain are nearby. Other technical adjuncts that may be helpful include the use of an ultrasound device for tumor localization and cortical electrophysiological monitoring to outline contiguous eloquent areas of the brain.

Since, in many instances, it is quite difficult for the surgeon to determine the precise location of a low-grade tumor at surgery, these tumors are usually ideal for a *stereotactic craniotomy*. In this instance, the quite clear delineation of the tumor as seen on the CT or MRI scan can be used to allow one stereotactically to pass a catheter into the center of the lesion. At the time of craniotomy the surgeon then follows this catheter to the lesion and thus is certain that he or she is removing the abnormal area that has been seen on the radiologic study.

D. Stereotactic Biopsy

Many patients today have MRI or CT scans that show quite small lesions, with no evidence of mass effect. In such an instance, CT or MRI guided stereotactic biopsy is an excellent means of obtaining a definitive tissue diagnosis without subjecting the patient to the risks and inconvenience of a standard craniotomy. Many times, such patients may be discharged from the hospital on the following day. Within the last several years, stereotactic biopsy has proved itself to be an extremely accurate, low-risk technique that is, therefore, ideal for the definitive diagnosis of many low-grade astrocytomas. In the modern era, this certainly appears to be the procedure of choice over the previously used open biopsy technique.

IX. POSTOPERATIVE ADJUVANT THERAPY

A. Chemotherapy

Over the years there have been several anecdotal reports on the use of various chemotherapeutic agents in small numbers of patients with low-grade astrocytomas (32,33). Invariably, one has been unable to draw conclusions about efficacy from such case reports. There has been one recent large prospective, randomized cooperative study that evaluated the potential role of chemotherapy (lomustine; CCNU) when given in addition to radiation therapy in these patients. In this report, of 60 patients there was no increase in survival when CCNU chemotherapy was added to the treatment regimen postoperatively (34). Therefore, it now appears that there is no proved beneficial effect of postoperative chemotherapy in the treatment of patients with low-grade astrocytomas.

B. Radiation Therapy

Perhaps the most important question in the treatment of low-grade astrocytoma is whether postoperative radiation therapy should be used as an adjunctive form of treatment. Even if we agree that postoperative radiation therapy is effective, we must then ask questions concerning the type of radiation therapy that should be used (e.g., standard whole-brain, localized external beam, or brachytherapy. The answer to the radiation therapy question should be relatively easy to come by in a randomized controlled prospective clinical trial. Here one would have to carry out a multigroup, long-term (perhaps as long as 10 years) study in which two large groups of patients (containing individuals who are balanced relative to important variables such as age, tumor location, and such) would be treated identically in every respect (e.g., extent of operation, use of steroids), except that one group would receive a specified course of radiation therapy and the other would not. The presence of a statistically significant difference in the length or quality of survival between these two groups could then be determined. Such a project has never been completed, although several such studies are now being carried out by cooperative groups in the United States and Europe. Unfortunately, the results of these endeavors will not be available for many years to come.

1. Literature Review

Because no single neurosurgeon's experience is sufficient to answer properly how patients with low-grade astrocytomas should be treated postoperatively and because the results of present cooperative trials are not available, a review of the major English language retrospective studies may furnish some guidance. We must be aware, however, that the previously published reports have not satisfied even the minimal criteria that could be set forth for a study to properly answer this question. More specifically, the previous studies have been retrospective analyses in which the irradiated and nonirradiated groups of patients have not been similar in important characteristics (e.g., age, Karnofsky performance scores). The pathological classification of the lesions has been different (e.g., varying numbers of grade I and II tumors), the location and size of the tumors have not been matched, and the extent of surgery has not been uniform (e.g., biopsy vs complete resection). Finally, the parameters of the treatment being tested (i.e., radiation therapy) have not been standardized.

The early report of Levy and Elvidge (35) reviewed 176 cases treated at the Montreal Neurologic Institute between 1940 and 1949. These authors found what has been confirmed subsequently by many other authors: that the gemistocytic type of astrocytoma has a poorer prognosis than other variants and that patients with cerebellar astrocytomas fared better than those with cerebral lesions, even in the face of incomplete removal. Several years later Bouchard and Pierce (36) reviewed all patients seen at this same institution over a much longer period and compared the survival of 81 low-grade astrocytoma patients who had received radiation therapy with a group of 71 low-grade astrocytoma patients who had not. They found that although the 3-year survival rate was virtually identical (59 vs 62%), the 5-year survival statistics showed an increased longevity in those who had received radiation therapy (38 vs 49%). They concluded that ionizing radiation should play a major role in the treatment of such patients.

In 1961 Gol (37) reviewed 194 cases of cerebral astrocytoma treated at Baylor. Two thirds of the postoperative patients were given radiation therapy. He found that, irrespective of surgical procedure (biopsy or resection), the addition of radiation therapy was associated with an increase in survival (2 vs 10 months with biopsy; 23 vs 32 months with resection). In addition, this study was the first indicating that patients in whom tumor was resected, rather than only biopsied, had a better outcome, no matter what other therapy was utilized.

Uihlein et al. (38) published the first of four major studies drawing from the clinical material of the Mayo Clinic. They reviewed 83 patients with astrocytoma treated between 1955 and 1959. Thirty-three patients underwent surgery alone, and 50 were treated with surgery followed by radiation therapy. They found that 65% of those treated with surgery alone and only 54% of those treated by surgery and radiation therapy were alive at 5 years. If anything, this indicated a decreased survival after the addition of radiation therapy. However, when the authors separated the irradiated patients into those who had received 35 Gy or more and those who had received a lower dosage, the 5-year survival rates were 63 and 42%, respectively. From this analysis they concluded that there is a "suggestion" that irradiation may be helpful in the treatment of the low-grade astrocytoma.

In 1976 Stage and Stein (39) reviewed the UCLA experience with supratentorial brain tumors and found 6 patients with grade I lesions and 45 patients with grade II lesions. An analysis of their survival curves indicated approximately a 40% 5-year survival for those treated with resection and radiation therapy, compared with a 20% 5-year survival for those treated with surgery alone.

Marsa et al. (40) reviewed the survival data for all patients treated with radiation therapy at Stanford between 1957 and 1973. They found a 5-year survival rate of approximately 41% and a 10-year survival rate of approximately 22%. In addition, after comparing the initial surgical pathological diagnosis with that found at subsequent autopsy, they confirmed that dedifferentiation to a higher degree of malignancy seemed to occur in a substantial proportion of patients.

In 1975 Leibel et al. (41) reviewed the experience at the University of California at San

Francisco in the treatment of astrocytomas. There were 147 patients who were treated at their institution between 1942 and 1967. If the patients who had complete resection of the lesion were excluded from the analysis, there was a clear-cut increased survival in the radiation therapy group vs the group who did not receive radiation therapy (i.e., 5-year survival of 46 vs 19%; 10-year survival of 35 vs 11%). From their analysis, patients with complete tumor removal or patients with cerebellar lesions did well, irrespective of whether radiation therapy was given. Finally, the authors indicated that the quality of life was acceptable in long-term survivors and that there were no instances of radiation damage in those who experienced long-term survival.

Weir and Grace (21), in 1976, studied 107 patients with grade I and II supratentorial astrocytomas treated in the province of Alberta, Canada, between 1960 and 1970. They analyzed the patients for prognostic factors that might be related to survival and found that young age, clinical grade at surgery (grade I more than grade II), and the addition of radiation therapy correlated with an increased survival. Fazekas (42) in 1977 reviewed 68 patients with grade I or II lesions treated at the Geisinger Clinic between 1958 and 1974. He concluded that patients with completely excised lesions and lesions in the cerebellum did well whether or not radiation was given. For those with incomplete resection, radiation increased the 5-year survival from 32 to 54%, although by 10 years this difference (26 vs 32%) was not thought to be significant.

Scanlon and Taylor (43), in 1979, published a second report from Mayo Clinic in which they reviewed 134 cases of low-grade gliomas treated between 1960 and 1969. Specifically eliminated were patients who had complete resection of the lesion, because they were not referred for radiation therapy. After analysing their data, they concluded that young age and location of the lesion in the cerebellum were important positive prognostic factors. In contrast with previous findings, they were able to show no advantage of subtotal resection over biopsy. In addition, they found that patients receiving <1400 rad equivalent therapy (ret) did just as well as those receiving a larger dose and that there was a worsening of survival when whole-brain radiation therapy, rather than localized radiation therapy was given.

In 1980, Bloom (44) reviewed the experience at the Royal Marsden Hospital in treating brain tumors with radiation therapy. His treatment group consisted of 120 patients with grade I or II lesions. Although survival data are given only for those treated with surgery and radiation therapy (grade I: 5-year survival 33%, 10-year 16%; grade II: 5-year 21%, 10-year 6%), he concluded that "delay of recurrence and greater survival can be expected following postoperative radiotherapy than after surgery alone."

In 1984, Laws et al. (19) again used the patient population at the Mayo Clinic to review 461 astrocytoma patients treated between 1915 and 1975. These cases were selected from a much larger group of patients and represented only those with supratentorial tumors who survived at least 30 days postoperatively and for whom follow-up data were available. Multiple prognostic factors were analyzed for possible correlation with increased survival. They found that patient age was the most important variable and surpassed all others in its positive correlation with long-term survival. In addition, they interpreted the data as supporting radical surgery and indicating a beneficial effect of radiation therapy only in those patients with poor prognostic factors (e.g., older age). Their data have been reinterpreted by Sheline (45), however, as showing a survival advantage for the irradiated group if one considers only those receiving >4000 rad as having been adequately irradiated.

In 1985, Garcia and associates (46) undertook a retrospective study of 86 adults treated at Washington University between 1950 and 1970. Although the number of patients with well-differentiated astrocytomas was small, they found that those with a juvenile pilocytic type did well, regardless of treatment, and did not require radiation therapy, a conclusion that has been confirmed in other recent studies.

In 1987, Piepmeier (7) reviewed the records of 60 patients with low-grade astrocytomas seen at the Yale–New Haven Hospital between 1975 and 1985. In this retrospective review, there was no significant difference in survival found between those patients who received radiation therapy in addition to surgery and those who did not. What is important in this study is that all patients who were irradiated received between 50 and 60 Gy, delivered over 5–6 weeks to fields that were delineated through CT scanning to include the tumor plus a wide margin of surrounding brain. The author cautioned that since the patient population was treated over the last decade, the mean follow-up time was slightly less than 5 years and, thus, might not be sufficient for evaluating the potential long-term beneficial effects of radiation therapy. However, most previous studies that indicated a beneficial effect of radiation therapy found this to occur at 5 years, with such beneficial effect decreasing at 10 years and longer.

In 1988, Medbery and colleagues (47) reviewed 60 patients with low-grade astrocytomas who were treated at the Bethesda Naval Hospital between 1960 and 1986. The series compared 50 patients who received postoperative radiation therapy with 10 patients who did not. Although the numbers are small, there appeared to be a survival advantage at 5 years for those patients with incompletely resected lesions who received radiation therapy.

In 1989, Shaw et al. (23) once again reviewed the patients at the Mayo Clinic and reported on 167 patients, of whom 139 (83%) received surgery plus radiation therapy, with a mean tumor dose of 50 Gy. The 5-year survival rate for those receiving high-dose (>53 Gy) radiation therapy was 68%, whereas the survival rate was 47% for those who received low-dose irradiation (<53 Gy), and 32% for those who had surgery, but were not irradiated. The comparable 10-year survival rates were 39, 21, and 11%, respectively. In contrast with these data for the grade I and II astrocytomas indicating a beneficial effect of radiation therapy, they found that postoperatively irradiation was not associated with improved survival in the patients with pilocytic astrocytomas.

Hirsch et al. (48), in 1989, reported on 22 pediatric patients (≤ 15 years old) who were operated on for grade I or II astrocytomas. None of these patients were initially given radiation therapy. Since only 3 recurrences (8%) were seen in the entire group of 42 patients (which included 8 patients with oligodendroglioma and 12 patients with oligoastrocytoma), the authors concluded that postoperative radiation therapy should not be given to pediatric patients with low-grade cerebral gliomas.

In 1990, North et al. (49) reported on a series of 77 patients from the Johns Hopkins School of Medicine who were treated with a uniform radiation therapy dose of 50–55 Gy over a period of 5½–6 weeks. Most importantly, in this study, quality of life was determined at 1–2 years postoperatively and at last follow-up at 2½ years after surgery. They observed that mental retardation was observed in 50% of the children who had received radiation therapy. Overall, however, 80% of short-term survivors and 67% of adult long-term survivors were intellectually and physically intact and without major neurological deficit.

Also, in 1990, Whitton and Bloom (50) reviewed 88 adults with cerebral low-grade gliomas who were treated with postoperative radiotherapy at the Royal Marsden Hospital between 1960 and 1985. Treatments were given five times a week for a total dose of 50–55 Gy. They were able to confirm that age was a very important prognostic factor, but indicated that it was still unclear whether or not postoperative radiotherapy was effective.

In 1991, Vertosick et al. (22) analyzed treatment results in 25 patients with well-differentiated cerebral astrocytomas. The median survival for their entire group of patients was 8.2 years, which was the longest that has yet been reported. They attributed this long-term survival to earlier diagnosis in the CT/MRI scan era rather than to the specific efficacy of any modern form of adjuvant therapy. Approximately 70% of their patients received postoperative radiation therapy, whereas 30% did not. In this series, the use of radiotherapy did not have a significant effect on the time to dedifferentiation or the time to death, although they cautioned that the number of patients in each group was small.

In 1992, McCormack et al. (8) carried out a retrospective review of 53 patients with supratentorial astrocytomas. Since fully 98% of their patients received postoperative radiation therapy, it could not be determined whether or not such patients lived longer than those who did not receive such adjuvant therapy.

There has been one report on the use of interstitial permanent radiation with low-intensity ^{125}I in 45 patients with low-grade astrocytomas (51). Although this report is encouraging, we are unable to evaluate the effectiveness of the technique. In 1991, Mundinger et al. (52) reported on the use of interstitial radiation in 89 patients harboring nonresectable low-grade brain stem astrocytomas. Since these tumors differ from cerebral tumors in many respects, one cannot extrapolate on the possible effectiveness of this technique in the treatment of cerebral astrocytomas. However, a paper such as this does indicate that interstitial radiation therapy with ^{125}I, when carried out through an implanted catheter, is a safe and feasible technique.

Given the results of careful histological studies, such as those reported by Kelly (10), in which isolated tumor cells are seen at a distance from the primary enhancing tumor nodule as seen on neuroradiologic studies, it would appear that the production of a relatively small, well-circumscribed necrotic volume by a technique such as stereotactic radiosurgery does not offer great promise from a theoretical point of view.

Most of the major English-language studies have found that radiation therapy is beneficial as an adjunct to surgery in the treatment of cerebral astrocytomas (Table 1). However, since, as we have indicated, these studies have all been flawed in one or more ways, we must consider the conclusion on the beneficial effect of radiation therapy reached from this literature review to be tentative, at best.

Future advances in technology may allow a subgroup of patients with low-grade atrocytomas to be selected who would most benefit from receiving postoperative radiation therapy. Currently, procedures have been developed that can measure the proliferative potential of low-grade astrocytomas, using immunohistochemical techniques such as in vivo (16) or in vitro (53) labeling with 5-bromodeoxyuridine (BRDU) or labeling with the monoclonal antibody Ki-67. A more simple technique may involve the measurement of nucleolar organizer regions (54). Preliminary data appear to reveal a correlation between a poor prognosis and an increase in proliferative potential. Furthermore, a study of 12 patients, with low-grade astrocytomas, who underwent PET scanning with [^{18}F]fluorodeoxyglucose (FDG) indicated that malignant change may be associated with a focal area of hypermetabolism that develops within an area that, in general, is hypometabolic (12). If this is confirmed in other studies, then perhaps only those patients whose tumors have a labeling index above a certain level or who have a hypermetabolic area on PET scanning should receive radiation therapy.

The issue of whether or not radiation therapy should be used in these patients is not one that can be taken lightly. In patients with anaplastic astrocytomas or glioblastoma multiforme, it is probable that the relatively short survival time prevents the long-term deleterious effects of radiation therapy from becoming manifest. This would not be true in patients with low-grade lesions, who have a much longer postoperative survival rate.

There have been many studies of complications produced by cerebral radiation therapy. One such study reported on patients in whom malignant gliomas developed after radiation therapy that had been previously administered for other conditions (55). At least seven such cases have been documented; patients who experienced this complication tended to be young, as is true for most patients with low-grade astrocytomas who are given radiation therapy. A recent review from the Mount Sinai Hospital in New York City found seven cases of radiation-induced meningiomas (56). The overwhelming majority of these patients had received low-dose radiation therapy (8 Gy) to the scalp for tinea capitis. The second largest group, however, were patients who received high-dose radiation for primary brain tumors.

Table 1 Treatment of Cerebral Astrocytoma

Refs.	Years of study	Type of astrocytoma	No. of cases	Radiation dose	3 yr Surgery	3 yr Surgery and radiation	5 yr Surgery	5 yr Surgery and radiation	10 yr Surgery	10 yr Surgery and radiation
35	1940–1949	Astrocytomas grade I and II	176	?	52	62	26	36		
36	1939–1958	Astrocytomas	152	5000–6000 Gy	59	61.7	38	49		
37	?	Astrocytomas grade I and II	194	?		*Median survival:*	Biopsy alone: 2 mo Biopsy + RT: 10 mo		Resection alone: 23 mo Resection + RT: 32 mo	
38	1955–1959	Astrocytomas grade I and II	83	2000–6000 Gy	63.6	64	65	54		
39	1956–1970	Cerebral astrocytomas grade II	45	3500–6500 Gy			20	42		
40	1957–1973	Astrocytomas	40	4900–6650 Gy		62		~41		~22
41	1942–1967	Astrocytomas grade I and II	147	3500–5000 Gy	27	59	19	46	11	35
21	1960–1970	Astrocytomas grade I and II	107	?	*Average survival:*	Surgery: 28 mo Surgery + RT: 35 mo	Surgery + RT: 35 mo			
42	1958–1974	Astrocytomas grade I and II	68	850–1400 ret			32	54	32	26
43	1960–1969	Astrocytomas grade I and II	134	1400 ret				64		

Table 1 (continued)

Refs.	Years of study	Type of astrocytoma	No. of cases	Radiation dose	Survival (%)					
					3 yr		5 yr		10 yr	
					Surgery	Surgery and radiation	Surgery	Surgery and radiation	Surgery	Surgery and radiation
44	1952–1970	Astrocytomas grade I and II	120 (adults)				Grade I: 33 Grade II: 21			Grade I: 16 Grade II: 6
19	1915–1975	Astrocytomas low-grade	461	4000–7900 rad			~35	~50	~10	~15
46	1950–1979	Astrocytomas grade I, II, III	86	3500–6100 rad	35	61	22	40	9	9
7	1975–1985	Astrocytomas low-grade	60 (adults)	5000–6000 rad			*Mean survival:* Biopsy alone: 6.67 yr; STR alone: 5.10 yr; TR alone: 9.58 yr Biopsy + RT: 6.01 yr; TR + RT: 6.34 yr; TR + RT: 7.65 yr			
47	1960–1986	Astrocytomas grade I and II	60	3200–6480 rad	58		STR:	25	43	**3**
20	1950–1982	Astrocytomas "well differentiated"	85	?	58	>4000 rad = 73 <4000 rad = 40	TR: 30	100 >4000 rad = 9 <4000 rad = 25	67 7	>4000 rad = 9 <4000 rad = 0

Ref	Dates	Histology	No. of patients	Radiation dose				
23	1960–1982	Astrocytomas grades I and II; Pilocytic astrocytomas and oligoastrocytomas	167	600–6500 rad		32	>5300 rad = 68, <5300 rad = 47	11 >5300 rad = 39, <5300 rad = 21
50	1960–1985	Astrocytomas grade I and II	60	5000–5500 rads	62		36	28
49	1975–1984	Astrocytoma grade I and II	77 (25 children)	5000–5500 rad			55	43
22	1978–1988	Astrocytoma grade I and II	25	5400–6000 rad	(all pts: median = 8.2 yr)		all pts. 65	all pts. 36
8	1977–1988	Astrocytoma grade I and II	53	2400–6800 rad	(all pts: median = 7.5 yr)		64	48

Although the reported incidence of radiation necrosis varies widely, white matter changes are being seen more and more frequently on MRI scans of patients who have previously undergone radiation therapy. A recent study indicates the presence of radiation necrosis in 9% of a series of 76 patients treated with whole-brain radiation for various intrinsic brain tumors (57). It is of interest that a review of 371 irradiated brain tumor patients by Marks and Wong (58) found the incidence of radiation necrosis to be 1.5% at 55 Gy and 4% at 60 Gy, with a substantial increase for higher doses. Since it is generally accepted that the risk of untoward sequelae from radiation therapy is greater after whole-brain radiation therapy than after more localized treatment, it would seem most prudent to carry out only localized radiation, if one decides to use this adjuvant form of therapy.

X. TREATMENT AT RECURRENCE

Failures of the previously described treatment modalities are almost always due to local recurrence. This can be the result either of the continued growth of the low-grade neoplasm (which can result in the death of the patient if this tumor is located in the deeper part of the brain), or to dedifferentiation of a low-grade tumor into a malignant glioma.

The treatment of such a recurrence depends on establishing the tumor grade. This implies that repeat biopsy will be necessary in most cases. If the tumor remains low-grade, then the patient may be followed by periodic CT, MRI, or PET scans, or a combination thereof. Observation may also be warranted if the patient's clinical status is stable. If such a tumor is enlarging and causing significant mass effect or cerebrospinal fluid obstruction, then repeat resection alone should be considered. On the other hand, if the neuroradiologic studies, clinical course, or biopsy indiate that malignant transformation has occurred, a more aggressive course consisting of repeat surgical resection, interstitial radiation therapy or chemotherapy, or a combination of such, may be considered. Since the time period between the initial radiation that may have been given and the recurrence may be quite long, reirradiation may even be considered. A good result after reirradiation has recently been described in a patient whose tumor recurred 8½ years after the initial treatment (59).

XI. OUTCOME

A review of the several series that were carried out before 1990 would indicate a 5-year survival rate of approximately 40–50% and a 10-year survival rate of approximately 20–30%. However, the two most recent series that included patients who were diagnosed solely within the CT scan era indicate a current median survival for the entire group of patients of approximately 7½ years, with a 5-year survival of approximately 65%, and a 10-year survival of approximately 40% (8,22).

XII. CONCLUSIONS

Because the prospective randomized studies that are presently being carried out have not been completed, the optimal treatment of the patient with a low-grade astrocytoma remains controversial. Until more definitive data become available, certain tentative conclusions may be drawn:

1. An attempt should be made to obtain pathological confirmation of the nature of a supratentorial lesion that is seen on CT or MRI scan and has at least some of the features of an intrinsic brain tumor.
2. Consistent with sound neurosurgical judgment for postoperative sequelae, an attempt should be made to carry out gross total removal of a hemispheric astrocytoma or to remove as much tumor as possible.

3. In the event of such a gross total surgical removal (and even in its absence for the cerebral pilocytic astrocytoma) radiation therapy can be withheld and the patient carefully followed-up with periodic CT or MRI scans. If the lesion does not show definitive evidence of recurrence, then radiation therapy should be withheld. If the cerebral low-grade astrocytoma is present in a pediatric patient (even if the resection has not been complete), then radiation should be withheld and the patient carefully followed with CT, MRI, and possibly PET scans.

4. It is likely that in the near future new techniques employing monoclonal antibodies and PET scanning will allow us to select a subpopulation of patients who would most likely benefit from postoperative radiation therapy.

5. However, currently, in cases where total removal cannot be accomplished, postoperative radiation therapy may be warranted.

6. Such radiation therapy should be given in a conventional fractionation schedule to a dose not exceeding 55 Gy. This radiation therapy should be given to a limited volume, as determined by CT or MRI studies, rather than to the whole brain. As future studies become available, it is quite possible that interstitial radiation therapy will play a role in the treatment of this tumor.

7. With present-day techniques, an optimal treatment regimen for the patient whose diagnosis is a low-grade astrocytoma will lead to a median survival of approximately 7½ years with a 5-year survival of approximately 65% and a 10-year survival of approximately 40%. A more precise estimate of survival time can be made if the particular prognostic variables of the individual patient are known.

REFERENCES

1. Kernohan JW, Mabon RF, Svien HJ, Adson AW. A simplified classification of the gliomas. Mayo Clin Proc 1949; 24:71–75.

2. Daumas-Duport C, Scheithauer BW, O'Fallon J, et al. Grading astrocytomas. A simple and reproducible method. Cancer 1988; 62:2152–2165.

3. Kim TS, Holliday AL, Hedley-Whyte ET, et al. Correlates of survival and the Daumas-Duport grading system for astrocytomas. J Neurosurg 1991; 74:27–37.

4. Krouwer HG, Davis RL, Silver P, et al. Gemistocytic astrocytomas: a reappraisal. J Neurosurg 1991; 74:399–406.

5. Schoenberg BS, Christine BW, Whisnant JP. The descriptive epidemiology of primary intracranial neoplasms: the Connecticut experience. Am J Epidemiol 1976; 104:499–510.

6. Silverman C, Marks JE. Prognostic significance of contrast enhancement in the low-grade astrocytomas of the adult cerebrum. Radiology 1981; 139:211–213.

7. Piepmeier JM. Observations on the current treatment of low-grade astrocytic tumors of the cerebral hemispheres. J Neurosurg 1987; 67:177–181.

8. McCormack B, Miller D, Budzilovich G, et al. Treatment and survival in adults with low-grade astrocytomas. Neurosurgery 1992; 31:636–642.

9. Guthrie BL, Laws ER. Supratentorial low-grade gliomas. Neurosurg Clin North Am 1990; 1:37–48.

10. Kelly PJ, Daumas-Duport C, Scheithauer BW, et al. Stereotactic histologic correlations of computed tomography and magnetic resonance imaging defined abnormalities in patients with glial neoplasms. Mayo Clin Proc 1987; 62:450–459.

11. Worthington C, Tyler JL, Villemure JG. Stereotactic biopsy and positron emission tomography correlation of cerebral gliomas. Surg Neurol 1987; 27:87–92.

12. Francavilla TL, Miletich RS, Dichiro G, et al. Positron emission tomography in the detection of malignant degeneration of low-grade gliomas. Neurosurgery 1989; 26:1–5.

13. Hoshino T, Wilson CB. Cell kinetic analysis of human malignant brain tumors (gliomas). Cancer 1979; 44:956–962.

14. Yoshii Y, Maki Y, Tsuboi K, et al. Estimation of growth fraction with bromodeoxyuridine in human central nervous system tumor. J Neurosurg 1986; 65:659–663.

15. Hoshino TA. A commentary on the biology and growth kinetics of low-grade and high-grade gliomas. J Neurosurg 1984; 61:895–900.
16. Hoshino T, Rodriguez LA, Cho KG, et al. Prognostic implications of the proliferative potential of low-grade astrocytomas. J Neurosurg 1988; 69:839–842.
17. Garcia CM, Fulling KH. Juvenile pilocytic astrocytomas of the cerebral hemispheres. J Neurosurg 1985; 63:382–386.
18. Palma L, Guidetti B. Cystic pilocytic astrocytomas of the cerebral hemispheres. J Neurosurg 1985; 62:811–815.
19. Laws ER, Taylor WF, Clifton MB, Okazaki H. Neurosurgical management of low-grade astrocytomas of the cerebral hemispheres. J Neurosurg 1984; 61:665–673.
20. Soffietti R, Chio A, Giordana MT, Vasario E, Schiffer D. Prognostic factors in well-differentiated cerebral astrocytomas in adults. Neurosurgery 1989; 24:686–692.
21. Weir B, Grace M. The relative significance of factors affecting postoperative survival in astrocytomas grade one and two. Can J Neurol Sci 1976; 3:47–50.
22. Vertosick FT, Selker RG, Arena VC. Survival of patients with well-differentiated astrocytomas diagnosed in the era of computed tomography. Neurosurgery 1991; 28:496–501.
23. Shaw EG, Daumas-Duport C, Scheithauer BW, et al. Radiation therapy in the management of low-grade supratentorial astrocytomas. J Neurosurg 1989; 70:853–861.
24. Scherer JH. Cerebral astrocytomas and their derivatives. Am J Cancer 1940; 40:159–198.
25. Russell DS, Rubinstein LJ. Pathology of tumors of the nervous system, 4th ed. Baltimore: Williams & Wilkins, 1977.
26. Winger MJ, MacDonald DR, Cairncross JG. Supratentorial anaplastic gliomas in adults—the prognostic importance of extent of resection and prior low-grade glioma. J Neurosurg 1989; 71:487–493.
27. Muller W, Afra D, Schroder R. Supratentorial recurrences of gliomas: morphological studies in relation to time intervals with astrocytomas. Acta Neurochir (Wien) 1977; 37:75–91.
28. Fults D, Brockmeyer D, Tullous MW, Pedone CA, Cawthon, RM. p53 Mutation and loss of heterozygosity on chromosomes 17 and 10 during human astrocytoma progression. Cancer Res 1992; 52:674–679.
29. Schiffer D, Giordana MT, Soffietti R, et al. Effects of radiotherapy on the astrocytomatous areas of malignant gliomas. J Neurooncol 1984; 2:167–175.
30. Cairncross JG, Laperrier NJ. Low-grade glioma: to treat or not to treat? Arch Neurol 1989; 46:1238–1239.
31. Salcman M. Radical surgery for low grade gliomas. Clin Neurosurg 1990; 36:353–366.
32. Djerassi I, Kim JS, Rigger A. Response of astrocytomas to high-dose methotrexate with citrovorum factor rescue. Cancer 1985; 55:2741–2747.
33. Eagan RT, Dinapoli RP, Herman RC, et al. Combination carmustine (BCNU) and dihydrogalactilol in the treatment of primary brain tumors recurring after irradiation. Cancer Treat Rep 1982; 66:1647–1649.
34. Eyre HJ, Eltringham JR, Crowley J, Morantz RA. A randomized trial of radiotherapy versus radiotherapy plus CCNU for incompletely resected low-grade gliomas: a Southwest Oncology Group study J Neurosurg (in press).
35. Levy LF, Elvidge AR. Astrocytoma of the brain and spinal cord: a review of 176 cases, 1940–1949. J Neurosurg 1956; 13:413–443.
36. Bouchard J, Pierce CB. Radiation therapy in the management of neoplasms of the central nervous system with a special note in regard to children: twenty years' experience, 1939–1958. AJR 1960; 84:610–628.
37. Gol A. The relatively benign astrocytomas of the cerebrum: a clinical study of 194 verified cases. J Neurosurg 1961; 18:501–506.
38. Uihlein A, Colby Y, Layton DD, Parsons WR, Carter TL. Comparison of surgery and surgery plus irradiation in the treatment of supratentorial gliomas. Acta Radiol 1966; 5:67–78.
39. Stage WS, Stein JJ. Treatment of malignant astrocytomas. AJR 1976; 120:7–18.
40. Marsa GW, Goffinet DR, Rubinstein LJ, Bagshaw MA. Megavoltage irradiation in the treatment of gliomas of the brain and spinal cord. Cancer 1975; 36:1681–1689.

41. Leibel SA, Sheline GE, Wara WM, Boldrey EB, Nielson SL. The role of radiation therapy in the treatment of astrocytomas. Cancer 1975; 35:1551–1557.
42. Fazekas JT. Treatment of grades I and II brain astrocytomas: the role of radiotherapy. Int J Radiat Oncol Biol Phys 1977; 2:661–666.
43. Scanlon PW, Taylor WF. Radiotherapy of intracranial astrocytomas: analysis of 417 cases treated from 1960 through 1969. Neurosurgery 1979; 5:301–307.
44. Bloom HJC. Intracranial tumors: response and resistance to therapeutic endeavors. Int J Radiat Oncol Biol Phys 1982; 8:1083–1113.
45. Sheline GE. The role of radiation therapy in the treatment of low-grade gliomas. Clin Neurosurg 1985; 33:563–574.
46. Garcia DM, Fulling KH, Marks JE. The value of radiation therapy in addition to surgery for astrocytomas of the adult cerebrum. Cancer 1985; 55:919–927.
47. Medbery CA, Straus KL, Steinberg SM, Cotelingam JD, Fisher WS. Low-grade astrocytomas: treatment results and prognostic variables. Int J Radiat Oncol Biol Phys 1988; 15:837–841.
48. Hirsch J-F, Sainte Rose C, Pierre-Kahn A, et al. Benign astrocytic and oligodendrocytic tumors of the cerebral hemispheres in children. J. Neurosurg 1989; 70:568–572.
49. North, CA, North RB, Epstein JA, et al. Low-grade cerebral astrocytomas. Survival and quality of life after radiation therapy. Cancer 1990; 66:6–14.
50. Whitton AC, Bloom HJG. Low grade glioma of the cerebral hemispheres in adults: a retrospective study of 88 cases. Int J Radiat Oncol Biol Phys 1990; 18:783–786.
51. Frank F, Fabrizi AP, Gaist G, Frank-Ricci R, Piazzi M, Spagnolli F. Late consideration in the treatment of low-grade malignancy cerebral tumors with iodine-125 brachytherapy. Appl Neurophysiol 1987; 50:302–309.
52. Mundinger F, Braus DF, Krauss JK. Long-term outcome of 89 low-grade brain stem gliomas after interstitial radiation therapy. J Neurosurg 1991; 75:740–746.
53. Nishizak T, Orita T, Saiki M, Furutani Y, Aoki H. Cell kinetic studies of human brain tumors by in vitro labeling using anti-BUDR monoclonal antibody. J Neurosurg 1988; 69:371–374.
54. Hara A, Hirayoma H, Sakai N. Correlation between nucleolar organizer region staining and Ki-67 immunostaining in human gliomas. Surg Neurol 1990; 33:320–324.
55. Shapiro S, Mealey J Jr, Sartorius C. Radiation-induced intracranial malignant gliomas. J Neurosurg 1989; 71:77–82.
56. Harrison MJ, Wolfe DE, Lau TS. Radiation induced meningiomas: experience at the Mount Sinai Hospital and review of the literature. J Neurosurg 1991; 75:564–574.
57. Hohwieler ML, Lo TC, Silverman ML, Friedberg SR. Brain necrosis after radiotherapy for primary intracerebral tumor. Neurosurgery 1986; 18:67–74.
58. Marks JE, Wong I. The risk of cerebral radionecrosis in relation to dose, time and fractionation: a follow-up study. Prog Exp Tumor Res 1985; 29:210–218.
59. Selbergeld D, Griffin BR, Vjemann GA. Reirradiation for recurrent cerebral astrocytoma. J Neurooncol 1992; 12:145–151.

13

Surgery for Malignant Gliomas

Michael Salcman
George Washington University, Washington, D.C.

I. INTRODUCTION

Patients with malignant glioma provide the clinician with an almost bewildering array of treatment options, primarily because of the lack of a truly effective therapy and secondarily because of the biological variability displayed by the tumor and its host (1,57). A surgical recommendation for the treatment of a grade 2 astrocytoma in the temporal lobe of a 22-year-old man will necessarily differ from that given to a 64-year-old woman with a grade 4 astrocytoma or glioblastoma multiforme centered in the body of the corpus callosum. In the treatment of malignant gliomas of all types, surgery is almost never the sole modality, and its use is usually embedded within the context of a total treatment plan (2,3). The effectiveness or practicality of some surgical options may depend as much on the availability or efficacy of other treatments as it does on the age and general condition of the patient or the site and histological character of the lesion. Malignant gliomas arise in all portions of the nervous system and at all ages; the signs and symptoms, as well as the risks of surgery, are usually conditioned by the age of the patient and the site of origin. Histologically, these tumors comprise a broad spectrum of lesions thought to arise through the dedifferentiation of adult astrocytes, ependymal cells, oligodendroglia, or their primitive precursors. Taken together, the variables of tumor site, patient age, and tumor histological type roughly circumscribe a prognostic range within which the likely benefit of a particular surgical option and treatment plan will be found (Table 1). Recommendations for surgery should never be made without an adequate knowledge of the relevant prognostic variables in an individual patient (4). We shall begin by discussing the available surgical options and their rationale in a relatively nontechnical manner and close with a discussion of how appropriate recommendations can be made in individual patients.

II. OPEN SURGERY OR CRANIOTOMY

It is now possible to safely remove the greater portion of glial tumors from virtually every location in the cerebral hemispheres as well as from many sites within the ventricles and in close proximity to the thalami and basal ganglia (5). As a practical definition, a *radical excision* of a glioma may be said to be the removal of its enhancing rim, as demonstrated either by computed tomography (CT)

Table 1 Prognostic Variables for Survival in Glioblastoma

Variable	Probability of survival
Patient	
Age	$p < 0.0002–0.00001$
Sex	NS
Performance preoperatively	$p < 0.001–0.00001$
Performance postoperatively	$p < 0.005$
Blood type	$p = 0.05$
Tumor	
Kernohan grade	$p < 0.00001$
Neovascularity	$p < 0.001$
Necrosis	$p < 0.001$
Lymphocytes	NS to $p < 0.01$
Therapy	
Extent of resection	$p < 0.001–0.0001$
Post-RT[a] volume	$p < 0.0001–0.00001$

[a]RT, radiotherapy.

or by magnetic resonance imaging (MRI) as well as all of the tissue contained within that boundary. There is a good correlation between the enhancing rim and the boundary of resectable tissue (6). However, a radical excision cannot remove the scattered nests of malignant cells that extend for variable distances into the surrounding neuropil, without endangering the functional capacity of the patient (7). As a practical matter, the neurosurgeon should always endeavor to resect the maximal amount of tumor, with the least possible mechanical disturbance to the brain or spinal cord (5). The safety and "completeness" of such removals have been increased by several technological advances. Large tumors in deep sites can be safely approached through narrow tunnels, with the aid of the magnification and illumination provided by the operating microscope and its attendant instrumentation. Bipolar coagulation and the use of the carbon dioxide laser can control the vascularity of the tumor. The lesion can be vaporized by the laser, or emulsified and removed by the ultrasonic aspirator, with minimal damage to surrounding structures (8). The use of the microscope emphasizes gentleness of technique and often provides the surgeon with a better view of the apparent margin (i.e., the enhancing rim) between the tumor and the subjacent brain. Edema fluid in the surrounding neuropil may be seen to glisten beneath the microscope, and subtle changes in tissue color and consistency are more easily identified. Intraoperative measurements are also frequently taken to determine the final size and shape of the resection bed; at the close of the operation, these measurements should closely match the ones obtained during preoperative scrutiny of the MRI or CT scan (5).

Some tumors in especially critical locations require microsurgical dissection within a natural fissure, sulcus, or ventricle for their exposure (9). The limits of safe resection can also be defined by functional testing of the language or motor areas in a manner similar to that employed in cortical and subcortical resections carried out for epilepsy (10,11). This method is to be preferred to the preoperative use of measurements to obtain the approximate location of eloquent areas in the brain, despite the fact that the motor strip can frequently be identified on contemporary MRI scans. Stereotactic techniques (see later) can also be used in combination with open craniotomy to safely lead the surgeon to deep targets through short incisions in critical areas of the overlying cortex (12). Intraoperative ultrasound can also be used for this purpose (13). Despite this impressive technological armamentarium, it is not clear that a radical excision can safely be carried out in most patients, and it is not known whether it is of benefit under all prognostic circumstances (14,15).

The biological and clinical rationale for the radical excision of glial tumors is summarized in Table 2. Almost all the data on the survival value of tumor resection is retrospective and uncontrolled. Nevertheless, a number of clinical points seem quite persuasive. Unlike lymphomas and leukemias, malignant gliomas are solid tumors composed of highly heterogeneous cell populations. The survival of patients with solid tumors outside the nervous system is usually a direct function of the surgical or anatomical stage of the disease (16). The survival of patients with a variety of benign and low-grade tumors within the nervous system, including meningiomas, chordomas, and low-grade astrocytomas, has also been shown to correlate with the extent of resection (17–20). Similar data have been put forth for medulloblastoma, a highly malignant neuroectodermal tumor of childhood (21). The available retrospective data for malignant astrocytoma and glioblastoma indicate a rough correlation between survival and the extent of resection for patients not receiving any other forms of therapy (Fig. 1) and a beneficial effect on the length and quality of survival when the postoperative CT scan has been cleared of all enhancing tumor (22–24) (Figs. 2 and 3). In a prospective randomized trial of radiation and chemotherapy carried out by the Brain Tumor Study Group, stratification of the patients by the extent of surgery, as defined by the postoperative CT-scan, revealed a statistically significant inverse relation (Fig. 4) between residual tumor burden and survival (25). This has been confirmed in several prognostic factor studies not specifically addressed to this variable (26–28).

From a theoretical point of view, mechanical cytoreduction is the most rapid and effective means for reducing tumor burden and for eliminating those cellular compartments of the tumor mass that are inherently resistant to virtually all other forms of therapy (2,3,12). The slowly dividing, poorly vascularized and underoxygenated cells in the center of the tumor are the least likely to respond to ionizing radiation and chemotherapy. In addition, surgery can alter the susceptibility of the remaining cells to these modalities by decreasing population pressure and altering cell kinetics (29), by changing the immunologic status of the host (30), and by improving the access of drugs and biologicals to the remaining mass (31,32). Surgery can be used on a repetitive basis to "set up" changes in therapy, to improve the neurological function of the patient (33), and to avoid the life-threatening effects of intractable intracranial hypertension (34). The

Table 2 Theoretical and Practical Benefits of Open-Tumor Resection

Mechanical cytoreduction
   Produces a rapid 2-log cell kill
   Removes resistant cells
   Prolongs survival

Amelioration of symptoms
   Improved neurological status
   Decreased intracranial pressure

Treatment interactions
   Can potentiate or facilitate radiotherapy, chemotherapy, and immunotherapy

Diagnostic precision
   Extensive tissue sampling
   Routine and special studies
   Tissue culture

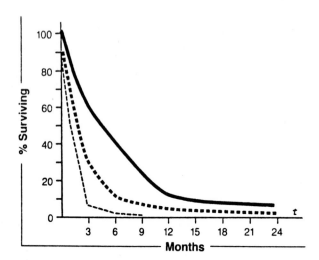

Figure 1   Effect of time and type of surgery on survival. The curves are based on 603 glioblastoma patients drawn from the literature in whom extensive surgical resection (solid line, 172 cases), partial surgical resection (heavy broken line, 301 cases), or simple biopsy (light broken line, 130 cases) was performed without subsequent irradiation or chemotherapy (From Ref. 3)

neurological status of the patient almost always improves or remains stable after reoperation, and such procedures can be used to prolong survival up to 37 weeks after radiographic or clinical recurrence (35–38) (Fig. 5). Before the advent of modern surgical techniques, reoperations were only infrequently and selectively performed (39–43). Local wound care and bone flap infections are among the most important postoperative considerations in patients with previously irradiated and devitalized tissues (44).

From a practical point of view, many more tumors are now susceptible to radical excision, irrespective of their size and location, because of recent advances in surgical technique and technology. In at least one series of patients treated by conventional craniotomy, 86% of the

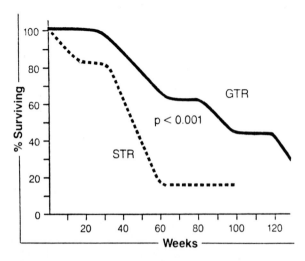

Figure 2   Cumulative survival rate after operation related to extent of surgical resection: GTR, gross total tumor resection; STR, subtotal tumor resection. (From Ref. 22)

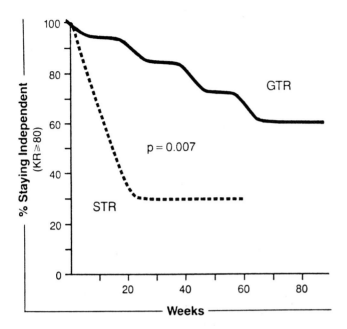

Figure 3 Extent of resection affects Karnofsky rating. The cumulative postoperative time spent in an independent status is dependent on the extent of the surgery. KR, Karnofsky rating; GTR, gross total tumor resection; STR, subtotal tumor resection. (From Ref. 22)

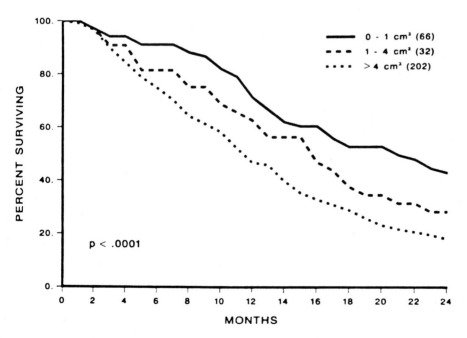

Figure 4 Survival curves of 300 patients in a valid study group relating survival to size of residual tumor on postoperative contrast-enhanced CT scans. The patients were divided into three groups based on tumor area (0–1, 1–4, and > 4 cm²). There is a significant ordering of the survival curves based on the residual tumor burden. (From Ref. 25)

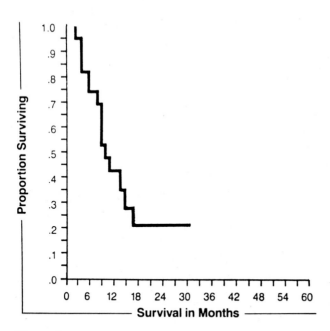

Figure 5 Kaplan–Meier survival curve after reoperation for malignant astrocytoma. The calculated probability of survival from the time of the second operation is plotted for 40 consecutive patients reoperated on in a consecutive series of 74 in whom reoperation was prospectively used during aggressive multimodality therapy; the median additional survival time until death or until the third operation is 37 weeks. (From Ref. 37)

postoperative CT scans were normalized (24), with an improved or stable neurological status in 97% and no operative mortality. The risk of postoperative complications is no greater following gross total resections than with subtotal tumor removals (45). Even in the basal ganglia and thalamus, computer-based stereotactic laser resections have successfully achieved gross total removals in many patients (46). Nevertheless, it is not at all clear that once a tumor has invaded the corpus callosum, the brain stem, or has shown evidence of subependymal spread, that removal of its grearter portion has any survival advantage over simple biopsy alone.

III.   STEREOTACTIC AND COMBINED PROCEDURES

Contemporary neurosurgery has benefited greatly from two important technical revolutions; the first was the advent of the operating microscope and the second, the mating of traditional stereotactic frames to imaging devices such as CT and MRI scanners (see also Chap. 16). In image-based stereotaxy, a mechanical device is bolted to the patient's head, and an MRI or CT scan is obtained in the usual fashion. The computer in the scanner is used to determine the three-dimensional coordinates of any point inside the head in relation to the "stereotactic space" delimited by the frame. These coordinates are then entered on the micrometers attached to the frame in the operating room, and probes of various types can be driven through small twist-drill holes in the skull to any intracranial location. The probes can be biopsy instruments to obtain tissue, endoscopes for the visualization of intraventricular disease, or catheters for the delivery of interstitial radiation or microwave hyperthermia (47–51). The procedures are carried out under local anesthesia and often employ small puncture holes in the skin through which stereotactic drills can be used to penetrate the skull (52). In some clinics, stereotactic procedures represent 20–30%

of the operations carried out for supratentorial tumors (12,53). Tissue can be safely obtained from the thalamus, the basal ganglia, and the brain stem with less than a 2.3% mortality, a 3% risk of hemorrhage, and a 1% morbidity (47,49). The small pieces of tissue are diagnostic in more than 90% of patients, and the procedure can be safely repeated in debilitated patients and through devitalized tissue. Except under extraordinary circumstances and through the use of expensive equipment (see later), stereotactic procedures cannot actually remove tumor tissue in therapeutically significant amounts. As indicated earlier, however, stereotactic probes can be used to deliver other treatment modalities, such as radiation and hyperthermia, to the tumor volume defined by the scan. Experimental techniques being developed include the stereotactic delivery of laser light for the photoactivation chemotherapy (54), endoscopic laser ablation of intraventricular masses, and catheter deposition of immunological reagents and other biologicals. A recent development has been the application of stereotactic radiosurgery to the treatment of malignant gliomas (55) (see Chap. 26). In this technique, the stereotactic frame and target calculation are carried out in the usual fashion, but instead of a probe being delivered to the tumor, the target is positioned at the intersection of multiple cobalt beams in the gamma knife or at the epicenter of rotation of a linear accelerator. Stereotactic radiosurgery has achieved some success in the treatment of acoustic schwannomas, pituitary tumors, and metastatic lesions; it is too early to know what its role will be in the therapy of intrinsic brain tumors.

Within just the past few years, combined approaches have emerged as an important technical strategy for the safe removal of glial tumors (12). In a combined approach, a stereotactic technique is used to guide the performance of an open craniotomy. Typically, a stereotactic frame is bolted to the patient's head, and a scan is performed to obtain the geometric coordinates of the tumor. The patient is then returned to the operating room and the electrode holder or the probe carrier of the frame is attached. A blunt probe is then stereotactically lowered to the surface of the scalp and used as the guide for outlining a relatively small scalp incision. A similar maneuver is used in designing the bone flap and in opening the dura. The stereotactic probe is then used to select the appropriate gyrus or sulcus for microsurgical incision, and the probe can be used as a guide to orient a transcortical tunnel all the way down to the target. When the tumor has been reached, the operating microscope is moved into place and the stereotactic arc can be removed. Variations on this theme include the use of a robotic arm to mark the incision points, so-called frameless stereotaxy (58), and computer-directed vaporization of the tumor by a laser attached to the stereotactic frame and guided by a stacked-slice reconstruction of the tumor volume stored in the computer's memory (56). This latter technique, when applied to a wide variety of lesions, can have an overall morbidity and mortality as low as 9.3 and 1%, respectively (56). Through the use of such combined approaches, it is possible to remove small lesions in relatively dangerous or poorly demarcated locations, lesions that formerly would have been subjected to stereotactic biopsy alone.

IV. SELECTION OF A SURGICAL APPROACH

All other things being equal, the size and location of the tumor should determine the type of surgical approach selected (Table 3). Large glial tumors in lateral sites should undergo open resection, with the aim of minimally disturbing the brain while achieving a maximal removal of the lesion. Sometimes this can best be accomplished by combining the advantages of open craniotomy with the precision of stereotactic surgery. When the tumor is more centrally located, when it is small and likely to be missed at open surgery, or when the tumor margins are poorly demarcated on the enhanced scan, it is better to subject the patient to a stereotactic biopsy. These considerations are especially important in patients who are neurologically intact and suffering from an initial seizure or other symptom brought on by a low-grade glioma with infiltrating margins (Table 4). Patients who are clinically ill from a large tumor, with potentially reversible focal deficits, or those

Table 3 Factors Influencing Technical Operability for Craniotomy

---

Tumor
 Size
 Location
 Histological type
 Vascularity
 Multiplicity

Patient
 Age
 Performance status
 Neurological deficits
 Prior therapy

Surgeon
 Ability
 Experience
 Technical resources

---

patients who are suffering from intracranial hypertension should be offered the benefits of open craniotomy. Elderly patients with mutifocal lesions or those in whom bilateral spread through the corpus callosum or the cerebrospinal fluid pathways have made meaningful resection impossible should be offered a stereotactic biopsy instead. For reasons that have nothing to do with the physiological ability of older patients to withstand the rigors of general anesthesia and craniotomy, the results of treating glial tumors in the elderly are so poor that the morbidity of open resection cannot be justified unless the tumor is unifocal, free from midline structures, and the host is in excellent neurological condition.

As with many situations in medicine, the selection of an appropriate surgical procedure for a

Table 4 Indications for Stereotactic Surgery

Tumor
 Is centrally located
 Is poorly demarcated by CT or MRI
 Is extremely small
 Is primarily cystic
 Has changed character

Patient
 Is too ill for craniotomy
 Is neurologically intact

Therapy
 Interstitial radiation
 Interstitial hyperthermia
 Stereotactic radiosurgery
 Requires repeat tissue sampling

---

given patient is really the selection of an appropriate patient for an available technique; guidelines and recommendations that we have given here to aid the selection process consist of relative contraindications, rather than hard and fast rules employed without exception. The role of the surgeon in tumor management is to establish a diagnosis, preserve life and function, and effect a cure if possible. Since virtually no malignant glial tumor can be cured by surgical resection alone, the type and extent of surgery offered to a patient should be considered in the context of other therapeutic options and should be consistent with the technical resources of the physician and the psychosocial resources of the patient and his or her family. In most cases, some combination of open resection or stereotactic surgery can produce a diagnosis, ameliorate symptoms, decrease the intracranial pressure, improve neurological status, remove most of the tumor, and deliver other therapeutic agents.

REFERENCES

1. Salcman M, ed. Neurobiology of brain tumors. Vol. 4. Concepts in neurosurgery. Baltimore: Williams & Wilkins, 1991:386 pp.
2. Salcman M. Resection and reoperation in neurooncology. Rationale and approach. Neurol Clin 1985; 3:831–842.
3. Salcman M. The role of surgical resection in the treatment of malignant brain tumors: who benefits? Oncology 1988; 2:47–59.
4. Salcman M. Epidemiology and factors affecting survival. In: Apuzzo MLJ, ed. Malignant cerebral glioma. Park Ridge, IL: American Association Neurological Surgery, 1990:95–109.
5. Salcman M. Supratentorial gliomas: clinical features and surgical therapy. In: Wilkins RH, Rengachary SS, eds. Neurosurgery. New York: McGraw-Hill, 1985:579–550.
6. Burger PC. Pathologic anatomy and CT correlations in the glioblastoma multiforme. Appl Neurophysiol 1983; 46:180–187.
7. Kelly PJ, Daumas-Duport C, Kispert DB, et al. Imaging-based stereotaxic serial biopsies in untreated intracranial glial neoplasms. J Neurosurg 1987; 66:865–874.
8. Salcman M, Robinson W, Montgomery E. Laser microsurgery: a review of 105 intracranial tumors. J Neurooncol 1986; 3:363–371.
9. Pia HW. Microsurgery of gliomas. Acta Neurochir 1986; 80:1–11.
10. Berger MS, Cohen WA, Ojemman GA. Correlation of motor cortex brain mapping data with magnetic resonance imaging. J Neurosurg 1990; 72:383–387.
11. Rostomily RC, Berger MS, Ojemann GA, Lettich E. Postoperative deficits and functional recovery following removal of tumors involving the dominant hemisphere supplementary motor area. J Neurosurg 1991; 75:62–68.
12. Salcman M. Malignant glioma management. Neurosurg Clin North Am 1990; 1:49–63.
13. Rubin JM, Dohrmann G. Intraoperative neurosurgical ultrasound in the localization and characterization of intracranial masses. Radiology 1983; 148:519–524.
14. Coffey RJ, Lunsford LD, Taylor FH. Survival after stereotactic biopsy of malignant gliomas. Neurosurgery 1988; 22:465–473.
15. Quigley MR, Maroon JC. The relationship between survival and the extent of the resection in patients with supratentorial malignant gliomas. Neurosurgery 1991; 29:385–389.
16. Gastrointestinal tumor study group. Adjuvant therapy of colon cancer: results of a prospectively randomized trial. N Engl J Med 1984; 310:737–743.
17. Adegbite AB, Khan MI, Paine KWE, et al. The recurrence of intracranial meningioma after surgical treatment. J Neurosurg 1983; 58:51–56.
18. Laws ER, Taylor WF, Clifton MB, et al. Neurosurgical management of low grade astrocytoma of the cerebral hemispheres. J Neurosurg 1984; 61:665–673.
19. Mirimanoff RO, Dosoretz DE, Linggood RM, et al. Meningioma: analysis of recurrence and progression following neurosurgical resection. J Neurosurg 1985; 62:18–24.
20. Salcman M. Radical surgery for low-grade glioma. Clin Neurosurg 1990; 36:353–366.

21. Park TS, Hoffman HJ, Hendrick EB, et al. Medulloblastoma: clinical presentation and management: experience at the Hospital for Sick Children, Toronto, 1950–1980. J Neurosurg 1983; 58:543–552.

22. Ammirati M, Vick N, Liao Y, et al. Effect of the extent of surgical resection on survival and quality of life in patients with supratentorial glioblastomas and anaplastic astrocytomas. Neurosurgery 1987; 21:201–206.

23. Andreou J, George AE, Wise A, et al. CT prognostic criteria of survival after malignant glioma surgery. Am J Neuroradiol 1983; 4:488–490.

24. Ciric I, Ammirati M, Vick N, et al. Supratentorial gliomas: surgical considerations and immediate postoperative results. Gross total resection versus partial resection. Neurosurgery 1987; 21:21–26.

25. Wood JR, Greene SB, Shapiro WR. The prognostic importance of tumor size in malignant gliomas: a computed tomographic scan study by the Brain Tumor Cooperative Group. J Clin Oncol 1988; 6:338–343.

26. Cohadon F, Aouad N, Rougier A, et al. Histologic and nonhistologic factors correlated with survival time in supratentorial astrocytic tumors. J Neurooncol 1985; 3:105–111, 1985.

27. Hirakawa K, Suzuki K, Ueda S, et al. Multivariate analysis of factors affecting postoperative survival in malignant astrocytoma. J Neurooncol 1984; 2:331–340.

28. Nelson DF, Nelson JS, Davis DR, et al. Survival and prognosis of patients with astrocytoma with atypical or anaplastic features. J Neurooncol 1985; 3:99–103.

29. Hoshino T. A commentary on the biology and growth kinetics of low grade and high grade gliomas. J Neurosurg 1984; 61:895–900.

30. Brooks WH, Roszman TL. Cellular immune responsiveness of patients with primary intracranial tumors. In: Thomas DGT, Graham DI, eds. Brain tumors: scientific basis, clinical investigation, and current therapy. London: Butterworth, 1980:121–132.

31. Salcman M, Broadwell RD. The blood–brain barrier. In: Salcman M, ed. Neurobiology of brain tumors. Vol. 4. Concepts in neurosurgery. Baltimore: Williams & Wilkins, 1991:229–249.

32. Tel E, Hoshino T, Barker M, et al. Effect of surgery on BCNU chemotherapy in a rat brain tumor model. J Neurosurg 1980; 52:529–532.

33. Beaney RP, Brooks DJ, Leenders KL, et al. Blood flow and oxygen utilization in the contralateral cerebral cortex of patients with untreated intracranial tumors as studied by positron emission tomography, with observations on the effect of decompressive surgery. J Neurol Neurosurg Psychiatry 1985; 48:310–319.

34. Shapiro WR. Treatment of neuroectodermal brain tumors. Ann Neurol 1982; 12:231–237.

35. Ammirati M, Galicich JH, Arbit E, et al. Reoperation in the treatment of recurrent intracranial malignant gliomas. Neurosurgery 1987; 21:601–614.

36. Harsh GR IV, Levin VA, Gutin PH, et al. Reoperation for recurrent glioblastoma and anaplastic astrocytoma. Neurosurgery 1987; 21:615–621.

37. Salcman M, Kaplan RS, Ducker TB, et al. Effect of age and reoperation on survival in the combined modality treatment of malignant astrocytoma. Neurosurgery 1982; 10:454–463.

38. Young B, Oldfield EH, Markesbery WR, et al. Reoperation for glioblastoma. J Neurosurg 1981; 55:917–921.

39. Frankel SA, German WJ. Glioblastoma multiforme: review of 219 cases with regard to natural history, pathology, diagnostic methods and treatment. J Neurosurg 1958; 15:489–503.

40. Hitchcock E, Sato F. Treatment of malignant gliomata. J Neurosurg 1964; 21:497–505.

41. Jelsma R, Bucy PC. Treatment of glioblastoma multiforme of the brain. J Neurosurg 1967; 27:388–400.

42. McKeran RO, Thomas DGT. The clinical study of gliomas. In: Thomas DGT, Graham DI, eds. Brain tumors: scientific basis, clinical investigation, and current therapy. London: Butterworth, 1980:194–230.

43. Roth JG, Elvidge AR. Glioblastoma multiforme: a clinical survey. J Neurosurg 1960; 17:736–750.

44. Tenney JH, Vlahov D, Salcman M, et al. Wide variation in risk of wound infection following clean neurosurgery: implications for perioperative antibiotic prophylaxis. J Neurosurg 1985; 62:243–247.

45. Fadul C, Wood J, Thaler H, Galicich J, Patterson RH, Posner JB. Morbidity and mortality of craniotomy for excision of supratentorial gliomas. Neurology 1988; 38:1374–1379.

46. Kelly PJ, Kall BA, Goerss S, et al. Computer-assisted stereotaxic laser resection of intra-axial brain neoplasms. J Neurosurg 1986; 64:427–439.

47. Apuzzo MLJ, Chandrasoma PT, Cohen D, et al. Computed imaging stereotaxy: experience and perspective related to 500 procedures applied to brain masses. Neurosurgery 1987; 20:930–937.
48. Gutin PH, Leibel SA, Wara WM, et al. Recurrent malignant gliomas: survival following interstitial brachytherapy with high-activity iodine-125 sources. J Neurosurg 1987; 67:864–973.
49. Ostertag CB, Mennel HD, Kiessling M. Stereotactic biopsy of brain tumors. Surg Neurol 1980; 14:275–283.
50. Salcman M, Samaras GM. Interstitial microwave hyperthermia for brain tumors. J Neurooncol. 1983; 1:225–236.
51. Salcman M, Sewchand W, Amin PP, et al. Technique and preliminary results of interstitial irradiation for primary brain tumors. J Neurooncol 1986; 4:141–149.
52. Salcman M, Bellis EH, Sewchand W, et al. Technical aids for the flexible use of the Leksell stereotactic system. Neurol Res 1989; 11:89–96.
53. Bosch DA. Indications for stereotactic biopsy in brain tumors. Acta Neurochir 1980; 54:167–179.
54. Powers SK, Cush SS, Walstad DL, Kwock L. Stereotactic intratumoral photodynamic therapy for recurrent malignant brain tumors. Neurosurgery 1991; 29:688–696.
55. Coffey RJ, Lunsford D, Flinkinger JC. The role of radiosurgery in the treatment of malignant brain tumors. Neurosurg Clin North Am 1991; 3:231–244.
56. Kelly PJ. Volumetric stereotactic surgical resection of intra-axial brain mass lesions. Mayo Clin Proc 1988; 63:1186–1198.
57. Salcman M. Survival in glioblastoma: historical perspective. Neurosurgery 1980; 7:435–439.
58. Watanabe E, Mayanagi Y, Kosugi Y, Manaka S, Takakura K. Open surgery assisted by the neuronavigator, a stereotactic, articulated, sensitive arm. Neurosurgery 1991; 28:792–800.

14

Surgery of Benign Brain Tumors

Byron Young
University of Kentucky, Lexington, Kentucky

I. MENINGIOMAS

A. Introduction

The term *meningioma* was coined by Cushing and Eisenhardt in their classic text describing these tumors (1). Meningiomas are benign tumors arising from the meninges that surround the brain. The meninges are composed of the dura mater and the arachnoid, the origin of which is probably mesodermal and neuroectodermal. Projecting from the arachnoid are the arachnoid villi, the channels through which cerebrospinal fluid (CSF) drains from the ventricular and subarachnoid spaces into the intracranial venous sinuses. The arachnoid villi are the most common location from which meningiomas arise, although a few also originate from fibroblasts and cells from the epithelial layer of the dura. The arachnoid cells provide covering for the central nervous system structures and also have fibroblastic, phagocytic, and secretory functions. The ectomesenchymal origin and the multiple functions of these cells may account for the great diversity of types of meningiomas (2).

Meningiomas account for about 15% of intracranial tumors (3). The review by Rohringer et al. of meningiomas diagnosed in Manitoba, Canada, from 1980–1987 showed that the crude incidence rate was 2.3:100,000 for all meningiomas, and 0.71:100,000 for malignant meningiomas. The age-specific annual incidence rate increased with age; by the eighth decade the age-specific annual incidence rate was 8.4:100,000. As in other series, this study reported that 71% of the tumors were meningotheliomas or transitional. Seven percent were malignant (4). Ninety percent of intracranial meningiomas are supratentorial (5). The incidence of meningiomas peaks in the fifth, sixth, and seventh decades. Intracranial meningiomas are very uncommon in children. Incidental asymptomatic meningiomas are not uncommonly found at autopsy in the elderly. These meningiomas may be multiple and are usually small. Possible etiological factors that have been suggested for meningiomas include head injury, radiation, and the contrast material thorium dioxide. An association between type 1 and type 2 neurofibromatosis and intracranial meningiomas also exists (2).

Meningiomas commonly demonstrate an abnormality at chromosome 22 that may be a component of meningioma tumor genesis (2,6). Meningiomas occur more commonly in females than males by a 2:1 ratio (4). Consequently, studies of hormonal receptor sites have been of interest. Progesterone receptors commonly occur; estrogen receptors occur much less frequently (2). Martuza and colleagues detected specific estradiol binding in seven of ten meningiomas. Progestin-binding sites were detected in two of five meningiomas studied (7).

B. Locations

Meningiomas are described by their location. Falx meningiomas arise from the dura dividing the two cerebral hemispheres. Parasagittal meningiomas arise at the junction of the falx and the dura overlying the brain near the midline. Both falx and parasagittal meningiomas are often contiguous with the sagittal sinus. Convexity meningiomas occur lateral to parasagittal meningiomas and extend to the lateral sphenoid wing. Meningiomas underneath the brain, arising from the dura at the skull base, are olfactory groove meningiomas, sphenoid wing meningiomas, and tuberculum sellar meningiomas. Meningiomas can arise from the meninges of the optic nerve, but this is an unusual occurrence. Meningiomas occurring in the posterior fossa are discussed in the chapter on skull-base tumors (Chap. 15). Intraventricular meningiomas are similarly uncommon. These tumors may arise either from the tela choroidea or the choroid plexus and occur preponderantly in the left ventricle.

C. Pathology

The World Health Organization (WHO) categorizes meningiomas into the following nine groups (8):

1. Meningotheliomatous (endotheliomatous, syncytial, arachnotheliomatous)
2. Fibrous (fibroblastic)
3. Transitional (mixed)
4. Psammomatous
5. Angiomatous
6. Hemangioblastic
7. Hemangiopericytic
8. Papillary
9. Anaplastic (malignant)

Russell and Rubinstein categorize meningiomas into three main groups: classic meningiomas (meningothelial, transitional, and fibroblastic types); angioblastic meningiomas; and malignant meningiomas (2). About two-thirds of meningiomas are of the meningotheliomatous, fibroblastic, or transitional types. The architecture of the transitional meningiomas consists of whorls or circles of meningothelial cells around a blood vessel, collagen fiber, or another meningothelial cell. Some of the whorls become *psammoma bodies* composed of calcium or apatite crystals within the circle of collagen fibers (Fig. 4) (2). Thickened portions of the arachnoid cell layer contain cap cell clusters. Cap cell cluster areas contain whorls and psammoma bodies (9). The cap cells of the arachnoid villi are thought to be the cells of origin of most meningiomas.

Angioblastic meningiomas, which consist of numerous, thin-walled vessels (Fig. 3), are distinguished from the other types of benign meningiomas by their more aggressive growth and tendency to recur after surgical resection. The cell of origin of these tumors remains debatable. Burger and Vogel suggest that these neoplasms derive from pericytes, rather than from arachnoid cells (10).

D. Clinical Presentation

The location of tumors determines their initial symptoms. Meningiomas occurring anterior to the coronal suture often become quite large before becoming symptomatic (11). Presenting symptoms are dementia, lethargy, and apathy. Urinary incontinence may occur because of the loss of cerebral inhibitory influence over bladder control. If the tumor becomes large enough to increase intracranial pressure, headaches and visual symptoms associated with the papilledema may develop. Seizures are not an infrequent initial sign. Tumors located more posteriorly over the primary motor cortex are often heralded by focal motor seizures or hemiparesis. Tumors occurring even more posteriorly over the primary sensory cortex present with focal sensory seizures or contralateral hemisensory symptoms. Falcine interhemispheric tumors may become so large that contralateral symptoms occur. Meningiomas located in the occipital area are uncommon and present with homonymous hemianopia and other visual phenomena (12).

Intraventricular meningiomas are rare and are not uncommonly quite large before becoming symptomatic. The most common site for intraventricular tumors is the trigone of the left lateral ventricle. The symptoms may be due to compression of adjacent cortex by the tumor or to an enlarged ventricle horn in which the tumor has occluded CSF outflow. The most common presentation for lesions in the trigone is homonymous hemianopia. Dysphasia may occur when the dominant hemisphere is involved. These tumors have a considerable blood supply from the anterior and posterior choroidal arteries (13).

E. Radiologic Evaluation

In the past, plain skull films have played an important role in establishing a preoperative diagnosis of meningioma. Meningiomas may have a certain characteristic appearance on plain skull films, such as hyperostosis or dense calcification. Computed tomography (CT) scanning or magnetic resonance imaging (MRI), however, have largely replaced plain skull film studies because they are far more informative. The CT windows for bone are even superior to plain skull films for showing bony invasion and hyperostosis. Meningiomas frequently contain calcium, are associated with peritumoral edema, and have a necrotic core. Computed tomography scans, with and without contrast administered, show these features and clearly delineate the size and location of the tumor. Aoki et al. observed by CT a linear enhancement (flare sign) along the dural margin of meningiomas. These authors attributed the flare sign to hypervascularity of the dura contiguous with the tumor. Thirteen of the 18 meningiomas they studied showed a flare sign. Three surgical specimens showed tumor cells beyond the attachment of the tumor. The tumor invasion was not distant enough, however, to fully account for the extent of the linear enhancement shown on the contrast MRI (14).

Magnetic resonance imaging of meningiomas shows the changes that are characteristic of extra-axial masses, such as "arcuate bowing of the white matter due to compression of the brain" and "a low-signal-intensity vascular rim caused by the circumferential displacement of pial vessels" (15). The signal intensity changes of meningiomas on MRI are highly variable. At field strengths between 0.05 and 1.0 T, fewer than 50% of lesions may be identified on the basis of signal intensity changes alone. A small lesion without secondary changes, such as edema, could thereby be missed by MRI without contrast enhancement. Contrast administration, however, provides an intensity-enhancing abnormality. Breger et al. showed an average of 180% enhancement of meningiomas on T1 images with gadolinium-diethylenetriamine pentaacetic acid (DTPA) (16). According to Wilms et al. prominent dural enhancement with contrast-enhanced MRI images occurs more frequently with meningiomas than with malignant tumors (17). An MRI scan is better than either a CT scan or angiography in detecting dural sinus invasion of the sagittal sinus (18). Magnetic resonance imaging angiography or special angiographic views to demonstrate the entire extent of sinus involvement are important preoperatively when the tumor is near the sagittal sinus or important draining veins.

Classic angiographic features of meningiomas include enlargement of the feeding arteries. Since meningiomas arise from the dura, the arteries that are enlarged are those supplying the dura, such as the middle meningeal artery and the tentorial artery. Meningiomas often have an intense "blush" caused by the hypervascularity of the tumors. Occasionally meningiomas can appear cystic and can be confused with metastatic tumors or cystic gliomas (19). Parisi et al. demonstrate that angiography, including external carotid artery injection, may be helpful in establishing an accurate preoperative diagnosis (20).

I obtain preoperative angiography on almost all patients presumed to have a meningioma. Angiography is not essential, however, to remove all meningiomas, particularly those that are small and not adjacent to the major draining veins. One of the major reasons for preoperative angiography is to determine both the intracranial and extracranial arterial supply of the tumor. Embolization of extracranial feeding vessels can greatly ease the removal of these tumors and reduce intraoperative blood loss. The major intracranial feeding vessels must also be identified so that the most important accessible major contributors can be divided early in the course of the operation.

Jelinek et al. developed an algorithm for the differential diagnosis of lateral ventricular tumors. The important criteria for differential diagnosis were age, location of the lesion within the lateral ventricle, and CT scan density of the lesion before contrast media. Use of MRI did not aid in the differential diagnosis, but did demonstrate the location and the extent of the tumor. Contrast material, however, was not administered to the patients receiving MRI scanning in this series. In all eight patients older than 30 years, lesions occurring in the trigone of the lateral ventricle were meningiomas. In patients between 6 and 30 years of age, the lesions were ependymoma and oligodendroglioma. In patients from birth to 5 years, all lesions in the trigone were choroid plexus papillomas. When the lesion is in the body of the lateral ventricle, rather than in the trigone, less specific data for correctly predicting the type of tumor were found. Patients older than 30 had two glioblastomas, one lymphoma, one metastasis, and six ependymomas. The patients aged 6–30 had one mixed glioma, one ependymoma, and one pilocytic astrocytoma. The patients aged 0–5 had two primitive neuroectodermal tumors, one teratoma, and one choroid plexus papilloma (21).

F. Operative Technique

1. General Principles

Preoperative planning and sound surgical judgment during the procedure are prerequisites for the successful outcome of any surgical procedure, but they are perhaps even more important if meningiomas are to be safely and completely excised. Dexamethasone is routinely administered for 24–48 h preoperatively to decrease cerebral edema and lessen postoperative edema from surgical manipulation.

The exact steps involved in removing a meningioma are dependent on the location, size, and blood supply of the tumor. For removal of meningiomas, I usually develop a larger scalp and bony opening than is necessary for the removal of primary malignant tumors. For primary malignant tumors, particularly when stereotactic approaches are made, a large bony opening is not necessary. With falcine and parasagittal meningiomas, however, greater exposure is needed because the exact extent of sinus involvement often cannot be determined preoperatively. A large U-shaped scalp flap overlying the tumor is first developed. When scalp arteries, such as the superficial temporal or occipital, are important contributors to the blood supply of the tumor, the scalp flap is designed to enable occlusion of these vessels before opening the skull. The skull opening is just slightly smaller than the scalp opening. Adequate skull exposure of the sinus beyond the area of the tumor attachment is needed for completely excising the tumor and readily gaining hemostasis if the sinus is entered during tumor removal. When the tumor involves the sagittal sinus, the bony opening is made across the midline to expose the sagittal sinus bilaterally in the region of tumor resection so that hemostasis can be quickly obtained if hemorrhage occurs during tumor removal (Fig. 6). Furthermore, a wide opening is necessary because convincing evidence is now available showing that wide dural excision beyond the base of the meningioma is followed by fewer recurrences (Fig. 7). Borovich and Doron pointed out that the dural involvement may extend far beyond the globular

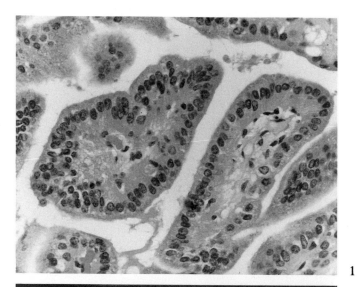

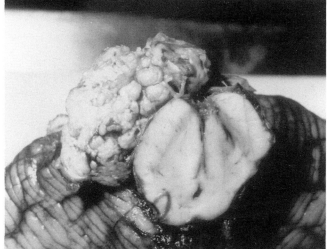

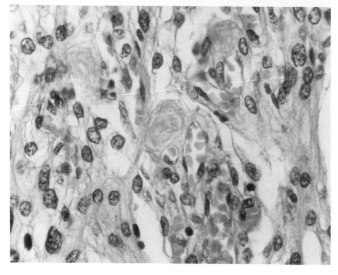

(See next page for legend.)

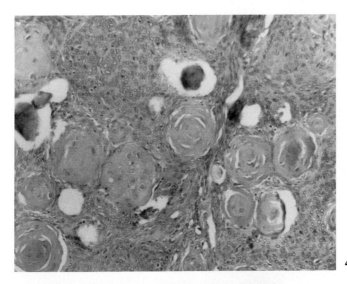

4

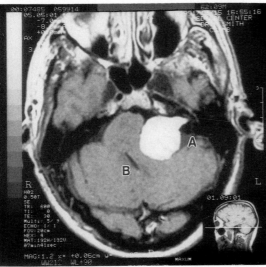

5

Figure 1   Choroid plexus papilloma with mostly uniform epithelial cells in papillary configurations.
Figure 2   Epidermoid in cerebellopontine angle causing brain stem compression.
Figure 3   Angioblastic meningiomas with distinctive numerous vascular channels.
Figure 4   Meningioma with classic psammoma bodies.
Figure 5   Contrast MRI of an acoustic neuroma filling the porous acusticus. The brain stem is displaced (A) and the fourth ventricle is s-like (B).

tumor. These authors recommend a wide excision of the dura surrounding the globular meningioma to reduce the recurrence rate (22). When meningiomas are located near the motor or sensory cortex, a large opening may enable less manipulation and retraction of contiguous normal brain.

Some meningiomas are very adherent to the bone. In this situation I perform a conventional removal of a rectangle of bone square of rectangular bone plate incision and then circumferentially open a smaller bony plate around the base of the tumor attachment in a fashion that allows the adherent bone to remain attached to the dura.

The dural opening is just slightly smaller than the bony opening. A U-shaped dural incision is made, which is usually based on the sagittal sinus to preserve the draining veins. When the dural attachment to the meningioma is very adherent and the dura is deeply infiltrated, a circumferential incision is made around the dural attachment of the tumor so that the larger dural flap can be reflected. The dural attachment can aid in dissecting the tumor from surrounding brain.

Some tumors, particularly smaller ones, have virtually no ingrowth of blood vessels or attachment to the underlying pial surface and come out with the elevated dura. Small tumors can be removed by developing the pial plane between the tumor and the brain. Large tumors are usually most safely removed by first debulking the core of the tumor. This is accomplished with a laser, an ultrasonic aspirator, or cautery loops. Reducing the central core of the lesion lessens manipulation of the contiguous brain during dissection. I routinely use the operating microscope to meticulously identify, divide, and coagulate the feeding vessels of tumors that have considerable vascularity (Fig. 8). When these vessels are torn during dissection, efforts to obtain hemostasis may injure normal adjacent brain and cause a neurological deficit or contribute to the development of postoperative epilepsy. To diminish injury to normal brain, self-retaining stationary brain retractors are used to gain exposure, rather than hand-held retractors.

2. Parasagittal and Falx Meningiomas

Meningiomas involving the sagittal or lateral sinus offer the surgeon unique challenges and opportunities. Because meningiomas are benign tumors and the associated symptoms are due to compression or edema of the surrounding brain, rather than to invasion and destruction, as with malignant primary tumors, a cure with no or little neurological deficit is possible. Complete excision of meningiomas that have invaded the sagittal or lateral sinuses may not be possible, however, because the risk of postoperative neurological deficit caused by occlusion of the venous outflow of critical or large areas of normal brain may be unacceptably high. The sagittal sinus anterior to the coronal suture can be divided without causing a neurological deficit. The sagittal sinus posterior to the coronal suture cannot be safely divided unless tumor invasion has already caused complete occlusion of the sinus. Sudden occlusion of the midportion of the sagittal sinus may result in paraparesis, and abrupt occlusion of the posterior portion of the sagittal sinus may result in death. Therefore, detailed angiographic studies should be performed for meningiomas that are attached to the sagittal sinus, at or posterior to the coronal suture, to determine whether the sinus is patent, totally occluded, or partially occluded. The sinus, when totally occluded, can be divided and removed along with the meningioma. Meningiomas that are attached to the sinus, but easily dissected from it, can be treated by superficial desiccation of the remaining sinus wall with a laser or by coagulation with monopolar and bipolar electrocautery units. When the wall of the deeply infiltrated sinus is still patent, the conventional method employed for many years has been to incompletely excise the tumor and leave the sinus area of involvement in place. Additional surgery or radiation therapy can then be provided if the tumor again becomes symptomatic. In time, the sinus may become completely obliterated by the tumor. Neurological deficit rarely occurs with gradual complete obliteration of the sinus. Because the relatively slow growth of the tumor provides adequate time for the development of collateral circulation, the tumor can be totally excised along with the occluded sinus.

Meningiomas are usually located on the surface of the brain and adjacent to the sagittal or lateral sinuses; therefore, they are intimately associated with important veins providing drainage to eloquent areas of the brain into the sagittal and venous sinuses. The superficial vessels that drain into the adjacent sagittal sinus often cannot be sacrificed without causing a neurological deficit. Sacrifice of patent veins draining the motor or sensory cortex may cause paralysis or hemisensory loss. Often the meningioma is quite adherent to the draining vessel. Great care must be taken to preserve these vessels.

If the proliferative index is low, which indicates a low recurrence rate for the tumor, and the patient is elderly, serial neurological examinations and MRI scans can be performed to determine the most appropriate treatment when the lesion becomes symptomatic or shows definite enlargement. Several techiques that have been described for completely excising the tumor involving a sinus that remains patent; my opinion is that these complex procedures carry more risk than waiting to perform repeat surgery when the sinus becomes occluded or treating residual tumor with stereotactic radiosurgery.

3. *Interventricular Meningiomas*

According to Fornari et al., intraventricular meningiomas in the lateral ventricles account for about 1% of intracranial meningiomas. The authors recommended a parietal occipital approach for these tumors so that the choroidal arteries supplying the tumor can be occluded before tumor resection. The operative death rate was 22% (13). Guidetti et al. recommended a parietal occipital approach to remove meningioma of the lateral ventricle (23). Jun and Nutik recommended a modification of transcallosal approach of Kempe and Blaylock for some cases of intraventricular meningioma of the trigone (24). Instead of completely dividing the splenium of the corpus collosum, Jun and Nutik partially sectioned the splenium to spare the interhemispheric visual transfer. Complete division of the splenium to remove a tumor in the dominant hemisphere causing a right homonymous hemianopia results in a verbal–visual disconnection syndrome, which is extremely disabling. Jun and Nutik's approach does cause auditory disconnection, which they indicated is not consequential, however. Jun and Nutik recommended piecemeal excision of these tumors (24).

The common surgical approaches to the tumor described by Spencer and coauthors include those through the lateral temporal parietal, middle temporal gyrus, occipital area, parietal occipital fissure, posterior portion of the corpus callosum, and temporal horn and occipital temporal gyrus (25). The array of approaches points out the considerable risk for postoperative neurological deficit, the need to exercise considerable clinical judgment in deciding on the preferred approach, and the necessity of an extensive preoperative evaluation to determine the safest avenue to remove these tumors. The exact approach taken to the tumor depends on the patient's neurological status, whether the tumor is located in the dominant hemisphere, the size of the tumor, and the source and quantity of blood supply to the tumor. Both MRI and angiography are essential preoperative studies. The side of the dominant hemisphere for language is determined by injection of amobarbital sodium (Amytal Sodium) into the carotid artery. My recommendation is stereotactic computer-assisted volumetric removal of these tumors as developed by Kelly (26).

G. Results of Surgery for Meningiomas

Perhaps the first successful complete removal of intracranial meningiomas was accomplished by Professor Pecchioli of Siena, Italy, in 1835. The patient was followed for 30 months and "he never showed any sign of recurrence and was in the best of health" (27).

Meningiomas are cured if complete surgical excision is achieved. Because meningiomas are benign neoplasms, completeness of surgical excision is the determining factor in recurrence rate.

Simpson proposed a system for grading the extent of resection of meningiomas (28).

Grade 1   Total resection of tumor plus dural insertion and infiltrated bone
Grade II   Dural tumor completely resected and dural attachment cauterized
Grade III Complete removal of the tumor without resection or coagulation of the dural attachment
Grade IV   Partial removal
Grade V   Simple decompression

Borovich and Doron demonstrated zones of microscopic meningotheliomatous neuronodules and fibrous sheet cell structures about 4 cm away from the insertion of meningioma to the dura (22)

Borovich et al. added a grade to Simpson's grading system, which included a wide dural incision 4 cm beyond the insertion of the tumor when possible (29).

Recurrence of the meningioma after surgery probably occurs in 10–20% of cases. Studies with the longest follow-up usually report the highest recurrence rates. In the study by Simpson, the average time of recurrence was 5 years postoperatively. In Simpson's series of 242 patients, 9% of the meningiomas recurred when the tumor and the dural attachment were completely excised; 19% recurred when the tumor alone was resected; and 40% of subtotally excised tumors recurred (28).

Even after a grade I resection, Adegbite et al. reported a recurrence rate of 10% at 5 years, 22% at 10 years, and 55% at 20 years. These authors used Simpson's grading system to study the recurrence patterns of intracranial meningiomas after surgical resection. In their study only the Simpson grade of the completeness of resection was statistically significant in relation to recurrence. Sex, site, tumor histology, and postoperative radiation therapy were not significant predictors of recurrence. The authors did not, however, include angioblastic or malignant meningiomas in their analysis. Four cases of angioblastic and malignant meningiomas recurred quickly (30).

In the series of meningiomas reported by Mirimanoff et al., convexity meningiomas accounted for 23% of the intracranial tumors, and parasagittal falx tumors accounted for 19% (31). The authors achieved complete excision of 96% of the convexity meningiomas and 76% of parasagittal falx meningiomas. Their overall complete excision rate for all tumors was 64% (31). In Chan and Thompson's series, the recurrence rates after a "complete resection" were 6% after 5 yeas, 15% after 10 years, and 20% after 15 years (32). The authors excluded malignant meningiomas and multiple meningiomas. Meningiomas along the sphenoid ridge had a total resection rate of 28% and had a recurrence progression probability of 34% within 5 years and 54% within 10 years (32). In the series by Mirimanoff et al., if a second resection was necessary, the probability of requiring a third resection was 42% within 5 years and 56% within 10 years (31). Convexity meningiomas have a recurrence rate of 9% (33). In the series by Lusins and Nakagawa, 8.9% of the patients had multiple meningiomas (34).

Guidetti and associates reported their series of 61 patients with tentorial meningiomas. Tentorial meningiomas accounted for 4.8% of all intracranial meningiomas (35). Other series have indicated an incidence of 2–3%. The mortality rate was 9.8% in the series by Guidetti et al. The authors reported good long-term results in 26 patients (61.9%), fair results in 11 (26.2%), and poor results in 5 (11.9%). The postoperative complication rate was 34%, but in 27% of the cases the deficit resolved. Tumors arising in the posterior fossa were approached from a medial or retromastoid approach. Tumors that were mainly supratentorial were approached from a temporal, occipital, or parietal occipital approach. The authors accomplished total removal in 84% of cases. None of their patients received postoperative radiotherapy (35).

When meningiomas occur in children, the recurrence rate seems to be at least double that of adults. Deen and associates reported a recurrence rate of 39% in patients younger than 21 years of age (33). Globus and co-workers reported that meningiomas occurring in children are more likely to have sarcomalike features (36).

In the series by Chan and Thompson, the 30-day perioperative mortality rate was 4% (32). The authors found that the perioperative death rate and the poor quality of survival postoperatively were related to whether or not the preoperative Karnofsky rating scale was 70 or above. In their series the recurrence rate was 11% when total tumor removal was accomplished, but 22% when cauterization of the dural attachment was performed. When partial tumor removal was accomplished, the recurrence rate was 37%. In this series patients with parasagittal falx meningiomas had a recurrence rate of 29% (32).

In Chan and Thompson's series of 257 cases, of which 80 were parasagittal falx meningiomas, the average survival was 9 years; the Karnofsky rating remained at 70 or above for 8.3 years (32).

Of their 53 cases of convexity meningiomas, the average survival was 9.6 years, and the Karnofsky rating remained at 70 or above for 9.1 years. Forty-one patients with posterior fossa meningiomas had an average survival rate of 6.8 years, with a Karnofsky score of 70 or above for 5.9 years (32).

Aoki et al. reported results of surgery performed on 342 patients with parasagittal falx meningiomas (14). Most of these operations were done without the aid of the operating microscope. The perioperative mortality was 7.3% for patients with parasagittal meningiomas and 14.3% for falx meningiomas. Five years after operation, only 47% of the patients had returned to work. Six percent were completely disabled (14).

In the series by Giombini et al., reporting 207 cases of meningiomas, no mortality occurred in the last 100 patients. In this series, approximately one-fourth of the survivors had postoperative neurological deficits that were not present before surgery or had a severe deficit after surgery. One-third of the patients were partially or totally disabled, most often by hemiparesis or hemiplegia (37).

H. Results of Radiotherapy for Meningiomas

The series reported by Carella et al. shows significant benefit of radiation therapy postoperatively (38). The authors studied the results of 68 patients who received radiation therapy for treatment of meningiomas: 43 received radiation therapy postoperatively, 14 had radiation for recurrence after the surgery, and the rest had radiation treatment alone. From this experience the authors reached the following conclusions:

1. Completely resected benign meningiomas should not be treated with radiation therapy.
2. Early postoperative radiation therapy should be used for all malignant meningiomas, even if the tumors are presumed to be completely resected.
3. Incomplete tumor resection should be followed by radiation therapy.

The possible exception to their recommendation is that radiation therapy could be given for small, residual tumors only after demonstrated growth (38).

In the foregoing series, the patients were divided into three groups: those treated by total resection without postoperative radiation therapy; patients treated with subtotal resections plus radiation therapy; and patients treated with subtotal resection following radiation therapy (38). The recurrence rate in the totally resected group was 4%. In the subtotally resected group with no postoperative radiation therapy, the recurrence rate was 60%. In patients treated with subtotal resection plus radiation therapy, the recurrence rate was only 32%. The patients where were not treated with radiation had a significantly shorter time for recurrence than those who were so treated. The authors concluded that their results proved that radiation therapy is beneficial treatment for partially resected meningiomas (38).

In the series by Barbaro et al. of patients treated with subtotal resection, the recurrence rates were significantly better if the patient received radiation therapy. Only 32% of the patients treated with radiation experienced tumor recurrence, whereas 60% of those not treated with radiation experienced recurrence (39). In the series by Petty and associates of 12 patients who had meningiomas treated with subtotal resection, only 3 patients had findings after radiation therapy; the median follow-up for these patients was 54.5 months (40).

Kondziolka et al. reported the results of treating 50 patients with meningiomas with stereotactic radiosurgery (41). They treated only elderly patients, those whose medical condition did not allow surgical treatment, patients with persistent tumor after surgical treatment, and those with tumors in locations that precluded surgical removal because of the high potential of complications. Sixteen of their patients previously underwent nonskull base tumor surgery. These authors reported no further tumor growth in this group of patients following radiosurgery. These 16 patients all had skull base tumors. The authors also treated 34 patients who had recurrence of tumors and controlled the progression of those tumors. Twenty-four of the patients were followed from 6 to 12 months, 16 from 12 to 24 months, and 10 from 24 to 36 months. Three of these patients suffered delayed radiation injury to the brain. The authors suggested that stereotactic radiosurgery may be beneficial in lesions that have been subtotally resected or for patients with high surgical risk (41).

The long-term risk of radiation therapy for treatment of meningiomas may be substantial. In the series by Al-Mefty et al. of 51 patients, 22 experienced delayed complications of radiotherapy. Two developed visual deficits, 6 had hypopituitarism, and 17 had radiation injuries to the brain (3).

I. Hormonal Therapy for Meningioma

Grunberg et al. reported their experience using the antiprogesterone mifepristone (RU486) as treatment for patients with unresectable meningioma. Five of 14 patients showed objective signs of reduced tumor size or improvement in the visual field examination, and 5 subjectively improved. About 70% of meningiomas have progesterone receptors, whereas only 30% have estrogen receptors. Mifepristone blocks the progesterone receptors. Too few patients were included in this trial to allow the authors to reach conclusions about the efficacy of this antiprogesterone drug (42).

J. Relation of Seizures and Meningiomas

In Chan and Thompson's series of patients, 39% had preoperative seizures (32). Forty percent of those patients continued to have seizures postoperatively. Nineteen percent of patients without preoperative seizures had at least one seizure postoperatively. The highest percentage of patients having seizures preoperatively were those with tumors located in the convexity parasagittal regions: 48% of these patients had seizures; 29% had preoperative seizures when the meningioma was located elsewhere. Forty-four of the patients with convexity parasagittal meningiomas had seizures postoperatively; 9% of patients with meningiomas in other locations had seizures post-operatively. If one or more of the major venous draining veins was sacrificed to resect the parasagittal falx meningiomas, 80% of patients developed seizures postoperatively. In contrast, only 12% of the patients had postoperative seizures when the draining veins were saved (32).

In the series by Aoki et al., 57% of the patients had had preoperative epilepsy, and 35% of those with epilepsy before surgery had persisting epilepsy after surgery. Fifteen percent had postoperative seizures. Twenty-five percent of the total had seizures after surgical treatment (14). Giombini et al report that 17% of their patients with convexity meningiomas had epilepsy after surgery (37), and 43% of the patients with parasagittal and falx meningiomas had seizures after surgery (43).

K. Radiation Induction of Meningiomas and the Hemangiopericytoma

Meningiomas are the most frequent neoplasm induced by radiation. These meningiomas differ in location, number, and aggressiveness from noninduced meningiomas (44). Al-Mefty et al. reviewed 45 patients who had received radiation during adulthood and who developed lesions presumably as a late secondary effect of cranial radiation. In adults who have had cranial radiation, sarcomas and malignant astrocytomas occur more frequently than do meningiomas (3).

Guthrie et al. reported an average survival of 94 months for patients with supratentorial angioblastic meningiomas (meningeal hemangiopericytoma) (45). In contrast, the average survival was 64 months when the tumor was attached to the tentorium or in the posterior fossa. The authors strongly recommend radiation therapy for these tumors, even after total resection, "particularly if the tumor is at a difficult operative site" (46). They also recommend obtaining chest films at frequent postoperative sessions (6- to 12-month intervals) for early detection of metastasis.

L.   Factors Affecting Recurrence and Regrowth Rate

Borovich and Doron examined dural strips taken radially along the margin of resected globular meningiomas (22). In 64% they found macroscopic nodules on the inner surface of the dura extending from 1 to 3 cm from the base of the globular meningioma. The diameter of the nodules varied from 1 to 8 mm. The nodule was solitary in four of the nine cases, but multiple in five. In eight cases (57%), microscopic islets or linear aggregates of meningothelial cells were found. In five of the cases only microscopic meningothelial cell islets were identified. Borovich and Doron proposed that tumor recurrence may be due to the growth of these microscopic or macroscopic regionally multiple tumors surrounding a completely excised globular meningioma. Borovich and Doron advocated a wide dural resection beyond the margin of tumor. Failure to remove the regional macroscopic and microscopic tumors may account for the unexpected "recurrences" in the core from which the globular tumor is completely excised (22).

Whether the histological features predict the recurrence rate for meningiomas is unsettled. Most studies report a higher incidence of recurrence for angioblastic meningiomas and, indeed, separate this type of meningioma from the other benign forms (47). With the exception of the papillary and angioblastic meningioma, the histological type of the tumor probably does not influence the recurrence rate (28). Boker and co-workers reported that mitosis, evidence of brain invasion, and focal necrosis were predictive of high recurrence rates (48).

Jaaskelainen et al. studied the growth rate of meningiomas from 43 patients who had recurrences after a radical primary operation. The authors used serial volume measurements obtained by CT scans to determine the relation between histological anaplasia and growth rate of the tumor. They concluded that atypical and anaplastic meningiomas had a faster growth rate than "benign meningiomas." All 43 patients had recurrences after a radical primary operation. The volume of the recurrent lesion was determined by CT scanning or by weighing the tumor removed at the second operation (49).

Domenicucci et al. attribute multiple meningiomas to "multicentricity of dural foci" and suggest that multiple symptomatic meningiomas are uncommon because only a small portion of these foci develop into tumors large enough to become symptomatic (50).

Firsching et al. reported 17 patients with incidentally discovered meningiomas and reviewed the literature discussing the growth rate of these tumors (51). The growth rate in this series was 3.6%, which supported the contention that these lesions have a very slow annual growth rate. The authors suggested CT scans, within 6 months after the original discovery of the tumor, to assess and determine its growth rate. They suggested that observation without surgical intervention is justified in selected asymptomatic patient, depending on the age of the patients, their overall physical health, and the location of the tumor. Most of these tumors had volumes of less than 2 cm, but some were considerably larger. In this small series there was no relation between the growth rate and the initial volume of the tumor (51).

May et al. reported the use of flow cytometry to assess the DNA content of tumor cells to predict their growth rate (52). This study assessed whether there was a correlation between the percentage of cells in the S and G_2M phases of the cell cycle and growth rate. The percentage of cells in the S and G_2M phases is called the *proliferative index*. The studies by May et al. show that the proliferative index of recurrent meningiomas is significantly higher than that of nonrecurrent tumors. The authors studied the tumors removed from 40 patients at the first operation: 20 patients subsequently developed recurrent neoplasms and 20 did not. From the results of DNA analysis by flow cytometry, these authors suggested that the tumor is more likely to recur when the proliferative index is 20% or greater (52).

M.   Tumors of the Choroid Plexus

Choroid plexus tumors are of two types: papillomas and carcinomas. This chapter will discuss the benign papillomatous lesions (Fig. 1). Posterior fossa choroid plexus papillomas are more common

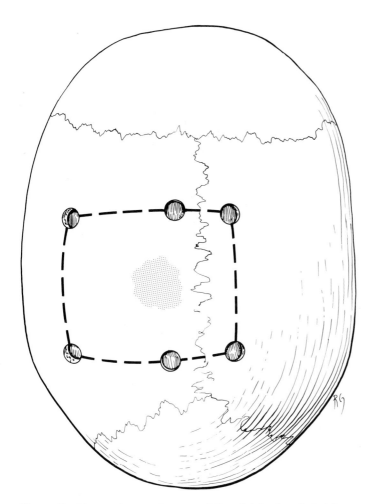

Figure 6 The craniotomy (interrupted lines joining burr holes) is approximately 4 cm beyond the tumor (stippled area) to allow wide dural excision. The sagittal sinus, underlying the midline sagittal suture, is exposed by this large craniotomy.

in adults, but are more commonly located in the lateral ventricles of children. Ellenbogen and colleagues reviewed their series of 40 patients treated surgically (53). The most common symptom was increased intracranial pressure. Benign papillomatous lesions are frequently associated with hydrocephalus, caused by either overproduction of CSF or by obstruction of venticular outlets. The second most common symptom was focal or generalized seizures. In this series males were affected more commonly than females at a ratio of 3:2. The papillomas presented most frequently in the first 2 years of life. The authors reported a 5-year survival rate of 84% for papillomas (53). The surgical approaches for these lesions are the same as those discussed in the section on intraventricular meningiomas.

McGirr et al. reviewed the 26 patients with choroid plexus papillomas who underwent surgery at the Mayo Clinic (54). Four patients died preoperatively; in 14 patients, total removal of the tumor was obtained; and in 12 patients, the tumor was subtotally removed. Two of the patients who underwent subtotal resection were not treated with radiation therapy and did not have evidence of recurrent disease 6 and 8 years postoperatively. Four of the patients who received radiation therapy were alive at last follow-up, and four had died. Sixty-nine percent of the patients in this series presented with hydrocephalus, and 76% were adults. Males were more often affected than females. All of the adults had posterior fossa choroid plexus papilloma, and all of the patients with lesions located in the lateral ventricle were younger than 16 years of age. These authors concluded that "radiation therapy probably is best reserved for recurrent disease after the most complete surgical resection possible" (55).

Hawkins reviewed a 20-year experience of 17 choroid plexus papillomas (56). The operative mortality in his series was 4 of 17 (24%). Three others died within a few months of surgery. Six patients were well and attended school, and 4 were moderately handicapped.

N. Epidermoids

Epidermoids occur most frequently in the parapontine region, the cerebellopontine angle, and the parapituitary region (Fig. 2). Intracerebral epidermoids are rare (57). Chandler et al. reviewed 332 cases, of which only 5.8% were intracerebral (58). The authors excluded intraventricular meningiomas from the analysis. In another study Chandler et al. postulated that intraventricular, intracerebral, and surface epidermoids occur when the neural tube closes and divides from the cutaneous ectoderm during embryological development; rests of ectoderm are left on the inner or outer surface or within the neural tube. In their review of the literature, the authors found that 36% of the patients with intracerebral epidermoids presented with "mental changes" (59).

O. Intracranial Lipomas

Intracranial lipomas are extremely rare lesions. Kazner et al. found 11 intracranial lipomas in 17,500 patients examined by cranial CT scan. The incidence of lipomas in this series of CT scans was 0.06% (60). In a series of 3200 patients with brain tumors studied by CT scan, only 11 lipomas (0.34%) were detected. Lipomas occur most commonly in the corpus callosum, but are also found

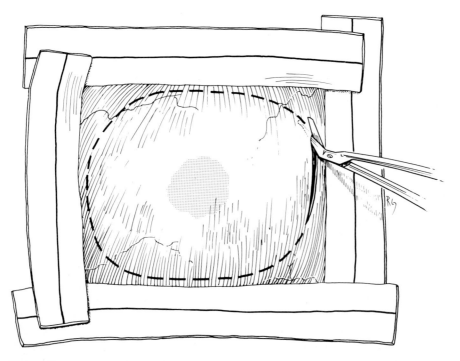

Figure 7 Dural excision (interrupted lines) 4 cm beyond tumor margin (stippled area).

in the tuber cinereum, quadrigeminal plate, and ambient cistern. These rare lesions are rarely symptomatic and very infrequently require surgical intervention. Lipomas are heterotopic lesions and do not have the growth potential of neoplasms. On CT scan, lipomas have a calcified outer shell and an inner core of low density. In the rare instances in which a lipoma causes hydrocephalus, shunting is usually indicated, rather than excision of the lipoma (60).

In the series by Truwit and Barkovich, interhemispheric lipomas accounted for 75% of their cases (61). Twenty-five percent were near the quadrigeminal–superior cerebellar area; 14% were suprasellar–interpeduncular; 9% were in the cerebellopontine angle; and 5% were in the sylvian fissure. From their MRI studies, Truwit and Barkovich concluded that lipomas are "congenital malformations that result from abnormal persistence and maldifferentiation of meninx primitiva during the development of the subarachnoid cisterns" (62).

II. INTRACRANIAL SCHWANNOMAS

A. Site of Origin

Intracranial schwannomas are benign tumors that arise almost exclusively from the sensory portion of the eighth cranial nerve. Although designated for many decades as acoustic neuromas or neurinomas, the tumors actually arise from the vestibular portion of the eighth cranial nerve. The superior branch of the vestibular nerve is the most common specific site of origin. Accordingly, some authors now refer to these tumors as vestibular schwannomas. The trigeminal nerve is the next most common site of origin, but origination from this nerve is very rare. Origin from a motor nerve is even rarer. The facial nerve is the most common motor nerve involved. The glossopharyngeal, vagus, and accessory nerves are extremely rarely involved (8).

Schwannomas arise at the transition zone between Schwann cells and oligodendroglia. This zone is located approximately 10 mm from the pial surface when the eighth cranial nerve is the site of origin (10). Acoustic neuromas begin in or near the internal auditory meatus; they expand the internal auditory meatus and grow in the cerebellopontine angle. Acoustic neuromas usually cause a funnel-shaped enlargement of the medial portion of the internal auditory meatus (8).

Schwannomas occur most commonly in the third through sixth decades. The peak incidence occurs in the fifth decade. Acoustic neuromas afflict women more often than men by a ratio of 3:1–2:1 (8).

B. Clinical Presentation

The symptoms associated with acoustic neuromas depend primarily on the size of the tumor, the cranial nerve of origin, and mass effect on contiguous structures. A few tumors are discovered incidentally while they are still asymptomatic. The most common presentation of an acoustic neuroma is slowly progressive hearing loss and tinnitus. Episodic vertigo and imbalance are common symptoms. Facial dysesthesia occurs as the tumor becomes large enough to compress the trigeminal nerve. Facial nerve palsy is usually a late sign because full facial function is preserved, even when the nerve is tightly stretched and markedly thinned over a large tumor and only a few fibers appear to remain in continuity. An asymmetric blink is often an early subtle sign of facial nerve compression. Trigeminal schwannomas present with facial numbness and pain. Hemiparesis, quadriparesis, spasticity, gaze disturbances, and decreased level of consciousness may occur with brain stem compression.

C. Gross and Histological Features

Schwannomas are benign tumors composed of Schwann cells that provide covering for the cranial nerves. Most schwannomas are circumscribed; larger tumors are lobulated. The distinctive architecture of the schwannomas consists of two types of tissue. Antoni type A tissue is compact and composed of tightly bunched Schwann cells. Antoni type B tissue is loosely meshed. These two different types of tissues are well demarcated from each other (Fig. 9). The tumors' consistency is variable; from firm to very soft (8). In the series reported by Kasantiku et al. (63), the tumors were "usually encapsulated, gray, brown, or red in color, and firm, rubbery, soft or mixed in consistency" (64). Intracranial malignant schwannomas are extremely rare (8).

D. Diagnostic Studies

Until the development of CT and MRI, the diagnosis of acoustic neuromas was based on the patient's symptoms and signs, pure tone audiography, speech discrimination testing, demonstration of enlargement of the internal auditory canal by plain skull films or polytomography, and pneumoencephalography. These lesions are now diagnosed by CT scanning and MRI with demonstration of an extra-axial mass in the cerebellopontine angle associated with enlargement of the porous acusticus (Fig. 5). An MRI scan is the diagnostic test of choice.

Enhancement is greater for acoustic neuromas than for other intracranial tumors (16). According to Runge, the other changes include enlargement of the nerve sheath, an extracanalicular mass, and ISO-to-increased intensity of both nerve and tumor on T2-weighted images. Both precontrast and postcontrast scans must be performed to prevent false-positive and false-negative results (18).

E. Growth Rates

Schwannomas are usually extremely slow-growing tumors. Bederson et al. (65) assessed the growth rate of acoutsic neuromas in 70 patients who were treated conservatively either because they were asymptomatic or because observation only was the patient's desire. The average length of follow-up was 26 months. The average tumor growth rate was 1.6 mm in the first year and 1.9

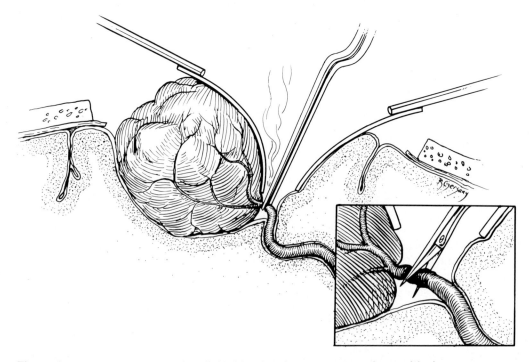

Figure 8 A major feeding vessel is divided in plane between tumor and normal brain.

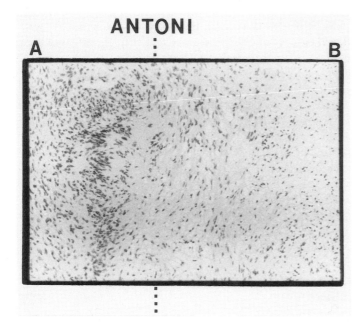

Figure 9 Compact texture and spindle cells comprising Antoni A tissue on left and the loose meshed Antoni B tissue on right.

mm in the second, although considerable variation occurred between cases. The tumor growth rate of individual patients on CT scan, however, was not highly variable. In 53% of these patients the tumor enlarged, in 40% no growth was evident, and in 6% the tumor decreased in size. Thirteen percent of their patients subsequently required surgery because of rapid tumor growth and neurological deficit. The average size upon detection of tumors that subsequently required surgery was larger than the size of those that did not, which suggests that large tumors will more likely require surgery. The average follow-up for these patient was 26 months. The author suggested yearly follow-up intervals to detect tumors growing more rapidly.

F.   Results of Surgical Series

Recent reports of large surgical series of acoustic neuromas show that total tumor removal and high preservation of facial function are achieved with very low mortality rates. As acoustic neuromas are benign tumors, total removal results in cure; and should be the goal along with preservation of facial nerve function. Serviceable hearing can be preserved in a few selected cases. Excellent discussions of current surgical treatment of these lesions have been published (66–70).

Cushing markedly decreased the extremely high mortality rate associated with surgical resection at the turn of this century by performing subtotal intracapsular removal (71). He wrote the classic text on acoustic neuromas. To avoid the high recurrence rate associated with subtotal removal, Dandy totally removed these tumors with sacrifice of the facial nerve (72). House pioneered the translabyrinth approach (73). Before the 1950s, most neurosurgeons removed acoustic neuromas by the suboccipital approach. House used a transtemporal approach and microsurgical technique to achieve facial nerve preservation in 95% of his patients, with a mortality rate of 5.4%.

Several approaches have been described for removing acoustic neuromas. These approaches are based on the surgeon's experience and on whether or not an attempt is made to preserve postoperative hearing. Hearing cannot be preserved when the translabyrinthine approach is used. The translabyrinthine, suboccipital, and retrosigmoid approaches, as well as combinations of these approaches, are currently being used.

Preservation of the facial and auditory nerves requires clear identification of the arachnoid–tumor interface and the important blood supply to the auditory structures, the pons, and the auditory nerve. These procedures are performed with the operating microscope and neurophysiological monitoring of facial and auditory nerve function.

Ebersold et al. used a retrosigmoid approach in 255 patients and accomplished total tumor removal in 249 of 256 procedures (92.6%) (67). In six of the seven patients not undergoing complete tumor removal, only microscopic deposits were left on the facial nerve. Two postoperative deaths occurred in this series, both from pulmonary embolus. The anatomical continuity of the facial nerve was preserved in 92.6% of cases. Ninety-six percent of the 160 patients examined 1 year after surgery had some facial function. Hearing was preserved in 23.5% of those who had had hearing preoperatively. When the tumor was 2 cm in diameter or smaller, hearing was preserved in almost 50% of the patients. Postoperative CSF leak, which occurred in 11%, was the most common complication (67). Bederson et al. reported anatomical preservation of the facial nerve in 96% of their cases (65). Partial facial paresis and facial palsy developed postoperatively in 31 and 5%, retrospectively. Hearing was worsened in 57%; 13% retained useful or normal hearing postoperatively.

Glasscock et al. used the translabyrinthine, middle fossa, suboccipital, and combined translabyrinthine and suboccipital approaches to excise cerebellopontine angle tumors (68). Most of these procedures were performed using either the translabyrinthine or the combined suboccipital translabyrinthine approach. Ninety-two percent of the tumors were acoustic neuromas, and 5% were meningiomas. Total resection was accomplished in 99% of the patients, with a mortality rate of only 1%. The facial nerve was preserved in 86% of cases. Seventy-one percent of the tumors were between 0.3 and 5 cm in diameter. The most common postoperative complication was CSF leak, which occurred in 14% of cases. Lownie and Drake performed radical intracapsular, rather than complete, removal of acoustic neuromas on 12 patients because of the patients' advanced age, unwillingness to accept the risk of facial palsy or deafness (74). Eighteen percent of the tumors recurred within 3 years of surgery, but after 3 years there was no further recurrence. The facial nerve was preserved in 80% of these patients, all of whom had tumors 3 cm in diameter or larger. The authors suggested that subtotal resection may be acceptable under certain circumstances as an alternative to stereotactic radiosurgery.

G. Hearing Preservation

As these series demonstrate, hearing can be preserved in a few patients. Some disagreement exists about the criteria for serviceable hearing and selection of patients in whom hearing preservation should be attempted. Glasscock defines *serviceable hearing*, in the presence of normal hearing contralaterally, as a speech discrimination score of greater than 70% (75). By using this definition, Whittaker and Luetje (76) analyzed the data of Fischer and co-workers (69), and Ebersold et al. (67), and concluded that 15% of Fischer's patients and 7% of Ebersold's had serviceable hearing postoperatively. Whittaker and Luetje recommended that attempts at hearing preservation should be undertaken if the tumor is smaller than 20 mm in diameter, if the preoperative speech discrimination score is 70% or better, and if the patient is fully informed about the potential results (76).

Fischer et al. reported the results of their attempts to preserve hearing in 99 patients who were not deaf before surgery (69). They obtained a macroscopic complete removal in 92 of their cases; in 30 of these cases the tumor was larger than 30 mm in diameter. Hearing was preserved in 29.3%

of patients with schwannomas smaller than 30 mm and in 20% of those larger than 30 mm in diameter. Some hearing was preserved in 29 cases and was categorized as good in 8 (speech reception threshold [SRT] less than 30 dB; speech discrimination score (SDS) greater than 70%), serviceable in 4 (SRT < 50 dB and SDS > 50%), and measurable in 17 (any measurable hearing). Hearing was preserved in 20% of patients with tumors 20 mm or larger in diameter. Hearing preservation was good in 4, serviceable in 3, and measurable in 9 of these 14 patients. The preoperative factors significantly related to hearing preservation were good auditory level for low frequencies and preoperative tumor diameter smaller than 20 mm. They recommended that, regardless of tumor size, hearing preservation should be attempted in all patients with residual hearing before surgery (69).

H. Stereotactic Radiosurgery

Linskey et al. reported the results of 92 patients with acoustic neuromas treated with stereotactic radiosurgery (77). These patients were elderly, had medical conditions making the risk of surgery unacceptable, or had bilateral tumors, unilateral tumor with contralateral deafness, or recurrent tumor after surgical resection. These authors considered absence of tumor growth or tumor shrinkage the criterion for satisfactory response to stereotactic radiosurgery. No tumor growth during follow-up was demonstrated in 97% of the patients. The tumors were smaller in 23% of the patients and unchanged in 74%. The median time to objective tumor shrinkage was 12 months. Useful hearing preservation was achieved in 50% at 6 months and in 38% at 1 year. Thirty-four percent of the patients with normal preoperative facial nerve function had delayed facial dysfunction postoperatively. Delayed trigeminal nerve dysfunction occurred in 32%. Linskey et al. indicated that "if cranial neuropathies occur, they are usually partial and tend to improve or resolve with time" (78).

I. von Recklinghausen's Neurofibromatosis

Patients with von Recklinghausen's neurofibromatosis have multiple schwannomas. In the central form the cranial nerves are primarily involved. In the peripheral form the tumors primarily affect the peipheral nerves. Although bilateral acoustic neuromas are a classic feature of von Rechlinghausen's neurofibromatosis, bilateral acoustic neuromas do not exclusively occur in individuals with neurofibromatosis. Martuza and Ojemann reported a series of 15 patients with bilateral acoustic neuromas in whom the average age of symptom onset was 23 years (79). Their review suggested that bilateral acoustic neuromas are an autosomal dominant trait or may be the result of spontaneous mutation. Bilateral acoustic neuromas usually occur with neurofibromatosis, but can occur with or without other intracranial tumors or the cutaneous stigmata of neurofibromatosis. Eleven of their patients had no family history of neurofibromatosis. Martuza and Ojemann pointed out that the facial and cochlear nerves go directly into and are surrounded by tumor in bilateral acoustic neuromas. Postoperative loss of hearing and facial nerve dysfunction are consequently higher in patients who undergo surgery for bilateral acoustic neuromas.

ACKNOWLEDGMENTS

Daron Davis, M.D., and Dianne Wilson, M.D., of the University of Kentucky Department of Pathology prepared the photography of the tumor specimens.

The exacting chore of proofreading has been willingly undertaken by Flo Witte, of the Publications Office, whose attention to detail and constructive suggestions have been invaluable.

To Christy Thompson has fallen the laborious task of preparing the chapter. Her patience, good humor, and skill are acknowledged with the deepest gratitude.

The author expresses his profound appreciation to others making significant contributions to the preparation of the manuscript.

REFERENCES

1. Cushing H, Eisenhardt L. Meningiomas. Their classification, regional behavior, life history, and surgical end results. Springfield: Charles C Thomas, 1938.
2. Russell D, Rubinstein L. Pathology of tumors of the nervous system. 5th ed. Baltimore: Williams & Wilkins, 1989:449–532.
3. Al-Mefty O, Kersh JE, Routh A, Smith RR. The long-term side effects of radiation therapy for benign brain tumors in adults. J Neurosurg 1990; 73:502–512.
4. Rohringer M, Sutherland GR, Louw DF, Sima AA. Incidence and clinicopathological features of meningioma. J Neurosurg 1989; 71:665–672.
5. Maxwell R, Chou S. Pre-operative evaluation and management of meningiomas. In: Schmidek HH, ed. Meningiomas and their surgical management. Philadelphia: WB Saunders, 1991:109–117.
6. Atkinson LL, Schmidek HH. Genetic aspects of meningiomas. In: Schmidek HH, ed. Meningiomas and their surgical management. Philadelphia: WB Saunders, 1991:42–47.
7. Martuza RL, MacLaughlin DT, Ojemann RG. Specific estradiol binding in schwannomas, meningiomas, and neurofibromas. Neurosurgery 1981; 9:665–671.
8. Russell D, Rubinstein L. Pathology of tumors of the nervous system. 5th ed. Baltimore: Williams & Wilkins, 1989:465.
9. Kida S, Yamashima Y, Kubota T, Ito H, Yamamoto S. A light and electron microscopic and immunohistochemical study of human arachnoid villi. J Neurosurg 1988; 69:429–435.
10. Burger PC, Vogel FS. Surgical pathology of the nervous system and its coverings. 2nd ed. New York: John Wiley & Sons, 1982.
11. Maxwell R, Chou S. Convexity meningioma surgery. In: Schmidek HH, ed. Meningiomas and their surgical management. Philadelphia: WB Saunders, 1991:203–210.
12. Maxwell RE, Chou SN. Parasagittal and falx meningiomas. In: Schmidek HH, ed. Meningiomas and their surgical management. Philadelphia: WB Saunders, 1991:211–220.
13. Fornari M, Savoiardo M, Morello G, Solero CL. Meningiomas of the lateral ventricles. Neuroradiological and surgical considerations in 18 cases. J Neurosurg 1981; 54:64–74.
14. Aoki S, Sasaki Y, Machida T, Tanioka H. Contrast-enhanced MR images in patients with meningioma: importance of enhancement of the dura adjacent to the tumor. AJNR 1990; 11:935–938.
15. Price AC, Runge VM, Babigian GV. Brain: neoplastic disease. In: Runge VM, ed. Clinical magnetic resonance imaging. Philadelphia: JB Lippincott, 1990:141–142.
16. Breger RK, Papke RA, Pojunas KW, Haughton VM, Williams AL, Daniels DL. Benign extraaxial tumors: contrast enhancement with Gd-DTPA. Radiology 1987; 163:427–429.
17. Wilms G, Lammens M, Marchal G, Demaerel P, Verplancke J, Van Calenbergh F, Goffin J, Plets C. Baert AL. Prominent dural enhancement adjacent to nonmeningiomatous malignant lesions on contrast-enhanced MR images. AJNR 1991; 12:761–764.
18. Price AC, Runge VM, Babigian GV. Brain: neoplastic disease. In: Runge VM, ed. Clinical magnetic resonance imaging. Philadelphia: JB Lippincott, 1990:113–176.
19. Dell S, Ganti SR, Steinberger A, McMurtry J 3rd. Cystic meningiomas: a clinicoradiological study. J Neurosurg 1982; 57:8–13.
20. Parisi G, Tropea R, Guiffrida S, Lorribardo M, Guiffre F. Cystic meningiomas. Report of seven cases. J Neurosurg 1986; 64:35–38.
21. Jelinek J, Smirniotopoulos JG, Parisi JE, Kanzer M. Lateral ventricular neoplasms of the brain: differential diagnosis based on clinical, CT, and MR findings. AJNR 1990; 11:567–574.
22. Borovich B, Doron Y. Recurrence of intracranial meningiomas: the role played by regional multicentricity. J Neurosurg 1986; 64:58–63.
23. Guidetti B, Delfini R, Gagliardi FM, Vagnozzi R. Meningiomas of the lateral ventricles: clinical, neuroradiologic, and surgical considerations in 19 cases. Surg Neurol 1985; 24:364–370.
24. Jun CL, Nutik SL. Surgical approaches to intraventricular meningiomas of the trigone. Neurosurgery 1985; 16:416–420.

25. Spencer DD, Collins W, Sass KJ. Surgical management of lateral intraventricular tumors. In: Schmidek HH, ed. Meningiomas and their surgical management. Philadelphia: WB Saunders, 1991:343–358.
26. Kelly PJ. Tumor stereotaxis. Philadelphia: WB Saunders, 1991.
27. Giuffre R. Successful radical removal of an intracranial meningioma in 1835 by Professor Pecchioli of Siena. J Neurosurg 1984; 60:50.
28. Simpson D. The recurrence of intracranial meningiomas after surgical treatment. J Neurol Neurosurg Psychiatry 1957; 20:22–39.
29. Borovich B, Doron Y, Braun J, Guilburd JN, Zaaroor M, Goldsher D, Lemberger A, Gruszkiewicz J, Feinsod M. Recurrence of intracranial meningiomas: the role played by regional multicentricity: part 2: clinical and radiological aspects. J Neurosurg 1986; 65:168–171.
30. Adegbite AB, Khan MI, Paine KW, Tan LK. The recurrence of intracranial meningiomas after surgical treatment. J Neurosurg 1983; 58:51–56.
31. Mirimanoff RO, Dosoretz DE, Linggood RM, Ojemann RG, Martuza RL. Meningioma: analysis of recurrence and progression following neurosurgical resection. J Neurosurg 1985; 62:18–24.
32. Chan RC, Thompson GB. Morbidity, mortality, and quality of life following surgery for intracranial meningiomas: a retrospective study in 257 cases. J Neurosurg 1984; 60:52–60.
33. Deen HG Jr, Scheithauer BW, Ebersold MJ. Clinical and pathological study of meningiomas of the first two decades of life. J Neurosurg 1982; 56:317–322.
34. Lusins JO, Nakagawa H. Multiple meningiomas evaluated by computed tomography. Neurosurgery 1981; 9:137–141.
35. Guidetti B, Ciappetta P, Domenicucci M. Tentorial meningiomas: surgical experience with 61 cases and long-term results. J Neurosurg 1988; 69:183–187.
36. Globus JH, Zucker JM, Rubinstein JM. Tumors of the brain in children and adolescents: a clinical and anatomic survey of ninety-two verified cases. Am J Dis Child 1943; 65:604–663.
37. Giombini S, Solero CL, Morello G. Late outcome of operations for supratentorial convexity meningiomas: report on 207 cases. Surg Neurol 1984; 22:588–594.
38. Carella RJ, Ransohoff J, Newall J. Role of radiation therapy in the management of meningioma. Neurosurgery 1982; 10:332–339.
39. Barbaro NM, Gutin PH, Wilson CB, Sheline GE, Boldrey EB, Wara WM. Radiation therapy in the treatment of partially resected meningiomas. Neurosurgery 1987; 20:525–528.
40. Petty AM, Kun LE, Meyer GA. Radiation therapy for incompletely resected meningiomas. J Neurosurg 1985; 62:502–507.
41. Kondziolka D, Lunsford L, Coffey RJ, Flickinger JC. Stereotactic radiosurgery of meningiomas. J Neurosurg 1991; 74:552–559.
42. Grunberg SM, Weiss MH, Spitz IM, Ahmadi J, Sadun A, Russell CA, Lucci L, Stevenson LL. Treatment of unresectable meningiomas with the antiprogesterone agent mifepristone. J Neurosurg 1991; 74:861–866.
43. Giombini S, Solero CL, Lasio G, Morello G. Immediate and late outcome of operations for parasagittal and falx meningiomas: report of 342 cases. Surg Neurol 1984; 21:427–435.
44. Rubenstein AB, Shalit MN, Cohen ML, Zandbank U, Reichenthal E. Radiation-induced meningioma: a recognizable entity. J Neurosurg 1984; 61:966–971.
45. Guthrie BL, Ebersold MJ, Scheithauer BW, Shaw EG. Meningeal hemangiopericytoma: histopathological features, treatment, and long-term follow-up of 44 cases. Neurosurgery 1989; 25:514–522.
46. Guthrie BL, Ebersold MJ, Scheithauer BW, Shaw EG. Meningeal hemangiopericytoma: histopathological features, treatment, and long-term follow-up of 44 cases. Neurosurgery 1989; 25:521.
47. Skullerud K, Loken AC. The prognosis in meningiomas. Acta Neuropathol 1974; 29:337–344.
48. Boker DK, Meuer H, Gullotta F. Recurring intracranial meningiomas. Evaluation of some factors predisposing for tumor recurrence. J Neurosurg Sci 1985; 29:11–17.
49. Jaakelainen J, Haltia M, Laasonen E, Wahlstrom T, Valtonen S. The growth rate of intracranial meningiomas and its relation to histology. An analysis of 43 patients. Surg Neurol 1985; 24:165–172.
50. Domenicucci M, Santoro A, D'Osvaldo DH, Delfini R, Cantore GP, Guidetti B. Multiple intracranial meningiomas. J Neurosurg 1989; 70 :41–44.
51. Firsching RP, Fischer A, Peters R, Thun F, Klug N. Growth rate of incidental meningiomas. J Neurosurg 1990; 73:545–547.

52. May R, Broome JC, Lawry J, Buxton RA, Battersby RD. The prediction of recurrence in meningiomas. A flow cytometric study of paraffin-embedded archival material. J Neurosurg 1989; 71:347–351.

53. Ellenbogen RG, Winston KR, Kupsky WJ. Tumors of the choroid plexus in children. Neurosurgery 1989; 25:327–335.

54. McGirr SJ, Ebersold MJ, Scheithauer BW, Quast LM, Shaw EG. Choroid plexus papillomas: long-term follow-up results in a surgically treated series. J Neurosurg 1988; 69:843–849.

55. McGirr SJ, Ebersold MJ, Scheithauer BW, Quast LM, Shaw EG. Choroid plexus papillomas: long-term follow-up results in a surgically treated series. J Neurosurg 1988; 69:848.

56. Hawkins JC III. Treatment of choroid plexus papillomas in children: a brief analysis of twenty years' experience. Neurosurgery 1980; 6:380–384.

57. Netsky MG. Epidermoid tumors. Review of the literature. Surg Neurol 1988; 29:477–483.

58. Chandler WF, Farhat SM, Pauli FJ. Intrathalamic epidermoid tumor: case report. J Neurosurg 1975; 43:614–617.

59. Chandler WF, Farhat SM, Pauli FJ. Intrathalamic epidermoid tumor: case report. J Neurosurg 1975; 43:617.

60. Kazner E, Stochdorph O, Wende S, Grumme T. Intracranial lipoma. Diagnostic and therapeutic considerations. J Neurosurg 1980; 52:234–245.

61. Truwit CL, Barkovich AJ. Pathogenesis of intracranial lipoma: an MR study in 42 patients. AJNR 1990; 11:665–674.

62. Truwit CL, Barkovich AJ. Pathogenesis of intracranial lipoma: an MR study in 42 patients. AJNR 1990; 11:673–674.

63. Kazantikul V, Netsky MG, Glasscock ME 3d, Hays JW. Acoustic neurilemmoma. Clinicoanatomical study of 103 patients. J Neurosurg 1980; 52:28–35.

64. Kazantikul V, Netsky MG, Glasscock ME 3d, Hays JW. Acoustic neurilemmoma. Clinicoanatomical study of 103 patients. J Neurosurg 1980; 52:30.

65. Bederson JB, von Ammon K, Wichmann WW, Yasargil MG. Conservative treatment of patients with acoustic tumors. Neurosurgery 1991; 28:646–651.

66. Rhoton AL Jr. Microsurgical removal of acoustic neuromas. Surg Neurol 1976; 6:211–219.

67. Ebersold MJ, Harner SG, Beatty CW, Harper CM, Quast LM. Current results of the retrosigmoid approach to acoustic neurinoma. J Neurosurg 1992; 76:901–909.

68. Glasscock ME 3d, Kveton JF, Jackson CG, Levine SC, McKennan KX. A systematic approach to the surgical management of acoustic neuroma. Laryngoscope 1986; 96:1088–1094.

69. Fischer G, Fischer C, Rémond J. Hearing preservation in acoustic neurinoma surgery. J Neurosurg 1992; 76:910–917.

70. Silverstein H, Rosenberg S. Surgical techniques of the temporal bone and skull base. Philadelphia: Lea & Febiger, 1992.

71. Cushing H. Tumors of the nervous acusticus and the syndrome of the cerebellopontine angle. New York: Hafner Publishing, 1963.

72. Dandy WE. An operation for the total removal of cerebellopontine (acoustic) tumors. Surg Gynecol Obstet 1925; 41:129–148.

73. House WF. Trans-temporal bone microsurgical removal of acoustic neuromas: report of cases. Arch Otolaryngol 1964; 80:617–67.

74. Lownie SP, Drake CG. Radical intracapsular removal of acoustic neurinomas. Long-term follow-up review of 11 patients. J Neurosurg 1991; 74:422–425.

75. Glasscock ME. Surgical management. Audio Dig. Otolaryngol Head Neck Surg 1991; 24(22).

76. Whittaker CK, Luetje CM. Vestibular schwannomas. J Neurosurg 1992; 76:897–900.

77. Linsky ME, Lunsford D, Flickinger JC, Kondzidka D. Stereotactic radiosurgery for acoustic tumors. Neurosurg Clin North Am 1992; 3:191–205.

78. Linsky ME, Lunsford D, Flickinger JC, Kondzidka D. Stereotactic radiosurgery for acoustic tumors. Neurosurg Clin North Am 1992; 3:200.

79. Martuza RL, Ojemann RG. Bilateral acoustic neuromas: clinical aspects, pathogenesis, and treatment. Neurosurgery 1982; 10:1–12.

15

Surgery of Cranial Base Tumors

Gail L. Rosseau
Chicago Neurosurgical Center, Chicago, Illinois

Laligam N. Sekhar
George Washington University Medical Center, Washington, DC

I. INTRODUCTION

Surgery of cranial base lesions owes much to several advances that occurred during the past decade. These advances include improved understanding of the complex anatomy of the skull base, recognition of the special problems of this group of lesions, increased collaboration among different disciplines, improved radiologic diagnosis and development of interventional radiology, advanced neuroanesthetic technique including intraoperative neurophysiological monitoring, and improved microsurgical and adjunctive operative techniques.

II. ANATOMICAL AND PATHOLOGICAL CLASSIFICATION

The skull base is traditionally divided anatomically into three regions: the anterior, middle, and posterior cranial base, according to the confines of the different fossae. The anterior cranial base is composed of the frontal bone, ethmoid bone (lamina cribrosa and crista galli), and sphenoid bone (anterior upper body of the sphenoid and the lesser wing). Important neural structures in this region include the olfactory nerve, which begins at the lamina cribrosa, and the optic nerves, which run in the optic canal. The floor of the anterior fossa is also the roof of the orbit.

The middle cranial base region includes the sella turcica and the floor of the middle cranial fossa. The sella turcica is formed by the body of the sphenoid bone, which cradles the pituitary gland. The bony floor of the middle fossa extends from the posterior border of the lateral wing of the sphenoid bone to the anterior surface of the petrous portion of the temporal bone. Medially, the middle fossa is bordered by the cavernous sinus, and laterally by an H-shaped suture zone called the pterion, which is the junction of the frontal, parietal, and squamous temporal bones with the greater wing of the sphenoid bone. Important neurovascular structures found in this region of the skull base include those that pass through the superior orbital fissure (cranial nerves III, IV, V_1, and VI), the foramen rotundum (V_2), foramen ovale (V_3), foramen spinosum (middle meningeal artery), and the carotid canal (internal carotid artery). Traversing the cavernous sinus are cranial nerves (CN) III, IV, V_1, VI, the carotid artery and its sympathetic nerve.

The posterior cranial base is composed of a central area, the clivus, and a lateral area, which is the posterior face of the petrous bone. The upper clivus develops from the sphenoid bone, whereas the lower clivus is part of the occipital bone. The petrous portion of the temporal bone is perforated by several openings through which travel important neural and vascular structures. These include the porous acousticus (cranial nerves VII and VIII), the jugular foramen (cranial nerves IX, X, and XI, and the internal jugular vein), and the hypoglossal canal (cranial nerve XII). The posterior fossa houses the brain stem and cerebellum.

Tumors of the cranial base may thus arise from the cranium itself, from intracranial tissues above the cranium (dural-based or intradurally), or from distant tissues, with subsequent spread to the skull base. In addition to this anatomical classification, cranial base tumors may also be described in terms of a pathological classification. Thus, these tumors may be benign, such as meningiomas and epidermoid tumors, or malignant. The malignant tumors may be further divided into slow-growing neoplasms (e.g., chordomas), rapidly growing cancers (e.g., adenocarcinomas), and metastatic lesions. Many of the malignant skull base tumors remain locally confined for a long time and metastasize relatively late in their course. Therefore, surgical excision combined with radiotherapy offers the best hope of a long-term control or cure (Table 1). Alternative treatment modalities, such as radiosurgery, are being tested for certain benign lesions. In the future, many such tumors may be treated by gene therapy.

III. TECHNIQUES OF RADIOLOGICAL EXAMINATIONS

A. Plain Films

Plain skull films give only a gross overview of bony anatomy and are of limited usefulness in these patients, owing to the complexity of the bony anatomy of the skull base. Gross bone destruction will be detected, as in clival chordomas or invasive pituitary adenomas.

B. Computed Tomography

Computed tomography (CT) scanning is the imaging modality of choice for definition of bony anatomy of the skull base. In addition to thin-section axial scans, direct coronal scans are also useful, especially in the evaluation of the pituitary, cavernous sinus, and cribriform plate. The use of intravenous contrast media aids in structuring a differential diagnosis (e.g., distinguishing suprasellar meningioma from carotid aneurysm).

Computed tomographic cisternography involves the placement of water-soluble contrast material such as metrizamide into the thecal sac, running the contrast into the intracranial subarachnoid cisterns, then scanning in axial or coronal planes, or both. This technique may allow the detection of a mass which effaces a cerebrospinal fluid (CSF)-filled space, such as an optic chiasm glioma or a hamartoma of the tuber cinereum. Finally, CT scanning is useful in the volumetric determination of a soft-tissue mass for subsequent external beam or intracystic radiation therapy.

C. Magnetic Resonance Imaging

Magnetic resonance imaging (MRI) is currently the modality of choice for demonstrating soft-tissue anatomy. Its abilities to directly image multiple projections and to demonstrate both static and flowing blood in vascular structures are particularly useful. This latter characteristic may allow the exclusion of aneurysm as the cause of an enhancing mass on CT scan. The T1 and T2

Table 1 Characteristics of Skull Base Tumors

	Meningioma	Chordoma	Nasopharyngeal carcinoma	Chondrosarcoma	Esthesio-neuroblastoma	Glomus jugulare
Frequency	8% of all intracranial tumors	1% of all intracranial tumors	25% of NPCs affect skull base	6% of all skull base tumors	3% of all nasal tumors	1% of all intracranial tumors
M/F ratio	1:3	2:1	3:1	1:1	2:1	1:6
Genetics	von Recklinghausen's		HLA A2, BW46, D, DR			Familial clustering
Age at onset	20–60 yr	40 yr	45 yr	30–40 yr	Bimodal: 20–30, 50–60	55 yr
X-ray appearance	Hyperostosis	Erosion of bone, tumor Ca^{2+}, sphenoid mass	Destruction of bone	Erosion of bone, tumor Ca^{2+}	Erosion of cribriform plate	Destruction of bone
Survival	Less than normal population at 15 years	30–50%, 5-yr	20–40%, 5-yr	40–60%, 5-yr	40%, 5-yr	93%, 10-yr
Metastases	Rare	10%	55%	Rare	20–40%	Rare
Radiosensitivity	Probably radiosensitive	Unknown	Radioresistant except lymphoepithelioma	Radioresistant	Radiosensitive	Local control frequent
Other	Sex steroid hormones	Chondroid chordoma variant	Chinese, EBV		Long survival with RT	

characteristics permit the distinction of fat, CSF, and cystic or necrotic regions. Images enhanced with Gd-DTPA (gadolinium dimeglumine) aid the differential diagnosis. Vascular enhancement is best revealed by MRI. It may also show important changes, such as pial invasion by tumor, and the consistency and vascularity of the tumor.

Today, these two imaging techniques are complementary in the evaluation of skull base tumors. Magnetic resonance imaging is used for evaluation of the soft-tissue components of these tumors, followed by CT to demonstrate bony anatomy.

D. Cerebral Angiography

Standard cerebral angiography has four major roles in the evaluation of skull base lesions: (1) defining the relation of the mass to important vascular structures, such as the carotid and basilar arteries and the cavernous sinus; (2) detailing the angioarchitecture of a soft-tissue mass, (e.g., meningioma), thereby confirming the CT or MRI diagnosis; (3) determining the need and the feasibility of preoperative embolization; and (4) test occlusion of the ipsilateral internal carotid artery in tumors that involve the internal carotid artery (1).

E. Balloon Test Occlusion—Xenon Computed Tomographic Cerebral Blood Flow Determination

In patients for whom the temporary or permanent occlusion of the internal carotid artery (ICA) is anticipated during surgery, a preoperative test occlusion of the ipsilateral internal carotid artery allows evaluation of the competency of the circle of Willis. Intracarotid placement of a Swan–Ganz catheter and systemic heparinization is followed by balloon inflation for 15 min, with continuous monitoring of the neurological examination. Any suggestion of neurological deficit results in immediate balloon deflation and catheter withdrawal. The lack of such a deficit, however, does not mean the patient has adequate cerebral circulatory reserve. An additional test, the xenon–CT cerebral blood flow (CBF) technique, allows determination of the adequacy of cerebral blood flow if, for example, postoperative hypotension occurs or intraoperative carotid ligation becomes necessary. In this technique, the balloon is deflated and the patient is moved to the CT scanner where for 4 min he or she is allowed to breathe a mixture of 31% xenon, 68% oxygen, and 1% CO_2. During this time, multiple scans are obtained at each of two or three levels. A computer produces a blood flow map for each cubic centimeter of brain scanned. The balloon is then reinflated and the process is repeated. Comparison of the blood flow maps before and after test occlusion gives evidence for the degree of risk that interruption of the carotid circulation may produce (Fig. 1a–d). Approximately 10% of patients fail the clinical test and are at high risk for a massive stroke in the event of ICA occlusion. Approximately 15% of the patients have CBF <35 cc/100 g per min and are at moderate risk for stroke in the event of ICA occlusion. Seventy-five percent of the patients tested pass both components of the test and are at minimal risk for stroke in the event of permanent ICA occlusion. In young patients, however, ICA reconstruction is always preferred, to avoid the long-term problems of ICA sacrifice. Such reconstruction is mandatory in the high-risk and moderate-risk patients. In those patients, the brain must be protected during temporary ICA occlusion with hypothermia and barbiturates. Balloon test occlusion (BTO) does not predict problems caused by thromboembolism. Occlusion of additional collaterals must be avoided.

F. Embolization

Embolization is most commonly used 2–15 days preoperatively to prevent excessive intraoperative bleeding. Superselective angiography is preferred to clearly disclose all feeding vessels as well as

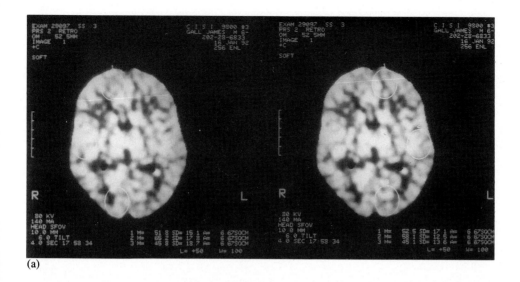

(a)

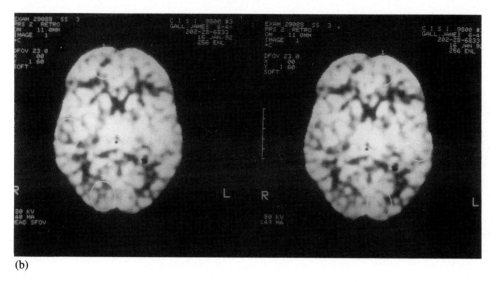

(b)

Figure 1 (a,b) Xenon-enhanced two-level CT/CBF study with balloon deflated. CBF is symmetric. (c,d) Balloon test occlusion caused marked decrease in left hemispheric CBF. During this period, the patient was clinically asymptomatic.

small, but potentially threatening, anastomoses in the skull base that are not easily visualized by conventional angiography. Feeders may be from the ICA, external carotid artery (ECA), or vertebral arteries. Staged embolization may be necessary. Provocative testing with amobarbital sodium (Amytal Sodium) or lidocaine is used to assess safety before embolization with small particles of polyvinyl alcohol foam (PVA) or absorbable gelatin powder (Upjohn, Kalamazoo, Michigan) (2). Palliative embolization is occasionally considered when the patient's poor health or the extent or type of lesion do not warrant surgery.

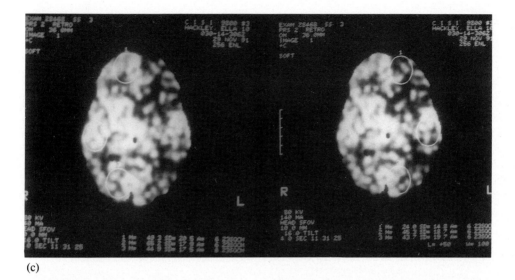

(c)

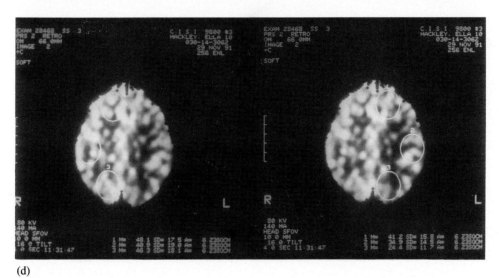

(d)

Figure 1   (continued)

IV.   DIFFERENTIAL DIAGNOSIS BY AREA

Table 2 summarizes the differential diagnoses by area.

A.   Planum Sphenoidale, Tuberculum Sellae, Olfactory Groove, Cribriform Plate

Meningiomas are the most common tumors in this region. They are extra-axial in location, and may exhibit bony change in the form of hyperostosis or "scalloped" deformity of the underlying bone. The MRI signal is often isointense with surrounding brain, but these tumors enhance intensely with contrast agents on both MRI and CT scans. Esthesioneuroblastomas (olfactory

Table 2 Differential Radiologic Diagnosis by Area

Planum sphenoidale, tuberculum sella,
olfactory groove, and cribriform plate
  Meningioma
  Esthesioneuroblastoma
  Osteochondroma
  Chondrosarcoma
  Encephalocele
  Nasal carcinoma
Intrasellar–sellar masses
  Pituitary adenoma
  Craniopharyngioma
  Meningioma
  Optic glioma
  Hypothalamic glioma
  Germinoma
  Arachnoid cyst
  Dermoid
  Histiocytosis
  Hamartoma
  Metastatic tumors
Parasellar masses
  Meningioma
  Schwannoma
  Aneurysm
  Large pituitary adenoma
  Metastatic tumors
Tumors of the sphenoid body and sinus
  Chordoma
  Mucocele
  Encephalocele
  Osteochondroma
  Chondrosarcoma
  Sphenoid sinus carcinoma
  Hematopoietic tumors
   Plasmocytoma
   Lymphoma
   Chloroma
  Direct extension
   Rhabdomyosarcoma
   Nasopharyngeal carcinoma
   Angiofibroma
  Metastatic tumors, especially neuroblastoma
Tumors of the clivus and foramen magnum
  Chordoma
  Meningioma
  Giant basilar artery aneurysm
  Chondrosarcoma
  Paraganglioma
  Metastatic tumors
External ear canal
  Carcinomas
  "Malignant external otitis"

Middle ear and jugular bulb
  Cholesteatoma
  Paragangliomas
  Glomus jugulare
  Glomus tympanicum
  Glomus vagale
  Encephalocele
Petrous apex
  Neurilemoma
  Paraganglioma
  Epidermoid
  Cholesterol cyst
  Mucocele
  Arachnoid cyst
  Hemangioma
  Chondroma
Internal auditory canal–cerebellopontine angle
(CPA)
  Acoustic neurinoma
  Meningioma
  Facial neurinoma
  Epidermoid
Parapharyngeal space–infratemporal fossa
  Paraganglioma
  Neurilemoma
  Sarcoma
  Juvenile angiofibroma
Sinuses and nasal cavity
  Carcinoma
  Mucocele
  Encephalocele
Pterygopalatine fossa
  Adenocystic carcinoma
  Squamous cell carcinoma
  Lymphoma

neuroblastoma) arise from the ganglion cells below the cribriform plate. These tumors are also extra-axial. They may produce bone destruction similar to that seen with malignant nasal tumors. Tumors of bony origin may be seen in this region, such as osteochondroma and chondrosarcoma. An encephalocele is detected as a soft mass near the glabella, generally involving the cribriform plate. Squamous cell carcinoma of the ethmoid sinus, frontal sinus mucocele, and fibrous dysplasia of the cranial base are other lesions that may involve the anterior cranial base.

B. Intrasellar or Suprasellar Masses

Pituitary tumors that extend beyond the confines of the sella turcica are labeled as *invasive* tumors. These generally produce no angiographic stain, but may markedly displace the carotid arteries. A thrombosed aneurysm may be distinguished on MRI or cerebral angiogram from a parasellar neoplasm, such as a meningioma or schwannoma. A craniopharyngioma most commonly appears as a suprasellar mass containing chunklike calcification and both solid and cystic components. Other lesions found in this region include optic nerve and hypothalamic gliomas, arachnoid cysts, dermoids, histiocytosis, hamartoma, and bony metastases.

C. Parasellar Masses

The parasellar lesions commonly involve the cavernous sinus. They include meningiomas, schwannomas, and lateral extension of invasive pituitary adenomas. In addition, aneurysms and local or perineural extension of a nasopharyngeal carcinoma may be seen in this location.

D. Tumors of the Sphenoid Body and Sinus

The most common tumor of the sphenoid body is the chordoma, a slow-growing, avascular mass that produces extensive bone destruction and commonly extends into the nasopharynx. Mucoceles are uncommon lesions of the sphenoid sinus and are caused by obstruction of the sphenoid ostium by inflammatory disease or a mass lesion. A bony defect through the body of the sphenoid, in combination with a mass in the nasopharynx, usually represents a transsphenoidal or sphenoethmoidal encephalocele. Osteochondromas and chondrosarcomas may be seen in this region, identified by peripheral areas of calcification. The more unusual sphenoid sinus carcinoma produces destruction of the sellar floor without expansion of the sella turcica, which is a finding commonly seen in pituitary tumors. Hematopoietic tumors all enhance homogeneously on CT scan, and include plasmocytoma, lymphoma, and chloroma (leukemic deposit). Hematogenous spread to the sphenoid bone may occur with any adult malignancy and is particularly common with neuroblastomas in children (3). Direct extension of parapharyngeal tumors is common and may occur with carcinoma in the adult and with angiofibroma or rhabdomyosarcoma in the child. The sphenoid sinus may also be involved secondarily by meningiomas.

E. Tumors of the Clivus and Foramen Magnum

Tumors in this area are classified anatomically into intradural and extradural lesions. Common intradural neoplasms include meningioma, epidermoid cyst, vertebrobasilar aneurysm, and neurilemoma, which may be derived from cranial nerves V, VII, IX, X, or XII.

Extradural clival tumors are divided into benign and malignant neoplasms. The benign lesions in this location include cholesterol granuloma and neurilemoma. Malignant neoplasms located in this area include chordoma, chondrosarcoma, adenocystic carcinoma, and basal cell carcinoma.

F.   External Ear Canal

Malignancies are the most common neoplasms of the external ear. In elderly diabetics, however, a chronic *Pseudomonas aeruginosa* infection, known as "malignant external otitis" may present a very similar appearance. The superficial location of masses in this region make them very amenable to biopsy.

G.   Middle Ear and Jugular Bulb

Cholesteatoma and paraganglioma are the most common neoplasms in this region. The bony wall separating the jugular bulb and carotid artery from the middle ear is smooth in a glomus tympanicum tumor, but eroded in a glomus jugulare or vagale one. The latter tumors are generally larger, more vascular, and more difficult to remove. Defects in the tegmen tympani or posterior wall of the mastoid may be clues to the presence of an encephalocele in the middle ear or attic.

H.   Petrous Apex

Common lesions in this region are neurilemomas and paragangliomas, both of which markedly enhance on CT scan. The key to differential diagnosis of these lesions is the region of the jugular foramen, where neurilemomas are more likely to erode the medial wall, while paragangliomas are more likely to erode the lateral wall. The most common hypodense lesion on CT scan of this region is a cholesterol granuloma. They are caused by obstruction to the outflow of petrous air cells. These lesions produce increased signals on T1- and T2-weighted MRI scans. A CT scan with thin-section images is the initial study in evaluation of facial nerve dysfunction and may disclose the presence of neurilemomas, meningiomas, and hemangiomas.

I.   Internal Auditory Canal and Cerebellopontine Angle

Most enhancing masses in the cerebellopontine angle (CPA) are acoustic neurinomas. The internal auditory canal (IAC) is usually enlarged by this mass, which tends to be rounded, forming an acute angle with the petrous bone. The second most common tumor of the CPA is the meningioma, which tends to enhance more uniformly, to be flattened at the junction with the posterior surface of the petrous bone, to cause hyperostosis of the underlying bone, and is more likely to be calcified than the neurilemoma. Epidermoid tumors and arachnoid cysts in this region present a low-density appearance on CT scan. The occasional aneurysm or arteriovenous malformation (AVM) may mimic a neoplasm in this region.

J.   Parapharyngeal Space–Infratemporal Fossa

The origin of a tumor in this region can usually be identified by the mass effect the neoplasm exerts on the parapharyngeal fat. This tissue, which is of low attenuation on CT and high signal on MRI T1 images, separates the masticator muscles from the deglutitional muscles in this region. The parapharyngeal space is itself separated by a thin layer of fascia into prestyloid (actually anterolateral) and poststyloid (posteromedial) compartments. Prestyloid masses are usually derived from the salivary gland. Poststyloid lesions arise in the jugular vein, carotid artery, or the cranial nerves (IX–XII), which pass through this space. Thus, paragangliomas and neurilemomas are the most common neoplasms in this region. In the masticator space, sarcomas and undifferentiated tumors are commonly seen. They push the parapharyngeal fat posteriorly and medially and tend to follow the mandibular nerve (V_3) through the foramen ovale. Squamous cell carcinoma and other malignancies of mucosal origin tend to arise medially and push the parapharyngeal fat laterally. Juvenile angiofibroma, a neoplasm found in adolescent males, involves the nasopharynx, the pterygopalatine fossa, and may extend posteriorly into the basisphenoid (4).

K. Sinuses and Nasal Cavity

The most common masses of the nasal cavity sinuses are carcinomas and mucoceles. Mucoceles may be produced by blockage caused by inflammatory or tumorous obstruction. Bone demineralization and destruction are more commonly observed in neoplastic sinus obstruction, but this may be difficult to evaluate. Encephaloceles may be the result of midline cranial base defects in this region.

L. Perineural Extension into Pterygopalatine Fossa

The pterygopalatine fossa (PPF) is a small fat-filled space between the posterior wall of the maxillary sinus and the pterygoid plates. Obliteration of this space is a sensitive sign of perineural extension of head and neck carcinomas, which tend to follow nerves through cranial base foramina. This behavior is characteristic of adenocystic carcinoma of the minor salivary glands and is also observed with squamous cell carcinoma and lymphoma.

Advances in radiologic imaging and increased collaboration with diagnostic and interventional neuroradiologists permit more detailed and accurate preoperative planning. This, in turn, facilitates decreased morbidity and increased thoroughness in the resection of tumors of the cranial base.

V. ANESTHETIC MANAGEMENT

Special anesthetic considerations during skull base surgery include a very slack brain to minimize retraction-induced damage; allowance of cranial nerve monitoring in some patients; replacement of packed red cells, fresh-frozen plasma, platelets, and other coagulation factors in the event of extensive blood loss; the protection of the brain in the event of temporary vascular occlusion; and airway management (5,6).

A. Brain Relaxation

Hyperventilation before intubation is standard. Intravenous thiopental is used for all patients: mannitol and furosemide is used in selected cases. Small doses of inhalation agents such as isoflurane are used. A low-dose thiopental infusion (2–3 mg/kg/h is maintained. Spinal drainage is reserved for extradural procedures without a mass in the tentorial notch or foramen magnum. The surgeon supplements these measures with basal approaches, cisternal drainage of CSF, and minimal or no brain retraction.

B. Airway

An armored endotracheal tube is often used. If the head will be turned, the endotracheal tube is wired interdentally. Some patients may need to be left intubated if lower cranial nerve function is questionable at the end of the procedure. Tracheotomy is reserved for selected cases, as in cases of difficult intubation or if cranial nerves IX–X dysfunction is certain.

C. Monitoring

Cranial nerve monitoring requires that the patient not be paralyzed, but the use of volatile agents must be minimal. Options include a thiopental drip and partial paralytic technique. Somatosensory-evoked potentials (SSEP) disappear if a high dose of isoflurane is used. Selected cases require monitoring of lower cranial nerves.

D. Brain Protection

The anesthesiologist must be aware of BTO results and vascular risk during surgery. For example, resection of cavernous sinus tumors may require cross-clamping of the carotid artery. Adequate cerebral perfusion pressure (CPP) must be maintained during this period if ischemic neurological deficits are to be avoided. Mild to moderate hypothermia (32–34°C), induced hypertension, barbiturate or etomidate protection when major vessels are occluded, and constant communication with the neurophysiologists are critical. Intraoperative electroencephalographic (EEG) monitoring may be useful to evaluate the adequacy of these interventions.

Several potential complications specific to cranial base surgery warrant attention. Direct operative stimulation of the trigeminal or vagal nerve may produce sudden profound bradycardia. This is generally reversed when stimulation stops, and antiarrhythmic treatment is usually unnecessary unless consequent changes in blood pressure are life-threatening.

Air embolism may occur in any craniotomy, but is particularly likely to occur with operations on the posterior fossa. Even the lateral position has been reported to be associated with an 8% incidence of air embolism (7). Continuous Doppler ultrasound is the most sensitive method in the detection of air emboli. Increases in pulmonary artery pressure and decreases in end tidal CO_2 imply larger volumes of air emboli. Prompt treatment is effective, and includes (1) surgical elimination of the source by coagulation or waxing of the open venous channel; (2) elevation of venous pressure by lowering the head, Valsalva maneuver, or jugular venous compression; (3) withdrawal of air through a central venous catheter; and (4) appropriate treatment of systemic hypotension.

Finally, significant blood loss is common in cranial base surgery, with the attendant requirement for transfusion of large volumes of blood products. Coagulation disorders may result. Most common is the need for fresh-frozen plasma (FFP) and, occasionally, platelets. Regular monitoring of prothrombin time (PT), partial thromboplastin time (PTT), platelet count, and thromboelastogram is necessary. The transfusion of fresh-frozen plasma and platelets should accompany any significant replacement of packed red blood cells. The rule followed at this institution is 2 units of fresh plasma and 8–10 units of platelet concentrate for every 6 units of packed red blood cells transfused, to restore diluted clotting elements (8).

VI. SURGICAL TECHNIQUE

The removal of a tumor has three important parts or phases: approach, resection, and reconstruction. The approaches used for cranial base surgery emphasize bone removal to minimize brain retraction. In addition to craniotomy, facial bone osteotomies or removal of temporal bone or occipital condyle may be employed. The resection phase is the most critical part of the operation. In this phase, the surgeon must avoid injury to brain parenchyma, arteries, and important veins and sinuses, and must be prepared to reconstruct these vascular structures should damage occur. Finally, meticulous attention to detail during the reconstructive phase is critical to a successful operation and postoperative course. Layered reconstruction is the key, using dural grafts, autologous fat as fillers, and vascularized regional or distant muscular grafts. For convenience, these approaches have been organized anatomically into the following groups: anterior, anterolateral, lateral, and posterior. In reality, tumors often traverse multiple fossae and, therefore, require a combination of approaches. These combined approaches may be performed in a single setting or in multiple stages.

VII. SURGICAL APPROACHES

A.   Anterior Approach to Tumors of the Cranial Base

The anterior approaches to reach tumors in the anterior cranial base are (1) transseptal, (2) transethmoidal, (3) transmaxillary, (4) extended frontal, (5) anterior craniofacial resection, (6) facial translocation, (7) transoral, and (8) transmandibular–transcervical. A brief description of these operative approaches follows.

1. The Transseptal Approach

The transsphenoidal approach offers the least morbidity and most acceptable cosmetic result. Its use is limited, however, to lesions of the midline nasal cavity, sphenoid sinus, sella turcica, and upper clivus, and will seldom provide the necessary exposure for total removal of an extensive skull base lesion. This approach is most often performed for surgery on the pituitary gland. A classification system has been devised that is based on the MRI appearance of the structures in this region (Table 3). Incisions may be totally endonasal, sublabial–transseptal, or endonasal with unilateral alotomy (Fig. 2).

2. The Transethmoidal Approach

The transethmoidal approach is designed for neoplasms of the pituitary gland. It is performed through a 3-cm incision that is located halfway between the dorsum of the nose and the medial canthus of the eye. After retraction of the intracanthal ligament and anterior lacrimal sac, the anterior and posterior ethmoid arteries are identified. After incision of the lateral nasal mucosa, the middle turbinate is removed. Further removal of the ethmoid mucosa and uncapping of the posterior ethmoid cell allow the identification of the sphenoid ostium and subsequent entrance into the sphenoid sinus. With the aid of the operating microscope, the floor of the sella turcica is removed, revealing the dura of the pituitary fossa.

   Advantages of this technique over the transseptal approach are (1) shorter anatomical distance to enter the sphenoid sinus, (2) no risk of septal mucosal perforation, (3) no risk of contamination from the oral cavity, and (4) devitalization of the teeth is avoided. Disadvantages of this approach include the necessity of an external scar and that the procedure is not a midline approach. This

Table 3   Classification of Pituitary Adenomas

Grade/Stage	Characteristic
Grade I	Smaller than 10 mm, sella normal or focally expanded
Grade II	Larger than 10 mm, sella enlarged
Grade III	Focal perforation of the sellar floor
Grade IV	Diffuse perforation of sellar floor
Grade V	Spread of the tumor by CSF or hematogenous pathways
Stage O	No suprasellar extension
Stage A	Suprasellar extension, without deformation of the third ventricle
Stage B	Suprasellar extension, with obliteration of the anterior recess of the third ventricle
Stage C	Suprasellar extension, with elevation of the floor of the third ventricle
Stage D	Intracranial extension into the:
	1. Anterior fossa
	2. Middle fossa
	3. Posterior fossa.
Stage E	Invasion of cavernous sinus

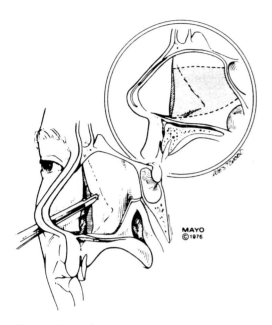

Figure 2   Resection of the bony portion of the nasal septum. Shaded area is the region occupied by retractor in the transsphenoidal approach.

paramedian approach creates the possibility of operator error in identification of the floor of the sella turcica.

3. The Transmaxillary Approach

The transmaxillary approach provides access to lesions of the upper and middle third of the clivus. As with the transoral approach, it is especially suited for extradural lesions, but some surgeons have used this approach for some intradural lesions, including basilar artery aneurysms. Preoperative measures usually necessary with this approach include the placement of a tracheostomy tube, which remains in place 2–3 days, and a pharyngogastric tube, which remains at least 5 days.

The incision is along the upper alveolar margin. Titanium plates are positioned for screw placement during opening, so that bony reconstruction of the maxilla will be precise at the end of surgery, providing perfect dental occlusion. The advantage of this procedure is that no major vessel or cranial nerve is at risk during this anteroinferior approach. Disadvantages are the same as described for the transoral approach, as well as the added potential for dental malocclusion.

A modification of this approach, the extended maxillectomy, has been devised to provide exposure of the craniocervical junction. It is suitable for treatment of basilar invagination or extensive tumors in this region. This approach adds a Le Fort I osteotomy to the midline hard and soft palate incisions, providing extensive exposure. The primary disadvantage is the potential for malocclusion and improper palatal function postoperatively (9) (Fig. 3a–c).

4. The Extended Frontal Approach

The extended frontal approach (basal frontal approach) is used in midline tumors involving the skull base between the ethmoid sinuses and the clivus. The transethmoid approach provides similar exposure, but the view of the optic nerves and orbital apex is more limited by that approach. A major advantage of the extended frontal approach is that it causes minimal violation of the upper aerodigestive tract, making reconstruction relatively simple. The major disadvantage to patients is

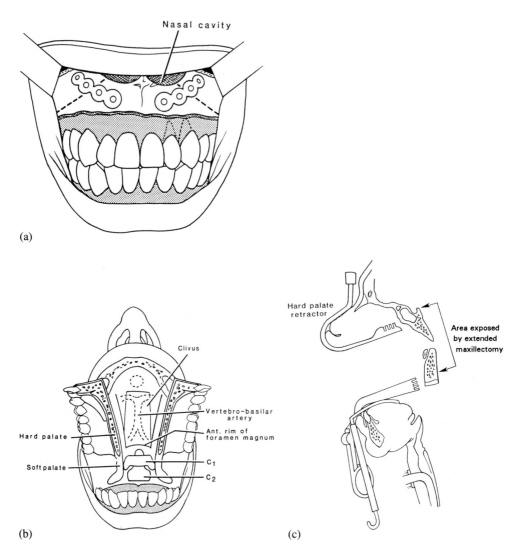

Figure 3 Schematic representation of the transmaxillary and extended maxillectomy approaches. (a) After superior alveolar mucosal incision and periosteal elevation, the position of the fixation plates on the maxillary buttresses is determined before the saw cut to provide perfect dental occlusion. (b,c) Extended maxillectomy: (b) transoral and (c) sagittal views.

the loss of olfaction, with the consequent decrease in taste sensation. The scalp incision is bicoronal, and the temporary bone removal includes orbito–frontal–ethmoidal osteotomies, the performance of which minimizes frontal lobe retraction (10) (Fig. 4a,b).

4. The Anterior Craniofacial Resection Approach

The anterior craniofacial resection approach may be used for almost any disease involving the nasal cavity or sinuses, the facial skin, or the bone or meninges of the anterior cranial base. It is commonly used for meningiomas, esthesioneuroblastomas, and nasal malignancies. The approach is accomplished through a combination of bicoronal and lateral rhinotomy incisions. In addition,

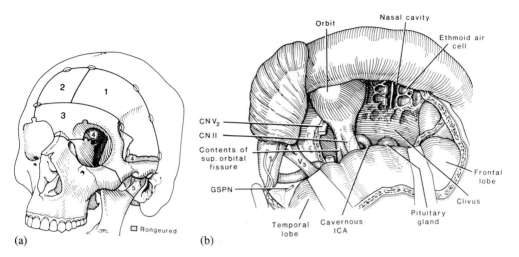

Orbit — Nasal cavity — Ethmoid air cell

CN V₂ — CN II — Contents of sup. orbital fissure — V₃ — GSPN — Temporal lobe — Cavernous ICA — Pituitary gland — Clivus — Frontal lobe — Rongeured

(a) (b)

Figure 4 The extended frontal approach, used for midline tumors of the skull base between the ethmoid sinuses and the clivus. (a) Diagrammatic representation of craniotomies and osteotomies used in the extended frontal approach. (b) Exposure provided by this approach.

the lip may be split if palatine excision is necessary. Depending on the requirements of each patient, facial exposure may be increased to allow orbital exenteration, maxillectomy, rhinectomy, or other, as indicated.

Disadvantages of this approach are permanent anosmia and temporary loss of forehead sensation. The surgeon must pay attention to details of closure to avoid obstruction of the lacrimal sac or drooping of the medial canthus of the eye. Advantages include wide exposure, a complication rate of less than 10%, and a good prognosis for patients with differentiated squamous cell carcinoma treated by craniofacial resection (11) (Fig. 5a,b).

5. The Facial Translocation Approach

The facial translocation approach provides simultaneous direct access to the nasopharynx, clivus, and infratemporal fossa. The sphenoid sinus, cavernous sinus, orbital fissures, anterior and middle cranial fossae are also reachable. This approach is especially useful in the treatment of extensive angiofibromas and parotid salivary gland neoplasms, nasopharyngeal carcinomas, clival chordomas, sphenoid rostrum sarcomas, and transcranial lesions. The paranasal, conjunctival, and temporal facial incisions join the hemicoronal and preauricular incisions which may be extended into the cervical region when necessary. Forehead branches of the facial nerve are electively sectioned and reapproximated at the end of the procedure by a slight telescoping of the silicon tubing in which the transected ends are placed. Recovery of forehead function begins at 6–9 months. The temporal muscle is important in the reconstructive phase of this approach, as it is used to provide vascularized protection of the temporal dura, and to eliminate dead space created by tumor and maxillary sinus removal.

Late complications of this procedure may include enophthalmos or full nasolacrimal duct obstruction. The latter may require surgical treatment with modified dacryocystorhinostomy. Advantages of this approach are the wide exposure, simplified control of essential structures, and functional and esthetic features of the cranial and facial reconstruction (12) (Fig. 6).

6. The Transoral Approach

The transoral approach is recommended for removal of lesions of the lower third of the clivus, the craniocervical junction, and the anterior segments of the first two cervical vertebrae. It is especially

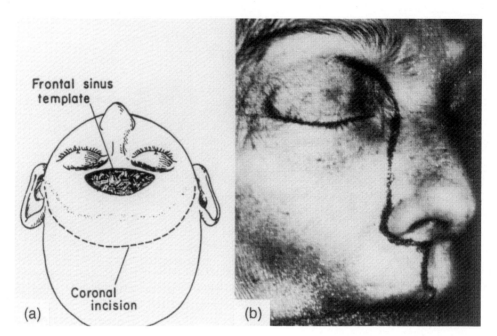

Figure 5   (a) Diagrammatic representation of bicoronal incision, demonstrating the location of the frontal sinus template. (b) Lateral rhinotomy incision marked on a cadaver specimen.

useful in the treatment of extradural lesions, as the risk of developing meningitis is far less when the intradural space is not entered. Nevertheless, with meticulous attention to details of the augmented closure technique, this approach may be used to remove intradural lesions, clip aneurysms, and perform occipitocervical fusions. Preoperative evaluation for this approach must include inspection of the jaw. If the jaws do not open more than 25 mm, the approach may not be done without splitting the mandible. The state of the teeth, oropharynx, and respiratory system are particularly important when contemplating this approach.

Incisions are midline intraoral. If the lesion extends above the foramen magnum, the soft and hard palates must be split; if below the foramen magnum soft palate retraction will suffice. Advantages of this approach include direct access to lesions within 11–14 mm of midline and anterior to the neuraxis. Disadvantages include depth of surgical field, poor access to intradural posterior fossa hemorrhage if it should occur, occasionally significant bony clival venous bleeding, and postoperative problems associated with airway management or mucosal wound breakdown (13) (Fig. 7a,b).

7.   The Transmandibular–Transcervical Approach

The transmandibular–transcervical approach provides exposure of the middle compartment of the skull base, from the foramen magnum to the sphenoid sinus, infratemporal fossa, inferior surface of the petrous bone, and the parapharyngeal space.

After tracheostomy, an incision is created that extends from the mastoid tip to the submental region, continuing superiorly to include the lip in the midline (Fig. 8a,b). Mandibulotomy, lateral retraction of the tongue, and partial posterior palatectomy or maxillectomy, as well as meticulous dissection of important neurovascular and glandular duct structures, provide exposure of the cranial base.

Advantages include wide exposure along planes very familiar to otolaryngologists. Disadvantages include conductive hearing loss (treated with tympanostomy tubes) and the potential for dysphagia and recurrent aspiration (14).

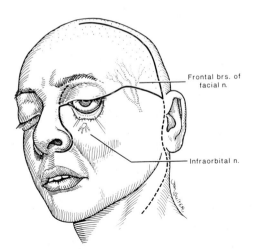

Figure 6 Outline of incisions used in the facial translocation approach.

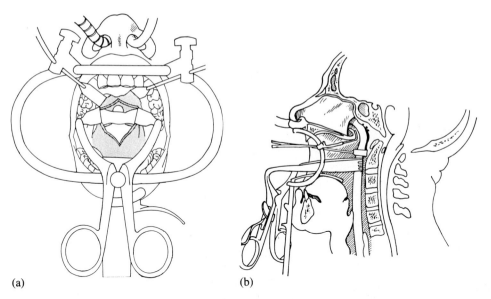

(a)   (b)

Figure 7 Diagrammatic representation of the transoral approach. This example demonstrates soft palate retraction without division, used for lesions below the clivus. (a) Transoral view; (b) sagittal view.

8. Illustrative Cases

Patient RW: Tuberculum Sellae Meningioma.   A 70-year-old man presented with progressive visual loss. He had previously undergone three craniotomies and a course of radiotherapy in an attempt to control a meningioma of the anterior and middle cranial base. Imaging studies demonstrated recurrent tumor with new extradural extension into the sphenoid and ethmoid sinuses (Fig. 9a,b).

By an extended subfrontal approach, the tumor was totally removed and reconstruction was carried out with fascia lata and vascularized pericranial grafts. Postoperatively, his vision was unchanged, but worsened 6 months later despite lack of any evidence of tumor recurrence. The

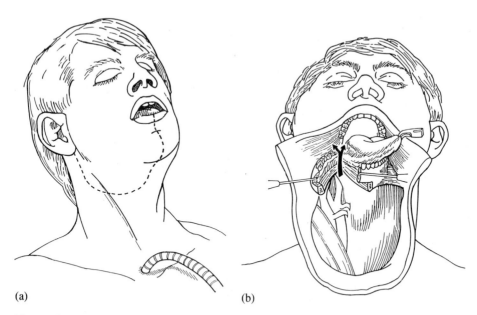

(a)   (b)

Figure 8 (a,b) Illustration of the transmandibular–transcervical approach: (a) the cervical incision and dissection is performed initially, followed by the splitting of the lip and stair-step median mandibulotomy; (b) basic exposure. Dissection may proceed in a medial or lateral direction, as dictated by the tumor.

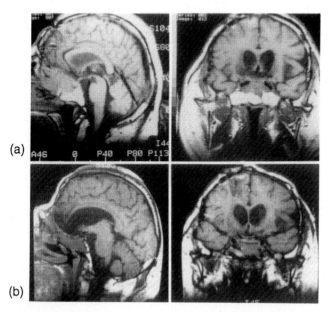

Figure 9 (a) Preoperative MRI sagittal (left) and coronal (right) images that demonstrate a meningioma involving the anterior and middle cranial base. Sphenoid sinus obstruction has resulted in the formation of a mucocele. (b) Postoperative sagittal (left) and coronal (right) T1-weighted images demonstrate total tumor removal. Despite bony reconstruction of the anterior cranial base, there is some prolapse because of multiple previous operations and radiation therapy.

visual loss was presumed to be a delayed ischemic event caused by prior radiotherapy. Four years later, he lives independently with no sign of recurrence.

Patient FD: Esthesioneuroblastoma.   A 59-year-old woman presented with a several-month history of bilateral visual loss progressing to left eye blindness. She also reported anosmia and decreased appetite. Imaging studies revealed the presence of a large soft-tissue mass involving the nasopharynx, ethmoid, cribriform plate, planum sphenoidale, sphenoid and right maxillary sinuses, and both optic canals. Transnasal biopsy confirmed the diagnosis of esthesioneuroblastoma.

Through combined extended frontal and transfacial approaches, a gross total removal of the tumor was achieved. The vision in her right eye stabilized, but did not improve. Owing to the malignant nature of the lesion, she underwent a course of postoperative radiation therapy. Three years later, she lives independently and has no sign of tumor recurrence (Fig. 10a–d).

B.   Anterolateral Approaches to Tumors of the Cranial Base

Approaches useful in the removal of tumors in the middle cranial base are (1) subtemporal and preauricular infratemporal fossa, (2) middle fossa, (3) orbitozygomatic and transzygomatic, and (4) transpetrous apex. A brief description of these operative approaches follows.

1.   The Subtemporal–Preauricular Infratemporal Fossa Approach

The subtemporal-preauricular infratemporal fossa approach has been useful for the removal of neoplasms not only involving the middle fossa, but also the sphenoid area, petrous apex, orbit, cavernous sinus, clivus, infratemporal fossa, and the retro- and parapharyngeal areas. The incision begins in the preauricular region, then extends behind the hairline to or past the midline, depending on the needed exposure for a particular tumor. A frontotemporal craniotomy is performed, followed by zygomatic or orbitozygomatic osteotomies which allow maximal anteroinferior reflection of the temporalis muscle. The mandibular condyle and the capsule of the temporomandibular joint are dislocated anteroinferiorly after dividing the attachment of the stylomandibular and sphenomandibular ligaments to the mandible. If, however, more space is needed or if free muscle flap reconstruction is used, the condyle of the mandible is incised.

The greater wing of the sphenoid bone is then rongeured to unroof the foramen ovale laterally and posteriorly, the foramen rotundum laterally and the superior orbital fissure inferiorly. Further dissection exposes the eustachian tube, which is permanently occluded in both its bony and cartilaginous segments. The genu of the petrous ICA lies just medial to the eustachian tube. Mobilization or reconstruction of the ICA are then carried out, depending on the nature of the involvement of the artery by tumor.

Medial petrous bone, including the petrous apex, may then be drilled from the floor of the middle fossa. This exposes the clivus, allowing tumor removal inferiorly to the level of the foramen magnum.

The advantage of this approach is the extensive exposure it provides. A disadvantage of the approach is the occasional problem with jaw drift in those few patients with tumors that require excision of the mandibular condyle, but this is a minimal disability (15) (Fig. 11a,b and 12).

2.   The Middle Fossa Approach

The middle fossa approach is designed primarily for the removal of medially placed extradural lesions of the skull base. The incision starts at the zygomatic root and extends 7–8 cm superiorly (Fig. 13). The advantage of this approach is access to the petrous apex and internal auditory canal, with preservation of cochlear or vestibular function. It is indicated for (1) removal of small,

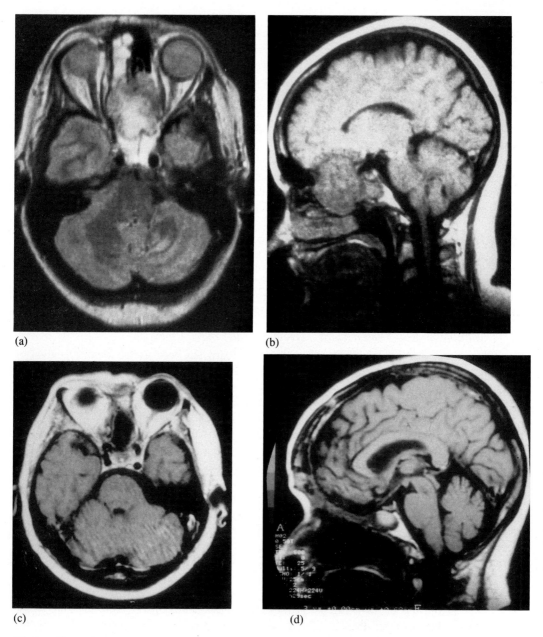

(a)   (b)

(c)   (d)

Figure 10   (a,b) Preoperative (a) axial and (b) sagittal MRI demonstrating esthesioneuroblastoma that involved the maxillary, ethmoid, and sphenoid sinuses, nasopharynx, cribriform plate, planum sphenoidale, and both optic canals. (c,d) Postoperative (c) axial and (d) sagittal MRI demonstrating tumor removal.

laterally placed acoustic neuromas; (2) exposure of the facial nerve (labyrinthine and upper tympanic segments) for treatment of temporal bone fractures, idiopathic facial palsy, or tumor removal; (3) selective vestibular nerve section; and (4) decompression of the internal auditory canal (IAC) in patients with neurofibromatosis type II who have bilateral acoustic neurinomas. The disadvantage is that exposure is too limited for large tumors (16).

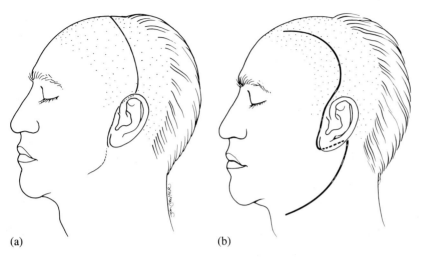

(a)　　　　　　　　　　　　　　(b)

Figure 11 (a,b) The two types of skin incision for the subtemporal–preauricular infratemporal fossa approach are shown. (a) The bicoronal incision; with extension into the preauricular area is preferred. (b) If neck dissection is desired for tumor removal or cervical ICA control, a preauricular incision with cervical extension may be employed, as demonstrated.

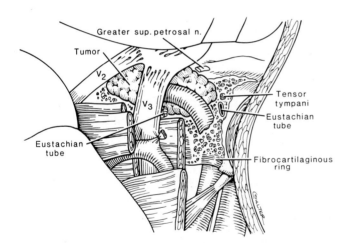

Figure 12 Extensive exposure provided by the subtemporal–infratemporal fossa approach.

3. The Orbitozygomatic and Transzygomatic Approaches

The orbitozygomatic approach was designed to provide good exposure to the infratemporal fossa, the parasellar region, and the interpeduncular fossa. The procedure is performed through a bicoronal scalp incision. The temporal muscle is mobilized, separating it from both the temporal fossa and the zygoma. The superior and lateral orbital margins are exposed. A frontotemporal craniotomy is then created, which includes the superior and lateral orbital rim, as well as the frontal process of the zygoma and the zygomatic arch. This wide bone removal allows excellent exposure of, for example, parasellar tumors and basilar tip aneurysms, without the need for excessive brain retraction. It has been estimated that the working distance to these lesions in the parasellar region and the interpeduncular fossa is shortened by about 3 cm by the addition of the orbitozygomatic osteotomies to the frontotemporal craniotomy.

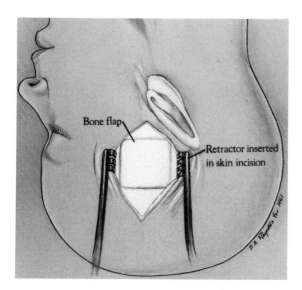

Figure 13   The skin incision for the middle fossa approach extends 7–8 cm superiorly from the hairline and is 0.5 cm anterior to the helix. The bone flap is situated so that ⅔ cm of the exposure is anterior to the EAC.

4.   The Transpetrous Apex Approach

The transpetrous apex approach was originally designed to provide access to aneurysms of the vertebrobasilar artery junction and the origin of the anterior inferior cerebellar artery (AICA). Its use has been expanded to include tumors of the petroclival region. A periauricular skin incision is followed by mobilization of the temporalis muscle. A subtemporal craniotomy is then performed, centered low over the petrous ridge. The lower part of the squamous temporal bone is removed with rongeurs until the cranial window is nearly flush with the floor of the middle fossa. Next, the middle meningeal artery is coagulated and divided. The anterior part of the parameatal bone is then drilled away; the area of drilling is surrounded by the trigeminal ganglion anteriorly, the cochlea posteriorly, the sphenopetrosal groove laterally, and the carotid canal and internal auditory canal inferiorly. Next, dural incisions are made and the superior petrosal sinus is divided. The dural incision may be extended into the tentorium to further enlarge the surgical field.

The petrous apex may also be removed from an intradural approach, after defining the landmarks in the middle cranial fossa extradurally. The lower limit of clival exposure facilitated by this technique is the horizonal segment of the petrous internal carotid artery. If further exposure is desired, a subtemporal–infratemporal fossa approach is necessary with displacement of the entire petrous ICA and further removal of clival bone. This technique allows access as low as the hypoglossal foramen (17).

5.   Illustrative Cases

Patient WZ: Cavernous Sinus Meningioma.   A 55-year-old man complained of left eyelid drooping for 18 months, restriction of visual field on left upward gaze, and numbness over the left

---

Figure 14   (a) Preoperative MRI demonstrating tumor involvement in the cavernous and sphenoid sinuses and petroclival region. (b) Preoperative arteriogram demonstrating left grade IV cavernous sinus meningioma. Encasement and narrowing of the left ICA are demonstrated. (c) Postoperative CT showing gross total removal of tumor and patent left petrous–supraclinoid (P–S) saphenous vein interposition graft.

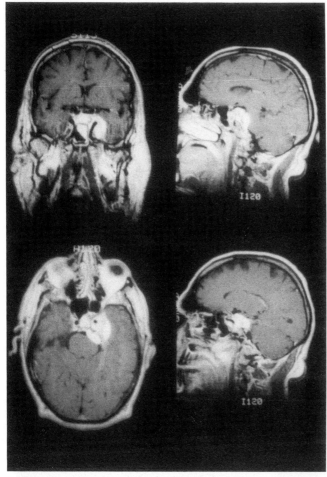

(a)

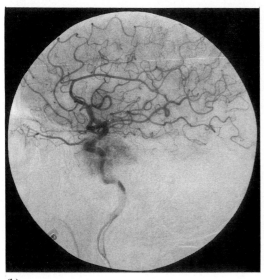

(b)

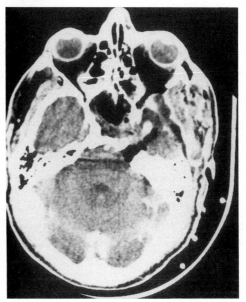

(c)

mandible. Physical examination revealed partial left cranial nerve IV and VI palsies. The CT and MRI scans demonstrated a left grade IV cavernous sinus mass, encasing the cavernous carotid artery and extending to the sphenoid sinus and petroclival region, where it caused both hyperostosis of the petrous apex and pressure on the brain stem (Fig. 14a). Cerebral arteriography demonstrated carotid artery narrowing and vascular tumor blush from branches of the meningohypophyseal trunk (see Fig. 14b).

Total tumor removal was accomplished in two stages by left frontotemporal craniotomy with orbitozygomatic osteotomy. During the first stage, tumor was removed from the tentorial notch, but could not be dissected from the intracavernous carotid artery. Thus, a saphenous vein interposition graft was placed from the petrous to the supracavernous portion of the ICA.

During the second stage, the remaining tumor within the cavernous sinus (including carotid artery), sphenoid bone and sinus, and petroclival area was completely removed.

Postoperatively, the patient had partial left cranial nerve III and V palsies, total left fourth and sixth nerve palsies, and conductive hearing loss. Temporary CSF leakage was treated with additional sutures and a lumbar drain. Postoperative-imaging studies demonstrated graft patency and no residual tumor (see Fig. 14c). By 4-months follow-up, hearing was nearly normal after the insertion of a myringotomy tube, and the left eye was centered by the injection of botulinum toxin into the medial rectus muscle.

Patient AM: Giant Pituitary Tumor. A 43-year-old man presented with an 8-month history of headache, deteriorating vision, and left facial numbness. Physical examination was significant for visual acuity 20/30 OU.

The MRI scan demonstrated a large mass involving the sphenoid and cavernous sinuses, nasopharynx, petroclival region, and CPA (Fig. 15 a,b).

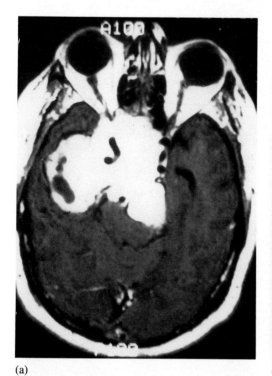
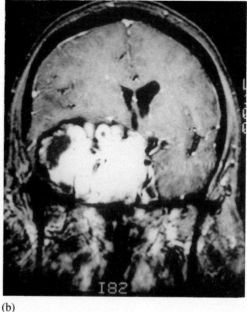

(a)   (b)

Figure 15 (a,b) (a) Axial and (b) coronal MRI demonstrating large mass in the sphenoid and cavernous sinuses, nasopharynx, petroclival region, and CPA. (c) CT scan demonstrating near-total tumor removal.

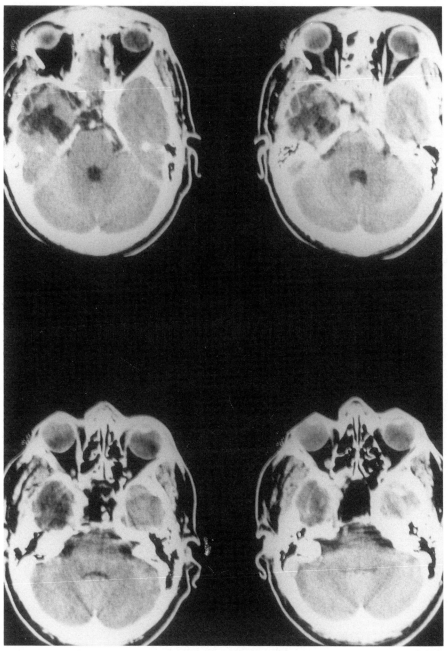

(c)

Cerebral angiography revealed displacement of the basilar and right internal carotid arteries without narrowing. The patient passed the clinical and xenon blood flow portions of the balloon test occlusion.

By a combination of subtemporal–preauricular–infratemporal fossa, subtemporal, and transsylvian approaches, a subtotal resection of a giant prolactin-secreting pituitary adenoma was achieved.

Postoperatively, the patient developed an intermittent CSF leak. Through a previous bicoronal incision, residual tumor was removed from the sella tucica, sphenoid sinus, and both cavernous sinuses, followed by reconstruction with fascia lata, autologous fat, and a pericranial flap.

Physical examination at the 9-month follow-up visit revealed mild right abducens and trochlear nerve paresis. Visual acuity was 20/40 OD, 20/25 OS. A CT scan revealed near-total tumor removal (see Fig. 15c).

Neuroendocrine evaluation was normal. Bromocriptine therapy was initiated for control of the small residue of tumor, and strabismus surgery is planned to improve the diplopia.

Patient RD: Cavernous Sinus Meningioma with Extension into the Infratemporal Fossa, Sphenoid Sinus, and Maxillary Sinus.   A 40-year-old man presented 5 years after a left pterional craniotomy for partial resection of a sphenoid wing meningioma with complaints of progressive left jaw drift and painful swelling, proptosis, diplopia, and V_2 distribution paresthesia. Examination revealed left-sided cranial nerve palsies, including III, IV, V_{2-3}, and VI, and obvious proptosis. The CT and MRI scans revealed the presence of recurrent tumor involving the cavernous sinus, middle fossa, infratemporal fossa, sphenoid and maxillary sinuses (Fig. 16a,b). Three days before the operation, embolization of the left internal maxillary artery was performed. At surgery, a near-total resection was accomplished through a transfacial approach. The tumor resection cavity in the infratemporal space was occluded with a rectus abdominus free flap. Postoperatively, the patient developed CSF rhinorrhea, probably related to both hydrocephalus and some sagging of the flap by gravity effect. At reexploration, the flap was adjusted to totally eliminate epidural dead space, and external ventricular drainage was instituted. After the meningitis resolved, a ventriculoperitoneal shunt was placed.

At discharge, the patient was cognitively normal, and had cranial nerve palsies that included III, IV, V, VI, and partial VII on the left. At 6-months follow-up, facial nerve function was normal and the oculomotor and abducens nerve palsies were improving. Enhanced MR images revealed no evidence of residual tumor (see Fig. 16c,d). External beam radiotherapy is being considered to ensure destruction of any possible microscopic tumor residue.

C.   Lateral Approaches to Tumors of the Cranial Base

A variety of lateral surgical approaches to this area have been employed. These include (1) translabyrinthine–transcochlear, (2) petrosal, and (3) total petrosectomy.

1.   *Translabyrinthine–Transcochlear Approach*

The translabyrinthine and transcochlear approaches are used to treat tumors causing more temporal bone involvement, as in large acoustic neurinomas. This incision is also postauricular (Fig. 17a–c). The additional exposure gained by the translabyrinthine approach is through the labyrinth, causing permanent total ipsilateral hearing loss. This usually represents no new deficit, as it is used primarily in patients with large acoustic neurinomas who have already markedly reduced or absent hearing. The transcochlear approach is essentially an extension of the translabyrinthine approach, and involves the exposure and temporary posterior displacement of the facial nerve. The use of this approach may result in a prolonged facial paralysis, with potential for incomplete recovery and

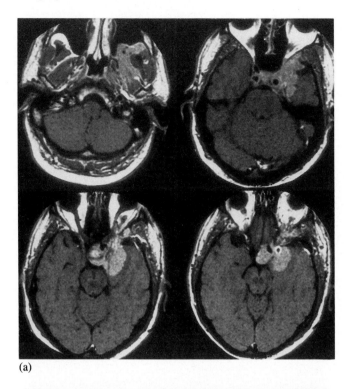

(a)

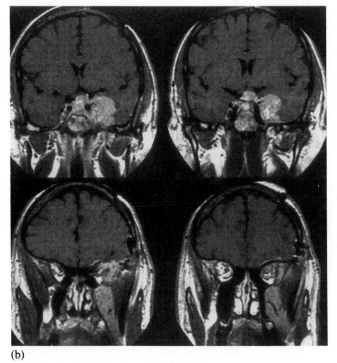

(b)

Figure 16 (a,b) Preoperative (a) axial and (b) coronal MRI, demonstrating recurrent tumor involving the cavernous sinus, middle fossa, infratemporal fossa, sphenoid and maxillary sinuses. (c,d) Postoperative (c) axial and (d) coronal MRI, reveal no evidence of residual tumor.

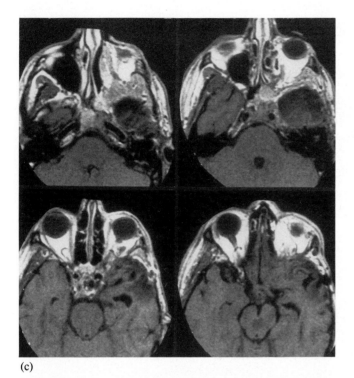

(c)

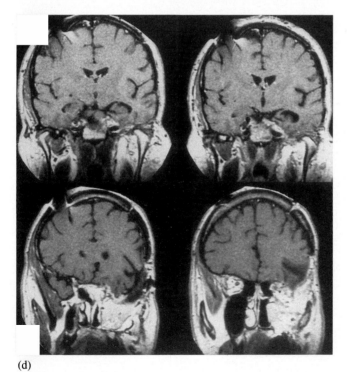

(d)

Figure 16   (continued)

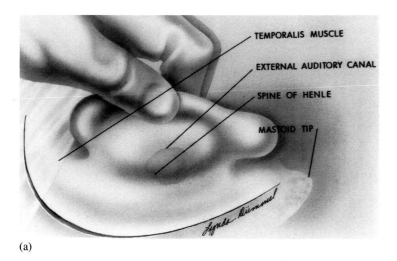

(a)

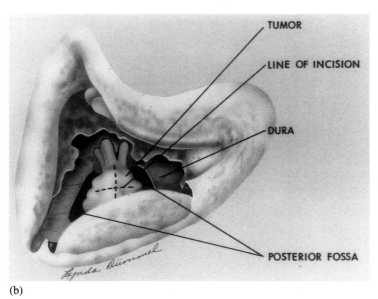

(b)

Figure 17 Diagrammatic representation of translabyrinthine and transcochlear approaches. (a) Skin incision 2 cm behind the postauricular sulcus. (b) Translabyrinthine approach: The small acoustic neurinoma is exposed by incising the dura covering the IAC and posterior fossa. (c) Transcochlear approach: Bone removal to this point includes the entire tympanic bone and labyrinth. The facial nerve has been rerouted posteriorly. Removal of the cochlea has begun.

synkinesis (18). In these approaches, as in many of the skull base surgery approaches, an additional incision is required, so that adipose tissue from elsewhere in the subcutaneous tissues may be packed into the mastoidectomy site to prevent a cutaneous CSF fistula.

2. The Petrosal Approach

The petrosal approach is centered on the petrous ridge, reminiscent of the pterional approach, which is centered on the sphenoid ridge. The approach is useful for tumors in the petroclival area, with or without extension into the middle and posterior cranial fossae. The incision is in the shape of a reverse question mark, starting in the preauricular area at the root of the zygoma, encircling the

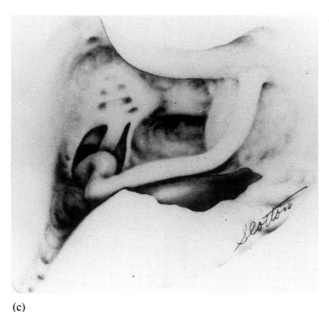

(c)

Figure 17 (continued)

pinna, and descending posteriorly to 1 cm behind the mastoid process (Fig. 18). Advantages of the approach include shortening of the distance to clivus by 3 cm, preservation of otologic structures (e.g., cochlea, labyrinth) and basal venous channels (e.g., transverse and sigmoid sinuses, basal and occipital veins, vein of Labbé), and early interruption of the tumor's vascular supply. Disadvantages include potential injury to the vein of Labbé, with subsequent venous infarction, and trochlear nerve injury during splitting of the tentorium. This latter complication causes minimal morbidity (19).

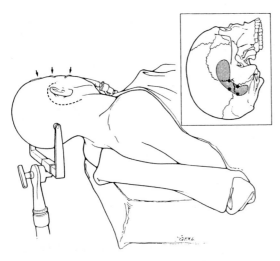

Figure 18 Position of patient and location of incision for right-sided petrosal approach. (Inset) Burr holes bridging the transverse sinus and extent of bone flap.

3. The Total Petrosectomy

Total petrosectomy refers to both a surgical approach and an operation. As an approach, it is used to resect tumors of the petroclival region and tentorium. The total petrosectomy operation is used to remove en bloc tumors of the temporal bone. It is applicable with modifications to all classes of invasive petrous bone neoplasms (Table 4).

Preoperative evaluation includes special attention to cerebral angiography. If the patient with malignant involvement of the ICA clinically fails the BTO, or if a dominant or noncollateralized sigmoid sinus is involved by tumor, surgery is not performed.

The incision extends from the frontotemporal hairline, behind the ear and ends onto the neck (Fig. 19a–c). The external auditory canal is transected and oversewn, providing broad lateral cranial base exposure. Lateral bone removal includes mastoidectomy with skeletonization of the sigmoid sinus, temporal and suboccipital craniotomies, mandibular condylectomy, and zygomatic osteotomy. In benign and low-grade malignancy tumors, the petrous bone resection may be done in piecemeal fashion, sparing neural and vascular structures wherever possible. Reconstrutive challenges require meticulous attention to detail (see Fig. 19D–F). A formal total petrosectomy accomplishes en bloc resection of highly malignant neoplasms. Such an en bloc resection necessarily includes the seventh and eighth cranial nerves and in some patients, cranial nerves IX–XI as well, to achieve complete tumor resection.

The prognosis for tumor-free survival is good after radical petrous bone resection in two-thirds of patients with low-grade malignancies (average period of follow-up, 20 months). In one-fourth of patients with large petrous malignancies, a similarly good prognosis can be anticipated after radical surgery and adjuvant therapy (average follow-up, 29 months) (20).

The advantage of this challenging surgical approach is the potential for long-term tumor-free survival, especially in patients treated early or with low-grade malignancies. Disadvantages specific to this approach include approximately 40% conductive hearing deficit owing to oversewing of the EAC and potential temporomandibular joint problems from joint resection. The fact that many of these patients have had prior surgery and radiation increases the potential for problems of wound healing.

4. Illustrative Case

Patient RR: Epidermoid. A 35-year-old man presented with an 18-month history of progressive difficulties with gait and speech, blurred vision, and memory loss. Physical examination was significant for gait and speech dyspraxias. An MRI scan revealed a large extra-axial mass involving the left CPA, medial temporal lobe, and cavernous sinus, encasing the superior cerebellar (SCA) and left posterior cerebral (PCA) arteries and displacing the basilar and left internal

Table 4 Classification of Anatomical Tumor Spread in Petrous Bone Tumors

Grade	Area
1	Partial petrous bone (two of these three areas: inner ear, middle ear, and around the external canal)
2	Entire petrous bone (all three of above areas)
2a	Petrous ICA infiltration
3	Entire petrous bone
3a	Adjacent cranial base bone (i.e., middle fossa, osseous floor, clivus, occipital condyle . . .)
3b	Dural infiltration
3c	Infratemporal upper cervical soft tissue
3d	Cavernous sinus infiltration

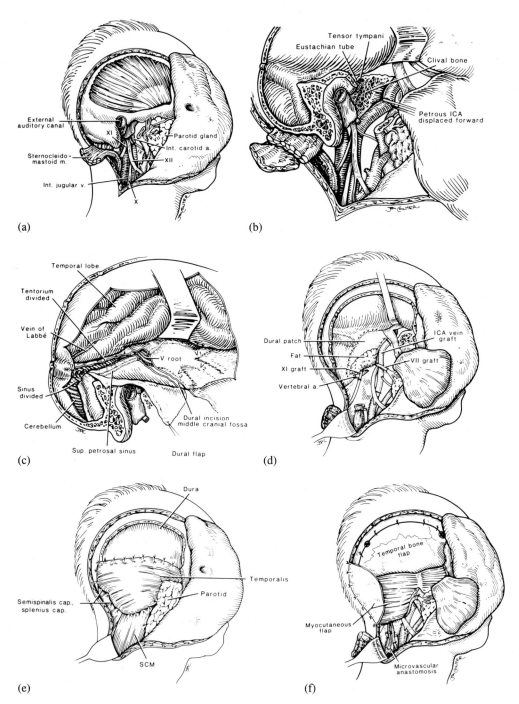

Figure 19 (a–c) Progressive steps in exposure using the total petrosectomy approach: (a) Forward rotation of the frontotemporal, retroauricular, and cervical skin flap; (b) resection of the bony floor of the middle cranial fossa; and (c) dural opening, exposing the temporal lobe and cerebellum. (d–f) Progressive steps in reconstruction after total petrosectomy (composite reconstruction; not every feature will be required in each case): (d) Reconstruction of carotid artery with a saphenous vein interposition graft, CN VII and XI with cable grafts, and of the dura with autogenous adipose and fascia lata patch graft. (e); further dural reconstruction, using temporalis, sternocleidomastoid, semispinalis, and splenius capitus muscles; and (f) position of microanastomosed rectus abdominus free flap to provide further support to dural repair and fill surgical defect.

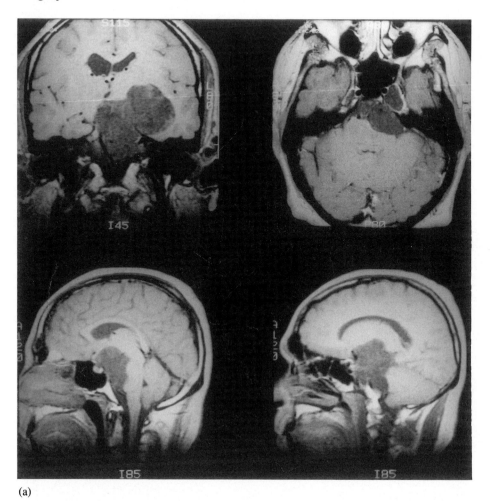

(a)

Figure 20 (a) Preoperative MRI reveals large extra-axial mass involving the left CPA, medial temporal lobe, and cavernous sinus, encasing the superior cerebellar (SCA) and the posterior cerebral (PCA) arteries. (b) The cerebral arteriogram demonstrates displacement of the basilar and left internal carotid arteries. (c) Postoperative CT demonstrates total tumor removal.

carotid arteries (Fig. 20a). The cerebral arteriogram further illustrates the displacement of the basilar and left internal carotid arteries (see Fig. 20b).

With use of a petrosal approach, a gross total removal of a large epidermoid cyst was achieved (see Fig. 20c).

At 6-weeks follow-up, he displayed mild but improving dysphasia, dyspraxia with his right hand, and no cranial neuropathy.

D. Posterolateral Approaches to Tumors of the Cranial Base

Tumors that distort the brain stem and involve important lower cranial nerves are among the most difficult challenges to the skull base surgeon. Posterolateral approaches to these neoplasms include (1) retromastoid craniectomy, (2) extreme lateral transcondylar, and (3) transjugular.

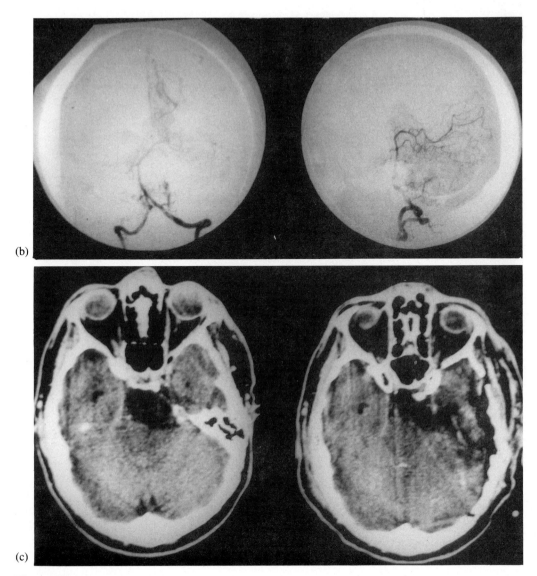

Figure 20   (continued)

1. Retromastoid Craniectomy

Retromastoid craniectomy is a modification of a standard neurosurgical approach, the suboccipital craniotomy. This approach provides the exposure of the cerebellopontine angle, and is commonly used to remove acoustic neurinomas. The incision is in the postauricular area, behind the hairline.

2. The Extreme Lateral Transcondylar Approach

The extreme lateral approach was developed as an approach for resection of neoplasms ventral or ventrolateral to the spinal cord and medulla, especially intradural extramedullary tumors, such as meningiomas and neurofibromas. Its advantages over transoral and transcervical approaches is the superior lateral exposure, allowing complete tumor removal and subsequent fusion where necessary. In addition, it is useful for treatment of aneurysms arising from the vertebral artery.

The incision extends from the lateral aspect of the neck rostrally to the base of the mastoid process, where it curves posteriorly. The vertebral artery (VA) is identified between the first and second cervical vertebrae. Bone removal includes a retromastoid craniectomy and lateral partial hemilaminectomy–facetectomy of posterior vertebral elements as required (Fig. 21). The advantages of this approach are the direct visualization of the tumor–cord–brain stem interface, control of the involved vertebral artery, and tumor devascularization early in the procedure. It does not cause spinal instability, but may be used as a route for fusion if mandated by the absence of other elements of the spinal column. As with other lateral approaches, potential injury to radicular vessels and nerve roots must be avoided (21).

3. The Transjugular Approach

The transjugular approach is a modification of the combined lateral suboccipital (retromastoid) infralabyrinthine approach. It is used to remove tumors located in the jugular foramen that extend intra- and extracranially. The retroauricular incision extends from the anterior border of the sternocleidomastoid to the hyoid bone. Advantages of this approach include preservation of hearing and vestibular function, improved exposure by mobilization of the sigmoid and transverse sinuses, preservation of the facial nerve within the bony fallopian canal, and reconstructive potential within the exposure should the spinal accessory nerve be injured or sacrificed because of tumor invasion. Disadvantages are the same as any surgical approach to tumors in this region, and primarily involves the risk of pharyngeal paresis and aspiration pneumonia (22) (Fig. 22a,b).

4. Illustrative Case

Patient L.S.: Petroclival Meningioma. A 51-year-old woman presented with a 6-month history of left-sided hearing loss and intermittent tinnitus. Examination was significant for the left cranial nerve VIII deficit, as well as decreased corneal and gag reflexes on the left. The MRI scan revealed a mass in the left petroclival region, with broad dural base, distorting the brain stem and partially encircling the basilar artery (Fig. 23a,b). Preoperative arteriography included embolization of feeding vessels from the ipsilateral ascending pharyngeal artery.

A large petroclival meningioma was removed in two stages. The first stage provided the exposure, and included retromastoid and temporal craniotomies, zygomatic osteotomy, and trans-

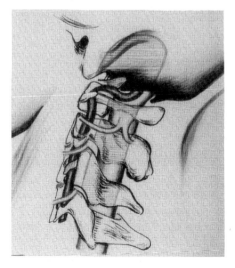

Figure 21 Illustration of the extreme lateral approach, indicating extent of bone removal and exposure of the vertebral artery.

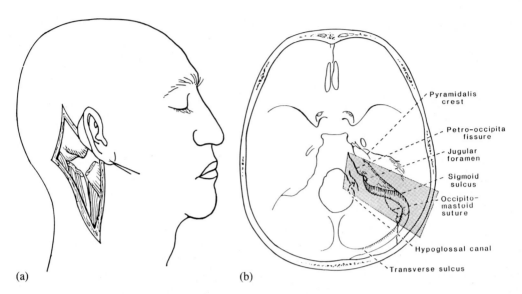

Figure 22 (a,b) Illustration of the surgical approach to the jugular foramen: (a) skin incision and initial soft-tissue exposure and (b) corridor accessed by this approach.

labyrinthine approach. Four days later, during the second stage, the sigmoid sinus was transsected, exposing the tumor. The abducens nerve, anterior inferior cerebellar artery (AICA), and one of its perforating vessels were completely encased.

In the immediate postoperative period, she has additional abducens and facial nerve paresis, a partial trigeminal nerve deficit, and the expected operative hearing loss. The sixth and seventh nerve palsies are expected to improve over time. No tumor residual was identified on postoperative imaging studies (see Fig. 23c,d).

VIII. COMPLICATIONS OF SKULL BASE OPERATIONS

Surgical treatment of skull base lesions poses a variety of special problems. Despite preventive measures and extreme vigilance, complications do occasionally arise. These may be divided into the following broad categories: (1) neurological, (2) cerebrospinal fluid leakage, (3) vascular, (4) infections, and (5) systemic.

A. Neurological Complications

The most serious potential complications are neurological. This results from brain edema and contusion caused by prolonged retraction during lengthly cranial base operations. Direct brain injury and ischemic injury owing to arterial or venous occlusion may also lead to serious complications. Prevention is the best way to address this potential problem area and involves careful choice of surgical approach. In general, cranial base surgery approaches are based on the principle that operative exposure is most safely provided by bone removal, rather than brain retraction. Postoperatively, CT scans are performed at frequent, regular intervals to provide early detection of edema, contusion, pneumocephalus, or hematoma before they cause clinical manifestations.

Temporary or permanent cranial nerve palsies do occur and are one of the major causes of

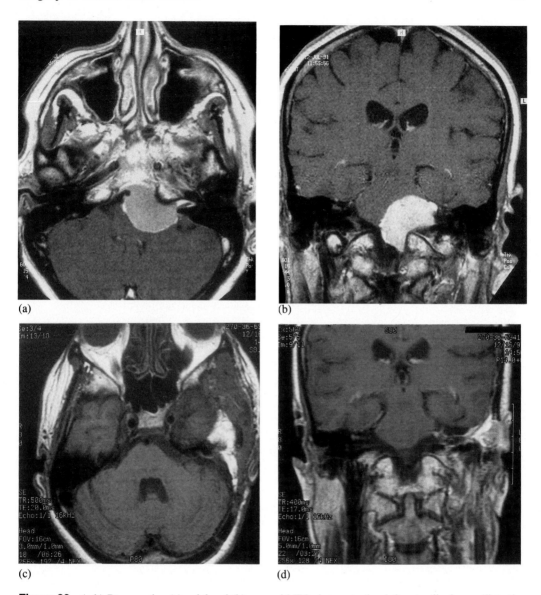

(a) (b)

(c) (d)

Figure 23 (a,b) Preoperative (a) axial and (b) coronal MRI, demonstrating left petroclival mass distorting the brain stem and partially encasing the basilar artery. (c,d) Postoperative (c) axial and (d) coronal MRI, showing gross total tumor removal.

morbidity in cranial base surgery. Motor nerves tend to recover more than sensory nerves. The oculomotor nerve is of primary concern, as it innervates several muscles of the eye. Even a slight degree of function during the postoperative period greatly improves the prognosis for recovery.

The function of the ophthalmic division of the trigeminal nerve (V_1) is very important, as injury to an insensate cornea is a potential cause of blindness. Facial nerve dysfunction causes both physical and emotional disabilities. Those patients whose facial nerves require partial excision at surgery because of tumor invasion or who fail to improve after 12 months, should be offered cable grafting. A House-Brackmann grade III functional result may be expected after recovery (Table 5).

Table 5 House-Brackmann Facial Nerve Grading System

Grade	Description	Characteristics
I	Normal	Normal facial function in all areas
II	Mild dysfunction	Gross: slight weakness noticeable on close inspection; may have very slight synkinesis At rest: normal symmetry and tone Motion 　Forehead: moderate to good function 　Eye: complete closure with minimum effort 　Mouth: slight asymmetry
III	Moderate dysfunction	Gross: obvious, but not disfiguring difference between two sides; noticeable but not severe synkinesis, contracture, or hemifacial spasm At rest: normal symmetry and tone Motion 　Forehead: slight to moderate movement 　Eye: complete closure with movement 　Mouth: slightly weak with maximum effort
IV	Moderately severe dysfunction	Gross: obvious weakness or disfiguring asymmetry At rest: normal symmetry and tone Motion 　Forehead: none 　Eye: incomplete closure 　Mouth: asymmetric with maximum effort
V	Severe dysfunction	Gross: only barely perceptible motion At rest: asymmetry Motion 　Forehead: none 　Eye: incomplete closure 　Mouth: slight movement
VI	Total paralysis	No movement

Injury to the glossopharyngeal and vagus nerves may cause significant problems with airway protection and swallowing, with consequent aspiration pneumonia and poor nutrition. Early placement of temporary tracheostomy or gastrostomy tubes is recommended in these patients.

Finally, disabling chronic shoulder joint arthropathy can be avoided by direct repair of the inadvertently transected spinal accessory nerve.

Temporary hypopituitarism may occur if tumor resection is in the region of the hypophysis. Diabetes insipidus is quite common, but usually transient. Pre- and postoperative endocrine testing is the rule when the surgical plan includes dissection in the region of the sella turcica.

The extensive bone removal required and proximity to paranasal sinuses of skull base lesions places patients at risk for the development of CSF leaks. Meticulous attention to the details of cranial base reconstruction will prevent many leaks. Nevertheless, CSF leakage may occur through the sphenoid sinus, temporal bone, or eustachian tube. Most leaks occur in the immediate postoperative period, while the patient is still hospitalized. Any suspicious fluid discharged from nose, mouth, or ear is analyzed for the presence of β_2-transferrin, a definitive protein marker for CSF (23). Small leaks are treated by lumbar spinal drainage, but large or persistent leaks require surgical reexploration. Associated pneumocephalus may be a source of severe headache or mental status change.

Vascular complications are related to technical problems encountered when a major vessel is encased by tumor. In the subarachnoid space, vessels are delineated by an arachnoid plane, facilitating the dissection of vessels from tumor. In the skull base and cavernous sinus, however, this protective encircling membrane around the vessels is absent. Techniques basic to vascular surgery are rigorously adhered to, such as early attainment of proximal and distal control, and sharp dissection to avoid difficult-to-repair irregular tears. The skull base surgeon must be thoroughly versed in the techniques of cerebral revascularization. Even when vessel occlusion or interruption is not anticipated preoperatively, unforseen technical difficulties may require immediate revascularization to avoid massive ischemic deficit or death.

Infections occur in skull base surgery patients, and may be life-threatening. Extradural abscess, meningitis, and osteomyelitis are feared complications. They are best treated by prevention. Interestingly, the prolonged length of these operations and need for staged procedures would seem to predispose these patients to an increased occurrence of infection, but this was not borne out in our current series.

Finally, systemic complications are similar to those to which many neurosurgical patients are predisposed: deep vein thrombosis (DVT), pneumonia, seizures, and debilitation secondary to poor nutrition (24).

IX. SPECIALIZED SURGICAL TREATMENT MODALITIES

A. Stereotactic Radiosurgery

Stereotactic techniques involve cranial attachment of a guiding device that allows an instrument or radiation beam to reach the depths of the brain or skull base with 1-mm precision. Combination of stereotactic devices with CT offers increased accuracy in target definition and in planning an anatomically safe trajectory.

Stereotactic radiosurgery (see Chap. 26) uses focused beam radiation by one of three currently available techniques: (1) multisource radioactive cobalt (the gamma knife), (2) proton beam utilizing the Bragg peak effect, and (3) the linear accelerator. The largest experience and longest follow-up is available for patients treated with gamma knife. In this technique, treatment is done under local anesthesia, without an incision, and frequently in approximately 1 h. Morbidity and mortality are negligible. The technique is generally limited to lesions smaller than 3 cm and with a clearance of at least 3 mm from the optic nerves.

Adjunctive stereotactic treatments for skull base lesions include intracavitary placement of radioactive isotopes (usually ^{32}P) for cystic neoplasms and interstitial brachytherapy. The latter offers a means of local, relatively long-term, low-dose-rate, high-dose intratumoral radiation therapy of unresectable tumors. Its role in the care of patients with skull base tumors remains to be defined (25).

X. FUTURE CONSIDERATIONS

Surgery of skull base tumors has rapidly emerged within the last decade as a separate neurosurgical subspecialty. The formation of multidisciplinary cranial base surgery teams and the concentration of patients at centers that support such teams, has allowed increasing opportunities to optimize care of patients with uncommon neoplasms.

In the future, new surgical approaches and microsurgical instruments will permit increasingly safe tumor removal. Alternative or adjuvant therapies, particularly radiosurgery, offer the potential for tumor control or cure. Finally, advances in molecular genetics may one day offer preventive treatment for some of these skull base tumors.

REFERENCES

1. deVries EJ, Sekhar LN, Horton JA, et al. A new method to predict safe resection of the internal carotid artery. Laryngoscope 1990; 100:88–95.
2. Jungreis CA, Horton JA. Interventional radiology: embolization. In: Sekhar LN, Janecka IP, eds. Surgery of cranial base tumors: a color atlas. New York: Raven Press, 1992 (in press).
3. Latchaw RE. Imaging of tumors at the base of the skull: the sphenoid bone. In: Sekhar LN, Schramm VL, eds. Tumors of the cranial base. Mt Kisco, NY: Futura Publishing Company, 1987:39–64.
4. Curtin HD. Radiology of skull base lesions. In: Sekhar LN, Schramm VL, eds. Tumors of the cranial base. Mt Kisco, NY: Futura Publishing Company, 1987:81–84.
5. Domino KB. Anesthesia for cranial base tumor operations. In: Sekhar LN, Schramm VL, eds. Tumors of the cranial base. Mt Kisco, NY: Futura Publishing Company, 1987:107–114.
6. Gonzalez RM. Special anesthetic considerations in cranial base tumor surgery. In: Sekhar LN, Janecka IP, eds. Surgery of cranial base tumors: a color atlas. New York: Raven Press, 1992 (in press).
7. Albin MS, Carroll RG, Maroon JC. Clinical considerations concerning the detection of venous air embolism. Neurosurgery 1978; 3:380–384.
8. Domino KB. Anesthesia for cranial base tumor operations. In: Sekhar LN, Schramm VL, eds. Tumors of the cranial base. Mt Kisco, NY: Futura Publishing Company, 1987:112–121.
9. Crockard A. Transmaxillary approach to the clivus. In: Sekhar LN, Janecka IP, eds. Surgery of cranial base tumors: a color atlas. New York: Raven Press, 1993.
10. Sekhar LN, Nanda A, Snyderman CH, Janecka IP. The extended frontal approach to midline tumors of the anterior, middle, and posterior cranial base. J Neurosurg 1992; 76:198–206.
11. Schramm VL. Anterior craniofacial resection. In: Sekhar LN, Schramm VL, eds. Tumors of the cranial base. Mt. Kisco, NY: Futura Publishing Company, 1987:265–278.
12. Janecka IP, Sen CN, Sekhar LN, Arriaga MA. Facial translocation: a new approach to the cranial base. Otolaryngol Head Neck Surg 1990; 103:413–419.
13. Crockard A. Transoral approaches to intra/extradural tumors. In: Sekhar LN, Janecka IP, eds. Surgery of cranial base tumors: a color atlas. New York: Raven Press, 1993.
14. Krespi YP, Har-El G. The transmandibular–transcervical approach to the skull base. In: Sekhar LN, Janecka IP, eds. Surgery of cranial base tumors: a color atlas. New York: Raven Press, 1993.
15. Sekhar LN, Schramm VL Jr, Jones NF. Subtemporal–preauricular infratemporal fossa approach to large and posterior cranial base neoplasms. 1987; J Neurosurg 67:488–497.
16. Brackmann DE. The middle fossa approach. In: Sekhar LN, Janecka IP, eds. Surgery of cranial base tumors: a color atlas. New York: Raven Press, 1993.
17. Kawase T, Shiobara R, Toya S. Anterior transpetrosal–transtentorial approach for sphenopetroclival meningiomas: surgical method and results in ten patients. Neurosurgery 1991; 28:869–876.
18. Brackmann DE. Translabyrinthine/transcochlear approach. In: Sekhar LN, Janecka IP, eds. Surgery of cranial base tumors: a color atlas. New York: Raven Press, 1993.
19. Al-Mefty O. Petrosal approach for petroclival meningiomas. Neurosurgery 1988; 22:510–517.
20. Sekhar LN, Pomeranz S, Janecka IP, Hirsch B, Ramasastry S. Classification, technique, and results of surgical resection of petrous bone tumors. In: Sekhar LN, Janecka IP, eds. Surgery of cranial base tumors: a color atlas. New York: Raven Press, 1993.
21. Sen CN, Sekhar LN. An extreme lateral approach to intradural lesions of the cervical spine and foramen magnum. Neurosurgery 1990; 27:197–204.
22. Samii M, Draf W. The diagnosis and operative strategy of large glomus tumors. In: Scheunemann H, Schürmann K, Helms J, eds. Tumors of the skull base. New York: De Guyer Publishers, 1986:237–244.

23. Reisinger PWM, Hochstrasser K. The diagnosis of CSF fistulae on the basis of detection of β_2-transferrin by polyacrylamide gel electrophoresis and immunoblotting. J Clin Chem Clin Biochem 1989; 27:169–172.
24. Sen CN, Snyderman CH, Sekhar LN. Complications of skull base operations. In: Sekhar LN, Janecka IP, eds. Surgery of cranial base tumors: a color atlas. New York: Raven Press, 1993.
25. Lunsford LD. Stereotactic methods for diagnosis and treatment of skull base lesions. In: Sekhar LN, Schramm VL, eds. Tumors of the cranial base. Mt Kisco, NY: Futura Publishing Company, 1987:151–162.

16

Stereotactic Surgery in the Diagnosis and Treatment of Brain Tumors

**Nayef R. F. Al-Rodhan and
Patrick J. Kelly**
Mayo Clinic and Mayo Graduate School of Medicine,
Rochester, Minnesota

I. INTRODUCTION

Even though there were sporadic reports of stereotactic techniques in the 19th century (1,2), credit for the development of modern stereotactic concepts is usually given to Robert Henry Clarke (3,4). Clarke foresaw the use of stereotactic techniques for the diagnosis and treatment of brain neoplasms. He proposed this concept (5) to his collaborator, neurosurgeon Victor Horsley. However, Horsely did not feel that stereotaxis had any application beyond the laboratory.

Human stereotaxis was not employed until 1947, when Spiegel and colleagues of Philadelphia reported its use for dorsal median thalamotomy in an attempt to provide an alternative to frontal lobotomy, which was popular at the time (6). Interestingly, these authors did propose the use of stereotactic methods in the management of intracranial tumors. Others soon developed stereotactic instruments and procedures, most notably Talaraich in Paris (1949) and Leksell in Stockholm (1949). Although the original use of stereotaxis was psychosurgical, interest in ablative procedures for pain and movement disorders was sparked.

After a promising initiation, interest in stereotactic neurosurgery waned after the introduction of L-dopa in the late 1960s. Even though its pioneers had suggested the use of stereotactic techniques in the management of intracranial neoplasms, not much interest in tumor stereotaxis was generated until the advent of computed tomography (CT) scanning. Computed tomography scanning provides a precise three-dimensional data base that can be easily incorporated into a stereotactic coordinate system. In addition, surgeons could actually *see* the tumor on CT images and were no longer required to infer the position of tumors from visual shifts on angiograms or displacement of parts of the ventricular system. Tumors could now be targeted directly and many neurosurgeons began rethinking their approaches to intracranial neoplasms. The incorporation of imaging technology, CT, and later magnetic resonance imaging (MRI), into stereotactic technique signaled the rebirth of stereotactic neurosurgery for the biopsy and resection of not only previously unresectable lesions, but also lesions that were considered to be within the realm of routine conventional neurosurgery.

II. STEREOTACTIC PROCEDURES

A. Stereotactic Approaches in Intracranial Tumors

In general, stereotactic methods allow a surgeon to (1) find the lesion, (2) identify the CT and MRI interface between tumor and surrounding brain tissue, (3) delineate the relations between tumor and normal vascular and neuroanatomic structures, (4) be more selective in the surgical approach in attempts to establish the histological diagnosis or resect the tumor while preserving normal structures. Stereotactic approaches are not appropriate for all intracranial tumors. Obviously, there is little difficulty in finding or defining the histological limits of most extra-axial lesions. In addition, certain intra-axial lesions can be operated on using nonstereotactic methods. For example, glial neoplasms located in the frontal, temporal, or occipital poles can undergo lobectomy employing classic neurosurgical methods. In general, stereotactic procedures are less extensive than classic craniotomy. They have a greater assurance of achieving the goals of the procedure (e.g., obtaining a tissue diagnosis or achieving a significant cytoreduction). In many subcortical locations, stereotactic procedures are associated with lower morbidity than nonstereotactic methods.

Stereotactic methods can be used to biopsy tumors, to drain intracranial cysts, implant radioactive substances within tumor cysts, and implant interstitial radionuclides into solid neoplasms. In addition, stereotactic third ventriculostomy can be employed to relieve obstructive hydrocephalus. Furthermore, CT- and MRI-defined tumors can be radically extirpated by volumetric stereotactic resection.

B. Stereotactic Biopsy

Freehand methods for CT-directed needle biopsy have been described. However, stereotactic biopsy is superior because of the increased accuracy, and the ability to combine CT with other data sources, such as stereotactic angiography, to augment the safety of the procedure. In addition, stereotactic biopsy has a slightly higher diagnostic yield than CT-directed free-hand procedures. Mortality and morbidity for stereotactic biopsy procedures are low; usually between 1 and 4%.

The primary goal of a stereotactic biopsy procedure is to obtain a tissue diagnosis. In glial neoplasms, multiple samples within a heterogeneous tumor can provide a spectrum of pathology to the pathologist for accurate classification of the neoplasm as to the histological subtype and grade.

A stereotactic biopsy can be obtained with several instruments, including pediatric bronchoscopy forceps or specially designed devices, such as the corkscrew biopsy instrument originally described by Backlund, or the side-biting window cannula of the Sedan type. In addition, there are a variety of imaging-compatible stereotactic frames available to direct the instrument to a CT- or MRI-defined target point within the lesion.

In planning a stereotactic biopsy, it is best to avoid essential brain tissue within the biopsy trajectory. In addition, knowledge of the location of important blood vessels is important to select a safe biopsy trajectory. For this reason stereotactic arteriography is recommended; however, occasionally the standard angiogram can provide the required information.

Many report doing stereotactic biopsy under local anesthesia. We prefer general anesthesia at our institution, for several reasons. First, it may be less traumatic to the patient psychologically. Second, biopsy of subcortical lesions can occasionally be associated with a seizure in patients under local anesthesia, even with adequate levels of anticonvulsants. And third, a rare biopsy procedure is complicated by hemorrhage, especially in vascular tumors. This event occasionally requires craniotomy to stop the bleeding. Although possible, this is not conveniently done under local anesthesia.

Biopsy procedures are associated with few complications. These include hemorrhage, seizures, and local infections at the scalp entry site. Hemorrhage is frequently identified after taking the biopsy specimen from a vascular tumor. Arterial or venous bleeding can be noted extending out of the biopsy cannula. It is important to keep the biopsy cannula clear, for as long as this is clear the blood will extend out the cannula and not form a local parenchymal hematoma. The cannula is kept clear by a constant stream of saline irrigation. Bleeding should stop within 20 min. If it has not stopped by that time, a stereotactic craniotomy may be necessary to coagulate the bleeding point. The appearance of a clinically significant hematoma following a stereotactic biopsy procedure is rare (< 1%) in our experience, and half of these patients ultimately recover to their preoperative baselines as the clot absorbs.

There are several contraindications to stereotactic biopsy. These include vascular lesions that are now usually identified on preoperative MRI studies. The surgeon should be very reluctant to perform stereotactic biopsy on an intensely enhancing, discretely circumscribed lesion on CT scanning. An MRI should be performed to exclude the possibility of thrombosed arteriovenous malformation or cavernous hemangioma which are angiographically occult. A stereotactic craniotomy should be considered to resect very vascular lesions seen on arteriography, as opposed to performing a stereotactic biopsy.

The second contraindication to performing stereotactic biopsy is represented by a lesion with significant mass effect and midline shift. Although biopsy can be tolerated in these patients, edema or a small hemorrhage complicating the procedure could result in neurological decompensation and herniation. Lesions with significant mass effect are best treated by stereotactic resection, lobectomy, or other means of internal decompression.

C. Stereotactic Management of Cystic Lesions

Certain gliomas, hemangioblastomas, metastatic tumors, and craniopharyngiomas can produce symptoms by the development of a tumor cyst. Ideally, the best treatment for this is to excise the lesions and, in some instances, the cyst wall as well. Occasionally, drainage of the cyst and excision of a mural nodule, for example, in certain pilocytic astrocytomas and hemangioblastomas, will cure the cyst. Nevertheless, the anatomical location of some of these lesions or the medical condition of the patient may not warrant an aggressive surgical procedure. Significant palliation can be obtained by aspirating the contents of the cyst.

In general, stereotactic cyst aspirations are performed employing a method very similar to a stereotactic biopsy procedure. A target point in the most dependent portion of the cyst is chosen and access is obtained by means of a biopsy cannula. Frequently, these procedures are done under local anesthesia, such that the cyst fluid can be slowly withdrawn while talking to the patient. Cyst fluid should be withdrawn slowly. If the patient develops headache while aspirating the cyst, the surgeon should wait until the headache has virtually resolved before resuming slow aspiration of the cyst contents. Rapid decompression by means of a syringe of a lesion causing increased intracranial pressure can result in a reversed shift and possibly secondary brain stem vascular injury. In general it is best to perform aspirations of more than 70–80 ml in two or more stages.

If a biopsy is to be combined with cyst aspiration, it is best to perform the biopsy first before aspirating the cyst. The reason for this should be obvious: aspirating the cyst will change intracranial anatomical relations, rendering the biopsy target point calculations inaccurate. One can choose a trajectory that traverses the cyst into the lesion, obtain the biopsy, then back the biopsy cannula back a measured number of millimeters which would place it in the cyst cavity, and then proceed with the cyst aspiration. Alternatively, two separate trajectories, one to biopsy the lesion and a second to aspirate the cyst, could be employed.

Tumor cysts merely undergoing aspiration will usually recur within several weeks to months. When aspirating a cyst, one must decide on how this is going to be managed on a long-term basis. In craniopharyngiomas, metastatic tumors, and some glial neoplasms, aspiration of the cyst may allow a patient to complete radiation therapy. External beam radiation therapy may prevent the cyst from recurring. In addition, aspiration of a cyst may neurologically stabilize a patient with a view toward performing surgical removal of the lesion and cyst wall at a later date. In malignant lesions a catheter connected to a subcutaneous Ommaya reservoir can be employed, such that the cyst can be drained percutaneously by puncture of the reservoir with a 25-gauge needle when the patient becomes symptomatic. In our experience, this is rarely a long-term solution, as the catheters may become blocked or infected.

D. Intracavitary Irradiation

Recurrent tumor cysts can be treated by the instillation of a beta-emitting colloid. The beta-irradiation is transmitted only a short distance (0.5–1 mm) into tissue. This is adequate to radiate the wall of a cyst, but delivers minimal radiation to the brain tissues surrounding the cyst cavity. Nonetheless, this is frequently adequate to prevent a cyst from reaccumulation. There are a variety of beta-emitting colloids available: ytrium-90 (^{90}Y), rhenium-196 (^{186}Re), and phosphorus-32 (^{32}P). The only one approved by the Food and Drug Administration at this juncture for use intracranially in the United States is phosphorus-32. Its penetrance into soft tissues is approximately 1.7 mm, it is a pure beta-emitter, with a mean energy of 0.69 MeV, and a half life of 14.2 days. The dose of ^{32}P to be injected will depend on the volume of the cyst calculated by a variety of techniques, but typically a dose between 200 and 250 cGy is delivered to the inner surface wall of a tumor cyst.

It is best to inject a radioactive colloid into a cyst that has been expanded by the cyst fluid. Not infrequently this requires three separate operations for a patient presenting with an intracranial cystic lesion. The first procedure is usually done to drain the cyst, reverse neurological problems, and biopsy the lesion. The cyst is allowed to reaccumulate as judged by serial CT or MRI examinations, but not to the extent of producing neurological symptoms. At this point, the radioactive colloid may be instilled in a stereotactic procedure. After approximately 3–4 weeks (1½–2 half lives), the cyst is tapped a third time and the remaining cyst fluid and residual radioactive ^{32}P is withdrawn.

This form of therapy is simple and usually effective. However, it is occasionally necessary to treat a cyst a second time if the first instillation of ^{32}P is not effective in arresting the secretion of cyst fluid.

E. Stereotactic Volumetric Craniotomy

As more advanced computer hardware and software became available, stereotaxy evolved from point-in-space targets, a concept associated with functional procedures in the 1950s and 1960s, to volumetric targets that proved more appropriate and useful in tumor stereotaxis. In the latter technique, volumes interpolated from tumor contours defined by stereotactic-imaging techniques (CT, MRI) are reconstructed in stereotactic space. These volumes can be resected by employing stereotactically directed instruments and computer interactive methods. Techniques have been developed for the resection of superficial as well as deep-seated intra-axial lesions (7,8).

In this section we review our methods and our clinical experience with volumetric stereotactic resection of intracranial lesions over a 6-year period.

III. VOLUMETRIC STEREOTACTIC SURGERY: MATERIALS AND METHODS

Volumetric stereotactic resections of intracranial neoplasms are performed in three separate stages: (1) data base acquisition phase, (2) surgical planning, and (3) the interactive surgical procedure. A replaceable stereotactic headframe allows all of the foregoing to be performed in a single operative day or the data acquisition to be done on one day and the interactive surgery to be performed on another day in a separate procedure.

A. Data Acquisition

The techniques and methods of data base acquisition have been described extensively elsewhere (8). In the following account, a brief outline is discussed. The patient is fitted initially with a CT and MRI-compatible stereotactic headframe (the COMPASS system), which is applied under local anesthesia and mild intravenous sedation. This is secured to the skull by carbon fiber pins that are inserted into twist drill holes (1/8 in.) drilled through the outer table of the skull into the diploe. Detachable micrometers are employed to measure the carbon fiber fixation points relative to the vertical supports of the headframe (Fig. 1). These micrometer readings are reproduced in reap-

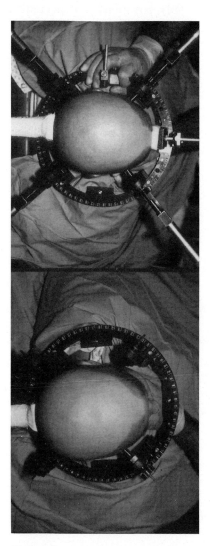

Figure 1 Stereotactic headframe with micrometers attached to its vertical support elements. These micrometers are used to measure the length of the carbon fiber fixation pin extending beyond the vertical support. This provides a mechanism for the accurate reapplication of the frame.

plications of the frame for the surgical procedures. Following placement of the stereotactic headframe, the patient is transferred to the neuroradiology suite where stereotactic CT, MRI, and digital angiograms are performed (Fig. 2).

1. Stereotactic Computed Tomography Scanning

The stereotactic frame is secured to a CT table adaptation plate. Then, nine reference marks on each CT slice are obtained using a CT-localization system that has nine carbon fiber localization rods arranged in the shape of the letter N and located on either side of the head and anteriorly. The CT scanning is performed on a General Electric 9800 CT scanning unit focusing on 5-mm adjacent slices throughout the lesion.

2. Stereotactic Magnetic Resonance Imaging

The MRI localization system consists of capillary tubes filled with copper sulfate solution arranged in an N-shaped configuration. These are located bilaterally, anteriorly, posteriorly, and superiorly, and result in at least nine reference marks on each axial coronal or sagittal MR image from which stereotactic coordinates are calculated.

3. Stereotactic Digital Angiography

Stereotactic stereoscopic digital angiography (DSA) is used for the spatial localization of intracranial vessels (arteries and veins) relevant to the location of the lesion and the surgical approach. In addition the stereotactic localization of the sulci and fissures of the brain surface are established by the identification of the deep vascular segments on the orthogonal view of the stereoscopic pair. Angiography is performed using the femoral catheterization technique. Orthogonal and 6° oblique arterial and venous phases are obtained in orthogonal and 6° stereoscopic pairs. The stereotactic headframe is placed on a digital fluoroscopy table adaptation plate on the General Electric 3000 or 5000 digital angiographic units. The angiographic localization system consists of nine radiopaque reference marks on Lucite plates that are located on either side of the head

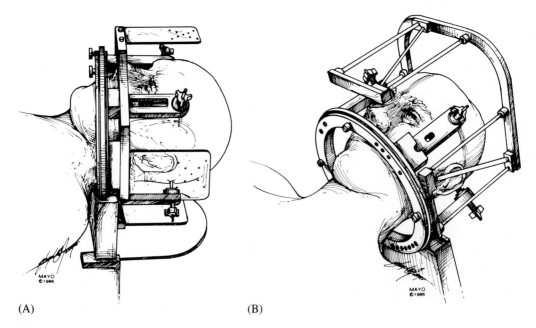

(A)   (B)

Figure 2 Stereotactic data acquisition localization systems for (A) planar images such as CT and MRI, and (B) projection images such as digital angiography.

anteriorly and posteriorly, resulting in 18 reference marks on each anteroposterior (AP) and lateral angiographic image. The relations between the fiducial marks and their location on the digital angiographic images form the basis for calculations of stereotactic coordinates for intracranial vessels. A 6° indexing mark on the base ring of the stereotactic headframe is used for precise rotation of the headframe on the DSA base unit to obtain an exact 6° rotation for the oblique images of the stereotactic pairs.

B. Surgical Planning

The stereotactic surgical approach to the lesion is planned at the computer console after data acquisition (CT, MRI, digital angiography) has been completed and the archived tapes from the CT, MRI, or DSA host computer system have been loaded onto the surgical computer system (Fig. 3). The outline of the lesion defined by CT (contrast enhancement and hypodensity) and MRI (T1, T2, and gadolinium) is traced by the surgeon from these digitized outlines. The computer creates separate volumes from CT- and MRI-defined data bases.

In planning the surgical approach, two considerations are important: (1) the three-dimensional shape of the tumor since an effort is made to approach the tumor along its long axis; (2) the three-dimensional anatomical relation of the lesion to vascular structures, subcortical white matter pathways, and overlying cortical tissue. This surgical approach to the target is defined by two stereotactic frame parameters: (1) the collar (angle from the horizontal plane) and (2) arc (angle from the vertical plane). The computer will slice through the CT- or MRI-defined three-dimensional lesional volume in a plane perpendicular to the intended surgical approach. These slices are displayed on video monitors in the operating room or directly into the operating microscope by means of a "heads-up" display monitor in which the image can also be scaled to the exact size of the surgical field.

1. Stereotactic Instrumentation

The patient's head, fixed in the stereotactic headframe, is moved in three-dimensional space by means of a stepper motor-controlled three-axis (X,Y,Z) slide system with optical encoder feedback (COMPASS Stereotactic System; Stereotactic Medical Systems, New Hartford, New York). The

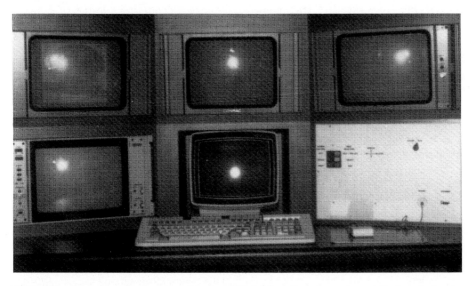

Figure 3 Computer-planning console where CT, MRI, and angiography are displayed after data acquisition for use during surgical planning.

three-axis stepper motors (*X*, *Y*, and *Z*) are activated manually by switches on a control panel or automatically by computer. The COMPASS stereotactic instrument employs the arc-quadrant principle: the slide system is used to place an intracranial target point in the center of the sphere defined by the fixed arc and quadrant. Instruments or probes directed perpendicular to a tangent of the arc-quadrant will always pass through the focal point or center of the sphere.

The heads-up display unit is attached to the operating microscope. This projects the computer-generated stereotactic tumor slice images derived from CT or MRI into the microscope, which are scaled to the exact size of the surgical field visualized under amplification and reflects these images into the surgeon's eyes. The computer-generated images are thus superimposed over the actual surgical field. The slice images are displayed in conjunction with a circular image that corresponds to the configuration of a stereotactically directed cylindrical retractor for deep lesions or a stereotactically placed trephine in the resection of superficial lesions.

2. Surgical Procedure

If the surgical procedure is planned immediately following the data acquisition procedure, the patient returns to the operating room directly from the neuroradiology suite. If, however, surgery and data acquisition are to be done on two separate days, the stereotactic headframe is removed and reapplied on the day of surgery. Accurate duplication of headframe reposition is ensured by micrometer readings obtained during the initial headframe placement. It is important to note that the round base ring of the stereotactic headframe and the fact that it can be detached from the positioning slide system allows a patient to undergo data acquisition in the most comfortable position (supine) and to be operated on in a position that will be comfortable and convenient for the surgeon. Computer software will account for this rotation and update stereotactic frame coordinates and image displays accordingly.

After anesthesia and replacement of the stereotactic headframe, the patient is positioned on the operating table and the base ring of the headframe is rotated to the appropriate setting, as planned by the surgeon on the computer console.

Superficial Lesions. In the resection of superficial lesions, the stereotactic instrument is used to center a circular trephine that is only slightly larger than the lesion, the computer display of the circular trephine is superimposed by the heads-up display onto the actual trephine in the surgical field (Fig. 4). The displayed CT- and MRI-defined slice images demonstrate to the surgeon the relation of the tumor boundaries to the edges of the trephine. The surgeon uses these images to recognize and create a plane around the tumor to circumscribe before removing the lesion. It should be noted that this procedure is considerably different from standard "internal decompression" operations in which the surgeon enters the center of the lesion and works peripherally.

In computer-assisted stereotactic resection the surgeon first isolates the lesion from surrounding brain tissue before resecting the tumor as a single specimen or piecemeal. This departure from conventional technique prevents intracranial tumor shifts that may be encountered when the lesion is debulked, as in conventional technique. A positive by-product of the *isolation-before-removal* method, as proposed here, is that the tumor is separated from its blood supply before it is entered. Blood loss is frequently much less with volumetric stereotactic resection than with conventional tumor surgery.

Deep Lesions. Deep tumors are approached through a 1.5-in. (3.8-cm) cranial trephine and a laser-produced incision in nonessential cortical and subcortical white matter pathways (Fig. 5). This technique employs a stereotactically directed cylindrically shaped retractor 0.8 in. (2 cm) in diameter that is introduced through the cortical incision. The retractor not only maintains the exposure from the surface of the brain to the superficial aspect of the lesion, but also provides a fixed reference structure within the surgical field to which the computer-generated slice images can be related.

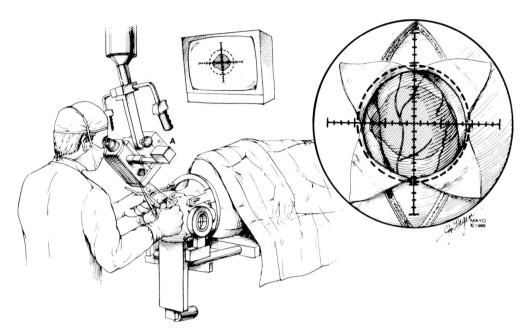

Figure 4   Method for stereotactic resection of superficial tumor. The trephine has been placed stereotactically. The computer displays the position of a tumor volume slice at a specified distance along the viewline on a display monitor and into the HUD unit of the operating microscope (A). The image is scaled until the configuration of the trephine in the image display is exactly the same size and aligns to the trephine. The surgeon then uses the tumor slice image as a template that will aid in the isolation of the tumor from surrounding brain tissue. (From Ref. 7)

The surgeon uses computer-generated information of the tumor slice that corresponds to each depth of the retractor to develop a plane between the tumor and surrounding brain tissue. This plane is then separated with the use of a carbon dioxide laser. The lesion itself is removed with laser, suction, and bipolar cautery.

There are, in general, several stereotactic approaches that can be employed in the resection of deep subcortical lesions. These include transcortical (for tumors within 5–10 mm of the brain surface), transsulcal, transsylvian, and interhemispheric approaches. For lesions in the posterior fossa, the patient is operated on with the stereotactic headframe placed in the inverted position, thereby providing unlimited access to the posterior fossa (data acquisition is also performed with the head frame inverted) (Fig. 6). Midline lesions in the cerebellum are approached through the inferior vermis, whereas lateral cerebellar lesions are approached through a lateral craniectomy, and pontine lesions are approached in a lateral oblique trajectory that traverses the middle cerebellar peduncle.

After resection, the dura is closed primarily, the bone flap is replaced and secured with nylon suture, and the skin is closed in layers. The stereotactic frame is removed at the end of the procedure and a head dressing is applied.

IV.   RESULTS

A.   Overall Results and Complications

Our surgical data comprise 500 consecutive patients operated on at the Mayo Clinic between 1984 and 1990. This includes 458 supratentorial lesions and 52 infratentorial lesions in patients having

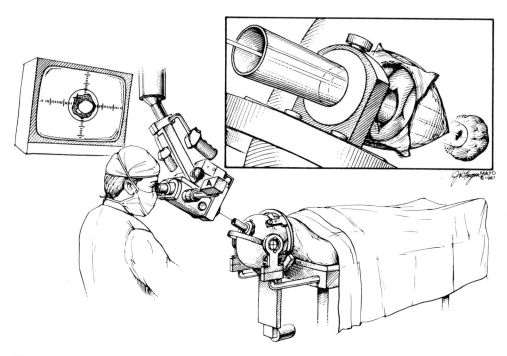

Figure 5 Stereotactic resection of deep tumors employs a stereotactically directed cylindrical retractor, operating microscope, and surgical laser. The computer displays the configuration of the retractor with reference to its end and slices through the tumor volume cut perpendicular to the surgical viewline. This is displayed on the computer monitor as well as in the HUD unit of the operating microscope (A). (From Ref. 7)

an age range between 2 and 78 years (Table 1). There were 272 glial tumors (which included 191 astrocytomas), 54 nonglial tumors, and 74 nonneoplastic mass lesions (Table 2). There were 252 patients with normal preoperative examinations, including 85 cases with single or multiple seizures as the presenting symptom. The other 248 cases presented with a neurological deficit. Postoperative neurological examinations revealed improvement in 225 cases, in comparison with preoperative examinations, whereas 238 cases were neurologically unchanged. Of these 238 cases that did not change, 25 had a deficit that did not change, whereas 213 started out as normal and stayed normal. Thirty-seven patients were neurologically worse postoperatively. Eleven of these had been neurologically normal preoperatively, whereas 26 were noted to have worsening of existing neurological deficits. Of these 26 patients, 13 had a deficit that was consistent with trauma related to the approach used. For example, one patient had postoperative worsening of a preoperatively noted gait ataxia after a transvermian approach to a deep-seated midline cerebellar thrombosed arteriovenous malformation. Another patient had dyspraxia of the right upper extremity following transsylvian removal of a metastatic lesion located under the left insular cortex. Nine other patients had contralateral superior quadrantopia, and two had homonymous hemianopia after posterior temporo-occipital approach to resect mesial temporal or ventral posterior thalamic lesions. The remaining 24 patients had neurological complications caused by perilesional trauma to surrounding functional parenchyma during gross total resection of deep lesions. This was most frequently noted following resection of lesions with an infiltrating component, such as high-grade (10 cases), grade 2 astrocytoma (5 cases), oligoastrocytoma (1 case), oligodendroglioma (1 case), lymphoma (1 case), as well as 1 case having a centrally located metastatic tumor and 1 case with a suprasylvian

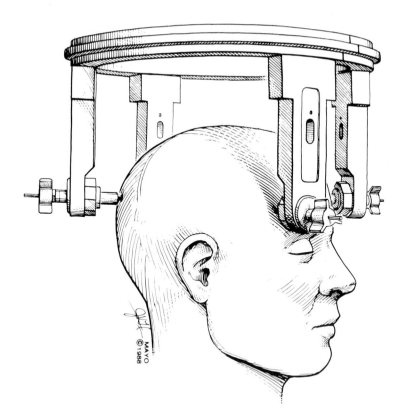

Figure 6 Inverted placement of the stereotactic headframe for posterior fossa procedures.

vascular malformation. However, 4 patients with thalamic pilocytic astrocytoma also had mild postoperative deficits related to trauma of the internal capsule in tumor removal.

Six patients died within 30 days following surgery. Causes of death included pulmonary embolism (2 cases), progressive edema following resection of a partially infiltrating thalamic astrocytoma in the brain stem (1 case), disseminated intravascular coagulation (DIC) (1 case), entrapment of temporal horn by rapid growth of a high-grade glioma for which the patient's family did not want any further intervention (1 case), and rapid preresection deterioration from mass effect in a high-grade glioma (1 case).

The overall morbidity was 7.4% and mortality 1.2%.

B. Results in Specific Histological Groups

The following is a summary of the preoperative, postoperative neurological status, and results in all patients who underwent stereotactic resection of lesions of various histological types.

1. Results in Glial Neoplasm Group

High-Grade Gliomas.   Complete removal of the portion of the tumor manifest as contrast enhancement in nearly all grade 3 (20 patients) and grade 4 (93 patients) astrocytomas was documented on postoperative scans. Thirteen patients with grade 4 astrocytomas had normal preoperative examination while 80 had a deficit. Postoperatively 46 improved, 9 were worse, and 38 remained the same. Four patients died within 30 days of surgery. The overall morbidity of resecting these grade 4 tumors was 10%, and the mortality was 3%.

Table 1 Locations of 500 Intra-Axial Brain Mass Lesions

Site	Right	Left	Total
Supratentorial			
Central	26	24	50
Basal ganglia	12	8	20
Thalamus	14	26	40
Third ventricle			29
Posterior/deep frontal	49	54	103
Parietal	41	46	87
Occipital	8	13	21
Temporal	27	25	52
Temporo-occipital	4	6	10
Temporoparietal	6	12	18
Parieto-occipital	5	4	9
Corpus callosum			2
Lateral ventricle	12	5	17
Total			458
Infratentorial			
Deep cerebellar hemisphere			20
Cerebral vermis			4
Pons			9
Midbrain			4
Medulla			5
Total			42

A retrospective comparison of survival times in patients with grade 4 astrocytomas who had undergone stereotactic resection and radiation therapy with a consecutive series of patients who underwent radiation therapy following biopsy alone is illustrated Figure 7. Mean survival following radiation was 42 weeks in the resection group and 22 weeks in the biopsy group. It should be noted that this is a retrospective series in which surgical selection bias cannot be completely excluded. Furthermore, this is a homogeneous group of patients with grade 4 astrocytomas (Daumas-Duport system) and not a series of "glioblastomas." This is an important point since the term *glioblastoma* in the usual three-tiered classification system frequently includes patients with lesions that would be considered grade 3 in a four-tiered numerical grading system (Kernohan, Daumas-Duport). Necrosis is the factor that separates *glioblastoma* from *anaplastic astrocytoma* in the three-tiered system, but can be found in grade 3 and grade 4 neoplasms in the four-tiered systems, which stratify by means of factors in addition to and including the presence or absence of necrosis. We have found that grade 3 lesions tend to be more infiltrative than grade 4, do not as frequently present a discrete contrast-enhancing mass lesion that can be resected and, because of this, biopsies, rather than resections are usually performed. However, grade 3 lesions have a much better prognosis than grade 4 lesions (Fig. 8).

Twenty patients had grade 3 astrocytomas. Nine of these had a normal preoperative examination; 11 had a preoperative deficit. Eight of these patients noted improvement of their preoperative neurological deficit, whereas 2 were worse postoperatively.

As stated in the previous paragraph, grade 3 tumors tend to be more infiltrative and do not

Table 2 Histological Findings in 500 Intra-axial Brain Mass Lesions

Histological type		Number of lesions
Glial Tumors		272
Astrocytoma	191	
Grade IV	93	
Grade III	20	
Grade II	19	
Grade I	6	
Pilocytic astrocytoma	53	
Oligodendroglioma	42	
Oligoastrocytoma	26	
Subependymoma	3	
Ependymoma	5	
Medulloblastoma	3	
Neurocytoma	2	
Nonglial tumors		154
Metastatic	91	
Meningioma	19	
Lymphoma	9	
Choroid plexus papilloma	1	
Ganglioglioma	8	
Colloid cyst	22	
Hemangioblastoma	3	
Teratoma	1	
Nonneoplastic Mass Lesions		74
Vascular lesions	43	
Abscess	3	
Cystocercosis	1	
Hematoma	3	
Tuberous sclerosis	8	
Glial scar (epilepsy)	7	
Radiation necrosis	7	
Arachnoid cyst	1	
Pleomorphic xanthoastrocytoma	1	
		500

usually present the significant contrast-enhancing mass lesion most frequently noted with grade 4 gliomas; therefore, a lower number of these patients undergo resection procedures in favor of stereotactic biopsy. Nevertheless, if we compare survival following stereotactic resection and radiation therapy with survival following biopsy alone and radiation, excluding in the latter group all patients with a primarily infiltrating lesion, survival is prolonged in grade 3 astrocytoma patients following resection of a mass lesion in comparison with those who undergo biopsy only.

Nineteen patients had grade 2 astrocytomas (11 normal examinations, and 8 had a deficit preoperative); postoperatively 5 of these improved neurologically and 5 were worse. The rest remained the same. Of the 6 grade 1 astrocytomas (all had normal examination preoperatively), seizures in 1 patient improved and 5 remained the same. In lower grade gliomas, mixed oligas-

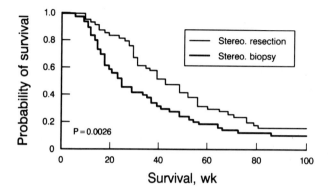

Figure 7 Comparison of survival in grade 4 astrocytoma patients undergoing stereotactic biopsy and stereotactic resection.

trocytomas and oligodendrogliomas the CT-defined hypodensity in nonessential brain areas was targeted and completely resected.

Pilocytic Astrocytomas. In the pilocytic astrocytoma group, comprising 53 cases (21 with normal preoperative examination and 32 with deficit), neurologic improvement was noted in 27 patients, but 4 were worse following surgery. One of these patients died 8 days postoperatively. Therefore, overall morbidity in the 53 pilocytic astrocytomas was 8%, and mortality was 2%. In general, pilocytic astrocytomas are histologically circumscribed and can be completely resected (Fig. 9). They should not be included with the usual "low-grade" astrocytomas of the fibrillary, gemistocytic, or protoplasmic type, as their prognosis is much better, in general, and following surgical resection, in particular.

2. Results in Nonglial Neoplasm Group

There were 154 nonglial tumors. These include 91 metastatic tumors. The metastatic tumors were completely resected as confirmed by postoperative CT scans. Of these, 36 patients had a normal preoperative examination, whereas 55 presented with a deficit. Postoperatively 38 patients showed neurological improvement, 48 remained the same, and 5 patients were worse.

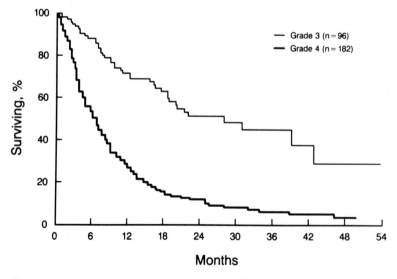

Figure 8 Kaplan–Meier survival curves in grades 3 and 4 astrocytomas.

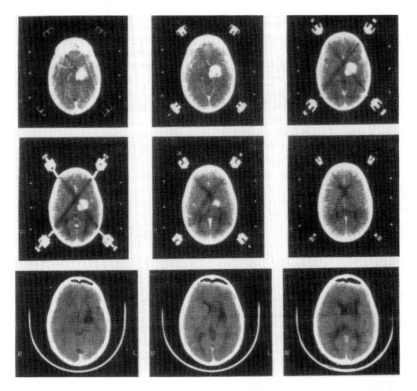

Figure 9 (Top) Preoperative CT scan in a 6-year-old boy with a left thalamic pilocytic astrocytoma. (Bottom) Postoperative CT scan showing complete resection.

Other nonglial neoplasms resected utilizing the CT- or MRI-based volumetric technique included 19 meningiomas (Fig. 10) (2 were worse after surgery and 1 of these died), 9 lymphomas (1 worse), 1 choroid plexus papilloma (none worse), 8 gangliogliomas (3 improved, none worse), 22 colloid cysts (Fig. 11) (none of these were neurologically worse postoperatively), 3 hemangioblastomas (2 improved neurologically, 1 same), and 1 teratoma (same). In general, this group of nonglial neoplasms, basically circumscribed tumors, were completely resected with good postoperative neurological results.

V. DISCUSSION

We believe that there are several broad advantages to the use of computer-assisted stereotactic resection of intra-axial brain lesions, which include (1) the surgeon maintains the ability to monitor the surgical field as is done with conventional surgery, but has the added advantage of monitoring the computer-generated image of the surgical field from CT and MRI; (2) continuous awareness and orientation throughout surgery of the position of the stereotactically directed surgical instruments relative to the imaging data base; thus providing (3) the confidence and security in the ability to perform a more complete resection of deep-seated and centrally located lesions than would be the case with conventional techniques; (4) minimal and least-invasive exposure of desired location of lesions (small linear incision, small cranial trephine directed exactly over the lesion,

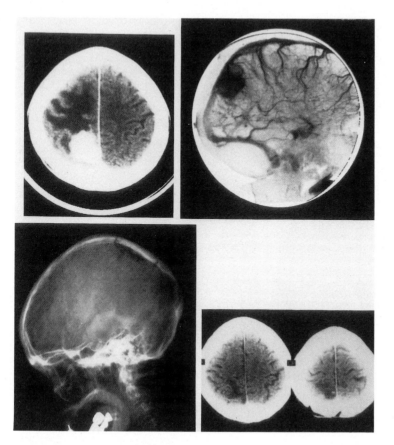

Figure 10 (Top) CT and angiogram of an anaplastic meningioma in a 72-year-old woman. (Bottom) Skull radiograph showing the stereotactic trephine and postoperative CT head scan showing complete resection of the tumor.

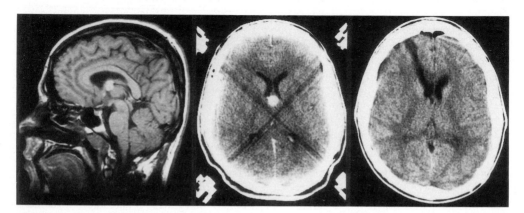

Figure 11 (Left) MRI and CT scans showing a colloid cyst in a 29-year-old man. (Right) Postoperative CT scan showing complete removal of the cyst.

and minimal or no exposure of surrounding brain tissue) and, therefore, minimal morbidity and a shorter hospital stay (8).

Identification of the plane between the lesion and the surrounding essential parenchyma is a major advantage of this technique by virtue of the computer display in cross sections of the digitized lesion volume. Although some surgeons believe that the plane should be identifiable with the usual magnification of the operating microscope, it is not infrequent that surgical trauma, bleeding, and edema can obscure the borders and make it very difficult to identify planes, thereby either resulting in a neurological deficit or in a less aggressive resection.

It has been our experience that the results of stereotactic resection of intra-axial lesions were more dependent on the histological type of the lesion, rather than their location.

Computer-assisted stereotactic resection, although employed for all intra-axial mass lesions, is more useful for histologically circumscribed types of lesions than for lesions with infiltrating and solid tumor tissue, such as fibrillary astrocytomas.

Examples of histologically circumscribed tumors include pilocytic astrocytomas and metastases. Pilocytic astrocytomas (unlike other low-grade gliomas) are very amenable to complete and safe resection because they consist of largely solid tumor tissue that displaces brain parenchyma. These lesions, the borders of which can be defined by contrast enhancement on CT scanning (9), can be resected, regardless of their location, with excellent postoperative results (10,11). Single metastatic lesions in patients with stable systemic disease are also excellent candidates for stereotactic resection whether superficial or deep. Stereotactic resection is accomplished with minimal morbidity and good palliative gross total resection of the lesion. Postoperatively CT scanning has confirmed total resection in all our patients with metastatic lesions, which is much higher than the 30% resection accomplished in one conventional series (12). Also the 0% mortality and 5% morbidity in this series of 91 metastatic tumors compares favorably with other reported conventional series with an 11% mortality rate (12,13).

Similarly, cavenous hemangiomas that are well circumscribed can be resected safely and completely from any location (14). In this series of 43 cases, there was no mortality and 12% morbidity, even though many of these lesions were located within essential brain tissue (thalamus, third ventricle).

An important distinction should be made between the aforementioned histological types and low-grade gliomas (other than pilocytic astrocytomas). Low-grade gliomas (grade 1 or 2 fibrillary astrocytomas, oligodendrogliomas, and mixed gliomas) consist of isolated tumor cells infiltrating intact brain parenchyma, with little true tumor tissue (15,16). Therefore, resection of these lesions (hypodensity on CT scan, signal prolongation on MRI) results in neurological deficits (10,17,18). Therefore, the resection of these lesions (except in nonessential brain tissue) is inadvisable.

High-grade gliomas (grade 4), although not curable, can be helped with stereotactic resection. The rate of complications from the resection of the CT-contrasting part of these tumors in essential brain tissue has been acceptable (19). Serial stereotactic biopsies from high-grade gliomas through CT hypodense and MRI T2-prolonged signal areas peripheral to areas of CT contrast enhancement have revealed isolated tumor cells within edematous brain parenchyma (15,16,20–24). After the resection of the CT-contrasting region of the tumor, patients eventually will show tumor "recurrence" within several months. In our current series, consisting of 93 cases of grade 4 fibrillary astrocytomas, there was a 4% mortality and a 10% morbidity. Although the mean postoperative survival in our series (resection plus radiation and occasionally chemotherapy) is only slightly better than the mean survival times of older series (37 weeks; 20, 25–27), it is difficult to make direct comparisons. This is because, in most series, glioblastomas (i.e., grade 3 and grade 4) are grouped together and, second, unlike previous series (20,26), our cases tend to be located in central or deep-seated locations, with more polar lesions being treated with conventional lobectomies and, therefore, more complete resections. Nonstereotactic resection of these deep lesions has been associated with higher complications (26). Thus, stereotactic resection of the CT-enhancing portion of high-grade gliomas in deep and central locations permits a more aggressive palliative resection, with reduction of tumor burden and preservation of neurological function. Other studies have suggested that postoperative survival and prognosis were directly related to the completeness of the surgical removal (22).

Computer-assisted stereotactic resection of intraventricular lesions can be done with more direct and smaller approaches through nonepileptogenic, nonessential cortex and fiber tracts. The brain and ventricular incisions need only be large enough to introduce and manipulate a cylindrical retractor that measures 2 cm (through a 3.8-cm cranial trephine), even for large intraventricular lesions. This is also true for third ventricular lesions such as colloid cysts (28).

Serial stereotactic biopsy techniques have allowed safe and accurate diagnosis of lesions before resection as well as added insight into the behavior of glial neoplasms (15,16,29). Stereotactic surgical techniques have evolved from limited functional procedures to more elaborate definitive resection techniques that should become more widely used in the future (8).

There are clear and distinct advantages to the use of CT stereotactic techniques in the treatment of brain tumors. With this technology, the surgeon is able to take a biopsy of the lesion or perform a more direct, confident, and complete resection of tumors in areas that are relatively inaccessible to conventional nonstereotactic craniotomy. There are also advantages for the patient: minimal invasive cranial exposure, less morbidity, a shorter hospital stay, a more complete neurological palliation and, in some cases, cure.

ACKNOWLEDGMENTS

The authors gratefully acknowledge the help of Cathy Hunt, R.N. for her diligent and tireless help, and the expert secretarial assistance of Mary Hanenberger.

REFERENCES

1. Ditmar C. Uber die Lage des sogenannten Gefafszentrums in der Medulla oblongata. Ber Saechs Ges Wiss Leipzig (Math Phys) 1873; 25:449–469.
2. Zernov DN. L'encephalometre. Proc Gen Clin Ther 1890; 19:302.
3. Clarke RH, Horsley V. On a method of investigating the deep ganglia and tracts of the central nervous system (cerebellum). Br Med J 19806; 2:1799–1800.
4. Horsely V, Clarke RH. The stucture and function of the cerebellum examined by a new method. Brain 1908; 31:45–124.
5. Clarke RH. Investigations of the central nervous system. Methods and instruments. Johns Hopkins Hosp Rep 1920; special volume:1–162.
6. Spiegel EA, Wycis HT, Marks M, Lee A. Stereotactic apparatus for operations on the human brain. Science 1947; 106:349–350.
7. Kelly PJ. Volumetric stereotactic surgical resection of intra-axial brain mass lesions. Mayo Clin Proc 1988; 63:1186–1198.
8. Kelly PJ. Tumor stereotaxis. Philadelphia: WB Saunders, 1991.
9. Daumas-Duport C, Monsaingeon V, Szenthe L, Szikla G. Serial stereotactic biopsies: a double histological code of gliomas accroding to malignancy and 3-D configuration, as an aid to therapeutic decision and assessment of results. Appl Neurophysiol 1982; 45:431–437.
10. Kelly PJ, Kall BA, Goerss S, Earnest F IV. Computer-assisted stereotaxic laser resection of intra-axial brain neoplasms. J Neurosurg 1986; 64:427–439.
11. McGirr SJ, Kelly PJ, Scheithauer BW. Stereotactic resection of juvenile pilocytic astrocytomas of the thalamus and basal ganglia. Neurosurgery 1987; 20:447–452.
12. Haar F, Patterson RH Jr. Surgery for metatastic intracranial neoplasm. Cancer 1982; 30:1241–1245.

13. MacGee EE. Surgical treatment of cerebral metastases from lung cancer: the effect on quality and duration of survival. J Neurosurg 1971; 35:416–420.
14. Davis DH, Kelly PJ. Stereotactic resection of occult vascular malformations. J Neurosurg 1990; 72:698–702.
15. Kelly PJ, Daumas-Duport C, Kispert DB, Kall BA, Scheithauer BW, Illig JJ. Imaging-based stereotaxic serial biopsies in untreated intracranial glial neoplasms. J Neurosurg 1987; 66:865–874.
16. Kelly PJ, Daumas-Duport C, Scheithauer BW, Kall BA, Kispert DB. Stereotactic histologic correlations of computed tomography- and magnetic resonance imaging-defined abnormalities in patients with glial neoplasms. Mayo Clin Proc 1987; 62:450–459.
17. Kelly PJ. Computer-assisted stereotaxis: new approaches for the management of intracranial intra-axial tumors. Neurology 1986; 36:535–541.
18. Kelly PJ, Kall BA, Goerss S. Computer-assisted stereotactic resection of posterior fossa lesions. Surg Neurol 1986; 25:530–534.
19. Kelly PJ, Kall BA, Goerss SJ, Earnest F. Computer-assisted stereotactic resection of intra-axial brain neoplasms. J Neurosurg 1986; 64:427–439.
20. Jelsma R, Bucy PC. The treatment of glioblastoma multiforme of the brain. J Neurosurg 1967; 27:388–400.
21. Green SB, Byar DP, Walker MD, Pistenmaa DA, Alexander E Jr, Batzdorf U, Brooks WH, Hunt WE, Mealey J Jr, Odom GL, Paoletti P, Ransonoff J II, Robertson JT, Selker RG, Shapiro WR, Smith KR Jr, Wilson CB, Strike TA. Comparisons of carmustine, procarbazine, and high-dose methylprednisolone as additions to surgery and radiotherapy for the treatment of malignant glioma. Cancer Treat Rep 1983; 67:121–132.
22. Wood JR, Green SB, Shapiro WR. The prognostic importance of tumor size in malignant gliomas: a computed tomographic scan study by the Brain Tumor Cooperative Group. J Clin Oncol 1988; 6:338–343.
23. Burger PC. Pathologic anatomy and CT correlations in the glioblastoma multiforme. Appl Neurophysiol 1983; 46:180–187.
24. Burger PC, Dubois PJ, Schold SC Jr, Smith KR Jr, Odom GL, Crafts DC, Giangaspero F. Computerized tomographic and pathologic studies of the untreated, quiescent, and recurrent glioblastoma multiforme. J Neurosurg 1983; 58:159–169.
25. Frankel SA, German WJ. Glioblastoma multiforme: review of 219 cases with regard to natural history, pathology, diagnostic methods, and treatment. J Neurosurg 1958; 15:489–503.
26. Gehan EA, Walker MD. Prognostic factors for patients with brain tumors. Natl Cancer Inst Monogr 1977; 46:189–195.
27. Hitchcock E, Sato F. Treatment of malignant gliomata. J Neurosurg 1964; 21:498–505.
28. Abernathey CD, Davis DH, Kelly PJ. Treatment of colloid cysts of the third ventricle by stereotactic microsurgical laser craniotomy. J Neurosurg 1989; 70:525–529.
29. Daumas-Duport C, Scheithauer BW, Kelly PJ. A histologic and cytologic method for the spatial definition of gliomas. Mayo Clin Proc 1987; 62:435–449.

17

Primary Central Nervous System Lymphoma

James Baumgartner and Brian T. Andrews
School of Medicine, University of California,
San Francisco, California

Mark L. Rosenblum
Henry Ford Health Sciences Center, Detroit, Michigan

I. INTRODUCTION

Primary central nervous system lymphomas (PCNSLs) are non-Hodgkin's lymphomas that are mostly of B-cell origin. Previously a rare disease, accounting for 1–1.5% of all primary brain tumors, PCNSL has increased rapidly in incidence over the past 15 years. Although the increase has been greatest in patients with the acquired immunodeficiency syndrome (AIDS) (1), it has been substantial in patients without AIDS as well (2). Left untreated, PCNSLs are rapidly fatal. They are extremely sensitive to radiation, but tend to recur after treatment; the median duration of survival is 13 months, and the 5-year survival rate is less than 5% (3). Recent experience with neoadjuvant chemotherapy followed by radiation therapy for tumor recurrence has been more encouraging, with median survival up to 44.5 months (4–9). This chapter reviews the history, presentation, diagnosis, and treatment of PCNSLs and discusses the findings of immunohistochemical and molecular studies, which have shown an association between these tumors and Epstein–Barr virus (EBV) (2,10–16).

II. HISTORY

The tumors now classified as PCNSL were first described by Bailey (17), who called them *perithelial sarcomas* because of the perivascular location of tumor cells. He noted that in one case (reviewed by F. B. Mallory), the tumor resembled a "lymphosarcoma or malignant lymphoma." In 1938, Yuile (18) also noted the resemblance to tumors of lymph node origin, then called reticulum-cell sarcomas (RCS). Yuile used this term to describe his case, but postulated that, in the brain, these tumors arose from nonlymphocytic microglial cells. One group of pathologists, including Russel and associates (19), preferred to call PCNSL "microgliomatosis" because silver carbonate stain, which they felt was specific for microglial cells, was not well taken up by extracranial RCS (20). Some used the term *RCS* (21–23), whereas still others, including Rubinstein (24), used the terms interchangeably or together (RCS–microglioma) (25–27). This controversy occupied pathologists for nearly 50 years until it became clear that these tumors were indeed lymphomas (28–30).

The International Working Formulation sponsored by the National Cancer Institute (31) classifies PCNSLs with other non-Hodgkin's lymphomas. Scattered cases of primary intracranial T-cell lymphomas have been reported (32–35), but most PCNSLs are small or large B-cell non-Hodgkin's lymphomas (2,5,6,36–45).

III. DEMOGRAPHICS AND PREDISPOSING FACTORS

The incidence of PCNSL is now at least 1:1 million persons in the general population, 1:1000 among transplant recipients, and 1:50 among patients with AIDS. Recent studies suggest that the incidence of this tumor is increasing.

A. Non-Acquired Immunodeficiency Syndrome Primary Central Nervous System Lymphoma

Hochberg and Miller, in their excellent review of non-AIDS PCNSL, report a slow, but steady, increase in this diagnosis since 1960 (2). At the Massachusetts General Hospital, PCNSL accounted for 0.6% of brain tumor admissions before 1975 and 2.3% since. Modeling, using the National Cancer Institute's Surveillance, Epidemiology and End Results Program, suggests that non-AIDS PCNSL increased threefold during the period 1973–1984. The average age at diagnosis is 55 years, with a male preponderance of 1.4–1.7:1. Women tend to be slightly older than men at diagnosis (45).

The risk of developing PCNSL is approximately 1:1000 among renal transplant recipients and may be slightly higher among cardiac transplant patients (46–48). The risk increases with the duration and severity of immunosuppression (48–51). The median time from transplantation to tumor development is 9 months, and the median age at presentation is 37 years (50,52).

Several congenital immunodeficiency syndromes are associated with an increased incidence of PCNSL, including the Wiskott–Aldrich syndrome (53–56), severe combined immunodeficiency (57), immunoglobulin (Ig)A deficiency and elevated IgE with defective chemotaxis (58). These syndromes predispose patients to infection and abnormal immunoglobulin production. T-cell function may also be abnormal, although it is usually normal in IgA deficiency (59). Primary CNS lymphoma accounted for 18% of the 78 cases of cancer reported to the Immunodeficiency Cancer Registry in patients with the Wiskott–Aldrich syndrome (57). Among children with these syndromes, the median age at presentation with PCNSL is 10 years (57,60).

Primary CNS lymphoma has also been associated with a number of diseases that alter immune function or the treatment of which causes immunosuppression. These include systemic lupus erythematosus (61), idiopathic thrombocytopenic purpura (30), Sjögren's syndrome (62), sarcoidosis (63), progressive multifocal leukoencephalopathy (PML) (64), multiple sclerosis (65), and glioblastoma multiforme (66).

B. Acquired Immunodeficiency Syndrome-Associated Primary Central Nervous System Lymphoma

In early studies, the reported incidence of AIDS-associated PCNSL was 2.5% (67). In nearly one-fourth (0.6%) of these patients, PCNSL was the first manifestation of AIDS (67); however, subsequent studies have suggested that such patients constitute only 6–16% of AIDS-related

PCNSL (36,68). The AIDS-associated PCNSL tends to occur late in the course of the human immunodeficiency virus (HIV) infection, when CD4-positive cell counts are very low, frequently fewer than 34/dl (43,69). The overwhelming majority of patients are men and the average age at presentation is 35 years (36,68). Independent modeling using the University of California, San Francisco (UCSF) AIDS data base and a predictive model developed by the Centers for Disease Control (CDC) both estimated that approximately 1848 cases of AIDS-associated PCNSL occurred in 1991 (36,67). Thus, the annual incidence of AIDS-related PCNSL now approaches that of meningioma (22,50).

IV. PRESENTATION

Hochberg and Miller describe four distributions of lesions in patients with PCNSL (2): solitary or multiple discrete intracranial nodules (30–50% of cases); diffuse meningeal or periventricular lesions (10–25%); uveal or vitreous deposits (10–20%); and localized intradural spinal masses (very rare). The pattern of CNS involvement determines the presenting symptoms (2).

A. Non-Acquired Immunodeficiency Syndrome Primary Central Nervous System Lymphoma

Most PCNSLs are solitary or multiple discrete intracranial masses. Roughly 67% of lesions are supratentorial, 33% are infratentorial; 30–45% are multifocal, and 18% involve both supra- and infratentorial spaces (2,45). Helle and colleagues found a lower incidence of multifocal lesions, ranging from 0 to 33%, in series reported before 1980 (45); this may reflect the less reliable neuroimaging techniques used in earlier years. Symptoms associated with discrete intracranial nodules include headache, seizures, motor and sensory deficits, cerebellar deficits, visual field deficits, and changes in personality and memory.

Diffuse meningeal or periventricular involvement was found in 24% of Hochberg's cases and in 23% of Helle's, but in only 13% of Jiddane's (2,68,70). Some of these cases may be metastatic disease from occult peripheral lymphoma. Symptoms associated with meningeal involvement include meningismus, abducens palsy, and cervical or thoracic radiculopathy. Periventricular lesions, including those in the thalamus or corpus callosum, cause personality changes, depression, memory loss, and psychosis.

Uveal or vitreous deposits of lymphoma can cause cloudly or blurred vision and altered visual acuity (71–73). Uveal or vitreal involvement usually precedes CNS involvement by 7 months, but can occur after PCNSL has been documented (2). The age at presentation and the male/female ratio are the same as in other patients with non-AIDS PCNSL (71).

Localized intramedullary intradural spinal masses, usually in the thoracic or lower cervical region, occur in fewer than 1% of patients with non-AIDS PCNSL (74). The initial symptoms are asymmetric leg weakness, followed shortly by a complete sensory level; cerebral spinal fluid (CSF) pleocytosis is not seen (75–77). The presenting signs and symptoms in two large series of non-AIDS PCNSL are listed in Table 1.

B. Acquired Immunodeficiency Syndrome-Associated Primary Central Nervous System Lymphoma

The general distribution of lesions in AIDS-associated PCNSL is similar to that in non-AIDS PCNSL. Multifocal discrete intracranial nodules were found at presentation in 67% of patients in our series (36) and in 59% of patients in the series of Goldstein et al. (68). This finding is

Table 1 Presenting Signs and Symptoms of Non-AIDS PCNSL

Symptoms/signs	Hochberg and Miller (n = 66) (%)	Helle et al. (n = 22) (%)
Personality/memory change	24	36
Cerebellar signs	21	14
Headache/meningismus	15	28
Seizures	13	9
Motor dysfunction	11	28
Visual changes	8	18
Cranial nerve deficits		4

Source: Refs. 2 and 45.

confounded by the possibility, in AIDS patients, of coexisting multiple intracranial diseases, either separately or in the same mass lesion (36). The AIDS-associated PCNSLs cause a mass effect and tend to be deep-seated. The exact percentage of periventricular lesions is not readily discernible from published reports. Meningeal involvement is distinctly unusual at presentation and is usually found only in dura overlying intracerebral lymphomas located near the subarachnoid space (36). In our experience, symptomatic meningeal lymphoma in AIDS patients is almost always metastatic from a systemic lymphoma. Uveal and vitreal deposits of lymphoma have not been reported in large series of AIDS-associated PCNSL. Only one case of intramedullary spinal cord lymphoma has been described in a patient with AIDS. This lesion grew just below the inferior extent of the radiation field after successful treatment of an intracranial PCNSL with whole-brain radiation therapy (36). The presenting signs and symptoms in two recent series of AIDS-associated PCNSL are listed in Table 2.

V.   RADIOGRAPHIC FINDINGS

The radiographic findings of PCNSL are suggestive rather than diagnostic. Tissue diagnosis is required before therapy can be started.

A.   Non-Acquired Immunodeficiency Syndrome Primary Central Nervous System Lymphoma

On noncontrast computed tomography (CT) scans, non-AIDS PCNSLs are hyper- or isodense, compared with normal brain, and cause edema and mass effect. The lesions are generally

Table 2 Presenting Signs and Symptoms of AIDS-Associated PCNSL

Symptoms/signs	Baumgartner et al. (n = 55) (%)	Goldstein et al. (n = 17) (%)
Headache/lethargy	53	65
Hemiparesis/hemisensory loss	31	71
Cranial nerve deficits	18	18
Seizures	20	41

Source: Refs. 36 and 68.

deep-seated and are more frequently unifocal than multifocal. After administration of contrast material, dense enhancement is typical, although ring enhancement may be seen (78). Subependymal growth and a butterfly pattern of growth across the corpus callosum are strongly suggestive of PCNSL (Fig. 1).

Magnetic resonance imaging (MRI) shows non-AIDS PCNSLs as slightly hypointense lesions (relative to gray matter) on T1-weighted images and as slightly hyperintense on T2-weighted images (79). There is usually dense contrast enhancement after administration of gadolinium dimeglumine (Gd-DTPA) (79). The lesions tend to be solitary and larger than 2 cm in diameter (79). On angiograms, PCNSLs appear as a homogeneous vascular stain, with a meningiomalike pattern in the late arterial or early venous phase (80) or as an avascular intra-axial mass (70).

B. Acquired Immunodeficiency Syndrome-Associated Primary Central Nervous System Lymphoma

The differential diagnosis of CNS space-occupying lesions in AIDS patients includes toxoplasmosis (50–70%), PCNSL (20–30%), PML (10–20%), and several less frequent diseases. Multiple diseases may be found in different lesions or in a single lesion (36). In addition, the signal characteristics of CNS lesions in AIDS patients may be different from those in patients without AIDS. Several of these characteristics are suggestive of AIDS-associated PCNSL. On CT scans, AIDS-associated PCNSLs are typically hypodense and surrounded by mild to moderate edema.

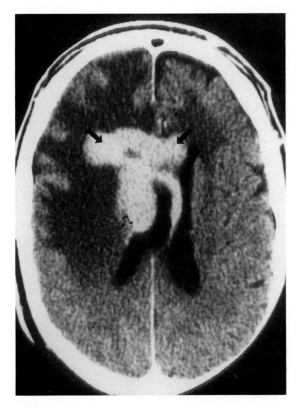

Figure 1 Axial, contrast-enhanced CT brain scan showing subependymal (open arrow) and "butterfly" (solid arrows) growth typical of PCNSL. Note the surrounding edema.

The lesions exert less mass effect than would be anticipated for the size of the enhancing lesion, suggesting an infiltrative process. Contrast-enhanced CT scans usually show ring enhancement and an irregular contour. T2-weighted MR images often show areas of central hyperintensity surrounded by areas of hypointensity, forming a ring or target. The lesions tend to be smaller than 2 cm in diameter at presentation (79) (Fig. 2). The number of lesions detected by MRI may also suggest the diagnosis. In a series of 275 patients with AIDS, Ciricillo and Rosenblum found that 57% of patients with solitary lesions on MRI had lymphoma, 35% had toxoplasmosis, and 8% had PML (81,82).

VI. DIAGNOSTIC STUDIES
A. Lumbar Puncture

In cases of meningeal or periventricular PCNSL, cells can enter the CSF. Rarely, these have been identified as "malignant" non-Hodgkin's cells (2,68,70,83,84). The sensitivity of CSF cytological analysis can be increased by staining centrifuged cells for cell surface markers. The identification of monoclonal B-cell populations in CSF is sufficient to diagnose lymphoma (2,68,74,85, 86).

B. Surgery

Surgical biopsy is usually necessary to establish the diagnosis of PCNSL. This can be accomplished by an open craniotomy to expose the tumor, or by CT-guided or ultrasound-guided stereotactic biopsy.

1. Open Craniotomy

The PCNSLs can be approached directly; subtotal or total resection is possible, especially if the lesion is superficial. Resection of deep-seated PCNSLs is associated with significant perioperative morbidity, primarily caused by postoperative edema, which can be difficult to control (87). In AIDS-associated PCNSL, the diagnostic accuracy of open resection techniques was 87% (36). However, resection provides no significant increase in survival or response to therapy compared with biopsy only (37,78,88). Therefore, it is difficult to justify the higher morbidity of open craniotomy over stereotactic biopsy in the treatment of PCNSL.

2. Computed Tomography-Guided Stereotactic Biopsy

A CT-guided stereotactic biopsy is an effective method for diagnosing PCNSL in patients with and without AIDS (5,36,37,68,88–91). It can be performed under local anesthesia, with minimal morbidity, and the diagnostic accuracy is greater than 84%. The diagnostic accuracy can be increased by selecting target points at the edges of mass lesions, since tissue from central areas is often necrotic and nondiagnostic. The CT-guided stereotactic biopsy is particularly well suited for deep-seated lesions and is the method we prefer for obtaining diagnostic material in cases of suspected PCNSL.

3. Ultrasound-Guided Stereotactic Biopsy

Ultrasound-guided stereotaxy can be used in patients who are unwilling or unable to cooperate with the CT-guided stereotactic procedure, such as mildly demented AIDS patients who cannot tolerate the stereotactic head frame. The procedure allows real-time imaging of the biopsy, but requires general anesthesia and a craniotomy large enough to accommodate an ultrasound probe (5 cm in diameter). In our series, the diagnostic accuracy was 100%; there was no perioperative morbidity, and patients could usually be discharged in less than 48 h (36).

VII. PATHOLOGY

Pathological analysis of PCNSLs from patients with and without AIDS usually shows high-grade, non-Hodgkin's B-cell lymphoma (Table 3). In general, the histological grade is higher in AIDS-associated PCNSLs. In non-AIDS patients, it has been suggested that the histological type is prognostic of the outcome with treatment: small-cell, cleaved tumors have the longest survival (36.5 months) and slowest progression of disease, and large-cell, immunoblastic tumors have the worst prognosis (11.25 months) (2,92). No correlation between histological type and outcome has been demonstrated in AIDS patients (36).

VIII. TREATMENT

A. Natural History

Survival data from patients who undergo no treatment other than diagnostic procedures suggest the natural history of PCNSL. The average duration of survival after presentation was 4.6 months in patients without AIDS treated surgically (3) and only 6 weeks in patients with AIDS who had a biopsy (36). In both groups, radiologic and postmortem studies demonstrated rapid tumor enlargement that correlated with the neurological decline. In some patients without AIDS and most of those with AIDS, multiple intracranial foci of tumor developed. Patients receiving surgical treatment alone almost always died from tumor progression (3,36).

B. Corticosteroids

Corticosteroid treatment can cause a partial or complete regression of the CT abnormalities in patients with non-AIDS PCNSL (2,93). Hochberg et al. found this phenomenon in 37% of 48 patients treated with dexamethasone following in doses of 24 mg/day for 10 days (2). Even preoperative treatment overnight with dexamethasone can decrease the enhancement seen on CT scans and make accurate stereotactic biopsy difficult. This phenomenon, thought to represent both a decrease in enhancement owing to an alteration in the leakiness of vessels and a toxic effect of glucocorticoids on lymphoma cells, is usually transient, typically lasting months (94–97). With recurrent lesions, it has been seen serially as many as five times (Gutin PH, personal communication). In patients already receiving glucocorticoids, recurrent lesions may show decreased enhancement when the dose is increased (2).

In AIDS-associated PCNSL, a similar effect from glucocorticoids has been noted. In our series, treatment with glucocorticoids did not increase survival (36).

C. Surgery and Whole-Brain Radiation Therapy

Early experience showed increased survival after radiation therapy for non-AIDS PCNSL. Henry et al. reported a median survival of 4.6 months after surgical excision and 15.2 months after postoperative radiation (3). Although the initial response to radiation therapy was good, the relatively short survival time was discouraging. Tumor recurrence or progression was most common at the original site.

In patients with AIDS-associated PCNSL, whole-brain radiation therapy also causes tumor regression (Fig. 3) and increases survival, although only slightly. With whole-brain radiation (3000–5000 cGy), the duration of survival is 2.5–4.3 months after presentation (36,68,69). The use of a radiation boost to the tumor bed is controversial. Remick et al. reported an average survival time of 4.2 months after presentation in six patients treated with whole-brain radiation therapy (3000–4000 cGy) and a boost to the tumor bed (1000–1800 cGy) (43); three additional

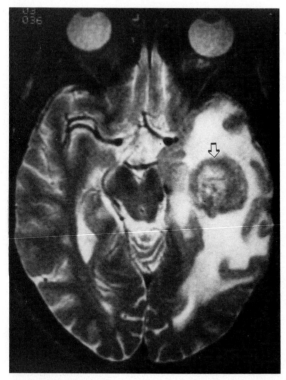

2

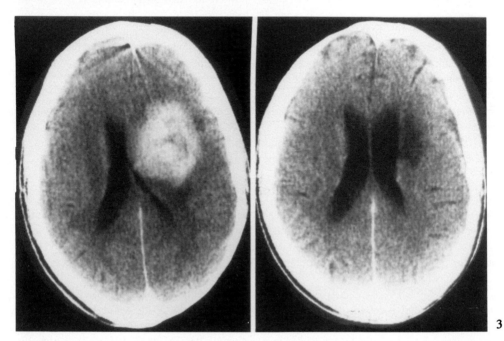

3

Figure 2 Axial T2-weighted MR image of brain showing the target lesion (arrow) typical of AIDS-associated PCNSL. Note the surrounding edema.

Figure 3 Axial, contrast-enhanced CT brain scans, obtained before (left) and 1 month after (right) whole-brain radiation therapy, showing a complete response to treatment.

Table 3 Pathologic Findings in Two Series of PCNSL

Type of lymphoma	AIDS ($n = 55$)[a] (%)	Non-AIDS ($n = 61$)[b] (%)
Small-cell, cleaved		18.0
Small-cell, noncleaved	33	8.2
Large-cell, cleaved		9.8
Large-cell, noncleaved	12	14.9
Large-cell, immunoblastic	31	39.3
Lymphoma, not otherwise classified	18	9.8
Lymphoma and toxoplasmosis	4	
Lymphoma and *Mycobacterium avium-intracellulare*	2	

[a]Ref. 36.
[b]Ref. 2.

patients treated with whole-brain radiation therapy, without a boost, survived an average of 8.3 months. The data of Goldstein et al. suggest that a boost to the tumor bed after whole-brain radiation therapy increased survival from 72 to 167 days (68). In all reported series, the patients usually died of AIDS-related opportunistic infections, rather than tumor progression. Better control of these infections should increase the duration of survival.

D. Surgery, Whole-Brain Radiation Therapy, and Adjuvant Chemotherapy

Several investigators have suggested that adjuvant chemotherapy after whole-brain irradiation increases the response to therapy and the duration of both overall and disease-free survival in patients with non-AIDS PCNSL (6,38,41,88,98). Chamberlain and Levin reported an increase in median survival from 13 to 30 months when adjuvant chemotherapy (procarbazine, lomustine, and vincristine) was added to surgery and radiation therapy (with hydroxyurea as radiation sensitizer) (6). In the series of Pollack et al., 5-year survival increased from 27–78% when patients received some form of chemotherapy in addition to radiation therapy (88). Shibamoto et al. reported average survivals of 35.8 months in ten patients who received chemotherapy (vincristine, doxorubicin, cyclophosphamide, and prednisolone) after surgery and radiation therapy (30–40 Gy to the whole brain and a local boost up to 60 Gy) and 11.8 months in 16 patients who had surgery and radiation therapy only; eight of the ten patients treated with chemotherapy were alive at the time of the report (98). DeAngelis et al. used a regimen of systemic methotrexate therapy, with or without intrathecal methotrexate, followed by 4000 cGy of whole-brain radiaton therapy with a 1440 cGy boost and two courses of high-dose cytarabine (cytosine arabinoside) (7). The response rate to methotrexate before radiation therapy was 63%, and the survival rate was 75% at a median follow-up of 25.4 months.

Postirradiation chemotherapy may also improve survival in AIDS patients wth PCNSL, particularly those with less depressed CD4 cell counts. In our series, the three longest survivors (122, 245, and 380+ days) received high-dose methotrexate in addition to whole-brain radiation therapy (36). Hochberg et al. also reported improved response and survival in AIDS-associated PCNSL treated with methotrexate after radiation therapy, and the treatment was surprisingly well tolerated (5). Since AIDS patients with PCNSL usually die from opportunistic infections, the apparent beneficial effect of methotrexate is difficult to explain.

E. Surgery and Neoadjuvant Chemotherapy Followed by Whole-Brain Radiation Therapy

Treatment with high-dose methotrexate and leucovorin rescue has long been known to be useful in treating PCNSLs that fail to respond to radiation therapy (99–101). Unfortunately, methotrexate administration after whole-brain radiation therapy has been associated with an encephalopathy characterized by dementia and myoclonic jerks as well as by leukoencephalopathy and calcification of small intracranial arterioles that can be seen on MRI (102). Methotrexate administration before CNS radiation rarely causes encephalopathy and is thought by some to protect against late-occurring radiation toxicity (5). Primary treatment of PCNSL with chemotherapeutic regimens that include methotrexate has yielded encouraging results. Cohen et al. reported a complete tumor response, improved clinical status, and more than 3-year survival in a child treated with vincristine, carmustine, methotrexate, and dexamethasone (9). Gabbai et al. treated 22 patients with three courses of methotrexate (3.5 g/m² for 1–3 weeks) before radiation therapy (8). Twenty-one patients responded completely or partially before radiation therapy, and the median Karnofsky performance score increased from 50 before treatment to 90 immediately before radiation therapy. The median survival was more than 27 months. Vitreous and retinal disease did not respond to chemotherapy and required radiation to the orbits. Neuwelt et al. (4) used a regimen in which cyclophosphamide was given intravenously, the blood–brain barrier was transiently opened with mannitol, and methotrexate was infused under general anesthesia; the patients also received oral procarbazine and intravenous vincristine. The median survival was 44.5 months when this regimen was used as the sole therapy and 17.8 months when it was used after whole-brain radiation therapy. Detailed neuropsychological evaluation of patients who had a complete response and survived at least 1 year after treatment showed only mild deterioration in short-term memory and good preservation of global neuropsychological function (103).

IX. PROGNOSTIC FACTORS

A. Non-Acquired Immunodeficiency Syndrome Primary Central Nervous System Lymphoma

The histopathological diagnosis is strongly predictive of survival among non-AIDS patients with PCNSL. Small-cell cleaved and noncleaved tumors appear to have the best prognosis (median survival with treatment, 36.5 and 35.0 months, respectively), and large-cell immunoblastic tumors have the worst prognosis (median survival with treatment, 11.25 months) (2). Neither Hochberg and Miller (2) nor Bogdhan et al. (92) found age to be a determinant of survival time, although patients younger than 50 years of age without a history of immunosuppression appeared to fare better than older patients. From multivariant analysis, Pollack et al. found that age younger than 60 years at presentation, preoperative Karnofsky performance score greater than 70, and strictly hemispheric tumor location all were associated with longer survival (88).

B. Acquired Immunodeficiency Syndrome-Associated Primary Central Nervous System Lymphoma

The histopathological diagnosis has not been shown to correlate with the duration of survival in AIDS patients with PCNSL. A Karnofsky performance score greater than 70 at presentation has been associated with a better response to therapy and longer survival (68). Several authors suggest that patients with PCNSL as the first manifestation of AIDS survive longer than those previously diagnosed with AIDS (68,69). The effect of hemispheric versus diffuse tumor on survival has not been adequately examined.

X. TREATMENT RECOMMENDATIONS

A. Non-Acquired Immunodeficiency Syndrome Primary Central Nervous System Lymphoma

At UCSF, the regimen used to treat non-AIDS PCNSL consists of neoadjuvant chemotherapy, followed by radiation therapy. Postbiopsy patients are staged by slit-lamp examination, MRI of the neuraxis with and without gadolinium, lumbar puncture with cytological examination of CSF, HIV testing, and, when systemic disease is suspected, bone marrow biopsy and CT of the chest and abdomen. After initial staging, chemotherapy consisting of high-dose methotrexate (3.5 g/m^2) and three cycles of CHOD [cyclophosphamide 750 mg/m^2, doxorubicin (Adriamycin) 50 mg/m^2, and vincristine 1.4 mg/m^2 on day 1, and dexamethasone 6 mg/m^2 on days 1–5] is given. After the second cycle of CHOD, patients are restaged; if no progression of disease is found, a third cycle is started. After the third cycle of CHOD or if staging is positive after the second cycle, patients receive whole-brain radiation therapy in split fractions to a total dose of 4140 cGy. Thereafter, patients are followed with serial brain MRI, with and without gadolinium.

B. Acquired Immunodeficiency Syndrome-Associated Primary Central Nervous System Lymphoma

In AIDS patients, the decision to proceed with biopsy for suspected PCNSL is complicated by the differential diagnosis of mass lesions in this population. Approximately 50% of space-occupying lesions are toxoplasmosis, 25% are PCNSL, and 10% are PML; a mass lesion is most likely to be a toxoplasma abscess or PCNSL. The initial treatment is based on the assumption that most mass lesions are toxoplasmosis. Once a mass lesion has been diagnosed, blood is drawn for anti-toxoplasma titers, and an empirical trial of pyrimethamine and sulfadiazine is begun. Corticosteroids can be administered if there is life-threatening cerebral edema, since steroids themselves can decrease the CT contrast enhancement and reduce the mass effect produced by PCNSLs. Therefore, if the mass begins to resolve after institution of combined therapy, the steroids should be gradually withdrawn.

Persistence of the beneficial effect of treatment confirms that the mass lesion was toxoplasmosis. If antitoxoplasma titers are negative or if the patient deteriorates, stereotactic biopsy is performed urgently unless the patient is severely debilitated from systemic AIDS-related illnesses. If the titers are positive, the antitoxoplasma therapy continues, and CT scans or MR images are obtained weekly. A biopsy is performed if any lesion enlarges or if the patient declines clinically. The most accessible lesion in the least eloquent brain region is selected for biopsy; although multiple lesions can be biopsied during a single procedure, we have usually sampled only one location. If the biopsy is positive, treatment consisting of whole-brain radiation therapy (4000 cGy) and corticosteroids is started. When multiple lesions are present, most respond to this therapy. If any mass enlarges during radiation therapy, it is probably not PCNSL, and another biopsy should be considered. Clinical deterioration after radiation therapy is generally due to AIDS-related opportunistic infections. Treatment is based on the location and type of infection identified.

XI. BASIC SCIENCE

Epstein-Barr virus has been found in associaton with non-AIDS and AIDS-associated PCNSL (2,10–14). Whether EBV is a causative agent or merely facilitates the malignant transformation of B-cells remains controversial (15,16). A clinical link between EBV infection and malignant lymphoma exists in the X-linked lymphoproliferative syndrome (Duncan's syndrome).

This syndrome is characterized by a selective deficiency in the control of EBV-mediated infection and an increased incidence of malignant lymphomas, including PCNSL (14,104–107).

An association between non-Hodgkin's lymphomas, EBV, and rearrangement of the c-*myc* protooncogene has long been known. Several investigators have identified EBV DNA sequences in PCNSL by Southern blotting (2,10,11,108,109), in situ hybridization (13,110,111), and polymerase chain reaction (PCR)-enhanced Southern blotting (10,12). Even though positive results using all three techniques are convincing, it is difficult to know with certainty the significance of negative in situ hybridization–PCR results obtained from paraffin blocks. The limited data available suggest that the pathogenesis of PCNSL in immunocompetent patients is different from that in patients with a history of immunocompromise.

In AIDS-associated large-cell immunoblastic PCNSL, Meeker et al. (11) have shown both the presence of EBV sequences and the absence of c-*myc* rearrangement; all of the tumors were monoclonal. In contrast, most (70%) peripheral AIDS-associated non-Hodgkin's lymphomas are EBV-negative, are frequently polyclonal, and show c-*myc* rearrangement (108,112). Human immunodeficiency virus sequences have not been identified or extracted from PCNSL specimens from AIDS patients. The clinical presentation of PCNSL is markedly different from peripheral non-Hodgkin's lymphoma in AIDS patients. Ziegler et al. found diffuse lymphadenopathy in 40% of AIDS patients with peripheral non-Hodgkin's lymphoma (113). Generalized lymphadenopathy was not found in our series of AIDS-associated PCNSL (36). The data from both clinical and molecular studies suggest a different pathogenesis for PCNSL and peripheral non-Hodgkin's lymphoma in AIDS patients. MacMahon et al. have shown nonprotein-coding EBV transcripts in 21 of 21 AIDS-associated PCNSLs by in situ hybridization (114).

In non-AIDS PCNSL, the presence of EBV sequences has been related to a history of immunocompromise. Nakhleh et al. found EBV sequences in one renal transplant recipient with non-AIDS PCNSL and in only one of eight patients without a history of immunocompromise (13). With PCR and in situ hybridization, Rouah et al. found EBV sequences in only two of nine cases of PCNSL without a history of immunocompromise; however, both patients had a history of secondary immunocompromise (diabetes mellitus and alcohol abuse) (12). Bashir et al. found EBV sequences in four of four cases of non-AIDS PCNSL with a history of immunocompromise and in none of four patients without a history of immunocompromise (115). Therefore, it is difficult to implicate EBV as an etiological or associated agent in non-AIDS PCNSL without a history of immunocompromise. The role of c-*myc* and the degree of monoclonality remain unknown. Detailed Southern blot studies of fresh non-AIDS PCNSL would be useful in the analysis of these tumors.

ACKNOWLEDGMENT

Supported in part by grants CA 13525 and 1R01 CA 55514-01 from the National Institutes of Health. The authors thank Stephen Ordway for editorial assistance.

REFERENCES

1. Rosenblum ML, Levy RM, Bredesen DE, et al. Primary central nervous system lymphomas in patients with AIDS. Ann Neurol 1988; 23(suppl):13–16.
2. Hochberg FH, Miller DC. Primary central nervous system lymphoma. J Neurosurg 1988; 68:835–853.
3. Henry JM, Heffner RR Jr, Dillard SH, et al. Primary malignant lymphoma of the central nervous system. Cancer 1974; 34:1293–1302.
4. Neuwelt EA, Goldman DL, Dahlborg SA, et al. Primary CNS lymphoma treated with osmotic blood–brain barrier disruption: prolonged survival and preservation of cognitive function. J Clin Oncol 1991; 9:1580–1590.

5. Hochberg FH, Loeffler JS, Prados M. The therapy of primary brain lymphoma. J Neurooncol 1991; 10:191–201.
6. Chamberlain MC, Levin VA. Adjuvant chemotherapy for primary lymphoma of the central nervous system. Arch Neurol 1990; 47:1113–1116.
7. DeAngelis LM, Yahalom J, Heinemann MH, et al. Primary CNS lymphoma: combined treatment with chemotherapy and radiotherapy. Neurology 1990; 40:80–86.
8. Gabbai AA, Hochberg FH, Lingood RM, et al. High-dose methotrexate for non-AIDS primary central nervous system lymphoma. Report of 13 cases. J Neurosurg 1989; 70:190–194.
9. Cohen IJ, Voger R, Matz S, et al. Successful non-neurotoxic therapy (without radiation) of a multifocal primary brain lymphoma with a methotrexate, vincristine, and BCNU protocol (DEMOB). Cancer 1986; 57:6–11.
10. Hochberg FH, Miller G, Schooley RT. Central nervous system lymphoma related to Epstein–Barr virus. N Engl J Med 1983; 309:745–748.
11. Meeker TC, Shiramizu B, Kaplan L, et al. Evidence for molecular subtypes of HIV-associated lymphoma: division into peripheral monoclonal, polyclonal and central nervous system. AIDS 1991; 5:669–674.
12. Rouah E, Rogers BB, Wilson DR, et al. Demonstration of Epstein–Barr virus in primary central nervous system lymphomas by the polymerase chain reaction and in situ hybridization. Hum Pathol 1990; 21:545–550.
13. Nakhleh RE, Manivel JC, Copenhaver CM, et al. In situ hybridization for detection of Epstein-Barr virus in central nervous system lymphomas. Cancer 1991; 67:444–448.
14. Pattengale PK, Taylor CR, Panke T, et al. Selective immunodeficiency and malignant lymphoma of the central nervous system. Possible relationship to the Epstein–Barr virus. Acta Neuropathol 1979; 48:165–169.
15. List AF, Greco FA, Vogler LB. Lymphoproliferative diseases in immunocompromised hosts: the role of Epstein–Barr virus. J Clin Oncol 1987; 5:1673–1689.
16. Shapiro RS, McClain K, Frizzera G, et al. Epstein–Barr virus associated B cell lymphoproliferative disorders following bone marrow transplantation. Blood 1988; 71:1234–1243.
17. Bailey P. Intracranial sarcomatous tumors of leptomeningeal origin. Arch Surg 1929; 18:1359–1402.
18. Yuile CL. Case of primary reticulum cell sarcoma of the brain. Relation of microglial cells to histiocytes. Arch Pathol 1938; 26:1037–1044.
19. Russel DS, Marshall AHE, Smith FB. Microgliomatosis: a form of reticulosis affecting the brain. Brain 1948; 7:1–15.
20. Ganderson CH, Henry J, Malamud N. Plasma globulin determinations in patients with microglioma. Report of five cases. J Neurosurg 1971; 35:406–415.
21. Char DH, Margolis L, Newman AB. Occular reticulum cell sarcoma. Am J Ophthalmol 1981; 91:480–483.
22. Doak PB, Montogomerie JZ, North JDK, et al. Reticulum cell sarcoma after renal homotransplantation and azathioprine and prednisone therapy. Br Med J 1968; 4:746–748.
23. Enzmann DR, Krikorian J, Norman D, et al. Computed tomography in primary reticulum cell sarcoma of the brain. Radiology 1979; 130:165–170.
24. Rubinstein LJ. Tumors of the central nervous system. Washington DC: Armed Forces Institute of Pathology, 1972:215–234.
25. Benjamin I, Case MES. Primary reticulum-cell sarcoma (microglioma) of the brain with massive cardiac metastasis. Case report. J Neurosurg 1980; 53:714–716.
26. Horvat B, Pena C, Fischer ER. Primary reticulum cell sarcoma (microglioma) of brain. An electron microscopic study. Arch Pathol 1969; 87:609–616.
27. Schaumburg HH, Plank CR, Adams RD. The reticulum cell sarcoma–microglioma group of brain tumours. A consideration of their clinical features and therapy. Brain 1972; 95:199–212.
28. Houthoff HJ, Poppema S, Ebels EJ, et al. Intracranial malignant lymphomas: a morphologic and immunocytologic study of twenty cases. Acta Neuropathol (Berl) 1978; 44:203–210.
29. Miyoshi I, Kubonishi I, Yoshimoto S, et al. Characteristics of a brain lymphoma cell line derived from primary intracranial lymphoma. Cancer 1982; 49:456–459.

30. Varadachari C, Palutke M, Climie ARW, et al. Immunoblastic sarcoma (histiocytic lymphoma) of the brain with B cell markers. Case report. J Neurosurg 1978; 49:887–892.

31. The non-Hodgkin's lymphoma pathologic classification project: the National Cancer Institute sponsored study of classifications of non-Hodgkin's lymphomas. Summary and description of a working formulation for clinical usage. Cancer 1982; 49:2112–2139.

32. Bednar MM, Salerni A, Flanagan M, et al. Primary central nervous system T-cell lymphoma. J Neurosurg 1991; 74:668–672.

33. Morgello S, Maiese K, Petito CK. T-cell lymphoma in the CNS. Clinical and pathologic features. Neurology 1989; 39:1190–1196.

34. Grant JW, von Deimling A. Primary T-cell lymphoma of the central nervous system. Arch Pathol Lab Med 1990; 114:24–27.

35. Kuwata T, Funahashi K, Itakura T, et al. [T cell type primary lymphoma of the central nervous system: a case report.] (Jpn) No Shinkei Geka 1987; 15:657–661.

36. Baumgartner JE, Rachlin JR, Beckstead JH, et al. Primary central nervous system lymphomas: natural history and response to radiation therapy in 55 patients with acquired immunodeficiency syndrome. J Neurosurg 1990; 73:206–211.

37. Pittman KB, Olweny CLM, North JB, et al. Primary central nervous system lymphoma. A report of 9 cases and review of the literature. Oncology 1991; 48:184–187.

38. Amadori M, Maltoni M, Ravaioli A, et al. Primary lymphoma of the central nervous system. Tumori 1991; 77:32–35.

39. Epstein LG, DiCarlo FJ Jr, Joshi VV, et al. Primary lymphoma of the central nervous system in children with acquired immunodeficiency syndrome. Pediatrics 1988; 82:355–363.

40. Socie G, Pirot-Chauffat C, Schlienger M, et al. Primary lymphoma of the central nervous system. An unresolved therapeutic problem. Cancer 1990; 65:322–326.

41. Goldstein J, Dickson DW, Rubenstein A, et al. Primary central nervous system lymphoma in a pediatric patient with acquired immune deficiency syndrome. Treatment with radiation therapy. Cancer 1990; 66:2503–2508.

42. Egerter DA, Beckstead JH. Malignant lymphomas in the acquired immunodeficiency syndrome. Additional evidence for a B-cell origin. Arch Pathol Lab Med 1988; 112:602–606.

43. Remick SC, Diamond C, Migliozzi JA, et al. Primary central nervous system lymphoma in patients with and without the acquired immune deficiency syndrome. A retrospective analysis and review of the literature. Medicine 1990; 69:345–360.

44. Ahmed T, Wormser GP, Stahl RE, et al. Malignant lymphomas in a population at risk of acquired immune deficiency syndrome. Cancer 1987; 60:719–723.

45. Helle TL, Britt RH, Colby TV. Primary lymphoma of the central nervous system. Clinicopathological study of experience at Stanford. J Neurosurg 1984; 60:94–103.

46. Hoover R, Fraumeni JF Jr. Risk of cancer in renal transplant recipients. Lancet 1973; 2:55–57.

47. Penn I. Development of cancer as a complication of clinical transplantation. Transplant Proc 1977; 9:1121–1127.

48. Weintraub J, Warnke RA. Lymphoma in cardiac allotransplant recipients. Clinical and histological features and immunological phenotypes. Transplantation 1982; 33:347–351.

49. Cho ES, Connolly E, Porro ES. Primary reticulum cell sarcoma of the brain in a renal transplantation recipient. Case report. J Neurosurg 1974; 41:235–239.

50. Schneck SA, Penn I. De novo brain tumors in renal transplant recipients. Lancet 1971; 1:983–986.

51. Sheil AGR. Cancer in renal allograft recipients in Australia and New Zealand. Transplant Proc 1977; 9:1133–1136.

52. Penn I. The incidence of malignancies in transplant recipients. Transplant Proc 1975; 7:323–326.

53. Brand MM, Marrinkovich VA. Primary malignant reticulosis of the brain in Wiskott–Aldrich syndrome. Report of a case. Arch Dis Child 1969; 44:536–542.

54. Hutter JJ Jr, Jones JF. Results of a thymic epithelial transplant in a child with Wiskott–Aldrich syndrome and central nervous system lymphoma. Clin Immunol Immunopathol 1981; 18:121–125.

55. Kinney TD, Adams RD. Reticulum cell sarcoma of the brain. Arch Neurol Psychiatry 1943; 50:552–564.

56. Model LM. Primary reticulum cell sarcoma of the brain in Wiskott Aldrich syndrome. Arch Neurol 1977; 34:633–635.

57. Filiovich AH, Heinitz KJ, Robison LL, et al. The Immunodeficiency Cancer Registry. A research resource. Am J Pediatr Hematol Oncol 1987; 9:183–184.

58. Bale JF Jr, Wilson JF, Hill HR. Fatal histiocytic lymphoma of the brain associated with hyperimmunoglobulinemia-E and recurrent infections. Cancer 1977; 39:2386–2390.

59. Wara DW. Immunologic disorders. In: Rudolph A, ed. Rudolph's pediatrics. 19th ed. San Mateo: Appleton & Lange, 1991: 451–476, 1148.

60. Perry GS III, Spector BD, Schuman LM, et al. The Wiskott Aldrich syndrome in the United States and Canada (1892–1979). J Pediatr 1980; 97:72–78.

61. Lipsmeyer EA. Development of malignant cerebral lymphoma in a patient with systemic lupus erythematosis treated with immunosuppression. Arthritis Rheum 1972; 15:183–186.

62. Talal M, Bunim JJ. The development of malignant lymphoma in the course of Sjögren's syndrome. Am J Med 1964; 36:529–540.

63. Trillet M, Pialat J, Chazot G, et al. Lymphome non Hodgkin "primitif" de l'encephale. Sarcoidose. Cancer thyroidien. Deficit immunitaire cellulaire. Rev Neurol 1982; 138:241–248.

64. Ho K, Garancis JC, Paegle RD, et al. Progressive multifocal leukoencephalopathy and malignant lymphoma of the brain in a patient with immunosuppressive therapy. Acta Neuropathol 1980; 52:81–83.

65. Castaigne P, Excourolle R, Brunet P, et al. Reticulosarcome cerebral primitif associé à de lésions de sclérose en plaques. Rev Neurol 1974; 130:181–188.

66. Giromini D, Peiffer J, Tzonos T. Occurrence of a primary Burkitt-type lymphoma of the central nervous system in an astrocytoma patient. A case report. Acta Neuropathol 1981; 54:165–167.

67. Levy RM, Jannssen RS, Bush TJ, et al. Neuroepidemiology of acquired immunodeficiency syndrome. In: Rosenblum ML, Levy RM, Bredesen DE, eds. AIDS and the nervous system. New York: Raven Press, 1988: 13–27.

68. Goldstein JD, Dickson DW, Moser F, et al. Primary central nervous system lymphoma in acquired immune deficiency syndrome. A clinical and pathologic study with results of treatment with radiation. Cancer 1991; 67:2756–2765.

69. Levine AM, Sullivan-Halley J, Pike MC, et al. Human immunodeficiency virus-related lymphoma. Cancer 1991; 68:2466–2472.

70. Jiddane M, Nicole F, Diaz P, et al. Intracranial malignant lymphoma. Report of 30 cases and review of the literature. J Neurosurg 1986; 65:592–599.

71. Rockwood EJ, Zakov ZN, Bay JW. Combined malignant lymphoma of the eye and CNS (reticulum cell sarcoma). Report of 3 cases. J Neurosurg 1984; 61:369–374.

72. Parver LM, Font RL. Malignant lymphoma of the retina and brain. Initial diagnosis by cytologic examination of vitreous aspirate. Arch Ophthalmol 1979; 97:1505–1507.

73. Kattah JC, Jenkins RB, Pilkerton AR, et al. Multifocal primary ocular and central nervous system malignant lymphoma. Ann Ophthalmol 1982; 13:589–593.

74. Jellinger K, Radaskiewicz TH, Slowik F. Primary malignant lymphoma of the central nervous system in man. Acta Neuropathol [Suppl] 1975; 6:95–102.

75. Hautzer NW, Aiyesimoju A, Robitaille Y. "Primary" spinal intramedullary lymphomas: a review. Ann Neurol 1983; 14:62–66.

76. Bruni J, Bilbao JM, Gray T. Primary intramedullary malignant lymphoma of the spinal cord. Neurology 1977; 27:846–898.

77. Mitsumoto H, Breuer AC, Lederman RJ. Malignant lymphoma of the central nervous system: a case of primary spinal intramedullary involvement. Cancer 1980; 46:1258–1262.

78. Mendenhall NP, Thar TL, Agee OF, et al. Primary lymphoma of the central nervous system. Computerized tomography scan characteristics and results for 12 cases. Cancer 1983; 52:1993–2000.

79. Schwaighofer BW, Hesselink JR, Press GA, et al. Primary intracranial CNS lymphoma: MR manifestations. AJNR 1989; 10:725–729.

80. Jack CR, Reese DF, Scheithauer BW. Radiographic findings in 32 cases of primary CNS lymphoma. AJR 1986; 146:271–276.

81. Ciricillo SF, Rosenblum ML. Use of CT and MR imaging to distinguish intracranial lesions and to define the need for biopsy in AIDS patients. J Neurosurg 1990; 73:720–724.

82. Ciricillo SF, Rosenblum ML. Imaging of solitary lesions in AIDS [letter]. J Neurosurg 1991; 74:1029.

83. Berry MP, Simpson WJ. Radiation therapy in the management of primary malignant lymphoma of the brain. Int J Radiat Oncol Biol Phys 1981; 7:55–59.

84. Jellinger K, Slowik F, Sluga E. Primary intracranial malignant lymphomas. A fine structural, cytochemical and CSF immunological study. Clin Neurol Neurosurg 1979; 83:173–186.

85. Ezrin-Waters C, Klein M, Deck J, et al. Diagnostic importance of immunological markers in lymphoma involving the central nervous system. Ann Neurol 1984; 16:668–672.

86. Jones GR, Mason WH, Fishman LS, et al. Primary central nervous system lymphoma without intracranial mass in a child. Diagnosis by documentation of monoclonality. Cancer 1985; 56:2804–2808.

87. Littman P, Wang CC. Reticulum cell sarcoma of brain. Cancer 1975; 35:1412–1420.

88. Pollack IF, Lunsford LD, Flickinger JC, et al. Prognostic factors in the diagnosis and treatment of primary central nervous system lymphoma. Cancer 1989; 63:939–947.

89. Danavaros P, Mikol J, Nemeth J, et al. Stereotactic biopsy diagnosis of primary non-Hodgkin's lymphoma of the central nervous system. A histological and immunohistochemical study. Pathol Res Pract 1990; 186:459–466.

90. Nakamine H, Yokote H, Itakura T, et al. Non-Hodgkin's lymphoma involving the brain. Diagnostic usefulness of stereotactic needle biopsy in combination with paraffin-section immunohistochemistry. Acta Neuropathol 1989; 78:462–471.

91. Sherman ME, Erozan YS, Mann RB, et al. Stereotactic brain biopsy in the diagnosis of malignant lymphoma. Am J Clin Pathol 1991; 95:878–883.

92. Bogdhan U, Bogdahn S, Mertens HG, et al. Primary non-Hodgkin's lymphoma of the CNS. Acta Neurol Scand 1986; 73:602–614.

93. Sugita Y, Shigemori M, Yuge T, et al. Spontaneous regression of primary malignant intracranial lymphoma. Surg Neurol 1988; 30:148–152.

94. Homo-Delarche F. Glucocorticoid receptors and steroid sensitivity in normal and neoplastic human lymphoma tissues. A review. Cancer Res 1984; 44:431–437.

95. Vaquero J, Martinez R, Rossi E, Lopez R. Primary cerebral lymphoma: the "ghost tumor." J Neurosurg 1984; 60:174–176.

96. Baxter JD, Harris AW, Tomkins GM, et al. Glucocorticoid receptors in lymphoma cells in culture: relationship to glucocorticoid killing activity. Science 1971; 171:189–191.

97. Claman HN. Corticosteroids and lymphoid cells. N Engl J Med 1972; 287:388–397.

98. Shibamoto Y, Tsutsui K, Dodo Y, et al. Improved survival in primary intracranial lymphoma treated by high dose radiation and systemic vincristine–doxorubicin–cyclophosphamide–prednisolone chemotherapy. Cancer 1990; 65:1907–1912.

99. Ervin T, Canellos GP. Successful treatment of recurrent primary central nervous system lymphoma with high dose methotrexate. Cancer 1980; 45:1556–1557.

100. Herbst KD, Corder MP, Justice GR. Successful therapy with methotrexate of the multicentric mixed lymphoma of the central nervous system. Cancer 1976; 38:1476–1478.

101. Abelson HT, Kufe DW, Skarin AT, et al. Treatment of central nervous system tumors with methotrexate. Cancer Treat Rep 1981; 65:137–140.

102. Lui HM, Maurer HS, Vongsivut S, Conway JJ. Methotrexate encephalopathy. Hum Pathol 1978; 9:636–649.

103. Crossen J, Goldman DL, Dahlborg SA, Neuwelt EA. Neuropsychological assessment outcomes of nonacquired immunodeficiency syndrome patients with primary central nervous system lymphoma before and after blood–brain barrier disruption chemotherapy. Neurosurgery 1992; 30:23–29.

104. Purtilo DT. Immune deficiency predisposing to Epstein–Barr virus-induced lymphoproliferative syndrome as a model. Adv Cancer Res 1981; 34:279–312.

105. Purtilo DT. Pathogenesis and phenotypes of an X-linked recessive lymphoproliferative syndrome. Lancet 1976; 2:882–885.

106. Purtilo DT, De Florio D Jr, Hutt LM. Variable phenotypic expression of an X-linked recessive lymphoproliferative syndrome. N Engl J Med 1977; 297:1077–1081.

107. Purtilo DT, Hutt L, Bhawan J, et al. Immunodeficiency to the Epstein–Barr virus in the X-linked recessive lymphoproliferative syndrome. Clin Immunol Immunopathol 1978; 9:147–156.
108. Shiramizu B, McGrath MS. Molecular pathogenesis of AIDS-associated non-Hodgkin's lymphoma. Hematol Oncol Clin North Am 1991; 5:323–330.
109. Ambinder RF. Human lymphotrophic viruses associated with lymphoid malignancy: Epstein–Barr and HTLV-1. Hematol Oncol Clin North Am 1991; 4:821–833.
110. Weiss LM, Movahed LA, Warnke RA, Sklar J. Detection of Epstein–Barr viral genomes in Reed–Sternberg cells of Hodgkin's disease. N Engl J Med 1989; 320:502–506.
111. Weiss LM, Movahed LA. In situ demonstration of Epstein–Barr viral genomes in viral-associated B-cell lymphoproliferations. Am J Pathol 1989; 134:651–659.
112. Subar M, Neri A, Inghirami G, et al. Frequent c-*myc* oncogene activation and infrequent presence of Epstein–Barr virus genome in AIDS-associated lymphoma. Blood 1988; 72:667–671.
113. Ziegler JL, Drew WL, Miner RC, et al. Outbreak of Burkitt's-like lymphoma in homosexual men. Lancet 1982; 2:631–633.
114. MacMahon EM, Glass, JD, Hayward SD, et al. Epstein–Barr virus in AIDS-related primary central nervous system lymphoma. Lancet 1991; 338:969–973.
115. Bashir RM, Harris NL, Hochberg FH, et al. Detection of Epstein–Barr virus in CNS lymphomas by in situ hybridization. Neurology 1989; 39:813–817.

18

Tumors Associated with the Phakomatoses

Ronald E. Warnick
University of Cincinnati Medical Center,
Cincinnati, Ohio

I. INTRODUCTION

The phakomatoses are a heterogeneous group of disorders that are characterized by their involvement of the skin, eyes, viscera, and central nervous system (CNS). The term *phakomatoses* was coined in 1923 by van der Hoeve to describe the syndromes of neurofibromatosis and tuberous sclerosis, and was derived from the Greek word *phakos*, meaning mother spot (1). The phakomata, or mother spots, described the multiple hamartomas involving the skin and other organs in these two syndromes. Subsequently, these and other multisystem disorders were encompassed by the broad term *neurocutaneous syndromes*, despite the fact that one major syndrome, von Hippel–Lindau disease, has no apparent dermatological manifestations. For practical reasons, both terms will be used interchangeably in this chapter, recognizing their inadequacy as descriptive terms.

The three most common neurocutaneous syndromes are neurofibromatosis, tuberous sclerosis, and von Hippel–Lindau disease. All three disorders share an autosomal dominant pattern of inheritance, and recent molecular studies have identified the chromosomal abnormality associated with each syndrome. The importance of these disorders to neuro-oncologists lies in the frequent, and often multifocal, neoplastic involvement of the central nervous system. The broad range of brain tumors associated with the phakomatoses will be the focus of this chapter.

II. NEUROFIBROMATOSIS

A. History and Nomenclature

The clinical entity of multiple cutaneous tumors was first recognized by Tilesius in 1793 and called molluscum fibrosum (2). Nearly a century later (1882), Frederick David von Recklinghausen described two patients with cutaneous and subcutaneous tumors, introducing the term multiple neurofibromatosis (3). Since these early clinical descriptions, two distinct forms of neurofibromatosis have been recognized: (1) neurofibromatosis type 1 (NF-1, von Recklinghausen's neurofibromatosis) and (2) neurofibromatosis type 2 (NF-2, bilateral acoustic neurofibromatosis). The terms peripheral and central neurofibromatosis have previously been used to describe the patterns of nervous system involvement in these two syndromes but have been abandoned as inaccurate.

B. Neurofibromatosis Type 1

1. Epidemiology and Genetics

Neurofibromatosis type 1 (NF-1) affects 1 of every 3000 individuals and represents 90% of all cases of neurofibromatosis (4,5). Inheritance is autosomal dominant, with complete penetrance by age 5; however, the clinical expression is highly variable even within the same family (4,6). Surprisingly, nearly half of affected individuals have a negative family history and are thought to represent spontaneous mutations (4).

Recent advances in molecular biology have allowed the localization and characterization of the gene responsible for the NF-1 syndrome. The NF-1 gene is located on the long arm of chromosome 17 near the centromere (7). It is uncertain whether the NF-1 gene acts as a tumor suppressor gene, or as a growth promoter (8). Closely linked DNA markers have been identified and are presently being evaluated for use in prenatal and early childhood (presymptomatic) testing of affected families (9). It must be recognized that this form of genetic screening can accurately detect only the presence of the NF-1 gene, but cannot predict the severity of the disease (i.e., the expression of the gene).

2. Clinical Syndrome

The expression of NF-1 is usually apparent by age 5 and is characterized by early involvement of the skin (cafe au lait macules, cutaneous neurofibromas), the eyes (Lisch nodules), and the peripheral and central nervous system (plexiform and spinal neurofibromas, hamartomas, gliomas). Diagnostic criteria for NF-1 were established in 1987 by a National Institutes of Health (NIH) Consensus Development Conference and are listed in Table 1 (10).

Systemic Features.   Dermatological signs are consistent and early manifestations of NF-1. Cafe au lait macules are often present at birth and tend to enlarge with age. By age 6, 97% of children with NF-1 have six or more cafe au lait macules (5). Axillary and inguinal freckles are merely cafe au lait spots occurring in areas of skin lacking sun exposure and generally are apparent by middle childhood in 80% of patients (5). Cutaneous or subcutaneous neurofibromas are encapsulated tumors containing connective tissue, Schwann cells, and neural elements (11). They arise along the course of peripheral and autonomic nerves, most frequently over the trunk, and are usually of variable number and size. In most series, 25–30% of patients with NF-1 have peripheral

---

Table 1   Diagnostic Criteria for Neurofibromatosis Type 1

The diagnostic criteria are met if a person has two or more of the following:

1. Six or more cafe au lait macules larger than 5 mm in greatest diameter in prepubertal persons, or larger than 15 mm in greatest diameter in postpubertal persons
2. Two or more neurofibromas of any type, or one plexiform neurofibroma
3. Freckling in the axillary or inguinal regions
4. Optic glioma
5. Two or more Lisch nodules (iris hamartomas)
6. A distinctive osseous lesion such as sphenoid dysplasia or thinning of long-bone cortex, with or without pseudoarthrosis
7. A first-degree relative with neurofibromatosis type 1 by the above criteria

Source: Ref. 52.

neurofibromas, with most lesions appearing during puberty (4). Plexiform neurofibromas are sessile masses arising from larger peripheral, cranial, or sympathetic nerves with involvement of both cutaneous and subcutaneous layers. They often involve the face with invasion of the orbit. Malignant transformation to neurofibrosarcoma occurs in approximately 5% of cases (11).

Hamartomas of the iris (Lisch nodules) are diagnosed by slit-lamp examination in over 90% of postpubertal NF-1 patients, but are apparent in only 30% of patients younger than 6 years (5). They do not result in ophthalmological complications, but are important, since their presence is diagnostic of NF-1 (12). Other less frequent ocular findings include pulsatile exophthalmos, which is caused by sphenoid wing dysplasia, and buphthalmos ("ox eye"), which describes enlargement of the globe secondary to congenital glaucoma.

Visceral involvement in NF-1 may be reflected clinically by systemic hypertension resulting from either pheochromocytoma or renal vascular stenosis. Congenital pseudoarthrosis (usually tibial), or scoliosis typify the skeletal disorders seen in NF-1 (5).

Central Nervous System Involvement. The hallmark of NF-1 is the multifocal involvement of the neuraxis by low-grade neoplasms and hamartomatous lesions. Overall, there is a 15–20% incidence of brain tumors in the NF-1 syndrome, with optic pathway gliomas constituting most of these tumors (13,14). Spinal tumors are less common and may be either intrinsic gliomas or neurofibromas arising from the dorsal nerve roots. In addition, the advent of magnetic resonance imaging (MRI) has allowed demonstration of brain heterotopias in as many as 60% of NF-1 patients (15).

Optic pathway gliomas. Gliomas involving the optic pathway are the most frequent CNS tumors in NF-1, occurring in up to 15% of children affected with this syndrome (6). However, only one-third of affected patients are symptomatic (6). This is mainly a disease of young children: 75% of tumors occur in the first decade, with a peak incidence at age 5 (16). No sex propensity has been noted.

Two distinct subsets of optic pathway gliomas are recognized: (1) isolated tumors involving the optic nerve, and (2) tumors involving the optic chiasm and the hypothalamic region. This anatomical distinction is important because of the different modes of presentation, treatment options, and outcome.

Pathologically, these tumors are usually low-grade fibrillary or pilocytic astrocytomas, some of which contain foci of oligodendroglioma (17). Although the cellular appearance of these tumors is similar, regardless of position along the optic pathway, two distinct patterns of growth have been identified for optic nerve gliomas. In patients with NF-1, the growth of optic nerve gliomas is typically circumferential, with frequent microscopic involvement of the leptomeninges (18). This is in contrast with sporadic optic nerve gliomas unrelated to NF, which generally demonstrate an intraneural growth pattern (18). Although the overall proliferative potential of optic pathway gliomas is low, these tumors may have erratic, unpredictable growth.

Optic nerve gliomas are usually unilateral, but may present with bilateral involvement in up to 15% of affected patients (6). These tumors produce symptoms of progressive proptosis and monocular visual loss over 6–12 months (19). Funduscopy often reveals an edematous optic disc resulting from venous obstruction. The MRI scan after gadolinium infusion shows fusiform enlargement of the optic nerve within the orbit (Fig. 1) (20). Magnetic resonance imaging is superior to computed tomography (CT) in the detection of intracranial extension of optic nerve gliomas.

The therapeutic management of optic nerve gliomas in NF patients remains controversial. These tumors generally exhibit indolent growth and even spontaneous regression (21). However, caudal extension to involve the optic chiasm and hypothalamus, malignant transformation, and rarely cerebrospinal fluid (CSF) spread, all may occur (21). There is general agreement that surgery is warranted when progressive proptosis causes disabling pain or endangers the globe, or for cosmetic reasons (19). In patients with optic nerve glioma and minimal or no symptoms, expectant management with serial visual and radiographic studies is indicated (19). However, the approach to patients with unilateral optic nerve glioma and progressive visual loss remains controversial. For such patients, en bloc resection of the tumor and adjacent optic nerve has been suggested to prevent intracranial extension of the tumor (19). When gross total resection can be accomplished, the 5-year disease-free survival is approximately 95% (22). Postoperative irradiation has been reserved for patients with incomplete resection and has resulted in a 5-year disease-free survival of nearly 90% (23). Others have advocated a nonsurgical approach to patients with unilateral tumors and failing vision, since the specific radiographic appearance obviates the need for biopsy, and posterior extension of these tumors is rare (24). Primary irradiation of these tumors has produced 10-year local control rates of 90% in some series (25). Visual function remains stable in most patients after radiotherapy, with improvement noted in 30–40% of patients (25,26). However, irradiation of optic pathway tumors has been associated with late sequelae including pituitary dysfunction, intellectual decline, and vascular disease (17). For these reasons, neoadjuvant chemotherapy has been recommended to obviate, or at least delay, the need for radiation therapy. Preliminary experience with the regimen of dactinomycin (actinomycin D) and vincristine has demonstrated a beneficial response in young children with optic nerve gliomas (24). However, more experience and longer follow-up are necessary to determine the role of chemotherapy in the initial treatment of these tumors.

Patients with gliomas involving the optic chiasm or hypothalamus are distinct from patients with isolated optic nerve gliomas. The prognosis for patients with chiasmatic–hypothalamic glioma is less predictable, reflecting both the anatomical location and the proliferative potential of these tumors. Patients with NF-1 may harbor an asymptomatic chiasmatic–hypothalamic glioma that is discovered incidentally on a screening MRI scan. Children younger than 2 years old may have abnormal eye movements and developmental delay at presentation. Diencephalic dysfunction may be manifest in severe failure to thrive and in hyperkinetic behavior (Russell's syndrome) (27). Older children often have progressive visual defects and endocrine dysfunction, including growth failure and precocious puberty (28). Headaches and signs of increased intracranial pressure may reflect obstruction of the third ventricle, producing hydrocephalus.

Magnetic resonance imaging provides excellent resolution of the suprasellar structures, and coronal views are particularly helpful in defining the diencephalic component. Chiasmatic–hypothalamic gliomas are hypointense compared with normal brain tissue on T1-weighted MRI and usually enhance homogeneously with gadolinium (Fig. 2a) (29). Signal abnormality in the optic tracts may course posteriorly as far as the lateral geniculate bodies (see Fig. 2b) (26). The differential diagnosis includes solid craniopharyngioma, pituitary adenoma with suprasellar extension, and suprasellar germinoma.

Patients with NF-1 who have small chiasmal tumors, minimal or no symptoms, and a classic radiographic appearance do not require treatment and can be managed expectantly with serial neuroimaging and ophthalmological examinations (28). Surgery should be performed to confirm the pathology if the radiographic diagnosis is uncertain. Craniotomy may also be indicated for cyst drainage and cytoreduction of large tumors (28). For symptomatic patients with tumors having a substantial exophytic component, an aggressive surgical approach has been advocated to delay or avert the need for adjuvant treatment (30). Patients with diencephalic involvement may also require shunting (28).

The adjuvant treatment of patients with chiasmatic–hypothalamic gliomas remains controversial. As mentioned earlier, a subset of patients can be followed expectantly. Because many of these patients remain stable without treatment, the long-term morbidity of radiation therapy may outweigh its possible benefit. In contrast, patients with larger tumors causing symptoms usually require treatment to prevent tumor progression. Most studies evaluating the efficacy of adjuvant

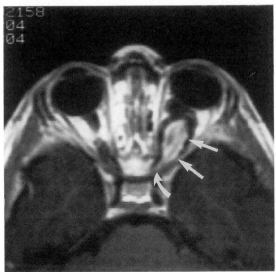

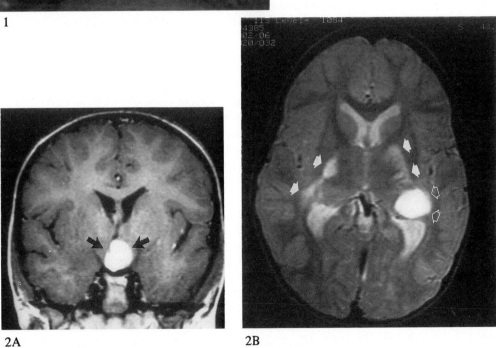

Figure 1 Optic nerve glioma. Axial MR image, with gadolinium, demonstrates a fusiform, enhancing mass within the orbit (straight arrows) with extension through the optic canal (curved arrow).

Figure 2 Hypothalamic glioma: (A) coronal MR image after gadolinium infusion shows a lobulated, suprasellar mass (arrows) that extends superiorly to the third ventricle; (B) axial T2-weighted MR image demonstrates signal abnormalities within both optic tracts (closed arrows) and involvement of the lateral geniculate (open arrows).

radiation therapy show that postoperative irradiation decreases recurrence rates (25,26,28). In another study, however, this improvement was not accompanied by an increase in long-term survival (21). Clinically, the visual function of 30–40% of patients improves after radiation therapy (25,26). Irradiation of the suprasellar region, however, may produce significant morbidity, including intellectual decline, delayed vascular injury, and excessive or insufficient production of hormones (23).

The morbidity associated with radiation therapy has prompted investigations of neoadjuvant chemotherapy. Dactinomycin (actinomycin D) combined with vincristine has been used as primary treatment of chiasmatic–hypothalamic gliomas in children younger than 5 years old (31). This regimen results in lessened or stable disease in approximately two-thirds of patients. Among the patients whose tumors progressed, the median time to progression was 3 years. Chemotherapy, therefore, was successful in delaying the initiation of radiation therapy. Most importantly, the long-term cognitive function of these children remained normal. At the University of California, San Francisco, a five-drug, nitrosourea-based regimen was used as primary treatment for all children under 18 years of age who had optic pathway gliomas (32). This regimen included lomustine (CCNU), 6-thioguanine, procarbazine, dibromodulcitol, and vincristine. An initial radiographic response was seen in 11 of 15 evaluable patients, and the scans of 3 children were stable at the first evaluation. Three patients ultimately experienced progressive disease (1 initially and 2 after a partial response), and all of these remained stable after focal radiation therapy. In addition, the visual function of most patients stabilized or improved during treatment. Therefore, considerable evidence supports the use of primary chemotherapy in the treatment of children with chiasmatic–hypothalamic glioma.

The 5-year survival rate of patients with chiasmatic–hypothalamic glioma is 80–95% (23,26). Significantly lower 10-year survival survival rates of 60–80% emphasize the slow growth rate of these tumors and the need for long-term follow-up study (33). Patients with purely chiasmal lesions (86% survival at 15 years) generally fare better than those with extensive hypothalamic involvement (57%) (23). The prognostic importance of neurofibromatosis remains controversial, although most studies describe a favorable outcome in patients with this syndrome compared with sporadic optic pathway glioma (22,34).

Recurrent chiasmatic–hypothalamic gliomas may require reoperation when removal of a well-defined cystic or exophytic component is considered likely to improve the neurological condition. Focal radiation therapy is indicated for patients who have not previously received radiation treatment. Otherwise, chemotherapy with the drug combinations described earlier has been successful in salvage treatment for optic pathway glioma.

Other gliomas. Although the vast majority of gliomas associated with NF-1 are situated along the visual pathway, nearly 15% of gliomas associated with this syndrome are located in the cerebellum, cerebral cortex, or brain stem (15,35). These gliomas have a similar anatomical distribution compared with those occurring in the general population; however, there are important differences in histological type and prognosis. Cerebellar gliomas associated with NF-1 are almost solely astrocytomas, with ependymomas and oligodendrogliomas being extremely rare (36). Histologically, 50% of these cerebellar astrocytomas exhibit anaplastic changes (36). This is in sharp contrast to the classic juvenile pilocytic astrocytoma, which makes up 85% of cerebellar astrocytomas in the general pediatric population (17). This difference in histology helps explain the poorer outcome of cerebellar astrocytoma in NF-1: 50% 5-year survival, compared with over 90% 5-year survival for cerebellar astrocytoma in non-NF patients (17,36). The poor prognosis of cerebellar anaplastic astrocytomas in NF patients warrants aggressive adjuvant therapy, including postoperative irradiation (5500–6000 cGy), with the field of treatment determined by the results of neuraxis staging, and possibly the addition of nitrosourea-based chemotherapy, which may also be beneficial in this setting (37). The majority of cerebral gliomas in NF-1 patients are histologically malignant, which is the reverse of what is the case in the general pediatric population (36). The benefit of adjuvant radiation therapy for patients with high-grade astrocytoma has been demonstrated, and most available evidence supports the use of focal field of irradiation to a total dose of 5400–6000 cGy (38,39). Recent data from the Children's Cancer Study Group (CCSG) support the role of adjuvant nitrosourea-based chemotherapy following radiation therapy in the treatment of high-grade gliomas (41). The postoperative management of low-grade gliomas of the cerebral cortex remains controversial, since there has been no randomized study evaluating the role of adjuvant radiotherapy in this group. Given the available evidence, patients with radiographically confirmed complete resection can be observed with serial imaging studies (17). The decision whether or not to treat a patient with a partially resected low-grade astrocytoma should be based on age, duration of preoperative symptoms, and extent of resection (17). Brain stem gliomas associated with NF-1 may occur at any level of the brain stem. The few reports discussing this association have noted that most of these brain stem lesions are focal or exophytic. Therefore, they are associated with a generally favorable outcome, compared with brain stem gliomas in the general population, which mainly consist of diffuse, malignant gliomas (17,41,42). The indolent nature of most brain stem gliomas in NF has led to the recommendation that treatment be withheld unless there is unequivocal clinical or radiographic evidence of tumor progression (42).

Nonneoplastic lesions. Cranial MRI has revealed foci of signal abnormality in as many as 60% of asymptomatic NF-1 patients (15,35,43). These lesions appear as high-signal areas on T2-weighted images and generally are not associated with significant mass effect (15). The incidence of these "unidentified bright objects" increases with age and in association with chiasmatic–hypothalamic gliomas (15). They commonly appear in the basal ganglia, cerebellar penduncles, brain stem and, less frequently, the subcortical white matter (Fig. 3) (15,35). Surprisingly, the location and number of these MRI abnormalities do not correlate with the neurological examination, developmental status, or electrophysiological studies (43,44). Limited clinicopathological correlation suggests that these MRI abnormalities represent either glial nodules or hamartomatous lesions (45). Because of their histological appearance of glial proliferation, and the frequent proximity to areas of true glial neoplasm, it has been suggested that these abnormal areas have the potential for neoplastic growth (45). From a clinical viewpoint, patients with these MRI abnormalities should be followed with serial MRI studies to assess the growth potential of these lesions.

C. Neurofibromatosis Type 2

1. Epidemiology and Genetics

Neurofibromatosis type 2 (NF-2) affects 1 of every 50,000 individuals and represents only 10% of all cases of neurofibromatosis (4,5). It is also inherited in an autosomal dominant fashion with high penetrance, but unlike NF-1, it has a consistent clinical expression (bilateral acoustic neuromas).

Molecular studies have demonstrated deletions on the long arm of chromosome 22 in sporadic acoustic neuromas and meningiomas (46,47). Subsequent cytogenetic analyses of acoustic neuromas, meningiomas, and neurofibromas in NF-2 families have revealed loss of specific alleles on chromosome 22 as the common pathogenesis of this clinical syndrome (48). The NF-2 locus is postulated to encode a tumor suppressor gene the loss of which promotes the development of multiple CNS tumors in NF-2 (49). The recent identification of flanking DNA markers on chromosome 22 will soon allow prenatal and presymptomatic diagnosis of NF-2 (50).

2. Clinical Syndrome

Neurofibromatosis type 2 has a mean age of presentation of approximately 20 years old and is characterized by limited skin involvement (less than six cafe au lait macules), ocular pathology (presenile cataracts), and tumors of the central nervous system (bilateral acoustic neuromas, meningiomas, and schwannomas) (51). The diagnostic criteria for NF-2 were established by the NIH in 1987 (Table 2), and recently revised to include modern neuroimaging criteria (10,52).

Systemic Features.   Dermatological signs are less pronounced in NF-2. Cafe au lait macules are present in up to 40% of patients, but usually number fewer than six (51). Cutaneous and subcutaneous neurofibromas are found in nearly one-third of NF-2 patients (51). Ocular findings are limited to presenile cataracts, which affect 85% of NF-2 patients (53). In contrast with NF-1, visceral disease is extremely rare.

Central Nervous System Involvement.   By definition, all patients with NF-2 have central nervous system involvement. Although the NF-2 syndrome is characterized by bilateral acoustic neuromas, these may coexist with other cranial nerve schwannomas, as well as multiple meningiomas (49). Just as bilateral acoustic neuromas may occur in NF-1, glial neoplasms may be associated with the NF-2 syndrome. Spinal nerve sheath tumors arise from dorsal nerve roots and are often multiple. Pathologically these are true schwannomas, in contrast with spinal nerve sheath tumors in NF-1, which are neurofibromas (54).

Bilateral acoustic neuromas.   Symptoms referable to bilateral acoustic neuromas appear at a mean age of 20 years (51). This is in contrast with the nonhereditary forms of acoustic neuroma, which most frequently occur in the fifth and sixth decades. Over half of patients with NF-2 also have schwannomas involving the trigeminal or lower cranial nerves (15).

Pathologically, the term *acoustic neuroma* is a misnomer, since these tumors are actually schwannomas arising from the vestibular (not cochlear) division of the eighth cranial nerve (55). These tumors arise from Schwann cells that invest the cranial nerves as they penetrate the pia. Schwannomas are usually well encapsulated and microscopically exhibit alternating regions of compact (Antoni type A) and loose (Antoni type B) tissue architecture (55). Significant vascularity and evidence of microscopic hemorrhages are often present (55). As noted earlier, allelic deletions on chromosome 22 have been identified in acoustic neuromas associated with NF-2 (46).

Most patients present with unilateral or bilateral hearing loss, tinnitus, and cerebellar findings (51). Headache and altered mental status may be signs of hydrocephalus. Cranial nerve dysfunction may reflect direct neural compression by the acoustic neuroma or the presence of other cranial nerve schwannomas (15).

Magnetic resonance images typically show a well-demarcated extra-axial mass in the cerebellopontine angle that is hypo- to isointense to brain on T1-weighted sequences and hyperintense on T2-weighted images (2). These tumors generally enhance uniformly after gadolinium infusion, although they may appear heterogeneous secondary to necrosis or cystic degeneration (Fig. 4a). Calcification may be present, but is best visualized by CT. An MRI scan is extremely sensitive in the detection of purely intracanalicular tumors. Large tumors may compress the fourth ventricle and cause obstructive hydrocephalus. An MRI of the complete spine with gadolinium is essential in the detection of spinal schwannomas (See Fig. 4b).

The role and timing of surgery for bilateral acoustic neuromas has remained controversial, mainly because the growth rate of these tumors is quite variable. Previously, surgery was reserved for patients with progressive cranial nerve and brain stem dysfunction. However, late surgery was rarely associated with preservation of cranial nerve function (56). In 1987, the NIH Consensus Committee recommended consideration of early surgery for patients with small acoustic neuromas, in whom cranial nerve preservation would be more likely (10). Recently, Martuza and Eldridge have published general guidelines to help in the surgical management of these patients (49): (1) Patients who are asymptomatic, or who have mild hearing loss, should be followed expectantly with serial audiological and radiographic studies, since many of these tumors will exhibit indolent growth. (2) Patients with impaired but functional hearing, associated with contralateral hearing loss, should be closely observed. Preoperative deaf rehabilitation should be initiated. (3) Patients

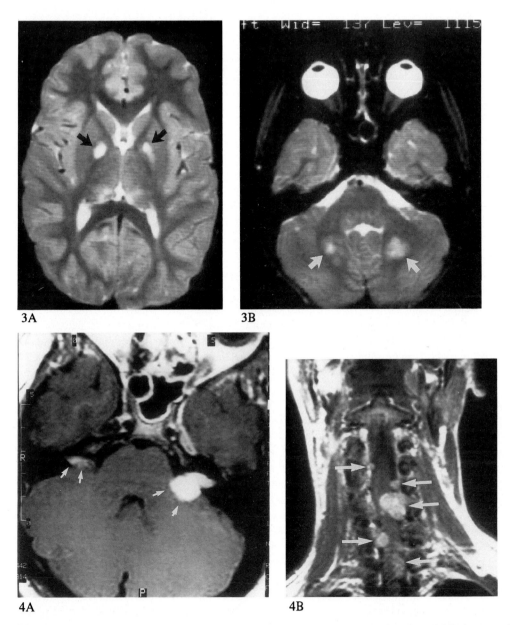

3A   3B

4A   4B

Figure 3 Heterotopias associated with neurofibromatosis type 1. Axial T2-weighted MR images show bilateral signal abnormalities within (A) the basal ganglia and (B) the cerebellum.

Figure 4 Neurofibromatosis type 2: (A) axial MR image with gadolinium demonstrates bilateral acoustic neuromas (arrows), which are pathognomonic of this syndrome; (B) coronal MR image after gadolinium infusion reveals multiple schwannomas within the cervical canal (arrows).

Table 2 Diagnostic Criteria for Neurofibromatosis Type 2

The diagnostic criteria are met if a person has either of the following:

1. Bilateral eighth nerve masses seen with appropriate imaging techniques (for example, CT or MRI)
2. A first-degree relative with neurofibromatosis type 2 and either a unilateral eighth nerve mass or two of the following:
   Neurofibroma
   Meningioma
   Glioma
   Schwannoma
   Presenile cataract

Source: Ref. 52.

with clinical or radiographic evidence of tumor progression, and who have functional hearing in the contralateral ear, should undergo microsurgical resection, with neurophysiological monitoring to preserve cranial nerve function. (4) Large tumors causing brain stem compression and neurological dysfunction should be debulked, regardless of the hearing status of the opposite ear.

The role of adjuvant external beam radiotherapy in the treatment of acoustic neuromas is unknown. Certainly, patients with partially resected tumors benefit from the addition of postoperative radiation therapy. In one study, patients with residual tumor treated with at least 4500 cGy had a 10-year disease-free survival of 94%, compared with 54% for patients not receiving radiotherapy (57). Recently, stereotactic radiosurgery has been used as primary treatment in a few patients with bilateral acoustic neuromas. Over half of the treated patients showed a reduction in tumor volume on radiographic studies (58). However, the follow-up period was too short (median 13 months) to assess long-term tumor control. In addition, several patients with serviceable hearing preoperatively experienced complete hearing loss, and there was a significant incidence of delayed trigeminal and facial nerve dysfunction, which was generally reversible (58). Thus, the efficacy and safety of stereotactic radiosurgery in the treatment of bilateral acoustic neuromas has not been fully defined and it therefore remains an experimental modality.

Meningiomas. Multiple meningiomas are a common feature of NF-2, occurring in up to half of these patients (15). Conversely, nearly 25% of meningiomas occurring before age 21 are associated with NF (59). Meningiomas arise from arachnoidal cells of the leptomeninges and choroid plexus. Although most have a dural attachment and grow as extra-axial masses, as many as one-third of meningiomas associated with NF grow within the ventricles (15).

Meningiomas associated with NF-2 are often asymptomatic and found incidentally. Focal neurological symptoms and seizures may occur in patients with parasagittal lesions and those of the convexity, and the specific features vary with location. Intraventricular tumors may cause only signs and symptoms of increased intracranial pressure secondary to hydrocephalus (60).

The MR images generally show a dural-based mass that is isotense with gray matter on both T1- and T2-weighted sequences (29). Gadolinium enhancement is usually homogeneous and helps define the frequent occurrence of multiple meningiomas (Fig. 5) (15). Although dense calcifications can be seen on MRI, CT is more sensitive in the detection of tumor mineralization and hypertrophy of the adjacent skull (hyperostosis) (29).

Asymptomatic meningiomas associated with NF-2 generally do not require surgical intervention, since their growth is often indolent. The surgical approach to symptomatic lesions is based on multiple considerations, including tumor size and location, growth rate, and patient's age. The exact surgical approach is dictated by anatomical location (e.g., convexity, base of skull, intraventricular). As extra-axial masses, most meningiomas retain an arachnoidal plane along the brain interface, which allows en bloc resection, causing minimal brain disruption.

Patients with partially resected meningiomas may benefit from the addition of postoperative radiation therapy (61–63). In one series, the recurrence rate was halved and the mean disease-free interval doubled by the addition of adjuvant radiation therapy (63). The appropriate timing of radiation therapy, however, remains controversial. Most advocate adjuvant treatment beginning within 3 months of surgery, whereas others withhold treatment until there is evidence of disease progression (61–64). In the pediatric population, age is an important determinant of the timing of radiation therapy after subtotal resection.

II. TUBEROUS SCLEROSIS

A. History

The syndrome of tuberous sclerosis (TS) has been described in the medical literature for more than 100 years; first by von Recklinghausen, and later by Bourneville, whose name is often associated with this syndrome (65). Then, at the turn of the century, Vogt described the triad of facial adenoma, mental retardation, and epilepsy that has become the hallmark of this disease.

B. Epidemiology and Genetics

Tuberous sclerosis (TS) affects 1 of every 10,000 births and, therefore, is the second most common phakomatosis (67). Inheritance is autosomal dominant, with near complete penetrance, but highly variable expression. However, most cases of TS are sporadic and reflect somatic mutations (67). Some of these sporadic cases may actually have a parent who is an unrecognized carrier of this disease because of minimal expression.

Molecular studies of the genome families affected by TS have yielded conflicting results. The gene responsible for TS was initially localized to the distal long arm of chromosome 9, based on an analysis of 19 families (68). A subsequent report implicated a locus on the long arm of chromosome 11, using linkage analysis (67). Recently, independent linkage analysis has demonstrated that TS is genetically heterogeneous, in that deletions at either the chromosome 9 or 11 loci may result in the clinical syndrome (69). It is unknown whether or not the clinical expression of this syndrome varies with the site of chromosomal loss.

C. Clinical Syndrome

Tuberous sclerosis is a syndrome characterized by multiple hamartomas affecting the skin, eyes, brain, and viscera. Central nervous system involvement is the rule, with as many as 80% of patients exhibiting mental retardation and epilepsy (66,70). More than half of patients present during the first year of life (65,71). The triad of adenoma sebaceum, mental retardation, and epilepsy is sufficient to make the clinical diagnosis of TS (Table 3). Radiographically, subependymal tubers are pathognomonic for this disease.

Dermatological manifestations of TS are prominent. Areas of hypopigmentation ("ash leaf" spots) are seen at birth in 70% of patients (66). Adenoma sebaceum are facial hamartomas that appear in a butterfly distribution during midchildhood in over 80% of patients (66). Less common lesions include shagreen patches, cafe au lait macules, and subungual fibromas. Ocular pathology is limited to retinal hamartomas, which are found in approximately one-half of TS patients and are generally asymptomatic (66). Common visceral manifestations include angiomyolipoma of the kidney, cardiac rhabdomyoma, and cystic lung disease.

1. Central Nervous System Involvement

Tubers.   The classic clinicopathologic finding in TS is the periventricular glial nodule, or subependymal tuber, which can be demonstrated in nearly all patients with the clinical diagnosis of TS (65). Subpial nodules, or cortical tubers, are also present in most TS patients (65).

Pathologically, tubers are hamartomas of the subependymal or subpial regions of the brain. They consist of foci of gliosis, which include both glial cells and neurons, and have both abnormal cell structure and tissue architecture (72).

Seizures are a common presenting symptom and usually appear during the first 6 months of life (73). The seizure may have a focal component, but is most commonly a myoclonic spasm (73). The electroencephalogram demonstrates the typical hypsarrhythmic tracing found in infantile spasms (73). Rarely, the seizure focus can be localized to a particular cortical tuber visualized on radiographic studies.

The incidence of significant mental retardation among TS patients varies from 50 to 80% (70). Early radiographic screening of noninstitutionalized seizure patients has demonstrated radiographic findings typical of TS in patients with normal intelligence (66). The degree of retardation does not appear to be correlated with ventricular size or cortical atrophy (66). Although patients with the largest number of subependymal and subpial nodules generally exhibit more profound retardation, there is no definite correlation between the number of lesions and intelligence (70). Thus, a retarded patient may have only one demonstrable lesion on imaging studies, whereas another patient may exhibit multiple lesions and have normal intelligence (70). A CT scan is still the most sensitive modality for the detection of subependymal tubers. These lesions appear as small calcific nodules projecting into the lateral ventricle, most commonly in the region of the caudate nucleus ("candle guttering") (Fig. 6a). They do not enhance after contrast administration. On MRI, tubers are slightly hyperintense to the periventricular gray matter on T1-weighted images and are contrasted by the surrounding low-intensity CSF (74). These lesions are less easily visualized on T2-weighted images because they have an intensity similar to the adjacent CSF, although large areas of calcification are more apparent on this sequence (75). Unlike CT, subependymal nodules may show patchy enhancement on MRI after gadolinium infusion (75). Subpial nodules are typically located in the cortex or subcortical white matter, and appear hypointense on T1-weighted images and hyperintense on T2-weighted images (74). The incidence of calcification within subpial tubers is approximately 50% and increases with age (65). Contrast enhancement is rare.

Subependymal and subpial tubers are benign lesions that do not require surgical intervention. Rarely, an intractable seizure focus can be localized to a particular cortical tuber and resection may be indicated to improve seizure control (66). The concern about periventricular tubers is the risk of transformation to a subependymal giant-cell astrocytoma (see next section).

Subependymal Giant-Cell Astrocytoma.   Subependymal giant-cell astrocytoma (SGCA) is the second most common CNS lesion in TS, affecting as many as 5% of patients (76). This frequency contrasts with the 15 and 100% incidence of brain tumors associated with NF-1 and NF-2, respectively. The mean age of presentation of SGCA is the early to midteens and there is no sex predisposition (76).

Pathologically, SGCA consists of bizarre spindle cells, gemistocytes, and occasionally giant ganglion cells (77). Arrangement of glial cells around vascular structures is often prominent and may be associated with microscopic hemorrhage (77). Focal areas of necrosis and mitoses are common and do not reflect malignant potential (78). An origin of these tumors from subependymal tubers has been postulated, based on two observations: (1) histological evidence of transitional forms between subependymal tuber and SGCA has been demonstrated (72), and (2) serial CT studies of individual patients have documented the transition from subependymal nodule to symptomatic tumor (79). Thus, it seems certain that a small percentage of subependymal tubers will transform to a true subependymal neoplasm.

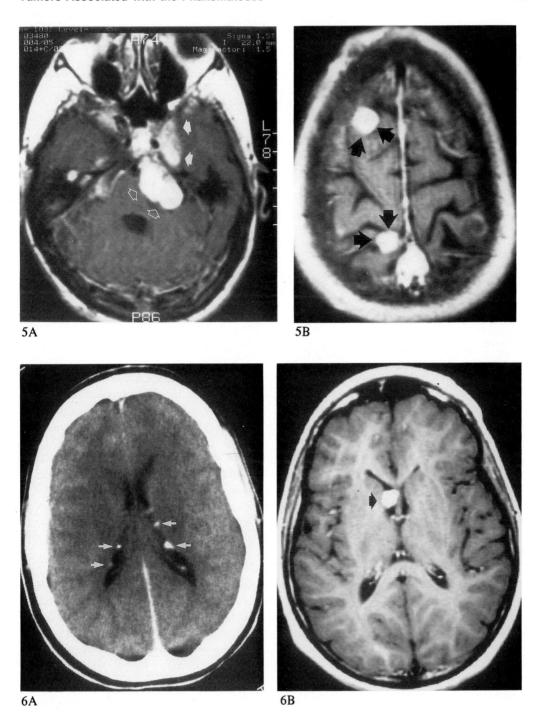

Figure 5 Multiple meningiomas in a patient with neurofibromatosis type 2: (A) axial MR image with gadolinium demonstrates dural-based, enhancing tumors within the temporal fossa (closed arrows) and adjacent to the brain stem (open arrows); (B) gadolinium-enhanced axial MR image near the vertex reveals additional convexity meningiomas (arrows).

Figure 6 Tuberous sclerosis: (A) axial CT image shows multiple calcified subependymal tubers lining the lateral ventricles (arrows); (B) axial MR image with gadolinium demonstrates an enhancing subependymal giant-cell astrocytoma within the frontal horn of the lateral ventricle (arrow).

Table 3 Diagnostic Features of Tuberous Sclerosis

Dermatologic
  Adenoma sebaceum[a]
  Shagreen patches
  Subungal fibromas
  Cafe au lait macules
Ocular
  Retinal hamartomas
Visceral
  Angiomyolipoma of kidney
  Cardiac rhabdomyoma
  Cystic lung disease
Central nervous system
Clinical
  Mental retardation[a]
  Myoclonic seizures[a]
Radiographic
  Subependymal tubers
  Subpial tubers
  Subependymal giant cell astrocytoma

[a]Represents Vogt's triad for the clinical diagnosis of tuberous sclerosis.

The SGCAs typically occur in the region of the foramen of Monro and obstruct CSF outflow, thereby producing signs and symptoms of increased intracranial pressure. Symptoms in infants include an enlarging head, irritability, vomiting, and lethargy, whereas those in older children or adults are intermittent headaches, nausea, and vomiting. Development of intractable seizures may also occur (79).

Radiographically, SCGAs are usually located near the foramen of Monro and may be multiple (2). Obstructive hydrocephalus is often present and may be asymmetric, reflecting unilateral foraminal obstruction (2). On MRI, SGCA appears as an enlarging intraventricular mass that has signal characteristics similar to the subependymal tuber. However, in comparison with tubers, SGCA appears more heterogeneous and enhances with contrast (see Fig. 6b) (75). Thus, an enlarging intraventricular mass that is contrast-enhancing usually signals the transition from glial nodule to neoplasm.

The surgical management of SGCA is based on the patient's neurological condition and the growth rate on imaging studies. An asymptomatic patient with a slowly enlarging intraventricular enhancing mass can be followed expectantly with serial radiographic studies (80). Patients who are symptomatic from obstructive hydrocephalus require surgical intervention. In the past, this consisted of unilateral or bilateral shunting procedures, without attempts at tumor resection (66). The development of modern neurosurgical techniques and improved neuroanesthetic support have allowed resection of these tumors through a transcallosal approach, with acceptable morbidity (80). Complete resection usually obviates the need for a shunting procedure. Large, vascular tumors may be amenable to only a partial resection. However, fenestration of the septum pallucidum at surgery will provide communication between the lateral ventricles and eliminate the need for a shunt. Newly developed endoscopic procedures allow biopsy of symptomatic periventricular nodules (to differentiate between subependymal tuber and SGCA), fenestration of the septum, and shunt placement through a single burr hole (Crone K, personal communication).

There is no modern study analyzing the possible benefit of megavoltage radiation therapy in the adjuvant treatment of SGCA, or at recurrence. Overall, the frequency of tumor recurrence is low, as evidenced by a 10-year survival of 80% after surgery (78).

III. VON HIPPEL–LINDAU DISEASE

A. History

Eugene von Hippel described hereditary hemangioblastomas involving the retina in 1904 (81). However, it was not until 1926 that Arvid Lindau recognized the association between retinal, cerebellar, and visceral hemangioblastomas (81). This syndrome was later termed *von Hippel–Lindau disease* by van der Hoeve as a tribute to both contributions in the understanding of this disease (81). Despite its inclusion in the group of neurocutaneous syndromes, there are no dermatological manifestations of von Hippel–Lindau disease.

B. Epidemiology and Genetics

von Hippel–Lindau (VHL) is an autosomal dominant disease that exhibits variable penetrance and expression. A positive family history can be obtained in up to 75% of patients when detailed pedigrees are constructed (85). Recognition of affected family members is further enhanced by the use of modern-imaging studies to screen at-risk family members (83).

Molecular studies have accurately mapped the gene responsible for VHL disease to the short arm of chromosome 3 (84). Closely linked DNA markers have been identified and should allow presymptomatic testing of patients at risk in the near future (84).

C. Clinical Syndrome

von Hippel–Lindau disease is characterized by hemangioblastomas involving the retina, viscera, and central nervous system. Diagnostic criteria advanced by Melman and Rosen in 1964 require two sites of involvement, with a negative family history, and one site when there is at least one other affected family member (Table 4) (85). The diagnosis of VHL is often difficult to establish in a patient with an isolated lesion, because the expression and age of onset of this disease is so highly variable. Because of the late onset of many features of VHL, it has been recommended that at-risk relatives receive regular screening with ophthalmological examination and imaging studies (81).

1. Systemic Features

As noted before, there are no dermatological manifestations of VHL disease. Ocular involvement by retinal hemangioblastomas occurs in as many as two-thirds of VHL patients and generally

Table 4 Diagnostic Features of von Hippel–Lindau Disease[a]

Ocular
  Retinal hemangioblastomas
Visceral
  Multicystic renal disease
  Renal cell carcinoma
  Pheochromocytoma
  Pancreatic cysts
  Epididymal cysts
Central nervous system
  Cerebellar hemangioblastomas
  Hemangioblastomas of other CNS locations (cortex, brain stem, spinal cord)

[a]*If negative family history*: Two anatomical sites of involvement are required for the diagnosis of von Hippel–Lindau disease. *If positive family history*: One anatomical site of involvement is required for the diagnosis of von Hippel–Lindau disease.

appears before involvement of other organs (mean age 21) (81). Approximately one-half of affected patients have multiple lesions, which are frequently bilateral (82). Although retinal hemangioblastomas may be asymptomatic, they usually pursue a progressive course, leading to retinal detachment and blindness (82). Early treatment of progressive lesions with cryotherapy or laser photocoagulation may prevent visual loss (81,82).

Visceral cysts commonly affect the kidney, pancreas, and epididymis. Multicystic renal disease occurs in 50% of patients and is usually asymptomatic (86). However, nearly one-fourth of VHL patients will progress to renal cell carcinoma (81). Renal cell carcinoma associated with VHL disease occurs at a younger age (mean age 43) and without sex predisposition, compared with sporadic cases (81). This tumor is frequently multifocal, metastasizes in 50% of patients, and is a significant cause of mortality in VHL patients (81). Pheochromocytomas occur in 10% of patients and may be bilateral (87).

2. Central Nervous System Involvement

Hemangioblastomas of the CNS can be demonstrated in as many as 72% of VHL patients when careful screening with modern imaging studies is performed (88). The sites of predilection include the cerebellum (52% of patients), spinal cord (44%), and brain stem (18%) (88). Supratentorial lesions are much less common.

Cerebellar Hemangioblastoma.   Cerebellar hemangioblastomas often present in the first or second decade (mean age 32), and there is a strong male preponderance (81,89). It should be noted that only 40% of patients with cerebellar hemangioblastomas are affected by VHL disease (81). The remainder are sporadic cases not part of a hereditary syndrome, and this group is generally older (fifth to sixth decades).

Hemangioblastomas are highly vascularized tumors that consist of three cellular components: lipid stromal cells, endothelial cells lining a capillary network, and pericytes (90). The numerous vascular channels and foamy stromal cells are reminiscent of renal cell carcinoma (86). As many as 75% of cerebellar hemangioblastomas are cystic and consist of a smooth cyst filled with xanthochromic fluid and a solid mural nodule (86). The polycythemia that frequently accompanies cerebellar hemangioblastoma is attributable to erythropoietinlike activity, which can be assayed from solid tumor, cyst contents, and even CSF (91). Immunohistochemical studies have identified small granular cells within hemangioblastomas that are responsible for the production of this hematopoietic factor (91).

Patients with cerebellar hemangioblastoma present with a duration of symptoms averaging 1 year (86). Occipital headaches and cerebellar symptoms are seen in 75% of patients (86). The specific cerebellar signs vary with location: midline tumors cause truncal ataxia, whereas dysmetria is more common in patients with laterally situated tumors. Specific cranial neuropathies reflect brain stem hemangioblastomas, and symptoms of increased intracranial pressure may result from obstructive hydrocephalus. As many as 30% of patients will demonstrate laboratory evidence of polycythemia (86). Although the absolute hemoglobin level is not generally informative, changes in this baseline value with treatment may correlate with tumor status (86).

Approximately 75% of cerebellar hemangioblastomas are cystic (86). On MRI, the cyst fluid is hyperintense to CSF, reflecting increased protein content. The mural nodule may be hypo- to isointense to brain on T1-weighted images and hyperintense on T2-weighted sequences (2). After gadolinium infusion, the mural nodule enhances uniformly; however, the cyst wall remains nonenhancing unless there is neoplastic involvement (Fig. 7a) (2). Solid tumors are best imaged after contrast infusion, and often areas of signal void are seen within the tumor, reflecting large vascular channels (see Fig. 7b) (92). Multiple lesions within the cerebellum, brain stem, or cervicomedullary junction are often visualized with gadolinium-enhanced MRI (88).

Surgery is indicated for symptomatic hemangioblastomas that are accessible by modern

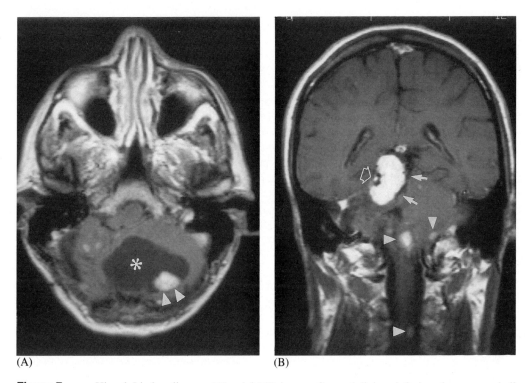

(A)   (B)

Figure 7   von Hippel–Lindau disease: (A) axial MR image after gadolinium infusion shows a cerebellar hemangioblastoma with a large cystic component (asterisk) and an enhancing mural nodule (arrowheads); (B) coronal MR image with gadolinium demonstrates a solid hemangioblastoma (closed arrows) arising at the tentorium, which contains areas of signal void representing large vascular channels (open arrow). Other cerebellar and cervical cord hemangioblastomas are also visualized (arrow heads).

microsurgical techniques. The classic cystic lesion of the cerebellar hemisphere is approached with the goals of cyst drainage and complete resection of the mural nodule. The cyst wall rarely exhibits neoplasic involvement and, therefore, can be left undisturbed. Large, solid tumors are frequently extremely vascular and require the intraoperative use of the neodymium:yttrium–aluminum–garnet (Nd:YAG) laser to devascularize the tumor during removal. Hemangioblastomas within the brain stem, or those that involve the exiting cranial nerves, may not be amenable to complete resection with acceptable neurological deficit.

Recurrence after previous complete resection is unusual and can be managed by repeat surgical resection (90). The role of radiation therapy in the treatment of hemangioblastoma is not fully defined. In one anecdotal report, preoperative irradiation produced a striking reduction in tumor volume (93). In addition, retrospective studies have demonstrated statistically significant improvement in local disease control when patients with residual disease were treated with at least 5000 cGy (90). Therefore, patients with unresectable or recurrent hemangioblastomas probably benefit from focal irradiation. The role of stereotactic radiosurgery in the treatment of primary or recurrent disease is unknown.

It must be emphasized that the spectrum of disease expression varies greatly among individuals. Therefore, patients diagnosed with VHL disease must be followed on a regular basis with ophthalmological examinations, MRI with gadolinium of the neuraxis, and CT or MRI of the abdomen.

V. SUMMARY

The phakomatoses, or neurocutaneous syndromes, are important clinical entities to all medical practitioners because of their multisystem involvement of the skin, eyes, viscera, and central nervous system. Knowledge of the pathognomonic skin, ocular, and visceral features of each syndrome will help identify patients who are at risk for the development of CNS neoplasms. This recognition will prompt early screening of these patients with MRI and allow earlier detection of CNS tumors. Conversely, all patients with a newly diagnosed brain tumor should be carefully evaluated for any stigmata suggesting the diagnosis of a neurocutaneous syndrome, since this would influence the diagnosis, treatment, and prognosis of the patient's tumor. In addition, recognition of a hereditary syndrome will allow screening of at-risk relatives by clinical examination, imaging studies, and DNA linkage studies. Lastly, optimal management of patients with phakomatoses requires a multidisciplinary approach to maximize the duration and quality of life of each patient and to advance our basic science and clinical understanding of these complex diseases.

ACKNOWLEDGMENTS

The author is indebted to William Ball, M.D. and Robert Lukin, M.D. for providing many of the MRI scans used in this chapter.

REFERENCES

1. Gomez MR. Preface. In: Gomez MR, ed. Neurocutaneous diseases. A practical approach. Boston: Butterworths, 1987:xi.
2. Braffman BH, Bilaniuk LT, Zimmerman RA, MR of central nervous system neoplasia of the phakomatoses. Semin Roentgenol 1990; 25:198–217.
3. Rubenstein AE. Neurofibromatosis. A review of the clinical problems. Ann NY Acad Sci 1986; 486:1–13.
4. Huson SM. Recent developments in the diagnosis and management of neurofibromatosis. Arch Dis Child 1989; 64:745–749.
5. Listernick R, Charrow J. Neurofibromatosis type 1 in childhood. J Pediatr 1990; 116:845–853.
6. Lewis RA, Gerson LP, Axelson KA, Riccardi VM, Whitford RP. von Recklinghausen neurofibromatosis. II. Incidence of optic gliomata. Ophthalmology 1984; 91:929–935.
7. Barker D, Wright E, Nguyen K, Cannon L, Fain P, Goldgar D, Bishop DT, Carey J, Baty B, Kivlin J, Willard H, Waye JS, Greig G, Leinwand L, Nakamura Y, O'Connell P, Leppert M, Lalouel J-M, White R, Skolnick M. Gene for von Recklinghausen neurofibromatosis is in the pericentromeric region of chromosome 17. Science 1987; 236:1100–1102.
8. Collins FS, Ponder BAJ, Seizinger BR, Epstein CJ. The von Recklinghausen neurofibromatosis region on chromosome 17. Genetic and physical maps come into focus. Am J Hum Genet 1989; 44:1–5.
9. Ward K, O'Connell P, Carey JC, Leppert M, Jolley S, Plaetke R, Ogden B, White R. Diagnosis of neurofibromatosis 1 by using tightly linked, flanking DNA markers. Am J Hum Genet 1990; 46:943–949.
10. Neurofibromatosis Conference Statement. National Institutes of Health consensus development conference. Arch Neurol 1988; 45:575–578.
11. Russell DS, Rubinstein LJ. Pathology of tumors of the nervous system. 5th ed. Baltimore: Williams & Wilkins, 1989:560–568.
12. Lubs M-LE, Bauer MS, Formas, ME, Djokic B. Lisch nodules in neurofibromatosis type 1. N Engl J Med 1991; 324:1264–1283.
13. Blatt J, Jaffe R, Deutsch M, Adkins JC. Neurofibromatosis and childhood tumors. Cancer 1986; 57:1225–1229.
14. Hochstrasser H, Boltshauser E, Valavanis A. Brain tumors in children with von Recklinghausen neurofibromatosis. Neurofibromatosis 1988; 1:233–239.

15. Aoki S, Barkovich AJ, Nishimura K, Kjos BO, Machida T, Cogen P, Edwards M, Norman D. Neurofibromatosis types 1 and 2. Cranial MR findings. Radiology 1989; 172:527–534.

16. Heideman RL, Packer RJ, Albright LA, Freeman CR, Rorke LB. Tumors of the central nervous system. In: Pizzo PA, Poplack DG, eds. Principles and practice of pediatric oncology. Philadelphia: JB Lippincott, 1989:505–553.

17. Warnick RE, Edwards MSB. Pediatric brain tumors. Curr Probl Pediatr 1991; 21:129–173.

18. Stern J, Jakobiel FA, Housepian EM. The architecture of optic nerve gliomas with and without neurofibromatosis. Arch Ophthalmol 1980; 98:505–511.

19. Tenny RT, Laws ER, Younge BR, Rush JA. The neurosurgical management of optic glioma. Results in 104 patients. J Neurosurg 1982; 57:452–458.

20. Hendrix LE, Kneeland JB, Haughton VM, Daniels DL, Szumowski J, Williams AL, Mark LP, Czervionke LF. MR imaging of optic nerve lesions. Value of gadopentetate dimeglumine and fat-suppression technique. AJNR 1990; 11:749–754.

21. Wong JYC, Uhl V, Wara WM, Sheline GE. Optic gliomas. A reanalysis of the University of California, San Francisco experience. Cancer 60; 1987:1847–1855.

22. Alford EC, Lofton S. Gliomas of the optic nerve or chiasm. Outcome by patient's age, tumor site, and treatment. J Neurosurg 1988; 68:85–98.

23. Kovalic JJ, Grigsby PW, Shepard MJ, Fineberg BB, Thomas PR. Radiation therapy for gliomas of the optic nerve and chiasm. Int J Radiat Oncol Biol Phys 1990; 18:927–932.

24. Packer RJ, Bilaniuk LT, Cohen BH, Braffman BH, Obringer AC, Zimmerman RA, Seiger KR, Sutton LN, Savino PJ, Zackai EH, Meadows AT. Intracranial visual pathway gliomas in children with neurofibromatosis. Neurofibromatosis 1988; 1:212–222.

25. Horwich A, Bloom HJG. Optic gliomas. Radiation therapy and prognosis. Int J Radiat Oncol Biol Phys 1985; 11:1067–1079.

26. Danoff BF, Kramer S, Thompson N. The radiotherapeutic management of optic gliomas in children. Int J Radiat Oncol Biol Phys 1980; 6:45–50.

27. DeSousa AL, Kalsbeck JE, Mealey J, Fitzgerald J. Diencephalic syndrome and its relation to opticochiasmatic glioma. Review of twelve cases. Neurosurgery 1979; 4:207–209.

28. Rodriguez LA, Edwards MSB, Levin VA. Management of hypothalamic gliomas in children. An analysis of 33 cases. Neurosurgery 1990; 26:242–247.

29. Barkovich AJ, Edwards MSB. Brain tumors in childhood. In: Barkovich AJ, ed. Pediatric neuroimaging. Vol. 1. New York: Raven Press, 1990:149–203.

30. Wisoff JH, Abbott R, Epstein F. Surgical management of exophytic chiasmatic–hypothalamic tumors in childhood. J Neurosurg 1990; 73:661–667.

31. Packer RJ, Sutton LN, Bilaniuk LT, Radcliffe J, Rosenstock JG, Siegel KR, Bunin GR, Savino PJ, Bruce DA, Schut L. Treatment of chiasmatic/hypothalamic gliomas of childhood with chemotherapy. An update. Ann Neurol 1988; 23:79–85.

32. Petronio J, Edwards MSB, Prados M, Freyberger S, Rabbitt J, Silber P, Levin VA. Management of chiasmal and hypothalamic gliomas of infancy and childhood with chemotherapy. J Neurosurg 1991; 74:701–708.

33. Bloom HJG, Glees J, Bell J. The treatment and long-term prognosis of children with intracranial tumors. A study of 610 cases, 1950–1981. Int J Radiat Oncol Biol Phys 1990; 18:723–745.

34. Rush JA, Younge BR, Campbell RJ, MacCarty CS. Optic glioma. Long-term follow-up of 85 histopathologically verified cases. Ophthalmology 1982; 89:1213–1219.

35. Bognanno JR, Edwards MK, Lee TA, Dunn DW, Roos KL, Klatte EC. Cranial MR imaging in neurofibromatosis. AJR 1988; 151:381–388.

36. Ilgren EB, Kinnier-Wilson LM, Stiller CA. Gliomas in neurofibromatosis: a series of 89 cases with evidence for enhanced malignancy in associated cerebellar astrocytomas. Pathol Annu, 1985; 20(part 1):331–358.

37. Chamberlain ML, Silver P, Levin VA. Poorly differentiated gliomas of the cerebellum. A study of 18 patients. Cancer 1990; 65:337–340.

38. Dohrmann GJ, Farnell JR, Flannery JT. Glioblastoma multiforme in children. J Neurosurg 1976; 44:442–448.

39. Marchese MJ, Chang CH. Malignant astrocytic gliomas in children. Cancer 1990; 65:2771–2778.
40. Sposto R, Ertel IJ, Jenkin RDT, Boesel CP, Venes JL, Ortega JA, Evans AE, Wara W, Hammond D. The effectiveness of chemotherapy for treatment of high grade astrocytoma in children. Results of a randomized trial. J Neurooncol 1989; 7:165–177.
41. Milstein JM, Geyer JR, Berger MS, Bleyer WA. Favorable prognosis for brainstem gliomas of neurofibromatosis. J Neurooncol 1989; 7:367–371.
42. Raffell C, McComb JG, Bodner S, Gilles FE. Benign brain stem lesions in pediatric patients with neurofibromatosis. Case reports. Neurosurgery 1989; 25:959–964.
43. Duffner PK, Cohen ME, Seidel FG, Shucard DW. The significance of MRI abnormalities in children with neurofibromatosis. Neurology 1989; 39:373–378.
44. Goldstein SM, Curless RG, Post JD, Quencer RM. A new sign of neurofibromatosis on magnetic resonance imaging of children. Arch Neurol 1989; 46:1222–1224.
45. Rubinstein LJ. The malformative central nervous system lesions in the central and peripheral forms of neurofibromatosis. A neuropathological study of 22 cases. Ann NY Acad Sci 1986; 486:14–29.
46. Seizinger BR, Martuza RL, Gusella JF. Loss of genes on chromosome 22 in tumorigenesis of human acoustic neuroma. Nature 1986; 322:644–647.
47. Seizinger BR, De La Monte S, Atkins L, Gusella JF, Martuza RL. Molecular genetic approach to human meningioma. Loss of genes on chromosome 22. Proc Natl Acad Sci USA 1987; 84:5419–5423.
48. Seizinger BR, Rouleau G, Ozelius LJ, Lane AH, St George-Hyslop P, Huson S, Gusella JF, Martuza RL. Common pathogenetic mechanism for three tumor types in bilateral acoustic neurofibromatosis. Science 1987; 236:317–319.
49. Martuza RL, Eldridge R. Neurofibromatosis 2 (bilateral acoustic neurofibromatosis). N Engl J Med 1988; 11:684–688.
50. Rouleau GA, Seizinger BR, Wertelecki W, Haines JL, Superneau DW, Martuza RL, Gusella JF. Flanking markers bracket the neurofibromatosis type 2 (*NF2*) gene on chromosome 22. Am J Hum Genet 1990; 46:323–328.
51. Kanter WR, Eldridge R, Fabricant R, Allen JC, Koerber T. Central neurofibromatosis with bilateral acoustic neuroma. Genetic, clinical and biochemical distinctions from peripheral neurofibromatosis. Neurology 1979; 30:851–859.
52. Mulvihill JJ. Background and biologic perspective. In: Mulvihill JJ, moderator. Neurofibromatosis 1 (Recklinghausen disease and neurofibromatosis 2 (bilateral acoustic neurofibromatosis). An update. Ann Intern Med 1990; 11:39–52.
53. Kaiser-Kupfer MI. Ophthalmic manifestations. In: Mulvihill JJ, moderator. Neurofibromatosis 1 (Recklinghausen disease and neurofibromatosis 2 (bilateral acoustic neurofibromatosis). An update. Ann Intern Med 1990; 11:39–52.
54. Halliday AL, Sobel RA, Matuza RL. Benign spinal nerve sheath tumors. Their ocurrence sporadically and in NF types 1 and 2. J Neurosurg 1991; 74:248–253.
55. Russell DS, Rubinstein LJ. Pathology of tumors of the nervous system. 5th ed. Baltimore: Williams & Wilkins, 1989:537–544.
56. Martuza RL, Ojemann RG. Bilateral acoustic neuromas. Clinical aspects, pathogenesis, and treatment. Neurosurgery 1982; 10:1–12.
57. Wallner KE, Sheline GE, Pitts LH, Wara WM, Davis RL, Boldrey EB. Efficacy of irradiation for incompletely excised acoustic neurilemomas. J Neurosurg 1987; 67:858–863.
58. Linskey ME, Lunsford LD, Flickinger JC. Radiosurgery for acoustic neurinomas. Early experience. Neurosurgery 1990; 26:736–745.
59. Deen GH, Scheithauer BW, Ebersold MJ. Clinical and pathological study of meningiomas of the first two decades of life. J Neurosurg 1982; 56:317–322.
60. Ferrante L, Acqui M, Artico M, Mastronardi L, Rocchi G, Fortuna A. Cerebral meningiomas in children. Childs Nerve Syst 1989; 5:83–86.
61. Taylor BW, Marcus RB, Friedman WA, Ballinger WE, Million RR. The meningioma controversy. Postoperative radiation therapy. Int J Radiat Oncol Biol Phys 1988; 15:299–304.
62. Carella RJ, Ransohoff J, Newall J. Role of radiation therapy in the management of meningioma. Neurosurgery 1982; 10:332–339.

63. Barbaro NM, Gutin PH, Wilson CB, Sheline GE, Boldrey EB, Wara WM. Radiation therapy in the treatment of partially resected meningiomas. Neurosurgery 1987; 20:525–528.

64. Solan MJ, Kramer S. The role of radiation therapy in the management of intracranial meningiomas. Int J Radiat Oncol Biol Phys 1985; 11:675–677.

65. Altman NR, Purser RK, Post MJD. Tuberous sclerosis. Characteristics of CT and MR imaging. Radiology 1988; 167:527–532.

66. Nagib MG, Haines SJ, Erickson DL, Mastri AR. Tuberous sclerosis. A review for the neurosurgeon. Neurosurgery 1984; 14:93–98.

67. Smith M, Smalley S, Cantor R, Pandolfo M, Gomez MI, Baumann R, Flodman P, Yoshiyama K, Nakamura Y, Julier C, Dumars K, Haines J, Trofatter J, Spence MA, Weeks D, Conneally M. Mapping of a gene determining tuberous sclerosis to human chromosome 11q14–11q23. Genomics 1990; 6:105–114.

68. Fryer AE, Connor JM, Povey S, Yates JRW, Chalmers A, Fraser I, Yates AD, Osborne JP. Evidence that the gene for tuberous sclerosis is on chromosome 9. Lancet 1987; 1:659–661.

69. Janssen LAJ, Sandkuyl LA, Merkens EC, Maat-Kievit JA, Sampson JR, Fleury P, Hennekam RCM, Grosveld GC, Lindhout D, Halley JJ. Genetic heterogeneity in tuberous sclerosis. Genomics 1990; 8:237–242.

70. Kingsley DPE, Kendall BE, Fitz CR. Tuberous sclerosis. A clinicoradiological evaluation of 110 cases with particular reference to atypical presentation. Neuroradiology 1986; 28:38–46.

71. Conzen M, Oppel F. Tuberous sclerosis in neurosurgery. An analysis of 18 patients. Acta Neurochir 106:106–109.

72. Russell DS, Rubinstein LJ. Pathology of tumors of the nervous system. 5th ed. Baltimore: Williams & Wilkins, 1989:767–768.

73. Curatolo P, Cusmai R, Pruna D. Tuberous sclerosis. Diagnostic and prognostic problems. Pediatr Neurosci 1985–86; 12:123–125.

74. Nixon Jr, Houser OW, Gomez MR, Okazaki H. Cerebral tuberous sclerosis. MR imaging. Radiology 1989; 170:869–873.

75. Martin N, Debussche C, DeBroucker T, Mompoint D, Marsault C, Nahum H. Gadolinium-DTPA enhanced MR imaging in tuberous sclerosis. Neuroradiology 1990; 31:492–497.

76. Frerebeau P, Benezech J, Segnarbieux F, Harbi H, Desy A, Marty-Double C. Intraventricular tumors in tuberous sclerosis. Childs Nerv Syst 1985; 1:45–48.

77. Russell DS, Rubinstein LJ. Pathology of tumors of the nervous system. 5th ed. Baltimore: Williams & Wilkins, 1989:116–117.

78. Shepherd CW, Scheithauer BW, Gomez MR, Altermatt HJ, Katzmann JA. Subependymal giant cell astrocytoma. A clinical, pathological, and flow cytometric study. Neurosurgery 1991; 28:864–868.

79. Morimoto K, Mogami H. Sequential CT study of subependymal giant-cell astrocytoma associated with tuberous sclerosis. Case report. J Neurosurg 1986; 65:874–877.

80. McLaurin RL, Towbin RB. Tuberous sclerosis. Diagnostic and surgical considerations. Pediatr Neurosci 1985–86; 12:43–48.

81. Huson SM, Harper PS, Hourihan MD, Cole G, Weeks RD, Compston DAS. Cerebellar haemangioblastoma and von Hippel–Lindau disease. Brain 1986; 109:1297–1310.

82. Hardwig P, Robertson DM. von Hippel–Lindau disease. A familial, often lethal, multi-system phakomatosis. Ophthalmology 1984; 91:263–270.

83. Neumann HPH, Eggert HR, Weigel K, Friedburg H, Wiestler OD, Schollmeyer P. Hemangioblastomas of the central nervous system. J Neurosurg 1989; 70:24–30.

84. Seizinger BR, Smith DI, Filling-Katz MR, Neumann H, Green JS, Choyke PL, Anderson KM, Freiman RN, Klauck SM, Whaley J, Decker HJH, Hsia YE, Collins D, Halperin J, Lamiell JM, Oostra B, Waziri MH, Gorin MB, Scherer G, Drabkin HA, Aronin N, Schinzel A, Martuza RL, Gusella JF, Haines JL. Genetic flanking markers refine diagnostic criteria and provide insights into the genetics of von Hippel–Lindau disease. Proc Natl Acad Sci USA 1991; 88:2864–2868.

85. Melmon KL, Rosen SW. Lindau's disease. Review of the literature and study of a large kindred. Am J Med 1964; 36:595–617.

86. Lamiell JM, Salazar FG, Hsia YE. von Hippel–Lindau disease affecting 43 members of a single kindred. Medicine 1989; 68:1–29.
87. Horton WA, Wong V, Eldridge R. von Hippel–Lindau disease. Clinical and pathological manifestations in nine families with 50 affected members. Arch Intern Med 1976; 136:769–777.
88. Filling-Katz MR, Choyke PL, Oldfield E, Charnas L, Patronas NJ, Glenn GM, Gorin MB, Morgan JK, Linehan WM, Seizinger BR, Zbar B. Central nervous system involvement in von Hippel–Lindau disease. Neurology 1991; 41:41–46.
89. De la Monte SM, Horowitz SA. Hemangioblastomas. Clinical and histopathological factors correlated with recurrence. Neurosurgery 1989; 25:695–698.
90. Smalley SR, Schomberg PJ, Earle JD, Laws ER, Scheithauer BW, O'Fallon JR. Radiotherapeutic considerations in the treatment of hemangioblastomas of the central nervous system. Int J Radiat Oncol Biol Phys 1990; 18:1165–1171.
91. Bohling T, Haltia M, Rosenlof K, Fyhrquist F. Erythropoietin in capillary hemangioblastoma. An immunohistochemical study. Acta Neuropathol 1987; 74:324–328.
92. Anson JA, Glick RP, Crowell RM. Use of gadolinium-enhanced magnetic resonance imaging in the diagnosis and management of posterior fossa hemangioblastomas. Surg Neurol 1991; 35:300–304.
93. Helle TL, Conley FK, Britt RH. Effect of radiation therapy on hemangioblastoma. A case report and review of the literature. Neurosurgery 1980; 6:82–86.
94. Sung DI, Chang CH, Harisiadis L. Cerebellar hemangioblastomas. Cancer 1982; 49:553–555.

19

Brain Metastases

**Alex J. Tikhtman and
Roy A. Patchell**
University of Kentucky, Lexington, Kentucky

I. INTRODUCTION

Metastasis to the brain is a deadly and debilitating condition developing at some point in 20–40% of the general cancer population. The grave prognosis of disseminated malignancy, with involvement of the central nervous system (CNS) has bred frustration and a sense of futility about treatment, with occasional arguments that therapy only prolongs the patient's suffering, if it prolongs life at all (35). However, we believe that such opinion reflects only a failure to select the group of patients for whom treatment holds the promise of a meaningful prolongation of life. Alternatively, research in the past at times has produced enthusiastic reports of therapeutic successes based on individual experience, anecdotal data, and uncontrolled trials, complicating the job of deciding what is best for one's patient.

Currently, many answers are incomplete owing to a lack of definitive randomized trials, especially concerning the role of chemotherapy and stereotactic radiosurgery for treatment of brain metastases. In this chapter, we will attempt to review the existing data on the management of parenchymal brain metastases and to develop a rational approach to diagnosis and therapy of this problem.

Systemic adrenocorticosteroids, whole-brain radiotherapy (WBRT) and surgery for single accessible metastases have established value in reversing neurological dysfunction and increasing survival. However, even after the use of these modalities, the median survival remains short, largely due to the progression of systemic disease or its complications. The average patient with brain metastases requires expeditious workup and therapy to enhance the quality of remaining life and to avoid prolonged hospitalization.

II. INCIDENCE

A marked discrepancy exists in the frequency of the intracranial metastases found in autopsy studies of cancer patients. Earlier studies reported the prevalence of about 5–10% (29,35).

This figure has risen dramatically over the years, and is currently at 20–40% for the adult cancer population (11,21,24) and 10–15% for pediatric cancer patients (36) at the time of death. Possible explanations accounting for this increased incidence of intracranial metastases include improved autopsy technique, increased premortem diagnosis owing to the advent of computed tomography (CT) and magnetic resonance imaging (MRI); longer survival of cancer patients, and changes in the incidence of tumor types, with an increase in lung cancer and malignant melanoma seen during the last three decades. Older neurosurgical series also tended to underestimate the actual prevalence of brain metastases because of a selection bias against surgery for patients with known systemic cancer.

Intracranial metastases currently represent slightly more than 50% of all malignant brain tumors (100). Most of these are intraparenchymal, with other sites involving the skull, dura, and leptomeninges. These lesions may produce symptoms by expanding in the brain parenchyma, or by occluding the cerebrospinal fluid (CSF) channels with secondary hydrocephalus.

From CT scan evidence, about 50% of brain metastases are single (21). These are defined as single intracranial lesions, with or without evidence of metastatic spread elsewhere in the body. When a single metastasis occurs as the only site of disease in the body, the term *solitary metastasis* is used, describing a rare entity. The exclusion of multiple brain metastases, possibly small and asymptomatic, depends on the sensitivity of imaging studies. Thus, with the use of a contrast-enhanced MRI, the population of patients thought to have single brain metastases may significantly shrink (18).

The histological type of the primary tumor usually dictates the frequency and pattern of intracranial spread, the clinical course and the response to therapy. In the United States, the most common sources of brain metastases currently are the lung, breast, gastrointestinal tract (mostly colon), genitourinary tract (mostly kidney), and skin (malignant melanoma), in that order (68,106). In the younger population (<21), brain metastases arise most commonly from sarcomas (osteogenic sarcoma, rhabdomyosarcoma, and Ewing's sarcoma), and germ cell tumors (97).

Multiple metastases usually occur in malignant melanoma (8) and to a lesser degree, in lung cancer. Metastases from colon, breast, and renal cell carcinoma are more often single.

III. PATHOPHYSIOLOGY

The mechanism by which most solid tumors produce brain metastases most likely involves hematogenous spread from primary or secondary sites in the lung. The distribution of these lesions within the brain, in numbers proportional to the relative blood flow to specific areas of the brain, supports this route of spread. Thus, 80% of metastases are found in the cerebral hemispheres, 15% in the cerebellum, and about 3% in the brain stem (21,77). In approximately 90% of patients with brain metastases of all tumor types, autopsy reveals lung involvement. Additional supportive evidence derives from the observation that primary lung cancer produces earlier brain involvement than other tumor types. Invasion of the pulmonary vasculature by an enlarging mass as well as the structurally abnormal capillary endothelium in the tumor tissue may allow the entry of malignant cells into the arterial circulation (11).

To account for the cases in which the lung is not invaded by cancer, spread to the brain by the passage of tumor emboli through a patent foramen ovale or Batson's vertebral venous plexus has been proposed. The role of Batson's plexus may be important in the production of brain metastases from gastrointestinal and pelvic primaries, accounting for the greater frequency of subtentorial lesions (three times that of other tumors) seen with these cancers (3,12,18).

Tumor cells tend to lodge at the gray–white junction and arterial watershed zones (21) and cause extensive vasogenic edema as the metastases enlarge, owing to the disruption of the capillary endothelium, which in turn allows the entry of fluid into the tumor tissue and surrounding brain parenchyma.

IV. THE CLINICAL PICTURE

Two-thirds of patients with brain metastases develop neurological symptoms during the course of their illness (11). Whether gradual or acute in onset, the symptoms are seldom specific enough to permit making a definite diagnosis. The progressive neurological dysfunction is usually related to the gradually expanding tumor mass and the associated edema, or to the development of obstructive hydrocephalus. Occasionally, a more acute onset may occur secondary to a seizure, hemorrhage into a metastasis, invasion or compression of an artery by tumor, or stroke caused by embolization from tumor foci in other organs (77).

The four most common presenting complaints are headache, focal weakness, cognitive dysfunction, and seizures. Less commonly, problems with gait, speech, or vision may be the sole complaints (77).

Headaches occur in 50% (43). These are often mild, diffuse, or bifrontal, having no localizing value. However, when focal, the headache may be localized to the site of the lesion in up to 70% of cases (89). The occurrence of an early-morning headache, thought to be associated with increased intracranial pressure, is described by 40% of tumor patients with headaches. Headaches are more common in patients with multiple metastases or with single ones in the posterior fossa. Their occurrence implies increased intracranial pressure secondary to brain edema or hydrocephalus, with traction exerted upon pain-sensitive structures, such as the venous sinuses or the dura at the base of the skull. However, papilledema, the classic hallmark of raised intracranial pressure, is now seen in fewer than 25% of patients upon presentation (77). This is due to earlier diagnosis using neuroimaging. The headaches may become more intense upon postural changes or straining and be associated with other symptoms characteristic of increased intracranial pressure (ICP), such as vomiting, visual blurring, confusion and, rarely, syncope.

Focal weakness is the presenting complaint of 18–40% of patients. Usually gradual in onset, a hemiparesis may be subtle and go unnoticed by the patient. One series found focal weakness in 67% of patients at the time of diagnosis, whereas only 18% complained of it upon presentation (77). The discrepancy in the frequency of signs and symptoms may be explained by the slowness with which the signs develop, frank denial, or the neglect seen with nondominant hemisphere involvement. The presence of hemiparesis often points toward tumor involvement of the contralateral hemisphere, with compromise of the motor cortex by tumor invasion or, more frequently, by edema caused by a more distant lesion.

Complaints of problems with memory, mood, and personality are made by one-third of the patients, whereas cognitive dysfunction, as evidenced by standard tests of mental status, may be present in as many as 75% (77).

Seizures occur in about 10% of patients as the first sign of metastases. However, up to 40% of patients develop seizures in the course of their disease (8,77,89). Seizures are usually focal or secondarily generalized after a focal onset. Malignant melanoma is the most common tumor type presenting with seizures, probably because of the cortical involvement often seen with multiple melanoma metastases (8,62).

The frequency of abnormal signs found in the absence of symptoms reflects the importance of a complete neurological examination for the early diagnosis of cerebral metastases.

V. DIAGNOSIS

Patients suspected of harboring brain metastases should undergo neuroimaging before therapy (such as steroids) is started. Steroids restore the blood–brain barrier and reduce the peritumoral edema. Thus, if started before imaging, they may preclude the entry of contrast agent into the tumor tissue, possibly causing a false-negative scan and a delaying in the diagnosis (88).

The diagnostic techniques used for the detection of brain metastases in the pre-CT era, including skull films, radionuclide scan, electroencephalogram (EEG), cerebral angiography, and pneumoencephalography, are less sensitive and less specific than CT and MRI and seldom contribute to the diagnosis when the latter are inconclusive (11). All patients should at least have a contrast CT. The addition of a precontrast scan adds improved ability to detect hemorrhage within the tumor, which otherwise may be obscured by contrast. The use of high-dose contrast and delayed imaging (double-dose delayed; DDD CT) further increases the sensitivity, yielding additional information in 67% of cases and revealing the lesions in 11.5% of patients with suspected brain metastases and negative contrast standard CT, according to one study (18).

MRI, especially when combined with the infusion of gadolinium (contrast MR) identifies nearly twice the number of definite metastases seen with DDD-CT (18). The advantages of CT include the lower cost, greater availability, often faster scan time, greater sensitivity to acute hemorrhage, tolerance to the presence of metal (life-support equipment, pacemakers, surgical clips) which precludes MRI, and the greater ease of administration to patients who are unstable or uncooperative (4,18).

As many as one-third of patients presenting with brain metastases do not have a prior diagnosis of cancer (68). The initial workup should include a thorough history, with a review of systems, which in 25% will suggest the primary site of cancer; a complete physical; routine chemistry analyses, liver function tests, blood smear, urinalysis, stool guaiac test, sputum cytologic evaluation, and a chest x-ray film. The latter will produce findings in up to 70% of cases, reflecting the high incidence of primary and secondary lung involvement in patients with metastases (4,68). If results of the initial workup are negative, on occasion, CT of the chest, abdomen, and pelvis will localize the primary, or suggest its source by the pattern of lymph node involvement. However, in spite of an extensive workup, at least 15% of patients with brain metastases may be expected to remain without a definite primary cancer site (68,99). Among the patients in whom the primary is found, most have lung cancer, with gastrointestinal tumors next most common (68). Patients in whom the primary is not found should have a brain biopsy to make a definitive diagnosis.

VI. DIFFERENTIAL DIAGNOSIS

A high level of suspicion for alternative diagnoses should be maintained in patients with presumed brain metastases, even when they already have cancer elsewhere. This is especially true for single brain lesions. A recent study showed an 11% rate of misdiagnosis of brain metastases in patients with a typical single lesion on CT and MRI of the head and a known primary (74). Primary brain tumors, hemorrhagic and ischemic infarcts, granulomas, and abscesses may mimic the clinical and imaging picture of metastases. When cancer patients show progressive neurological deterioration, but the CT of the head remains normal, additional possibilities to consider include metabolic encephalopathy, medication toxicity, leptomeningeal metastases, carcinomatous and infectious meningitis, progressive multifocal leukoencephalopathy, and degenerative changes related to radiotherapy.

On CT, brain metastases favor peripheral sites at the gray–white junction. Most are hypodense (except some adenocarcinomas, which may be hyperdense), have a round appearance, avid contrast enhancement, and significant peritumoral edema. The larger lesions may have a heterogeneous enhancement, producing a mottled appearance, whereas the smaller ones are often ring-enhancing. Hemorrhage within and around the tumor is often seen with metastases from malignant melanoma, choriocarcinoma and, to a smaller extent, from lung, kidney, and colon primaries. Calcifications are rarely seen within metastases, but are more common in the slower-growing primary brain tumors (4).

Primary brain tumors are usually single and larger than metastases upon presentation, possibly owing to a slower growth and less perifocal edema, although as many as 10% of gliomas are multifocal. Meningiomas are highly vascular, always adjacent to the meninges, and may occur at a higher rate in patients with breast cancer. If CT and MRI scans are inconclusive, angiography may show a vascular pattern characteristic of a meningioma or a glioblastoma, but usually a biopsy will be needed to resolve the issue (4).

Brain abscesses occur more often in cancer patients than in the general population. Patients at a higher risk are those with lymphomas, immunosuppression from chemotherapy, prior surgery and radiotherapy (because of the facilitated entry of microorganisms from the skin and sinuses). These patients may not have a fever or other signs of infection owing to the immunosuppression. The CT appearance may be identical with that of metastases, except for the tendency toward sites uncommon with metastases, such as the basal ganglia (4). A biopsy is indicated when any doubt exists about the nature of the lesion (11).

Ischemic infarction, at times, may be difficult to distinguish from tumor, especially in the subacute phase when accompanied with edema and contrast enhancement. An MRI scan may be of help in demonstrating a mass, or the CT scan may be repeated in 4 weeks, at which point most infarcts will "mature," showing sharper margins and a resolution of edema and enhancement. Infarcts are common in cancer patients, occurring in 15% at autopsy. Apart from the usual causes of stroke in the aging population, patients with a disseminated malignancy may develop a hypercoagulable state predisposing to cerebral thromboses, or a nonbacterial endocarditis with subsequent emboli to the cerebral circulation (11).

Thrombocytopenia in cancer patients with bone marrow suppression from chemotherapy and disseminated intravascular coagulation (DIC) increases the risk of intracranial hemorrhage, including intracerebral and subdural hematomas. When a cancer patient presents with an intracerebral hemorrhage, the diagnosis may be delayed, since the suspected presence of a metastases leading to the event often cannot be excluded by CT owing to the hyperdense appearance of the acute bleed. A contrast CT may show abnormal enhancement, raising the suspicion of an embedded mass, although within several days after a primary hemorrhage, some enhancement usually will develop even if tumor is not present. An MRI scan done hours to several days after the bleed may aid the diagnosis. Alternatively, the diagnosis may become apparent if the hematoma is evacuated or the scans repeated are in several weeks (11).

VII. TREATMENT

Without any specific therapy, patients with brain metastases develop progressive cognitive and motor dysfunction and increasing symptoms of raised intracranial pressure, with eventual obtundation and death. This will usually occur at about 4 weeks after the clinical diagnosis, usually as the direct result of neurological decompensation from brain herniation (26,42,48,66,83).

Current means of treatment for brain metastases include steroids, radiation therapy, conventional neurosurgery, chemotherapy, radiosurgery, and brachytherapy. The usefulness of these approaches to the individual patient may be limited by the extent of the intracranial and systemic metastases, as well as the tumor type.

A. Adrenocorticosteroids

Steroids are useful for reversing the neurological dysfunction caused by the vasogenic brain edema associated with brain metastases. These agents act by decreasing the permeability of the capillary endothelium, thereby reestablishing the blood–brain barrier (10,37). Occasionally, direct oncolytic effects have been noted in metastatic and primary CNS lymphoma but, in general, steroids are not cytotoxic. A prompt neurological improvement from the effects of the raised intracranial pressure and, to a lesser degree, from focal motor dysfunction usually occurs within several hours to 2 days after the medication is started. The favored agent is dexamethasone owing to its minimal mineralo-corticoid activity and a lower frequency of steroid-induced psychosis (11). The usual starting dose is 10 mg, iv or po, followed by 4 mg every 6 h. Occasional patients require higher doses to effect improvement. In the acutely neurologically decompensating patient with herniation, doses as high as 100 mg are indicated, coupled with additional emergency measures, such as hyperventilation, osmotic diuretics, and surgical decompression (7,11).

Treatment with regular doses of steroids for several days preoperatively or before starting radiation therapy may reduce postoperative brain swelling and decrease the frequency of adverse reactions to brain radiotherapy, although conclusive proof of a radioprotective role for steroids is lacking.

The common adverse acute side effects of steroid therapy include mental status changes (such as euphoria, confusion, occasionally delirium), hyperglycemia, sodium and water retention, and hypokalemia. Prolonged use may result in suppressed immune function, with increased rate of infection, peptic ulcer disease, increased catabolism, proximal muscle weakness caused by steroid-induced myopathy, and poor wound healing. A prophylactic H_2 blocker may be started to avoid gastrointestinal complications of steroid therapy.

The dose of dexamethasone should be tapered gradually over several weeks, upon the completion of brain radiotherapy or surgery to minimize long-term toxicity. Some patients may not tolerate the taper and redevelop the signs of brain edema. In such cases, the lowest effective dose may be continued. Steroid dependence is often an indication of an incomplete response to radiation therapy or surgery. During the taper, the patients may develop a steroid withdrawal syndrome, with symptoms of nausea, vomiting, and confusion. A repeat CT would help distinguish this problem from similar complaints caused by recurrent brain edema (11).

When steroids are used as the sole palliative treatment for brain metastases, the median survival is doubled from 1 to about 2 months, as compared with no treatment (42,47,62,82). This modest improvement in survival, however, attesting to the favorable risk/benefit ratio of therapy, does not reflect the frequently dramatic functional improvement and greater patient independence imparted by steroid therapy. Unfortunately, without additional treatment, after initial recovery most of these patients will experience a progression of neurological decline caused by tumor growth, and many will die of neurological causes.

B. Radiation Therapy

The palliative effects of radiation therapy for brain metastases were first reported in 1954 by Chao et al. (9). Since then, radiation therapy has become the treatment of choice for most patient with brain metastases. About two-thirds of treated patients show neurological improvement. The median survival is increased modestly, to 3–6 months (6,10,48,66,69,72,106). Over half of the patients treated with whole-brain radiation therapy die of progressive systemic disease, with stable neurological function. Thus, whole-brain radiation therapy provides adequate control of in-tracranial metastases in most patients. Although rare, sterilization of cerebral metastases by radiation therapy alone has been observed (10). Usually, radiation therapy begins after the patient has been started on a regimen of corticosteroids, which are continued until the patient completes radiotherapy. Whether the steroids prevent the occasional transient worsening of symptoms seen during radiotherapy has never been proven.

The optimum total radiation dose, the number of subfractions, and the schedule of treatments has not been determined. Several large multi-institutional trials performed by the Radiation Therapy Oncology Group (RTOG) (6,34,43,55) reported no significant difference in the neurological control of disease or the length of survival among various total doses, ranging from 2000 to 5000 cGy. Total doses lower than 2000 cGy appear to be less effective. Increased focal radiation to the tumor site has not been effective (48). Typical radiation treatment schedules used for brain metastases consist of short courses (7–15 days) of whole-brain radiation with relatively high doses per fraction (150–400 cGy/day), and total doses usually in the range of 3000–5000 cGy. Such regimens decrease the time spent in therapy while delivering adequate amounts of radiation. The daily dose should be reduced in patients with good prognosis (e.g., solitary resectable metastases), since a large proportion of long-term survivors may otherwise have some degree of dementia and leukoencephalopathy related to high-dose/fractionation schedules (19,73).

The role of radiation therapy when given to patients who have had an apparent complete surgical resection is controversial. The several currently existing uncontrolled nonrandomized, retrospective trials that examine the question (18,25,35,82) have found no increase in survival from the addition of postoperative radiation therapy. However, in most of the studies, there has been a small increase observed in the number of recurrent brain metastases in the patients who were not irradiated. This question is currently being examined in a large multigroup national trial, although it will be several years before the definitive answer is known. At present, patients who have had a complete resection and who have long expected survivals may benefit from not receiving immediate radiation therapy. On the other hand, patients with any suggestion of residual disease should get postoperative whole-brain radiation therapy.

C. Surgery

Despite the possible palliative advantages of surgical treatment, until recently the efficacy of surgery for brain metastases in improving survival of cancer patients has been unclear because of the lack of controlled trials. Numerous uncontrolled surgical series have shown longer survival of surgically treated patients when compared with historical controls treated with whole-brain radiotherapy alone (15,24,26,63,93,101,102). Retrospective reports of uncontrolled studies of patients treated with whole-brain radiotherapy only and surgery plus whole-brain radiotherapy have also generally shown an increased survival in the surgically treated patients (65).

A recent prospective randomized trial was performed at the University of Kentucky (74) in which 48 patients with known systemic cancer and a single brain lesion were treated with either biopsy of the suspected brain metastasis plus whole-brain radiation or complete surgical resection of the metastasis plus whole-brain radiation. The radiation doses were the same in both groups and consisted of a total dose of 3600 cGy given as 12 daily fractions of 300-cGy each. There was a statistically significant increase in survival in the surgical group (40 versus 15 weeks). In addition, the time to recurrence of brain metastases and the duration of functional independence were significantly longer in the resection group.

Although the data came from a relatively small study, the results clearly demonstrated that surgical resection was of benefit. Surgery plus postoperative whole-brain radiotherapy is now the treatment of choice for a single accessible brain metastasis.

Surgical resection of brain metatases is unfortunately not an option for most patients with this problem. Since approximately 50% of patients with brain metastases have a single lesion, and half of these are not surgical candidates because of extensive systemic disease or the inaccessibility of the lesion, only 25% of all patients with brain metastases may benefit from surgery as the initial treatment (75). Other potential roles of surgery include exploration to establish a tissue diagnosis, palliation of an unresectable large tumor by debulking, and emergency decompression in patients with impending herniation.

D. Radiosurgery

An increasingly available option in the United States is the technique of delivering high doses of ionizing radiation to discrete small intracranial targets using stereotactically directed beams of radiation, which was pioneered by Leksell and Larsson in Sweden in the 1950s (55). The gamma knife and the linear accelerator are the two types of units in current use (54,58). The first gamma knife in the United States started operation in 1987 in Pittsburgh, where its major application has been directed against vascular lesions and benign tumors (57).

Despite the use of stereotactic radiosurgery in the treatment of tumors for almost 40 years, no controlled studies exist that examine whether the radiosurgery is of any benefit in the treatment of brain metastases. To date, the literature consists of small series and individual case reports of highly selected patients (see also Chap. 26). There has been almost no quantitative survival data or toxicity data presented. More recently, there have been a few studies that appear to show that some shrinkage of metastatic lesions occurs after treatment with the gamma knife. Whether a shrinkage of lesions will translate into a meaningful increase in survival or decrease in neurological mobidity and mortality remains to be demonstrated. An ongoing randomized trial (Joint Center for Radiation Therapy, Boston) will compare the actual effectiveness of radiosurgery as initial therapy against conventional surgery, both followed by whole-brain irradiation. Radiosurgery now remains an unproved but possibly effective treatment for those patients who are not surgical candidates or have unresectable disease.

E. Chemotherapy

The results of chemotherapy in the treatment of brain metastases have been disappointing (11,37,88). Although the disrupted tumoral blood–brain barrier may permit more effective entry for chemotherapeutic agents, the technical difficulties of delivering chemotherapeutic at an adequate dose to all parts of the tumor have been a limitation. Corticosteroids, frequently used early in the management of brain metastases, tend to reconstitute the blood–brain barrier and to further decrease penetration into drug the tumor (88).

Patients with brain metastases from certain tumor types, such as breast cancer (80), germ cell tumors (88) and small-cell lung cancer (61), appear to respond to chemotherapy more frequently than patients with other solid tumors (1). However, chemotherapy is fraught with many potential side effects, including significant neurotoxicity, which can be detrimental to the quality of life (51). Efforts to study the effect of chemotherapy on the survival of patients with brain metastases have been inconclusive, secondary to the lack of randomized, controlled trials.

Currently, chemotherapy is probably best reserved for the management of patients with brain metastases from chemosensitive primaries who are not surgical candidates because of multiple brain metastases or extensive systemic disease.

F. Interstitial Brachytherapy

The use of interstitial brachytherapy (see also Chap. 25), a technique involving the placement of radioactive implants within the area of tumor, has been advocated in selected patients. The implants allow delivery of high-dose focal radiation to the tumor, while minimizing the risk of significant radiation exposure to the surrounding normal brain tissue because of the rapid falloff of radiation intensity at the margins of the precalculated target area. Both permanent and removable implants have been used. The placement may be accomplished stereotactically or during surgery. In one series, a median survival of 80 weeks after brachytherapy was achieved in patients with controlled systemic disease at the time of treatment (78). The major complication of brachytherapy is radiation necrosis, which may present with the clinical and imaging picture of an expanding mass months after treatment. A biopsy at times is required to differentiate tumor necrosis from recurrence; steroids and surgical resection may help to reverse the neurological progression secondary to the radiation necrosis. The incidence of this complication appears to vary with the total dose of radiation given (46).

Along with radiosurgery, this technique may offer an additional treatment option for patients with nonresectable metastases or prior maximal doses of whole-brain radiotherapy.

VIII. TREATMENT OF RECURRENT BRAIN METASTASES

Another difficult and frequently encountered clinical problem is the treatment of recurrent brain metastases. The recurrence of brain metastases is often complicated by the fact that many of these patients also have extensive systemic disease. In general, the same types of treatment used for newly diagnosed brain metastases are also available for recurrences. However, the type of previous therapy may limit the therapeutic options available for treatment of the recurrence.

In the patient with a recurrence, who initially had a single metastasis treated by surgery alone (without postoperative radiotherapy), all methods of treatment (including a full course of whole-brain radiation therapy) are available, and the situation is virtually identical to a newly diagnosed metastasis. More commonly, patients with recurrence have already received radiation therapy to the brain, and the previous radiation therapy limits the amount of subsequent radiation that can be safely given. In these patients, the amount of additional radiation that can be given is usually in the range of 1500–2500 cGy, and this dose range is usually too low to control the tumor (41,88). Several uncontrolled studies have found no meaningful increase in survival or control of neurological symptoms in patients who were reirradiated following recurrence of brain metastases. However, these studies consisted of relatively heterogeneous patient groups with extensive disease and a large proportion of radioresistant tumors. A recent study by Cooper et al. (17) suggests that reirradiation may be somewhat more beneficial in the subpopulation of patients who had an initial favorable response to radiotherapy and were in good general condition when they developed the recurrence in the brain. However, even in this favorable subgroup, only 42% of patients had symptomatic improvement, and the median survival after reirradiation was only 5 months. Despite the relatively poor results with reirradiation, additional radiotherapy is frequently the only treatment option for patients with recurrent disease.

Stereotactic radiosurgery, using either a linear accelerator or a gamma knife, has been used to treat recurrent brain metastases. Radiosurgery has the theoretical advantage of being able to deliver large doses of additional radiation to small areas of the brain. Loeffler et al. (56) reported a series of 18 patients with recurrent tumors who were treated with a linear accelerator. The treated lesions were apparently controlled with a decrease in size or stabilization posttreatment. Quantitative survival data were not reported, however. Further studies are therefore needed to determine the true value of stereotactic radiosurgery in the management of recurrent brain metastases.

Conventional surgery for recurrent tumors is an option only in patients who have a single recurrence and who are in reasonably good general condition. The experience with reoperation is limited. Sundaresan et al. (94) reported a series of 21 patients, who were treated with craniotomy for their initial brain metastases and underwent a second craniotomy for recurrence. After the second operation, two-thirds experienced neurological improvement, and the median survival after surgery for the recurrence was 9 months. These patients were a select group with relatively little systemic disease and a recurrent single metastasis. The results in patients who received only radiotherapy as the treatment of the initial brain metastases and who were then treated with surgery at recurrence appear to be less favorable. A study from Memorial Sloan–Kettering Cancer Center included patients who were treated with surgery after failing whole–brain radiation therapy as initial therapy (75). The median survival after surgery for recurrence was 5 months, but the group as a whole had a shorter overall survival than comparable patients treated with surgery plus whole-brain radiation therapy as the initial treatment of newly diagnosed brain metastases. The value of brachytherapy for recurrent metastases is unclear. Chemotherapy has also been used to treat recurrent metastatic tumors but its benefits have not been documented.

REFERENCES

1. Athanassiou A, Begent RHJ, Newlands ES, Parker D, Rustin GJS, Bagshawe KD. Central nervous system metastases of choriocarcinoma. Cancer 1983; 52:1728–1735.
2. Bakay L. Results of surgical treatment of intracranial metastasis from pulmonary cancer. J Neurosurg 1958; 15:338–341.
3. Batson OV. The function of the vertebral veins and their role in the spread of metastases. Ann Surg 1940; 112:138–149.
4. Benton JR, Steckel RJ, Kagan AR. Diagnostic imaging in clinical cancer management: brain metastases. Invest Radiol 1988; 23:335–341.
5. Berry HC, Parker RG, Gerdes AJ. Irradiation of brain metastases. Acta Radiol Ther 1974; 13:535–544.
6. Borgelt B, Gelber R, Kramer S, Brady LW, Chang CH, Davis LW, Perez CA, Hendrickson FR. The palliation of brain metastases: final results of the first two studies by the Radiation Therapy Oncology Group. Int J Radiat Oncol Biol Phys 1980; 6:1–9.
7. Black P. Brain metastasis: current status and recommended guidelines for management. Neurosurgery 1979; 5:617–631.
8. Byrne TN, Cascino TL, Posner JB. Brain metastasis from melanoma. J Neurooncol 1983; 1:313–317.
9. Chao J-H, Phillips R, Nickson JJ. Roentgen-ray therapy of cerebral metastases. Cancer 1954; 7:682–688.
10. Cairncross JG, Kim J-H, Posner JB. Radiation therapy for brain metastases. Ann Neurol 1980; 7:529–541.
11. Cairncross JG, Posner JB. The management of brain metastases. In: Walker, ed. Oncology of the nervous system. Boston: Martinus Nijhoff, 1983:341–377.
12. Cairncross JG, Cheenik NL, Kim J-H, Posner JB. Sterilization of cerebral metastases by radiation therapy. Neurology 1979; 29:1195–1202.
13. Cascino TL, Byrne TN, Deck MDF, Posner JB. Intra-arterial BCNU in the treatment of metastatic brain tumors. J Neurooncol 1983; 1:211–118.
14. Castaldo JE, Bernat JL, Meier FA, Schned AR. Intracranial metastases due to prostatic carcinoma. Cancer 1983; 52:1739–1747.
15. Catinella FP, Kittle CF, Faber LP, Milloy FJ, Warren WH, Von Roenn KA. Surgical treatment of primary lung cancer and solitary intracranial metastasis. Chest 1989; 95:972–975.
16. Chu FCH, Hilaris BB. Value of radiation therapy in the management of intracranial metastases. 1961; Cancer 14:577–581.
17. Cooper JS, Steinfeld AD, Lerch IA. Cerebral metastases: value of re-irradiation in selected patients. Radiology 1990; 174:883–885.
18. Davis PC, Fludgins PA, Peterman SB, Hoffman JC. Diagnosis of cerebral metastases: double-dose delayed CT vs contrast-enhanced MR imaging. AJNR 1991; 12:293–300.
19. DeAngelis CM, Delattre JY, Posner JB. Radiation-induced dementia in patient cured of brain metastases. Neurology 1989; 39:789–796.
20. DeAngelis LM, Mandell LR, Thaler HT, et al. The role of postoperative radiotherapy after resection of single brain metastases. Neurosurgery 1989; 24:798–805.
21. Delattre JY, Krol G, Thaler HT, Posner, JR. Distribution of brain metastases. Arch Neurol 1988; 45:741–744.
22. Derby BM, Guiang RL. Spectrum of symptomatic brain-stem metastasis. J Neuro–Neurosrug Psychiatry 1975; 38:888–895.

23. Deutsch M, Parsons JA, Mercado R. Radiotherapy for intracranial metastases. Cancer 1974; 34:1607–1611.

24. Deviri E, Schachner A, Halevy A, Shalit M, Levy MJ. Carcinoma of lung with a solitary cerebral metastasis. Cancer 1983; 52:1507–1509.

25. Diener-West M, Dobbins TW, Phillips TL, Nelson DF. Identification of an optimal subgroup for treatment evaluation of patients with brain metastases using RTOG study 7916. Int J Radiat Oncol Biol Phys 1989; 16:669–673.

26. DiStefano A, Yap HY, Hortobagyi GN, Blumenschein GR. The natural history of breast cancer patients with brain metastases. Cancer 1979; 44:1913–1918.

27. Dosoretz DE, Blitzer PH, Russell AH, Wang CC. Management of solitary metastasis to the brain: The role of elective brain irradiation following complete surgical resection. Int J Radiat Oncol Biol Phys 1980; 6:1727–1730.

28. Doyle TJ. Brain metastasis in the natural history of small-cell lung cancer. Cancer 1982; 50:752–754.

29. Earle KM. Metastatic and primary intracranial tumors of the adult male. J Neuropathol Exp Neurol 1954; 13:448–454.

30. Egawa S, Tukiyama I, Akine Y, Kajiura Y, Yanagawa S, Watai K, Nomura K. Radiotherapy of brain metastases. Int J Radiat Oncol Biol Phys 1986; 12:1621–1625.

31. Eyre HJ, Ohlsen JD, Frank J, LoBuglio AF, Cracken JD, Waterall JJ, Mansfield CM. Randomized trial of radiotherapy versus radiotherapy plus metronidazole for the treatment metastatic cancer to the brain. J Neurooncol 1984. 2:325–330.

32. Galicich JH, Sundaresan N, Arbit C, Passe S. Surgical treatment of single brain metastasis: factors associated with survival. Cancer 1980; 45:381–386.

33. Gamache FW, Galicich JH, Posner JB. Treatment of brain metastases by surgical extirpation. In: Weiss L, Gilbert H, Posner J, eds. Brain metastasis. Boston: GK Hall & Co, 1980:390–414.

34. Gelber RD, Larson M, Borgett BB, Kramer S. Equivalence of radiation schedules for the palliative treatment of brain metastases in patients with favorable prognosis. Cancer 1981; 48:1749–1753.

35. Grant FC. Concerning intracranial malignant metastases: their frequency and the value of surgery in their treatment. Ann Surg 1926; 84:635–646.

36. Graus F, Walker RW, Allen JC. Brain metastases in children. J Pediatr 1983; 103:635–646.

37. Greig NH. Chemotherapy of brain metastases: current status. London: Academic Press, 1984:157–186.

38. Haft H, Wang GC. Metastatic liposarcoma of the brain with response to chemotherapy: case report. Neurosurgery 1988; 23:777–780.

39. Hagen N, Cirrincione C, DeAngelis LM. The role of radiotherapy after resection of single brain metastases from melanoma. Neurology 1989; (suppl. 1): 39–262.

40. Hasse J. Surgery in bronchial carcinoma with metastasis. Lung 1990; (suppl): 1145–1152.

41. Hazuka MB, Kinzie JJ. Brain metastases: results and effects of re-irradiation. Int J Radiat Oncol Biol Phys 1988; 15:433–437.

42. Hazra T, Mullins GM, Lott S. Management of cerebral metastasis from bronchogenic carcinoma. Johns Hopkins Med J 1972; 130:377–383.

43. Hendrickson FR. The optimum schedule for palliative radiotherapy for metastatic brain cancer. Int J Radiat Oncol Biol Phys 1977; 2:165–168.

44. Hendrickson FR. Radiation therapy of metastatic tumors. Semin Oncol 1975; 2:43–46.

45. Hendrickson FR, Lee M-S, Larson M, Gelber RD. The influence of surgery and radiation therapy on patients with brain metastases. Int J Radiat Oncol Biol Phys 1983; 9:623–627.

46. Heros DO, Kasdon DL, Chun M. Brachytherapy in the treatment of recurrent solitary brain metastases. Neurosurgery 1988; 23:733–737.

47. Horton J, Baxter DH, Olson KB. The management of metastases to the brain by irradiation and corticosteroids. Am J Radium Ther Nuclear Med 1971; 3:334–335.

48. Hoskin PJ, Crow J, Ford HT. The influence of extent and local management on the outcome of radiotherapy for brain metastases. Int J Radiat Oncol Biol Phys 1990; 19:111–115.

49. Ichinose Y, Hara N, Ohta M, Motohiro A, Hata K, Yagawa K. Brain metastases in patients with limited small cell lung cancer achieving complete remission. Chest 1989; 96:1332–1335.

50. Ishizuka T, Tomoda Y, Kaseki S, Gotto S, Hara T, Kobayashi T. Intracranial metastasis of choriocarcinoma. Cancer 1983; 1896–1903.

51. Kleisbauer JP, Vesco D, Orehek J, Blaive B, Clary C, Poirer R, Saretto S, Carles P, Dongay G, Guerin JC, Martinal Y. Treatment of brain metastases of lung cancer with high doses of etoposide (VP16-213). Eur J Cancer Clin Oncol 1988; 24:131–135.

52. Komaki R, Cox JD, Stark R. Frequency of brain metastasis in adenocarcinoma and large cell carcinoma of the lung: correlation with survival. Int J Radiat Oncol Biol Phys 1983; 9:

53. Kurtz JM, Gelber R, Brady LW, Carella RJ, Cooper JS. The palliation of brain metastases in a favorable patient population: a randomized clinical trial by the Radiation Therapy Oncology Group. Int J Radiat Oncol Biol Phys 1981; 7:891–895.

54. Leksell L. Stereotactic radiosurgery. J Neurol Neurosurg Psychiatry 1983; 46:797–803.

55. Loeffler JS, Alexander E III, Kooy HM, Wen PY, Fine HA, Black PM. Radiosurgery for brain metastases. Principles Pract Oncol 1991; 5:1–11.

56. Loeffler JS, Kooy HM, Wen PY, Fine HA, Cheng C-W, Mannarino EG, Tsai JS, Alexander E III. The treatment of recurrent brain metastases with stereotactic radiosurgery. J Clin Oncol 1990; 8:576–582.

57. Lunsford LD, Flickinger J, Coffey RH. Stereotactic gamma knife radiosurgery. Arch Neurol 1990; 47:169–175.

58. Lutz W, Winslou KR, Maleki PV. A system for stereotactic radiosurgery with a linear accelerator. Int J Radiat Oncol Biol Phys 1988; 14:373–381.

59. MacGee EE. Surgical treatment of cerebral metastases from lung cancer. J Neurosurg 1971; 35:416–420.

60. McIntosh R, Thatcher N. Management of the solitary metastasis. Thorax 1990; 45:909–911.

61. Madajewicz S, West CR, Park HC, Ghoorah J, et al. Phase II study—intra-arterial BCNU therapy for metastatic brain tumors. Cancer 1981; 47:653–657.

62. Madajewicz S, Karakousis C, West CR, Caracandas J, Avellanosa AM. Malignant melanoma brain metastases. Cancer 1984; 53:2550–2255.

63. Magilligan DJ, Duvernoy C, Malik G, Lewis JW, Knighton R, Ausman JI. Surgical approach to lung cancer with solitary cerebral metastasis: twenty-five year experience. Ann Thorac Surg 1986; 42:360–364.

64. Mahaley MS Jr. Commentary on diagnosis and surgical management of metastatic brain tumors. J Neurooncol 1987; 4:193–193.

65. Mandell L, Hilaris B, Sullivan M, Sundaresan N, et al. The treatment of single brain metastasis from non-oat cell lung carcinoma. Surgery and radiation versus radiation therapy alone. Cancer 1986; 58:641–649.

66. Markesbery WR, Brooks WH, Gupta GD, Young AB. Treatment for patients with cerebral metastases. Arch Neurol 1978; 35:754–756.

67. Martini N. Rationale for surgical treatment of brain metastasis in non-small cell lung cancer. Ann Thorac Surg 1986; 42:357–358.

68. Merchut MP. Brain metastases from undiagnosed systemic neoplasms. Arch Intern Med 1989; 149:1076–1180.

69. Montana GS, Meacham WF, Caldwell WL. Brain irradiation for metastatic disease of lung origin. Cancer 1972; 29:1477–1480.

70. Neuwelt EA, Specht HD, Barnett PA, Dahlborg SA, et al. Increased delivery of tumor-specific monoconal antibodies to brain after osmotic blood–brain barrier modification in patients with melanoma metastatic to the central nervous system. Neurosurgery 1987; 20:885–895.

71. Newman SJ, Hansen HH. Frequency, diagnosis and treatment of brain metastases in 247 consecutive patients with bronchogenic carcinoma. Cancer 1974; 33:492–496.

72. Order SE, Hellman S, Von Essen CF, Kligerman MM. Improvement in quality of survival following whole brain irradiation for brain metastasis. Neurology 1968; 91:149–153.

73. Paleologos NA, Imperato JP, Vick NA. Brain metastases. Effects of radiotherapy on long-term survivors. Neurology 1991; 41(suppl 1):129.

74. Patchell, RA, Tibbs PA, Walsh JW, Dempsey RJ, et al. A randomized trial of surgery in the treatment of single metastases to the brain. N Engl J Med 1990; 322:494–500.

75. Patchell RA, Cirrincione C, Thaler HT, Galicich JH, Kim J-H, Posner JB. Single brain metastases: surgery plus radiation or radiation alone. Neurology 1986; 36:447–453.

76. Patchell RA. Brain metastases. Neurol Clin 1991; 9:1–8.

77. Posner JB. Clinical manifestations of brain metastasis. In: Weiss L, Gilbert H, Posner J, eds. Brain metastasis. Boston: GK Hall & Co., 1980:189–207.

78. Prados M, Leibel S, Barnett CM, Gutin P. Interstitial brachytherapy for metastatic brain tumors. Cancer 1989; 63:657–660.

79. Rosen ST, Makuch RW, Lichter AS, Ihde DC, et al. Role of prophylactic cranial irradiation in the prevention of central nervous system metastases in small cell lung cancer. Potential benefit restricted to patients with complete response. Am J Med 1983; 74:615–623.

80. Rosner D, Nemoto T, Lane WW. Chemotherapy induces regression of brain metastases in breast carcinoma. Cancer 1986; 58:836–839.

81. Rossi NP, Zavala DC, Van Gilder. A combined surgical approach to non–oat-cell pulmonary carcinoma with single cerebral metastasis. Respiration 1987; 51:170–178.

82. Ruderman D, Hall TC. Use of glucocorticoids in the palliative treatment of metastatic brain tumors. Cancer 1965; 18:298–306.

83. Sause WT, Crowley JJ, Morantz R, Rotman M, et al. Solitary brain metastasis: results of an RTOG/SWOG protocol evaluation surgery plus RT versus RT alone. Am J Clin Oncol 1990; 13:427–432.

84. Schold SC, Vurgrin D, Golbey RB, Posner JB. Central nervous system metastases from germ cell carcinoma of testis. Semin Oncol 1979; 6:102–108.

85. Sculier J-P, Feld R, Evans WK, DeBoer G, et al. Neurologic disorders in patients with small cell lung cancer. Cancer 1987; 60:2275–2283.

86. Sharr MM. Intracranial metastases. Management and the place of the CT scan in patients who are treated with surgery only. J Neurooncol 1983; 1:307–312.

87. Sheline GE, Brady LW. Radiation therapy for brain metastases. J Neurooncol 1987; 4:219–225.

88. Siegers HP. Chemotherapy for brain metastases: recent developments and clinical considerations. Cancer Treat Rev 1990; 17:63–73.

89. Simionescu MD. Metastatic tumors of the brain. A follow-up study of 195 patients with neurosurgical considerations. J Neurosurg 1960; 17:361–373.

90. Smalley SR, Schray MF, Lews ER, O'Fallon JR. Adjuvant radiation therapy after surgical resection of solitary brain metastasis: association with pattern of failure and survival. Int J Radiat Oncol Biol Phys 1987; 13:1611–1616.

91. Stortebecker TP. Metastatic tumors of the brain from a neurosurgical point of view. J Neurosurg 1954; 11:84–111.

92. Suit HD, Todoroki T. Rationale for combining surgery and radiation therapy. Cancer 1985; 55:2246–2249.

93. Sundaresan N, Galicich JH, Beattie EJ. Surgical treatment of brain metastases from lung cancer. J Neurosurg 1983; 58:666–671.

94. Sundaresan N, Sachdev VP, Di Giacinto, Hughes JEO. Reoperation for brain metastases. J Clin Oncol 1988; 6:1625–1629.

95. Taylor HG, Lefkowitz M, Skoog SJ, Miles BJ, et al. Intracranial metastases in prostate cancer. 1984. Cancer 53:2728–2730.

96. Torre M, Quaini E, Chiesa G, Rewini M, et al. Synchronous brain metastasis from lung cancer. Result of surgical treatment in combined resection. J Thorac Cardiovasc Surg 1988; 95:994–997.

97. Vannucci RC, Baten M. Cerebral metastatic disease in childhood. Neurology 1974; 24:981–985.

98. Vugrin D, Cvitkovic E, Posner J, Hajdu S, Geldey B. Neurological complications of malignant germ call tumors of testis. Cancer 1979; 44:2349–2353.

99. Vieth RG, Odem GL. Intracranial metastases and their neurosurgical treatment. J Neurosurg 1965; 23:375–383.

100. Walker AE, Robins M, Weinfeld FD. Epidemiology of brain tumors: the national survey of intracranial neoplasms. Neurology 1985; 35:219–226.

101. White KT, Fleming TR, Laws ER. Single metastasis to the brain. Surgical treatment in 122 consecutive patients. Mayo Clin Proc 1981; 56:424–428.

102. Winston KR, Walsh TW, Fisher EG. Results of operative treatment of intracranial metastatic tumors. Cancer 1980; 45:2639–2645.

103. Wroe SJ, Foy PM, Shaw MDM, Williams IR, et al. Differences between neurological and neurosurgical approaches in the management of malignant brain tumors. Br Med J 1986; 293:1015–1018.

104. Young B, Patchell RA. Surgery for a single metastasis. In Wilkins RH, Rengachary SS, eds. Neurosurgery update I. New York: McGraw-Hill, 1990:473–476.

105. Young DF, Posner JB, Chu F, Nisce L. Rapid course radiation therapy of cerebral metastases: results and complications. Cancer 1974; 34:1060–1076.

106. Zimm S, Wampler GI, Stablein D, et al. Intracranial metastases in solid tumor patients: natural history and results of treatment. Cancer 1981; 48:384–394.

20

Pediatric Brain Tumors: Classification, Presentation, and Radiology

Mark J. Kotapka
Hospital of the University of Pennsylvania,
Philadelphia, Pennsylvania

Luis Schut
University of Pennsylvania and Children's Hospital
of Philadelphia, Philadelphia, Pennsylvania

I. INTRODUCTION

Brain tumors are the most frequent solid tumor of childhood and, after leukemia, the most common malignancy of the pediatric population (1). Brain tumors occur at a rate of 2.4:100,000 children at risk per year (2). Approximately 50% of childhood brain tumors occur supratentorially, with the remainder occurring in the posterior fossa and spinal cord (3). The distribution of primary central nervous system (CNS) tumors diagnosed during a 7-year period at the Children's Hospital of Philadelphia is presented in Table 1. The frequency of specific types of brain tumors in this series is presented in Table 2.

The prognosis for both long-term survival and preservation of neurological function in children with brain tumors has improved dramatically in recent years (4). Currently, more than 50% of children with brain tumors that are treated survive at least 5 years (Table 3).

In pediatric patients it is necessary to consider long-term functional outcome in addition to survival. This is particularly important in the treatment and postreatment evaluation of young children with brain tumors. For example, a 3-year-old patient treated for a malignant brain tumor must attain normal adult cerebral function with minimal change, based on his or her inherent potential, to be considered to have had really a satisfactory result. To achieve this outcome, it is important that a team approach be employed in the treatment and follow-up of children with brain tumors. One role of the team is to assist the patient's family in preparing for the death of a child (see Chap. 33). Although, this is an extraordinarily painful event for the family, they can be helped in dealing with this tragedy. Families of a child surviving treatment for a pediatric brain tumor, as well as the child, may require assistance in dealing with the social, emotional, and educational problems that may occur in these patients. Coping with the fear of recurrence, dealing with the use of the illness as an excuse for failure, and avoidance of unrealistic goal-setting all require external support so that the family unit remains functional and the patient's ultimate development is optimized. Such support and appropriate interventions, when needed, are all part of the care of the child with a pediatric brain tumor. In addition to these neuropsychiatric

Table 1 The Distribution of 382 Primary Central Nervous System Neoplasms Diagnosed at Children's Hospital of Philadelphia 1979–1986

Location	Number	Percentage
Supratentorial	205	53.7
Infratentorial	156	40.8
Spinal cord	21	5.5

and social issues, the child with a brain tumor requires comprehensive medical management for myriad complicating and associated conditions that may ensue during or following therapy.

Many brain tumors in the pediatric population cannot be cured by surgery alone, but require a combination of surgery, radiotherapy, and chemotherapy. The occurrence of glioblastoma multiforme in children is rare. The most malignant lesions in children (primitive neuroectodermal tumors and anaplastic astrocytomas) have proved sensitive to such combined therapeutic approaches. The surgical resection of childhood tumors often may be aggressive, even in eloquent brain regions, owing to the plasticity and recuperative ability of the immature nervous system. Thus, even when surgical cure is not possible, a significant reduction in tumor volume may be attained, allowing more effective adjuvant therapy to be employed. This approach may be particularly useful in cases of very young children for whom a delay of radiotherapy, until the child is older, offers the best chance for normal intellectual development. In these cases, surgical resection, followed by chemotherapy, is often the treatment of choice. Repeat surgery, chemotherapy, and radiotherapy reserved for possible future recurrence.

II. CLASSIFICATION

The classification of childhood brain tumors continues to be debated. The lack of a uniformly accepted classification system has been a major problem in the evaluation of various therapeutic modalities employed in the treatment of children with brain tumors. Many pediatric brain tumors are composed of poorly differentiated cells that manifest considerable histological diversity.

Table 2 The Frequency of Tumor Types in 361 Primary Brain Tumors Diagnosed at Children's Hospital of Philadelphia 1979–1986

Tumor	%
Astrocytoma	32.1
Primitive neuroectodermal tumor	19.4
Ganglioglioma	6.7
Craniopharyngioma	6.7
Ependymoma	5.5
Germ cell tumor	5.3
Mixed glioma	4.7
Oligodendroglioma	2.8
Meningioma	2.8
Choroid plexus tumors	2.2
Pineocytoma	1.4
Other	1.0

Table 3 Survival of Patients with Brain Tumors Diagnosed at Children's Hospital of Philadelphia: 1974–1980

Tumor	Patients	Alive at 5 yrs
Anaplastic glioma	4	1
Low-grade glioma	60	48
Ependymoma	18	5
Brain stem glioma	27	2
Craniopharyngioma	10	8
Primitive neuroectodermal tumors	35	15
Germ cell tumors	9	5
Total	163	84 (52%)

In the posterior fossa, most such tumors have traditionally been called medulloblastomas, although the stem cell of this tumor, the medulloblast, has not been well characterized. A recent classification system by Rorke and co-workers recommended that all childhood tumors composed of primitive undifferentiated cells be termed *primitive neuroectodermal tumors* (5).

Within the category of primitive neuroectodermal tumors are childhood brain tumors in different regions of the neuraxis, which have previously been called medulloblastoma, ependymoblastoma, pineoblastoma, and central neuroblastoma. Furthermore, Rorke and co-workers suggested that, since these poorly differentiated tumors frequently show considerable histological diversity, they be subdivided according to evidence of differentiation along identifiable cellular lines, such as astrocytic, neuronal, or ependymal. This type of subclassification system has clinical importance, since the more differentiated lesions tend to be less responsive to standard therapies.

This classification system has not been uniformly accepted. Objections to it include the fact that it is an oversimplification and thus provides only a loose framework for grouping primitive tumors. In addition, it fails to distinguish between tumors that have been well studied, such as medulloblastoma, and those that need to have their biology better defined, such as central neuroblastoma. Until markers such as monoclonal antibodies that are specific to each tumor type are developed, this controversy will not rest.

Primarily based on light microscopic criteria, a modification of the World Health Organization (WHO) classification of brain tumors has recently been proposed for use in childhood brain tumors (Table 4, Ref. 6). This classification system employs the term *primitive neuroectodermal tumor* to describe all small-cell tumors of the posterior fossa.

Ependymoblastomas are considered a subset of primitive neuroectodermal tumors and are distinct from other forms of ependymoma. The modified World Health Organization classification of childhood tumors of the central nervous system will be used for the remainder of this chapter.

III. SIGNS AND SYMPTOMS

Children with brain tumors frequently have symptoms and signs that strongly suggest the appropriate diagnosis. Early in the course of the illness complaints may be vague and consist of intermittent headache, fatigue, personality change, decreased school performance, or, in infants, plateauing or loss of developmental milestones. Late in the course of the illness, complaints related to raised intracranial pressure may predominate.

The clinical triad of symptoms associated with increased intracranial pressure—headache, vomiting, and blurred or double vision—is the hallmark of brain tumors in childhood. These symptoms occur more frequently with infratentorial tumors owing to the propensity of lesions in

Table 4 Childhood Brain Tumors (Revised World Health Organization Classification)

  I. Tumors of neuroepithelial tissue
      A. Glial tumors
          1. Astocytic tumors
              a. Astrocytoma
              b. Anaplastic astrocytoma
              c. Subependymal giant cell tumors
              d. Gigantocellular glioma
          2. Oligodendroglial tumors
          3. Ependymal tumors
              a. Ependymomas
              b. Anaplastic ependymoma
              c. Myxopapillary ependymoma
          4. Choroid plexus tumors
          5. Mixed gliomas
      B. Neuronal tumors
      C. Primitive neuroectodermal tumors
          1. Primitive neuroectodermal tumor, not specified
          2. Primitive neuroectodermal tumor, with
              a. Astrocytes
              b. Oligodendrocytes
              c. Ependymal cells
              d. Neuronal cells
              e. Other (melanocytic, mesenchymal)
              f. Mixed cellular elements
          3. Medulloepithelioma
      D. Pineal cell tumors
          1. Primitive neuroectodermal tumor (pineoblastoma)
          2. Pineocytoma
 II. Tumors of meningeal and related tissues
      A. Meningiomas
      B. Meningeal sarcomatous tumors
      C. Primary melanocytic tumors
III. Tumors of nerve sheath cells
 IV. Primary malignant lymphomas
  V. Tumors of blood vessel origin
 VI. Germ cell tumors
VII. Malformative tumors (craniopharyngiomas, lipomas)
VIII. Local extension from regional tumors
 IX. Metastatic tumors
  X. Unclassified tumors

this location to cause obstructive hydrocephalus, even with small- to medium-sized tumors. In supratentorial lesions, such symptoms also may occur, but usually indicate the presence of a large tumor of the hemispheres or a tumor located in the third ventricle.

A. Headache

Headache is probably the most common but least diagnostically helpful symptom of childhood brain tumors. The characteristic headache of increased intracranial pressure is head pain that is present on arising, may be relieved by vomiting, and improves during the day. This headache pattern is believed to be due to the antigravity effects of recumbency during sleep, which decreases cardiac venous return and cerebrospinal fluid (CSF) drainage, thereby increasing intracranial pressure during sleep and leading to more severe symptoms in the morning hours. Headache tends to be bifrontal or bitemporal and is usually without localizing value. In very young children unable to verbalize their complaints, irritability may be the only manifestation of headache. A focal headache, although implying local cranial disease, is rarely due to increased intracranial pressure. Headache that awakens the child from sleep is suggestive of raised intracranial pressure, but may also occur with migraine.

Headache is quite common in childhood and is a frequent reason to seek neurological consultation. Although most brain tumors will cause additional symptoms within 4–6 months after the onset of headache and although clinical suspicion of brain tumors should be greatest in children with recent onset of headache, these general guidelines are not particularly helpful early in the course of the illness (7). In our experience, headaches have been present for longer than 6 months before diagnosis in 10% of patients with brain tumors.

By far the most important determinant of the significance of nonspecific headaches is a careful neurological examination. Obviously, any focal neurological abnormalities should suggest the presence of an intracranial lesion. However, the absence of deficits does not exclude the possibility of a mass lesion. The symptoms of headache should be taken seriously in any child, and additional diagnostic studies should be strongly considered (even in the absence of focal deficits) particularly in children with associated changes in behavior or personality.

B. Vomiting

Vomiting frequently occurs in children with brain tumors. In patients with increased intracranial pressure, vomiting usually occurs in the morning and is associated with, and usually relieves, the headache. When caused by raised intracranial pressure, vomiting may occur infrequently, if at all, during the rest of the day. It is not necessarily associated with nausea or anorexia, and often the child is hungry soon after the vomiting attack. These features tend to distinguish vomiting on a central nervous system basis from vomiting secondary to gastrointestinal disease, which is usually associated with nausea and abdominal pain and is temporally related to eating.

Less frequently, vomiting may occur secondary to tumors that invade or compress the floor of the fourth ventricle. The vomiting patterns in such lesions are different, usually being more constant during the day, and are associated with persistent nausea, anorexia, and significant weight loss. In infiltrative gliomas of the lower brain stem, vomiting may be the predominant feature of the illness for months before other symptoms become evident. Children with such lesions are often incorrectly considered to have psychogenic vomiting.

C. Visual Difficulties

Visual symptoms are not infrequent in children with brain tumors. By far the most common complaint is blurring of vision, which may be the young child's way of describing double vision. In the older child, complaints of double vision are more frequent. Most commonly, diplopia is caused by stretching and paresis of one or both of the abducens nerves, secondary to increased intracranial pressure. The older child may be able to describe two objects lying horizontally, side by side. Parents most frequently observe that one or both eyes intermittently turn inward, especially when the child is fatigued. Examination will usually show an inability to deviate the eye laterally with an associated gaze paretic nystagmus.

Other ocular motor deficits may occur and are of more localizing value. Internuclear ophthalmoplegia or a gaze palsy accompanied by other cranial nerve dysfunction may indicate the presence of an infiltrative lesion of the brain stem. Vertical nystagmus may indicate the presence of a lesion at the cervicomedullary junction.

Decreased vision is infrequent in children with brain tumors, but when it occurs, it necessitates diagnostic evaluation. Tumors of the sellar or suprasellar region, such as craniopharyngiomas and chiasmatic–hypothalamic gliomas, frequently cause visual deficits owing to either direct compression or invasion of the optic nerves or chiasm. Other types of brain tumors may cause impairment of vision secondary to raised intracranial pressure and subsequent papilledema. Initially, visual examination may reveal enlargement of the blind spot. However, even with existing modern health care systems, an occasional child will still present with full-blown papilledema, or even optic atrophy, secondary to long-standing visual complaints that had not been investigated.

D. Head Size

Expanding head size may be the predominant sign of increased intracranial pressure in infants harboring brain tumors. As these children have unfused cranial sutures and open fontanelles, rapid head growth may be the only sign of raised intracranial pressure. Careful serial head circumference measurements will show the head to "cross percentiles" on standard growth charts before the development of macrocephaly. In addition to a tense fontanelle and split cranial sutures, limitation of upgaze (sunset sign) and optic pallor may be present at the time of diagnosis. Although focal neurological deficits may be difficult to elicit, a history of developmental delay may be elicited in most infants.

E. Other Signs and Symptoms

Seizures are not common in children with brain tumors. However, for specific types of tumor, seizures may be the most common presenting complaint (8). One such tumor is the ganglioglioma. Seizures also occur with astrocytomas of the cerebral hemispheres and with oligodendrogliomas.

Cerebellar deficits and ataxia are frequently noted in children with tumors of the posterior fossa. In midline lesions of the cerebellum, truncal and gait ataxia are usually found. In cerebellar hemispheric lesions, limb ataxia is common. Difficulty in reaching for objects (dysmetria), an intention tremor, or difficulties in rapid-alternating movements suggest lateralizing cerebellar damage.

Meningismus may occur in children with tumors of the posterior fossa. The posterior cranial fossa is innervated by ascending meningeal branches from the upper three cervical nerves, which enter the skull through the foramen magnum, jugular foramen, and hypoglossal canal. Herniation of the cerebellar tonsils or tumor through the foramen magnum leads to stretch and irritation of these nerves and subsequent neck pain and rigidity. Attempts to passively flex the head forward are actively resisted and result in severe pain. Infants not infrequently assume an arched opisthotonic posture.

Focal neurological deficits, other than those already mentioned, are uncommon in pediatric brain tumors. An occasional patient with a large hemispheric tumor may present with hemiparesis or with hemisensory complaints. This is in marked contrast with the situation in adults, in whom focal neurological deficits are frequently noted on presentation.

IV. NEURODIAGNOSTIC STUDIES

Before the mid-1970s, confirmatory studies in children with brain tumors were far from optimal. With the appropriate use of skull radiography, ventriculography, and cerebral angiography, the presence of a mass lesion could usually be established, but little other information was obtained preoperatively. The development of computed tomography (CT) has supplanted the need for these other tests in most cases. More recently, magnetic resonance imaging has even further improved our neurodiagnostic capabilities.

A. Computed Tomography

Computed tomography is currently the most widely used imaging technique in the diagnosis and follow-up evaluation of children with brain tumors (9). When performed before and after the infusion of intravenous contrast, computed tomography detects nearly 100% of childhood tumors. The direct effect of the mass, especially obstruction of cerebrospinal fluid (CSF) flow and ventricular dilatation, can easily be appreciated. Additionally, this technique is widely available, is easily adapted to the special needs of imaging infants and children, and is generally well tolerated. A vast experience has been accumulated with computed tomography of childhood brain tumors, such that certain patterns of abnormalities have become recognized as nearly diagnostic of tumor type. These characteristics will be reviewed in the latter discussion of individual tumors. This information allows exact presurgical planning and negates the need for more invasive tests, such as angiography.

However, computed tomography does have some limitations. It may not adequately visualize basal structures, such as the hypothalamus, pituitary, and visual pathway. Small lesions in the third ventricle and pineal region may also be difficult to detect or fully characterize. In the posterior fossa, surrounding bone artifact may make the visualization of intrinsic brain stem lesions less than optimal (10).

B. Magnetic Resonance Imaging

The last decade has witnessed the development of magnetic resonance imaging (10,11). This technique provides unsurpassed imaging detail of the nervous system, both in health and in disease. Additionally, the technique avoids the use of ionizing radiation, and it provides images in all three anatomical planes. However, the experience with magnetic resonance imaging is not yet as great as with computed tomography, it is not yet as widely available, and it is more difficult to adapt to the needs of the pediatric patient.

In the experience to date, magnetic resonance imaging appears to be even more sensitive than computed tomography in the detection of pediatric brain tumors. Furthermore, the signal and contrast-enhancing characteristics of the various brain tumors are, in many cases, highly specific to tumor type. Magnetic resonance imaging is clearly superior, because of its greater resolution, in the detection of small midline or basal supratentorial lesions. Likewise, the posterior fossa is visualized without artifact, making even focal intrinsic brain stem lesions readily identifiable. In some situations, it remains difficult, just as with computed tomography, to differentiate tumor from reactive changes that are nonneoplastic in the postoperative or irradiated patient.

At present, computed tomography and magnetic resonance imaging are complementary diagnostic procedures in the evaluation of a pediatric patient suspected of harboring a brain tumor or in the follow-up of a child after such a tumor has been treated.

V. SPECIFIC COMMON BRAIN TUMORS IN CHILDREN

A. Supratentorial Tumors

1. Astrocytoma

Differentiation between low-grade astrocytomas and anaplastic gliomas has prognostic signifiance, regardless of the location of the lesion. In addition to histological grading, the location of the tumor affects prognosis based on its relative resectability, spread along white matter tracts (e.g., into the brain stem and across the corpus callosum), and even response to therapy. Because the deeper diencephalic and mesencephalic tumors often cannot be resected, but can only be biopsied, the lack of correlation between tumor histological features and clinical course may be the result of inadequate tissue specimens from heterogeneous tumors. It is valuable to consider glial tumors both by histological type and by location. Low-grade gliomas of the cerebral hemispheres account for approximately 50% of astrocytic tumors in children (12). These tumors may be cystic or solid. The cortical and subcortical lesions are frequently of low-density and are not contrast-enhancing on computed tomographic scans, but are well demonstrated by magnetic resonance imaging. Presentation may be associated with seizures, focal neurological deficits, or signs of elevated intracranial pressure. More deeply located lesions in the white matter or deep gray nuclei often become very large, are frequently cystic, and are intensely enhancing on imaging studies. In adults this would imply malignancy; however, in children these tumors may behave less aggressively.

Optic Chiasmatic and Hypothalamic Gliomas. In children, these lesions are usually low-grade astrocytomas that involve the visual pathways and hypothalamus. In our experience, younger children tend to have larger tumors that are frequently cystic, with greater visual deficits at presentation and poorer response to therapy. Although 10–20% of children with these lesions have neurofibromatosis, it is yet to be determined if this condition affects outcome (13). The differential diagnosis includes germinomas, craniopharyngiomas, and pituitary tumors. Presentation in the first year of life is generally characterized by unusual eye movements, growing head size, and irritability. Occasionally, the tumor is manifested by a stroke, the result of compression or occlusion of the intracranial internal carotid artery. In older children, precocious puberty is not an uncommon presentation. Evaluation of a patient with a suspected hypothalamic–visual pathway glioma must include complete ophthalmological evaluation. In children in the first year of life, it can be extremely difficult to obtain good measurements of visual acuity and almost impossible to assess the visual fields. Because of this, caution must be exercised in the long-term prognosis for vision. In older children, vision will frequently stabilize following therapy, but rarely improve.

Gliomas in this anatomical location are easily identified with current neuroradiologic techniques. Computed tomography typically demonstrates a hypodense mass that will brightly enhance on contrast administration (Fig. 1). Central necrosis is frequently found. Magnetic resonance imaging better demonstrates the full extent of these lesions (Fig. 2). Visual pathway involvement, frequently extending along the optic radiations and sometimes even to the lateral geniculate bodies, may be identified. Angiography is rarely of benefit, provided adequate magnetic resonance images of the internal carotid arteries and their major branches have been obtained. The major differential diagnosis is that of an optic sheath meningioma. This usually may be distinguished from an optic glioma because in meningiomas the intact optic nerve is frequently seen running through the tumor.

2. Ganglioglioma

Gangliogliomas occur primarily in cortical or subcortical locations. They most frequently present with seizures (14). There often may be a history of gradual intellectual deterioration. Gangliogliomas are usually hypodense and nonenhancing on computed tomography scans, but are usually easily detected with magnetic resonance imaging.

3. Craniopharyngioma

The craniopharyngiomas are the most common nonneuroepithelial tumors of the central nervous system in childhood and account for approximately 6–8% of pediatric brain tumors (15). They

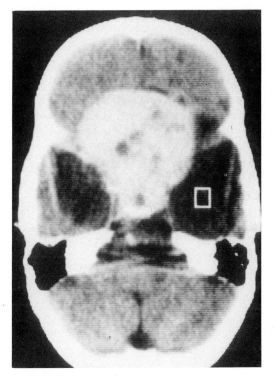

Figure 1 A CT scan with contrast, demonstrating a large hypothalamic—chiasmatic glioma with bilateral temporal fossa cysts.

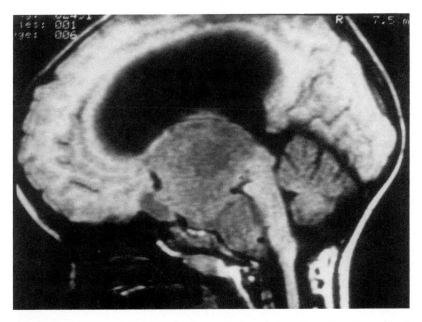

Figure 2 Midline sagittal MRI demonstrating a large hypothalamic–chiasmatic glioma with accompanying hydrocepahlus.

arise in the sellar or suprasellar area within the pituitary gland or in the pituitary stalk. Although efforts are made to differentiate Rathke's cleft cyst from the true craniopharyngioma, and craniopharyngioma from epithelial epidermoid tumors, it is not uncommon to see elements of all these lesions within a single tumor. The tumor is first manifested by hormonal dysfunction, visual disturbances, or symptoms and signs of raised intracranial pressure. Most patients have abnormal visual acuity or field deficits on ophthalmological testing. Extraocular movements may be disturbed, if the tumor is large, either by direct compression of the third nerve or by the effects of raised intracranial pressure on the sixth cranial nerve.

Plain skull films frequently demonstrate a calcified lesion in the sellar region, enlargement of the sella, or erosion of the clinoids. Computed tomography demonstrates a lesion in the sellar region that may contain calcium, may be cystic or solid, and usually enhances with intravenous contrast. Magnetic resonance imaging also is useful in the evaluation of these lesions and also gives additional information concerning the vascular anatomy of the region. The differential diagnosis includes hypothalamic–optic glioma, germinoma, and pituitary tumors.

B. Infratentorial Tumors

1. Primitive Neuroectodermal Tumors

Primitive neuroectodermal tumors (PNET), also known as medulloblastomas, are the most common malignant primary central nervous system tumor in children and constitute approximately one-third of childhood posterior fossa tumors (5). These tumors are composed of primarily small round or oval-shaped cells, with hyperchromic nuclei and poorly defined cytoplasm. The cell of origin of these tumors has not been well defined. Some authorities have suggested that the tumor is derived from remnants of fetal external granular cells of the cerebellum or from small-cell rests in the posterior medullary velum. Most childhood tumors of this type involve the cerebellar vermis, fill the cavity of the fourth ventricle, and infiltrate the floor of the fourth ventricle by local extension (16).

Children with PNETs present most commonly with symptoms of increased intracranial pressure, including vomiting, lethargy, and morning headache. These symptoms may be associated with unsteadiness of gait and diplopia. The clinical course is usually short, with diagnosis in most patients within 3–4 months of the onset of symptoms.

Computed tomography reveals an isodense or hyperdense midline posterior fossa mass (Fig. 3) that frequently enhances homogeneously (17). The appearance of these tumors on magnetic resonance imaging is also that of a brightly enhancing tumor (Fig. 4) that may contain microcysts or foci of hemorrhage. Seeding of the tumor throughout the intracranial cerebrospinal fluid spaces may also be demonstrated. Hydrocephalus is frequently noted.

2. Cerebellar Astrocytoma

Low-grade astrocytomas of the cerebellar hemispheres constitute approximately 30–40% of childhood posterior fossa tumors (18). Cerebellar astrocytomas peak in incidence in the beginning of the second decade of life. These tumors usually arise in the cerebellar hemispheres, but may occur in the vermis. Cerebellar astrocytomas may be primarily cystic, solid, or mixed. Most cerebellar astrocytomas are histologically benign lesions. The most common histological type, the juvenile pilocytic cerebellar astrocytoma, is composed of areas of compact, fibrillated cells, alternating with looser, more spongy areas. The compact areas often contain an abundance of eosinophilic, beaded, or cigar-shaped structures, called Rosenthal fibers (19). Less frequently, cerebellar astrocytomas contain areas that suggest increased malignancy, including necrosis and mitosis. Tumors with a favorable prognosis tend to contain microcysts, Rosenthal fibers, and foci of oligodendroglia. Tumors with a less favorable outcome tend to contain perivascular rosettes, have a high cell density, and have foci of frank anaplasia.

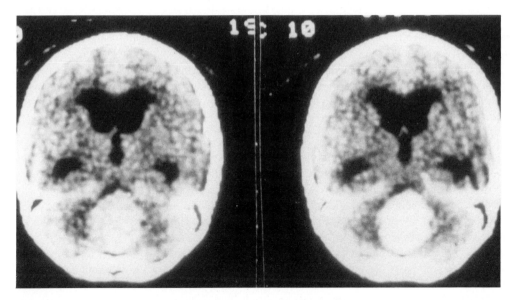

Figure 3 A CT scan without (left) and with (right) contrast administration demonstrating a large PNET of the posterior fossa with hydrocephalus.

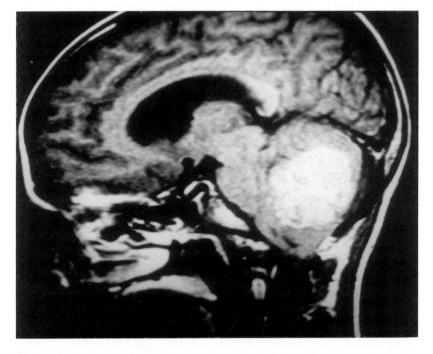

Figure 4 Midline sagittal MRI, demonstrating a large PNET of the posterior fossa.

Cerebellar astrocytomas present with progressive clumsiness and ataxia, primarily of the extremities. Subsequently, symptoms and signs of raised intracranial pressure, truncal ataxia, and head tilt may occur.

Both computed tomography and magnetic resonance imaging demonstrate these lesions as cystic or solid hemispheric tumors (Figs. 5 and 6). Cystic lesions frequently demonstrate enhancing mural nodules or enhancement of the entire tumor capsule. Solid tumors may demonstrate inhomogeneous enhancement (20).

3. Brain Stem Gliomas

Brain stem gliomas constitute approximately 10–20% of childhood posterior fossa tumors. Although these tumors frequently are of low grade on histological examination, they carry a dire prognosis, with a 5-year survival rate of less than 30% (21). Brain stem gliomas cause neurological dysfunction by both compression and infiltration of the brain stem. These tumors tend to extend both superiorly and inferiorly, producing diffuse enlargement of the brain stem. A subgroup of brain stem gliomas are exophytic and may carry a better prognosis.

Children with brain stem gliomas usually develop symptoms insidiously, and a delay of 3–6 months between the onset of symptoms and diagnosis is not infrequent (22). Symptoms include involvement of any of the cranial nerves, motor difficulties, gait disturbances, nausea, vomiting, and headaches. Bulbar abnormalities, including swallowing and speech difficulties, are not unusual early in the course of the illness. The more exophytically placed lesions may cause little in the way of cranial nerve dysfunction, although such lesions located in the medulla seem to be associated more frequently with unsteadiness, nausea, and vomiting.

On computed tomography, low-density changes are usually seen in the brain stem, with associated compression and obliteration of the surrounding cisterns (23). The fourth ventricle may be distorted and displaced posteriorly. Commonly, there is minimal contrast enhancement. Some brain stem gliomas may be hyperdense, enhancing lesions, with cystic areas. Magnetic resonance imaging better demonstrates the rostral–caudal extent of the tumor, clearly outlines the normal brain stem border, and is more accurate in the postoperative evaluation of the extent of surgical resection (10).

4. Ependymoma

Ependymomas make up approximately 10–20% of posterior fossa tumors in children. These tumors most commonly arise from the floor of the fourth ventricle, but may arise more laterally and extend into the cerebellopontine angle. Ependymomas have a variable histological pattern, and microscopic findings may not correlate well with the clinical course.

The clinical symptoms of posterior fossa ependymomas are quite variable and depend on the location of the tumor within the posterior fossa. When the tumor arises in the fourth ventricle, hydrocephalus may occur with resultant signs and symptoms of increased intracranial pressure. Cranial nerve palsies from invasion of the brain stem or from compression as these nerves exit the brain stem are common. The duration of symptoms may be variable. In most patients, symptoms are present for longer than 9 months before diagnosis (24).

Computed tomography and magnetic resonance imaging both demonstrate ependymomas as enhancing tumors of the fourth ventricle. Magnetic resonance imaging also provides information concerning brain stem invasion, seeding within the intracranial cerebrospinal fluid pathways, and lateral tumor extension through the foramen of Luschka.

VII. SUMMARY

Central nervous system neoplasms represent an important disease entity in pediatrics. Childhood brain tumors occur throughout the neuraxis and consist of a variety of histological lesions with variable long-term responses to available therapies. Most childhood brain tumors present with

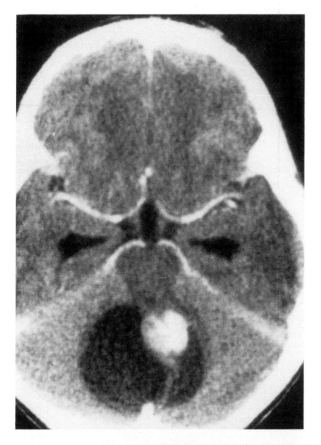

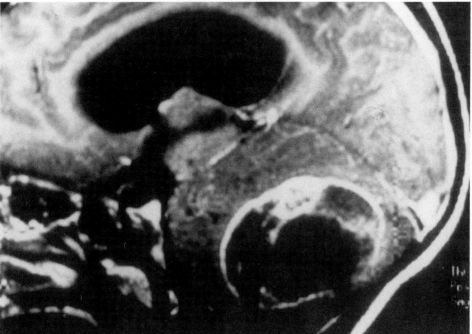

Figure 5 A CT scan with contrast, demonstrating a cystic low-grade astrocytoma of the cerebellum.
Figure 6 Sagittal MRI with contrast, demonstrating a cystic astrocytoma of the cerebellum. Note enhancement of entire tumor capsule. In such a case, operative resection must include the capsule to achieve a cure.

signs and symptoms of raised intracranial pressure, with or without focal neurological deficits, depending on location of the tumor and nature of the lesion. Modern neurodiagnostic techniques including computed tomography and magnetic resonance imaging may fully characterize these lesions in a noninvasive manner before treatment and allow close follow-up during and after therapy.

REFERENCES

1. Freeman AI. Introduction. Cancer 1985; 56:1743.
2. Silverberg E. Cancer statistics. CA 1983; 33:9–25.
3. Rorke LB, Schut L. Introductory survey of pediatric brain tumors. In: McLaurin RL, Schut L, Venes JL, Epstein F, eds. Pediatric neurosurgery. 2nd ed. Philadelphia: WB Saunders, 1989:335–337.
4. Bruce DA, Schut L, Sutton LN. Supratentorial brain tumors in children. In: Youmans JR, ed. Neurological surgery. 3rd ed. Philadelphia: WB Saunders, 1990:3000–3016.
5. Rorke LB. The cerebellar medulloblastoma and its relationship to primitive neuroectodermal tumors. J Neuropathol Exp Neurol 1983; 42:1–15.
6. Rorke LB, Gilles FM, Davis RL, Becker LE. Revision of the World Health Organization classification of brain tumors for childhood brain tumors. Cancer 1985; 56:1869–1886.
7. Honig PJ, Charney EB. Children with brain tumor headaches. Am J Dis Child 1982; 136:121–124.
8. Bakus RF, Millichap JG. The seizure as a manifestation of the intracranial tumor in childhood. Pediatrics 1962; 29:978–984.
9. Segall MD, Batzinsky S, Zee CS, et al. Computed tomography in the diagnosis of intracranial neoplasms in children. Cancer 1985; 56:1748–1755.
10. Packer RJ, Zimmerman RA, Luerson T, et al. Nuclear magnetic resonance in the evaluation of brain stem gliomas of childhood. Neurology 1985; 35:397–401.
11. Packer RJ, Batzinsky S, Cohen ME. Magnetic resonance imaging in the evaluation of intracranial tumors of childhood. Cancer 1985; 45:1767–1772.
12. Heideman RL, Packer RJ, Albright LA, Freeman CN. Central nervous system tumors. In: Pizzo PA, Poplack DG, eds. Principles and practice of pediatric oncology. Philadelphia: JB Lippincott (in press).
13. Packer RJ, Savino PJ, Bilaniuk LT. Chiasmatic gliomas of childhood: a reappraisal of natural history and effectiveness of cranial irradiation. Childs Brain 1983; 10:393–403.
14. Sutton LN, Packer RJ, Rorke LB, et al. Cerebral gangliogliomas in childhood. Neurosurgery 1983; 13:125–126.
15. Hoffman HJ, Raffel C. Craniopharyngiomas. In: McLaurin RL, Schut L, Venes JL, Epstein F, eds. Pediatric neurosurgery. 2nd ed. Philadelphia: WB Saunders, 1989:399–408.
16. Park TS, Hoffman HJ, Hendrich EB, et al. Medulloblastoma, clinical presentation and management. Experience at the Hospital for Sick Children, Toronto, 1950–1980. J Neurosurg 1983; 58:543–552.
17. Zimmerman RA, Bilaniuk LT, Pahlajanl H. Spectrum of medulloblastomas demonstrated by computed tomography. Radiology 1978; 126:137–141.
18. Laurent JP, Cheek WR. Brain tumors in children. J Pediatr Neurosci 1985; 1:1–31.
19. Gilles FM, Winston K, Fulchiero A, Leviton A. Histologic features and observation variation in cerebellar gliomas in children. JNCI 1977; 58:175–181.
20. Zimmerman RA, Bilaniuk LT, Bruno L, Rosenstock J. Computed tomography of cerebellar astrocytoma. AJR 1978; 130:929–933.
21. Littman P, Jarrett P, Bilaniuk LT, et al. Pediatric brain stem gliomas. Cancer 1980; 45:2787–2792.
22. Panitch MS, Berg BO. Brain stem tumors of childhood and adolescence. Am J Dis Child. 1970; 119:465–472.
23. Bilaniuk LT, Zimmerman RA, Littman P, et al. Computed tomography of brain stem gliomas in children. Radiology 1980; 134:89–95.
24. Pierre-Kahn A, Hirsch JF, Roux FX, et al. Intracranial ependymomas in childhood—survival and functional results of 47 cases. Childs Brain 1983; 10:145–156.

21

Management of Pediatric Brain Tumors

Jeffrey H. Wisoff and Fred J. Epstein
New York University Medical Center,
New York, New York

I. INTRODUCTION

Central nervous system (CNS) tumors are the second most common form of neoplasia to affect the pediatric population and the third leading cause of death in children younger than 16 years old (1–3). Brain and spinal cord tumors account for 20% of all pediatric cancers, compared with 1–2% of all adult malignancies (2). Their incidence appears to be increasing in frequency from 2.4 new cases per 100,000 children per year in 1973 to 3.3 cases per 100,000 children per year in 1986 (1, 4–12). There are approximately 1500 new central nervous system tumors annually (3, 7, 11).

Pediatric brain tumors can be part of the clinical manifestation of one of the phakomatoses. Tuberous sclerosis is associated with subependymal giant-cell astrocytomas. Optic pathway tumors, hemispheric astrocytomas and hamartomas, nerve sheath tumors, and meningiomas may be seen in children with neurofibromatosis. Cerebellar hemangioblastoma presenting in childhood is pathognomonic of von Hippel–Lindau disease (see Chap. 18).

Sixty to seventy percent of childhood brain tumors arise in the posterior fossa, including medulloblastomas, cerebellar astrocytomas, brain stem gliomas, and fourth ventricle ependymomas (2, 7, 13–16). Supratentorial tumors are most often low-grade astrocytomas. During the first 2 years of life the location and pathology of brain tumors differs: most are malignant supratentorial neoplasms, with a relatively high incidence of teratomas and choroid plexus tumors (14, 17–20). Although the pathogenesis of pediatric brain tumors remains obscure, recent advances in molecular biology and cytogenetics have begun to identify possible sites of oncogenesis. Chromosomal abnormalities associated with brain tumors include deletions of chromosome 22 (meningiomas, acoustic neuromas), alterations of chromosome 17 (medulloblastoma, astrocytoma), and loss on chromosome 10 (glioblastoma) (21–25).

This chapter will discuss the common brain tumors of childhood, their current treatment, long-term prognosis, late sequelae of therapy, and future directions in pediatric neuro-oncology.

II. MEDULLOBLASTOMA

Medulloblastoma (or posterior fossa PNET) is the most common malignant pediatric brain tumor, accounting for 20% of all CNS neoplasms of childhood (2, 14, 16, 26). Although the primitive undifferentiated cells that constitute the tumor have been traditionally thought to be of cerebellar origin, the revised World Health Organization (WHO) classification of pediatric CNS tumors considers all undifferentiated neoplasms, regardless of location, as derived from a common primitive neuroepithelial cell and categorizes them as primitive neuroectodermal tumors (PNET) (27). The prognostic importance of neuronal or glial differentiation is uncertain (28, 29).

Medulloblastomas are common throughout childhood, with a peak incidence between 5 and 10 years. A second smaller peak is seen in early adulthood (2, 14). They usually arise in the midline cerebellar vermis, with variable extension into the fourth ventricle, cerebellar hemisphere, and brain stem (Fig. 1). Involvement of the fourth ventricle explains the almost universal occurrence of hydrocephalus at diagnosis (30). In adolescents, the tumor may present laterally in the cerebellar hemisphere, eliciting a proliferative leptomeningeal reaction resembling a sarcoma ("desmoplastic medulloblastoma"). The location of the medulloblastomas adjacent to the fourth ventricle permits early dissemination of tumor along the cerebrospinal fluid (CSF) pathways (30). Twenty-five to forty-five percent of newly diagnosed patients will have laboratory or radiographic evidence of leptomeningeal metastasis (30–32).

A. Treatment

Surgical excision is the initial therapeutic intervention. The surgical objective is a gross total resection or near total resection with less than 1.5 cm^3 of residual tumor (32, 33). Both institutional and cooperative group studies have demonstrated a disease-free survival advantage in patients who have had a radical resection of their tumor. The routine use of advanced surgical technology, including the operating microscope, ultrasonic surgical aspirator, and the CO_2 laser has permitted radical resection of almost every medulloblastoma with decreased operative morbidity. Although some degree of hydrocephalus is universally present preoperatively, fewer than 30% of children who have received a radical resection of their tumor will ultimately require a shunt (33). In pediatric neurosurgical centers, surgical mortality is under 1%. Transient neurological deficits (ataxia, dysarthria, cranial nerve palsies, mutism, and aseptic meningitis) are not uncommon; however, permanent morbidity is seen in fewer than 10% of the children (32, 33).

The propensity for leptomeningeal dissemination mandates postoperative staging both for treatment planning and prognosis (31). Gadolinium-enhanced magnetic resonance imaging (MRI) determines the extent of surgical resection and the presence of residual disease. Gadolinium-enhanced MRI of the spine or a computed tomography (CT) myelogram and CSF cytological studies completes the CNS evaluation. Since 5% of patients may have systemic metastasis at diagnosis, a bone marrow aspirate and biopsy should be performed (32, 34).

For over 40 years craniospinal irradiation has been the mainstay of postoperative therapy (16, 30, 32, 35–40). Standard doses include 5000–5500 cGy to the posterior fossa and 3500–4500 cGy to the neuroaxis (spinal cord and remainder of the brain) with 5-year event-free survival ranging from 20 to 80% (16, 31, 32, 34, 37, 41). Several patient, tumor, and therapeutic factors have emerged that identify children at high risk for recurrence of their tumor following surgery and irradiation. Younger age (<3 years), presence of metastatic disease at diagnosis, and subtotal resection with >1.5 cm^3 of residual tumor have a significant adverse effect on survival and place the child in a poor-risk category (31, 32, 37). Tumor differentiation (4), size, and local extension of tumor (37); presence of massive hydrocephalus; and male sex have been implicated as negative prognostic variables; however, the large cooperative group studies have not yet provided a consistent or reliable correlation.

Although irradiation alone may be curative in most good-risk patients (16, 32, 37), long-term sequelae of treatment are common. Radiation therapy has been associated with intellectual deterioration, developmental delay, endocrine dysfunction, and the development of irradiation-induced tumors (42–54). These deleterious effects have been seen with as low as 1200–2400 cGy of whole-brain irradiation (46, 53, 55), far below the dose required for control of medulloblastomas. The incompletely myelinated nervous system of the younger child is more sensitive to the deleterious effects of ionizing radiation, with greater risk of long-term toxicity (49, 55–58).

Recent clinical trials have attempted to reduce the dose of craniospinal irradiation in good-risk patients. Although there were several initially encouraging single-institution reports, a recent joint Childrens Cancer Study Group (CCSG)–Pediatric Oncology Group (POG) study demonstrated an *increased* neuroaxis recurrence in children receiving low-dose (2500 cGy) craniospinal irradiation. Therefore, this lower dosage was abandoned. Future strategies now being developed to decrease radiation damage include combining low-dose neuroaxis irradiation with chemotherapy, delaying irradiation in the child younger than 3 years old with intensive chemotherapy, and the use of hyperfractionated irradiation.

In the child with additional risk factors for recurrence (poor-risk), combined craniospinal irradiation and multidrug chemotherapy has been demonstrated to offer a 10–20% increase in 5-year disease-free survival in several cooperative group trials conducted by CCSG, POG, and SIOP (International Society of Pediatric Oncology) (34, 37, 59). High-dose chemotherapy alone is currently undergoing evaluation in children younger than 2 years of age, this has the intent of delaying time to irradiation and ameliorating the severe toxicity of irradiating the immature nervous system. Preliminary information suggests that this neoadjuvant approach can be successful if the infant has had a radical surgical resection.

III. CEREBELLAR ASTROCYTOMAS

Ten to twenty percent of pediatric brain tumors will be astrocytomas of the cerebellum (2, 14, 60). Their incidence is relatively constant throughout childhood and adolescence. They are evenly divided between boys and girls. Their clinical presentation is similar to that of medulloblastomas, depending on the anatomical location for symptoms and signs. Cerebellar astrocytomas are unique among the intra-axial tumors, since they are one of the few tumors cured by surgical excision alone.

There are two histological types of cerebellar astrocytoma: 80–85% are juvenile pilocytic astrocytomas (JPAs), and the remainder are diffuse astrocytomas (2). The JPAs have a distinct pathological pattern, consisting of alternating areas of high and low cellularity, abundant Rosenthal fibers, and microcysts. They most often occur as a cystic tumor of the cerebellar hemisphere, with a mural nodule of tumor and an associated nonneoplastic reactive cyst (Fig. 2). The diffuse astrocytoma is histologically analogous to the supratentorial fibrillary astrocytoma. They are usually solid tumors that frequently present as midline cerebellar vermis masses indistinguishable from medulloblastoma on preoperative CT or MRI scanning. Diffuse astrocytomas are more common in younger children and patients with neurofibromatosis. They may undergo malignant degeneration in 10–15% of the cases.

A. Treatment

Cystic cerebellar JPAs are surgical lesions: gross total resection of the mural nodule is curative (61). Recurrence-free survival is greater than 95% at 10 and 20 years (61, 62). Children who have significant residual tumor on postoperative MRI should undergo repeat surgery if the tumor does not extend deep into the brain stem. Minimal residual disease may be carefully observed, since

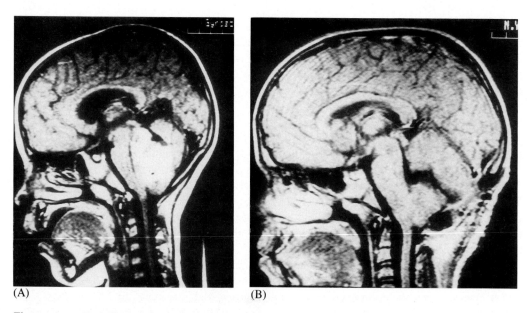

Figure 1   Medulloblastoma: (A) preoperative MRI, (B) postoperative MRI. Note gross total resection.

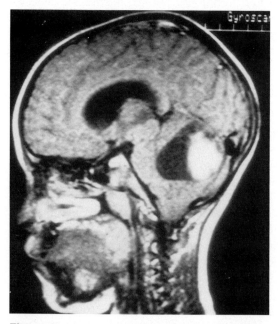

Figure 2   Cystic cerebellar astrocytoma: contrast enhanced MRI.

spontaneous involution of tumor after near gross total resection is common. Radiation therapy should not be considered as a primary adjunctive therapy. Even if the tumor recurs, repeat surgery can be curative if tumor burden is limited (62).

Although solid diffuse astrocytomas traditionally carry a worse prognosis, this may be a reflection of inadequate surgical resection, rather than of the tumor's more aggressive biological behavior. All midline vermian tumors should be radically resected, since the surgeon cannot intraoperatively distinguish histology. In our experience, we have not seen a totally resected solid diffuse astrocytoma recur in over 20 years of patient follow-up. Hydrocephalus, which often accompanies midline tumors, will usually resolve after a gross total tumor resection, with less than 20% of the children requiring shunt placement.

Permanent morbidity and mortality are rare in hemispheric tumors. Complications of resection of midline tumors are similar to medulloblastomas: increased cerebellar deficits, pseudobulbar palsy, and aseptic meningitis.

IV. BRAIN STEM GLIOMAS

Brain stem gliomas are the third most common tumor of the posterior fossa in childhood (8, 63, 64). In a manner similar to medulloblastomas, they occur most frequently between the ages of 5 and 10 years, although they are divided equally between the sexes. Intrinsic brain stem tumors have traditionally been treated with irradiation and, occasionally, adjunctive chemotherapy, with relatively little success (64). The neurological course may be transiently improved, but then tumor invariably progresses after a short remission. The location within the brain stem and usual malignant histology has resulted in a poor overall prognosis: mean survival is less than 1 year and there is a less than 30% 5-year survival (63–67).

As the routine use of CT and MRI scans allowed better visualization of the interior of the brain stem, it became obvious that brain stem tumors are a heterogeneous group of tumors that could be classified based on a combination of the clinical course, neurological examination, and the neurodiagnostic evaluation of location within the brain stem (66, 68–73). Intrinsic brain stem tumors may be classified into five general categories: diffuse, focal, cystic, exophytic, and cervicomedullary.

A. Classification

The diffuse brain stem tumor is the most common, having the CT scan appearance of hypodensity throughout the pons, often extending rostrally into the midbrain with variable tumor enhancement. The MRI characteristically discloses a more diffuse tumor than the CT scan, with extension into medulla, pons, midbrain, and even thalamus (66, 68, 74–76) (Fig. 3). Focal brain stem tumors are defined by an area of contrast enhancement smaller than 2.5 cm in diameter and by the absence of associated hypodensity on CT or edema on MRI. It is important to emphasize that in many neoplasms the MRI discloses that a tumor that appears to be "focal" on the CT scan is in fact diffuse (66).

Dorsally exophytic tumors fill the fourth ventricle and are indistinguishable from other vermian–fourth ventricle tumors clinically or radiographically (66, 71, 73) (Fig. 4). Cystic brain stem astrocytomas are rare. The gadolinium-enhanced MRI discloses only the mural nodule enhancing with contrast and a large cyst that excavates the brain stem (66). These tumors are commonly in the cerebral peduncle or pons. Tumors with ringlike enhancement are not cystic tumors, but rather, are malignant gliomas. Tumors of the cervicomedullary junction extend rostrally into the medulla and caudally into the cervical spinal cord (70). Although the rostral–caudal length of the tumors varies, these neoplasms rarely extend above the pontomedullary junction.

B. Presentation

The clinical manifestations of brain stem neoplasms are directly correlated with the anatomical classification, as noted on the neurodiagnostic studies (65, 66, 68–72). The diffuse tumor is the most common brain stem tumor and the one that is the historical model for brain stem gliomas. The clinical evolution is relatively rapid. Extraocular muscle paresis and diplopia, with or without obvious facial weakness, is the most common primary complaint. Neurological examination

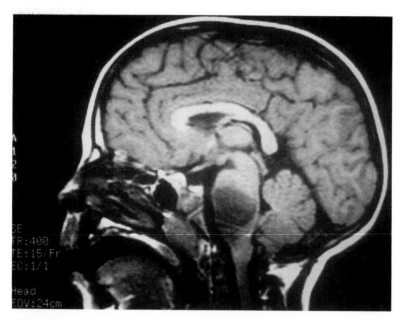

Figure 3 Diffuse brain stem glioma: note diffuse enlargement of pons.

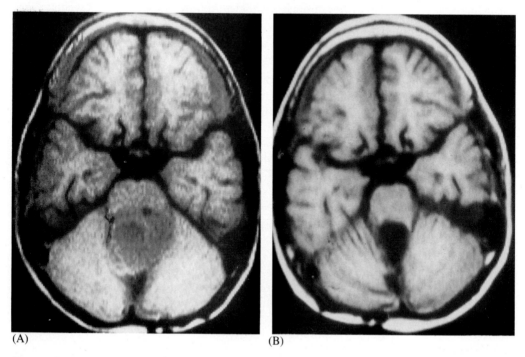

(A)   (B)

Figure 4 Dorsally exophytic brain stem glioma: (A) preoperative MRI; (B) postoperative MRI.

discloses bilateral multiple cranial nerve dysfunction, ataxia, and various degrees of spastic hemiparesis or quadriparesis.

Focal tumors that present in a manner identical with the diffuse neoplasm are usually malignant with a similar clinical course (66). In our experience, a tumor that appeared focal on the CT scan, but was associated with typical bilateral signs and symptoms, was invariably reclassified as diffuse, with the MRI scan demonstrating a more extensive neoplasm than the CT scan. The true focal tumors have an atypical history, with neurological symptoms present for 6–18 months before definitive diagnosis. The neurological examination discloses signs and symptoms referable to a single focus in the brain stem (i.e., unilateral, often single, cranial nerve dysfunction and contralateral hemiparesis).

Cystic astrocytomas are rare neoplasms that, in most circumstances, have a small mural nodule and a large cystic component that is responsible for the symptomatology. The clinical course is variable, with months to years passing between the first symptoms and the definitive diagnosis. Hemiparesis, with or without oculomotor dysfunction, is the earliest symptom.

Lower cranial nerve dysfunction associated with quadriparesis or hemiparesis is the primary symptom in cervicomedullary tumors. Occasionally, intractable neck pain and torticollis are the only complaints. Symptoms are commonly present for many months or even years before definitive diagnosis.

C. Treatment

1. Irradiation

Radiation therapy in doses larger than 5000 cGy produces clinical improvement and increased length of survival in children with diffuse brain stem gliomas (59, 77–79). Radiation portals are limited to the posterior fossa, since leptomeningeal dissemination at diagnosis is rare, occurring only after local recurrence (72, 80). Higher doses of radiation improve length of survival; however, the therapeutic window is narrow, with unacceptable toxicity when more than 6000 cGy of conventional therapy (single dose of 180 cGy/day) is administered.

Hyperfractionated irradiation is currently being evaluated as a means to administer higher doses of radiation (81, 82). Laboratory models of radiation therapy, using tissue cultures of malignant cells, demonstrate that small doses (fractions) of radiation administered more than once a day prevent tumor repopulation to greater extent than moderate doses delivered once a day. When the fractions are spaced 4–8 h apart (hyperfractionated or > one fraction per day), there is a redistribution of actively proliferating cell compartments through the cell cycle, with progression of tumor cells into radiosensitive phases. In nonproliferating or slowly proliferating tissues (e.g., normal CNS tissue), there is minimal redistribution of cells and, accordingly, no increase in sensitization. The net effect of hyperfractionated irradiation is increased tumor cell kill and greater tolerated doses, without increased toxicity (83, 84).

Institutional trials at NYU, University of California, San Francisco, and Childrens Hospital of Philadelphia (81, 82) established short-term efficacy, improved survival, and no increase in neurological sequelae with hyperfractionated irradiation to 7200 cGy, administered as 100 cGy twice daily. Current multiinstitutional protocols are being conducted by the CCSG and POG to confirm these preliminary results and to investigate the feasibility of escalating the dose to 7800 cGy. Although previous studies have not demonstrated enhanced quality or length of survival with standard irradiation and chemotherapy, combining hyperfractionated irradiation and chemotherapy or immunotherapy will be a future direction for investigation.

2. Biopsy

Although the goal of surgery is to reduce the tumor burden, the amount of neoplastic tissue that is actually removed is variable. Radical, thorough, subtotal excision of a slow-growing tumor offers the possibility of long-term clinical remission, whereas the same operation for a malignant tumor does not favorably affect the (dismal) prognosis. Some neurosurgeons and oncologists have suggested that it is essential to obtain histological grading of tissue before recommending a course of treatment (63, 65, 72). The biopsy specimens, from either stereotactic or open biopsy, are usually extremely small and may fail to identify the malignant component of the tumor. Review of autopsy and biopsy data from multiple large series demonstrates significant pathological discrepancies (85). Retrospective analysis of 94 patients treated at NYU indicated that only patients with low-grade tumors had sustained improvement following surgery, whereas all patients with malignant tumors died within 12–18 months (66). These results demonstrate a direct correlation of pathology to the clinical course and the neuroradiologic delineation of tumor extent and location (66, 74, 77). All diffuse brain stem tumors were malignant in our series. This is in agreement with autopsy findings as well as other recent clinical series. The combination of MRI scanning and clinical presentation is uniformly diagnostic of malignancy in diffuse tumors and obviates the need to inflict a surgical procedure on an already ill child.

3. Surgical Excision

Cystic, focal, exophytic, and cervicomedullary tumors are amenable to aggressive surgical intervention (66, 69–71). Exophytic tumors have been well documented to have a benign course following radical surgical excision (66, 71, 73) and were discussed with cerebellar astrocytomas.

Cystic and focal astrocytomas occur either in the pons or the midbrain. Because the exposure is relatively limited, the CO_2 laser is the ideal instrument for excising the solid nodular component of the neoplasm. In the pons, the mass bulges posteriorly into the fourth ventricle, and the laser is used to incise the overlying ependyma and enter the cyst, should one be present. A mural nodule can be excised through a large cyst cavity, whereas solid focal tumors are removed piecemeal with the laser or ultrasonic aspirator until a glial–tumor interface is reached.

Midbrain tumors are approached subtemporally through the lateral aspect of the cerebral peduncle. Cystic astrocytomas of the brain stem with mural-enhancing nodules and nonenhancing cyst walls are amenable to radical resection and carry a good prognosis. An enhancing cyst wall is pathognomonic of a malignant glioma. Short-term palliation may be obtained by evacuation of the necrotic tumor in the core of the cyst.

The CO_2 laser and ultrasonic aspirator are used to debulk the tumors occurring at the cervicomedullary junction. In most circumstances, it is possible to obtain a gross total excision of the cervical component of the tumor and a radical subtotal removal of the medullary component (70).

V. EPENDYMOMA

Ependymoma is the least common of the posterior fossa neoplasms, yet it still constitutes 8–10% of all CNS tumors of childhood (2). They have a propensity for younger children, with over half occurring before 2 years of age. They may arise in the fourth ventricle or supratentorially in either brain parenchyma or in the lateral ventricles.

Seventy percent of all ependymomas are located in the posterior fossa, originating from the ependyma of the fourth ventricle and growing to fill the fourth ventricle and extending through the foramena of Luschka and Magendie (34). They will commonly extend laterally into the cerebellopontine angle or, unlike other posterior fossa neoplasms, inferiorly over the dorsal cervical spinal cord to the C3–C5 level (Fig. 5). The tumor may envelop cranial nerves and branches of the vertebral and basilar arteries as it grows in the basal cisterns. The intimate relation of the tumor to CSF pathways permits early leptomeningeal dissemination. Ten to fifteen percent of children will have neuroaxis metastasis at diagnosis (86, 87).

Pathologically, the tumors are graded in a fashion analogous to astrocytomas. The low-grade tumors have features that recapitulate the normal ependymal cell morphology, whereas the anaplastic tumors have various degrees of pleomorphism, increased cellularity, mitotic activity, necrosis, and endothelial hyperplasia. The significance of histological grading is controversial, with most studies demonstrating a tendency toward a worse prognosis with increasing anaplasia. A primitive, extremely malignant neoplasm, the ependymoblastoma, is now considered to be a variant of PNET (27).

A. Presentation

The duration of symptoms and clinical presentation are related to the anatomical location, as with other posterior fossa tumors (16, 34, 88). With extension into the basal cisterns, cranial nerve dysfunction may become manifest. Neck pain and torticollis may occur as result of tumor in the cervical region. The MRI and CT scans demonstrate a mass filling the fourth ventricle that cannot be differentiated from medulloblastoma, solid vermis astrocytoma, or dorsally exophytic brain stem gliomas. The presence of tumor extension along the dorsal surface of the upper cervical spinal cord is highly suggestive, but not pathognomonic, of ependymoma.

Postoperative staging includes assessment of residual posterior fossa tumor, CSF cytology, and gadolinium-enhanced MRI of the spine. As with medulloblastoma, several prognostic factors have been identified: leptomeningeal dissemination, young age (<2–3 years), and subtotal surgical resection are associated with rapid tumor recurrence and poor survival (87, 89–92). As discussed earlier, histological grading of anaplasia has an uncertain influence on prognosis. Overall 5-year disease-free survival is between 40 and 60% (90–92). Children with gross total resection of their tumor (documented by no identifiable tumor on postoperative scans) have the best survival, approaching 80–85% 5-year survival in recent series (90, 92).

B. Treatment

Ependymomas of the fourth ventricle are the most surgically challenging of the posterior fossa tumors. Radical surgical excision should be attempted in all patients. With microsurgical technique, a gross total resection can be accomplished in 30–40% of the children (90, 92). Total resection may be limited by a broad attachment of the tumor to the floor of the fourth ventricle, with brain stem invasion or invasion of cranial nerves and vessels in the basal cisterns. Extension over the dorsal surface of the cervical spinal cord is usually not a major surgical problem: the tumor grows above the pia and can be peeled off the cord. Supratentorial tumors can be totally resected in most cases: involvement of thalamus, hypothalamus, and basal ganglia may preclude complete removal.

Adjuvant irradiation is clearly of benefit in patients with residual tumor, disseminated tumor, and anaplastic histological type (39, 87, 90, 91, 93). Between 5000 and 6000 cGy are required for tumor control. The incidence of dissemination is extremely low for supratentorial ependymoma, and involved field irradiation is adequate. Controversy exists about the propriety of craniospinal irradiation for posterior fossa ependymomas. Most centers recommend neuroaxis irradiation for anaplastic ependymomas because 80% of the patients who ultimately develop metastasis have a high-grade lesion (87, 91, 93). However, dissemination is almost never seen without recurrence at the primary site, suggesting that tumor spread is secondary to failure of local control of the ependymoma (89). A recent trial of local irradiation by POG identified no secondary dissemination (34). The issue of craniospinal irradiation is of particular importance, since most children with posterior fossa ependymoma are quite young and thus are the most prone to develop long-term sequelae.

Although recurrent ependymomas have been shown to be chemosensitive tumors, responding to the same agents as medulloblastomas, prospective trials combining craniospinal irradiation and chemotherapy by CCSG and SIOP have failed to demonstrate an increase in disease-free survial or overall survival with chemotherapy (94). Future innovations in treatment may include deferred irradiation for older children with totally resected tumors, increased tumor resectability using intraoperative neurophysiological monitoring to pursue tumors into the brain stem, and adjuvant chemotherapy in combination with either local irradiation, hyperfractionated irradiation, or reduced-dose neuroaxis irradiation.

VI. SUPRATENTORIAL GLIOMAS

Supratentorial gliomas are a heterogeneous assortment of neuroectodermal tumors that encompass approximately one-third of pediatric brain tumors (95, 96). The most common tumor is the low-grade astrocytoma [grade 1 and 2 of Kernohan (97) or grade 1 WHO (27)] composed of fibrillary or protoplasmic neoplastic astrocytes. Other low-grade tumors include the juvenile pilocytic astrocytoma, oligodendroglioma, mixed glioma, and ganglioglioma (2, 14). Approximately 20% of supratentorial gliomas will be malignant neoplasms: anaplastic astrocytomas and glioblastomas (2, 14).

Within each of these pathological entities, the biological behavior may be quite variable. Studies of cell cycle kinetics, cytogenetics, and cytometrics have demonstrated slow growth rates in most histologically well-differentiated gliomas (98–101). Clinical experience supports the indolent nature of many of these low-grade tumors, with prolonged survival occurring commonly (102–104).

In spite of benign histology, only 60–70% of children with low-grade gliomas will be long-term survivors (7, 11, 15, 39, 95, 103–105). The heterogeneity in location, treatment regimens, neurodiagnostic evaluation, and the unclear natural history have resulted in extensive controversy and debate in the literature, with 10-year survivals ranging from 10 to 94% (1, 7, 11, 15, 16, 40, 96, 104, 106, 107). In view of their unique presentation and clinical course, optic pathway tumors are discussed in a separate section.

In contrast with the low-grade tumors, malignant astrocytomas carry a poor prognosis, similar to adult tumors. Children with glioblastomas have a dismal outcome, with 5-year survival ranging from 5 to 15% (108–110). Anaplastic astrocytomas fare better with 20–40% long-term survival (109). Leptomeningeal dissemination may occur in approximately 10% of children with malignant astrocytomas, especially tumors located adjacent to the ventricles (111). Routine postoperative neuroaxis staging is recommended for these patients.

A. Presentation

The signs and symptoms of supratentorial gliomas are dependent on anatomical localization and histological grade. Brief prodromes are more characteristic of malignant gliomas. Symptoms of increased intracranial pressure occur in most patients, especially those with malignant tumors. Obstructive hydrocephalus is common with deep tumors of the basal ganglia and thalamus that impinge on the ventricles, whereas superficial hemispheric gliomas rarely present with hydrocephalus. Macrocrania may be the only sign of large cerebral tumors in infants. Among the older children, over one-half with hemispheric tumors complain of headache, usually worse in the morning and associated with emesis. Rarely, patients with chronic increased intracranial pressure and papilledema may present with intermittent visual obscurations, visual loss, or even blindness.

Focal signs and symptoms are related to the anatomical location of the neoplasm (96). Most children with hemispheric astrocytomas will have some involvement of the posterior frontal lobe (motor cortex) or basal ganglia, resulting in a monoparesis or hemiparesis. Occipital lobe tumors will often result in visual field abnormalities. Other neurological deficits may be more subtle and insidious, including sensory loss, personality changes, and deteriorating school performance. Seizures will occur in approximately 40–60% of children with hemispheric gliomas (34, 96). Similar to the focal neurological deficits, the seizure pattern will reflect the location of the tumor; for example, complex seizures with temporal lobe tumors and focal motor seizures with frontoparietal neoplasms. Since the advent of CT and especially MRI, unsuspected low-grade tumors have been frequently identified as the cause of chronic epilepsy (104, 107).

B. Treatment

1. Surgery

Surgical intervention has been the primary therapy for nearly all low-grade gliomas of childhood. Most pediatric neurosurgeons believe that gross total excision of low-grade tumors offers the potential for long-term event-free survival or possible cure. Approximately 30% of infratentorial and 18% of supratentorial low-grade gliomas are superficial in location and amenable to gross total surgical excision (16, 96, 103, 112–115). Long-term event-free survival following gross total resection (>10 years) ranges from 50 to 82% in recent retrospective series (103, 106, 107, 113, 115–117).

Unfortunately many low-grade gliomas of childhood extend into vital areas or arise in deep midline structures (e.g., chiasmatic–hypothalamic, thalamic, basal ganglia), rendering complete surgical excision impossible. The role of radical subtotal resection of these tumors is less clear. Laws et al. (103) found survival beyond 5 years similar for total resections and radical subtotal resections, but not for biopsy or partial resection. Radical subtotal resection of deep, midline tumors as the sole treatment modality has been promulgated for thalamic (118), septal (119), hypothalamic (120, 121), and dorsal exophytic brain stem tumors (71, 73).

Radical resection of malignant gliomas of childhood has been correlated with improved disease-free survival and overall survival in two prospective CCSG studies (110, CCSG-945: Wisoff JH, Boyett J, personal communication, 1992). This survival advantage is independent of adjuvant radiation, chemotherapy, and tumor location. A recent CCSG-945 study demonstrated the greatest benefit with greater than 90% tumor resection.

2. Irradiation

Although there is no consensus about the optimal treatment of subtotally resected low-grade tumors, therapeutic irradiation has been the traditional adjuvant treatment in these patients, in spite of conflicting reports concerning efficacy (7, 40, 79, 103, 106, 116, 118, 122–125). The use of irradiation is limited by a relatively narrow therapeutic window. Doses in excess of 4000 cGy are required to delay tumor progression (122, 123, 125). There is no prospective or randomized study examining long-term efficacy, late effect, or quality of survival following irradiation for low-grade gliomas. The question of efficacy is especially important, since tumors are being diagnosed at an earlier stage as a result of routine screening of minimally symptomatic children with MRI and CT scans.

There is a clear benefit of adjuvant irradiation for children with malignant gliomas (108, 109). Doses of 5400–6000 cGy appear to offer longer survival time than doses lower than 5000 cGy (109). Although whole-brain irradiation was frequently recommended in the past, most centers now treat a focal field with generous margins around the tumor (34, 109). As in medulloblastoma, irradiation has been associated with intellectual deterioration, developmental delay, endocrine dysfunction, and the development of irradiation-induced tumors (42–47, 50–54, 126).

3. Chemotherapy

Postirradiation adjuvant chemotherapy has been demonstrated to significantly increase survival in children with malignant astrocytomas (110). A randomized CCSG trial of a nitrosourea-based regimen increased 5-year survival to 43%, compared with children receiving only irradiation (110). This effect on survival was most significant for children with glioblastoma. Preirradiation chemotherapy has been proposed to facilitate the efficacy of radiotherapy by providing further tumor debulking. Several antineoplastic agents such as cisplatin have also demonstrated radiosensitizing properties that could potentially augment the efficacy of irradiation. Currently, there are several institutional and cooperative group trials of neoadjuvant intensive chemotherapy for children younger than 3 years of age that are intended to delay the initiation of irradiation, thereby protecting the immature brain.

VII. OPTIC PATHWAY TUMORS

Optic pathway gliomas comprise a broad spectrum of tumors, ranging from tubular thickening of the optic nerves and chiasm to massive exophytic lesions of the hypothalamus. Although infrequently seen in the adult, these neoplasms represent 3–6% of pediatric brain tumors, ocurring with equal frequency in boys and girls (127, 128). Approximately one-third of these tumors involve only the optic nerve, whereas two-thirds involve some combination of optic chiasm, hypothalamus, third ventricle, and optic tracts (127, 129). The association of these tumors with neurofibromatosis is well known (29, 128, 129–134): 20%–50% of patients with optic pathway gliomas will have neurofibromatosis, whereas 15% of patients with neurofibromatosis have a lesion of the visual pathways. The natural history of these tumors is variable: some behave similarly to hamartomas, with minimal or no growth for many years, whereas others progress with insidious visual loss, vegetative compromise, and death (58, 129, 130, 132, 135–139). Pathologically these tumors are low grade-astrocytomas, often with pilocytic features.

A. Classification and Presentation

The tremendous variability in outcome has made attempts to understand the natural history and analyze the response to treatment extremely difficult (137). The authors have used a three-tiered classification, based on the preoperative MRI, that guides surgical intervention and addresses the apparent increase in morbidity and mortality observed in more posteriorly located tumors (29, 129, 136, 140, 141): (1) prechiasmatic optic nerve gliomas, (2) diffuse chiasmatic gliomas, and (3) exophytic chiasmatic–hypothalamic gliomas.

   Prechiasmatic optic nerve gliomas (Fig. 6) on CT or MRI demonstrate fusiform enlargement of the nerve within the orbit, optic canal, or intracranially without enlargement of the chiasm. Bilateral lesions are occasionally demonstrated in patients with neurofibromatosis. *Diffuse chiasmatic gliomas* demonstrate diffuse enlargement of the chiasm, with variable extension into the optic nerve and tracts. They are usually diagnosed in children with neurofibromatosis. The gadolinium-enhanced MRI and T2 sequence are particularly helpful in delineating these tumors and their involvement of contiguous structures. *Exophytic chiasmatic–hypothalamic gliomas* (Fig. 7) are a unique subset of the posterior tumors that should be considered separately, since they are amenable to radical surgical excision (121, 127, 130, 133, 142). These patients present with large bulky exophytic hypothalamic–chiasmatic tumors.

B. Clinical Presentation

Prechiasmatic optic gliomas commonly present over a 6- to 9-month period with progressive visual loss and proptosis if the tumor involves the intraorbital nerve (78, 132, 133, 135, 143–145). In the infant, nystagmus and strabismus may be the first indication of visual deficits. Funduscopic evaluation usually demonstrates a swollen disc with venous engorgement, although atrophy may be

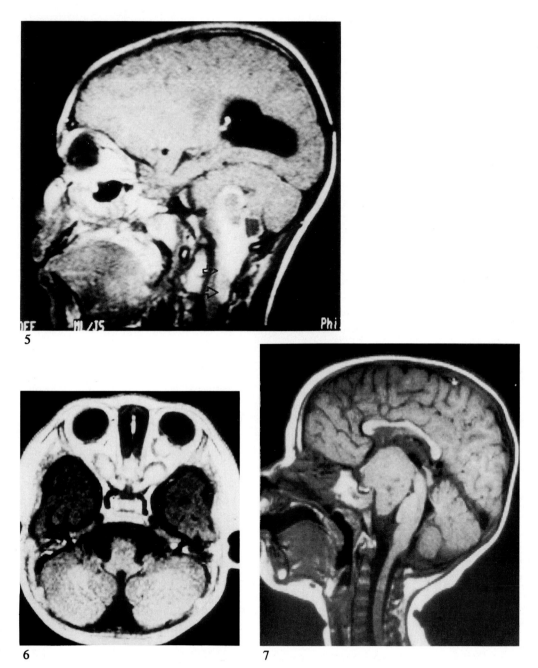

Figure 5 Fourth ventricle ependymoma: gadolinium-enhanced MRI. Note extension along dorsal surface of upper cervical spinal cord (arrows).

Figure 6 Contrast enhanced CT scan of bilateral optic nerve gliomas.

Figure 7 Gadolinium-enhanced MRI of exophytic hypothalamic–chiasmatic glioma.

seen with longer prodomes. Diffuse enlargement of the optic nerve on MRI is pathognomonic of optic nerve glioma in children with neurofibromatosis.

Diffuse chiasmatic gliomas usually present with a combination of diminished visual acuity and bilateral visual field deficits. Endocrinopathy and hydrocephalus are rare. Most of these children will have neurofibromatosis and may be diagnosed in a clinically asymptomatic child by surveillance CT or MRI scan. As with the prechiasmatic tumors, the MRI scan of these lesions is pathognomonic in the presence of a history of neurofibromatosis.

Among the chilren with exophytic chiasmatic–hypothalamic gliomas, there are three distinct age-related patterns of clinical presentation. *Infants* younger than 2 years old almost invariably present with macrocephaly, failure to thrive, diencephalic syndrome, and visual failure. Severe hydrocephalus, with signs of incipient herniation may require emergency CSF shunting. The CT and MRI scans demonstrated massive tumors (see Fig. 7). In *children 2–5 years* old, endocrine dysfunction is the most common presentation. Precocious puberty and growth hormone failure will often bring children to medical attention. Approximately half of the children have abnormal visual examinations. *Older children and young adults* will present with visual complaints and endocrinopathy.

Hypothalamic hamartomas should be briefly mentioned, since they may be difficult to differentiate from exophytic tumors on radiographic and clinical evaluation. They are rare congenital malformations—not true neoplasms (146–148). They may present only with precocious puberty or as part of a more generalized cerebral dysfunction, including gelastic and grand mal seizures, behavior disorder, and mental retardation (148, 149).

C. Treatment

1. Surgery

In the management of visual pathway gliomas, the only treatment that shows unequivocal benefit is the complete resection of *a glioma restricted to one optic nerve* (146). The goal of surgery is preservation of the globe and the prevention of tumor extension into the chiasm. Surgical excision of optic nerve tumors is indicated in patients with progressive proptosis, progressive visual loss; with radiographic evidence of tumor enlargement, and tumors associated with a blind eye. Proptosis alone is an indication for resection when it produces pain, endangers the health of the cornea or globe, or causes significant cosmetic disfigurement (127, 150).

The management of children with minimal or no symptoms is more controversial (34, 45, 103, 127, 132, 135, 137–140, 145, 150). Since these tumors frequently have an indolent course, especially in children with neurofibromatosis, most authors support a moderate approach of expectant management (34, 45, 103, 135, 137–140, 145). Serial visual acuity and field examinations, visual evoked potentials in younger children, and MRI permit deferral of therapy with a low risk to the child of significant visual loss or tumor extension into the chiasm.

Surgical intervention is rarely indicated for *diffuse chiasmatic tumors*. The characteristic MRI appearance in a setting of neurofibromatosis is pathognomonic of a chiasmal glioma and thus obviates the need for a biopsy for histological confirmation. The rare circumstances with an atypical clinical or radiographic presentation, in which a suprasellar germ cell tumor, craniopharyngioma, or dermoid is suspected, are an indication for obtaining a biopsy.

The observation that many gliomas present exophytically in the suprasellar region, with displacement of normal anatomy and the known long-term palliation that has followed radical subtotal resection of other low-grade midline astrocytomas (103, 119) encouraged several authors to explore the feasibility of performing radical subtotal resections of exophytic chiasmatic–hypothalamic tumors, with a good clinical response (120, 121, 133, 142).

2. Irradiation

Although there is no consensus about the optimal treatment of subtotally resected tumors, therapeutic irradiation has been the traditional adjuvant treatment for children with optic pathway gliomas and progressive symptomatic disease (20, 129, 131, 134, 136, 139, 140). Doses larger than 4500 cGy are required to delay tumor progression (129), with most authors recommending 5000–5500 cGy (20, 129, 131, 133). Stabilization of tumor size or diminished tumor volume following irradiation has been well documented (129, 131, 134, 140), although clinical improvements in visual function and neurological deficits occur in only few patients (151). Objective tumor shrinkage on CT scans is seen in most irradiated patients (20, 1341, 133). Recurrence appears to be significantly lower in irradiated patients but documentation of improved survival is lacking (133, 134, 138).

3. Chemotherapy

Chemotherapy has been advocated as an alternative to irradiation for young children with chiasmatic–hypothalamic tumors (34, 133, 151, 152). Packer et al. (151) treated 24 children, preponderantly younger than 3 years of age, with combination chemotherapy [vincristine and dactinomycin (actinomycin D)]. Fifteen of the children lacked evidence of progression, and all were alive after a median follow-up of 4.3 years.

A pilot study of the Children's Cancer Study Group is evaluating the combination of vincristine and carboplatin. Rodriquez et al. and Warnick and Edwards (133, 145) reported the initial results of a five-drug, nitrosourea-based regimen for the primary therapy of children younger than 18 years with optic pathway gliomas. Whether these protocols will allow us to postpone irradiation to permit brain maturation or obviate the need for radiotherapy remains uncertain.

VIII. CRANIOPHARYNGIOMAS

Craniopharyngiomas are the most common nonglial tumor of childhood, accounting for 6–8% of pediatric brain tumors (2). They arise from epithelial nests that are embryonic remnants of Rathke's pouch (2) located along an axis extending from the sella turcica along the pituitary stalk to the hypothalamus and the floor of the third ventricle. Histologically composed of stratified epithelium, they gradually enlarge and appear as partially calcified solid and cystic masses preponderantly in the suprasellar region. The cystic component can reach several centimeters in size. Craniopharyngiomas extend along the path of least resistance into the basal cisterns or can invaginate into the third ventricle. Depending on the direction of growth, the optic nerves and chiasm may be displaced posteriorly, with tumor extending into the frontal fossa, or anteriorly, with retrochiasmatic tumor involving the hypothalamus and upper brain stem. With continued growth superiorly into the third ventricle, hydrocephalus may develop.

Presenting signs and symptoms of craniopharyngiomas are related to pressure upon adjacent neural structures. The main presenting symptoms are raised intracranial pressure in 60–75% of the patients and visual disturbances in approximately half of the children (153). Endocrine dysfunction, including growth failure, delayed sexual maturation, excessive weight gain, and diabetes insipidus, is present in 20–50% of the children at diagnosis, but is rarely the symptom that brings the child to medical attention. The prodrome is usually less than 2 years (154).

Formal preoperative neuro-ophthalmological, endocrinological, and neuropsychological testing is mandatory. Seventy to eighty percent of children will demonstrate abnormal visual acuity or constricted visual fields on preoperative testing (153, 154). The specific ophthalmologic deficits reflect the direction of growth of the tumor and its compression of various portions of the visual apparatus: prechiasmatic extension will compress its optic nerves with loss of visual acuity,

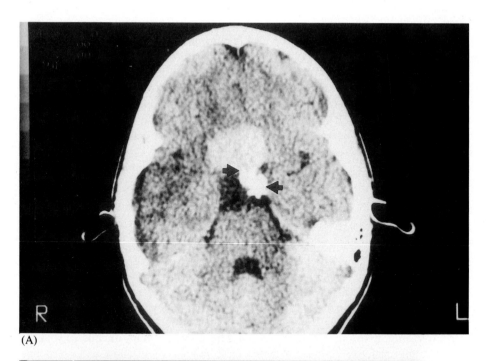

(A)

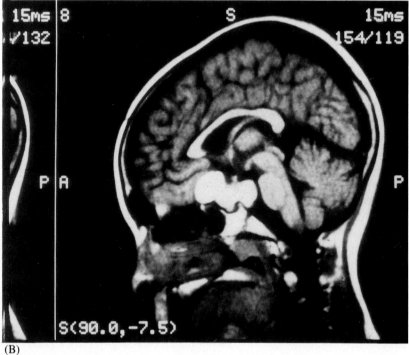

(B)

Figure 8 Craniopharyngioma: (A) CT scan, note calcification (arrows); (B) MRI preoperative; (C) MRI postoperative, note gross total resection.

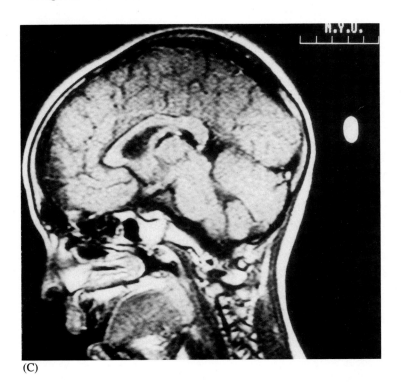

(C)

whereas posterior tumors cause chiasmatic compression with complex visual field defects. Endocrine evaluation shows growth hormone deficiency or gonadotropin deficiency in up to 60% of cases and thyroid or adrenal dysfunction in approximately one-third (153). Fewer than 30% are endocrinologically normal at diagnosis.

Neuroradiological evalution includes both CT and MRI. Tumor morphology and the distorted neural anatomy are best delineated by MRI (155, 156). However, since the MRI does not identify areas of calcification, a CT scan must be obtained for a complete preoperative evaluation (Fig. 8). Hydrocephalus may be noted in 30% of the patients, preponderantly those with larger tumors (34, 153).

A. Treatment

Initial preparation for all therapeutic interventions in craniopharyngiomas includes hormonal replacement, based on the endocrinological testing and, when surgery is anticipated, perioperative corticosteroids. The optimal treatment of craniopharyngiomas is controversial (157–167). The intimate association of these tumors with the visual pathways, hypothalamus, and limbic system can result in severe visual, endocrine, and cognitive deficits. Although most patients can compensate for neurological deficits and endocrinological deficiencies, the cognitive and psychosocial sequelae may be functionally devastating, interfering with education, limiting independence, and adversely affecting the quality of life as these children approach adulthood (161).

1. Surgery

Most pediatric neurosurgeons favor complete microsurgical resection as the treatment of choice for newly diagnosed craniopharyngiomas (153, 154, 159, 162, 165, 167). The surgical technique employs a frontal or frontotemporal (pterional) craniotomy and microsurgical dissection of the tumor from the optic apparatus, vessels of the circle of Willis, and hypothalamus. The pituitary stalk is often the site of origin of these tumors and must be sectioned in over 70% of the cases to achieve a potentially curative total resection. The extent of resection must be confirmed by a postoperative CT scan. Seventy to ninety percent of primary tumors are amenable to total resection (34, 159, 162, 165, 167). Rare intrasellar tumors or residual intrasellar tumor may be resected transphenoidally (105).

Endocrine disturbances are common after radical resection as a result of hypothalamic manipulation and pituitary stalk sectioning (153, 163, 165. 167, 168). Diabetes insipidus is almost universally present immediately following surgery. Over the course of the first week, diabetes insipidus may alternate with inappropriate antidiuretic hormone release (SIADH). Meticulous attention to fluid balance and electrolyte status is essential to avoid severe fluctuations from hypernatremia to hyponatremia. Permanent diabetes insipidus requiring replacement with synthetic vasopressin (desmopressin; DDAVP) will develop in approximately 75% of children. Other hormonal replacement therapy is required approximately 80% of the time (163, 167). Weight gain, with or without overt hyperphagia, may occur (168).

Following radiographically confirmed total resection, no adjuvant therapy is administered. A good outcome, with normal psychosocial integration and age-appropriate academic performance, is reported in over 70% of children (167) and was seen in 82% of our 23 patients who underwent radical resection since 1985. Total removal of the tumor offers the optimal ophthalmological recovery and outcome (153). Preoperative hydrocephalus will often resolve after radical tumor resection, thereby obviating the need for a shunt.

Recurrence rates range from 0 to 20% (153, 162, 165, 167, 169). Most recurrences occur within 2 years. Repeat surgery can be curative especially with solid tumors; however, scarring from previous surgery may increase the operation's technical difficulty. The morbidity following repeat surgery is high, with fewer than one-third having a good outcome (167).

2. Irradiation

Craniopharyngiomas are radiosensitive tumors. In the presence of gross residual disease, irradiation will decrease the disease progression rate from 75% to 20–30% (157). Doses of at least 5000 cGy are required to obtain clinical responses (170). Current technology minimizes radiation damage to adjacent neural structures; however, panhypopituitarism will occur almost universally. With large tumors, significant portions of the temporal and frontal lobes will be included in the radiation portals. Long-term sequelae of irradiation include secondary tumors, optic neuropathy, and vascular injury with the development of moyamoya disease (162).

3. Intracavitary Therapy

Local treatment with intracavitary irradiation utilizing colloidal ^{32}P (171) or intracavitary bleomycin (60) obliterates the cystic component in up to 90% of the cases, but will not affect solid tumor growth. Simple stereotactic aspiration of tumor cysts or placement of an Ommaya reservoir into the cyst for serial aspirations is never indicated as primary therapy in children and should be reserved for palliation when surgery and irradiation have failed.

The advantages of subtotal resection with irradiation versus radical surgery are unclear. Early retrospective reviews suggested equivalent or superior tumor control and less long-term morbidity with conservative surgery and irradiation (160, 161, 164, 166). Many of the data from these studies were obtained before the advent of CT scanning and the introduction of microsurgical technique, and of modern neuroanesthesia. As discussed earlier, recent reports of radical resection show excellent postoperative functional survival and low recurrence rates when surgery is performed by experienced surgeons in centers that provide comprehensive postoperative care (159, 162, 165, 167). An attempt at radical curative resection should be the initial treatment of craniopharyngiomas. Overall long-term survival for all patients and treatments approaches 90% at 5 years and 80% at 10 years (36, 162, 167).

IX. GERM CELL TUMORS

Primary intracranial germ cell tumors are a heterogeneous group of five related neoplasms that are histologically indistinguishable from germ cell tumors of the gonads (2, 172–174). Although rare among adult brain tumors, they constitute approximately 3–6.5% of central nervous system malignancies of childhood (172, 174), with the highest incidence occurring among the Japanese (175). Primary intracranial germ cell tumors represent almost 10% of all germ cell neoplasms diagnosed in the first 15 years of life (173). They are more common in boys [2.24:1 (172)], with a peak incidence in the second decade, coincident with the onset of puberty (172).

The histological variants of germ cell tumors, in descending order of frequency, are teratoma (including mature, immature, and malignant), germinoma, endodermal sinus (yolk sac) tumor, embryonal carcinoma, and choriocarcinoma (172, 176, 177). Combinations of two or more types within the same tumor are frequent (176, 178). Each of these represents neoplastic transformation of normal embryonic or extraembryonic tissues (172): the primordial germ cell (germinoma), the pluripotential stem cell (embryonal carcinoma), the differentiated embryo (teratoma), yolk sac endoderm (endodermal sinus tumor), and trophoblast (choriocarcinoma). These tumors may secrete several tumor markers that may be identified immunohistochemically on tumor tissue or serologically in blood or CSF. These markers include human chorionic gonadotropin (hCG), alpha-fetoprotein (AFP), and placental alkaline phosphatase (PLAP) (172, 174, 179).

From a clinical perspective, these tumors can be grouped as benign teratomas, germinomas, and nongerminomatous germ cell tumors (NGGCT). Except for the benign teratomas, all germ cell tumors are malignant and capable of metastasis.

A. Presentation

Intracranial germ cell tumors arise almost exclusively along an axis bisecting the third ventricle from above the sella turcica to suprasellar (37%), to the pineal gland (48%) (172) (Fig. 9). Ten percent of children may present with tumors in both pineal and suprasellar locations. Regardless of histological type, they manifest neurological, ophthalmological, and endocrinological signs and symptoms that are dependent on tumor location.

Most children with pineal region tumors present with increased intracranial pressure from obstruction of the aqueduct of Sylvius and subsequent hydrocephalus. Compression of the quadrigeminal plate in the dorsal midbrain by a pineal mass produces Parinaud's syndrome: paralysis of upward gaze and convergence. Rarely, movement disorders or corticospinal tract signs result from locally invasive tumors, and dementia or personality changes from long standing hydrocephalus.

Suprasellar tumors typically present with a triad of visual loss, diabetes insipidus, and panhypopituitarism. Two-thirds of the children have visual field defects resulting from compression of the optic chiasm. Diabetes insipidus occurs in 60–95% of cases and may precede other symptoms for a considerable period (174). All children with a diagnosis of diabetes insipidus should be evaluated with an MRI study.

The length and nature of the clinical prodrome may be related to specific histologies. Germinomas have the longest duration of preoperative symptoms and will most likely present as suprasellar masses with diabetes insipidus, visual loss, and panhypopituitarism. Hydrocephalus is the initial presentation in approximately 50% of NGGCTs (34, 174).

Precocious puberty is seen in up to 20% of intracranial germ cell tumors (174), with over half of choriocarcinomas presenting with this syndrome. Three mechanisms may lead to precocious

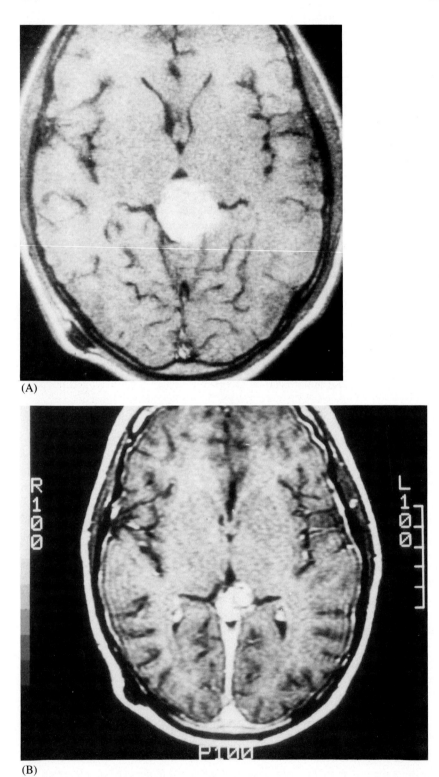

(A)

(B)

Figure 9 Nongerminomatous germ cell tumor of the pineal region: (A) gadolinium-enhanced MRI at diagnosis; (B) gadolinium-enhanced MRI after two courses of chemotherapy. Note 75% decrease in tumor volume.

puberty: pineal body destruction, with ablation of a gonadal inhibitory factor; hypothalamic nuclei damage resulting in a similar release of gonadal inhibition; and ectopic secretion of hCG and luteinizing hormone (LH) by the tumor (172, 174).

A relation among age, location, sex, and histological type has been noted (172). Suprasellar tumors are found in 75% of girls, whereas two-thirds of tumors in boys were primarily pineal. NGGCT, especially choriocarcinoma, is usually diagnosed between birth and 9 years. Teratomas are the most common congenital tumor. Germinomas are preponderantly tumors of preadolescent and teenaged boys.

Neuroradiologic evaluation should include both CT and MRI (156). Germinomas are hyperdense on precontrast CT and intensely enhancing with a gadolinium-enhanced MRI. Teratomas demonstrate a variegated appearance on both CT and MRI from the admixture of calcification, fat, and cysts, whereas contrast enhancement is suggestive of malignant variants. The presence of fat is almost pathognomonic of a teratoma. The NGGCTs have a heterogeneous appearance. The presence of intratumoral hemorrhage in a pineal or suprasellar mass is suggestive of choriocarcinoma. Preoperative evaluation includes measurement of serum and CSF tumor markers (172, 179–181): hCG (choriocarcinoma, embryonal carcinoma), AFP (endodermal sinus tumor, embryonal carcinoma), and PLAP (germinoma).

B. Treatment

1. Surgery

Before the introduction of modern neurosurgical techniques, surgical resection of germ cell tumors, particularly in the pineal region, was associated with a high operative morbidity and mortality. A tumor with the radiographic appearance of a germ cell tumor in a pubertal boy was often treated empirically with irradiation. With the advent of microsurgical technique and advances in neuroanesthesia, the risk following a direct surgical approach to pineal and other third ventricular masses has been dramatically reduced to 1% or less (172).

The reliance on MRI and CT for definitive diagnosis is dangerous, since many tumors in this location—the various germ cell as well as non–germ cell tumors—have a similar radiographic appearance. Although a radiosensitive germinoma has been presumed to be the most common pineal tumor, contemporary series with histological diagnosis have demonstrated pure germinoma in fewer than one-third of pineal masses (172, 182). Only a histological diagnosis permits the development of rational specific therapy (183). Focal, empiric irradiation could be suboptimal for malignant non–germ cell tumors (when craniospinal irradiation is indicated) and inappropriate for benign lesions, such as mature teratomas, that are curable by surgical resection alone (172, 182, 184, 185).

Most pediatric neurosurgeons currently believe that the initial treatment of germ cell tumors should be a craniotomy, open biopsy and, when technically feasible, a radical resection of the tumor (34, 180). Stereotactic procedures should be avoided for biopsy, since one-third of tumors may be of mixed histological type that can be missed by the limited tissue sampling of this technique. Intraoperative frozen-section histological assessment is essential: a diagnosis of mature teratoma mandates complete removal for cure, whereas with a germinoma or NGGCT, a radical subtotal resection is adequate, since postoperative irradiation or chemotherapy may allow a remission or cure to be obtained.

Several surgical approaches to the pineal region have been promulgated; occipital–transtentorial and infratentorial–supracerebellar being the most common (184, 185). The choice of approach is based on the direction of tumor growth and preference of the operating surgeon (180). The operative technique for suprasellar germ cell tumors is similar to the approach used for craniopharyngiomas and optic pathway tumors. Postoperative neuroaxis staging with a gadolinium-enhanced complete spinal MRI and CSF cytological study is mandatory. Dissemination at diagnosis is seen in at least 10% of all germ cell tumors and is significantly more common with NGGCT (34, 172, 180, 183).

2. Irradiation

Germinoma is a highly radiosensitive tumor that is potentially curable in over 80% of children with histologically confirmed germinoma who receive irradiation (186, 187). The optimal dose and extent of irradiation remains controversial; 5000 cGy appears to be the minimal dose required for cure. Although some reports have advocated craniospinal irradiation, based on reports of a high incidence of spinal metastasis in focally irradiated pateints (187), those studies lacked histological confirmation and neuroaxis staging. Most centers now irradiate the tumor site and ventricular system and reserve craniospinal irradiation for disseminated tumors (188, 189). There are institutional studies investigating reduced-dose irradiation and chemotherapy to offset the deleterious effects of large-volume and high-dose irradiation on the developing nervous system.

3. Chemotherapy

Disseminated germinoma and NGGCTs have a dismal prognosis following conventional treatment with surgery and irradiation (172, 177, 183, 190). Chemotherapy protocols employing synergistically cytotoxic drugs, including vinblastine, bleomycin, cyclophosphamide, and cisplatin, have achieved complete remission rates in 60–90% of localized and disseminated testicular carcinomas and seminomas (172, 191–196). Preliminary experience with analogous protocols for intracranial NGGCT is encouraging, with long-term disease-free survival reported in most cases (172, 183, 190, 197). Although the ultimate value of intensive chemotherapy as adjuvant or neoadjuvant therapy is uncertain, it would appear reasonable, given the poor prognosis with conventional therapy, to enter patients with these rare tumors in currently available prospective trials.

X. LATE EFFECTS OF RADIATION AND CHEMOTHERAPY

Meadows et al. (55) reviewed psychometric evaluations on 31 leukemic children who received 2400 cGy plus intrathecal methotrexate. Analysis by age group demonstrated an average IQ loss of 14 points in the 2-year 8-month to 3-year 3-month group, 21 points in the 3-year 9-month to 5-year 3-month group, and only a 7-point loss in the children over 6 years. Ochs (198) presented a group of 42 children: 22 received craniospinal irradiation and 20 had cranial irradiation plus methotrexate. Fifty percent of the patients younger than 5 years at the time of treatment required special education, compared with 26% of the whole group.

A Childrens Cancer Study Group (199) report examined neuropsychological impairment following prophylactic cranial irradiation in leukemic children. A direct correlation was established between age and impairment: younger children had greater IQ loss. Williams and Davis (200) reviewed 28 studies in the literature that have considered neuropsychological outcome of leukemic children receiving cranial irradiation. Of 20 studies that examined age, 13 found younger patients experienced greater neuropsychological deficits.

Evidence of anatomical damage is provided by Carli et al. (56). They reviewed CT scans, in 72 children receiving central nervous system irradiation, searching for radiographic correlates of radiation toxicity. Age younger than 5 years was the most significant factor predicting a CT scan abnormality.

A. Neuropsychological Evaluation

Although much has been published concerning the survival rates for children with brain tumors, relatively little has been published to evaluate and compare the quality of survival of children with specific types of tumors. Evaluation of survival has been by neurological examination using Bloom's or Bouchard's taxonomy (four categories ranging from incapable of self-care to no disability) (35, 201). These investigations indicate that more than 70% of surviving children experienced no disability or only mild handicaps (35, 86, 201). Studies of infants produced less-encouraging results, with fewer than 20% judged to be completely normal (18, 19, 54). These classifications provide gross evaluations of general functioning and do not attempt to address specific cognitive and behavioral changes.

More recent studies have begun to provide evaluations of changes in cognitive functioning through the use of well-established neuropsychological test instruments. These studies reveal cognitive deficits in survivors in excess of the distribution normally expected in the general population. Hirsch et al. (38) found that, in 28 survivors of medulloblastoma, only 12% had IQs above 90, and 26 of the 28 patients (93%) manifested behavioral disturbances. Danoff et al. (43) reported intelligence test scores demonstrating an IQ less than 79 (mentally defective to borderline) in 17 individuals (45%) out of 38 patients with primary brain tumors. The mean age at diagnosis of this group was 7.9 years; the mean follow-up interval to assessment was 9.3 years. Emotional problems or disturbances were noted in 14 patients (37%).

Kun and Mulhern et al. (47, 48) have serially followed a group of 26 pediatric patients with primary brain tumors of mixed etiology and localization. Of 15 children studied after cranial irradiation, 8 had subnormal IQ scores. Serial postirradiation testing in 10 patients showed improvement in 2, stability in 5, and further deterioration in 3. The only neuropsychological study involving irradiated astrocytoma patients (126) demonstrated instances of diffuse cortical dysfunction involving deficient problem-solving and an inability to cope with novel situations, whereas psychometric intelligence, as a whole, remained consistent with premorbid levels. Location of lesion and presence of hydrocephalus did not appear to be determining factors.

In a careful review of the literature on neuropsychological sequelae in children with brain tumors (47), several observations, based on the limited data, were presented: (1) overall, children with brain tumors display a high incidence of intellectual impairment and emotional/behavioral problems; (2) hydrocephalus preoperatively does not significantly affect postoperative functional outcome; (3) CNS irradiation, especially whole-brain radiation, is associated with decreased neuropsychological functioning; (4) younger children do not do as well neuropsychologically as their older counterparts; and (5) children with supratentorial tumors do not do as well as those with infratentorial tumors.

Although there is no universally accepted definition of quality of life, it is conceptualized as a multidimensional assessment, with functional status being a major component. Neuropsychological testing, together with periodic systems review and additional endocrine determinations, can provide interim assessments of change in the patient's clinical status and thereby monitor the development of damage to CNS functioning before disease recurrence or death. This allows appropriate intervention or remedial strategies to be instituted earlier, thereby directly affecting the patient's quality of survival. As long-term survival and possible cure become a reality for most children with brain tumors, a near-normal quality of life must remain the goal of these survivors.

REFERENCES

1. Kramer S, Meadows AT, Jarret P, et al. Incidence of childhood cancer: experience of a decade in a population-based registry. JNCI 1983; 70:49–55.
2. Russell DS, Rubinstein LJ. Pathology of tumors of the nervous system. 4th ed. Baltimore: Williams & Wilkins, 1977.
3. Silverberg E, Lubera J. Cancer statistics, 1986. CA 1986; 36:9–23.
4. Cancer Surveillance Program of Los Angeles. University of Southern California.

5. Carrea R, Zingale D. Epidemiology of neoplasms of the central nervous system in infancy and childhood. In: Amador LV, ed. Brain tumors in the young. Springfield: Charles C Thomas, 1983.

6. Children's Cancer Study Group. Registrations of CNS tumors, 1985–1986.

7. Farwell JR, Dohrmann GJ, Flannery JT. Central nervous system tumors in children. Cancer 1977; 40:3123–3132.

8. Horm JW, Asire AJ, Young IL, et al. SEER program: cancer incidence and mortality in the United States 1973–1981. Bethesda: National Institutes of Health Publication No. 85–1837, 1984.

9. Schoenberg BS, Schoenberg DG, Christine BW, et al. The epidemiology of primary intracranial neoplasms of childhood. Mayo Clin Proc 1976; 5:51–56.

10. US Department of Health and Human Services. National Cancer Institute Monograph 57: surveillance, epidemiology, and end results—incidence and mortality data 1973–77.

11. Young JL, Miller RW. Incidence of malignant tumors in US children. J Pediatr 1975; 86:254–258.

12. Young JL, Ries LG, Silverberg E, et al. Cancer incidence, survival, and mortality for children younger than age 15 years. Cancer 1986; 58:598–602.

13. Abramson I, Rabin M, Cavanaugh PJ. Brain tumors in children: analysis of 136 cases. Radiology 1974; 112:669–672.

14. Burger PC, Vogel FS. Surgical pathology of the nervous system and its coverings. 2nd ed. New York: John Wiley & Sons, 1982.

15. Haishamin O. Intracranial tumors of children. Childs Brain 1977; 31:69–78.

16. Humphreys RP. Posterior cranial fossa tumors in children. In: Youman JR, ed. Neurological surgery. Philadelphia: WB Saunders, 1982.

17. Albright AL. Brain tumors in neonates, infants, and toddlers. Contemp Neurosurg 1985; 7:1.

18. Farwell JR, Dohrman GJ. Intracranial neoplasms in infants. Arch Neurol 1978; 35:533–537.

19. Fessard C. Cerebral tumors in infancy: 66 clinicoanatomical case studies. Am J Dis Child 1968; 115:302–308.

20. Visot A, Rougerie J, Derome PJ, Evrard E. Gliomes opto-chiasmatiques. Neurochirurgie 1980; 26:181–192.

21. Cogen PH, Daneshvar L, Metzger AK, et al. Deletion mapping of the medulloblastoma locus on chromosome 17p. Genomics 1990; 8:279–285.

22. James CD, Carlbo, E, Dumanski JP, et al. Clonal genomic alterations in glioma malignancy stages. Cancer Res 1988; 48:5546–5551.

23. James CD, Carlbom E, Nordenskold M, et al. Mitotic recombination of chromosome 17 in astrocytomas. Proc Natl Acad Sci USA 1989; 86:2858–2862.

24. Seizinger BR, Martuza RL, Gusella JF. Loss of genes on chromosome 22 in tumorigenesis of human acoustic neuroma. Nature 1986; 322:644–647.

25. Seizinger BR, De La Monte S, Atkins L, et al. Molecular genetic approach to human meningioma: loss of genes on chromosome 22. Proc Natl Acad Sci USA 1987; 84:5419–5423.

26. Liu HM, Bailey OT. Neuropathology. In: Amador LV, ed. Brain tumors in the young. Springfield: Charles C Thomas, 1983.

27. Rorke LB, Gilles FH, Davis RL. Revision of the World Health Organization classification of brain tumors for childhood brain tumors. Cancer 1985; 56:1869–1886.

28. Caputy AJ, McCoullough DC, Manz HJ, et al. A review of the factors influencing prognosis of medulloblastoma: the importance of cellular differentiation. J Neurosurg 1987; 66:80–87.

29. Packer RJ, Savino PJ, Bilanuik LT, et al. Chiasmatic gliomas of childhood. A reappraisal of natural history and effectiveness of cranial radiation. Childs Brain 1983; 10:393–403.

30. Chin HW, Maruyama Y, Young AB. Medulloblastoma: recent advances and directions in diagnosis and management, part II. Curr Probl Cancer 1984; 8:1–54.

31. Allen JC, Epstein F. Medulloblastoma and other primary malignant neuroectodermal tumors of the CNS: the effect of patient's age and extent of disease on prognosis. J Neurosurg 1982; 57:446–451.

32. Edwards MSB, Hudgins RJ. Medulloblastoma and primitive neuroectodermal tumors of the posterior fossa. In: McLaurin RL, Schut L, Venes JL, et al, eds. Pediatric neurosurgery. 2nd ed. Philadelphia: WB Saunders, 1989:347–356.

33. Albright AL, Wisoff JH, Zeltzer PM, et al. Current neurosurgical treatment of medulloblastomas in children: a report of the Children's Cancer Study Group. Pediatr Neurosci 1989; 15:276–282.
34. Warnick RE, Edwards MSB. Pediatric brain tumors. Curr Prob Pediatr 1991; 21:129–173.
35. Bloom HJG, Wallace ENK, Henk JM. The treatment and prognosis of medulloblastoma in children. AJR 1969; 105:43–62.
36. Bloom HJG, Glees J, Bell J. The treatment and long term prognosis of children with intracranial tumors: a study of 610 cases. Int J Radiat Oncol Biol Phys 1990; 18:723–745.
37. Evans AE, Jenkin RDT, Sposto R, et al. The treatment of medulloblastoma: results of a prospective randomized trial of radiation with and without CCNU, vincristine and prednisone. J Neurosurg 1990; 72:572–582.
38. Hirsch JF, Renier D, Czernichow P. Medulloblastoma in childhood: survival and functional results. Acta Neurochir 1979; 48:1–15.
39. Leibel SA, Sheline GE. Radiation therapy for neoplasms of the brain. J Neurosurg 1987; 66:1–22
40. Sheline GE. Radiation therapy of brain tumors. Cancer 1977; 39:873–881.
41. Packer RJ, Sutton LN, Rorke LB, et al. Prognostic importance of cellular differentiation in medulloblastoma of childhood. J Neurosurg 1984; 61:296–301.
42. Bamford FN, Jones PM, Pearson D, Ribeiro GG, Shalet SM, Bearwell CG. Residual disabilities in children treated for intracranial space-occupying lesions. Cancer 1976; 37:1149–1151.
43. Danoff BF, Chowchock FS, Marquette C, et al. Assessment of the long-germ effects of primary radiation therapy for brain tumors in children. Cancer 1982; 49:1580–1586.
44. Duffner PK, Cohen MD, Thomas P. Late effects of treatment on the intelligence of children with posterior fossa tumors. Cancer 1983; 51:391–395.
45. Duffner Pk, Cohen ME, Thompson PRM, Lansky SB. The long term effects of cranial irradiation on the central nervous system. Cancer 1985; 56:841–1847.
46. Eiser C. Intellectual abilities among survivors of childhood leukemia as a function of CNS irradiation. Arch Dis Child 1978; 53:391–395.
47. Kun LE, Mulhern RK, Crisco JJ. Quality of life in children treated for brain tumors. Intellectual, emotional and academic function. J Neurosurg 1983; 58:1–6.
48. Kun LE, Mulhern RK. Neuropsychologic function in children with brain tumors: II. Serial studies of intellect and time after treatment. Am J Clin Oncol 1983; 6:651–656.
49. Mechanick JI, Hochberg FH, LaRocque A. Hypothalamic dysfunction following whole-brain irradiation. J Neurosurg 1986; 65:490–494.
50. Richards GE. Effects of irradiation on the hypothalamic and pituitary regions. In: Gilbert, Kagan, eds. Radiation damage to the nervous system. New York: Raven Press, 1980: 175–180.
51. Shalet SM, Beardwell CG, Aarons BM, et al. Growth impairment in children treated for brain tumors. Arch Dis Child 1978; 53:491–494.
52. Sheline GE, Wara WM, Smith V. Therapeutic irradiation and brain injury. Int J Radiat Oncol Biol Phys 1980; 6:1215–1228.
53. Soni SS, Marten GW, Pitner SE, et al. Effects of central nervous system irradiation on neurophysiologic functioning of children with acute lymphocytic leukemia. N Engl J Med 1973; 293:113–118.
54. Spunberg JJ Chang CH Goldman M, et al. Quality of long-term survival following irradiation for intracranial tumors in children under the age of two. Int J Radiat Oncol Biol Phys 1981; 7:727–736.
55. Meadow AT, Massari DJ, Fergusson J, et al. Decline in IQ scores and cognitive dysfunctions in children with acute lymphocytic leukaemia treated with cranial irradiation. Lancet 1981; 2:1015–1018.
56. Carli M, Periolongo G, Drigo P, et al. Risk factors in long-term sequelae of central nervous system prophylaxis in successfully treated children with acute lymphocytic leukemia. Med Pediatr Oncol 1985; 13:334–340.
57. Pfefferbaum-Levine B, Copeland DR, Fletcher JM, et al. Neuropsychologic assessment of long-term survivors of childhood leukemia. Am J Pediatr Hematol Oncol 1984; 6:123–128.
58. Roberson C, Till K. Hypothalamic gliomas in children. J Neurol Neurosurg Psychiatry 1974; 37:1047–1052.
59. Freeman CR, Suissa S. Brain stem tumors in children: results of a survey of 62 patients treated with radiotherapy. Int J Radiat Oncol Biol Phys 1986; 12:1823–1828.

60. Takahashi H, Nakazawa S, Shimura T. Evaluation of postoperative intratumoral injection of bleomycin for craniopharyngioma in children. J Neurosurg 1985; 62:120–127.

61. Sutton LN, Schut L. Cerebellar astrocytomas. In: McLaurin RL, Schut L, Venes JL, et al, eds. Pediatric neurosurgery. 2nd ed. Philadelphia: WB Saunders, 1989:338–346.

62. Ilgren EB, Stiller CA. Cerebellar astrocytomas: therapeutic management. Acta Neurochir 1986; 81:11–26.

63. Albright AL, Price RA, Guthkelch N. Brain stem gliomas of children: a clinicopathological study. Cancer 1983; 52:2313–2319.

64. Allen JC. Brain stem glioma. Neurol Neurosurg 1983; 4:2.

65. Albright AL, Guthkelch AN, Packer RJ, et al. Prognostic factors in pediatric brain stem gliomas. J Neurosurg 1986; 65:751–755.

66. Epstein FJ, Wisoff JH. Surgical management of brain stem tumors of childhood and adolescence. Neurosurg Clin North Am 1990; 1:111–121.

67. Littman P, Jarrett P, Bilaniuk, et al. Pediatric brainstem gliomas. Cancer 1980; 45:2787–2792.

68. Berger MS, Edwards MSB, LeMasters D, et al. Pediatric brainstem tumors: radiographic, pathological, and clinical correlations. Neurosurgery 1983; 12:298–302.

69. Epstein F, McCleary EL. Intrinsic brainstem tumors of childhood: surgical indications. J Neurosurg 1986; 64:11–15.

70. Epstein FJ, Wisoff JH. Intra-axial tumors of the cervicomedullary junction. J Neurosurg 1987; 67:483–487.

71. Hoffman HJ, Becker L, Craven MA. A clinically and pathologically distinct group of benign brainstem gliomas. Neurosurgery 1980; 7:243–248.

72. Stroink AR, Hoffman HJ, Hendrick EB, et al. Diagnosis and management of pediatric brain-stem gliomas. J Neurosurg 1986; 65:745–750.

73. Stroink AR, Hoffman HJ, Hendrick EB, et al. Transependymal benign dorsally exophytic brain-stem gliomas in childhood: diagnosis and treatment recommendations. Neurosurgery 1987; 20:439–444.

74. Bradac GB, Schorner W, Bender A, et al. MRI (NMR) in the diagnosis of brainstem tumors. Neuroradiology 1983; 27:208–213.

75. Lee BC, Kneeland JB, Walker RW, et al. MR Imaging of brainstem tumor AJNR 1985; 6:159–163.

76. Tsuchida T, Shimbo Y, Fukuda M, et al. Computed tomography and histological studies of pontine glioma. Childs Nerv Syst 1985; 1:223–229.

77. Kim TH, Chin HW, Pollan S, et al. Radiotherapy of primary brain stem tumors. Int J Radiat Oncol Biol Phys 1980; 6:51–57.

78. Little HL, Chambers JW, Walsh FB. Unilateral intracranial optic nerve involvement. Neurosurgical significance. Arch Ophthalmol 1965; 73:331–337.

79. Wara WM. Radiation therapy for brain tumors. Cancer 1985; 55:2291–2295.

80. Packer RJ, Allen J, Nielsen S, et al. Brainstem gliomas: clinical manifestations of meningeal gliomatosis. Ann Neurol 1983; 14:177–182.

81. Edwards MSB, Wara WM, Urtasun RC, et al. Hyperfractionated radiation therapy for brain-stem glioma: a phase I–II trial. J Neurosurg 1989; 70:691–700.

82. Packer RJ, Allen JC, Goldwein JL, et al. Hyperfractionated radiotherapy for children with brainstem gliomas: a pilot study using 7200 cGy. Ann Neurol 1990; 27:167–173.

83. Withers HR. Cell cycle redistribution as a factor in multifraction irradiation. Radiology 1975; 114:199–202.

84. Withers HR, Thames HD, Peters LJ, Fletcher GH. Normal tissue radioresistance in clinical radiotherapy. Biological bases and clinical implications of tumor radioresistance. In: Proceedings of the 2nd Rome international symposium, Sept 1980.

85. Tomita T, McClone DG, Naidich TP. Brain stem gliomas in childhood: rational approach and treatment. J Neurooncol 1984; 2:117–122.

86. Giuffre R, Caroli F, Delfini R, et al. Long-term follow-up of 440 children operated on for primary intracranial tumors. Neurochirurgia 1982; 25:119–123.

87. Salazar OM. A better understanding of CNS seeding and a brighter outlook for postoperatively irradiated patients with ependymomas. Int J Radiat Oncol Biol Phys 1983; 9:1231–1234.

88. Coulon RA, Till K. Intracranial ependymomas in children: a review of 43 cases. Childs Brain 1977; 3:154–168.
89. Goldwein JW, Glauser TA, Packer RJ. Recurrent intracranial ependymomas in children: survival, patterns of failure, and prognostic factors. Cancer 1990; 66:557–563.
90. Healey EA, Barnes PD, Kupsky WJ, et al. The prognostic significance of postoperative residual tumor in ependymoma. Neurosurgery 1991; 28:666–672.
91. Kun LE, Kovnar KH, Sanford RA. Ependymomas in children. Pediatr Neurosci 1988; 14:57–63.
92. Nazar GB, Hoffman HJ, Becker LE, et al. Infratentorial ependymomas in childhood: prognostic factors and treatment. J Neurosurg 1990; 72:408–417.
93. Wallner KE, Wara WM, Sheline GE, et al. Intracranial ependymomas: results of treatment with partial or whole brain irradiation without spinal irradiation. Int J Radiat Oncol Biol Phys 1986; 12:1937–1941.
94. Friedman HS, Oakes WJ. The chemotherapy of posterior fossa tumors in childhood. J Neurooncol 1987; 5:217–229.
95. Dohrman GJ, Farwell JR, Flannery JT. Astrocytomas in childhood: a population based study. Surg Neurol 1985; 23:64–68.
96. Hoffman HJ. Supratentorial brain tumors in children. In: Youman JR, ed. Neurological surgery. Philadelphia: WB Saunders, 1982.
97. Kernohan JW, Mabon RF, Svien HJ, et al. Symposium on new and simplified concept of gliomas. A simplified classification of the gliomas. Proc Mayo Clin Staff Meet 1949; 24:71–75.
98. Hoshino T. A commentary on the biology and growth kinetics of low-grade and high-grade gliomas. J Neurosurg 1984; 61:895–900.
99. Hoshino T, Nagashima T, Murovic J, et al. In situ cell kinetics studies on human neuroectodermal tumors with bromodeoxyuridine labeling. J Neurosurg 1986; 64:453–459.
100. Hoshino T, Wilson CB. Cell kinetic analysis of human malignant brain tumors (gliomas). Cancer 1979; 44:956–962.
101. Shitara N, McKeever PE, Whang-Peng J, et al. Flow-cytometric and cytogenetic analysis of human cultured cell lines derived from high- and low-grade astrocytomas. Acta Neuropathol 1983; 60:40–48.
102. Cohandon F, Aouad N, Rougier A, et al. Histologic and non-histologic factors correlated with survival time in supratentorial astrocytic tumors. J Neurooncol 1985; 3:105–111.
103. Laws ER, Taylor WF, Clifton MB, et al. Neurosurgical management of low-grade astrocytoma of the cerebral hemispheres. J Neurosurg 1984; 61:665–673.
104. Spencer DD, Spencer SS, Mattson RH, et al. Intracerebral masses in patients with intractable partial epilepsy. Neurology 1984; 34:432–136.
105. Laws ER. Transsphenoidal microsurgery in the management of craniopharyngiomas. J Neurosurg 1980; 52:661–666.
106. Cohen ME, Duffner PK. Brain tumors in children: principles of diagnosis and treatment. New York: Raven Press, 1984.
107. Hirsch JF, Sainte Rose C, Pierre-Kahn A, et al. Benign astrocytic and oligodendrocytic tumors of the cerebral hemispheres in children. J Neurosurg 1989; 70:568–572.
108. Dohrman GJ, Farwell JR, Flannery JT. Glioblastoma multiforme in children. J Neurosurg 1976; 44:442–448.
109. Marchese MJ, Chang CH. Malignant astrocytic gliomas in children. Cancer 1990; 65:2771–2778.
110. Sposto R, Ertel IJ, Jenkin RDT, et al. The effectiveness of chemotherapy for the treatment of high grade astrocytoma in children: results of a randomized trial. J Neurooncol 1989; 7:165–177.
111. Vertosick FT, Selker RG. Brain stem and spinal metastasis of supratentorial glioblastoma multiforme: a clinical series. Neurosurgery 1990; 27:516–522.
112. Mercuri S, Russo A, Palma L. Hemispheric supratentorial astrocytomas in children. J Neurosurg 1981; 55:170–173.
113. Palma L, Russo A, Mercuri S. Cystic cerebral astrocytomas in infancy and childhood: long-term results. Childs Brain 1983; 10:79–91.
114. Palma L, Guidetti B. Cystic pilocytic astrocytomas of the cerebral hemisphere. Surgical experience with 51 cases and long-term results. J Neurosurg 1985; 62:811–815.

115. Palma L, Russo A, Celli P. Prognosis of so-called "diffuse" cerebellar astrocytoma. Neurosurgery 1984; 15:315–317.
116. Scanion PW, Taylor WF. Radiotherapy of intracranial astrocytomas: analysis of 417 cases treated from 1960 through 1969. Neurosurgery 1979; 5:301–308.
117. Weir B, Grace M. The relative significance of factors affecting postoperative survival in astrocytomas. Grades one and two. Can J Neurol Sci 1976; 3:47–50.
118. Bernstein M, Hoffman HJ, Holliday WC, et al. Thalamic tumors in children. Long-term follow-up and treatment guidelines. J Neurosurg 1984; 61:649–656.
119. Page LK, Clark R. Gliomas of the septal area in children. Neurosurgery 1981; 8:651–655.
120. Gillet GR, Symon L. Hypothalamic glioma. Surg Neurol 1987; 28:291–300.
121. Wisoff JH, Abbott IR, Epstein F. Surgical management of exophytic chiasmatic–hypothalamic tumors of childhood. J Neurosurg 1990; 73:661–667.
122. Bloom HJG. Intracranial tumors: response and resistance to therapeutic endeavors, 1970–1980. Int J Radiat Oncol Biol Phys 1982; 8:1083–1113.
123. Deutsch M. Radiotherapy for primary brain tumors in very young children. Cancer 1982; 50:2785–2789.
124. Garcia DM, Fulling KH, Marks JE. The value of radiation therapy in addition to surgery for astrocytomas of the adult cerebrum. Cancer 1985; 55:919–927.
125. Marsa GW, Probert JC, Rubenstein LJ, Bagshaw MA. Radiation therapy in the treatment of childhood astrocytic gliomas. Cancer 1973; 32:646–656.
126. Hochberg FH, Slotnick B. Neuropsychologic impairment in astrocytoma survivors. Neurology 1980; 30:172–177.
127. Hoffman HJ. Optic pathway gliomas. In: Amador LV, ed. Brain tumors in the young. Springfield: Charles C Thomas, 1983; 622–633.
128. Koos WT, Miller MH. Intracranial tumors of infants and children. London: Churchill–Livingstone, 1971:172–188.
129. Alvord EC, Lofton S. Gliomas of the optic nerve or chiasm. Outcome by patients' age, tumor site and treatment. J Neurosurg 1988; 68–86–98.
130. Fletcher WA, Imes RK, Hoyt WF. Chiasmatic gliomas: appearance and long term changes demonstrated by computed tomography. J Neurosurg 1986; 65:154–159.
131. Gould RJ, Hilal SK, Chutorian AM. Efficacy of radiotherapy in optic gliomas. Pediatr Neurol 1987; 3:29–32.
132. Hoyt WF, Baghdassarian SA. Optic glioma of childhood. Natural history and rationale for conservative management. Br J Ophthalmol 1969; 53:793–798.
133. Rodriguez LA, Edwards MSB, Levin VA. Management of hypothalamic gliomas in children: an analysis of 33 cases. Neurosurgery 1990; 26:242–247.
134. Wong JY, Uhl V, Wara WM, Sheline GE. Optic gliomas. A reanalysis of the University of California, San Francisco experience. Cancer 1987; 60:1847–1855.
135. Borit A, Richardson EF Jr. The biological and clinical behavior of pilocytic astrocytomas of the optic pathways. Brain 1982; 105:161–187.
136. Danoff BF, Kramer S, Thompson N. The radiotherapeutic management of optic nerve gliomas in children. Int J Radiat Oncol Biol Phys 1980; 6:45–50.
137. Hoyt WF, Fletcher WA, Imes RK. Chiasmal gliomas: appearance and long-term changes demonstrated by computerized tomography. Prog Exp Tumor Res 1987; 30:113–121.
138. Imes RK, Hoyt WF. Childhood chiasmal gliomas: update on the fate of patients in the 1969 San Francisco study. Prog Exp Tumor Res 1987; 30:108–112.
139. Oxenhandler DC, Sayers MP. The dilemma of childhood optic glioma. J Neurosurg 1978; 48:34–41.
140. Brand WN, Hoover SV. Optic gliomas in children: review of 16 cases given megavoltage radiation therapy. Childs Brain 1979; 5:459–466.
141. Menezes AH, Bell WE, Perrett GE. Hypothalamic tumors in children. Childs Brain 1977; 3:265–280.
142. Albright AL, Sclabassi RJ. Cavitron ultrasonic surgical aspirator and visual evoked potentials for chiasmal gliomas in children: report of two cases. J Neurosurg 1985; 63:138–140.
143. Dandy WE. Prechiasmal intracranial tumors of the optic nervies. Am J Ophthalmol 1922; 5:169–188.

144. Lloyd LA. Gliomas of the optic nerve and chiasm in childhood. Trans Am Ophthalmol Soc 1973; 71:488–535.
145. Wright E, McDonald WI, Call NB. Management of optic nerve gliomas. Br J Ophthalmol 1980; 64:545–552.
146. Lin SR, Bryson MM, Gobien RP, Fitz CR, Lee YY. Radiologic findings of hamartomas of the tuber cinereum and hypothalamus. Radiology 1978; 127:697–703.
147. List CF, Dowmann, CE, Bagchi BK, Bebin J. Posterior hypothalamic harmartomas and gangliomas causing precocious puberty. Neurology 1958; 8:164–174.
148. Zuniga OF, Tanner SM, Wild WO, Mosier HD Jr. Hamartoma of CNS associated with precocious puberty. Am J Dis Child 1983; 137:127–133.
149. Sato M, Ushio Y, Arita N, Mogami H. Hypothalamic hamartoma: report of two cases. Neurosurgery 1985; 16:198–206.
150. McCoullough DC, Johnson DL. Optic nerve gliomas and other tumors involving the optic nerve and chiasm. In: McLaurin RL, Schut L, Venes JL, et al., eds. Pediatric neurosurgery: surgery of the developing nervous system. 2nd ed. Philadelphia: WB Saunders, 1989:391–198.
151. Packer RJ, Sutton LN, Bilaniuk LT, et al. Treatment of chiasmatic/hypothalamic gliomas of childhood with chemotherapy: an updated report. Ann Neurol 1988; 23:79–85.
152. Rosenstock JG, Packer RJ, Bilaniuk LT, et al. Chiasmatic optic glioma treated with chemotherapy. A preliminary report. J Neurosurg 1985; 63:862–866.
153. Choux M, Lena G, Genitori L. Le craniopharyngiome de l'enfant (craniopharyngioma in children). Neurochirurgie 1991; 37 (supp 1):7–10.
154. Hoffman HJ. Craniopharyngiomas. Can J Neurol Sci 1985; 12:348–352.
155. Pusey E, Kortman KE, Flannigan BD, et al. MR of craniopharyngiomas: tumor delineation and characterization. AJNR 1987; 8:439–444.
156. Zimmerman RA. Imaging of intrasellar, suprasellar, and parasellar tumors. Semin Roentgenol 1990; 25:174–197.
157. Amacher L. Craniopharyngioma: the controversy regarding radiotherapy. Childs Brain 1980; 6:57–64.
158. Baskin DS, Wilson CB. Surgical management of craniopharyngiomas: a review of 74 cases. J Neurosurg 1986; 65:22–27.
159. Carmel P, Antunes J, Chang C. Craniopharyngiomas in children. Neurosurgery 1982; 11:382–389.
160. Cavazzuti V, Fischer EG, Welch, et al. Neurological and psychological sequelae following different treatment of craniopharyngioma in children. J Neurosurg 1983; 59:409–417.
161. Fischer EG, Welch K Shillito J, et al. Craniopharyngiomas in children: long term effects of conservative procedures combined with radiation therapy. J Neurosurg 1990; 73:534–540.
162. Hoffman HJ, De Silva M, Humphreys RP, Drake JM, Smith ML, Blaser SI. Aggressive surgical management of craniopharyngiomas in children. J Neurosurg 1992; 76:47–52.
163. Lyen KR, Grant DB. Endocrine function, morbidity, and mortality after surgery for craniopharyngioma. Arch Dis Child 1982; 57:837–841.
164. Richmond IL, Wara WM, Wilson CB. Role of radiation therapy in the management of craniopharyngiomas in children. Neurosurgery 1980; 6:513–517.
165. Tomita T. Management of craniopharyngiomas in children. Pediatr Neurosci 1988; 14:204–211.
166. Wen B-C, Hussey DH, Staples, et al. A comparison of the roles of surgery and radiation therapy in the management of craniopharyngiomas. Int J Radiat Oncol Biol Phys 1989; 16:17–24.
167. Yasargil MG, Curcic M, Kis M, et al. Total removal of craniopharyngiomas: approaches and long-term results in 144 patients. J Neurosurg 1990; 73:3–11.
168. Shiminski-Maher T, Rosenberg M. Late effects associated with treatment of craniopharyngiomas in childhood. J Neurosci Nurs 1990; 22:220–226.
169. Sung KI, Chang CH, Harisiadis L, et al. Treatment results of craniopharyngiomas. Cancer 1981; 47:847–852.
170. Flickinger JC, Lunsford LD, Singer J, et al. Megavoltage external beam irradiation of craniopharyngiomas: analysis of tumor control and morbidity. Int J Radiat Oncol Biol Phys 1989; 19:117–122.
171. Coffey RJ, Lunsford LD. The role of stereotactic techniques in the management of craniopha-

ryngiomas. In: Rosenblum ML, ed. The role of surgery in brain tumor management. Philadelphia: WB Saunders, 1990:161–172.

172. Jennings MT, Gelman R, Hochberg F. Intracranial germ-cell tumors: natural history and pathogenesis. J Neurosurg 1985; 63:155–167.

173. Marsden HB, Buch JM, Swindell R. Germ cell tumors of childhood. A review of 137 cases. J Clin Pathol 1981; 34:879–883.

174. Rueda-Pedraza, ME, Heifetz SA, Sesterhenn IA, Clark GB. Primary intracranial germ cell tumors in the first two decades of life: a clinical, light-microscopic, and immunohistochemical analysis of 54 cases. Perspect Pediatr Pathol 1987; 10:160–207.

175. Koide O, Watanabe Y, Sato K. A pathological survey of intracranial germinoma and pinealoma in Japan. Cancer 1980; 42:2119–2130.

176. Jellinger K. Primary intracranial germ cell tumours. Acta Neuropathol 1973; 25:291–306.

177. Wara WM, Jenkin RDT, Evans A, et al. Tumors of the pineal and suprasellar region. Children's Cancer Study Group treatment results 1960–1975. Cancer 1979; 43:698–701.

178. Nishiyama RH, Batsakis JG, Weaver DK, et al. Germinal neoplasms of the central nervous system. Arch Surg 1966; 93:342–347.

179. Shinoda J, Yamada H, Sakai N, et al. Placental alkaline phosphatase as a tumor marker for primary intracranial germinoma. J Neurosurg 1988; 68:710–720.

180. Edwards MSB, Hudgins RJ, Wilson CB, et al. Pineal region tumors in children. J Neurosurg 1988; 68:689–697.

181. Naganuma H, Inoue H, Misumi S, et al. Intacranial germ cell tumors: immunohistochemical study of three autopsy cases. J Neurosurg 1984; 61:931–937.

182. Stein B. Surgical therapy of benign pineal tumors. In: Neuwelt EA, ed. Diagnosis and treatment of pineal region tumors. Baltimore: Williams & Wilkins, 1986:254–272.

183. Allen JC, Kim JH, Packer RJ. Neoadjuvant chemotherapy for newly diagnosed germ-cell tumors of the central nervous system. J Neurosurg 1987; 67:65–70.

184. Neuwelt EA, Batjer HH. Pre- and postoperative management of pineal region tumors and the occipital transtentorial approach. In: Neuwelt E, ed. Diagnosis and treatment of pineal region tumors. Baltimore: Williams & Wilkins, 1986:208–212.

185. Stein B. The suboccipital supracerebellar approach to the pineal region. In: Neuwelt EA, ed. Diagnosis and treatment of pineal region tumors. Baltimore: Williams & Wilkins, 1986:213–222.

186. Sano K, Matsutani M. Pinealoma (germinoma) treated by direct surgery and postoperative irradiation. A long-term follow-up. Childs Brain 1981; 8:81–97.

187. Sung DI, Harasiadis L, Chang CH. Midline pineal tumors and suprasellar germinomas: highly curable by irradiation. Radiology 1978; 128:745–751.

188. Danoff BF, Sheline GE. Radiotherapy of pineal tumors. In Neuwelt E, ed. Diagnosis and treatment of pineal region tumors. Baltimore. Williams & Wilkins, 1986:300–308.

189. Dattoli MJ, Newall J. Radiation therapy for intracranial germinoma: the case for limited volume treatment. Int J Radiat Oncol Biol Phys 1990; 19:429–433.

190. Allen JC, Bosl G, Walker R. Chemotherapy trials in recurrent primary intracranial germ cell tumors. J. Neurooncol 1985; 3:147–152.

191. Brodeur GM, Howarth CB, Pratt CB, et al. Malignant germ cell tumors in 57 children and adolescents. Cancer 1981; 48:1890–1898.

192. Einhorn LH. Testicular cancer as a model for a curable neoplasm: the Richard and Hilda Rosenthal Foundation Award Lecture. Cancer Res 1981; 41:3275–3280.

193. Fraley EE, Lange PH, Kennedy BJ. Germ-cell testicular cancer in adults (part 1). N Engl J Med 1979; 301:1370–1377.

194. Fraley EE, Lange PH, Kennedy BJ. Germ-cell testicular cancer in adults (part 2). N Engl J Med 1979;301:1420–1426.

195. Montie JE. Changing concepts in the management of testis cancer. Cleve Clin Q 1984; 51:381–385.

196. Williams S, Birch R, Einhorn L. Treatment of disseminated germ-cell tumors with cisplatin, bleomycin, and either vinblastine or etoposide. N Engl J Med 1987; 316:1435–1440.

197. Kobayashi T, Yoshida J, Ishiyama J, et al. Combination chemotherapy with cisplatin and etoposide for

malignant intracranial germ-cell tumors: an experimental and clinical study. J Neurosurg 1989; 70:676–681.

198. Ochs J. Proceedings of controversies in paediatric and adolescent haematology and oncology. 1981.

199. Robison LL, Nesbit ME Jr, Sather HN, et al. Factors associated with IQ scores in long-term survivors of childhood acute lymphoblastic leukemia. Am J Pediatr Hematol Oncol 1984; 6:115.

200. Williams JM, Davis KS. Central nervous system prophylactic treatment for childhood leukemia: neuropsychological outcome studies. Cancer Treat Rev 1986; 13:113–127.

201. Bouchard J, Pierce B. Radiation therapy in the management of neoplasms of the central nervous system with a special note in regard to children: twenty years experience, 1939–1958. AJR 1960; 84:610–628.

22

Radiotherapy of Brain Tumors: Basic Principles

Bruce F. Kimler
University of Kansas Medical Center,
Kansas City, Kansas

I. INTRODUCTION

The purpose of this chapter is to provide a basic understanding of the physical, chemical, and biological events that accompany the interaction of ionizing radiations with biological systems. Certain concepts of radiation physics required for the use of radiation therapy in the management of malignancies will be reviewed. The interaction of ionizing radiations with the mammalian cell will be followed sequentially through initial radiochemical reactions, biochemical interactions with critical macromolecules, subcellular effects, and finally expression of cell death. Clinical radiation biology will be discussed from the standpoint of the radiobiological rationale that explains why and how radiation therapy can be effective against tumors while avoiding unacceptable toxic effects on critical normal tissue structures, especially those of the central nervous system. Finally, a variety of developing approaches and novel therapeutic modalities will be introduced that offer potential avenues for ultimate improvement in the therapy and management of brain tumors.

II. THE BASIC PHYSICS OF IONIZING RADIATION

A. History, Terms, and Definitions

It has been slightly less than 100 years since William Conrad Roentgen announced his discovery of mysterious new emanations produced by passing an electrical current through an evacuated cathode ray tube. These invisible "x-rays" could pass through solid objects and allow one to "see" through skin and tissue to the bones beneath. With time, the potential of radiation in the basic physical sciences, in power production, and in biology and medicine has been increasingly realized. Despite the fact that radiation and its biological effects have been more thoroughly studied and characterized than any other similar agent or force, there remains a pervasive public misunderstanding and even fear (1). When used appropriately and with respect, radiation can be a powerful tool. Just as surely, if not used cautiously, radiation has a definite potential to do harm.

B. Types

As the names implies, *ionizing radiations* are those radiative processes that possess sufficient energy to produce ionizations when they interact with matter. Ionizing radiations can be either particulate or electromagnetic. *Particulate radiations* are either subatomic particles (electrons, protons, neutrons, π-mesons) or entire nuclei that are traveling at near light speed and, therefore, are highly energetic. *Electromagnetic radiation*, so-called because it possesses characteristics of both an electrical and a magnetic nature, consists of photons. The *photon* has properties of a wave propagating through a medium, but also possesses properties of a particle.

C. Production

Radiation can be either naturally occurring or man-made. Naturally occurring radiations result from the decay of an unstable nucleus to a more stable isotopic form, relieving the stress by the emission of energetic particles or photons. In addition to individual neutrons and protons, nuclear decay may also produce electrons (*β-particles*) or two protons plus two neutrons, equivalent to a helium atom nucleus and referred to as an *α-particle*. The photons emitted by radioactive decay are designated as *γ-rays*. Radioactive decay is a random process, but does follow logical and predictable kinetics. A mathematical description of the kinetics (probability) of radiation decay is provided by

$$\frac{N(t)}{N(o)} = e^{-\lambda t}$$

where $N(t)$ = number of atoms at time t, $N(o)$ = number of original atoms, and λ is a proportionality (decay) constant in units of reciprocal time. From this, one can determine the *half-life*, the time required for one-half of the unstable atoms to undergo a decay. Alternatively, it is the time after which one would have one-half of the original activity (disintegrations per unit time) remaining. Because of the exponential nature of radioactive decay, the actual number of atoms decaying per unit time will be constantly decreasing. That is, in the first half-life, one-half the atoms decay; in the second half-life, one-fourth of the original atoms decay (also one-fourth of the original atoms remain); and so on. Although it is mathematically valid to state that the last atom will "never" decay, a more useful approach is to consider that 95% of the atoms will have decayed (and released their energy) in a little more than four half-lives.

The same radiations can also be artificially produced. Electrons can be stripped from an atom and then accelerated through alternating electric fields. This is the basis for the x-ray machine and the linear accelerator. The resultant electron is described in terms of the potential difference through which it has been accelerated and, consequently, the amount of kinetic energy acquired. When these accelerated, energetic electrons are used to bombard a target (particularly a metal such as beryllium or tungsten), they interact with the electron shells of target atoms. There is a momentary increase in energy states, which is then relieved by the emission of photons with a characteristic energy (and, hence, wavelength). These photons are referred to as *x-rays* and are characterized by the potential difference (e.g., 250 kVp, kilovolt peak) through which the electrons were accelerated. Similarly, a whole host of positively charged particles (protons and entire nuclei) can be created by stripping off the electrons and then subjecting the remaining nucleus to the same accelerating fields as those used for electrons. Because of the substantially greater mass of protons and whole nuclei relative to electrons, these particles are highly energetic. They are simply referred to as the nuclei of their original atom (He^{+2}, C^{+6}, Ne^{+10}, and so on). Finally, it is possible to produce uncharged neutrons with similar high energy owing to their mass and momentum.

Other than referring to the particles as electrons, rather than β-particles, and to the photons as x-rays, instead of γ-rays, there is no fundamental difference in the physical nature of these radiations that allows one to determine their origin (natural or artificial). Certainly, there is no difference in their biological effects.

D. Interaction with Matter

When radiations, either particles or photons, travel through a medium, they interact with atoms, losing energy and depositing that energy in the medium. As a consequence, the intensity of the initial beam is diminished or attenuated. A mathematical description of the kinetics of this attenuation is provided by

$$I/I_o = e^{-\mu x}$$

where I_o = the original radiation intensity or flux, I = the intensity of the exiting radiation, x = thickness of the absorbing material, and μ = an attenuation coefficient in units of reciprocal length. It is the differential absorption, as determined by the average atomic number of different substances, that provides the diagnostic capability of x-rays. Unfortunately, it also complicates the problem of dose deposition and localization when one uses radiation for therapeutic purposes. For radiation safety purposes, it is often more convenient to characterize attenuation processes by the half-value layer. Analogous to the half-life, the half-value layer is that thickness of absorber that reduces the incident radiation intensity by one-half.

Turning now to the specifics of how ionizing radiation interacts with matter, we see that it will depend mostly on the dose rate and the radiation quality. Later, we will see that the subsequent chemical reactions will also be determined by the amount of water in the system, the presence of oxygen, and the chemical makeup of the medium.

When radiation interacts with matter, two processes occur that differ in the amount of energy transferred. *Excitation* is simply the raising of an electron from one energy state to a higher energy state by the absorption of the incident radiation. For the most part, this process does not contribute to any meaningful consequences in biological systems. On the other hand, *ionization*, basically the removal of an electron from an atom, has profound effects. The result of ionization is the production of two ions: a net positive and a net negative. Two processes that produce these two ions (that are of importance in the energy range encountered clinically) are the *photoelectric effect* and the *Compton effect*. In the photoelectric effect, the incident photon imparts all of its energy (kinetic) to an outer shell electron, breaking it away from the parent atom. In the *Compton effect* (Fig. 1), the incident photon imparts a portion of its energy (kinetic) to an outer-shell electron, breaking it away. The residual energy is released in the form of another photon, but of lower energy. Obviously, both processes cause ionization, fulfilling the requirement for ionizing radiation.

The interaction of radiation with matter is a probability function or a matter of chance; that is, an individual particle or photon may or may not interact and, if interaction occurs, definite damage may or may not be produced. The spatial distribution of this radiation interaction is nonselective—the energy from ionizing radiation is deposited randomly throughout the material. However, energy absorption is "discrete," occurring in quantal, isolated interactions, and not homogeneously deposited. Even though interactions occur on a random basis, they do follow a pattern of logical kinetics that can be mathematically described with exponential equations similar to those applied to radioactive decay and attenuation.

E. Dosimetry and Units

One of the first requirements in understanding the interactions of ionizing radiation with biological material is a system of units to describe what is happening at the physical level. The early

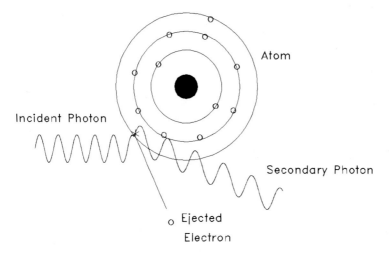

Figure 1   Interaction of an incident photon with an atom. An electron is ejected from the outer orbit, resulting in an ion pair consisting of a positively charged atom and a negatively charged electron. The residual energy remaining after overcoming the binding energy of the electron and providing kinetic energy to the electron is imparted to a secondary photon of lower energy than the original photon.

investigators and practitioners of ionizing radiations were restricted to phenomenological descriptions that, from our modern perspective, were often inadequate. For example, the output of an x-ray machine was once defined on the basis of the exposure time required to produce an erythematous reaction on the skin of a patient or the operator.

The first unit to be widely used, beginning about 1928, for the description of radiation interactions was the **roentgen** (R), after the discoverer of x-rays. A *roentgen* is defined as an exposure to electromagnetic radiation, such that the associated corpuscular emission per cubic centimeter of air (at standard temperature and pressure) produces ions carrying one electrostatic unit (ESU) of charge (1 ESU = 2.58×10^{-4} coulomb(C)/kg) of either sign. This unit applies only to electromagnetic radiation within the relatively narrow energy range of 0.2–3 MeV. This unit refers only to the incident exposure of some material to radiation, but does not address the more critical question of the actual energy absorbed.

For purposes of defining the actual dose absorption, the **rad** (radiation-absorbed dose) is used. This unit measures the amount of energy absorbed and does not depend on the type of radiation, the wavelength, the energy, or the nature of the material in which absorption takes place. Specifically, the *rad* was defined in 1956 as the absorption of 100 erg/g of material (2). For most biological tissues, an exposure to 1 R will result in a dose deposition of approximately 0.93–0.98 rad. Recently, the International Standard on Units has converted from the centimeter–gram–second (cgs) system of units to the meter–kilogram–second (MKS) system. Thus, the modern official scientific unit for radiation dose absorption is the gray (Gy), with *1 Gy* defined as 1 Joule deposited per kilogram of matter. Numerically, 1 Gy is 100 times larger than a rad, which has led to the common use of the cGy to replace the old, familiar rad unit. Typically, a brain tumor might be treated to a total dose of 50 Gy, or 5000 cGy, over a 5-week course of fractionated radiotherapy.

Macroscopically, *linear energy transfer* (LET) is a term that describes the rate at which energy is deposited as a charged particle travels through matter. The LET is expressed in keV/μ, or the energy deposited per unit distance of path traveled by the particle. In particular, LET is determined by two physical properties of the radiation: mass and charge. The usual electromagnetic radiations (x-rays and γ-rays) are termed low-LET radiation because, although having negligible mass and no charge, they produce fast electrons that then interact with additional atoms. The probability of an electron interaction with an atom is relatively small; therefore, the interactions of this primary agent of damage are sparse, and the ionizations produced are distant from each other. Highly ionizing radiations (e.g., α-particles neutrons) are high-LET radiations. Particulate radiations having an appreciable mass or charge have a greater probability of interaction with matter. These types of radiation lose energy rapidly, producing many ionizations in a very short distance.

Because of differences in the rate of energy loss and deposition, different LET radiations will produce varying biological responses. Generally, the greater the LET, the greater is the magnitude of the biological response. *Relative biological effect* (RBE) is a term relating the ability of radiations with different LET ranges to produce a specific biological response. The RBE has been defined as the ratio of the dose of a test radiation required to produce some defined level of effect, to the dose of 250 kVp x-rays, delivered under the same conditions, that are required to produce the same biological response for the same endpoint. It should be emphasized that, for the description of RBE, it is the biological response that is kept constant, not the dose of radiation. This is critical, because the RBE can change depending on the biological response or the test system employed. To convert units of dose to equivalent biological effect, one can multiply the RBE times the absorbed dose. Thus, the rad unit is converted to the *rem* (rad equivalent man); the corresponding unit in the mks system is the *sievert* (Sv). As for units of absorbed dose, 1 Sv is numerically equal to 100 rem. Generally, this is only of concern when one is considering the potential for carcinogenesis as a consequence of exposure to high LET radiations.

It is instructive to return to the aspect of the discrete, quantal deposition of energy when radiation interacts with matter. It can be easily shown by simple examples that the far-reaching biological effects produced cannot simply be the result of homogeneous deposition of energy in the system. Let us start with an absorbed dose of 4 Gy, a dose that we may assume (within reason) carries a 50% probability of killing either a typical mammalian cell or a typical human. By knowing the energy deposited and the average energy required to produce an ionization, we can calculate the total number of ionizations produced per gram. Assuming that, for the most part, the cell is composed of water, with a molecular weight of 18, we can determine the relative rate of ionization per molecule. We find that, at most, one molecule in every 5×10^7 molecules suffers any effect whatsoever. This cannot be considered a frequent perturbation, if homogeneous energy deposition is involved. In a similar fashion, we can convert the energy absorbed into thermal energy (calories) and determine that a lethal dose is capable of raising the temperature of the irradiated object by only 0.001°C. In other words, an amount of energy deposited throughout the body that is equivalent to that which we typically produce every 2 s as a result of normal metabolism.

Although the initial deposition of energy occurs very rapidly, in approximately 10^{-17} s, the biological changes resulting from radiation require a latent period before expression that may range from seconds to centuries, as we shall see (Table 1). It is instructive to bear in mind that the ultimate biological changes produced by radiation are not unique and, consequently, cannot be distinguished from similar damage produced by other agents or types of trauma.

III. THE BASICS OF RADIATION BIOLOGY

A. Radiation Chemistry

When ionizing radiation interacts with a biological system, ionizations are produced in molecules. Depending on the initial site of these ionizations, the action of radiation can be considered as either direct or indirect. *Direct action* is considered to produce damage by direct ionization of some critical biological macromolecule; *indirect action* produces damage through chemical reactions

Table 1 Sequences in the Development of Radiobiological Effects

Time(s)	Event
10^{-18} (as)	Absorption of ionizing radiation
10^{-15} (fs)	Physical events: Excitation of atoms
	Ionization of atoms, ion pair formed
10^{-12} (ps)	Physicochemical events: Dissociation of ion pair
	Formation of free radicals
	Hydration of electrons
10^{-9} (ns)	Physicochemical events: Breakage of chemical bonds
	Break macromolecular chains
10^{-6} (μs)	Chemical events: Restitution and chemical repair
	Abnormal reactions
	depolymerization
	enzyme inactivation
	DNA base changes
10^{-3} (ms)	Chemical events: DNA single-stranded breaks
	DNA double-stranded breaks
	DNA cross-linking
10^{0} (s)	Biochemical effects: Repair of DNA damage
	Fixation of DNA damage
10^{2} (min)	Cellular effects: Recovery—sublethal damage
	Recovery—potentially lethal damage
	Inhibition of metabolic synthesis
10^{4} (h)	Cell cycle division delay
	Point mutations
	Interphase death: necrosis, apoptosis
10^{5} (d)	Chromosomal aberrations
	Loss of reproductive integrity
	Cell death and lysis
10^{6}	Tissue effects: Breakdown of tissue organization
	Acute normal tissue effects
	Hyperplastic tissue recovery
10^{7}(mo)	Organ effects: Dysfunction, leading to organism death
10^{8}(y)	Chronic normal tissue effects
	Fibrosis, necrosis
10^{9}	Genetic effects: Somatic mutations (carcinogenesis)
10^{10}	Genetic mutations in next generations

initiated by ionizations in the surrounding milieu. Since the probability of any particular molecule being ionized depends on the size and the number (frequency or concentration) of that molecule, and since 70% of the typical cell is composed of water, the probability of an interaction occurring is greatest with water molecules. Thus, water will primarily mediate the indirect action of ionizing radiation in the cell.

1. Water Radiolysis

The absorption of radiation by a water molecule results in the ejection of an electron, leaving behind a positively charged water molecule. The free electron (e^-) is captured by another water molecule, forming the second ion, or is simply associated with a number of water molecules to form what is referred to as an aqueous electron. Ultimately, this leads to the production of an ion pair (HOH$^+$, HOH$^-$). The two ions produced by the foregoing reactions are unstable and rapidly dissociate, provided that normal water molecules are present, forming the hydrogen (H$^+$) and hydroxyl (OH$^-$) ions and the hydrogen (H·) and hydroxyl (OH·) free radicals (3). Free radicals contain a single unpaired orbital electron that renders them highly reactive because of the tendency of the unpaired electron to pair with another electron. The ultimate result of the interaction of radiation with water is the formation of an ion pair (H$^+$, OH$^-$) and free radicals (H·, OH·). Because they are extremely reactive owing to their chemical and physical properties, both ions and free radicals rapidly undergo a number of subsequent reactions. Because they are most likely to react in the immediate vicinity of where they were produced, they will usually simply recombine with other radiolytic species. Probably 90% of the time, there is a simple recombination and restitution of a normal water molecule, with no net effect on the biological system other than the liberation of a trivial amount of heat. Occasionally, new molecules (e.g., hydrogen peroxide) may be formed that may be damaging to the cell. Lastly, the immediate radiolytic species may react with simple molecules in the milieu, forming new radicals, such as the peroxyl radical, or they may react directly with a potentially critical macromolecule. All reactions are competitive, with the likelihood of any particular reaction determined by the reaction rate constant and the concentrations of the reactants and products. Because of their highly reactive nature, these free radicals have lifetimes on the order of only microseconds, and consequently must react within a few nanometers of their site of production (4).

2. Radiation Biochemistry

Although radiolytic species react only infrequently with molecules other than themselves or water, the consequences can be dramatic if it involves the alteration of biologically important molecules. In the simplest scenario, there is removal of a hydrogen atom, resulting in the formation of a biological free radical. The biological free radicals may combine with free hydrogen and return to the original molecule, resulting in no damage; or they may react further to create other reactive species that can eventually be expressed as damage. These reactive molecules are the ones that produce the critical damage on a crucial biological molecule. In particular, reaction with molecular oxygen will produce an organic oxyl radical, which is very reactive. The effects of free radicals in the cell are compounded by their ability to initiate chemical reactions, and thereby damage, at distant sites in the cell. Thus, ionizations can occur in the water milieu, but the defect can be transferred to a critical biological macromolecule, with subsequent far-reaching consequences. Still, most of the time, damage done to macromolecules is not expressed, owing to the processes of repair and restitution.

Reactions of radiation-induced radicals with carbohydrates and lipids are typically not critical in terms of long-lasting effects (5). First, large doses are required to produce effects. More importantly, carbohydrates and lipids are relatively simple structures, allowing a greater probability of proper and complete repair. If misrepaired, the probability of the altered structure being deleterious to the cell is not as likely. Finally, there are multiple copies of each type of molecule in the cell.

Although high doses are needed to achieve such effects in proteins, the damage here may be more critical (5). Not only are the structures more complex, and there are fewer copies of each protein in the cell, the damage induced (breakage of disulfide or hydrogen bonds) may produce a structural alteration that will functionally inactivate the protein.

Because the cell membrane is composed preponderantly of lipids and proteins, it is not surprising that the membrane can be affected by radiation. Permeability of the cell membrane may be altered, affecting the transport function of the membrane and its ability to keep molecules in or out of the cell. Alteration of membranes also can affect those organelles in the cell that are membrane-bound (e.g., nuclei, mitochondria, and lysosomes).

3. Damage to DNA

By far the most crucial of the biomolecules that can be damaged by xenobiotic attack are the nucleic acids, specifically, DNA (6). There is considerable evidence to indicate that the nucleus is much more sensitive to radiation damage than the cytoplasm, implying that the target for radiation is a nuclear constituent (7). Since DNA is the molecule in the nucleus that controls all cellular activities, it is reasonable to consider it as the most likely target for radiation effects (8). Each cell possesses, at most, only four copies of each molecule of DNA; therefore, loss or damage of less DNA may be critical. Moreover, the structure of DNA is not simple, with all genetic information existing in a particular sequence of base pairs. Thus, an ionization (either direct or indirect) in DNA may present a life-threatening situation to the cell.

Ionizations within the DNA bases can produce several types of chemical damage. These include the loss of a nucleotide base, a change in the identity of a base, or the breakage of hydrogen bonds between the two strands of the DNA double helix (Fig. 2). Typically, these are not as important as radical attack that results in damage to the backbone of the DNA. A single break in the sugar–phosphate linkage of the backbone of one strand of DNA (a single-stranded break) is also usually not critical. Such breaks are easily rejoined by passive processes, with no resultant damage to the cell. However, if there is further chemical reaction before proper rejoining, then the defect may be fixed (in the preservation sense, not the repair sense) and will be expressed as damage later.

Most critical of all is the situation in which breaks are produced in both strands of the DNA double helix. Not only is it more difficult for rejoining to occur properly, but physical continuity is lost for DNA replication or mRNA transcription. There may also be chemical cross-linking reactions between different regions of the same DNA molecule, between two separate DNA molecules, or between a DNA molecule and an adjacent protein in the chromatin

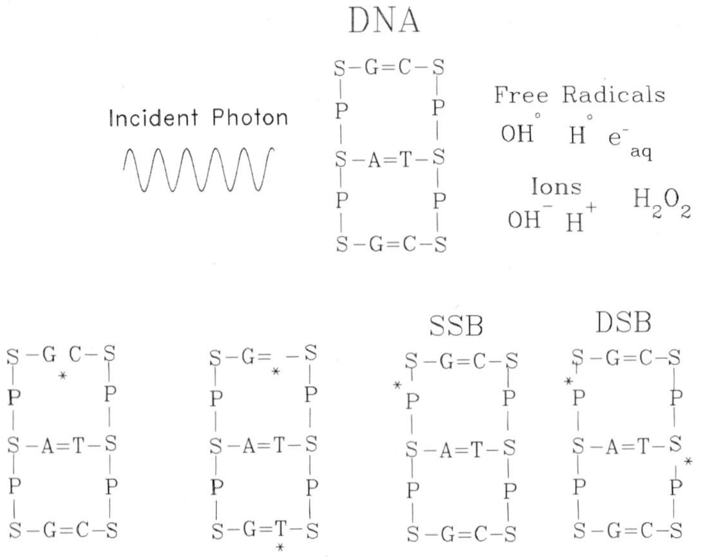

Figure 2 Schematic of biochemical damage produced in DNA as a result of either primary ionization in the DNA, or by interaction with free radicals or reactive chemical species. The upper structure represents the normal double-stranded structure of DNA. The lower-left structure shows a break in the hydrogen bonding between nitrogenous base pairs at the site of the asterisk. The next structure shows the loss of a nitrogenous base (upper) and a change in a nitrogenous base (lower). The next structure shows a break in a single strand of the DNA, and the final structure (right most) shows a double-stranded break in the DNA's double-helix structure.

complex. Overall, these chemical changes in DNA render it unable to function, either functionally or structurally, as a template for transcription or transmission of genetic information. Fortunately, much of this damage to DNA can be processed or otherwise repaired to return the molecule to its original state. In particular, 99% of the single-stranded breaks produced in DNA are rejoined within a matter of hours. Also, since much of the cellular DNA is not essential, the cell will not be affected by loss or alteration of such noncritical sequences. Some regions of DNA may be simply "filler" DNA between sequences of genetic coding. There may also be multiple copies of a particular gene sequence. Finally, not all genetic information is essential for each cell—a differentiated cell does not require the full genetic complement of a pluripotent cell. On the other hand, any residual change in the DNA molecule that is not repaired will persist as a mutation that may result in either minor consequences (the cell is alive, but has some functional impairment) or major consequences (death of the cell). Whereas genetic alterations in somatic cells will affect only the involved cells or, at worst, the individual (e.g., with carcinogenesis), mutations in germ cells have the potential to affect future generations.

B. Subcellular Effects

1. *Inhibition of Metabolic Syntheses*

As a consequence of radiation-induced damage to biological macromolecules, the synthesis of DNA, RNA, and protein can all be temporarily inhibited, provided sufficient doses are absorbed. The extent and duration of such inhibition is dose-dependent. Generally, the effects are transitory for low doses and synthesis resumes after some time. There may even be compensation for the "missing" synthesis, with levels returning to greater-than-control values. The inhibition of the different syntheses are generally independent effects. Unless the inhibition is for a very long time, there will be no lasting detrimental effects on the cell, once it recovers proper functioning.

2. *Chromosomal Damage*

Although changes in DNA molecules and the surrounding chromatin are discrete and do not necessarily result in structural changes in the chromosome, visible chromosomal aberrations may be produced. A chromosomal aberration is any observable change in the structure of a chromosome; it is also referred to as a lesion or anomaly. Some radiation-induced chromosomal breaks can be observed microscopically during the subsequent postirradiation cell division, particularly during metaphase and anaphase. What are observable are the consequences of the interaction of radiation with the chromosome (i.e., the gross or visible changes in chromosomal structure). It is assumed that there are many more changes in the chromosome that are not visible.

Structural changes in a chromosome can be produced by either direct ionization of the chromosome as ionizing radiation passes through it (direct action), or by an interaction with the products formed by the ionization of water (indirect action). The result of this interaction is the breakage of the chromosome, producing two or more chromosomal fragments, each having a broken end. These broken ends can join with other broken ends, forming new chromosomes, which may or may not appear structurally different from the original chromosome. With the development of new technqiues, such as fluorescence in situ hybridization (9, 10), we are no longer restricted to microscopic detection of chromosomal aberrations visible only when the cells are in mitosis. In particular, chromosomal aberrations such as deletions, translocations, and inversions can now be identified and have been correlated with neoplastic progression in several disease sites, including brain tumors.

The types of chromosomal aberrations formed will depend on how many breaks are involved; how many chromosomes are involved; where on the chromosome(s) the break(s) occur(s); and when in the cell cycle the ionizing event occurs (11). The random nature of the absorption of ionizing radiation can produce a single break in one chromosome or chromatid, two breaks in separate chromosomes or chromatids, or two or more breaks in the same chromosome or chromatid. The consequence to the cell of these structural changes may be loss of a part of the chromosome or chromatid, or rearrangement of the genetic material (i.e., DNA) within the chromosome set.

The most striking effect of chromosomal aberrations is when the disruption of the normal chromosomal structure is so severe that the cell is unable to complete the process of cell division. For example, a dicentric chromosome may be produced wherein each centromere is drawn to the pole of each daughter cell, but with the central portion of the chromosome stretched out between the two centrioles, restricting further movement. Here, the cell may be permanently arrested. Since the mitotic cell has very little capacity for metabolic synthesis, the cell will soon suffer a metabolic breakdown and begin to lyse. Alternatively, the chromosome may be stretched until it breaks at some random point, further disturbing the orderly distribution of equal chromatin content to the two daughter cells. With subsequent divisions, this process becomes exacerbated until the cell can no longer maintain vital functions and thus dies. Even if there is no visible alteration, there may still be a rearrangement or loss of genetic material that will result in death of both daughter cells once the cell has undergone one or more divisions.

Excellent correlations have been developed between the frequency of chromosomal aberrations produced and the extent of cell lethality observed (12). Typically, there are two possible reasons that chromosomal aberrations can result in the loss of survival: the inability to undergo an unlimited number of cell divisions and loss of reproductive integrity. There may be a functional defect in which genes that must be adjacent for proper transcription become separated (e.g., deletions, inversions), resulting in the loss of critical genetic information. Second, there may be physical defects (e.g., formation of ring chromosomes or dicentrics) that prevent the cell from completing division so that it will be held indefinitely (until it lyses) in mitosis. Even if the first division is completed, the chromosomal content may be so abnormal that both daughter cells will be blocked at the next or a subsequent attempted division (13).

C. Cellular Effects

1. Cell Cycle Perturbations and Progression Delay

When an asynchronously dividing population of mammalian cells is subjected to relatively low doses of radiation, there may be a blockade of cell progression through the cell cycle and a subsequent alteration of the cell cycle distribution. The sensitivity for delay (time delayed per unit dose) depends on the position in the cell cycle at the time of irradiation, but generally the sensitivity increases as one proceeds further into the cell cycle (13–15). As the likelihood for induction of delay increases, the effectiveness of delay (duration of delay per dose) also increases. Thus, although cells may be slowed down at several points in the cell cycle, they are usually arrested at some point in late G_2 or early mitosis. Typically, what is observed is that cells that are past some critical transition point in mitosis are refractory to delay in their present cycle (although they may be delayed in progressing through the next cycle) and will appear in mitosis on schedule (16). After a period of division delay, which tends to be transitory (except at very high doses), the duration of which is dose-dependent, cells will recover and once again proceed into mitosis. There are generally no long-term deleterious results from this temporary suspension of cell cycle progression. Once the cells resume their normal progression, they are indistinguishable from unirradiated or unaffected cells.

2. Interphase Death

A more serious cellular effect from ionizing radiation is the induction of what is termed *interphase death*. This involves the actual lysis and destruction of the cell, usually within a brief interval (1–4

h) following exposure. This form of cell death does not require the cell to complete (or even attempt to pass through) mitosis. As a consequence, cells break down and lyse during a phase other than mitosis.

Interphase death is not necessarily attributed to damage produced in the genetic compartments (DNA, chromosomes, nucleus) of the cell; rather, it is assumed that damage to cytoplasmic components is directly responsible. The most likely target for this damage is the membrane, either the cellular membrane, the nuclear membrane, or the membrane of specific subcellular organelles. It has been hypothesized that damage to the mitochondrial membranes may critically interfere with energy production. Likewise, damage to lysosomal membranes may lead to their breakdown and release of lytic enzymes, which would initiate an internal lysis of the cell. Consistent with this, there is usually microscopic evidence of large vacuoles, disrupted lysosomes, and such, that indicates severe damage has been done to the structural or functional state of the cell. Cells that have lost the ability to maintain a functional cell membrane will not be able to maintain the usual barrier to the entrance of foreign substances. This provides a common test and definition for cell viability. Normally, viable cells are able to prevent the dye trypan blue from entering the cell. Cells that cannot exclude the dye will appear stained and can be considered nonviable, with the assumption that they will soon lyse.

In addition to the typical expression of interphase cellular death through a cell necrosis process (loss of membrane integrity and cell lysis), an alternative process of *apoptosis* (programmed cell death) may occur (17, 18). This is characterized by production of specific endonucleases that cause nucleic acid degradation in the nucleus and the resultant death of the cell. Although this latter process does require protein synthesis, there is no requirement for DNA synthesis and the cell typically undergoes cellular disintegration before attempting a cell division.

Because of the requirement for a nongenetic mechanism for interphase cell death, and because of the rapidity with which it is expressed, there is usually a requirement for relatively large doses of radiation before one sees this effect. More typically, one will observe a mitotic form of cell death (see later) which can be induced by lower doses. However, interphase death can be expressed early on in all mammalian cells, and it is the only mechanism by which nondividing and terminally differentiated cells (such as neurons) can be killed by ionizing radiation.

3. Cell Survival and Reproductive Integrity

For those cells that do not undergo cellular necrosis or apoptosis immediately after exposure to ionizing radiation, there may still be expression of deleterious effects. Although a cell may still be metabolizing and quite functional (i.e., it appears intact), it may be "reproductively dead" if it has lost the ability to undergo an unlimited number of cell divisions. In fact, this form of death is referred to as *mitotic death,* since there is the requirement that the cell enter mitosis, and maybe even complete a number of mitoses before final expression of cell death and cell disruption. Thus, a cell that is reproductively dead may still undergo several cell divisions (and its daughter cells also) before they all stop dividing and lyse (13). Obviously, reproductive death cannot be expressed in a cell that has already lost the ability to divide. For example, a severely damaged chromosome, with altered genetic information that is no longer required, does not represent a threat to a cell as long as it does not attempt to divide.

Experimentally, reproductive death can be demonstrated only in assay systems that can show clonal expansion from single cells. Analysis of radiation-induced reproductive death in mammalian cells (either normal or tumor) was made possible by the development of an in vitro clonogenic assay system in 1956 (19). Whether using an in vitro or an in vivo assay system, the basic concept is that, for each surviving cell that retains the ability to divide an unlimited number of times, there will be one detectable colony. Pragmatically, it can be assumed that a cell that has undergone six divisions will continue to undergo divisions and, therefore, is a long-term survivor. Thus, a *surviving fraction* can be defined as the number of colonies formed following a prescribed dose, divided by the number of colonies formed in the absence of dose. If one plots the surviving fractions for several graded doses, one can produce a survival curve. Since the kinetics of radiation-induced cell kill are exponential, it is customary to plot the surviving fraction on a logarithmic axis to produce straight lines that are easier to analyze. It is important to remember that, with exponential killing, there is no dose that will guarantee the killing of the "last" cell. One may approach zero surviving cells, but will never reach it.

Two general theories have been developed to explain the shape of the mammalian cell survival curve and to characterize the kinetics of radiation-induced cell lethality. Historically, the first to be developed was that of *target theory* (20, 21), which postulates that direct action occurs when an ionizing particle interacts with and is absorbed by a biological macromolecule such as DNA, RNA, protein or any other macromolecule in the cell. Damage is produced by direct absorption of energy and the subsequent ionization of the biological macromolecule. When ionizing radiation interacts with a key molecule, or within a short distance around one of these key molecules, the name given to this sensitive area is *target*. The term target is based solely on the assumption that a random ionization occurring in this area will be of greater consequence to the life of the cell than an ionizing event occurring in another part of the cell. An ionization occurring within the target is called a *hit*. According to the definitions of target–hit, target theory applies only when radiation interacts with the target by direct action.

Several assumptions are made in the development of a target theory. It is assumed that the effect seen following radiation is due to an alteration of some particular site or target in the cell. For this, the ionizing radiation or event must directly involve this target (i.e., hit the target). As a consequence, all ionizing events that do not involve this target are wasted. A final aspect of target theory is that either single or multiple hits or targets can be considered as required to produce the ultimate expression of damage.

Because of the random and stochastic nature of the interaction of ionizing radiations with matter, mathematical descriptions for target theory can be developed that are similar to the exponential expressions previously derived for attenuation and radionuclide decay. For single-hit kinetics, in which only one event is necessary to inactivate the target, the equation

$$S/S_o = e^{-kD}$$

is derived, where S is the number of targets remaining that have not been hit, S_o is the original number of targets, D is the absorbed dose, and k is a proportionality constant (in units of reciprocal dose) that relates the probability of inactivation to the dose received. If we assume that there is only one such critical target per cell, then this equation becomes that of the probability of cell survival for a cell population. Note that the probability of survival (a number between 0 and 1) applies equally well to a single cell or to the entire population. That is, for a survival probability of 10%, we may state that, considering the population at large, 10% of the cells will survive and 90% will be killed. Alternatively, considering a single cell, we may state that any particular cell has a 10% chance of not being hit by an ionizing event and, therefore, will survive. This also carries with it a 90% chance that the cell will be hit and, consequently, will die. When this formula is plotted with surviving fraction (on a semilogarithmic axis) as a function of dose, a straight-line curve results.

However, most mammalian cell populations do not exhibit a straight-line survival curve. Instead, there is an initial portion of the curve where surviving fraction decreases less steeply than it does later on (19). This can be modeled with target theory by assuming that there are two or more targets per cell (or surviving unit) that must be inactivated. Thus, on the initial shoulder region of the curve (Fig. 3), one is accumulating the first of the required hits per target. This can be expressed as accumulation of sublethal damage, since it is insufficient to cause the death of the

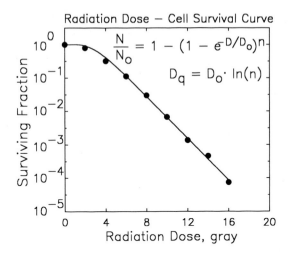

Radiation Dose — Cell Survival Curve

$$\frac{N}{N_o} = 1 - (1 - e^{-D/D_o})^n$$

$$D_q = D_o \cdot \ln(n)$$

Figure 3 A typical radiation dose–cell survival curve for mammalian cells. Surviving fraction is plotted on the logarithmic y-axis as a function of delivered dose on the x-axis. The actual observed data are represented by points; the calculated survival (line) is estimated by a single-hit–multiple-target model.

cell. Once the point is reached at which, on average, each cell has accumulated the requisite number of hits minus 1, then the survival curve will display exponential kinetics, as each additional hit has an equal likelihood of finally producing the death of a cell. A mathematical description of a shouldered mammalian cell survival curve is given by

$$N/N_o = 1 - (1 - e^{-kD})^n$$

where n is the numerical value obtained by extrapolating the straight line portion of the curve to the y-axis. This value is termed the extrapolation number. This is a graphic solution to experimental data and does not necessarily imply a particular mechanism of lethality.

Because it is somewhat difficult to think in terms of the reciprocal dose units of the inactivation constant k, a convention has developed of the *mean lethal dose*, or D_0. This is simply defined as the inverse of the linear slope of the survival curve. Pragmatically, it can be used to express the dose that, on the average, is required to kill each and every cell in the population. However, because of the exponential nature of cell kill, a D_0 dose will in fact kill only 63% of the cell population, leaving 37% still alive. For this reason, the D_0 is sometimes referred to as the D_{37}. Rewriting the survival equation, one obtains

$$N/N_o = 1 - (1 - e^{-D/D_0})^n$$

which is the form that is commonly seen. One can also calculate what is termed the *quasithreshold dose* (D_q) as a measure of the width of the shoulder on the survival curve. It is this dose that must be accumulated sublethally. Once this dose is exceeded, cells die with exponential kinetics. Mathematically, this is expresed as $D_q = D_0 (\ln n)$.

Alternately, a two-component (linear–quadratic) model is also popularly used to describe radiation-induced cell killing in mammalian cells (Fig. 4). The equation for cell survival is expressed as

$$N/N_o = e^{-(\alpha D + \beta D^2)}$$

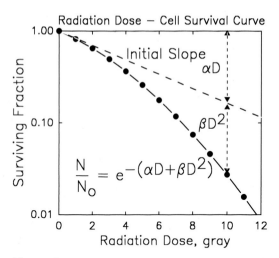

Figure 4   A typical radiation dose–cell survival curve for mammalian cells. Surviving fraction is plotted on the logarithmic *y*-axis as a function of delivered dose on the *x*-axis. The actual observed data are represented by points; the calculated survival (line) is estimated by the linear–quadratic model.

where α is in units of dose^{-1} and β is in units of dose $^{-2}$. Three lines of reasoning can be used as justification for multiple target–hit models or specifically for the linear–quadratic approach. If one assumes that double-stranded DNA breaks are the critical target for cell lethality, then there are two ways that ionizations can produce the required double-stranded break. First, there may be a single deposition of sufficient energy to simultaneously produce a break in two adjacent strands. Here, the production of damage will be directly (linearly) related to the dose (i.e., αD). Second, two separate and independent ionization events, each producing a one-strand break, occurring close enough together in time and space, will create the double-stranded break. Here, production of damage will be related to the square of the dose (quadratically) and expressed as βD^2. This is modeled schematically in Figure 5. An alternative model assumes that chromosomes represent the critical target and that chromosomal aberrations are the damage that results in lethality. The aberration can involve only one chromosome and result from only one ionizing interaction (αD); or it can involve two chromosomes and require two independent ionizing events (βD^2). Finally, one can choose not to define the critical target, but simply to use concepts of microdosimetry to postulate that there may be deposition of sufficient energy with a one-particle path (αD) to produce all the damage required for lethality, as with high-linear energy transfer (LET) radiations; or that two independent absorptions of energy (βD^2) are required to produce sufficient damage for lethality, as with low-LET radiations. Regardless of the approach that one employs, the model does adequately describe radiation-induced killing of mammalian cells, at least in tissue culture situations.

It is perhaps useful to compare the two approaches used to describe radiation-induced cell killing: the single-hit, multitarget model (D_0–n) and the linear–quadratic (α–β) model. In Figure 6, a representative set of data is shown for the survival observed subsequent to irradiation of 9L rat brain tumor cells in culture. As can be seen, both models provided calculated survivals (lines) that fit the observed data (points) quite reasonably. One would be hard-pressed to choose one model over the other for a data set such as this when survival is well-defined with little experimental variation. The problem becomes more severe when one considers the survival of cells in an organized tissue in which quite heterogeneous populations of cells are the norm.

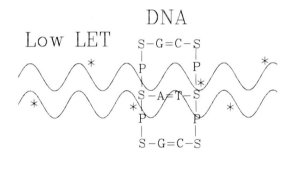

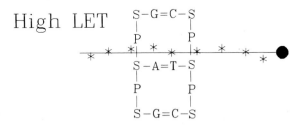

Figure 5 Schematic of double-stranded breaks produced in DNA as a result of two primary ionizations, resulting from either two low-LET photons, or from the passage of one high-LET particle through the DNA structure.

D. Effects on Organized Tissues

There is considerable variation in inherent radiosensitivity between the diverse cell types in the body. What has been termed the *law of Bergonie and Tribondeau* states that the inherent radiosensitivity of the typical mammalian cell is proportional to the mitotic activity, and is inversely proportional to the degree of differentiation. It is convenient to classify all mammalian cells into one of five categories (arranged here in order of decreasing radiation sensitivity with

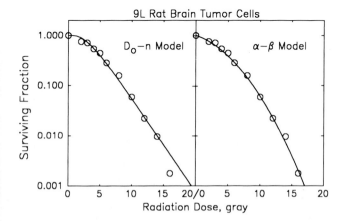

Figure 6 Radiation dose–cell survival curves for 9L rat brain tumor cells in vitro. Surviving fraction is plotted on the logarithmic *y*-axis as a function of delivered dose on the *x*-axis. The actual observed data are represented by circles; the calculated, expected survival by the lines. Both models provide an excellent fit to the experimental data.

examples): vegetative intermitotic cells (hematopoietic stem cells, basal germinal cells of the epidermis); differentiating intermitotic cells (intermediately differentiated cells in the hematopoietic series): multipurpose connective tissue cells (endothelial cells, fibroblasts, mesenchymal cells); reverting postmitotic cells (epithelial parenchymal cells of the liver, some smooth-muscle cells); and fixed postmitotic cells (erythrocytes, spermatids, striated muscle cells, neurons) (22). For the central nervous system, this presents a rather special situation. The primary functional parenchymal cells (the neurons) are among the most radioresistant cells known. They are completely differentiated and have zero potential for cell division. As such, it is impossible for them to suffer a reproductive death, although they may die through the process of interphase death. Typically, we assume that relatively large doses will be required to express this cellular effect. In contrast with the neurons, we have the (relatively) rapidly proliferating tumor cells that would be inherently more radiosensitive. If we only had to consider these two cell populations, radiation therapy of brain tumors would be straightforward and very effective. However, we must also take into account the wide variety of stromal elements that are critical in support of the neurons. The glial cells, the Schwann cells, and others all possess the potential for division and retain the ability for further differentiation. Add to this the relatively sensitive cells that constitute the endothelial linings of capillaries and blood vessels, and one has an organ that can be expected to respond unfavorably to radiation. It is these cells that present the critical cell populations that are at risk for the development of normal tissue complications. Even though, overall, the tolerance of the entire brain is rather high, it is not as high as we would project if only the fully differentiated neurons were at risk.

The pathological changes induced in brain depend on the radiation dose delivered and the volume of brain that is irradiated; and, to a smaller extent, the fractionation schedule, the dose rate, and the radiation quality (LET). For the most part, the dose-limiting toxic effects of radiation therapy to the brain are not expressed immediately, since there are few rapidly dividing cells in the brain. Rapid cell turnover rates are critical for acute toxicity in that they not only confer an inherent radiosensitivity to the cells, but also lead to an early expression of the toxicity, as it may take only a few days for the cells to undergo (or attempt to undergo) several cell divisions before dying and lysing. The acute syndromes (days to weeks) produced by brain irradiation may include nausea, vomiting, headache, and somnolence. Subsequently, long-term complications (months to years) may develop in irradiated brain tissue that are severe and dose-limiting.

As expected from the relative radioresistance of the cells involved, considerable doses (50–100 Gy) of whole-brain irradiation are required to produce cytological effects within a few hours (23). These changes consist of meningitis, choroid plexitis, cerebral vasculitis, and pyknosis of cerebellar granule cells. Inflammatory changes are observed within a few hours of irradiation, with perivascular and parenchymal infiltrates of granulocytes by 8 h. After 12–24 h, the infiltrate changes to mononuclear cells, with active phagocytosis and debris-filled macrophages. Throughout these processes, little effect, other than an occasional pyknosis, is observed in neurons. Finally, there are vascular changes expressed as blood vessel and capillary damage, with vasculitis, hemorrhage, and loss of permeability. This results in breakdown of the blood–brain barrier and may contribute to development of secondary effects. Fluid and electrolyte imbalance, parenchymal edema, and progressive damage to vascular structures and the supporting astrocytes can lead to extensive neuronal damage, especially in the brain stem and white matter. In radionecrosis of white matter, demyelination is related to impairment of oligodendrocytes and decreased synthesis of new myelin. The vascular deficiencies probably provide the foundation for the delayed expression of focal necrosis in the brain. If necrosis is secondary to vascular damage, then the greater susceptibility of white matter over gray matter may be explained by the decreased vascularity of the white matter (24). In addition to structural damage, there may also be functional deficits (memory and intellectual loss) and behavioral abnormalities expressed as long-term sequelae of brain irradiation, especially in pediatric patients in whom the brain is still developing.

Although most of what we know concerning acute and chronic radiation-induced toxicity of the central nervous system is based on administration of very large single doses (> 20 Gy), the individual small doses (2 Gy) used in daily fractionated radiotherapy may produce similar, but lower, toxicity. When delivered over several weeks (e.g., to total doses of 40 Gy or higher to the whole brain) fractionated radiation therapy can produce normal tissue damage as severe as that induced by large, single doses.

A final long-term complication that may need to be addressed is that of radiation-induced carcinogenesis and the production of a secondary malignancy. If radiation can produce sufficient damage to bring about death of tumor (and normal) cells, as required for therapeutic effect, then there will also be DNA or chromosomal damage induced in normal cells. If this damage is insufficient to kill the cell, but is instead passed along as a permanent, heritable mutation, there is a certain probability that a neoplastic transformation will occur that will eventually (perhaps years later) be expressed as a new primary tumor in the irradiated tissue.

IV. RADIOBIOLOGICAL CONCEPTS OF RADIATION THERAPY

A. General Considerations

Turning now to the clinical application of ionizing radiations to the management of cancer, we have available a very powerful cytotoxic (and cytostatic) agent. The problem, as with all other cancer treatment modalities, is that one must sterilize tumor cells, without incurring unacceptable toxicity in critical normal tissues. The first thing that must be taken into consideration is that there is no greater inherent radiosensitivity on the part of the neoplastic cell (compared with the normal cell) solely because it is neoplastic. In fact, a recent study (25) reports a wide range of in vitro intrinsic radiation sensitivities for glioblastoma multiforme cells that are not dissimilar to small-cell carcinoma or melanoma cells. On the other hand, there is also no greater radioresistance on the part of these cells in general. Therefore, we must balance the effects on the tumor cell population against the critical normal cell components. This is shown graphically in Figure 7 in

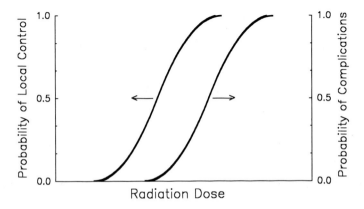

Figure 7 Probability of producing local control (left-hand axis and left-most curve) or complications (right-hand axis and right-most curve) is plotted as a function of radiation dose delivered.

which it is demonstrated that as one increases the dose delivered, one can produce an increase in the local control. The typical sigmoid shape of this curve is found in several radiobiologic settings. At low doses, the effect increases slowly, changes to an approximately linear increase between approximately 20 and 80%, and then plateaus, with decreasing effectiveness as the curve approaches 100%. As with other modalities, the dose to produce a 50% effect is quite often used for statistical analysis and for presentation of summary effects. This is because the slope of the line is steepest at 50%. This provides the most accurate values for a usable endpoint.

In addition to a curve for local control, one can also produce a similar curve for the local complications. Local complications will vary depending on the site and the normal tissues irradiated, but can range all the way from the trivial to the life-threatening and fatal. It is the relative positioning of these two curves that, more than anything else, influences the applicability of radiation therapy to the management of a particular tumor. For example, it does not matter how "sensitive" a particular tumor might be, as much as it matters whether the corresponding curve for complications is located to the left (in which case radiation therapy will not be very usable) or to the right (in which case radiation therapy is likely to be successful) of the control curve. Thus, rather than referring generically to tumors as being radiosensitive or radioresistant, it is more meaningful to refer to them as being radiocurable or radioincurable. This not only takes into account the absolute sensitivity of the tumor being addressed, but also the relative sensitivity of the critical surrounding normal tissues that are also at risk.

In the real world, we very seldom have two curves that are totally separated one from the other so that it would be possible to produce 100% control without any incidence of local complications. More typically, we have a displacement, as shown in Figure 8, for which there is significant overlap over a range of doses. This leads to the concept of a therapeutic window or therapeutic range, a range of doses within which one can hope to produce meaningful advantage against the tumor, without incurring too much toxicity. The logic for this is as follows. At doses to the left of the therapeutic range, one has a situation in which one can produce some benefit in the tumor, without incurring any risk of normal tissue complications. However, one would not be doing the most good for the greatest proportion of the patient population. On the other hand, delivery of doses to the right of the range will produce incremental increases in the percentage of local control, but at the cost of drastically increasing the local complication rate. The compromise is to use

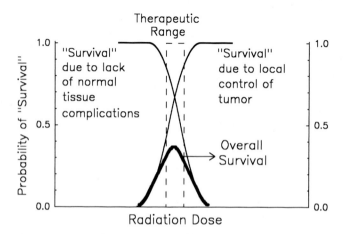

Figure 8   Probability of *survival* where survival refers to (1) the lack of fatal normal tissue complications and (2) successful eradication of tumor to achieve local control and cure. The overall probability of survival is the sum of these two reasons for survival (i.e., achieving local control without fatal complications).

doses within the therapeutic range. This is the range for which one produces overall the greatest degree of local control, without producing complications such that the results of local control are lost.

B. Increasing the Therapeutic Ratio

There are two approaches that can be employed in an attempt to separate the two critical curves to drive the control probability curve to the left or drive the complication probability curve to the right; that is, to produce sensitization of the tumor or protection of the normal tissues (Fig. 9). One can employ either physical means or biological means. Physically, this entails attempts to deliver dose accurately to the tumor volume and only the tumor volume. This starts with diagnosis to accurately and precisely define the location and extent of the tumor. If one wishes to confine the dose to the tumor, then one must first know where it is located. However, one also runs the risk of not treating a region of tumor if it is not included within the treatment volume. Thus, the more information that can be acquired about tumor localization, the better situated will be the radiation oncologist.

After having located the tumor and defined the volume that one wishes to treat, the next problem is to actually deliver the dose to that volume. Considerable efforts have been directed in the last 20 years to the refinement of the physical parameters of radiation therapy treatment machines. One area of improvement is in the use of more energetic treatment beams that are more tissue-penetrating. This means that one can deposit less dose in the peripheral surrounding normal tissues, while depositing more dose at the central region of the tumor. Conversely, the use of electron beams with limited and finite ranges can be used to avoid treating tissues at depths past the point of the tumor. Another approach is to use multiple fields and beams. Rather than direct a beam from only one orientation at a tumor, and thus treat the intervening normal tissues to a higher dose than can be delivered to the tumor, one uses several beams that all intersect at the tumor. Thus, any particular region of surrounding normal tissue receives only a fraction of the total dose being delivered to the tumor. The ultimate application of this approach is the use of rotational beam therapy during which the beam delivery unit is actually rotated about the patient throughout an entire 360° arc.

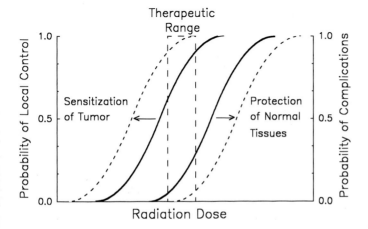

Figure 9 Approaches to increasing the probability of local control and cure (left-hand axis) by sensitizing the tumor, or decreasing the probability of complications (right-hand axis) by protecting the normal tissues. The arrows represent the desired direction of movement for the response curves that would improve patient outcome. By either means, the width of the therapeutic range is increased.

All of the foregoing techniques require very precise treatment-planning calculations. The use of computers and computer-assisted treatment planning to define doses in the various critical normal and tumor tissues have contributed greatly to the advances in this field. Finally, there have been many advances in the physical beams that are used for therapy. For example, high-LET radiations such as neutrons, π-mesons, and charged particles (accelerated nuclei stripped of their electrons) offer various advantages over the low-LET radiations (photons and electrons) that are commonly used in radiation therapy (26).

C.   Dose Fractionation

Historically, one of the earliest approaches that was employed to separate the control and complication probability curves, and thereby increase the therapeutic ratio, was the simple process of fractionating the dose delivered into numerous small dose increments (27). Early in this century Regaud and his colleagues (28, 29) noticed that if one delivered multiple small doses, instead of one large dose, one could decrease the damage induced in the normal tissues (at that time the skin was the most noticeable and the most affected normal tissue). It was also noticed that, although the effect on the tumor was diminished, there was less of a reduction than for the normal tissues. This means that with fractionation, one developed a greater therapeutic ratio between the effect on the tumor and the effect on normal tissues. This became a standard component of clinical radiation therapy practice and has been developed empirically ever since.

Initially, the enhanced success of fractionated radiation therapy was attributed simply to the concept that fractionation was less effective (allowing for an increase in the total dose tolerated) for tissues with rapid cell proliferation than for tissues with minimal or no cell turnover. Simplistically, one might expect a cancer cell to be more radiosensitive than its normal counterpart simply because it is either more rapidly progressing through the cell cycle or a greater fraction of the cell population is in a proliferating mode. For example, when compared with the fully differentiated, nondividing cells of the brain, the proliferating brain tumor cells would be more radiosensitive. However, even though tumor cell populations may, for the most part, be considered to be rapidly proliferating, numerous normal tissues also have a high proliferative capacity. Thus, additional explanations were required for the success of fractionated radiation therapy.

D.   The Four Rs of Fractionated Radiotherapy

On the basis of a half-century of radiobiological investigation and theoretical reasoning, certain radiobiological principles have evolved that provide a rationale for the concept of fractionated radiation therapy. It is important to realize that these have been derived, retrospectively, to explain the empirically developed clinical radiation therapy experience. These principles have been termed the *four Rs of radiotherapy* (30) and have been engraved indelibly on the brains of every resident in radiation oncology over the past two decades. The four Rs of repopulation, redistribution, repair, and reoxygenation will now be addressed.

Repopulation primarily refers to the ability of normal tissues to replenish themselves following injury. Because the dose increments are spread out over an extended time, fractionation also involves the element of protraction. The logic is that by protracting a course of radiation therapy over 5–6 weeks, one allows for hyperplastic compensation in some critically affected normal tissues. Although it is likely that no increase in tolerance will be obtained unless the protraction is extended to a period longer than 4 weeks, some benefit may be obtained from this. The reason for the 4-week requirement is that it may take this long for damaged cells to die, to go through the process of lysis, thereby creating a local depletion of cells; and for the remaining cells to mount a replacement proliferation. It is also likely that the tumor cells will continue to proliferate throughout this period. A possible improvement in therapeutic ratio is based on the assumption that the neoplastic cells are already proliferating out of normal control and, thus, depletion of these cells will not cause a corresponding increase in their growth rate. On the other hand, in normal tissues, cells with proliferative potential, but which are normally nondividing, will be stimulated to higher rates. Overall, it is hoped that this increase in the dose that normal tissues can tolerate will be greater than the additional dose one must deliver to compensate for tumor cell proliferation during protracted radiation therapy. As a rough rule of thumb, approximately 3 to 4 times more dose can be delivered by a conventional, daily fractionated schedule than if the dose were delivered in a single large fraction.

The second R, redistribution, reflects that a dose of radiation will have the greatest effect on the most sensitive cells in a population (31). One of the most important factors in determining the radioresistance or radiosensitivity of an individual cell is its position in the cell cycle (32–35). If cells are exposed to constant radiation doses at various temporal positions in the cell cycle, dramatic fluctuations and variations in survival will be observed (Fig. 10). Cells are most radiosensitive if treated while in mitosis, at the boundary between the G_1 and S-phases of the cell cycle, or in the G_2-phase. Cells in G_1 are less sensitive, with cells in S-phase being the most radioresistant (Fig. 11). Thus, an initial dose of radiation would be maximally effective against the sensitive cells, whereas cells located in the more radioresistant portions of the cycle would have a greater likelihood of surviving. If one were to irradiate immediately, one would be inefficiently delivering dose to a resistant population. However, with time, cells can progress from G_1 and S into more sensitive phases of cell cycles. Consequently, if one fractionates and protracts the doses, one provides an opportunity for the cells to redistribute throughout the cell cycle. The rationale is that, after a 24-h fractionation interval, one has regained the cell cycle distribution that was initially present before the first dose. Notice that we are only concerned with avoiding a cell cycle distribution for neoplastic cells that is enriched with cells located in radioresistant phases of the cell cycle. Normal cells, which we consider to be noncycling or cycling slowly, are not thought to be affected by redistribution.

The third R has to do with the repair of, or recovery from, radiation-induced damage. One

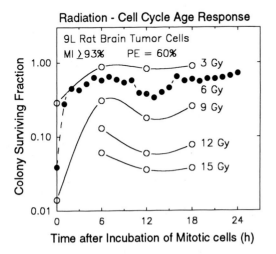

Figure 10 Cell cycle–age response to constant radiation doses for cultured 9L rat brain tumor cells selected in mitosis (32), incubated, and allowed to progress through the cell cycle before exposure to 3, 6, 9, 12, or 15 Gy. The mitotic index is greater than 93%, indicating the extreme purity of the population of mitotic cells selected; the plating efficiency is 60%. After 6-h incubation, cells are located in the mid-G_1 phase; by 12 h, at the boundary between G_1 and S phases; and by 18 h, in mid-to-late S-phase (35).

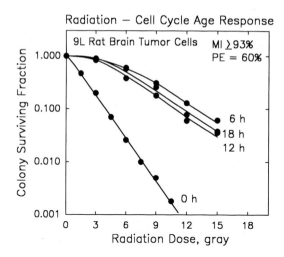

Figure 11   Radiation dose–cell survival curves for 9L rat brain tumor cells irradiated at different positions in the cell cycle. These data are redrawn from those in Figure 10. Note the extreme difference in survival between mitotic cells and cells located in other phases of the cell cycle.

aspect of this is the concept of sublethal damage. The shoulder in the initial portion of the radiation dose–cell survival curve (curve A of Fig. 12) implies the accumulation of what has been termed *sublethal damage*. In other words, one is depositing dose, but one is not producing cell lethality, or else one is producing lethality at a lower efficiency than what will be produced at a higher dose range. Subsequent to accumulation of sublethal damage, there is also the possibility that the cell will recover from this damage. Recovery or repair from sublethal damage is sometimes referred to as Elkind–Sutton recovery, or simply Elkind repair, after the investigators who first demonstrated this phenomenon in mammalian cells (36). As an example, if one considers the double-stranded DNA break to be the critical lethal lesion, then one can visualize a single-stranded break as a

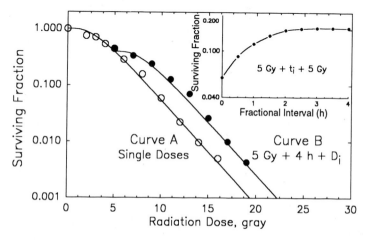

Figure 12   Theoretical radiation dose–cell survival curves for mammalian cells in vitro. Curve A represents survival of cells exposed to single radiation doses. Curve B represents the survival of cells given an initial dose of 5 Gy, and then variable additional doses following a fractionation interval of 4 h. The inset represents the increase in surviving fraction as a function of the fractionation interval between two doses of 5 Gy.

sublethal event. If another break is produced, a double-stranded break will ensue. However, if the first break is repaired before induction of the second break, then damage must again be accumulated sublethally. Phenomenologically, what is observed is a recovery of the shoulder region of the survival curve if one delivers two doses, separated by some fractionation interval (see curve B of Fig. 12). Since we are usually limited to an experimental observation of the reappearance of the shoulder region on a survival curve, without any specific knowledge about chemical or biochemical repair processes that might be occurring, it is more accurate to refer to this process as recovery from sublethal damage, than repair of sublethal damage. This recovery process occurs with definite kinetics, with recovery (hence, cell survival) increasing as the fractionation interval is increased. For most asynchronous populations of mammalian cells, the half-life for recovery is in the range of 15–60 min, so that most recovery has been accomplished by 4–6 h (see Fig. 12 inset). This time course for increase in cell survival is in the same range as the time course for rejoining of single-stranded DNA breaks and repair of chromosomal aberrations. Notice that the maximum recovery that can be obtained is limited by the amount of sublethal damage that was accumulated in the first place. Curve B will be displaced from curve A by, at most, a value equal to the D_q, the quasithreshold dose. The relative increase in surviving fraction will be at most equal to the value of n, the extrapolation number.

Another recovery process involves what has been termed *potentially lethal damage* (37, 38). Experimentally, if one holds irradiated mammalian cells for some time under conditions of growth inhibition (i.e., in plateau phase caused by contact inhibition, nutrient depletion, metabolic synthesis inhibition, hypoxia, cell cycle blockade), one will observe an increase in cell survival demonstrated over the entire range of the cell survival curve. Thus, damage that was potentially lethal (i.e., potentially capable of causing the death of the cell) has been rendered nonlethal. Recovery from potentially lethal damage occurs more slowly than recovery from sublethal damage: the half-life may be 1–4 h, and full recovery may require as much as 24 h. In contrast with recovery from sublethal damage, which is specifically a shoulder phenomenon, recovery from potentially lethal damage is a slope effect, as all damage is less effective at inducing the death of the cell. This also suggests that, whereas the extent of recovery from sublethal damage is fixed by the size of the shoulder, recovery from potentially lethal damage will be greater with larger doses and greater initial cell killing. Pragmatically, accumulation and recovery from sublethal damage is best demonstrated by small doses in the shoulder region of the survival curve; whereas recovery from potentially lethal damage is best expressed following large doses.

The therapeutic advantage that one would hope to gain from repair or recovery from sublethal or potentially lethal damage stems from the assumption that cells of normal tissues will be more capable of these processes than will cells in a tumor. With each dose fraction for which there is recovery from damage, the total dose that a normal tissue can tolerate will increase. Although we have no assurance that the dose a tumor can tolerate will not also increase proportionally, there are several aspects of the physiology and biochemistry of normal tissue versus tumor (e.g., relative fraction of proliferating cells, nutritional depletion in poorly vascularized solid tumors) that would suggest at least the potential for a therapeutic differential. However, we must accept that it could just as easily be the reverse, with more recovery occurring in tumor cells. In fact, Weischelbaum (39, 40) has postulated that it is the ability of human tumor cells in situ to recover from potentially lethal damage that is responsible and predictive for clinical outcome. Others would just as convincingly argue that it is accumulation and recovery from sublethal damage that is most critical (41).

The final R is that of reoxygenation (42). When neoplastic cells proliferate out of control, they frequently outgrow their available vascular supply. This may result in regions of central necrosis where cells do not receive sufficient nutrients to remain viable for any extended time. Between the necrotic core areas and healthy regions adjacent to the capillary beds, there may exist regions where cells remain viable, but under less than optimum conditions. The depletion of nutrients (including oxygen) will produce a population of cells that are growth-arrested, but which retain proliferative potential. The distance that oxygen can diffuse from the nearest capillary bed, through actively metabolizing cells, will depend on the oxygen partial pressure in the capillary and the metabolic rate of the cells, but is generally in the neighborhood of 100–200 μm (roughly 15 cell diameters). Thus, any solid tumor with a diameter greater than 400 μm potentially contains a population of hypoxic cells (43). These cells may be slightly radioresistant because of their quiescent status and decreased metabolism. More importantly, they will be radioresistant because oxygen acts at the radiochemical level to greatly increase the production of reactive radical species that can be damaging to critical biological macromolecules. Oxygen may also be involved in the fixation of damage on target molecules such that the damage is no longer amenable to repair processes. The net result is that cells irradiated under anoxic or hypoxic conditions will require approximately three times the dose of those under oxic conditions to produce the same level of cell kill (Fig. 13).

If a solid tumor is irradiated to a dose that is determined and limited by the tolerance of the surrounding normal tissues, the peripheral oxic tumor cells, adjacent to capillaries, should display approximately the same sensitivity as the well-oxygenated, radiosensitive normal cells. A dose that may kill nearly all the well-oxygenated cells will have little effect on the hypoxic cells. Thus, following the first radiation dose, most of the surviving cells will be in a hypoxic state and resistant to a subsequent dose. However, as the lethally damaged cells at the periphery of the tumor undergo the process of cell death and lysis, metabolism is shut down. Thus, oxygen and nutrients can now diffuse further into the tumor before being consumed. This process of reoxygenation operating between dose fractions will, one hopes, maintain the fraction of hypoxic viable cells at a level that is no greater than it was before initiation of therapy. The actual number of hypoxic cells will continually decline, but the proportion of hypoxic versus oxic cells will remain constant. If this does operate, then there is no need to actually kill the hypoxic tumor cells with radiation. Instead, one simply kills the oxic cells, allows them to die and be removed, and then converts the hypoxic cells back to oxic cells.

A critical aspect of the process of reoxygenation is that it has no effect on normal cells, since, with very rare exceptions, all normal tissues are fully oxygenated and maximally radiosensitive.

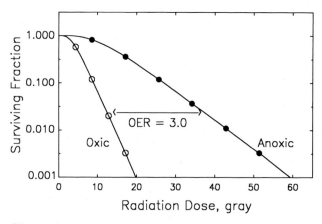

Figure 13 Representative radiation dose–cell survival curves for mammalian cells in vitro. The oxic curve represents survival of cells exposed under conditions of normal oxygenation. Curve B represents the survival of cells irradiated under hypoxic conditions. The oxygen enhancement ratio (OER) is the ratio of the doses required to produce the same level of cell lethality.

Thus, it is only the hypoxic tumor cell population that can be made more sensitive by allowing reoxygenation to occur between dose fractions. This is in contrast with the other three Rs for which there is no a priori guarantee that one will derive a greater dose–tolerance effect for normal tissues or a greater cytocidal effect for the tumor.

It is critical to bear in mind that although these four Rs provide a biological rationale for fractionated radiotherapy, they were developed in retrospect to explain the successes and failures of more than half a century of clinical radiotherapy, based mostly on empirical, pragmatic developments. It is only in the last 20–30 years that these biological bases have been used as guides to the development of new therapeutic approaches for the management of solid tumors. Even when new therapeutic efforts are not designed specifically on these biological rationales, there must still be an adherence to the basic concepts that underlie the response of tumors to radiation therapy. Considerable research effort is being directed toward efforts to improve the efficacy of radiation therapy (44). Although the magnitude of these efforts precludes a full discussion of their potential, a brief introduction can be provided that focuses on how they would take advantage of our increasing radiobiological knowledge.

V. AVENUES FOR IMPROVEMENT

A. Physics

As mentioned earlier, one approach to improving the therapeutic ratio (increasing the tumoricidal effect or reducing the damage done to normal tissues) is through improving the physical delivery of dose to the tumor while sparing the normal tissues. In addition to the technical improvement of existing megavoltage radiation therapy treatment machines that utilize photons and electrons, there is also better tumor localization and treatment planning. For example, stereotactic radiosurgery employs conventional photon therapy, but with the dose delivered to a small, well-defined volume, thereby avoiding the normal tissue complications observed when large volumes are irradiated with a large dose (see Chap. 26). This is already being used in the treatment of arteriovenous malformations as well as intracranial tumors. The same localization of tumor dose delivery is achievable through the technique of intraoperative radiation therapy, where the beam can be directed only to the volume to be treated. A similar approach is the use of interstitial implantation of radioactive sources to irradiate from within, sparing the surrounding normal tissues (see Chap. 25).

There are also efforts being made to exploit more esoteric radiation beams. Beams of protons, π-mesons, and accelerated charged nuclei offer certain advantages in terms of dose localization (45) on the tumor, while sparing surrounding normal tissues. For the high-LET radiations of π-mesons and charged nuclei, as well as for neutrons, there are also gains in radiobiological efficiency. Because of the nature of these densely ionizing radiations that deposit considerable dose in a small volume, several biological effects are produced that may be of therapeutic benefit. First, there is a reduction in the shoulder of the cell survival curve, compared with that produced by conventional, low-LET radiation. Along with the reduction in the accumulation of sublethal damage, there is also a decrease in the recovery from sublethal damage. A corresponding decrease in recovery from potentially lethal damage is also observed. Although this certainly decreases the tolerance of normal tissues, it may serve to remove any differential sensitivity between tumor and normal cells. There is also less cell cycle age-dependency with the high-LET beams. This could be an advantage in that one removes the peaks of cell resistance to radiation that may be present in tumor cells that are actively proliferating. Finally, and perhaps most importantly, the high-LET radiations demonstrate a lower value of the OER. This removes the inherent radioresistance that hypoxic cells enjoy. Since we assume that only tumor cells are hypoxic, this should provide a selective advantage in terms of increasing the therapeutic effect on tumors, without modifying the effect on normal tissues. Overall, the use of high-LET radiations could provide several advantages that would reduce the need for fractionated radiotherapy and its four Rs.

B. Radioimmunotherapy

A biological, rather than physical, approach to dose localization is offered by the recent emergence of radioimmunotherapy. Here, a monoclonal antibody specific for brain tumor cells (ideally) is coupled to a radioactive nuclide. Typically, a radionuclide is chosen that decays through emission of either an α-particle (a helium nucleus of two protons and two neutrons) or a β-particle (an electron). These have the advantage of depositing the dose within a short distance from the site of decay. The monoclonal antibody will home on and associate with the tumor, and thus only the tumor should receive any appreciable dose. There may also be additional gains in that the dose deposited may be of a high-LET and, consequently, a high-RBE, variety. There may also be an advantage, as might exist for interstitial implants of radionuclides, owing to the low-dose rate that is required (46).

C. Solutions to the Hypoxic Cell Problem

One area that has received considerable attention has been the problem of the radioresistant hypoxic tumor cell. There is a 30-year history of efforts to develop chemicals that will function as hypoxic cell radiosensitizers (47). These are compounds, such as nitroimidazoles, that will not be metabolically consumed and so will diffuse into hypoxic regions of tumors where oxygen cannot penetrate. There, they will act in an oxygen-mimetic fashion mediated through their electron affinity to sensitize the cells to radiation. Since well-oxygenated cells are already maximally radiosensitive, these compounds should function only to enhance tumor cell kill, without any effect on normal tissues. Interestingly, one of the few positive studies to date has been on the treatment of glioblastomas (48). However, because of toxicity problems with the nitroimidazoles now used, there is a need to develop better agents. Since some of the nitroimidazoles (e.g., misonidazole) undergo specific biochemical reactions that occur only under anaerobic conditions and lead to their retention within hypoxic cells, they have been used as markers of hypoxic regions in tumors. This concept, along with diagnostic techniques such as positron emission tomography (PET) and single-photon emission computed tomography (SPECT), may be used not only to confirm the presence of hypoxic cells within a tumor, but may also offer a means of monitoring the response of the tumor to the initial radiation therapy treatments.

Another approach to the problem of hypoxic tumor cells relies on simply delivering more oxygen to the tumor bed, to overcome the low oxygen tension in the capillaries within the central region of the tumor. Some patients have been irradiated while being treated with hyperbaric oxygen. Perfluorochemical emulsions, which can carry more oxygen than hemoglobin-mediated red blood cells, have been investigated. Pharmacological manipulation (e.g., nicotinamide, pentoxifylline, hydralazine) may offer some hope of physiologically altering blood flow to the tumor for therapeutic advantage. Metabolic manipulation (e.g., 2-deoxyglucose) or cytotoxic agents selective for hypoxic cells (e.g., mitomycin) may be directed to sterilize hypoxic tumor cells while sparing well-oxygenated cells. All of these approaches seek to remove the inherent radioresistance of hypoxic tumor cells, which makes them as sensitive as the adjacent normal tissue cells.

D. Adjuvant Hyperthermia

The use of hyperthermia (temperatures above 43°C) adjunctively with radiation therapy offers several advantages (49). First, hypoxic cells are no less sensitive to hyperthermia-induced cell killing than are well-oxygenated cells, thereby removing the selective disadvantage of hypoxic tumor cells. Second, the cell cycle age-dependencies of radiation and hyperthermia are complementary. Cells that survive radiation through being located in a radioresistant cell cycle phase will be sterilized by hyperthermia, and vice versa. Finally, hyperthermia administered simultaneously or sequentially with radiation therapy may cause a decrease in the cell's ability to recover from both sublethal and potentially lethal radiation damage.

E. Concomitant Chemotherapy

Another form of combined modality therapy is the concurrent use of radiation therapy and chemotherapy (50). This obviously includes the use of cytotoxic chemotherapeutic agents which provide at least additive cell kill from the two modalities. In addition, one may gain from complementary cell cycle age-dependencies to produce synergistic effects. Nontoxic chemicals can be used to enhance the efficacy of radiation therapy through a variety of mechanisms. Cell cycle progression inhibitors may allow accumulation of cells in radiosensitive regions of the cell cycle. Metabolic inhibitors may decrease the cell's ability to repair radical-induced damage. Specifically, attempts have been made to manipulate intracellular levels of glutathione, the major xenobiotic detoxifier of mammalian cells (51, 52). Inhibition of repair may function to decrease repair of DNA strand breaks, or phenomenologically to suppress accumulation and recovery from sublethal damage, or recovery from potentially lethal damage.

Another chemotherapeutic approach takes advantage of the enhanced proliferation of brain tumor cells compared with the mostly noncycling or slowing cycling critical cells of the brain (53, 54). Halogenated pyrimidines (bromo- or iododeoxyuridine) will be incorporated in place of thymidine only in cells that are actively synthesizing DNA. Once incorporated in DNA, these compounds have a radiosensitizing effect, in that a smaller radiation dose is required to produce DNA damage and cell kill.

F. Normal Tissue Radioprotection

In contrast with efforts to improve tumoricidal effect of radiation, there have also been attempts to diminish the effect of radiation on the normal tissues. One approach is to carry further the concept of fractionation (55). If one utilizes two even smaller doses per day (e.g., 1.2 Gy bid) instead of conventional daily fractionation (1.8–2.0 Gy per fraction), one observes a decrease in the damage produced in critical normal tissues, especially those composed of noncycling or slowly cycling cells and characterized as late-responding tissues (56, 57). This hyperfractionation achieves an increase in the tolerance dose of normal tissues, without a corresponding sparing of tumor cells, or rapidly dividing normal cells.

Normal tissue radioprotection can also be achieved by the use of compounds that function as radioprotective agents through interference with the production of structural changes at the basic chemical and biochemical levels (58). This requires differential uptake, with normal tissues accumulating and retaining more drug than the tumor. A number of aminothiol compounds (e.g., WR2721) have shown this property and are being developed clinically. Amelioration of normal tissue effects can also be accomplished by biological response modifiers that operate at the level of cell and tissue replacement (interleukins, colony-stimulating factors, and others). Finally, one can simply ameliorate the symptoms of radiation-induced damage, without actually altering the degree of damage that is produced.

The foregoing examples of efforts to improve upon the therapeutic use of ionizing radiations serve to indicate that much work remains to be done and that there is much to be gained in the arena of brain tumor therapy. The use of experimental model systems can provide a means to explore new and promising modalities and concepts. However, a certain caution is always required as one attempts to extrapolate from preclinical therapeutic experimentation to the reality of the clinic.

VI. CONCLUSION

In this chapter, we have followed the time course of ionizing radiation effects from the attosecond to the century. Along the way, we have covered the basics of radiation physics and radiation biology. We have examined the radiobiological rationales that explain the successes and failures of modern radiation therapy (59). We have also discussed how these radiobiological concepts can be used as a foundation on which to develop new and more efficient forms of radiation therapy and combined modality therapy.

It is worth reflecting that it has been less than 100 years since Roentgen first announced his discovery of the nature and properties of a mysterious new type of physical entity—the x-ray. In the intervening time, we have made great strides in our understanding and use of radiation. It remains for us to continue to develop better ways to apply this modality to the management of cancer, and especially to the treatment of malignant tumors of the central nervous system.

REFERENCES

1. Hall EJ. Radiation and life. Oxford: Pergamon Press. 1976.
2. Andrews HL. Radiation biophysics. Englewood Cliffs, NJ: Prentice-Hall, 1961.
3. Wardman P. Principles of radiation chemistry. In: Steel GG, Adams GE, Peckham MJ, eds. The biological basis of radiotherapy. New York: Elsevier, 1983:51–59.
4. Boag JW. The time scale in radiobiology. In: Nygaard OF, Adler HI, Sinclair WK, eds. Radiation research. Proceedings of 5th international congress of radiation research. New York: Academic Press, 1975:9–29.
5. Altman KI. Radiation chemistry. In: Dalrymple GV, Gaulden ME, Kollmorgen GM, Vogel HH, eds. Medical radiation biology. Philadelphia: WB Saunders, 1973:15–29.
6. Dalrymple GV, Baker ML. Molecular biology. In: Dalrymple GV, Gaulden ME, Kollmorgen GM, Vogel HH, eds. Medical radiation biology. Philadelphia: WB Saunders, 1973:30–43.
7. Grosch DS, Hopwood LE. Biological effects of radiations. New York: Academic Press, 1979: 71–92.
8. Elkind MM, Whitmore GF. The radiobiology of cultured mammalian cells. New York: Gordon and Breach Science, Publishers, 1967.
9. Gall JG, Pardue ML. Formation and detection of RNA–DNA hybrid molecule in cytological preparations. Proc Natl Acad Sci USA 1969; 64:600–604.
10. John H, Birnstiel ML, Jones KW. RNA–DNA hybrids at the cytological level. Nature 1969; 223:582–587.
11. Pizzarello DJ, Witcofski RL. Basic radiation biology. Philadelphia: Lea & Febiger, 1967:184–208.
12. Dewey WC, Firman SC, Nuller HH. Comparison of lethality and chromosome damage induced by x-rays in synchronized Chinese hamster cells in vitro. Radiat Res 1970; 43:561–568.
13. Elkind MM, Han A, Volz KW. Radiation response of mammalian cells grown in culture. IV. Dose dependence of division delay and postirradiation growth of surviving and nonsurviving Chinese hamster cells. JNCI 1963; 30:705.
14. Leeper DB, Schneiderman HS, Dewey WC. Radiation-induced division delay in synchronized Chinese hamster cells in monolayer culture. Radiat Res 1972; 50:401–417.
15. Leeper DB, Schneiderman HS, Dewey WC. Radiation-induced cycle delay in synchronized Chinese hamster cells: comparison between DNA synthesis and division. Radiat Res 1973; 53:326–337.
16. Schneiderman MH, Dewey WC, Leeper DB, Nagasawa H. Use of the mitotic selection procedure for cell cycle analysis. Comparison between the x-ray and cycloheximide G_2 markers. Exp Cell Res 1972; 74:430–438.
17. Kerr JFR, Wyllie AH, Currie AR. Apoptosis: a basic biological phenomenon with wide-ranging implications in tissue kinetics. Br J Cancer 1972; 26:239–257.

18. Searle J, Kerr JFR, Bishop CJ. Necrosis and apoptosis: distinct modes of cell death with fundamentally different significance. Pathol Annu 1982; 17:229–259.

19. Puck TT, Marcus PI. Action of x-rays on mammalian cells. J Exp Med 1956; 103:653–1666.

20. Lea DE. Actions of radiation on living cells. 2nd ed. London: Cambridge University Press, 1956.

21. Alper T. The target concept and target theory. In: Cellular radiobiology. London: Cambridge University Press, 1979:19–32.

22. Rubin P, Casarett GW. Clinical radiation pathology. vols 1 and 2. Philadelphia: WB Saunders, 1968.

23. Fabrikant JI. Radiobiology. Chicago: Year Book Medical Publishers, 1972:122–153.

24. Prasad KN. Human radiation biology. Hagerstown, Md: Harper & Row, 1974: 257–274.

25. Taghian A, Suit H, Pardo F, Gioioso D, Tomkinson K, Duboid W, Gerweck L. In vitro intrinsic radiation sensitivity of glioblastoma multiforme. Int J Radiat Oncol Biol Phys 1992; 23:55–62.

26. Raju MR. Heavy particle radiotherapy. New York: Academic Press, 1980.

27. Coutard H. Roentgenotherapy of epitheliomas of the tonsillar region, hypopharynx, and larynx from 1920 to 1926. AJR 1932; 28:313–331.

28. Regaud C. Sur les principles radiophysicologiques de la radiotherapie des cancers. Acta Radiol 1930; 11:456–486.

29. Regaud C, Ferroux R. Discordance des effets des rayons X, d'une part dans la peau, d'autro past dans le testicule, par le fractionement de la dosen. Diminution de l'effecacite dans le peau, maintion de l'eddicacite dans le testicule. CR Soc Biol 1927; 97:431–434.

30. Withers HR. The 4 R's of radiotherapy. In: Lett JT, Adler H, eds. Advances in radiation biology. vol 5. New York: Academic Press, 1975:241.

31. Withers HR. Cell cycle redistribution as a factor in multifraction irradiation. Radiology 1975; 114:199.

32. Terasima T, Tolmach LJ. Variations in several responses of HeLa cells to x-irradiation during the division cycle. Biophys J 1963; 3:11–33.

33. Sinclair WK, Morton RA. X-ray sensitivity during the cell generation cycle of cultured Chinese hamster cells. Radiat Res 1966; 29:450–474.

34. Kimler BF, Henderson SD. Cyclic responses of cultured 9L cells to radiation. Radiat Res 1982; 91:155–168.

35. Sinclair WK. Cell cycle dependence of the lethal radiation response in mammalian cells. Curr Top Radiat Res Q 1972; 7:264–285.

36. Elkind MM, Sutton H. X-ray damage and recovery in mammalian cells in culture. Nature 1959; 184:1293–1295.

37. Phillips RA, Tolmach LJ. Repair of potentially lethal damage in x-irradiated HeLa cells. Radiat Res 1966; 29:413–432.

38. Little JB, Hahn GM, Frindel E, Tubiana M. Repair of potentially lethal damage in vitro and in vivo. Radiol 1973; 106:689–694.

39. Weichselbaum RR. The role of DNA repair processes in the response of human tumors to fractionated radiotherapy. Int J Radiat Oncol Biol Phys 1984; 10:1127–1134.

40. Weichselbaum RR, Beckett M. The maximum recovery potential of human tumor cells may predict clinical outcome in radiotherapy. Int J Radiat Oncol Biol Phys 1987; 13:709–713.

41. Byfield JE. The role of radiation repair mechanisms in radiation treatment failures. Cancer Chemother Rep 1974; 58:527–538.

42. Kallman RF. The phenomenon of reoxygenation and its implication for fractionated radiotherapy. Radiology 1972; 105:135.

43. Thomlinson RH, Gray LH. The histological structure of some human lung cancer and the possible implications for radiotherapy. Br J Cancer 1955, 9:539–549.

44. Mitchell JB, Glatstein E. Radiation oncology: past achievements and ongoing controversies. Cancer Res 1991; 51(suppl):5065s–5073s.

45. Withers HR. Biological basis for high LET radiotherapy. Radiology 1973; 108:131–137.

46. Hall EJ. Radiation dose rate: a factor of importance in radiobiology and radiotherapy. Br J Radiol 1972; 45:81–97.

47. Brady LW, ed. Radiation sensitizers: their use in the clinical management of cancer. New York: Masson Publishing, 1980.

48. Urtasun RC, Band P, Chapman JD, Feldstein ML, Mielke B, Fryer C. Radiation and high dose metronidazole (Flagyl) in supratentorial glioblastomas. N Engl J Med 1976; 294:1364–1367.

49. Urano M, Double E. Hyperthermia and oncology: biology of thermal potentiation of radiotherapy, vol. 2 Utrecht: VSP BV Publications, 1989.

50. Hill BT, Bellamy AS, Antitumor drug-radiation interactions. Boca Raton: CRC Press, 1990.

51. Meister A, Anderson MA. Glutathione. Annu Rev Biochem 1983; 52:711–60.

52. Mitchell JB, Russo A. The role of glutathione in radiation and drug-induced cytotoxicity, Br J Cancer 1984; 55:96–104.

53. Mitchell JB, Russo A, Cook JA, Straus KL, Glatstein E. Radiobiology and clinical application of halogenated pyrimidine radiosensitizers. Int J Radiat Biol Phys 1989; 56:827–836.

54. Russo A, Gianni L, Kinsella TJ, Klecker RWJ, Jenkins J, Rowland J, Glatstein E, Mitchell JB, Collins J, Myers C. Pharmacological evaluation of intravenous delivery of 5-bromodeoxyuridine to patients with brain tumors. Cancer Res 1984; 44:1702–1705.

55. Withers HR. Biologic basis for altered fractionation schemes. Cancer 1985; 55:2086–2095.

56. Thames HG, Withers HR, Peters LJ, Fletcher GH. Changes in early and late radiation responses with altered dose fractionation: implications for dose–survival relationships. Int J Radiat Oncol Biol Phys 1982; 8:219–226.

57. Withers HR, Peters LJ, Kogelnik HD. The pathobiology of late effects of irradiation. In: Meyn RE, Withers HR, eds. Radiation biology in cancer research. Raven Press: New York. 1980:439–448.

58. Yuhas JM, Stroer JB. Differential chemoprotection of normal and malignant tissues. JNCI 1969; 42:331–335.

59. Withers HR. Biologic basis of radiation therapy. In: Perez CA, Brady LW, eds. Principles and practice of radiation oncology. Philadelphia: JB Lippincott, 1987:67–98.

23

The Role of Radiation Therapy in the Treatment of Adult Brain Tumors

Richard G. Evans
University of Kansas Medical Center, Kansas City, Kansas

I. INTRODUCTION

There are approximately 35,000 new brain tumors in the United States each year, including those that are metastatic to the brain. When cerebral metastases from solid primary tumors outside the central nervous system are not included, there is an increasing incidence of malignant glioma as a function of decade so that, in patients older than age 60 (an increasing portion of our population through the end of this century), over 90% of the tumors of the brain are astrocytomas, and half of these are glioblastoma multiforme. Table 1 illustrates the frequency of primary adult intracranial tumors and forms the basis for selection of the common tumors we will discuss. This chapter will be divided into five sections: low-grade primary tumors; high-grade primary tumors; recurrent brain tumors; radiation tolerance of the brain, including radiation necrosis; and recent and future approaches to the treatment of brain tumors using radiation.

There are several advantages to an open-tumor resection, including, particularly in gliomas for which there is known heterogeneity, obtaining a representative sampling of the tumor; reduction of intracranial pressure whenever necessary; and improvement of the neurological and subsequent Karnofsky performance of the patient before radiation. In addition, from a radiobiological stand-point, an open tumor resection decreases the tumor burden and also removes the hypoxic–radiation-resistant population of cells, the removal of which may possibly contribute to the improved survival in patients following radiation.

II. LOW-GRADE PRIMARY TUMORS

The low-grade primary tumors represent a heterogeneous group, and the gliomas, oligodendro-gliomas and mixed tumors will be dealt with in separate sections. No randomized trials have been

Table 1 Frequency of Adult Primary Brain Tumors

Tumor	Frequency (%)
Low-grade primary tumors	60
Gliomas	20
Oligodendrogliomas and mixed tumors	5
Ependymomas	5
Meningiomas	20
Pituitary tumors	5
Craniopharyngiomas, optic pathway gliomas, tumors of the pineal region, others	5
High-grade primary tumors	40
Anaplastic astrocytomas and glioblastoma multiforme	35
Tumors of brain stem	2–5
Primary CNS lymphoma	2–5

carried out on the role of postoperative radiation in low-grade astrocytomas, although there are several ongoing studies. The pilocytic astrocytomas and the cystic cerebellar astrocytomas are not included in these randomized studies, as these tumors are often amenable to complete surgical resection, and no postoperative radiation therapy is indicated. The remaining supratentorial gliomas, approximately 25% of the total, can be divided into low-grade gliomas, which make up 20%, and oligodendrogliomas and mixed tumors, which make up the remaining 5%.

A. Gliomas

A review by Shaw, carried out at the Mayo Clinic (1), showed that the 5- and 10-year survival rates for patients with low-grade astrocytomas treated by subtotal resection alone was in the range of 0–25%. Several retrospective reviews have indicated that postoperative radiation leads to improved survival, and Leibel et al. (2), examining data from the University of California, San Francisco (UCSF), found that the 5- and 10-year recurrence-free survival rates with incomplete resection alone were 19 and 11%, compared with 46 and 35% with the addition of postoperative radiation. Moreover, in the study from the Mayo Clinic (1), it was noted that patients who received at least 53 Gy had a significantly longer survival than those receiving less than this dose, suggesting a dose dependence. Most series that report on the use of surgery alone have 5-year survivals clustering near 20%, whereas, in series for which postoperative radiation has been used, 5-year survival rates range from 25 to 75%, with clustering near 50%. We can conclude, therefore, that there is at least a doubling in 5-year survival for this group of subtotally resected tumors by the addition of radiation therapy. A review of all the retrospective studies from this country and Europe led to the conclusion that postoperative radiation therapy should be given routinely to patients with low-grade astrocytomas, regardless of the extent of surgical resection, which led to initiation of the randomized clinical trials outlined in Table 2. The studies are basically a radiation dose-searching exercise, with the exception of the Brain Tumor Cooperative Group (BTCG)–Southwest Oncology Group (SWOG) study, which randomizes patients between observation or delayed treatment or immediate 54 Gy to a localized field. As discussed in Chapter 12, there is ample evidence in the literature indicating the tendency of partially resected low-grade gliomas not only to regrow, but often to undergo malignant transformation, so that the outcome following a second surgery at the time of recurrence and subsequent postoperative radiation therapy almost always leads to an inferior survival, compared with that achieved by treating the patients initially with radiation. In

Table 2 Current Randomized Studies in Supratentorial Low-Grade Gliomas

I.	BTCG/SWOG (US)	Astrocytomas Oligodendroglioma Mixed tumors	®⟨ Observation[a] / 54 Gy in 6 wk[b]
II.	NCCTG/Mayo RTOG/ECOG (US)	Astrocytoma Oligodendroglioma Mixed tumors Pilocytic—Bx only	®⟨ 50.4 Gy in 5½ wk[b] / 64.8 Gy in 7 wk[b]
III.	EORTC (Europe)	Astrocytoma Oligodendroglioma Mixed tumors	A ®⟨ Observation[a] / 54 Gy in 6 wk[b] B ®⟨ 45 Gy in 5 wk[b] / 59.4 Gy in 6½ wk[b]

[a]54 Gy if recurrence occurs.
[b]Partial brain only (tumor + 2- to 3-cm margins).
Studies I and II accept patients with any extent of surgical resection.
Study III accepts only patients with less than a total resection.

my view, the more important question is not if and when to treat with postoperative radiation, but what dose to use. It is hoped that the current trials will provide the answers to both the questions of when to treat with radiation and what dose range to use.

B. Oligodendrogliomas and Mixed Tumors

An unpublished review carried out in 1991 by Shaw at the Mayo Clinic (noted in Ref. 3) shows that the survival rates of 154 patients with supratentorial low-grade astrocytomas, mixed oligoastrocytomas, and oligodendrogliomas were no different in those receiving subtotal removal or biopsy than in those in whom a gross total or radical subtotal removal was obtained. Patients with oligodendrogliomas who underwent less than gross total removal had significantly improved survival with the addition of postoperative radiation therapy, provided it was greater than 50 Gy. These results confirm those of Wallner et al. (4) from UCSF, which showed that the 10-year survival rate for patients with oligodendrogliomas who received at least 45 Gy was 56% compared with 18% for those who were not irradiated. In addition, adjunctive radiation therapy increased the time to tumor recurrence, as well as the number of long-term survivors. However, series do exist that find no benefit to postoperative irradiation, as noted by Reedy et al. (5). It is hoped that the aforementioned current trials will throw light on this very important question. For mixed tumors, there is a suggestion from Mayo Clinic data (3) that there is an improvement in survival as the proportion of oligodendroglioma component increases, with the 5-year survival rate for mixed oligoastrocytomas being 63 compared with 72% for patients with pure oligodendrogliomas.

C. Ependymomas

Ependymomas in adults represent at most 5% of the total and, for a full discussion of the treatment of these tumors, the readers are referred to Chapter 21 on pediatric brain tumors. Although there are no randomized trials for this tumor type, the role of postoperative radiation therapy is well established by numerous studies. Many series divide patients into low- and high-grade ependymomas, and a review of the literature by Leibel and Sheline (6) indicates that, at 5 years, survivals are about 60–80% for low-grade tumors, whereas survivals in the range of 10–47% are noted for high-grade tumors. As we discussed in Chapter 20, the eventual degree of seeding is dependent not only on grade and location (infratentorial versus supratentorial), but also the degree of tumor control in the posterior fossa. The combination of high-grade and infratentorial location can result in seeding of the neuraxis in up to 15% of the patients, whereas a rate of only 5% is seen in low-grade infratentorial lesions. Recurrence at the primary site in the posterior fossa is by far the most frequent failure pattern. If the spinal magnetic resonance imaging (MRI) scan and cerebrospinal fluid (CSF) examination results are initially negative and the tumor is low-grade, I feel that either whole-brain irradiation, or irradiation over a large field encompassing the lesion, is appropriate. For high-grade or so-called anaplastic ependymomas, most authors recommend craniospinal irradiation, especially if the tumor is located in the infratentorial region. However, subarachnoid failure is very uncommon in the absence of local failure, and there remains the question of whether spinal metastases can be prevented by prophylactic treatment of the spinal axis, as discussed by Vanuytsel and Brauder (7).

D. Meningiomas

Meningiomas are more common in adults and represent about 20% of all brain tumors. Although there is a general perception that these tumors are benign and surgical treatment *only* is necessary, a significant proportion are very vascular and can surround important structures, such as cranial nerves and major arteries, making total removal impossible. In a series from the Massachusetts General Hospital, although the operative note indicated a total resection had been carried out, there was a 7% recurrence rate at 5 years, 20% at 10 years, and 32% at 15 years (8). An overview of the literature reveals that recurrence rates range from 35 to 60% following partial excision alone, which can be decreased to 2–30% if postoperative radiation therapy is given. One of the largest series, that from UCSF, by Barbaro et al. (9), shows that, following subtotal resection, 60% of the nonirradiated tumors recurred, compared with only 32% of those irradiated. Moreover, the median time to recurrence was significantly longer in the irradiated group (10 years versus 5 years in the nonirradiated group). In light of this, patients with so-called benign meningiomas, should receive postoperative radiation therapy following subtotal resection to doses of the order of 50–55 Gy with a 2-cm margin around the presurgical tumor volume. Although this view is not accepted by most neurosurgeons, I feel that the literature supports the use of immediate, rather than delayed, radiation, as patients treated at recurrence do significantly worse, usually because the tumor at recurrence is quite large and often nonresectable.

Malignant meningiomas, which represent approximately 5% of the total, definitely require postoperative radiation therapy to doses of at least 60 Gy to somewhat larger fields than the benign meningiomas, and this recommendation applies even to those patients who have undergone a total excision, as over three-quarters of these tumors eventually recur if they have not received postoperative radiation.

E. Pituitary Tumors

Approximately 80% of these tumors are endocrine-active and, of these, over half are prolactin-secreting, one-quarter growth hormone-secreting and approximately 20% corticotropin (ACTH)-secreting. It is generally considered that the hypersecreting adenomas should have an attempted complete resection, as their response to radiation therapy is somewhat slow and not always predictable. However, for the nonsecreting tumors, which are often large, surgical cure may be impossible and should not be attempted, as adjuvant radiation therapy in this subgroup is usually curative. The experience at UCSF with large nonfunctioning adenomas or prolactinomas showed a 60% recurrence rate within 5 years after incomplete resection, which was reduced to about 4% by the addition of radiation therapy. In the patients with visual field defects, there appeared to be a benefit from preradiotherapy surgical decompression. In patients with acromegaly following unsuccessful pituitary surgery, control rates above 60% can be obtained with radiotherapy, and a 50% reduction in the preirradiation level of growth hormone is obtained in most patients by 2 years following a dose of 45–50 Gy. In a large series by Grigsby et al. from Washington University School of Medicine (10) utilizing radiation only, 10-year disease-free survival was a function of the tumor type, with 69% for acromegaly, 83% for patients with amenorrhea or galactorrhea, and 80% for nonfunctioning adenomas. Only the presence of visual field defects at diagnosis conferred a poor prognosis. A report from the same institution using *both* surgery and radiation therapy showed some benefit to surgical decompression and tumor removal, in that the 10-year disease-free survival was approximately 76% for acromegaly, 93% for patients with amenorrhea or galactorrhea, and 90% for nonfunctioning adenomas. Both these reports indicated that there was a tendency to superior tumor control when radiation doses greater than 45 Gy were used.

III. HIGH-GRADE PRIMARY TUMORS

In this section, we will discuss the role of radiation in the anaplastic astrocytomas and glioblastomas, tumors of the brain stem, and lymphomas of the central nervous system.

A. Anaplastic Astrocytoma and Glioblastoma

Anaplastic astrocytoma and glioblastoma represent about 40% of the total of primary brain tumors in the decade between 40 and 49 years of age, but can represent close to 60% in patients older than age 60. In most series, the anaplastic astrocytomas make up approximately 10% and the glioblastomas 90% of the total. The role of postoperative radiation therapy was first established in a randomized trial carried out by the Brain Tumor Cooperative Group (BTCG) (11). In this study, the median survival time for patients undergoing surgery was only 14 weeks, whereas those treated with radiation therapy following surgery had a median survival time of 36 weeks. A series of subsequent trials carried out by the BTCG showed the benefit of increasing doses of radiation, with the median survival increasing from 28 weeks following a dose of 50 Gy to 42 weeks when 60 Gy was used. These and other trials have failed to demonstrate any survival advantage of doses greater than 60 Gy. Although several studies carried out over the last two decades have used whole-brain irradiation, the current wisdom now favors the use of 3-cm margins around the CT-defined contrast-enhancing lesion. Some authors use these margins around the MRI-defined T2 image, resulting in fields that often approach those of whole-brain irradiation. Several prognostic factors have been considered in the outcome of these patients, including age, performance status, location of tumor, degree of surgical resection, and preoperative tumor size. A recent report (12) dealing with anaplastic astrocytomas only, using combined data on over 100 patients from three RTOG malignant glioma trials, noted that the median survival time of patients undergoing partial or total resection was 49 months versus 18 months for those with a biopsy only. Patients whose tumors had a frontal location had a longer median survival time than those with nonfrontal lesions, but no survival difference was noted by univariate analysis of tumor size. Interestingly, when multivariate analysis was carried out, the extent of surgery was not predictive, and only younger age, frontal location, and smaller tumor size correlated significantly with extended survival.

A recent review by Quigley and Maroon (13) of 20 reports, totaling 5691 patients with supratentorial malignant gliomas, indicated that in only four reports was the extent of surgery related to survival. Moreover, in two of these four reports, the degree of resection followed age, histological grade, and performance status in importance. The improved prognosis as a function of younger age has been identified in patients with glioblastoma multiforme as well as anaplastic astrocytoma and, in a combined RTOG–ECOG study, survival at 18 months was 64% for patients younger than 40, compared with only 8% for those older than 60 years of age. Moreover, in almost all studies, age remains a significant factor, even after adjustment for histological type and performance status.

It seems clear from several studies that performance status is an independent prognostic factor, and patients with an initial Karnofsky performance status (KPS) of 70 or greater have a survival rate at 18 months of 34%, which falls to 13% or lower for patients with a Karnofsky status of 60 below. Because the degree of resection has not always been a stratification factor in most series, and anaplastic astrocytoma and glioblastoma patients are often pooled, it is difficult to draw concrete conclusions about the importance of degree of resection. However, what information is available would suggest that the degree of resection is not an independent prognostic factor. In a similar vein, there are few reliable data concerning the importance of preoperative tumor size; but many nonstratified studies indicate that size may be an important factor in anaplastic astrocytoma, but not for glioblastoma multiforme. An interesting observation made by Wood et al. (14) was that the *postoperative* tumor area was inversely related to survival and that patients with residual tumors smaller than 1 cm^3 had the longest survival times. Additionally, the prognostic importance of tumor area remaining after surgery was independent of histological type, age, and KPS. Unpublished data from analysis of several RTOG studies in glioblastoma patients confirm an advantage for patients with tumors in the frontal lobe, with a significantly longer median survival than those with lesions in the temporal or parietal lobes. Similar observations have been noted in patients with anaplastic astrocytoma.

B. Tumors of the Brain Stem

Tumors of the brain stem are uncommon to the adult age group, but represent approximately 10% of all pediatric brain tumors and are dealt with in more detail in Chapters 20 and 21. Although there is a paucity of data on grade, as a relatively small proportion of these tumors are biopsied, the larger studies indicate that approximately half the tumors are high-grade and half low-grade gliomas. Interestingly, if the tumor is well differentiated or even anaplastic, it more often involves the midbrain, whereas, if it is a glioblastoma, it is more frequently found in the medulla.

Historically, these patients have been treated with once-a-day fractionation to 50–55 Gy with a 2-cm margin around the tumor. Long-term survivals have been in the range of 25–40%, depending on the series, with most clustering around 30%. Modest improvements in outcome have been observed in children and also, more recently, in adults, using doses of about 72 Gy in twice-a-day fractions of 1 Gy each (hyperfractionation). In the series from UCSF (16), which has the largest number of adult patients, a recent update shows that the 3-year survival rate with doses of 66–78 Gy was 36% for children versus 60% for adults. There was no improvement in outcome when patients were treated to higher doses of 76 and 78 Gy with a twice-daily approach; therefore, 72 Gy has become the standard. The apparent improved outcome in adults should be interpreted with caution, in light of patient selection and differences in location of the tumor. We have discussed previously that location has definite prognostic value, with the patients whose tumors are in the midbrain or thalamus doing significantly better than those with lesions in the pons or medulla. A caveat is that different locations may harbor tumors of different grades. It is clear that most irradiated patients show rapid improvement in their neurological symptoms, and failure is almost always local. We have learned from the twice-a-day fractionation studies that doses higher than the 55 Gy used historically in single fractions can be safely given to both adults and children. However, it has been difficult, in a proportion of patients, to wean the patients from their steroid therapy.

C. Primary Central Nervous System Lymphoma

In the older literature, these tumors were referred to as microgliomas, but we now know that most are best described as B-cell lymphomas of the histiocytic type. Since the advent of immunosuppressive drug therapies in transplant patients and also the tremendous increase in patients with the acquired immunodeficiency syndrome (AIDS), the number of cases of primary CNS lymphoma appears to be on the increase. In addition, especially in the AIDS population, patients are presenting at an earlier age, more commonly in the second and third decades of life. Over half the cases are supratentorial in their presentation, and more than a third present with multiple lesions. The diagnosis is usually made from a CT-guided stereotaxic biopsy, and radiation therapy either alone or in combination with chemotherapy is the treatment of choice. As with lymphomas in other locations, there is a prompt improvement, both clinically and radiographically, in most patients. However, as Leibel and Sheline (17) noted, the duration of response is relatively short before local recurrence is noted, with median survival times of about 1 year. Whole-brain irradiation is preferred, and there appears to be a definite radiation dose response. A review of the literature by Murray et al. (18) showed that patients who received more than 50 Gy to the primary tumor site had a better outcome than those given less than 50 Gy. The RTOG conducted a study in which patients were given 40 Gy to the whole brain followed by an additional 20 Gy to the primary lesion (19). Although the 1- and 2-year survival rates were 48 and 28%, the median survival time of the 41 evaluable patients was just short of 1 year. As noted previously in several other brain tumor types, age and performance status were the most important predictors of outcome, with younger and higher-performance status patients having median survivals of the order of 2 years.

In addition to being radiation-sensitive, the lymphomas of the CNS also appear to be sensitive to various chemotherapeutic agents, which has led to a combined modality approach. In the 1990s, several planned studies will explore the benefit of adding chemotherapy, either before or after the radiation. A pattern appears to be emerging of two to three cycles of either a four- (cyclophosphamide, doxorubicin, vincristine, prednisolone; CHOP) or three-drug (procarbazine, lomustine (CCNU), vincristine; PCV) regimen before whole-brain irradiation. A randomized trial, however, will be necessary to confirm the early observation that a combined modality approach might be beneficial. It is doubtful that the AIDS patients with CNS lymphoma, because of their immunocompromised state and low white cell counts, would be candidates for such a combined regimen.

IV. RADIATION TREATMENT OF RECURRENT BRAIN TUMORS

The approach to a patient with a recurrent brain tumor depends, in great part, on whether the patient has received radiation as part of the initial treatment. In patients with low-grade brain tumors which recurred following observation only, as in the current BTCG–SWOG study, radiation therapy appears warranted, but the aggressiveness of such treatment needs to be tempered by the performance status and wishes of the patient. Whether or not they have received radiation or not as part of their initial treatment, approximately half of the patients can expect to recur, albeit several years after their initial treatment. In view of the paucity of data in the literature concerning prognosis following treatment, we recently carried out an analysis of patients with low-grade gliomas, who had local recurrence, and, with a median follow-up time of more than

7 years, we noted that, for the primary patients receiving radiation, the 5-year survival was 49% and the 10-year survival 22% (20). Moreover, of the 36 patients with locally recurrent tumors who underwent repeat surgery, one-third remained low-grade, whereas two-thirds had transformed into a high-grade tumor. This observation has been noted previously and is discussed elsewhere. Although each patient should be taken as an individual case, surgery represents the optimum method of removing the recurrent tumor, including the hypoxic radiation-resistant components and those that are poorly vascularized. This would be inappropriate if the patient's early death were inevitable or the benefits short-term. Even in selected patients, surgery is only a first step, and the only treatment of proved benefit for recurrent brain tumors is some type of radiation. In the foregoing review (20), the median survival of those patients receiving radiation as part of their treatment following recurrence was 20 months, whereas, in those not receiving radiation as part of their treatment, the median survival was only 6 months. These data must be viewed in the context that the patients who initially had low-grade tumors had undergone malignant transformation in two-thirds of the cases.

Unless the patient has not received radiation initially, the commonly used therapy for high-grade tumors that have recurred is either interstitial radiation (brachytherapy) or radiosurgery. There are certain size and location limitations to each of these procedures, and brachytherapy is suitable only for patients who have tumors no larger than approximately 5 cm, in a location that will tolerate radiation necrosis. This will occur in approximately half the patients, and requires surgery to remove the necrotic tissue, usually within 8–10 months from the time of the radioactive implant. In a similar vein, radiosurgery gives the best results in patients with a recurrent lesion that is localized and is 3 cm or smaller in diameter. A report from UCSF discussing survival and quality of life after interstitial brachytherapy in the treatment of patients with recurrent high-grade gliomas showed that, after a brachytherapy dose of approximately 70 Gy, a median survival of approximately 1 year after implantation could be expected (21). The success of brachytherapy in recurrent tumors has led to several studies in which it has been used as a boost procedure following external beam radiotherapy in patients with primary high-grade gliomas. The Joint Center for Radiation Therapy has used brachytherapy (50 Gy) boosts in a select group of patients, with performance status better than 70% and tumor size of about 5 cm, following approximately 60 Gy to the partial brain by external beam. Survival rates at 1 and 2 years after diagnosis were 87 and 57%, respectively, for those receiving brachytherapy versus the controls, who did not receive the implant. The 1- and 2-year survivals after diagnosis were 40 and 12.5%, respectively. However, focal radiation necrosis occurred in most patients undergoing brachytherapy, and surgical resection of the necrotic mass was required in these patients (22). A smaller number of patients have been treated with stereotactic radiosurgery, a somewhat more limited technique, in that only tumor recurrences 3 cm or smaller are suitable; doses between 10 and 20 Gy are given to these lesions at one sitting, using a modified linear accelerator, and it appears that many of these patients will also require additional surgery for radiation necrosis.

The pattern of failure following the use of stereotactic interstitial irradiation techniques as part of the primary treatment for malignant gliomas has changed in that there is an increased incidence of peripheral brain and distant CNS relapse (23). A word of caution is necesssary in regard to the selection of patients for these local techniques for recurrent or primary tumors, whether by radioactive seed implant or by radiosurgery: these procedures should be carried out in patients with good neurological function and a performance score in excess of 70, and patients with tumors in the cerebellum, midbrain, or other parts of the brain stem are not good candidates for such treatments because of the vital nature of these structures.

A final thought on selection bias: as we noted previously, in the 42 patients with glioblastoma mutliforme (22), the addition of brachytherapy to the primary treatment resulted in improvement of median survival to 27 months, compared with only 11 months for the controls. This may have been in part because 40% of the patients in the brachytherapy group underwent reoperation, compared within only 15% in the matched controls. This issue of selection bias has been addressed by Florell et al. (24). These authors noted that "eligible" patients for the brachytherapy boost, which is approximately a third of the patients in most series, tended to live longer, were younger, had a better Karnofsky functional status, and underwent more aggressive resections. The authors noted that the better outcome following adjuvant brachytherapy for malignant glioma was, at least in part, the result of patient selection.

V. RADIATION TOLERANCE OF THE BRAIN

This section will be divided into the following: radiation tolerance of the brain, radiation pathology, and the treatment of radiation necrosis.

A. Radiation Tolerance

The essentials are presented here, but, for a detailed discussion of this subject, readers are referred to an recent excellent text (25). Reactions of the brain to radiation can most conveniently be divided into (1) acute effects that might occur during treatment or within the few weeks following the completion of radiation therapy, (2) early delayed effects that appear from 1 to 3 months following completion of radiation, and (3) late, delayed effects, which can develop several months to many years following completion of radiation treatment.

When conventional (1.8–2 Gy/day) or hyper-fractionated (1 Gy twice daily) doses are delivered 5 days per week to a total dose of approximately 60 Gy to a large portion of the brain, some patients will describe symptoms of increased intracranial pressure, thought to be attributable to increased edema around the tumor; however, this phenomenon is difficult to detect on CT or MRI scans during the course of radiation. It is the wisdom of many radiation oncologists that the prophylactic use of dexamethasone during radiation treatment can minimize these acute effects. When seen in the radiation oncology department, most patients with malignant glioma have already been placed on a dexamethasone regimen, and it is my policy and that of many others to maintain these patients on at least 4 mg of dexamethasone per day during their radiation treatment. This is particularly important in light of the emerging approach of using 2- to 3-cm margins, either around the edema as seen on the T2 image or around the contrast-enhanced image on a T1 MRI study, which often results in rather large partial-brain fields. Many groups, however, prefer to use 2- to 3-cm margins around the contrast-enhancing ring on the CT scan, which leads to smaller brain fields.

The early delayed effects that appear 1–3 months following completion of radiation, marked by somnolence or an increase in signs and symptoms noted initially are self-limiting and usually resolve in 4–6 weeks. It is impossible to distinguish these effects seen uncommonly in brain tumor patients, from the possible progression of the tumor, as the CT and MRI findings are equivocal and should therefore not be used as evidence that there is tumor progression and that repeat surgical resection is necessary.

The third and most serious effects are those seen months to years after completion of treatment and are commonly described as late-delayed radiation injuries. As we will discuss in the section on pathology, the injury usually occurs after large partial volumes or the whole brain have been irradiated, with the changes in the white matter being quite diffuse. If, however, the CT scan reveals focal radiation necrosis, then localizing neurological signs may be noted. There is a paucity of data in the literature concerning late radiation changes as a function of the volume of brain treated, but it is clear that the radiation fraction size, rather than the overall time of dose delivery, is the key factor in the incidence of radiation necrosis. It is rare to note radiation necrosis following the delivery of 60 Gy of radiation, provided conventional fractionation is used. Leibel and Sheline (27) carried out a recalculation of the data of Marks et al. (26) for 139 patients who received conventional radiation dose fractions showed that the incidence of radiation necrosis was highly correlated with the total dose, in that no cases of necrosis were seen in 51 patients who received 57.6 Gy or less. There were 2 cases, or 3%, in 60 patients treated with doses of 57.6–64.8 Gy, and there was an 18% incidence of necrosis (5 patients) among 28 patients who received 64.8–75.6 Gy. Before these data are universally applied, there are several caveats, the first being that children younger than 3 years old have a higher incidence at each dose level than that just noted. The second is that the incidence of radiation necrosis can be increased if either concomitant or sequential chemotherapeutic agents are used. These late-radiation effects cannot be easily interpreted on diagnostic imaging, and a biopsy is required to confirm the diagnosis of either recurrent tumor or radiation necrosis.

B. Etiology and Pathology of Radiation Effects on the Brain

As we noted earlier, the acute phase of the delayed radiation effect on the brain can often be demonstrated by an expansile contrast-enhancing lesion on CT, largely confined to the white matter. There is some evidence that the brain in the peritumoral region, possibly because of edema, is more susceptible to radiation damage, which can be modified or partially alleviated by the use of dexamethasone during the radiation treatment. The supratentorial regions of the brain appear to be most sensitive to radiation, there being few reported instances of radiation necrosis to the brain stem and cerebellum. Autopsy studies have shown that the lesions are restricted largely to the white matter and typically show hemorrhagic coagulation necrosis. Exudation of fibrin from small blood vessels is also noted, and is demonstrated by classic fibrinoid necrosis. Vascular proliferation can also be noted, particularly in the acute phase of the delayed effect, but with time different from those changes seen with cerebral infarction. These vascular changes evolve, causing fibrin exudation and fibrinoid necrosis, with some evidence of vascular thickening. Although most changes are seen in or near the tumor bed, evidence of radiation necrosis has been noted in parts of the brain geographically removed from the neoplasm, which is clearly attributable to a complication occurring in the normal brain, rather than from the attempted therapeutic destruction of the tumor. In contrast, changes that constitute a desired therapeutic effect have been noted following the use of implanted radioactive sources (brachytherapy), and marked necrosis has been noted in this heavily irradiated region. Some observers believe that the early delayed effects can be ascribed to the interruption of myelin synthesis caused by radiation injury to the oligodendroglial cells, whereas the later effects are either attributed to injury to the vascular endothelial cells or to a direct effect on the glial cells themselves.

C. Treatment of Radiation Necrosis of the Brain

It is usually impossible to distinguish radiation necrosis from recurrent tumor on either CT or MRI and, when the necrosis is noted near the tumor bed, a neurosurgical procedure is necessary to detect possible tumor regrowth in regions removed from the zones of radiation necrosis. Most neurosurgeons would agree that the standard treatment for radiation-induced necrosis when indicated by the prognosis and performance status of the patient, is surgical excision of the mass. Although corticosteroids may be used initially to stabilize the symptoms, when the necrosis is favorably located, surgical resection is frequently beneficial. The long-term use of corticosteroid therapy has to be tempered by its effect on the stomach lining and muscles of the legs, as well as the ensuing immunosuppression and weight gain. There are scattered reports of attempts to reduce the use of high-dose steroids by treating patients with anticoagulants, such as heparin and warfarin.

Although corticosteroids can result in a dramatic improvement in the symptoms of radiation necrosis, and sometimes may be the only treatment necessary, in many patients the mass effect and neurological deterioration take on a relentlessly progressive course and in these instances, surgical excision of the necrotic mass becomes obligatory. Repeat craniotomy is not without its adverse side effects, as the possibility of poor wound healing from the previous radiation and adhesions in the brain from previous surgery can make the operation difficult. Often, however, the mass of necrotic tissue is well circumscribed from surrounding normal tissue, and it is my belief that an aggressive complete resection should be attempted when indicated by the overall status of the patient.

The importance and benefits of surgical intervention have been highlighted in those patients who have received either a brachytherapy or a radiosurgery boost, which has resulted in radiation necrosis in one-half to two-thirds of the patients. It is clear that patients who are selected for repeat surgery for focal radiation necrosis live significantly longer than those not undergoing a surgical procedure, as noted in the results from the UCSF patients (28). In this series, the median survival for patients with anaplastic astrocytoma who had repeat surgery was 124 weeks, compared with only 43 weeks for those who did not have such surgery. Similarly, in patients with glioblastoma multiforme, the patients who underwent repeat surgery had a median survival of 84 weeks, compared with only 36 weeks in those not undergoing such surgery. There exists a certain selection bias in those patients chosen to undergo reoperation; therefore, the benefits of reoperation must be interpreted with caution (24).

VI. RECENT AND FUTURE APPROACHES IN THE RADIATION TREATMENT OF BRAIN TUMORS

We have previously discussed the use of the implantation of radioactive seeds or radiosurgery as a boost technique following external beam radiation therapy for the treatment of malignant brain tumors (see Chaps. 25 and 26). The ultrahigh therapeutic doses that have been applied, using either brachytherapy or radiosurgery, would indicate that a plateau has probably been reached in terms of benefit from increased radiation doses. Moreover, the necessity of interventional neurosurgery to remove the foci of radiation necrosis following these boost techniques in one-half to two-thirds of the patients, together with the changed patterns of failure with new lesions being noted distant from the tumor bed, necessitates the exploration of newer approaches.

The prospects for radiation protection of the normal brain, carried out in animal models, have been disappointing, although studies of this nature should continue to be carried out in an attempt to develop a better therapeutic index between the tumor and the normal tissues of the brain. There have been a few scattered reports of the benefit of pentobarbital as a radiation protector of normal brain, but efforts in our laboratory have failed to confirm sufficient benefit to be explored in clinical studies. The prostaglandins have been investigated in animal models in an effort to augment the sulfhydryl radioprotection conferred by established radiation protectors such as amifostine (WR-2721), and efforts such as these should be continued.

In patients, most efforts have been directed at sensitizing tumors to radiation, and these will be discussed in this section. The radiation-resistance of primary brain tumors has been attributed, at least in part, to the existence of hypoxic fractions within tumors and the knowledge that well-oxygenated tissues are approximately three times more sensitive to radiation than anoxic tissues. The use of hypoxic cell sensitizers, such as misonidazole, in combination with radiation has been explored in a dozen randomized studies, all of which have shown no benefit in survival compared with conventional irradiation alone (29). In the same vein, we have explored, in a Phase I/II study, the use of the perfluorochemical emulsion Fluosol, with breathing of high-pressure oxygen in an attempt to oxygenate the hypoxic fractions of the tumor and, with conventional radiation, have noted a greater number of survivors at 3 years in patients with glioblastoma multiforme, compared with historical controls (30).

Recent reports from the University of California in San Francisco and the University of Arizona presented at the Ninth International Conference on Brain Tumor Research and Therapy in 1991, have reported on the use of interstitial irradiation with hyperthermia (31). Sneed et al. from the University of California in San Francisco reported on the treatment, by hyperthermia before and after brachytherapy, of 49 patients with recurrent brain tumors and noted a median survival of 44 weeks for recurrent glioblastoma multiforme (31). Stea et al. from the University of Arizona treated 30 patients with high-grade tumors in a Phase I/II clinical trial using interstitial ferromagnetic thermal radiotherapy as part of the primary treatment. Patients initially received 50 Gy of external beam radiation followed by an interstitial implant of iridium-192, with a 1-h hyperthermia treatment delivered before and after the interstitial radiation by means of thermally regulated ferromagnetic implants. Unfortunately, there were 12 acute toxic reactions in 24 patients, including seizures and transient neurological deficits, and 3 patients had major complications, including hydrocephalus, intracerebral hemorrhaging, and 1 death. Follow-up is short and, at the time of the report, 15 patients remained alive 6–38 months from diagnosis (31).

The halogenated pyrimidine analogues bromodeoxyuridine (BUDR) and idoxyuridine (IUDR) are known radiosensitizers that are selectively incorporated into rapidly dividing cells. The degree of radiosensitization is a function of the degree of replacement of thymidine by bromouridine or idoxyuridine, and sensitization up to a factor of three, compared with radiation alone, has been demonstrated in several animal systems. In a Phase I/II study carried out by the Northern California Oncology Group (NCOG), 310 patients with malignant gliomas received BUDR for 4 days during a 6-week course of radiation. This was followed by multiagent chemotherapy, and the median survival time for patients with anaplastic astrocytoma was 252 weeks, compared with 64 weeks for glioblastoma multiforme. To establish the role of BUDR, a randomized study is necessary, and this is currently being carried out at UCSF. The National Cancer Institute recently reported on long-term follow-up of a Phase I/II study of gliobastoma multiforme patients treated with IUDR and hyperfractionated irradiation. Forty-five patients were accrued to the study, and the results, with a minimum follow-up of 1 year, did not indicate a significant benefit of the use of the radiation sensitizer (median survival 11 months). Tumor biopsies at craniotomy showed relatively low sensitizer incorporation. The authors felt that the high inherent radiation resistance of gliobastoma multiforme, together with poor penetration and uptake of the sensitizer, was the cause of this disappointing result (32).

The approach that has been most extensively explored is the use of radiation treatments with altered fractionation. This has been of two types: first, *hyperfractionated* radiation when two or more treatments are given each day, with fraction sizes essentially half of that conventionally used, and second, so-called *accelerated* fractionation, in which the overall treatment time has been reduced by giving conventional-sized dose fractions two or sometimes three times per day. The use of hyperfractionated techniques is based on the rationale that by giving the radiation dose in a series of smaller, more frequent, fractions the radiation would preferentially affect the rapidly proliferating tumor cells when they enter the more radiosensitive phases of the cell cycle. In addition, as normal tissues have a slower rate of cell division and a greater capacity to repair sublethal radiation damage, there was hope that there would be greater control of the tumor, without increasing the rate of late complications in the normal brain. However, the results of several group trials using hyperfractionated radiation have been inconclusive, and none of the randomized trials have yet shown convincing improvement in outcome. The RTOG conducted a randomized Phase II trial of almost 500 patients for whom the doses were escalated from 64.8 to 81.6 Gy, using 1.2-Gy twice-daily fractions with an interval of 4–6 h between treatments. It was determined that patients in the 72-Gy arm had a longer median survival than those assigned lower doses or to the 81.6-Gy arm. The median survival was, in fact, reduced from 14.2 months to 11.7 months when the dose was increased from 72 to 81.6 Gy. It was felt that doses above 72 Gy resulted in an inferior outcome owing to excessive neurotoxicity. Given these studies, the RTOG is presently exploring the use of 72 Gy, given as 1.2-Gy fractions twice daily versus 60 Gy, given in one daily fraction of 2 Gy, with both arms using carmustine (BCNU), 80 mg/m^3 on days 1, 2, and 3 of radiotherapy, and then for 3 days every 8 weeks for 1 year following completion of radiation.

The rationale of accelerated fractionation is that the shortened overall treatment time would improve the therapeutic ratio by reducing the chance of tumor repopulation during treatment, which, it was hoped, would translate into greater tumor control. An RTOG Phase II trial accruing 300 patients was carried out, with patients receiving either 48 or 54.4 Gy at 1.6 Gy twice daily with BCNU. The median survival times were essentially the same as historical controls, being 11.7 months for the 48-Gy patients and 10.8 for those treated with 54.4 Gy. A similar trial was carried out in Europe by the EORTC in which patients were either treated with 60 Gy of conventionally fractionated radiation over 6 weeks or with accelerated fractionation using three fractions per day of 2 Gy each for 1 week. Following a 2-week break, the regimen was repeated for a total of 60 Gy in only 4 weeks. Although this accelerated fractionation schedule offered no survival advantage compared with conventional irradiation, it could be appropriate in patients with a relatively poor prognosis and a short survival expectancy, as it would reduce the treatment time from 6 weeks to 4 weeks.

Based on the success of bone marrow transplantation, both autologous and allogeneic, in the treatment of patients with lymphoma and leukemia, attempts have been made to use this rescue regimen in patients with solid tumors, including those of the brain. The majority of studies have been carried out in children and young adults with malignant brain tumors, using various combinations of chemotherapy, as the majority of patients were treated at recurrence and had already received full-dose radiation. In a pilot study of 25 adult patients with high-grade gliomas carried out at Lackland Air Force Base, extremely high-dose BCNU was followed by whole-brain irradiation and patients were then rescued with an autologous bone marrow transplant. The median survival of 26 months was most encouraging, resulting in a 44% two-year survival, but longer follow-up is needed before this approach can be recommended in more than a very selected group of patients (33).

An approach of even more limited application is the use of boron neutron capture therapy (BNCT). The rationale is based on the preferential uptake of ^{10}B into tumors compared to into normal tissues. Epithermal neutrons from a nuclear reactor are then focused on the brain when the ^{10}B captures a neutron, short-range, extremely energetic alpha particles are released and a therapeutic index is developed between the normal brain and the tumor tissue owing to the preferential concentration of ^{10}B in the tumor. After disappointing results of BNCT in this country several decades ago, there has been a resurgence of interest in Japan, brought about by better delivery systems of boron and the availability of epithermal neutrons. Hatanaka has treated over 100 glioblastoma patients in Japan, all of whom first received a surgical debulking procedure, followed by intra-arterial injection of a borate compound and subsequent irradiation with neutrons. This group has reported prolonged survivals of 50% at 5 years, with few complications in a highly selected group of patients with malignant glioma (34). A BNCT protocol has recently been developed by a team at the New England Medical Center in Boston in conjunction with a nuclear reactor group at MIT, and results should be forthcoming that will either support or refute the claims of the Japanese investigators.

REFERENCES

1. Shaw EG, Dumas-Dupont C, Scheithauer BW, et al. Radiation therapy in the management of low-grade supratentorial astrocytomas. J Neurosurg 1989; 70:853–861.
2. Leibel SA, Sheline GE, Wara WM, et al. The role of radiation therapy in the treatment of astrocytomas. Cancer 1975; 35:1551–1557.

3. Shaw EG, Scheithauer BW, O'Fallon JR, Tazelaar HD, Davis DH. Oligodendrogliomas: the Mayo Clinic experience. J Neurosurg 1992; 76:428–434.
4. Wallner KE, Gonzalez M, Sheline GE. Treatment of oligodendrogliomas with or without postoperative radiation. J Neurosurg 1988; 68:684–688.
5. Reedy DP, Bay JW, Hahn JR. Role of radiation therapy in the treatment of cerebral oligodendroglioma. Neurosurgery 1983; 13:499–503.
6. Leibel SA, Sheline GE. Radiation therapy for neoplasms of the brain. J Neurosurg 1987; 66:1–22.
7. Vanuytsel L, Brada M. The role of prophylactic spinal irradiation in localized intracranial ependymoma. Int J Radiat Oncol Biol. Phys 1991; 21:825–830.
8. Mirimanoff RO, Dosoretz DE, Linggwood RM, et al. Meningioma: analysis of recurrence and progression following neurosurgical resection. J Neurosurg 1985; 62:18.
9. Barbaro NM, Gutin PH, Wilson CB, Sheline GE, et al. Radiation therapy in the treatment of partially resected meningiomas. Neurosurgery 1987; 20:525–527.
10. Grigsby PW, Stokes S, Marks JE, Simpson JR. Prognostic factors and results of radiotherapy alone in the management of pituitary adenomas. Int J Radiat Oncol Biol Phys 1988; 15:1103–1110.
11. Walker MD, Alexander E, Hunt WE, et al. Evaluation of BCNU and/or radiotherapy in the treatment of anaplastic gliomas. J Neurosurg 1978; 49:333–343.
12. Curran WJ, Scott CB, Horton J, Nelson JS, et al. Does extent of surgery influence outcome for astrocytoma with atypical or anaplastic foci? J Neurooncol 1992; 12:219–227.
13. Quigley MR, Maroon JC. The relationship between survival and the extent of the resection in patients with supratentorial malignant gliomas. Neurosurgery 1991; 29:385–388.
14. Wood JR, Green SB, Shapiro WR. The prognostic importance of tumor size in malignant gliomas. J Clin Oncol 1988; 6:338–343.
15. Deutsch M, Green SB, Strike TA, et al. Results of a randomized trial comparing BCNU + radiotherapy, streptozotocin + radiotherapy, BCNU + hyperfractionated radiotherapy, and BCNU following misonidazole + radiotherapy in the postoperative treatment of malignant glioma. Int J Radiat Oncol Biol Phys 1989; 16:1389–1396.
16. Shrieve DC, Wara WM, Edwards MSB. Hyperfractionated radiation therapy for brain stem gliomas in children and adults [abstract]. Int J Radiat Oncol Biol Phys 1991; 21(suppl 1):120.
17. Leibel SA, Sheline GE. Radiation therapy for neoplasms of the brain. J Neurosurg 1987; 66:1–22.
18. Murray K, Kun L, Cox J. Primary malignant lymphoma of the central nervous system. J Neurosurg 1986; 65:600–607.
19. Nelson DF, Martz KL, Bonner H, et al. Definitive radiation therapy in the treatment of primary non-Hodgkin's lymphoma of the central nervous system, non–AIDS-related. J Neurosurg (in press).
20. DeWitt BL, Evans RG, Braun SD, Morantz RA, Wall TJ. Unpublished data, 1991.
21. Leibel SA, Gutin PH, Wara WM, et al. Survival and quality of life after interstitial implantation of removable high-activity iodine-125 sources for the treatment of patients with malignant gliomas. Int J Radiat Oncol Biol Phys 1989; 17:1129–1139.
22. Loeffler JS, Alexander E, Wen PJ, et al. Results of stereotactic brachytherapy used in the initial management of patients with glioblastoma. JNCI 1990; 82:1918–1921.
23. Loeffler JS, Alexander E, Hochberg FH, et al. Clinical patterns of failure following stereotactic interstitial irradiation for malignant gliomas. Int J Radiat Oncol Biol Phys 1990; 19:1455–1462.
24. Florell RD, McDonald DR, Irish WD, Berstein M, Leibel SA, Gutin PH, Cairncross JG. Selection bias, survival and brachytherapy for glioma. J Neurosurg 1992; 76:179–183.
25. Gutin PH, Leibel SA, Sheline GE, eds. Radiation injury to the nervous system. New York: Raven Press, 1991.
26. Marks JE, Baglan RJ, Prassad SC, et al. Cerebral radionecrosis: incidence and risk in relation to dose, time, fractionation and volume. Int J Radiat Oncol Biol Phys 1981; 7:243–252.
27. Leibel SA, Sheline GE. Radiation therapy for neoplasms of the brain. J Neurosurg 1987; 66:1–22.
28. Leibel SA, Gutin PH, Wara WM, et al. Survival and quality of life after interstitial implantation of removable high-activity sources for the treatment of patients with recurrent malignant gliomas. Int J Radiat Oncol Biol Phys 1989; 17:1129–1139.

29. Bleehen NM. Studies of high-grade cerebral gliomas. Int J Radiat Oncol Biol Phys 1990; 18:811–813.
30. Evans RG, Kimler BF, Morantz RA, Vats TS, Gemer LS, Liston V, Lowe N. A Phase I/II study of the use of Fluosol as an adjuvant to radiation therapy in the treatment of primary high-grade brain tumors. Int J Radiat Oncol Biol Phys 1990; 19:415–420.
31. Ninth International Conference on Brain Tumor Research and Therapy. Asilomar, California, 1991.
32. Goffman TE, Dachowski LJ, Bob H, Oldfield EH, et al. Long-term follow-up on National Cancer Institute Phase I/II study of glioblastoma multiforme treated with iododeoxyuridine and hyperfractionated irradiation. J Clin Oncol 1992; 10:264–268.
33. Johnson D, Thompson J, Corwin J et al. Prolongation of survival for high-grade malignant gliomas with adjuvant high-dose BCNU and autologous bone marrow transplantation. J Clin Oncol 1987; 5:783–789.
34. Hatanaka H. Experience of boron–neutron capture therapy for malignant brain tumors. Acta Neurochir 1988; 42:187–192.

The Role of Radiation Therapy in the Treatment of Brain Tumors in Children

Richard G. Evans

University of Kansas Medical Center, Kansas City, Kansas

I. INTRODUCTION

This chapter will be divided into four main sections: infratentorial primary tumors of childhood, supratentorial tumors, pediatric tumors seen in sellar and parasellar locations, and long-term side effects seen in children who have received radiation therapy.

It is appropriate for the reader to be aware of the questions raised by radiation oncologists when consulting on a pediatric patient with a brain tumor who has been referred to the department of radiation oncology. In the mind of the radiation oncologist, the roles of the neurosurgeon are manyfold and include, not necessarily in order of importance, the establishment of a tissue diagnosis, the relief of increased intracranial pressure and of the shift of any vital structures, the reestablishment of the circulation of the cerebrospinal fluid (CSF) if obstructed, the relief of any local compression of tumor on important functional regions and, finally, the extent to which the tumor has been resected. In reference to the degree of resection, I am reminded of a statement by Harvey Cushing, in 1931, which can be paraphrased as:

> When to take great risks; when to withdraw in the face of unexpected difficulties . . . takes surgical judgment, which is a matter of long experience and which can scarcely be transmitted by the written word.

Although the last quarter of a century has seen great advances in the overall prognosis of most pediatric patients with tumors, those seen in the prognosis of brain tumors, the second most common malignancy of childhood, have not been as substantial. However, the evolution of neurosurgical techniques and the better delineation of tumors through computed tomography (CT) and magnetic resonance imaging (MRI), along with the computed treatment planning of more restricted volumes for radiation therapy have allowed significant advances to be made in prognosis, particularly in patients with infratentorial tumors.

Table 1 illustrates the incidence of intracranial tumors in children and identifies the predominant tumors in children as being low-grade gliomas, medulloblastomas–ependymomas, and cranio-

Table 1 Incidence of Intracranial Tumors at All Ages and in Children Younger Than 15 Years of Age[a]

Tumor	All ages (%)	Children (%)
Glioma	45	70
Astrocytoma	15	30
Glioblastoma	15	5
Oligodendroglioma	8	1
Medulloblastoma	4	20
Ependymoma	4	10
Meningioma	15	1
Neurinoma	6	<0.5
Pituitary adenoma	6	1
Metastases	5–20	<0.5
Craniopharyngioma	3	10
Choroid plexus papilloma	0.5	3
Pinealoma	1	2
Hemangioma	3	1
Epidermoid	2	0.5
Dermoids–teratoma	<0.5	3
Sarcoma	2	4
Optic glioma	1	4

[a]The figures are approximate and are based on reports collected from the literature.
Source: Ref. 38.

pharyngiomas. Of note from Table 1 is that cerebral metastases from solid primary tumors outside the central nervous system (CNS) are rare in children. If cerebral metastases are not considered, then the information in Table 2 is more illustrative and describes the incidence of intracranial tumors as a function of decade of life. It also illustrates that medulloblastoma represents 21% of all cases in the first decade of life versus 10% in the second decade, whereas glioblastoma represents 1.3% of the tumors in the first decade, but rises to 7.4% by the second decade. Other differences of note between adult and childhood primary brain tumors are that the anatomical region most frequently involved in childhood brain tumors is the posterior fossa; brain stem gliomas are much more common in children; pituitary tumors are most uncommon in children, in whom the common tumor in this region is craniopharyngioma; and, finally, malignant CNS tumors of childhood, both malignant gliomas and medulloblastomas–ependymomas, have a tendency to metastasize by seeding throughout the subarachnoid space, whereas in adults this is an uncommon occurrence.

It is constructive when considering the differential diagnosis of tumors by location and age at onset of symptoms, to divide the tumors as described in Table 3, and we will first consider the common infratentorial tumors of childhood, followed by those in the supratentorial region, then craniopharyngiomas and optic pathway gliomas considering their sellar and parasellar locations, and finally, the long-term side effects of radiation.

For children younger than 3 years of age, special considerations need to be made of the long-term side effects of radiation on the developing brain, and therefore the approach to very young children will be considered separately at the end of this section.

Table 2 Frequency of Intracranial Tumors as a Function of Age Range

Histology	Age ranges						
	0–9	10–19	20–29	30–39	40–49	50–59	60–74
Astrocytoma	60	59	76	81	86	87	91
Low-grade	9.8	7.1	7.1	4.9	2.5	1.5	1.8
Astrocytoma	28.0	31.7	40.4	41.9	38.2	31.1	28.8
Anaplastic	18.5	10.9	11.0	12.8	9.6	8.3	11.0
Mixed	2.5	2.7	2.8	3.4	2.2	2.1	0.7
Glioblastoma	1.3	7.4	14.4	18.2	32.9	44.2	51.0
Medulloblastoma	21	10	5.5	2.3	1.0	0.1	0
Ependymoma[a]	8.7	2.7	4.3	1.8	0.8	1.3	0.5
Oligodendroglioma	1.1	4.0	5.0	6.4	6.2	3.6	1.6
Embryonal–teratoid[b]	1.0	1.3	0.3	0.3	0	0	0
Meningioma[c]	0.2	0.4	1.2	1.7	1.2	2.0	2.4

Data based on unpublished SEER program search 1978–1984.
[a]Includes differentiated and anaplastic ependymoma.
[b]Includes germinoma, mixed embryonal pinealomas, and malignant teratomas.
[c]Underestimate, since SEER does not include many "benign" tumors in its registry; these are probably malignant meningiomas.
Source: Ref. 39.

Table 3 Differential Diagnosis of Tumors by Location and Age at Onset of Symptoms

Location	Child	Adult
Supratentorial	Astrocytoma	Metastatic
	Glioblastoma	Glioblastoma
	Oligodendroglioma	Astrocytoma
	Sarcoma	Meningioma
	Neuroblastoma	Oligodendroglioma
	Mixed glioma	Mixed glioma
Infratentorial	Astrocytoma	Metastatic
	Medulloblastoma	Astrocytoma
	Ependymoma	Glioblastoma
	Brain stem glioma	Ependymoma
		Brain stem glioma
Sellar and parasellar	Craniopharyngioma	Pituitary
	Optic glioma	Meningioma
		Epidermoid
Base of skull		Neurinoma
		Meningioma
		Chordoma
		Carcinoma
		Dermoid, epidermoid

Source: Ref. 39.

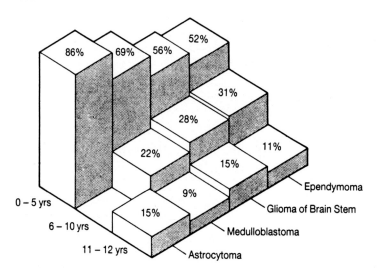

Figure 1 Age-related incidence of infratentorial primary tumors. (From Ref. 38)

II. INFRATENTORIAL PRIMARY TUMORS

The common tumors of childhood in this location are astrocytoma, medulloblastoma, brain stem glioma, and ependymoma; however, even within this location, there is a definite age-related incidence, as noted in Figure 1. This figure strikingly illustrates the high incidence of tumors of the posterior fossa in the first 5 years of life compared with ages 6 and older.

A. Astrocytoma

Approximately one-third of the tumors of the posterior fossa are low-grade cerebellar astrocytomas, and two-thirds of these are cystic. Most are amenable to complete resection as eloquently described by W. J. German in 1959, "Remember the lovely cysts with sparkling, yellow fluid and a nice mural nodule just begging to be taken from its nest." No adjuvant radiation therapy can be recommended in these situations, and cures approach 100%. However, when these low-grade tumors are incompletely removed, because of either extension into the brain stem or other factors and especially in those tumors in which poor prognostic histological features (high mitotic rate, necrosis, perivascular pseudorosettes; so-called glioma B tumors) are present, the prevailing data indicate that adjuvant radiation therapy is required. Doses of 50–55 Gy over 5–6 weeks, using 1.8-Gy fractions with 2-cm margins should be used. This combined modality approach should lead to 5-year survivals in the range of 80–90% and 10-year survivals of 70%, whereas, with subtotal resection alone, only one-third of the children remain recurrence-free. Although a few neurosurgeons prefer to perform repeat surgery on patients at the time of recurrence, it has been my experience and that of other authors that a high rate of malignant transformation occurs between operations and that the prognosis following radiation therapy after the second surgical removal is inferior to that when the radiation is employed following the first subtotal resection (1,2).

The prognosis of the very uncommon high-grade cerebellar astrocytomas is grim, and the treatment somewhat controversial, with some authors favoring craniospinal irradiation because of the propensity of these glioblastomas to seed the spinal tract. Even following aggressive doses of radiation to the whole brain and spinal column, with a boost to the posterior fossa, median survivals are less than 4 years.

B. Medulloblastoma

Medulloblastomas account for approximately one-third of the tumors in the posterior fossa, with at least a 2:1 male preponderance and with two-thirds of the cases arising in the first 5 years of life. Of all the pediatric brain tumors, the most dramatic improvements have been seen in this tumor, owing to multiple factors, including improved neurosurgical techniques, better staging of the tumor, and improved radiation therapy.

The use of shunts has led to spread of the tumor into the ventricular system and the CSF in up to 10% of cases (3). In evaluating possible dissemination to the spinal axis, although myelography remains the preferred technique, gadolinium-enhanced MRI of the spine has been effective in evaluating subarachnoid spread. As small pieces of this very fragile tumor can break off during surgery, most investigators have chosen to wait at least 2 weeks before obtaining CSF cytological samples and ordering an MRI of the spine to search for any tumor deposits that will require boost doses of radiation.

Very young patients appear to have a poorer prognosis, probably because of the higher incidence of advanced disease and the use of less intensive treatment. Generally speaking, the desmoplastic variant appears to have a better prognosis, whereas the primitive neuroectodermal tumors (PNET)–undifferentiated tumors appear to have a poorer prognosis. Patients who present with disease in the brain stem appear initially to do as well as other subgroups, but, by 7 years, more relapses are seen.

Most observers would agree that the role of surgery is key, but it has been difficult to study the importance of the degree of resection as an independent variable. There are conflicting data in the literature from both this country and Europe concerning differences in disease-free survival between children having a total versus a subtotal resection; however, it is my opinion that, provided no morbidity is likely to be encountered, a gross total resection should be attempted.

Although the operative staging system for medulloblastoma, as developed by Chang in 1969, has its limitations, it is the most widely accepted system in use and is shown in Table 4. Even if

Table 4 Operative Staging System for Cerebellar Medulloblastoma

Stage	Description
T1	Tumor less than 3 cm in diameter and limited to the classic midline position in the vermis, the roof of the fourth ventricle, and less frequently to the cerebellar hemispheres
T2	Tumor 3 cm or greater in diameter, further invading one adjacent structure or partially filling the fourth ventricle
T3A	Tumor further invading two adjacent structures or completely filling the fourth ventricle with extension into the aqueduct of Sylvius, foramen of Magendie, or foramen of Luschka, thus producing marked internal hydrocephalus
T3B	Tumor arising from the floor of the fourth ventricle or brain stem and filling the fourth ventricle
T4	Tumor spreading further through the aqueduct of Sylvius to involve the third ventricle or midbrain, or tumor extending to the upper cervical cord
M0	No evidence of gross subarachnoid or hematogenous metastasis
M1	Microscopic tumor cells found in cerebrospinal fluid
M2	Gross nodular seedings demonstrated in the cerebellar or cerebral subarachnoid space, or in the third or lateral ventricles
M3	Gross nodular seedings in spinal subarachnoid space
M4	Metastasis outside the cerebrospinal axis

Source: Ref. 40.

there are difficulties in comparing, retrospectively, data on staging before the modern era, it is clear that more recent studies indicate that the T3–T4 groups represent the majority and not the T1–T2s, as previously thought. In a recent study by the Children's Cancer Study Group (CCSG) of a very large number of patients (4), approximately one-third of the patients were in the T1–T2 grouping, two-thirds were in the T3–T4 grouping, 83% of the patients were M0, and the remaining 17% were in the M1–M3 group.

Medulloblastoma is a relatively radiosensitive tumor, and studies over the last two decades have shown a dose-dependence (5), with patients receiving more than 52 Gy to the posterior fossa, the most common site of relapse, having a significantly improved survival. The magnitude of the optimum dose to the craniospinal axis is somewhat more difficult to elucidate: the European studies recommend doses of approximately 30 Gy to the brain and spinal axis, and the studies in this country favor 36 Gy in 20 fractions of 1.8-Gy each and then delivery of a boost to the posterior fossa to bring this region up to 54 Gy. In patients with M1 (microscopic tumor cells in the CSF) and M2 (gross nodular seeding), somewhat higher doses, of about 40 Gy, are necessary and, in the presence of M3 disease (discrete areas of spinal subarachnoid seeding), these areas need to receive additional radiation up to spinal cord tolerance. In light of the observed growth failure (cranial irradiation) and effects on the sitting height of patients (spinal irradiation), a combined study by the Pediatric Oncology Group (POG) and the Children's Cancer Study Group (CCSG) randomized a large group of patients to either 36 or 24 Gy to the craniospinal axis. Unfortunately, this trial had to be aborted because of the observed failure of the lower dose to control neuraxis dissemination in a significant number of the early entrants into the study. This randomized study was attempted only in the so-called low-risk group of patients, that is, those with favorable factors including age younger than 5 years at presentation, T1–T2 tumors, and with gross total resection (6). Numerous studies in this country and in Europe have shown the efficacy of low-risk versus high-risk grouping; long-term survival in the low-risk group approaches 70%, in contrast with approximately half this value in the so-called high-risk group. In a recent study from Europe (7) reviewing the surgical aspects of medulloblastoma, it was noted that, although there was no difference in disease-free survival between children having total versus subtotal resections, disease-free survival was much poorer after biopsy or partial removal. More recent attempts to redefine the low-risk group have included postoperative MRI scans so that low-risk groups are considered in some studies as those with T1–T2 or T3a tumors with less than 1.5-cm^3 residual tumor. In a recent report from Germany of study HIT 88/89 (9th International Conference on Brain Tumor Research and Therapy, 1991), it was noted that 3 of 20 patients with MRI-documented residual tumor after surgery relapsed, despite the use of adequate radiation and multidrug chemotherapy.

The role of adjuvant chemotherapy is controversial, but it seems clear from numerous studies that multiagent chemotherapy cannot compensate for reduced doses of radiation to the spinal axis to prevent disease dissemination. However, adjuvant chemotherapy has been evaluated in two large prospectively randomized studies carried out in Europe and by the CCSG (4). Each trial included over 200 newly diagnosed and well-staged patients and each arm received identical radiotherapy. The overall disease-free survival at 5 years was 59% in the adjuvant chemotherapy arm versus 49% for the control arm in the CCSG study; in the European study (SIOP), the chemotherapy arm had a 55% disease-free survival versus 43% for the control, radiation therapy-only arm. In both studies, it was *only* in the groups with the T3–T4 lesions that a benefit from the chemotherapy was demonstrated. However, other studies (8) failed to reveal any benefit of adjuvant chemotherapy. Currently, the CCSG and POG are carrying out a prospective, randomized study, in the so-called high-risk medulloblastoma subset of patients, evaluating different adjunctive chemotherapy regimes in each of the two arms. It is hoped that the results of this study will delineate the role of chemotherapy in this poor-risk group; that is, for those with large primary tumors, dissemination at diagnosis or with residual tumor of greater than 1.5 cm^3 in the posterior fossa, as determined by MRI. The study may also reveal the prognosis of the subset of patients with initial brain stem involvement who have historically done poorly (9).

C. Ependymoma

Ependymomas represent fewer than 10% of tumors occurring in the posterior fossa, but make up two-thirds of the total group of CNS ependymomas. There is a male preponderance, as in medulloblastoma, with approximately half the patients in the infant to 5-year age group and another 30% in the 6- to 10-year age group. These tumors are similar to medulloblastoma in that they are relatively radiosensitive and tend to disseminate, but, whereas all medulloblastomas are considered to be high-grade, ependymomas are often divided into low- and high-grade groups. Svien and associates (10) have proposed a 4-grade system, while others have chosen to extend the Kernohan system and divide them into low-grade, that is grades I and II, and high-grade, III and IV. Although several authors have criticized the use of a grading system in ependymoma, the literature is replete with the importance of grade in determining prognosis of these patients. The POG has chosen to use the term *anaplastic* to describe the high-risk group. (There is a highly malignant variant called ependymoblastoma that tends to occur in the supratentorial region in infants and will be referred to in another section.) Svien's analysis is informative in that he noted that approximately 40% of supratentorial lesions were low-grade and 60% were high-grade, whereas, in the infratentorial region, the percentages were essentially reversed. It has been difficult to elucidate the influence of grade as an independent variable, for there are several other prognostic factors, such as location, size, and treatment, that need to be considered. However, most authorities agree that the more well-differentiated tumors need to be treated differently from the poorly differentiated ones and, even when the treatment is tailored to the degree of differentiation, a factor of up to 3 exists in terms of the length of survival in the two groups. Interestingly, supratentorial lesions tend to be larger and more anaplastic than the infratentorial lesions. In reviewing the literature, a range is found in the reported degree of seeding as a function of grade and location, but a reasonable estimate for infratentorial lesions appears to be 6% for the low-grade tumors compared with 16% in the high-grade or anaplastic tumors in terms of seeding the neuraxis. A review by Vanuytsel and Brada (11) has demonstrated that the degree of seeding is dependent on the control of the tumor in the posterior fossa, which may be more crucial than grade or location.

   In the approaches to treatment, the rationale for attempted gross total resection is similar to that described under medulloblastoma. In the series by Dohrmann and co-workers (12), it would appear that survival with surgery is, at best, only 20%, whereas a combined approach of surgery plus radiation results in long-term survivals in the 35–50% range (13).

   For doses of radiation and volumes to be used, the rationale is similar to that described under medulloblastoma. Again, local recurrence appears to be the main cause of failure, and doses of approximately 54 Gy are recommended to the posterior fossa. For the nonanaplastic tumors confined to the fourth ventricle, an ongoing study by POG, using posterior fossa radiation only, appears successful, in that seeding to the spinal axis (i.e., in the unirradiated region) was noted in an insignificant number of patients and, then, only in those with initial partial surgical removal of the tumor. Most authorities are in agreement that, for high-grade tumors, craniospinal irradiation is necessary, delivering approximately 40 Gy to the whole brain with a boost to the posterior fossa to 54 Gy and delivering 35 Gy to the spinal axis; this is being tested in a current single-arm POG protocol.

   The role of chemotherapy as adjuvant treatment for ependymomas is very unclear, and attempts so far using multiagent chemotherapy have met with limited success. A current CCSG study for patients with ependymoblastoma and malignant ependymoma is investigating any benefit from two different multiagent regimens used adjunctively with radiation.

D. Brain Stem Tumors

Tumors of the brain stem represent approximately 10% of all pediatric brain tumors, with 56% presenting in the first 5 years of life and a further 28% between the ages of 6 and 10. There appears to be no sex propensity, and almost all of the tumors are astrocytomas. Magnetic resonance imaging is probably superior to CT in the delineation of these tumors, but it is not possible to elucidate the grade from either MRI or CT. An increasing degree of tumor extension is seen with the higher-grade tumors. Albright and James (14) have suggested that tumors in the diencephalon, such as those in the thalamus or hypothalamus, be considered separately from those tumors in the brain stem proper (midbrain, pons, and medulla). However, others (15) have chosen to separate the tumors into thalamus–hypothalamus and midbrain versus those in the pons or medulla. The literature certainly supports this latter grouping, in that tumors of the midbrain and thalamic areas have a significantly better outcome than those in the pons and medulla; however, it is unclear whether this is attributable to tumor location per se or differences in the grade of the tumor in the different locations. Unlike the other major tumors of the posterior fossa—medulloblastoma and ependymoma—brain stem tumors show very little propensity for dissemination. The necessity of obtaining a tissue diagnosis in brain stem gliomas is rather controversial, although this is usually attempted if there is an exophytic component or if the patient is entered into a protocol for which the grade of the tumor could provide important research and prognostic information. In the larger series, of the proportion biopsied, 60% of the tumors have been low-grade or mixed gliomas, with the remainder being high-grade.

In almost all patients, failure is at the primary site. Studies in the last decade have sought to improve local control by using radiation doses higher than those used historically (50–55 Gy per day, as a single fraction) by applying twice-daily hyperfractionation techniques. In a series of dose-escalating studies carried out by several groups, including CCSG and POG, a trend toward increased survival has been noted when doses of 66 or 70.2 Gy have been used in a hyperfraction-ated manner, but an even higher dose of 75.6 Gy, also given twice a day, has failed to build on the marginal improvement noted with the other two doses. Location appears to be a definite prognostic factor in some reported series, with 5-year survivals reaching 50–60% in patients with tumors in the midbrain or thalamus, compared with only 15–25% for those with lesions in the pons and medulla. Whether this difference is due to the effects of tumor site, grade, or how diffusely the tumor has infiltrated, is unclear. Historically, mostly in patients who have not had biopsies, the use of a daily single-fraction technique and taking the brain stem to the radiation tolerance of 50–55 Gy, has yielded long-term survivals in the range of 25–40%, with most reports clustering near 30%. Attempts to improve these somewhat dismal survival rates following surgery and radiation by the addition of chemotherapy have as yet been ineffective. It is my opinion that the use of increased doses of radiation, despite being given in a hyperfractionated fashion to relatively large fields, has been taken to the limit of safety, without causing long-term effects, and that any future improvement will come from the use of prior or concomitant chemotherapy or possibly biological response modifiers, with the radiation given in a hyperfractionated fashion to avoid late effects.

E. Tumors in Children Younger Than Three Years of Age

The radiation tolerance of the brain begins to approach that of an adult by the time the child has reached the age of approximately 4 years. Most of the current studies being undertaken by the CCSG and POG have arbitrarily chosen the age of 3 in defining the term *baby* and, in fact, the first study carried out by the POG for children with tumors in this age group was affectionately known as "Baby POG." No group of patients in the field of oncology is as depressing, although challenging, to radiation oncologists, especially when attempting to explain to concerned parents that, if too low a dose is chosen, then the tumor is likely to recur, whereas, too aggressive doses of radiation can lead to complex developmental and mental problems in their surviving child. In 1986, Duffner et al. initiated within the POG a treatment, for children younger than the age of 3 with malignant brain tumors, in which cyclophosphamide (Cytoxan), vincristine, cisplatin, and etoposide (VP-16) were given in an attempt to delay radiation. This chemotherapy, in the absence of radiation, was associated with an overall 1-year progression-free survival of 47% in children diagnosed at 0–23 months and 42% diagnosed at 24–36 months. Most failures occurred within the first year, and a subset of patients in whom the chemotherapy failed were entered onto a sister POG protocol, using radiation, which resulted in an 80% survival at 1 year and 61% survival at 2 years. The major toxic effects of this chemotherapy included fevers, leukopenia, infection, high-frequency hearing loss, and two cases of second malignancies. In essence, therefore, the study demonstrated that postoperative chemotherapy could be used effectively to delay radiation in approximately half of the infants for at least 1 year, and that the progression-free survival of the children with ependymomas, medulloblastomas, and high-grade gliomas made up most of the favorably responding groups (16). Of concern to all oncologists who deal with pediatric patients with brain tumors are the long-term effects from 1 or 2 years of four cytotoxic chemotherapy agents given to these infants, although the long-term effects from radiation are well known.

III. SUPRATENTORIAL PRIMARY TUMORS

The major supratentorial brain tumors in the pediatric age group are shown in Table 5, and the major tumor types, low- and high-grade astrocytomas, ependymomas, oligodendrogliomas and mixed tumors, meningiomas, and pineal neoplasms, will be discussed in this section.

Whereas some observers follow the four-tier Kernohan system of grading astrocytic tumors others have found it more useful to subdivide these astrocytic neoplasms into three groups:

Table 5 Childhood Supratentorial Brain Tumors: Incidence, Age, and Sex Predilections

Neoplasm	Incidence[a]	Age predilection (median)	Sex ratio (M/F)
Low- and high-grade hemispheric astrocytomas	10–30%	9[c]	1
Ependymoma[b]	8–17%	2	1.3
Craniopharyngioma	5–16%	9	0.9
Pineal neoplasms	1–11%	1–16 yr	1.5–2
Meningioma	2–7%	7	4
Choroid plexus neoplasms	1–6%	<5 yr	Unclear
Optic pathway glioma	2–5%	5	0.7
Pituitary neoplasms	1–3%	17	3
Oligodendroglioma	1%	14	5
Primary cerebral neuroblastoma	1%	2–10 yr	1
Primary brain lymphoma	<1%	adults	1
Primitive neuroectodermal tumors	<1%	16 mo–10.8 yr	1–2

[a]As a percentage of all intracranial tumors of childhood
[b]Including infratentorial ependymomas
[c]Age varies as a function of histology
Source: Ref. 41.

well-differentiated astrocytoma, anaplastic astrocytoma, and glioblastoma multiforme (17). As in adult brain tumors, using both the Kernohan and Burger systems, there is a strong correlation of better prognosis with the low-grade tumors.

A. Low-Grade Supratentorial Astrocytomas

The group of low-grade and high-grade astrocytomas make up about one-quarter of the supratentorial tumors of childhood, with a slight preponderance of the high-grade variety. Most of the low-grade tumors are hypodense, as are approximately half of the anaplastic, whereas 80% of the glioblastoma multiforme cases are hyperdense. Of the anaplastic or intermediate-grade tumors, 80% show contrast enhancement, whereas almost all of the glioblastoma multiforme tumors show this feature. Peritumoral cerebral edema is very uncommon in the low-grade tumors, with approximately half of the anaplastic tumors showing edema and almost all glioblastoma multiforme demonstrating significant edema.

As in the cerebellar low-grade gliomas, surgery plays a major role and, in particular, is necessary for diagnosis and to relieve any mass effect or pressure. If total resection of these low-grade gliomas is possible, then there is no role for postoperative radiation therapy. In the subtotally resected cases, however, although there is a paucity of data for the pediatric age group, there appears to be a definite benefit from postoperative radiation, with the exception of pilocytic astrocytomas (18). In adult populations reported by Shaw et al. (19) and Leibel et al. (20), it was demonstrated that the addition of radiation improved the 5- and 10-year survivals from approximately 20 and 10% to 45 and 35% with the use of postoperative radiation. If one extrapolates from the adult literature and the little data available in the pediatric population, there appears to be a role for postoperative radiation in the subtotally resected group. Although this has never been demonstrated in a study setting, there are several current protocols being carried out by POG, the Radiation Therapy Oncology Group (RTOG), and the Brain Tumor Cooperative Group (BTCG). These groups are studying, in a randomized fashion, the benefit of 54 Gy within 3 weeks of subtotal resection, versus delivering the radiation at the time of progression. In my opinion, the danger of delaying radiation treatment, despite careful follow-up with CT and MRI studies, is that dedifferentiation of the tumor to a higher grade is a real possibility, as is the development of a large tumor at recurrence, requiring a second operation. Muller and co-workers (21), have reported that only 14% of the initial grade I astrocytomas were unchanged at recurrence, over half had progressed to grade II, and almost a third had progressed to glioblastoma multiforme. It has been my experience as well as that of others that patients definitely have a poorer prognosis when irradiated at the time of recurrence, compared with those treated after the first surgery.

There are several current randomized studies being carried out (in adults) evaluating the role of radiotherapy in adults with low-grade supratentorial tumors. In this country the Mayo North Central Cancer Study Group, together with RTOG and ECOG, are evaluating in all subtotally resected patients, 50.4 Gy versus 64.8 Gy and the European Organization for Research and Treatment of Cancer (EORTC) is carrying out a similar study randomizing patients between 45 and 59.4 Gy to a localized volume. Typically, radiation fields in this group of tumors would include a 2-cm margin around the tumor volume, as defined by the CT scan, or a 1-cm margin around the region of the high T2 signal on the MRI scan. The results of these studies are eagerly awaited by all those involved in brain tumor therapy.

B. High-Grade Astrocytomas

Anaplastic astrocytoma and glioblastoma occur less frequently in children than in adults and appear to have a somewhat better prognosis in children. Although several studies have demonstrated an improved survival, with an increased degree of resection, it is unclear whether this advantage is due to selection of patients; however, from the radiotherapy standpoint, it is more desirable to attempt to control a smaller bulk of tumor than a larger one.

There is a definite benefit of postoperative radiation therapy, particularly in patients with glioblastoma multiforme, with a range of reported 5-year survivals from as low as 10% to a high of 20% at 5 years. The question of whether these high-grade tumors are "local" is debatable, and the work of Kelly et al. at Mayo Clinic showing tumor cells as far out as 6 cm from the enhancing ring gives some indication of the infiltrating nature of these high-grade tumors. Historically, these patients were treated with whole-brain irradiation, but almost all current protocols are using more localized radiation therapy with a 2- to 3-cm margin around the T2 image or the CT ring plus edema. Certainly, more localized radiation treatment fields are much less morbid in children than whole-brain treatment. Although routine craniospinal radiotherapy is never indicated in the absence of proven tumor dissemination, a recent report by Kellie et al. (22) which showed radiographic or cytologic evidence of neuraxis dissemination in one-third of 29 children with glioblastoma at diagnosis, is especially thought-provoking. Several hundred adult patients with high-grade tumors have been treated with 60 Gy to the whole brain, which I do not currently recommend and, in view of the inability to show an improvement in adults for doses over 55 Gy to even localized fields, this would be the maximum I would recommend in children. Twice-a-day fractionation has been evaluated extensively by the BTSG and RTOG and, although this has not been evaluated in children, there appears to be no significant benefit in adults when compared with a conventional one-fraction-daily regimen.

The nitrosoureas appear to have some marginal efficacy when used adjuvantly in adults with high-grade tumors (see Chap. 28). In children, a prospective randomized trial carried out by the CCSG in high-grade tumors using 52 Gy in only one arm and chemotherapy during and following the same radiation in the other arm, demonstrated that the median disease-free survival was 9 months in the radiotherapy arm versus 25 months in the combined arm. This apparent benefit of chemotherapy in children is being further explored by the CCSG, using 54 Gy in both arms of the study and comparing two aggressive chemotherapy regimens added to the radiation to determine any possible advantage of adding chemotherapy to surgery plus radiation in high-grade supratentorial gliomas of childhood.

C. Ependymomas

Approximately 40% of childhood ependymomas occur above the tentorium, and we have already discussed the treatment of the remaining 60% that occur below the tentorium. Most series report that they represent 10–15% of the whole supratentorial group of tumors. We have discussed tumor grade previously and the observation that many authors now favor the use of the term anaplastic to describe the higher grade tumors. However, the older literature is replete with data reporting a very definite association of prognosis with grade, with the low-grade tumors having 5-year survivals of almost 70%, whereas the anaplastic variety show approximately half of this survival. Patients need to be evaluated in a fashion similar to those with medulloblastoma in terms of dissemination to the neuraxis. Although the degree of seeding does not approach that of the infratentorial ependymomas, and this problem is observed rarely in supratentorial low-grade tumors, seeding does occur in the anaplastic variety in as many as 12% of the cases, although the frequency appears to be related to the control of the primary tumor (11).

As in medulloblastoma, the data support the goal of complete resection, provided it is not a morbid procedure. The literature is somewhat controversial on the need for local, versus whole-brain, versus craniospinal radiotherapy, and recommendations depend on grade and likelihood of seeding the neuraxis. I interpret the data in the literature as supporting the use of whole-brain irradiation to approximately 40 Gy, with a boost of an additional 14 Gy to the tumor bed for the low-grade ependymomas, but in the anaplastic type, in view of the propensity for seeding, craniospinal irradiation is definitely indicated, taking the whole brain and the boost to the doses noted earlier, and adding 30–35 Gy to the spinal axis to S3 and then boosting any localized deposits to cord tolerance.

D. Oligodendrogliomas and Mixed Tumors

Oligodendrogliomas occur far more commonly in adults, and they represent only 1–5% of pediatric tumors in the supratentorial region. They are often mixed, usually with elements of high-grade astrocytoma. Over two-thirds of these tumors are hyperdense, but less than one-half enhance with contrast. Calcification is noted in approximately 70% of the cases. In almost all series, in which a significant number of children have been included, there appears to be a significant benefit of postoperative radiation therapy for subtotally resected patients. This group of tumors has been included in the EORTC study, in which randomization is between two different doses of radiation. I favor immediate postoperative radiation therapy to a localized field, with small margins to a minimum of 54 Gy, and caution against withholding radiation until the time of progression. In the review by Muller et al. (23), of 52 cases of oligodendroglioma that subsequently recurred, they noted that of 23 tumors initially grade I, 6 remained unchanged in grade, 15 were grade II, and 2 had converted to glioblastoma multiforme at the time of recurrence. Moreover, of the 29 initially grade II, 6 had converted to glioblastoma multiforme at the time of progression. Although "sampling error" at the time of initial resection needs to be considered, it is my belief that the foregoing study and others provides sufficient evidence for dedifferentiation to a higher grade in a significant proportion of cases, and my recommendation is immediate radiation treatment.

E. Meningiomas

The meningioma group of tumors is far less common in the pediatric age group and represents only about 5% of the total, with most being supratentorial, and an approximate 1:1 boy/girl ratio. In some series, 20% of the cases have associated neurofibromatosis. There is an increased incidence of meningioma following radiotherapy for a tinea capitas infection, at least in the studies from Israel; however, those from the United States fail to show such an association. In the meningiomas of childhood, the lateral ventricles seem to be a favored site. If the meningioma occurs in the posterior fossa, there is little or no associated edema, whereas in the supratentorial location, about one-half of the patients show moderate edema. Although historically, recurrences were thought to occur in only approximately 15% of the cases following surgical resection, with the advent of MRI and its associated sensitivity in detecting residual disease, this frequency is likely to be much higher in more recent series.

Complete resection is the initial goal of treatment, and in those children who have undergone an incomplete resection, there are only a few reported cases of long-term disease-free survival. Wara et al. (24), in a series of mostly adult patients, showed a 74% recurrence rate with subtotal resection when no postoperative radiation was given, compared with 29% when postoperative radiation was used adjuvantly. In addition, Taylor et al. (25) reports figures of 82% 10-year survival when radiation is added following subtotal excision, but only 18% with surgery alone. If one were to extrapolate these data to the pediatric situation, it would seem very appropriate to administer postoperative radiation therapy in every situation for which only a subtotal resection was obtained. Possibly in the young child under 3 years of age and with careful follow-up with CT or MRI, the radiation could be delayed. In the small group of patients with so-called malignant meningioma, postoperative radiation is definitely indicated. After review of the literature, I would recommend doses of approximately 54 Gy in 6 weeks to the tumor bed plus a 2-cm margin.

Although chemotherapy has not been explored in children with meningiomas, there are scattered reports in the adult population of the benefit of hormonal manipulation.

F. Tumors of the Pineal Region

The difficulty of taking biopsies of the pineal region, at least for the last decade or so, has given rise to some confusion concerning the distribution of tumors in this region. The data in Table 6 describe the frequency of occurrence of different types in histologically verified cases. Jennings et al. (26), from a series of almost 400 cases of pathologically verified germ cell tumors in this region, noted that 65% of germ cell tumors were germinomas, 18% teratomas, 5% embryonal carcinomas, 7% endodermal sinus tumors, and 5% choriocarcinomas. Additionally, approximately half of the germinomas arose in the suprasellar region and about one-third in the pineal, whereas 65% of the nongerminoma germ cell tumors arose in the pineal region, versus only 18% in the suprasellar area. Historically, in the belief that two-thirds of the pineal tumors were germinomas, a radiosensitive tumor, a typical approach was to use a small dose of radiation to the tumor and, if the response was a marked size reduction as judged by CT, then the patient either went on to whole-brain irradiation or craniospinal irradiation. If the so-called test dose showed no response on CT, then it was assumed that the patient had a nongerminoma, and local radiation therapy only was delivered. However, in the last 15 years, with the advent of tumor markers, improved CT, and the introduction of MRI, the management of tumors in the pineal region has been modified. In addition, neurosurgeons have been more successful in obtaining a tissue diagnosis, and attempts to obtain a biopsy are encouraged. The CSF should always be examined for cytological changes as well as for tumor markers; alpha-fetoprotein (AFP) and human chorionic gonadotropin (hCG). If significant amounts of either of these markers are present, that would strongly suggest a nongerminoma. In view of the intimate association of the pineal with the posterior part of the third ventricle and, therefore, the risks of spinal dissemination of pineal neoplasms, an MRI of the spine should always be obtained. Some authors report the added benefit of obtaining both serum and CSF values of AFP and hCG. If results of the CSF examination are positive or there has been spillage at the time of surgery, then craniospinal irradiation is usually recommended for patients with germi-

Table 6 Histologically Verified Pineal Region Tumors

	Sano and Matsutani	Lapras et al.	Bruce and Allen
Germ-cell tumors	77	20	10
Germinoma	58	10	2
Nongerminoma	19	10	8
Pineal-cell tumors	6	25	11
Pinocytoma		9	4
Pineoblastoma	6	16	7
Ependymoma	8	4	
Glioma	12	21	8
Other	3	16	1
Total	106	86	30

Source: Ref. 41.

noma, and some authors have proposed using chemotherapy before the radiation is initiated. If the CSF results are negative for cytological abnormalities and the MRI of the spine is also normal, then more local fields can be considered. I prefer whole-brain treatment, especially as there is little additional morbidity at the low doses required. Doses below 50 Gy to the primary are probably sufficient, but in the cases of dissemination to the spinal axis, 30 Gy should be delivered to this region, with additional boosts to control any documented spinal implants. Five-year survivals for pure germinoma, independent of site, should exceed 60% with the use of appropriate radiation fields and doses.

The nongerminoma germ cell tumors of this region (i.e., embryonal cell carcinomas, endodermal sinus tumors, and choriocarcinomas) are more aggressive tumors and 5-year survivals can be achieved only in about a quarter of the patients. Depending on the CSF and MRI findings, most authorities would recommend craniospinal irradiation using the doses noted earlier and consideration given to adjuvant chemotherapy.

IV. SELLAR AND PARASELLAR PRIMARY TUMORS OF CHILDHOOD

The two main tumors in this region are craniopharyngiomas, representing about 10% of all childhood CNS neoplasms, and optic pathway gliomas that represent 3–5%. Craniopharyngiomas are approximately twice as common in children as in adults, and over 90% of optic pathway tumors occur in the first two decades of life.

A. Craniopharyngiomas

Calcification is seen on skull x-ray films in almost all children with craniopharyngiomas, in contrast with approximately half of the adult group. In addition, radiographic findings include erosion of the dorum sellae and anterior clinoids and, on CT, approximately three-quarters of the lesions show contrast enhancement in children, compared with only a third in adults.

Many neurosurgeons favor discussing the management of these tumors in two groups, the predominantly solid and the predominantly cystic, and this approach will be taken here.

1. Predominantly Solid Craniopharyngioma

Most series report that total resection is attainable in only 50–60% of the children, as judged by a postoperative CT scan obtained 2–3 weeks following surgery. Pang (27) has reviewed all of the large series in the literature and reported that the recurrence rate following subtotal resection, without postoperative radiation therapy, is close to 75%, with most recurrences occurring within 3 years after surgery. The 10-year survival was 85% if total excision was achieved, but only 25% following subtotal resection only. In view of the morbidity associated with total resection, many neurosurgeons have changed to a policy of a planned subtotal resection, followed by postoperative radiation based on excellent early studies of Bloom et al. (28) and Kramer et al. (29). In a more recent series (30), 10-year survivals of 76% were achieved with planned postoperative radiation, versus 27% without radiation. By using multiple-field techniques to avoid overdosing normal structures lateral to the tumor and with relatively small fields of about 6 × 6 cm, doses in the range of 50–55 Gy appear adequate delivered over 6–7 weeks. The recent advent of stereotactic irradiation, either using the "gamma knife" or a modified linear accelerator, shows promise in controlling small solid tumors or recurrences following tumor aspiration.

2. Predominantly Cystic Tumors

Approximately 35% of craniopharyngiomas are predominantly cystic and there appears to be no clear indication in the literature whether the cystic tumors have a better prognosis than the solid types. It is well known to neurosurgeons that total excision is difficult to achieve, especially if the cyst wall is thin or the tumor has insinuated itself into the substance of the frontal and temporal lobes. There are proponents of cyst aspiration, followed by external beam irradiation, but this approach, or a simple tumor biopsy followed by radiation, is not recommended for children because of the high recurrence rate (31). The use of intracystic radioactive nuclides has found favor in some institutions, but it appears that case selection is extremely important. Doses of about 300–400 Gy have been delivered to the inner surface of the cyst, followed by decompression approximately 2 weeks later when the radionuclide has decayed. However, this method is unsuitable when the cyst wall is relatively thick or the cyst is multiloculated, as there are dosimetric problems with delivering sufficient doses of radiation through the thickness of the cyst wall and with obtaining uniform distribution of radionuclide through the whole tumor.

B.   Optic Pathway Gliomas

The optic pathway group of tumors of childhood represents fewer than 5% of the total cases of intracranial CNS tumors and has a very strong association with neurofibromatosis. In most recent series, approximately 20% of the children with visual pathway gliomas had associated neurofibromatosis, but more importantly from a diagnostic standpoint, neurofibromatosis is present in up to 50% of children with intraorbital gliomas. The recent introduction of screening of family members of patients with neurofibromatosis, using CT, will possibly lead to earlier diagnosis in asymptomatic patients. Typically however, delays of over 6 months are still commonly reported between the onset of symptoms and obtaining a diagnosis. Because of the lack of obscuration by surrounding bone, MRI imaging with the use of surface coils is the optimum study and preferable to CT, especially if there is infiltration of the chiasm. The advent of these exquisite diagnostic techniques has led most neurosurgeons to believe that surgical confirmation is probably unnecessary, especially if the child is known to have neurofibromatosis.

There appears to be a lack of agreement in the literature concerning the optimum management of this group of tumors. Authorities in the field have found it productive to discuss patients with isolated unilateral or bilateral optic nerve gliomas versus those in whom the tumor is confined to the chiasm or optic nerves. The wisdom, as gleaned from the literature, is that the optimum treatment for optic nerve tumors without chiasm extension, especially if there is visual loss, is surgical resection, with radiation or chemotherapy reserved for recurrent cases. If, however, the tumor is unresectable and there appears to be progression of the disease, then radiation therapy is the preferred treatment. Doses of close to 45–50 Gy appear to be appropriate from the reported studies of small groups of patients treated in this manner. If the glioma is limited to the optic nerve, then survival in excess of 90% can be expected if surgical removal is possible. It is the opinion of this observer that chiasmal tumors can be carefully followed, but on the first indication of progression, which eventually occurs in up to three-quarters of the patients, radiation therapy is indicated. With this regime survival rates in the range of 60–100% can be expected (32, 33). It is important to initiate radiation therapy as soon as possible when there are any signs of vision loss and, although vision can be improved with radiation in over a quarter of the patients, the damage to the nerve could be irreversible if the radiation is not started immediately. Unfortunately, as the median age at diagnosis of children with these visual pathway gliomas is younger than 5 years, and as many as a quarter of the patients are younger than 2 years, the radiation could result in growth failure as well as other endocrine deficits. In view of the potential risks of radiation, especially in those with large lesions, and young age, chemotherapy has been explored as a first attempt to stabilize or cause regression of the tumor, and in one small series, this has been possible in 80% of the patients. Even a delay of less than 1 year could be beneficial to allow further maturation of the child's nervous system and subsequent decreased sensitivity to radiation.

V. LONG-TERM SIDE EFFECTS

The approach to tumors in children less than 3 years of age has been discussed in Sec. I. E., and this section will discuss, in general terms, the known long-term side effects of children treated with radiation. Data on the long-term consequences of multiple-agent chemotherapy in children with brain tumors are currently unknown, as this approach has been fairly recent.

The last two decades have seen significant improvements in survival in many patients with pediatric brain tumors and, as children survive longer, the consequences of their radiation therapy to the brain and spinal cord are more likely to be revealed. Potential effects on both the physical and mental development of the child should be explored in the setting of a long-term follow-up clinic.

The degree and incidence of late effects in children treated for brain tumors with radiation is a complicated and multifactorial subject. As we have noted previously, the younger the child at the time of treatment, the more susceptible he or she is to delayed effects. It is also clear that there is a dose–response effect and also a fraction-size response, in that higher doses of radiation are likely to lead to more severe side effects, as are large fractions of radiation. The pediatric oncology community is constantly trying to determine the lowest effective radiation doses, although the study mentioned earlier in medulloblastoma patients in which an attempt was made to reduce the radiation dose to the brain and spinal cord met with failure. Although the worst side effect is tumor recurrence, studies like this deserve further exploration. My experience over the last 15 or so years is that most long-term survivors appeared to lead lives that are productive and of good quality, compared with their unirradiated counterparts. Although radiation oncologists need to assume responsibility for many of the late-term consequences, they cannot bear the sole burden, as it is impossible to exclude the influence of the tumor itself and the surgical manipulations that preceded the initiation of the radiation treatment. Whatever the etiology, the significant physical and neuropsychological problems in children treated for primary brain tumors with radiation are readily apparent. Many of the studies on long-term neuropsychological and intellectual deficits suffer from the lack of baseline information that predated the initiation of the radiation therapy. More recent studies have tried to remedy this problem by testing children before beginning radiation.

Relative to radiation necrosis of the *brain*, Burger et al. (34), reporting on patients treated with 50–60 Gy for intracranial gliomas, noted that the patients who developed radiation necrosis had not received dexamethasone (Decadron) during radiotherapy. Although the effect of edema surrounding the tumor is difficult to assess, it is possible that the use of corticosteroid therapy during radiation may decrease edema and protect against radiation necrosis. Provided the guidelines for craniospinal axis irradiation are followed in cases of medulloblastoma, ependymoma, or other, it is a very rare event to see radiation necrosis of the *spinal cord*. However, it is impossible to avoid including the *thyroid gland* during the spinal part of craniospinal irradiation, and the portion of the thyroid in the exiting beam may receive up to 50% of the dose delivered to the spine. However, as in patients treated for Hodgkin's disease in whom the effect is more common because of the higher dose used, the effect is chemical (increased thyroid-stimulating hormone; TSH), rather than clinical. Hypothyroidism can be easily corrected with small doses of daily thyroid replacement. When treating tumors that are situated near the *pituitary gland*, this often has to be included in the field of irradiation, and the resultant growth hormone deficiency has been well documented. Slowed growth and development can at least be partially reversed by the use of supplemental growth hormone initiated 2 years following completion of all treatment. Interestingly, growth hormone production appears to be the function of the pituitary region that is most sensitive to radiation, and decreased production is likely to result when doses above 20 Gy are delivered to this gland. There is clearly a combined effect on spinal bone growth in patients treated with cranio-spinal irradiation, for not only is the pituitary in the field (cranial portion), but also the bones themselves (spinal field). Changes in the *vertebral bodies*, although dependent on the age of the child at the time of irradiation, are usually severe when doses greater than 20–25 Gy are used. There is a definite dissociation between standing and sitting heights following spinal irradiation, and there appears to be some compensatory mechanism as the full-standing height is less affected than sitting height.

Although all efforts to avoid exposing the *eyes* during the whole-brain portion of craniospinal irradiation are taken, there is a danger of underdosing, and recurrences have been noted particularly in medulloblastoma patients in the region of the cribriform plate when the lateral eye blocks have shielded the inferior portion of the anterior cranial fossa and resulted in a suboptimum dose to this region. The *lens* is the most radiosensitive structure in the eye, and readers are referred to a chapter by this author on the effects of radiation on the lens, lacrimal gland, retina, and other eye structures, in the text, *Tumors of the Eye and Orbit* edited by Sagerman et al. (35).

Although much of our information on the long-term *neuropsychological* and intellectual side effects has come from studies in patients with acute lymphoblastic leukemia treated with whole-brain irradiation, there is sufficient data for patients with brain tumors to conclude that the more complex functions of the brain, such as mathematical manipulations, perceptual analysis, and abstract reasoning are the functions most commonly affected, particularly if the child was younger than 3 years old at time of treatment and in those who needed larger doses of radiation to control their tumors. Interestingly, Danoff et al. (36) found no correlation between the magnitude of the irradiated brain volume or the tumor type and the incidence of lowered IQ, although he confirms that children younger than 3 are the most likely to have severe problems. In the study by Hirsch et al. (37), comparing late effects in survivors who received surgical resection only for cerebellar astrocytoma or surgery plus craniospinal irradiation in patients treated for medulloblastoma, the latter group demonstrated a significantly higher incidence of lowered IQ scores. Although there is no doubt that significant intellectual and neuropsychological problems can be seen in children who have received brain irradiation, the radiation treatment per se is difficult to study as an independent factor. We noted earlier that a volume response has not been determined and, in addition, other effects caused by the tumor itself, surgical manipulation, damage to the hypothalamus, and blood flow changes, must be considered as contributing causes. The lowering of the radiation dose to the whole brain in leukemia patients, following the introduction of superior chemotherapy, had a very positive effect in terms of intellectual function, which could serve as a model in brain tumor patients. So far this approach has been disappointing, as several studies have shown that lowered doses to the spinal axis cannot be compensated for by the addition of chemotherapy.

Relative to the incidence of *second primary* tumors in patients undergoing, we have already noted the increased incidence in meningiomas from the treatment of tinea capitis infection in the studies reported from Israel. It is also well documented that certain groups of patients are genetically predisposed to developing multiple tumors, such as those with the nevoid basal cell carcinoma syndrome, neurofibromatosis, and retinoblastoma. It is entirely possible that radiation therapy potentiates, but is not necessarily the cause of, the development of second tumors in a genetically susceptible population of patients. The high incidence of osteosarcoma in retinoblastoma patients has been well documented, and note has been made that a significant proportion of the second malignancies are seen *outside* the radiation fields. Moreover, in those patients who were treated with radiation to the orbit for retinoblastoma, the high incidence of *infield* osteogenic sarcomas observed were in the era where low-voltage radiation was used and with which doses to the bone have been estimated to be at least three times greater than those that would be delivered to the bone with modern megavoltage radiotherapy equipment. There is no doubt that radiation certainly has *oncogenic potential*, as noted in the forgoing, in patients treated for tinea capitis and retinoblastoma, and we should add to this list, children irradiated for thymic enlargement who were placed at an increased risk of developing tumors within the thyroid gland. With the increasing use of multiple-agent chemotherapy, in addition to radiation, in the treatment of several groups of pediatriac brain tumor patients it is relevant that the nitrosoureas themselves may be leukemogenic. In a population of almost 300 patients followed by the Brain Tumor Study Group, a 25-fold increase in acute nonlymphocytic leukemia was noted in the survivors who had received multiple chemotherapeutic agents that included the nitrosoureas, together with procarbazine and other drugs.

With the more recent advent of preradiation chemotherapy in children younger than 3 years of age and the increasing use of combined modality treatment in children with brain tumors, it is essential that these patients be seen on a regular basis at a long-term follow-up clinic, not only for evaluation of any neuropsychological and endocrine problems, but also to detect any second malignancies at an early stage so that appropriate treatment can be initiated immediately.

REFERENCES

1. Griffin TW, Beaufait D, Blasko JC. Cystic cerebellar astrocytomas in childhood. Cancer 1979; 44:276–280.
2. Leibel SA, Sheline GE, Wara WM, Boldrey EB, Nielsen SL. The role of radiation therapy in the treatment of astrocytomas. Cancer 1975; 35:1551–1557.
3. Hoffman HJ, Hendricks EB, Humphreys RP. Metastases via ventricular–peritoneal shunt in patients with medulloblastoma. J Neurosurg 1976; 44:562.
4. Allen JC, Bloom J, Ertel I, Evans A, Hammond D, Jones H, Levin V, Jenkin D, Sposto R, Wara W. Brain tumors in children: current cooperation and institutional chemotherapy trials in newly diagnosed and recurrent disease. Semin Oncol 1986; 13:110–122.
5. Berry MP, Jenkin RDT, Keen CW, Nair BD, Simpson WJ. Radiation treatment for medulloblastoma: a 21 years review. J Neurosurg 1981; 55:43–51.
6. Brand WN, Schneider PA, Tokars RP. Long term results of a pilot study of low dose craniospinal irradiation for cerebellar medulloblastoma. Int J Radiat Oncol Biol Phys 1987; 13:1641–1645.
7. Albright AL. Surgical aspects of medulloblastoma. In: Zeltzer PM, Pochedly YC, eds. Medulloblastomas in children: new concepts in tumor biology diagnosis and treatment. New York: Praeger Publishers, 1986:155–163.
8. Deutsch M. Medulloblastoma: staging and treatment outcome. Int J Radiat Oncol Biol Phys 1988; 14:1103–1107.
9. Bloom HJG, Wallace ENK, Henk JM. The treatment and prognosis of medulloblastoma in children: a study of 82 verified cases. Am J Roentgenol Radium Ther Nucl Med 1969; 105:43–62.
10. Svien HJ, Mabon RF, Kernohan JW. Ependymomas of the brain: pathologic aspects. Neurology 1953; 3:1–15.
11. Vanuytsel L, Brada M. The role of prophylactic spinal irradiation in localized intracranial ependymoma. Int J Radiat Oncol Biol Phys 1991; 21:825–830.
12. Dohrmann GJ, Farwell JR, Flannery JT. Ependymomas and ependymoblastomas in children. J Neurosurg 1976; 45:273–283.
13. Shaw E, Evans RG, Scheithauer BW, Ilstrup DM, Earle JD. Radiotherapeutic management of pediatric and adult intracranial ependymomas. Int J Radiat Oncol Biol Phys 1987; 13:1457–1462.
14. Albright AL, James HE. Neurosurgical staging of mid-line intra-axial (nuclear) tumor. Cancer 1985; 56:1786–1788.
15. Grigsby DW, Thomas PRM. Irradiation of primary thalamic brain tumors in a pediatric population: A 33-year experience. Radiation Oncology Center scientific report 1985–1986. St. Louis: Mallinckrodt Institute of Radiology, 1987:45–47.
16. Duffner P, Horowitz M, Krischer J, Kun L, Cohen M, Friedman H, Sanford A, Burger P, Freeman C, James H, the Brain Tumor Committee of POG. Postoperative chemotherapy and delayed radiation therapy in infants with brain tumors: a Pediatric Oncology Group study. Presented at ninth international conference on brain tumor research and therapy, October 15–18, 1991, Asilomar, California.

17. Burger PC, Vogel FS. Surgical pathology of the central nervous system and its coverings. 2nd ed. New York: John Wiley & Sons, 1982.
18. Bloom HJG. Intracranial tumors: response and resistance to therapeutic endeavors, 1970–1980. Int J Radiat Oncol Biol Phys 1982; 8:1083–1113.
19. Shaw EG, Scheithauer BW, Gilbertson DT, Nichols DA, Laws ER, Earle JD, Dumas-Duport C, O'Fallon JR, Dinapoli RP. Post-operative radiotherapy of supratentorial low grade gliomas. Int J Radiat Oncol Biol Phys 1989; 16:663–668.
20. Leibel SA, Sheline GE, Wara WM, Boldrey EB, Nielson SL. The role of radiation therapy in the treatment of astrocytomas. Cancer 1975; 35:1551–1557.
21. Muller W, Afra D, Schroder R. Supratentorial recurrences of gliomas: morphological studies in relation to time intervals with astrocytomas. Acta Neurochir 1977; 37:75–91.
22. Kellie SJ, Kovnar EH, Kun LE, Horowitz ME, Heideman RL, Douglass EC, Langston JW, Sanford RA, Jenkins JJ, Fairclough DL, Ogle L. Neuraxis dissemination in pediatric brain tumors: response to preirradiation chemotherapy. Cancer 1992; 69:1061–1066.
23. Muller W, Afra D, Schroder R. Supratentorial recurrences of gliomas: morphological studies in relation to time intervals with oligodendrogliomas. Acta Neurochir 1977; 39:15–25.
24. Wara WM, Sheline GE, Newman H, Townsend JJ, Boldrey EB. Radiation therapy of meningiomas. Am J Roentgenol 1975; 123:453–458.
25. Taylor BW, Marcus RB, Friedman WA, Bollinger WE, Million RR. The meningioma controversy: postoperative radiation therapy. Int J Radiat Oncol Phys 1988; 15:299–304.
26. Jennings MT, Gelman R, Hochberg F. Intra-cranial germ cell tumors: natural history and pathogenesis. J Neurosurg 1985; 63:155–167.
27. Pang D. Craniopharyngiomas. In: Deutsch M, ed. Management of childhood brain tumors. Boston: Kluwer Academic Publishers, 1991:285–307.
28. Bloom HJG. Recent concepts in the conservative treatment of intracranial tumors in children. Acta Neurochir 1979; 50:103–116.
29. Kramer S, McKissock W, Concannon JP. Craniopharyngiomas, treatment by combined surgery and radiation therapy. J Neurosurg 1969; 18:217–226.
30. Manaka S, Teramoto A, Takakura K. The efficacy of radiotherapy for craniopharyngiomas. J Neurosurg 1985; 62:648–656.
31. Shapiro K, Till K, Grant N. Craniopharyngioma in childhood. J Neurosurg 1979; 50:617–623.
32. Flickinger JD, Torres C, Deutsch M. Management of low grade gliomas of the optic nerve and chiasm. Cancer 1988; 61:635–642.
33. Horwich A, Bloom HJG. Optic gliomas: radiation therapy and prognosis. Int J Radiat Oncol Biol Phys 1985; 11:1067–1079.
34. Burger PC, Mahaley MS, Dudka L, Vogel FS. The morphologic effects of radiation administered therapeutically for intracranial gliomas: A postmortem study of 25 cases. Cancer 1979; 44:1256–1272.
35. Evans RG. Radiotherapy of orbital lymphomas. In: Sagerman R, ed. Tumors of the eye and orbit. Basel: Springer-Verlag (in press).
36. Danoff BF, Cowchock S, Marquette C, Mulgrew L, Kramer S. Assessment of the long term effects of primary radiation therapy for brain tumors in children. Cancer 1982; 49:1580–1586.
37. Hirsch JF, Renier D, Czernichow P. Medulloblastoma in childhood, survival and functional results. Acta Neurochir 1979; 48:1–15.
38. Thomas DGT. eds Neuro-oncology: primary malignant brain tumors. Baltimore: Johns Hopkins University Press, 1990:165–167.
39. DeVita et al., eds. Cancer: principles and practice of oncology. vol. 2. Philadelphia: JB Lippincott, 1990: 1559, 1562.
40. Deutsch M, ed. Management of childhood brain tumors. Boston: Kluwer Academic Publishers, 1991:414.
41. Halperin et al, eds. Pediatric radiation oncology. New York: Raven Press, 1989:40, 384.

25

Interstitial Radiation Therapy of Brain Tumors

Penny K. Sneed and Philip H. Gutin
University of California, School of Medicine,
San Francisco, California

I. INTRODUCTION

There is a strong rationale for using interstitial radiotherapy in the treatment of high-grade gliomas. First, gliomas tend to remain localized (1–3). Second, radiation therapy is the single most effective modality in the treatment of malignant gliomas. This was demonstrated by a Brain Tumor Study Group (BTSG) prospective randomized trial for patients with malignant gliomas comparing supportive care alone (median survival 17 weeks), carmustine (BCNU) alone (median survival 25 weeks), and radiation alone or with BCNU (median survival 37.5 and 40.5 weeks, respectively) (4). Walker and associates reanalyzed results from three successive BTSG protocols conducted between 1966 and 1975 for patients with malignant gliomas and found stepwise increments in median survival with increasing radiation dose: 28 weeks for patients receiving 45.9–51.7 Gy, 36 weeks for 52.9–58.0 Gy, and 42 weeks for 58.5–62.0 Gy (5). Salazar et al. found a trend toward improved survival in patients with malignant gliomas treated with 70–80 Gy, compared with historical controls treated with 50–65 Gy (6).

However, Miller et al. recently analyzed 82 patients treated with external beam radiation therapy for high-grade gliomas and found no improvement in survival comparing the 50- to 60-Gy group (median survival 62 weeks) with the 60- to 70-Gy group (median survival 54 weeks) (7). It is generally accepted that high doses of conventionally fractionated external beam radiation result in a significant incidence of cerebral radiation necrosis (8,9). The use of interstitial radiotherapy allows the delivery of a high dose of radiation to a tumor while limiting the dose to surrounding brain tissue. A dose of 60 Gy or more can be given with a brain implant after 60-Gy external beam radiation therapy.

This chapter will discuss history, physics, and radiobiology relevant to interstitial radiotherapy of brain tumors. Patient selection, implantation technique, and results of interstitial radiotherapy for high-grade gliomas will be presented, based on experience gained at the University of California, San Francisco (UCSF).

II. HISTORY

Brachytherapy means treatment at short range and refers to the treatment of tumors with radiation sources placed directly adjacent to tumors (as in surface plaque or intracavity irradiation) or directly into tumors (as in interstitial irradiation). Shortly after Pierre and Marie Curie discovered radium in 1898, brachytherapy began to be used to treat cancer. In 1901, Pierre Curie gave a tube of radium to Danlos and suggested that he insert it into a tumor (10). Abbe, Stevenson, and Janeway were pioneers in interstitial irradiation in the early 1900s (11–13). Brachytherapy was in widespread use after World War I (14–17), but became less popular as the dangers of handling radioactive materials were better understood and as megavoltage teletherapy machines became available. In the last two decades, however, there has been a resurgence of interest in brachytherapy (18). Afterloading techniques minimize radiation exposure to health care personnel, and sophisticated computerized treatment-planning is now available. Brachytherapy is widely accepted to have an important role in the treatment of gynecological cancers and head and neck cancers and is used frequently in a broad spectrum of other tumors (12).

The first reported use of brachytherapy for brain tumors came from Hirsch, who inserted radium into the sella turcica to treat a pituitary adenoma in 1912 (19). Frazier implanted radioactive sources into parenchymal brain tumors beginning in 1914 (20). Over the next four decades, many authors reported on the use of interstitial radiation for various brain tumors (21). Two pioneers of stereotactic radioisotope implantation techniques were Talairach in Paris (22) and Mundinger in Freiburg, Germany (23). Between 1954 and 1982, Mundinger performed 472 permanent iridium-192 (^{192}Ir) or iodine-125 (^{125}I) brain implants for a variety of brain tumors, including 246 grade I and II astrocytomas, 63 grade III astrocytomas, and 36 glioblastomas (24).

Over the last two decades, brain implant techniques have improved substantially owing to the availability of computed tomography (CT) imaging and advances in stereotactic neurosurgery and radiation treatment planning.

III. PHYSICS

The dose distribution surrounding a radiation source implanted in tissue decreases rapidly with distance away from the source, owing to the inverse square law (intensity is inversely proportional to the square of the distance from a source) and to attenuation of the radiation as it passes through tissue. The most commonly used isotopes for interstitial irradiation include ^{192}Ir and ^{125}I. Iridium-192 emits 0.67 MeV β-particles and γ-rays with an average energy of 0.37 MeV (25). The half life of ^{192}Ir is 74.2 days (25). Iodine-125 has a half-life of 59.6 days and emits characteristic x-rays with an average energy of 28.5 keV (25). Brain implant arrays of either ^{192}Ir or high-activity ^{125}I sources can produce smooth isodose contours, conforming well to the shape of a tumor and delivering radiation at dose rates of about 40–60 cGy/h. We use ^{125}I exclusively for temporary brain implants because of the ease of radiation protection: ^{125}I implants can be shielded well with a 0.5-mm layer of lead, whereas a considerable thickness of lead is required for ^{192}Ir.

IV. RADIOBIOLOGY

A. Low-Dose-Rate Irradiation

Dose rates of about 30–100 cGy/h are typically used for brachytherapy, in contrast with a dose rate of at least 100 cGy/min for teletherapy. In general, the biological effect of radiation is lessened with decreasing dose rate, but normal cells may be spared to a greater extent than tumor cells. Low-dose-rate radiation tends to make proliferating tumor cells accumulate in G_2, a radiosensitive phase of the cell cycle. Normal, noncycling neuronal cells tend to remain in G_1, a radioresistant phase of the cell cycle (26).

It is believed that a significant proportion of the tumor cells comprising a malignant glioma may be hypoxic. In comparison with normally oxygenated cells, hypoxic cells are about three times more resistant to high-dose–rate irradiation. During low-dose–rate irradiation, this oxygen effect is much less, probably owing to decreased repair of sublethal radiation damage under hypoxic conditions (27, 28). Furthermore, there is an increase in biological effect, as a portion of the previously hypoxic cells become reoxygenated during the course of low-dose–rate irradiation (29).

These advantages of brachytherapy are nullified if the dose rate is so low that tumor cell repopulation exceeds tumor cell death (26). This may happen when high-grade gliomas are treated with permanent implants using low-activity ^{125}I sources. Therefore, high-grade gliomas are treated at UCSF at dose rates of about 40–60 cGy/h using temporary implants of high-activity ^{125}I sources.

B. Hyperthermia

There is much interest in *thermoradiotherapy*, the combination of hyperthermia with radiation therapy. Above temperatures of about 41–42°C, heat kills cells exponentially as a function of time and temperature, and heat inhibits the repair of sublethal and potentially lethal radiation damage. In addition, two classes of cells that tend to be radioresistant are particularly sensitive to heat: S phase cells and nutrient-deprived, low pH hypoxic cells (30).

Multiple nonrandomized clinical trials have compared radiation alone with radiation with superficial hyperthermia, demonstrating improved complete response rates and tumor control for superficial squamous cell carcinoma, adenocarcinoma, and melanoma lesions (31). Although more studies have reported on superficial hyperthermia than interstitial hyperthermia, there is reason to believe that interstitial hyperthermia may be more successful. Interstitial heating techniques allow excellent localization of heating at depth and are easily combined with brachytherapy (32–34).

V. PATIENT SELECTION

Brain tumors selected for removable interstitial implants are supratentorial, unifocal, well-circumscribed lesions smaller than 5–6 cm in diameter. Infratentorial tumors and those invading deep white matter are excluded on the basis of poor biological reserve in the event of radiation necrosis. Tumors invading the corpus callosum or spreading subependymally are excluded because they tend to rapidly disseminate. Karnofsky performance status (KPS) of at least 70 is generally required, as patients with KPS below 70 tend to have very poor survival.

VI. PRIOR SURGERY

At first diagnosis, patients with primary brain tumors undergo the most complete surgical resection deemed feasible without undue risk of compromising function, ranging from biopsy to gross total resection. In practice, most tumors are subtotally resected. Tumors are reresected 2–4 weeks before brachytherapy if tumor progression or recurrence has occurred since the primary external beam radiotherapy such that there is significant mass effect or edema.

VII. EXTERNAL BEAM RADIATION THERAPY

After initial surgical resection or biopsy, malignant gliomas are treated with external beam radiation therapy before brachytherapy. Focal radiation fields encompassing the tumor with a 3-cm margin are treated at 1.8 Gy per fraction, 5 days weekly to a total dose of 59.4 Gy.

VIII. CHEMOTHERAPY

Brain implant protocols for previously untreated malignant gliomas call for hydroxyurea (HU) to be given as a radiosensitizer during external beam radiation therapy at 300 mg/m^2 orally every 6 h on Mondays, Wednesdays, and Fridays. Following external beam radiotherapy and implant boost, most patients with malignant gliomas have been treated with six cycles of PCV combination chemotherapy, including procarbazine (60 mg/m^2 orally on days 8–21), lomustine (CCNU; 110 mg/m^2 orally on day 1), and vincristine (1.4 mg/m^2 intravenously on days 8 and 29) (35,36). A variety of chemotherapeutic agents are used at the time of treatment failure.

IX. IMPLANTATION TECHNIQUE

A. Preplanning

The Brown–Roberts–Wells (BRW) stereotactic system (Radionics, Burlington, Massachusetts) is used for placement of brain implant catheters after CT-based preplanning. First, the base ring is fixed to the patient's skull. A contrast-enhanced brain CT scan is performed with a graphite rod localizing system mounted on the base ring, providing axial images at 3-mm intervals.

A computer program named BRAIN was developed at UCSF to plan temporary brain implants on a VAX 11-780, or more recently, a VAX 4000, Model 300 computer (Digital Equipment Corporation, Maynard, Massachusetts) (37). The target volume is outlined on each axial CT image, including the contrast-enhanced tumor volume with a 0- to 5-mm margin. Catheter locations and angles and source positions and strengths are chosen empirically. Resulting radiation isodose lines may be displayed in any plane, and a dose–volume histogram gives data for normal tissue as well as the target volume. Catheters and sources are adjusted until a plan is created that encompasses the tumor with a 40- to 60-cGy/h isodose line conforming closely to the target volume. Depending on tumor size and geometry, the number of catheters used ranges from one to six, with one to four sources per catheter. A large inventory of sources is maintained, with activity ranging from about 3 to 40 mCi.

A different approach is to implant several parallel catheters, spaced evenly throughout the target volume, using a template. Although this gives a more uniform dose distribution within the target volume, we prefer to use fewer catheters to reduce the risk of bleeding and cerebral edema. Outside of the target volume, both techniques give very similar dose distributions (38).

At the end of the planning procedure, the BRAIN program prints out a description of the source loading, BRW frame angles, and the target location for each catheter. While the neurosurgeon inserts the brain implant catheters, the physicist calibrates the ^{125}I sources, and inserts the sources and spacers into smaller nylon catheters (1.04-mm inside diameter, 1.47-mm outside diameter). These loaded catheters are transported to the operating room in a lead-lined, covered tray to be sterilized and then afterloaded into the larger brain implant catheters.

B. Surgical Procedure

The brain implant procedure is performed under local anesthesia in adults or general anesthesia in children. Intravenous prophylactic antibiotics are routinely administered intraoperatively. Stereotactic coordinates for each catheter to be implanted are set on the BRW arc–ring system and verified with a phantom target, according to the coordinates supplied by the BRAIN program. A small scalp incision is made and a 3.4-mm–diameter hole is drilled through the skull with a twist drill passed through the guide on the arc–ring assembly. A purse-string suture is placed surrounding the skin incision to later prevent leakage of cerebrospinal fluid around the catheter. Each Silastic brain implant catheter (2.16-mm outside diameter and 1.57-mm inside diameter) with an inner stylet is passed through a plastic collar on the scalp surface, through the twist drill hole in the skull, to the target depth in the brain (Fig. 1). The plastic collar is glued to the catheter and sutured to the scalp and the scalp purse-string suture is tightened. Catheters are trimmed off 1–1.5 cm from the scalp surface. Burr holes are occasionally used in place of twist drill holes for sites felt to be at higher risk for bleeding.

After placement of all of the brain implant catheters, ^{125}I sources in smaller catheters are afterloaded in the operating room and fixed to each outer catheter with a hemostatic clip (Fig. 2). A sterile dressing is applied over the catheters.

C. Source Position Verification

Before removing the BRW base ring in the operating room, orthogonal radiographs are taken through a fiducial marker box mounted on the base ring. After the fiducial markers and ^{125}I source locations have been digitized into the computer, the BRAIN program displays actual source positions and radiation isodose lines on the preimplant CT images (Fig. 3) and makes available the actual dose–volume histogram. If the dose distribution is felt to be inadequate, a new plan can be created using the actual catheter locations, by altering the spacer lengths and source activities for one or more catheters as needed. The old inner catheters can then be replaced with new inner catheters at the bedside using sterile technique.

D. Radiation Protection

Because of its relatively low energy, ^{125}I is easily shielded by thin layers of lead. The sources may be transported to and from the isotope safe in a small lead container or a covered tray lined with lead. The surgeon loading the sources into brain implant catheters is protected with a lead apron,

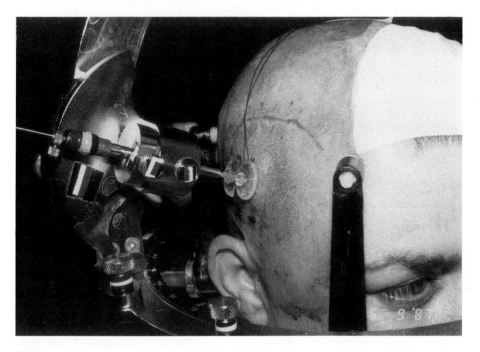

Figure 1 A patient undergoing catheter placement. One catheter has already been implanted. A second catheter with an inner stylet has just been passed through the guide on the arc–ring assembly and through a collar on the skin surface. The purse-string suture is ready to be tightened around the second catheter.

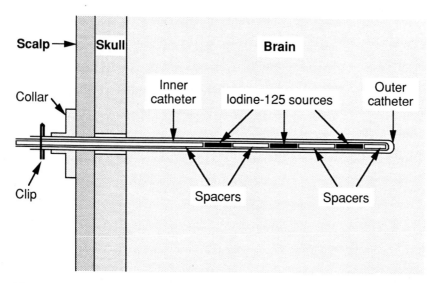

Figure 2 Schematic diagram of the implant unit. The outer catheter is glued to a plastic collar, which is sutured to the scalp. The inner catheter contains spacers and iodine-125 sources and is fixed to the outer catheter with a surgical clip.

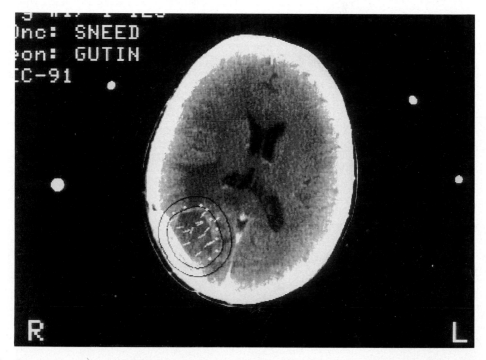

Figure 3 A CT scan showing a recurrent glioblastoma multiforme implanted with 13 iodine-125 sources in seven catheters. The target volume is marked with white "+" symbols. The actual source positions are superimposed on the CT image along with the resulting 50- and 25-cGy/h isodose contours. Tumor dose was prescribed at the 50-cGy/h line.

thyroid shield, leaded glasses, and reusable leaded vinyl rubber surgical gloves. Once the implant is in place, the exposure rates 1 m from the patient are reduced to less than 0.1 mR/h by a cloth hat containing removable 0.5-mm–thick lead panels within two or three of the hat's four compartments. While alone in his or her private hospital room, the patient does not need to wear the lead-lined hat. Hospital personnel and family members wear a lead apron during patient visits.

E. Implant Removal

Sources are usually left in place for 4–7 days. Implant removal is performed at the bedside by first removing the scalp and purse-string sutures and then withdrawing the catheters. Each catheter site in the scalp is sutured closed and a sterile dressing is applied. Patients are observed overnight and discharged from the hospital on the following morning.

F. Hyperthermia

Protocols combining interstitial hyperthermia with brain brachytherapy call for one hyperthermia treatment immediately before loading ^{125}I sources and a second hyperthermia treatment immediately after unloading the sources. The same catheters used to house the ^{125}I sources are used for the heating probes, but the catheters are placed more peripherally, about 3–5 mm within the boundary of the contrast-enhancing tumor mass, evenly spaced about 1.2–2.0 cm apart from each other. In addition, one to three extra catheters are implanted for multipoint thermometry. An example of a typical catheter arrangement for hyperthermia is shown in Figure 4 along with the resulting temperature distribution.

Dummy sources are loaded in the operating room to allow verification of the catheter positions before hyperthermia. The next morning, dummy sources are replaced with 915-MHz helical coil

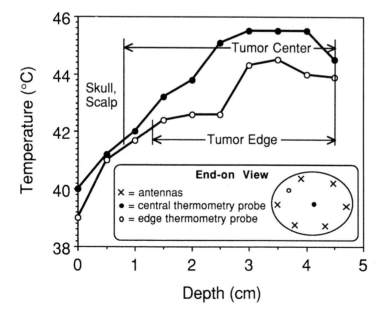

Figure 4 Graph of steady-state temperature versus depth for a recurrent glioblastoma multiforme heated with six microwave antennas. Temperatures were measured using two dedicated thermometry catheters, including one passing through the center of the tumor and one near the periphery of the tumor, as shown in the inset diagram. Vertical lines on the graph indicate the tumor boundaries for both catheters. The minimum tumor temperature was 42.0°C and the maximum 45.5°C.

microwave antennas (39,40). Multisensor fiber-optic or fluoroptic thermometry probes are inserted into the dedicated thermometry catheters. The goal of the hyperthermia treatment is to heat as much of the tumor as possible to at least 42.5°C for 30 min. Patients are monitored clinically for any acute side effects. If neurological changes are noted during hyperthermia, power levels are reduced until the changes resolve or treatment is terminated early if symptoms persist after power reduction.

X. FOLLOW-UP EVALUATION

The neuro-oncology service at UCSF performs or coordinates follow-up every 8 weeks, including neurological examination, contrast-enhanced CT, or gadolinium-enhanced MRI, and assessment of KPS and steroid requirement. In cases for whom it is difficult to distinguish between radiation necrosis and tumor progression on the basis of CT or MRI, positron emission tomography (PET) scans using rubidium-82 and [^{18}F1]-fluorodeoxyglucose are often useful (41).

XI. RESULTS

Removable high-activity ^{125}I implants have been performed in over 400 brain tumor patients at UCSF since December 1979. A review of this entire experience is in progress, but results are currently available for four subgroups, including 63 patients who underwent implant boost after external beam radiation therapy, 98 patients who underwent brain implant alone for recurrent gliomas, 48 patients who underwent thermoradiotherapy for recurrent primary or metastatic brain tumors, and 14 patients who underwent brain implant for initial or recurrent brain metastases.

A. Implant Boost for Malignant Gliomas

A total of 107 patients with previously untreated malignant gliomas were treated on a Northern California Oncology Group (NCOG) trial between January 1982 and January 1990 (35). The protocol called for surgery, focal external beam radiation therapy to a dose of 59.6 Gy at 1.8 Gy per fraction with concomitant hydroxyurea, followed by a 50- to 60-Gy brain implant boost, and then 1 year of PCV chemotherapy. There were 65 males and 42 females, with a median KPS of 90 (range 70–100). Patient age ranged from 19–74 years. The mean age was 51 years in patients with glioblastoma multiforme (GM), and 41 years in those with non-glioblastoma multiforme (NGM).

Of the 101 evaluable patients, 38 never underwent brain implant, most commonly because of tumor progression during external beam radiation therapy rendering the tumor no longer eligible for implant. The median survival from the date of diagnosis until death or last follow-up was 88 weeks for 34 implanted patients with GM, using a median brachytherapy dose of 51.9 Gy (range 42.0–66.1) at 30–60 cGy/h and 157 weeks for 29 implanted patients with NGM using a median dose of 55.0 Gy (range 46.0–75.9 Gy) at 30–60 cGy/h.

No major surgical complications occurred. There was a modest decrement in KPS with time. The mean KPS decreased from 86 to 75 at 24 months posttreatment for patients with GM, and from 91 to 78 at 30 months for patients with NGM. Approximately half of all patients required later reoperation for symptomatic necrosis of the tumor bed or tumor progression (35).

B. Implant Alone for Recurrent Malignant Gliomas

Between January 1980 and January 1988, 98 patients were treated with ^{125}I brachytherapy alone for recurrent malignant gliomas, having had tumor progression after prior external beam radiation therapy (42). Of 95 evaluable patients, 45 had GM and 50 had NGM. There were 55 males and 40 females, with a median KPS of 90 (range 70–100). Patient age ranged from 5 to 66 years, with a median age of 35 years for NGM and 50 years for GM.

One to six catheters (mean 2.7) were used to house 2–12 sources (mean 6.5). The dose delivered with brachytherapy ranged from 52.7 to 150.0 Gy, with a mean of 70.2 Gy for GM and 74.4 Gy for NGM, given at a mean dose rate of 42 cGy/h (range 20–90). The median survival from the time of the implant until death or last follow-up was 54 weeks for patients with GM and 81 weeks for those with NGM. Four patients with GM and 14 with NGM were living at least 3 years after implantation for recurrence.

Serious complications of the brain implant procedure included wound dehiscence in two patients, requiring skin grafting; cerebral edema in one patient, requiring management with mannitol and steroids; intracerebral hemorrhage in one patient; a brain abscess in the tumor bed and a case of meningitis, both of which were successfully treated with antibiotics. The mean KPS decreased from 86 at the time of implant to 79 at 18 months (33 patients) and to 76 at 3 years (18 patients). Similar to the experience with brain implant boost, about half of the patients required later repeat surgery, usually for a combination of tumor and necrosis (42).

C. Implant with Hyperthermia for Recurrent Tumors

A total of 49 recurrent tumors in 48 patients were treated with combined interstitial radiation therapy and ^{125}I brain implant between June 1987 and September 1990 (43). There were 29 men and 19 women. The median age was 43 years (range 18–71) and the median KPS was 90 (range 40–90). Tumors treated included 26 GMs, 16 NGMs, 4 adenocarcinomas, and 3 melanomas.

The median brachytherapy dose delivered was 57.9 Gy (range 47.6–63.3 Gy) except that one patient with a KPS of 40 was treated with only 32.6 Gy. A total of 3–11 catheters (median 6) were used to house one to three thermometry probes (median two) and one to eight heating antennas (median four). As expected, there was significant intratumoral and interpatient variation in temperatures achieved. The median maximum tumor temperature was 45.6°C (range 39.5–51.7°C), the median average tumor temperature was 43.2°C (range 39.2–47.4°C), and the median minimum tumor temperature was 40.1°C (range 37.0–45.7°C) (43).

Calculating actuarial survival from the date of the thermoradiotherapy until death or last follow-up, patients with GM had a 1-year survival of 45% and a median survival of 47 weeks. For NGM, the 1-year and 18-month probabilities of survival were 81 and 65%, respectively. Median survival has not yet been reached, with a median follow-up of 92 weeks in the living patients with NGM. All three treated melanoma brain metastases were locally controlled until the patients died of pulmonary metastases (two) or new brain metastases (one). Three of four patients treated for adenocarcinoma brain metastases died of the disease, whereas the remaining patient is living with local control at 59.6 weeks (43). Actuarial freedom from local tumor progression was significantly longer for the 23 patients in whom a minimum tumor temperature of at least 40.5°C was attained (median 52 weeks) than in the 25 patients with minimum tumor temperature less than 40.5°C (median 19 weeks) ($p = 0.001$).

D. Implant for Brain Metastases

Between December 1979 and July 1987, 14 patients had temporary ^{125}I brain implants for metastatic brain lesions, including 5 men and 9 women. The median patient age was 49 years (range 20–61 years). One patient had the implant 5 weeks before external beam radiation therapy, 4 had implant boost 2 weeks after whole-brain external beam radiotherapy, and 9 were implanted for tumor recurrence 4–16 months after whole-brain external beam radiotherapy. Primary tumor types included lung adenocarcinoma (5), lung squamous cell carcinoma (1), breast adenocarcinoma (4), melanoma (3), and uterine adenocarcinoma (1). The median tumor dose delivered with brachytherapy was 49.7 Gy (range 34.1–130.0 Gy). Median survival was 80 weeks. Eight patients were still alive at the time of analysis, with a median follow-up of 63 weeks (range 52–239 weeks) (44).

XII. DISCUSSION

Recognizing that radiation therapy has been the most effective treatment modality for malignant brain tumors, various radiotherapy techniques have been used without any meaningful improvement in survival so far, including accelerated fractionation, hyperfractionation, heavy-particle irradiation, and combination with radiosensitizers (45,46). Radiosurgery, like interstitial brachytherapy, makes possible the delivery of a high dose of localized radiation to the tumor, which may result in improved control. There are as yet few data for the use of radiosurgery for high-grade gliomas, although data are rapidly accumulating for this technique (47–49).

Extensive experience with brain brachytherapy has been gained over the last decade. Table 1 summarizes data from 11 reports, including two series from UCSF. Other authors have reported median survival ranging from 7 to 27 months for previously untreated ("primary") GM and 6 months to 58 weeks for recurrent GM (50–58), compared with the UCSF survival figures of 88 weeks (20.2 months) for primary GM (35) and 54 weeks (12.4 months) for recurrent GM (42). However, it is difficult to compare results among different series, because of variations in patient KPS, age, and other prognostic variables.

It is also difficult to compare results of brachytherapy series with published results for standard radiation therapy because of the necessary constraint that tumors to be implanted must be well circumscribed and limited in size. Florell et al. tried to assess the influence of these selection factors on expected survival (59). A retrospective review at the London Regional Cancer Center revealed that 32% of conventionally treated adults with malignant gliomas had a KPS of at least 70 and had technically implantable brain tumors, based on independent reviews of CT or MRI scans by Dr. Philip Gutin of UCSF and Dr. Mark Bernstein of the University of Toronto. Forty percent

Table 1 Brachytherapy Series

First author (Ref)	Isotope	Histology	No. patients	KPS range (median)	Median survival
Gutin (35)	^{125}I	1° GM	34	70–100 (90)	88 wk (20.2 mo)
		1° NGM	29	70–100 (90)	157 wk (36.1 mo)
Leibel (42)	^{125}I	Recurrent GM	45	70–100 (90)	54 wk (12.4 mo)
		Recurrent NGM	50	70–100 (90)	81 wk (18.6 mo)
Bernstein (50)	^{125}I	1° MG	23	70–100 (90)	60 wk
		Recurrent MG	18	50–100 (80)	44 wk
Chun (51)	^{192}Ir	1° GM	20	>70	14.5 mo
		1° AA	9	>70	15.5 mo
Fass (52)	^{125}I	20 recurrent GM /9 recurrent AA	29	50–100 (mean 73)	10 mo
Kumar (53)	^{60}Co	1° GM	30	Not stated	7 mo
		Recurrent GM	19	Not stated	6 mo
Larson (54)	^{198}Au	Recurrent GM	13	"Good"	9 mo
		Recurrent AA	20	"Good"	17 mo
Loeffler (55)	^{125}I	1° GM	35	70–90 (80)	27 mo
Mundinger (56)	^{192}Ir/^{125}I (permanent)	GM	17	Not stated	19% 2-yr surv
		AA	34	Not stated	47% 5-yr surv.
Patchell (57)	^{252}Cf	1° GM	48	>50	10 mo
		1° AA	8	>50	17 mo
Selker (58)	^{192}Ir	47 1° GM/8 1° AA	55	(80)	68 wk
		Recurrent GM	61	(70)	58 wk

of patients with GM were deemed eligible for brachytherapy. In these conventionally treated patients, the median survival was only 5.8 months for those who were not implant candidates, as opposed to 13.9 months for the implant candidates (59). Our results compare favorably, with an actuarial median survival of 20.2 months for patients with primary GM who underwent implant boost.

We compared results for our brachytherapy-treated patients with results of a Northern California Oncology Group trial of intravenous bromodeoxyuridine (BUDR) infusion with external beam radiotherapy followed by PCV chemotherapy. The BUDR trial yielded an actuarial median survival of 64 weeks for patients with GM and 252 weeks for patients with NGM, leading us to conclude that brachytherapy boost may be of value for primary GM, but not for primary NGM.

In attempt to assess the role of brachytherapy in the treatment of malignant gliomas, a Phase III prospective, randomized trial was instituted in 1987 by the Brain Tumor Cooperative Group. Patients are randomly assigned to implant (60 Gy) or no implant before external beam radiation therapy (60.2 Gy) with intravenous carmustine (BCNU). Another Phase III randomized trial is in progress at the University of Toronto. Until results of these trials are available, we can conclude only that results with brachytherapy appear very promising for the patients who have primary GM or recurrent malignant gliomas suitable for implantation, with longer median survival times, long-term survival in some patients, and low toxicity.

Strategies to improve results further are under investigation, including the combination of brachytherapy with BUDR or idoxyuridine (IUDR). In addition, a randomized trial is in progress at UCSF for implant candidates with GM, utilizing resection, external beam radiotherapy to 59.4 Gy with HU followed by implant boost to 60 Gy with or without interstitial hyperthermia. We hope that these efforts will impinge favorably on survival and quality of life for patients with malignant brain tumors.

REFERENCES

1. Choucair AK, Levin VA, Gutin PH, Davis RL, Silver P, Edwards MS, Wilson CB. Development of multiple lesions during radiation therapy and chemotherapy in patients with gliomas. J Neurosurg 1986; 65:654–658.
2. Hochberg FH, Pruitt A. Assumptions in the radiotherapy of glioblastoma. Neurology 1980; 30:907–911.
3. Wallner KE, Galicich JH, Krol G, Arbit E, Malkin MG. Patterns of failure following treatment for glioblastoma multiforme and anaplastic astrocytoma. Int J Radiat Oncol Biol Phys 1989; 16:1405–1409.
4. Walker MD, Alexander E Jr, Hunt WE, MacCarty CS, Mahaley MS Jr, Mealey J Jr, Norrell HA, Owens G, Ransohoff J, Wilson CB, Gehan EA, Strike TA. Evaluation of BCNU and/or radiotherapy in the treatment of anaplastic gliomas. J Neurosurg 1978; 49:333–343.
5. Walker MD, Strike TA, Sheline GE. An analysis of dose-effect relationship in the radiotherapy of malignant gliomas. Int J Radiat Oncol biol Phys 1979; 5:1725–1731.
6. Salazar OM, Rubin P, Feldstein ML, Pizzutiello R. High dose radiation therapy in the treatment of malignant gliomas: final report. Int J Radiat Oncol Biol Phys 1979; 5:1733–1740.
7. Miller PJ, Hassanein RS, Shankar Giri PG, Kimler BF, O'Boynick P, Evans RG. Univariate and multivariate statistical analysis of high-grade gliomas: the relationship of radiation dose and other prognostic factors. Int J Radiat Oncol Biol Phys 1990; 19:275–280.
8. Marks JE, Baglan RJ, Prassad SC, Blank WF. Cerebral radionecrosis: incidence and risk in relation to dose, time, fractionation and volume. Int J Radiat Oncol Biol Phys 1981; 7:243–252.
9. Sheline GE, Wara WW, Smith V. Therapeutic irradiation and brain injury. Int J Radiat Oncol Biol Phys 1980; 6:1215–1228.
10. Danlos H. Quelques considerationes sur le traitement des dermatoses par le radium. J Physiother (Paris) 1905; 3:98–106.
11. Abbe R. Radium's contribution to surgery. JAMA 1910; 55:97–100.

12. Hilaris BS. Handbook of interstitial brachytherapy. Acton, MA: Publishing Sciences Group, 1975.

13. Stevenson WC. Preliminary clinical report on a new and economical method of radium therapy by means of emanation needles. Br Med J 1914; 2:9–10.

14. Lenz M. The early workers in clinical radiotherapy of cancer at the Radium Institute of the Curie Foundation, Paris, France. Cancer 1973; 32:519–523.

15. Quick D. The value of interstitial radiation. AJR 1922; 9:161–166.

16. Quick D, Johnson FM. A new type of applicator for use with radium emanation. AJR 1922; 9:53–55.

17. Viol CH. A comparison of radiation dosages attainable by use of radium on and within tumors. AJR 1922; 9:56–57.

18. Hall EJ, Lam Y-M. The renaissance in low dose-rate interstitial implants. Front Radiat Ther Oncol 1978; 12:21–34.

19. Hirsch O. Die operative behandlung von hypophysistumoren: nach endonasalen methoden. Arch Laryngol Rhinol 1912; 26:529–686.

20. Frazier CH. The effects of radium emanations upon brain tumors. Surg Gynecol Obstet 1920; 31:236–239.

21. Bernstein M, Gutin PH. Interstitial irradiation of brain tumors: a review. Neurosurgery 1981; 9:741–750.

22. Talairach J, Ruggiero G, Aboulker J, David M. A new method of treatment of inoperable brain tumours by stereotaxic implantation of radioactive gold—a preliminary report. Br J Radiol 1955; 28:62–74.

23. Mundinger F. Die interstitielle radio-isotopen-bestrahlung von hirntumoren mit vergleichenden langzeitergebnissen zur rontgentiefentherapie. Acta Neurochir (Wien) 1964; 11:89–109.

24. Mundinger F, Weigel K. Long-term results of stereotactic interstitial curietherapy. Acta Neurochir [Suppl] 1984; 33:367–371.

25. Weaver KA, Anderson LL, Meli JA. Source characteristics. In: Anderson LL, Nath R, Weaver KA, et al, eds. Interstitial brachytherapy: physical, biological, and clinical considerations. New York: Raven Press, 1990:3–19.

26. Hall EJ. The biological basis of endocurietherapy: the Henschke memorial lecture 1984. Endocurie Hypertherm Oncol 1985; 1:141–152.

27. Hall EJ, Bedford JS, Oliver R. Extreme hypoxia; its effect on the survival of mammalian cells irradiated at high and low dose-rates. Br J Radiol 1966; 39:302–307.

28. Ling CC, Spiro IJ, Mitchell J, Stickler R. The variation of OER with dose rate. Int J Radiat Oncol Biol Phys 1985; 11:1367–1373.

29. Hall EJ. Radiobiology for the radiologist. Philadelphia: JB Lippincott, 1988:123,125.

30. Dewey WC, Freeman ML, Raaphorst GP, Clark EP, Wong RSL, Highfield DP, Spiro IJ. Tomasovic SP, Denman DL, Cross RA. Cell biology of hyperthermia and radiation. In: Meyn RE, Withers HR, eds. Radiation biology in cancer research. New York: Raven Press, 1980:589–621.

31. Overgaard J. The current and potential role of hyperthermia in radiotherapy. Int J Radiat Oncol Biol Phys 1990; 16:535–549.

32. Coughlin CT. Clinical hyperthermic practice: interstitial heating. In: Field SB, Hand JW, eds. An introduction to the practical aspects of clinical hyperthermia. London: Taylor & Francis, 1990:172–184.

33. Emami B, Perez CA. Interstitial thermoradiotherapy: an overview. Endocurie Hypertherm Oncol 1985;1:35–40.

34. Stauffer PR. Techniques for interstitial hyperthermia. In: Field SB, Hand JW, eds. An introduction to the practical aspects of clinical hyperthermia. London: Taylor & Francis, 1990:344–370.

35. Gutin PH, Prados MD, Phillips TL, Wara WM, Larson DA, Leibel SA, Sneed PK, Levin VA, Weaver KA, Silver P, Lamborn K, Lamb S, Ham B. External irradiation followed by an interstitial high activity iodine-125 implant "boost" in the initial treatment of malignant gliomas: NCOG study 6G-82-2. Int J Radiat Oncol Biol Phys 1991; 21:601–606.

36. Leibel S, Gutin P, Phillips T, et al. The integration of interstitial implantation into the primary management of patients with malignant gliomas: results of a phase II Northern California Oncology Group trial. Am J Clin Oncol 1987; 10:106.

37. Weaver K, Smith V, Lewis JD, Lulu B, Barnett CM, Leibel SA, Gutin P, Larson D, Phillips T. A CT-based computerized treatment planning system for I-125 stereotactic brain implants. Int J Radiat Oncol Biol Phys 1990; 18:445–454.

38. Saw CB, Suntharalingam N, Ayyangar KM, Tupchong L. Dosimetric considerations of stereotactic brain implants. Int J Radiat Oncol Biol Phys 1989; 17:887–891.
39. Satoh R, Stauffer PR, Fike JR. Thermal distribution studies of helical coil microwave antennas for interstitial hyperthermia. Int J Radiat Oncol Biol Phys 1988; 15:1209–1218.
40. Satoh T, Stauffer PR. Implantable helical coil microwave antenna for interstitial hyperthermia. Int J Hypertherm 1988; 4:497–512.
41. Valk PE, Budinger TF, Levin VA, Silver P, Gutin PH, Doyle WK. PET of malignant cerebral tumors after interstitial brachytherapy. J Neurosurg 1988; 69:830–838.
42. Leibel SA, Gutin PH, Wara WM, Silver PS, Larson DA, Edwards MSB, Lamb SA, Ham B, Weaver KA, Barnett C, Phillips TL. Survival and quality of life after interstitial implantation of removable high-activity iodine-125 sources for the treatment of patients with recurrent malignant gliomas. Int J Radiat Oncol Biol Phys 1989; 17:1129–1139.
43. Sneed PK, Gutin PH, Stauffer PR, Phillips TL, Prados MD, Weaver KA, Suen S, Lamb SA, Ham B, Ahn DK, Lamborn K, Larson DA, Wara WM. Thermoradiotherapy of recurrent malignant brain tumors. Int J Radiat Oncol Biol Phys 1992; 23:853–861.
44. Prados M, Leibel S, Barnett CM, Gutin P. Interstitial brachytherapy for metastatic brain tumors. Cancer 1989; 63:657–660.
45. Davis LW. Presidential address: malignant glioma—a nemesis which requires clinical and basic investigation in radiation oncology. Int J Radiat Oncol Biol Phys 1989; 16:1355–1365.
46. Nelson DF, Urtasun RC, Saunders WM, Gutin PH, Sheline GE. Recent and current investigations of radiation therapy of malignant gliomas. Semin Oncol 1986; 13:46–55.
47. Coffey RJ, Lunsford LD, Bissonette D, Flickinger JC. Stereotactic gamma radiosurgery for intracranial vascular malformations and tumors: report of the initial North American experience in 331 patients. Stereotact Funct Neurosurg 1990; 54–55:535–540.
48. Larson DA, Gutin PH, Leibel SA, Phillips TL, Sneed PK, Wara WM. Stereotaxic irradiation of brain tumors. Cancer 1990; 65:792–799.
49. Loeffler J. Stereotaxic radiosurgery for metastases and malignant gliomas. Second symposium on stereotactic treatment of brain tumors. New York, February 28–March 1, 1991:45–46.
50. Bernstein M, Laperriere N, Leung P, McKenzie S. Interstitial brachytherapy for malignant brain tumors: preliminary results. Neurosurgery 1990; 26:371–380.
51. Chun M, McKeough P, Wu A, Kasdon D, Heros D, Chang H. Interstitial iridium-192 implantation for malignant brain tumors. Br J Radiol 1989; 62:158–162.
52. Fass DE, Malkin MG, Arbit E, Anderson LL, Schupak KD, Lindsley KL, Leibel SA. MSKCC brachytherapy results. Second symposium on stereotactic treatment of brain tumors. New York, February 28–March 1, 1991:29.
53. Kumar PP, Good RR, Jones EO, Patil AA, Leibrock LG, McComb RD. Survival of patients with glioblastoma multiforme treated by intraoperative high-activity cobalt 60 endocurietherapy. Cancer 1989; 64:1409–1413.
54. Larson GL, Wilbanks JH, Dennis WS, Permenter WD, Easley JD. Interstitial radiogold implantation for the treatment of recurrent high-grade gliomas. Cancer 1990; 66:27–29.
55. Loeffler JS, Alexander E III, Wen PY, Shea WM, Coleman CN, Kooy HM, Fine HA, Nedzi LA, Silver B, Riese NE, Black PM. Results of stereotactic brachytherapy used in the initial management of patients with glioblastoma. JNCI 1990; 82:1918–1921.
56. Mundinger F, Ostertag CB, Birg W, Weigel K. Stereotactic treatment of brain lesions. Appl Neurophysiol 1980; 43:198–204.
57. Patchell RA, Maruyama Y, Tibbs PA, Beach JL, Kryscio RJ, Young AB. Neutron interstitial brachytherapy for malignant gliomas: a pilot study. J Neurosurg 1988; 68:67–72.
58. Selker RG, Eddy MS, Arena V. Pittsburgh brachytherapy experience. Second symposium on stereotactic treatment of brain tumors. New York, February 28–March 1, 1991:23–24.
59. Florell RC, Macdonald DR, Irish WD, Bernstein M, Leibel SA, Gutin PH, Cairncross JG. Selection bias, survival and brachytherapy for glioma. J Neurosurg 1992; 76:179–183.

26

Stereotactic Radiosurgery

John W. Walsh

**Hermann Hospital and the University of Texas Health Sciences
Center at Houston, Houston, Texas**

I. INTRODUCTION

Radiosurgery is a relatively newly developed treatment modality that employs stereotactic localization with focused beam ionizing radiation for the noninvasive destruction of small intracranial lesions. It is especially valuable for the eradication of a wide variety of benign and malignant brain tumors and has recently emerged as an effective alternative to microsurgery.

The term *stereotactic radiosurgery* was coined by Lars Leksell to describe the use of a single dose of precisely directed ionizing radiation "for the non-invasive destruction of intracranial tissues or lesions . . ." (1). It has been applied to this new technology because, in a manner similar to microsurgery, it enables the neurosurgeon to target and completely destroy only the tumor, to spare the surrounding normal tissue, and to accomplish this on a single occasion. It is similar to stereotactic craniotomy because the tumor is localized and targeted in three-dimensional space with modern neuroradiologic imaging and then inactivated under computer-assisted guidance. It differs from microsurgery in that destruction of the tumor is not seen at the time of treatment and takes place over a period of time.

Radiosurgery is markedly different from radiotherapy. Radiosurgery delivers very intense radiation to a very sharply delineated area, whereas radiotherapy uses less intense radiation per dose and, necessarily, includes substantial portions of surrounding normal brain, relying on the differences in susceptibility to radiation-induced injury between normal and tumor tissue for treatment results. Furthermore, although microsurgery and radiosurgery share the aim of complete eradication of the tumor, the aim of radiotherapy is generally the suppression of tumor growth.

The results of stereotactic radiosurgery have shown such efficacy and safety that it is now beginning to be considered for many tumors, even those that arise in young, healthy patients who would be considered treatable by other conventional means.

In this chapter, the currently available types of radiosurgery will be described, and the indications for treatment with radiosurgery and the results obtained for each of the various types of tumors treated will be discussed.

II. HISTORY

As early as 1946, it had been proposed that, based on their inherent physical characteristics, beams of positively charged particles (protons, deuterons, helium ions) could be focused by collimation and used to produce sharply defined lesions in the brain, and that this might be a method of treating certain brain disorders (2). At about the same time, methods for precise stereotactic localization of tumors and other intracranial lesions were being developed; and Lars Leksell, one such investigator, had developed a stereotactic frame for this purpose. It was Leksell who first proposed combining intraoperative stereotactic localization with the application of focused beam radiation. By 1951, he was investigating the advantages of using stereotactic radiosurgery to generate small lesions in humans for the treatment of certain involuntary movements and other functional disorders (3). This inquiry was the beginning of stereotactic and functional neurosurgery as a subspecialty field.

Leksell's first attempts at stereotactic radiosurgery were made using supervoltage x-ray beams, but he found that this did not generate sufficient energy to provide the necessary precision (4). His results were more encouraging with the use of charged-particle beams, but he recognized that the cost of making an instrument that would generate these particles was so high that it could not be produced in sufficient number to be widely used (5–7). Therefore, he turned to using γ-rays (spontaneously emitted x-radiation from naturally occurring radioisotopes) and devised an instrument, the Gamma Unit (now commonly called the gamma knife) that would give him the necessary intensity by providing multiple low-intensity sources of radiation to be focused on a single target.

This first Gamma Unit was completed in 1967 (8,9). It was designed to produce disk-shaped lesions at selected sites in deep cerebral nuclei (thalamus, basal ganglia) of patients with Parkinson's disease or intractable cancer pain. The first brain tumor to be treated with stereotactic radiosurgery, a craniopharyngioma, was treated with that gamma knife in late 1967 (9). However, the disk-shaped lesions were found not to be optimal for the treatment of tumors, so a second Gamma Unit, one that generated spherical lesions and was designed specifically for the eradication of brain tumors and vascular malformations, was built and installed in 1975 at the Karolinska Hospital in Stockholm (10,11).

The first Gamma Unit in the United States, an improved model, was installed at the University of Pittsburgh in 1987 (12).

During the 1980s, two types of preexisting instruments were being modified for application to stereotactic radiosurgery: charged-particle beam-generating instruments (CPBIs), the synchrocyclotron, the cyclotron, and the bevatron (13,14); and the x-ray-generating instrument, the linear accelerator (LINAC) (15–17). The modifications included methods for using stereotactic localization, collimating the charged particle or x-ray beam, and developing the necessary treatment parameters and dosimetry planning.

Of critical importance to the evolution of stereotactic radiosurgery are the innovations and improvements in imaging techniques. Before 1975, stereotactic localization of intracranial lesions was carried out with only pneumoencephalography or positive-contrast ventriculography. Today, stereotactic localization is performed with modern high-resolution computed tomography (CT) and magnetic resonance imaging (MRI). It is impossible to overstate the importance of this new technology to successful treatment with stereotactic radiosurgery.

III. BASIC PRINCIPLES AND CONSIDERATIONS

The essence of radiosurgery is the delivery of the gamma ray, x-ray, or charged-particle beams, with sufficient intensity to destroy a small tumor in a single application, without harm to adjacent normal structures. This has been accomplished by focusing multiple beams on a single target (gamma knife) or by moving a single beam so that in every position of its source the beam passes through a common point, the target (CPBI, modified LINAC). This can now be accomplished with a precision of less than 1 mm. In other words, the energy at the point of beam convergence or common passage is so intense that even the margin of the lesion, when treated at the 40th–90th percentile isodose line, receives enough radiation to inactivate it completely or destroy it, and yet, the falloff of radiation is so steep that normal brain structures less than 1 mm away receive virtually no radiation at all.

As a general principle, when the falloff of radiation is most steep, the distribution of radiation delivered to the tumor will not be homogeneous. This, of course, is the case with radiosurgery and is in marked contrast with what is generally desirable with radiotherapy, for which the radiation dose is deliberately kept low and for which it is important to maintain homogeneity in radiation intensity to assure that there will be no areas of tumor that receive larger or smaller amounts of radiation. With radiosurgery, this is never an issue because as long as the radiation dose is sufficient to destroy the tumor at the margin and the aim is complete destruction of the tumor, any greater dose reception more centrally is irrelevant. The risk that dose lack of homogeneity will produce intratumoral necrosis is also irrelevant, because such necrosis is expected after radiosurgery and generally indicates a favorable outcome.

The shape of the lesion produced by any single radiosurgical exposure is usually spherical or oval and, therefore, frequently will not coincide with the margins of the tumor to be treated, because most tumors (or other lesions) are highly irregular in configuration. Therefore, when a single exposure is used to cover a lesion, it is likely that normal structures will be included and subjected to the high dose of radiation used to destroy the tumor. For these reasons, it becomes the task of the stereotactic radiosurgery team to make certain that the shape of the radiation delivered fits, at least very closely, that of the tumor.

Some shaping of the radiation beam delivered to the tumor is available with the CPBIs and the modified LINAC. This is certainly useful, but it is usually insufficient for adequate tailoring of the radiation. The best tailoring is obtained by use of multiple overlapping isocenters. All three types of instruments provide for this, and it is the technique commonly used. Obviously, with irregularly shaped tumors, the greater the number of overlapping isocenters available, the better the fit that can be achieved in the tailoring. The CPBIs and modified LINACs frequently use two or three such isocenters, but are limited to this number by the length of time required to set up the equipment to generate them. The gamma knife, with present computer software, can generate up to 12 isocenters for a single treatment; and with the new Gammaplan software, it will be able to generate a much greater number.

Selection of the dose to be delivered is still the least standardized aspect of the treatment. It is still largely empirical and based on the radiosurgeon's training and experience and on the past experience of others in the field.

In an effort to establish common guidelines for the prediction of doses of radiation that would cause injury to adjacent normal brain structures, Kjellberg (18) analyzed his extensive experience with the radiosurgical treatment of arteriovenous malformations using the cyclotron and found that the minimum dose required to produce injury varies linearly and inversely with the volume of the lesion. He was, therefore, able to construct isoeffect lines for the doses associated with 91 and 99% likelihood of producing injury. This became the standard for radiosurgery and is still used by many radiosurgeons. However, it was soon found that these values were less accurate for the gamma knife and the modified LINAC and that the use of multiple isocenters and isocenters of different sizes in a given case could not be taken into account. Furthermore, a dose could not accurately be predicted from the line if external beam radiotherapy had been previously administered.

To address these concerns, Flickinger et al. (19) developed what they called an "integrated logistic formula." This is an adaptation for small targets of the standard equations used to determine doses for large-field external beam radiotherapy. The formula allows prediction of the minimum dose associated with a 3% risk of injury. This appears to be more closely related to experience with the gamma knife and modified LINAC and has now become the worldwide standard for dose–volume histogram analysis (20).

IV. RADIOSURGERY INSTRUMENTATION

A. Leksell Gamma Knife

Radiosurgery with the gamma knife involves focused beam radiation using γ-rays generated by cobalt-60 (^{60}Co) radioisotope. Two hundred and one sources of ^{60}Co are embedded in a cast iron dome (weighing approximately 18 tons) and situated in a hemispheric array. The gamma rays pass through finely machined channels to converge at the center of the dome, which is obviously a fixed point. For this reason, treatment requires that the patient's head be placed into the dome in such a manner that the tumor is placed exactly at the center, the point of beam convergence. This is accomplished by surgically attaching a stereotactic frame to the patient's head; localizing the tumor in three dimensions in relation to the center of the frame, using CT, MRI, or angiographic imaging; adjusting the frame settings according to this image-guided localization; and then placing the patient's head, with the now-adjusted frame, into the gamma knife dome so that the tumor becomes situated exactly in the center of the dome. Before the patient's head is moved into the dome, the frame (with the patient's head) is attached to one of four collimators, which is affixed to the side arms of the hydraulic table where the patient is now lying. When the hydraulic table is activated, the collimator–stereotactic frame–patent head assembly is moved into the dome bringing the tumor to its center for the specified period.

The gamma knife provides four ways to obtain a precise fit between the composite isodose configuration of the radiation and the three-dimensional shape of the tumor. First, as already mentioned, the composite isodose configuration can be shaped by using up to 12 small overlapping isocenters, rather than coverage with one to three larger isocenters (as is done with the other radiosurgical instruments). The coordinates for each isocenter can be repeatedly adjusted until an optimal dose fit is obtained. Second, the size of each isocenter can be varied by using one of four different collimators, each of which will generate 4-, 8-, 14-, or 18=mm areas of radiation injury. Further refinement can be achieved by separately selecting one of these for each isocenter. Third, in special circumstances, such as when a pituitary or other skull base tumor is being treated and is situated near the optic nerves or chiasm, the shape of the composite isodose lines can be adjusted from the spherical shape to several other shapes so that one side can be flattened to maximize the distance from the important structures. Finally, some isocenters can be given relatively greater weight than others; that is, they can be given a proportionally larger percentage of the radiation dose. It is this multifaceted facility to tailor the composite isodose lines so precisely to the configuration of the tumor that makes the gamma knife superior to any other radiosurgical instrument.

Because the gamma knife has virtually no moving parts, the large investment of time required with other radiosurgical instruments for calculation of the appropriate arc trajectories for the mobile gantry or couch is completely obviated, and the principal effort can be spent on obtaining optimal coverage of the tumor while maximally protecting adjacent normal brain structures. This function is best provided by the neurosurgeon and is the reason that all gamma knife centers are directed by a neurosurgeon.

The gamma knife is the same instrument worldwide. The only two models made are functionally identical, and the computer software (KULA or Gammaplan) and hardware (Digital

Microvax or Hewlett Packard), the stereotactic frame, and methods for dosimetry planning and treatment are uniform worldwide. This means that data from all the treatment centers can be accumulated and shared, and this provides a base for continuing innovation. There are now 11 Gamma Units in the United States and 41 worldwide.

B. Cyclotron, Bevatron, and Synchrocyclotron

These instruments are less common than the other two types because they require either an enormous capital investment or an affiliation with an existing nuclear science research center. There are approximately 30 sites worldwide where this affiliation has been possible or where development is in the active planning stage (21). As previously stated, these instruments use monoenergetic heavy-charged particles (protons, deuterons, or helium ions), propelled as a beam, and accelerated to a high-energy state for the inactivation of small tumors and other lesions. This type of radiation has several properties that set it apart from the other two types. The beams are very narrow, well collimated with little circumferential scattering, and have a finite range of tissue penetration. Also, treatment can be carried out by using either the fully or near fully energized beam passing through the lesion (plateau ionization region) or by using the greatly enhanced energy given off at the point of most rapid energy deceleration, the Bragg ionization peak. And finally, because the radiation energy ends after the Bragg peak, there is no danger of tissue damage past the range.

With Bragg-peak radiation, the increased energy transfer typically occurs over a very short distance, a distance shorter than the size of most tumors. So, unless beam characteristics are modified, the tumor will not be completely covered with the radiation. This modification is accomplished by enlarging and positioning the area of injury at Bragg's peak by the interposition of specific range-modifying absorbers and tissue equivalent compensators along the beam trajectory.

Stereotactic radiation, using the plateau ionization region, employs multiple coplanar or noncoplanar arcs or discrete stereotactically directed intersecting beams. Here, the high-dose regions at the site of beam convergence are usually quite sharply delineated and easily tailored to fit the exact configuration of the lesion. The Bragg-peak high-energy regions of individual beams develop beyond this point where they are harmlessly dissipated.

C. Modified Linear Accelerator

The instrument used for stereotactic radiosurgery is a modification of the standard LINAC. The standard LINAC is an instrument that generates beams of x-rays by directing a stream of electrons against a metallic target. These newly formed and widely scattered x-rays are focused, by using a primary and secondary collimator system, and directed toward a target lesion. It is a widely used and very important form of external beam radiation therapy. Most large and medium-sized hospitals and radiation therapy centers have acquired a LINAC, and it has become the primary means of treatment for many systemic tumors.

The principal advantage of the standard LINAC for external beam radiotherapy is that radiation of the target can be achieved with less injury to the overlying normal tissue by moving the x-ray-generating apparatus in its gantry along certain predetermined arcs during the exposure, arcs that are centered on the common predetermined target.

To modify a LINAC for radiosurgery, a special collimator must be added so that the beam of x-rays can be more precisely focused and the radiation intensity can be increased sufficiently to inactivate or destroy a tumor with a single treatment. This has been accomplished with a predicted accuracy of less than 1 mm, but a large commitment in time and personnel is required to recalibrate the now modified LINAC instrumentation each time the collimator is attached and to reestablish that the x-ray beam will be delivered with the intended precision. Usually only one patient can be treated per day. Furthermore, most of the day is spent by medical physicists and radiation oncologists to prepare the instrument for use, and the role of the neurosurgeon, who is most familiar with the relevant neuroanatomy and tumor biology may become secondary. This limitation of modified LINAC radiosurgery can be reduced substantially by acquiring one of the several modern, dedicated LINAC instruments and using it for only radiosurgery, but this is not often done.

Three different techniques have been used for treatment: single-plane rotation of the gantry, multiple, noncoplanar converging arcs, and simultaneous rotation of both the couch and gantry (22). Stereotactic localization of the lesion has most often been carried out using the Brown–Roberts–Wells (BRW) frame but the Talairach and Leksell frames have also been used. During dosimetry planning, adjustments of the isocenter location, gantry arc rotation interval, couch angle, and collimator field size are made. In addition, the type and number of treatment arcs, and the arc-start angle, arc-end angle, couch angle, and relative dose distribution have to be determined. Three to seven arcs are generally used for a total of 250–500° of arc rotation, and the total dose administered to the target is the sum of contributions from each arc. Dose–volume histograms are used to determine optimal composite radiation dose in relation to absolute volume of the lesion. Commercially prepared computer software for the more expensive, dedicated units is now available, but most modified LINAC centers use programs obtained from a variety of vendors and these vary in quality and reliability from one center to another.

As of January 1992, there were at least 61 modified LINAC programs in the United States alone (22) and many others worldwide.

V. INDICATIONS

Since randomized, prospective studies of the efficacy of radiosurgery for treatment of specific brain tumors have not yet been completed, no hard and fast indications for its use have been established.

Until about 5 years ago, radiosurgery was recommended only for patients for whom microsurgery was not an option. Up to that time, so few patients had been treated with this modality and their follow-up had been so brief that very little information about the mortality, morbidity, and rate of tumor recurrence associated with the procedure was available. The indications were any one of the following: advanced age or medical impairment sufficient to make the patient an unacceptably high risk for anesthesia or microsurgery; lesion located within a critical brain region (deep-seated or located within an area controlling a specialized neurological function, such as speech or movement); recurrent or persistent tumor not easily removable with conventional microsurgery and not highly responsive to external beam radiation; or progressive enlargement of a tumor in a patient who adamantly refuses microsurgery.

A few indications specific for individual tumor types were also advocated: bilateral cerebellopontine angle tumors in a patient with type 2 neurofibromatosis (NF-2); acoustic neuroma on the side of a patient's only hearing ear; or a tumor that involves a cavernous sinus or petrous apex and is not resectable with acceptable risk using skull base, transsphenoidal, or any other microsurgical approach.

Now that more than 6000 cases have been successfully treated with radiosurgery and very few deaths or complications have occurred, these guidelines are becoming much broader. This is especially so for certain benign tumors, such as meningiomas along the skull base and in the cerebellopontine angle, acoustic neuromas, and pituitary tumors. Follow-up studies are much better, and the results obtained are so encouraging that many radiosurgeons are now advocating radiosurgery as an alternative to microsurgery for most of these tumors, even when they arise in young healthy patients and in noncritical, microsurgically approachable regions of the brain.

Radiosurgery is now also generally accepted for malignant tumors as a good alternative to microsurgery in certain situations. For example, metastases lend themselves well to radiosurgical treatment because they are circumscribed and have been shown to respond well, with only rare recurrence. The treatment of two metastases is not uncommon.

Radiosurgery, like microsurgery, is now being advocated for destruction of the solid, CT or MRI contrast-enhancing portion of tumor in gliomas in an effort to potentiate subsequent adjunctive external beam radiotherapy or chemotherapy and, thereby, lengthen and improve the quality of survival of the patient. Small circumscribed areas of glioma recurrence after aggressive multimodality treatment are also often best handled by radiosurgery.

Generally accepted contraindications to radiosurgery include proximity to the special sensory nerves (because they are especially vulnerable to radiation), and the location of tumor too superficial or inferior to be brought into the point of beam convergence or common radiation passage.

The optic nerves and chiasm are the neural structures most easily injured by radiosurgery. A tumor should be at least 5 mm away from these structures, and no more than 8–9 Gy should spill over to them. The acoustic, vestibular, and trigeminal nerves also need special protection from radiation, but tumors adjacent to them can be managed if the dose is kept within acceptable levels. The vulnerability of all these structures to radiation injury is increased if prior external beam radiotherapy has been given.

Tumors situated laterally on the cortical surface, especially if they are also frontal or occipital, and those at or below the foramen magnum are often difficult or impossible to treat with radiosurgery, especially if the patient has a large head. Below the foramen magnum, movement of the odontoid process and cervical vertebrae makes such treatment impossible.

VI. TREATMENT

Candidates for radiosurgery are usually first identified by a review of CT, MRI, and angiography studies sent to the treatment centers for consultation. A thorough evaluation of the patient on an outpatient basis is then carried out, and specific consultations (ophthalmology, endocrinology, otolaryngology, audiology, or other), laboratory, and additional imaging and neurosensory studies are obtained.

On the morning of treatment, a stereotactic frame is attached to the patient's head under local anesthesia, using MRI-compatible pins or carbon fiber rods. Children younger than age 14 usually require general anesthesia. The stereotactic neuroradiologic studies are then obtained. In most centers, high-resolution stereotactic CT scan or digital subtraction angiography is preferred. Stereotactic MRI scanning is also possible; but until recently, it has not been used because standard T1- and T2-weighted and spin-echo images are frequently associated with substantial (3- to 4-mm) localization inaccuracies. Some correction for these errors has been proposed (23). We have recently used magnetization prepared–rapid gradient echo (MP-RAGE) sequencing (24,25) and are now able to generate serial 1-mm–thick contrast-enhanced axial, coronal, and sagittal sections through the tumor with 1-mm $\times$ 1-mm $\times$ 1-mm resolution and reproducible localization to within 1 mm of that obtained with high-resolution CT scan.

Dosimetry planning is then begun. This is often done by a radiosurgery team that consists of a neurosurgeon, a radiation oncologist, and one or more radiation physicists. This process often takes 1–2 h, and the treatment is not begun until the entire dosimetry plan is complete. As we have stated, multiple overlapping isocenters may be used. The center of the stereotactic frame is first established, and the coordinates for each isocenter are determined in reference to the frame center. The collimators needed to generate lesions just large enough to include all the tumor are then selected. Each set of coordinates and collimator size is entered into the computer and a set of isodose lines for the composite radiation profile is obtained. Radiation beam-blocking patterns, gantry and couch angle settings, or values for the weighting of some isocenters over others are added, and radiation dose and exposure times are specified.

For gamma knife treatment, the patient is then positioned on the hydraulic table so that the head, with attached stereotactic frame, can be secured to the selected collimator. The computer-specified isocenter coordinates and exposure times are then set on the stereotactic apparatus, and the treatment is begun. The hydraulic table moves the patient's head in and out of the gamma knife dome according to the specified time(s).

For CPBI and modified LINAC treatment, the patient is positioned on the couch, and the head with the stereotactic apparatus is secured. In addition to the isocenter coordinates and collimator size, the arc-start, arc-end, couch angle, gantry arc rotation interval, collimator field size, and other settings specific for the CPBI or modified LINAC are set.

The entire treatment is most often delivered on a single occasion and within a single day. Most patients treated in the United States are hospitalized overnight; in many other centers, they are treated as outpatients and released 1 or 2 h later.

VII. RADIOSURGERY OF SPECIFIC TUMORS

The following is a consideration of factors specific to the radiosurgical treatment of certain types of brain tumors and a summary of the results of treatment now published.

Evaluation of the results of radiosurgical treatment of tumors presents several special problems. It is a common dilemma in evaluation of the results of treatment of tumors that the cases with longest follow-up are the ones originally studied with diagnostic methods that are now outdated, whereas the more recent cases that have used current, state-of-the-art procedures have not been followed for sufficiently long periods to yield the most reliable data. Nowhere do we encounter this more than in radiosurgery. As we have previously mentioned, in the last 5 years we have seen major advances in the imaging and laboratory techniques so critical to successful treatment, and these not only significantly improve our ability to treat, but also enhance our ability to examine our results in follow-up. Treatment itself has also changed dramatically in the last 5 years. Of most significance here is the decrease in radiation doses now commonly given. It appears that with the reduction in radiation dose delivered to the tumor, the likelihood of complications is markedly reduced, without apparent change in the likelihood of tumor recurrence. Evaluation of the results of radiosurgery on tumors also presents special problems in terms of the time required to evaluate results. In this relatively new field, there is a period of months to years before the full benefit of the treatment itself is realized; and when we look at the special issues related to the treatment of tumors, such as regrowth, even more time is needed to establish our results. Finally, as with studies in any field, the early reports will necessarily be of only a few cases. Thus, the conclusions we draw from reports of the early work are important, but of limited predictive value, and reports on the more recent work still await long-term follow-up.

The results will be given here as one of two sets: those using the earlier imaging and laboratory techniques and having follow-up data for more than 3 years; and those using modern techniques and having follow-up data for up to 3 years.

A. Benign Tumors

1. *Meningiomas*

Meningiomas are often particularly suitable for radiosurgery because they frequently develop at sites at which complete microsurgical excision of the tumor is difficult or impossible and where the tumor involves critical structures, such as a carotid artery or its branches, a cavernous sinus, or one or more of the cranial nerves (Fig. 1). They often develop at such sites as the medial portion of the sphenoid wing, clivus, petrous apex, tentorium, or cerebellopontine angle. Attempts at complete microsurgical excision often lead to substantial neurological impairment or even death. For some of these patients, radiosurgery alone becomes a good alternative. For others, subtotal microsurgical removal of the tumor, followed by radiosurgery for destruction of the remnant is more effective.

More than 500 patients with meningiomas have now been treated with the gamma knife, and the results of treatment of approximately 150 of these have been reported.

One early study is a report of 30 cases with long-term follow-up (9 cases more than 10 years). The authors found a decrease in tumor size in 14; cessation of tumor growth in 12; and continued tumor growth in only 4 cases. Thus, for 86.7% of this admittedly small number of patients, tumor growth was stopped (26). These figures compare well with the relative rates of recurrence of meningioma after microsurgery when followed for similar lengths of time (27). Twenty of the 30 patients presented preoperatively with symptoms of cranial nerve dysfunction, 7 of these experienced complete resolution of these impairments, and 5 had partial resolution. Eighteen patients were clinically unchanged. No side effects or complications were observed (26).

Lunsford et al. have reported their results on 59 more recently treated patients followed for shorter periods. For patients followed for 12–36 months, tumor size had decreased in 31, was unchanged in 23, but was increased in 5. Intratumoral necrosis occurred in 22 of these patients (demonstrated by loss of contrast enhancement of follow-up imaging). Clinical improvement was observed in 9 patients and stabilization of neurological state in another 44. Only 6 patients deteriorated clinically. The results were similar for patients followed less than a year; but, because of the short follow-up period, reduced tumor size or clinical improvement was observed slightly less often (28,29). Reports of the few patients recently treated by Bunge et al. (followed for 6–36 months) and Forster et al. (followed for up to 24 months) show similar results (26).

Only one study of meningiomas treated with the modified LINAC has been published.

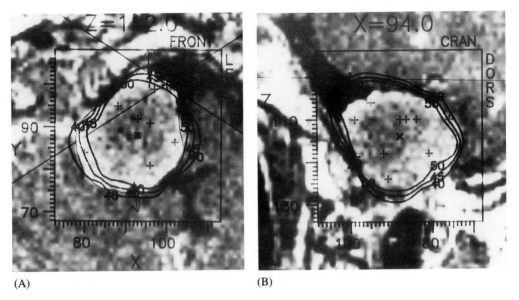

(A) (B)

Figure 1 Stereotactic MRI of 86-year-old woman with foramen magnum meningioma showing composite isodose distributions used for treatment. Nine overlapping isocenters required; MP-RAGE protocol with gadolinium-DTPA contrast enhancement: (A) axial and (B) sagittal projections.

Twenty-eight tumors were treated, 25 of which were located at the skull base. The patients were followed for 2–86 months (mean 27.3 months). Six were clinically improved, 17 were unchanged, and 2 were worse. Tumor size was distinctly smaller in 4 cases and unchanged in 19. Continued tumor growth was observed in 2 instances, and 1 patient experienced reduction in visual fields (30).

2. Acoustic and Other Neuromas

Acoustic neuromas constitute the largest group of tumors treated with radiosurgery. More than 800 have now been treated worldwide, and most were treated with the gamma knife. The microsurgical approach to these tumors is often difficult and associated with a high risk of injury to surrounding cranial nerves, vascular structures, brain stem, and cerebellum; hence, radiosurgery is an especially attractive alternative. The gamma knife is particularly useful here because complex dosimetry planning, using multiple overlapping isocenters, is usually required for a close fit to these highly irregularly shaped tumors (Figs. 2 and 3).

Two large series of patients with acoustic neuromas treated with gamma knife radiosurgery have recently been reported, one from the Karolinska Hospital in Sweden and one from the University of Pittsburgh.

Between 1969 and 1990, 227 procedures were done for acoustic neuroma at the Karolinska Hospital in patients who were followed postoperatively for 12–206 months (mean 54 months). Forty-nine patients had NF-2 with bilateral acoustic neuromas, and 10 of these underwent treatment of the tumors on both sides. One hundred and fourteen of these tumors decreased in size, and 79 showed no change. The remaining 34 showed continued growth over a 6- to 12-month period, but 13 of these stopped growing spontaneously after a year and remained inactive for the duration of the follow-up period. Nineteen of the 34 were given further treatment, either microsurgical excision (11 tumors) or a second gamma knife treatment (8 tumors) (31).

Patients with unilateral tumors fared better than those with the bilateral lesions associated with NF-2. Ninety-seven (56%) unilateral tumors decreased in size, and another 56 (32%) exhibited no change; whereas only 17 (32%) of bilateral NF-2 tumors decreased in size, and 23 (43%) showed no change. Only 21 (12%) of those that were unilateral continued to grow, but 13 (25%) of the bilateral NF-2 tumors showed continued growth.

The rate of complications compares favorably with that of published figures for microsurgery. Several patients developed facial paresis (16%) or numbness (12%) within the first 6–8 months of treatment, but this usually resolved completely over the next 6–12 months. Of 26 patients who had useful hearing before surgery, 7 (27%) retained useful hearing for at least 5 years; but in 2 (8%) patients, severe loss of hearing was observed by 1 year, and this was unchanged at 5 years. Some loss of vestibular function (caloric responses) was also seen. The incidence of transient facial weakness or numbness has recently been reduced to 5% or less, with no change in the likelihood of continued tumor growth, by the reduction in radiation dose (from 50–70 Gy to the center of the tumor and 25–35 Gy to the margin, to 15–25 Gy to the center and 10–15 Gy to the margin) (31). Whether this also reduces the incidence of hearing or vestibular function deficits has not yet been determined.

At the University of Pittsburgh 92 patients were treated and followed for up to 36 months (32–34). In this more recent series, radiation doses of 16–18 Gy to the tumor margin at or above the 50% isodose line were used to minimize complications. The tumor in 21 (23%) was decreased in size, was unchanged in 68 (74%), and larger in only 3 (3%) after an average period of 12 months following treatment. None of the 3 that measured larger has required microsurgical decompression. Loss of central tumor contrast enhancement (presumed central necrosis) was seen in 72 (78%) patients approximately 6 months following treatment. All these patients returned to the preoperative clinical level of function, as determined by Karnofsky performance score (KPS) rating.

Complications of cranial nerve dysfunction were also very uncommon. Facial (30%) and

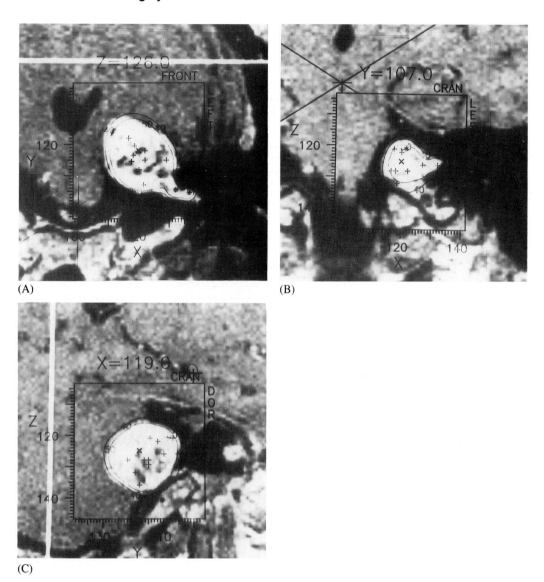

Figure 2 Stereotactic MRI of 35-year-old man with left acoustic neuroma showing composite isodose distributions used for treatment. Twelve overlapping isocenters used. Note tumor extending into porus acousticus and extension of isodose lines to include this; MP-RAGE protocol with gadolinium-DTPA contrast enhancement: (A) axial, (B) coronal, and (C) sagittal projections.

trigeminal (33%) neuropathies developed, but were partial at onset and improved notably with time. However, when the impairment was severe, recovery was usually incomplete. Useful hearing was preserved in 38% at 1 year, and no instance of further hearing loss was noted.

The treatment of acoustic neuromas with the CPBI and with the modified LINAC have recently been addressed (21,22,35), but information on the techniques and results have not yet been reported.

To date, there are no published reports on radiosurgery for the treatment of trigeminal, facial, or other nonacoustic neuromas. We have now treated, with the gamma knife, three patients with persistent trigeminal neuroma after craniotomy and one with persistent facial neuroma. Two of the trigeminal neuromas were within and adjacent to Meckel's cave and the third just rostral to the cerebellopontine angle and within the cavernous sinus. The facial neuroma was situated within the cerebellopontine angle. Three of the patients have now been followed for 6 months, including follow-up MRI scans, and the fourth—the posterior fossa and cavernous sinus trigeminal neuroma—for 3 months. In all four cases, the patients are neurologically at their preoperative level, and the tumor has not increased in size. We plan to continue with follow-up studies.

3. Sellar and Parasellar Tumors

Pituitary Adenomas. Pituitary adenomas were among the earliest to be treated with radiosurgery and are the only ones to have been treated in large number with the CPBIs. As of December 1990, 2710 patients with these tumors have received treatment at four sites, 475 at the Berkeley synchrocyclotron, 1083 at the Harvard cyclotron in Cambridge, 366 at the Burdenko Neurosurgical Institute in Moscow, and 312 at the Leningrad Institute of Nuclear Physics. The patients from these four centers include 1149 with acromegaly and growth hormone-secreting tumors, 535 with Cushing's disease and ACTH-secreting tumors, 264 with prolactinomas, 2 with thyrotropin-secreting tumors, and 220 for which no endocrine hypersecretion was identified (21).

For most patients with acromegaly, CPBI radiosurgery produced a reversal of clinical symptoms and reduction of growth hormone levels within 3–6 months, even though the charged particle radiation was administered at different centers and in different ways. At Berkeley, stereotactic helium ion plateau beam radiosurgery was used, with 30–50 Gy usually administered in four fractions over 5 days. For these patients, mean growth hormone levels decreased by 70% within the first year and further with time; and normal levels, achieved in some patients, were sustained for the long term (more than 10 years) follow-up (21,36). In Cambridge, Bragg-peak proton beam irradiation was used, with similar effectiveness. Clinical improvement was obtained in 90% of patients within 2 years, with 60% reduction of growth hormone levels (<10 ng/ml) (37). At the Moscow (38) and Leningrad (39) centers, plateau proton beam radiosurgery was administered, using single-fraction doses of 100–120 Gy, and partial or total remission was achieved in 89% of patients.

All four types of CPBI radiosurgery have also been effective in the treatment of Cushing's disease. The Berkeley team treated 83 such patients. The adult patients received 50–150 Gy to the pituitary gland in three or four fractions. More than 50% (44 patients) attained normal membrane cortisol levels within 1 year, and 35 patients attained normal dexamethasone suppression. All this was sustained for the 10-year follow-up period. Five of these patients were teenagers, who were treated with lower radiation doses (60–120 Gy), and all developed normal cortisol levels without hypopituitarism or neurological impairment. However 9 of 59 "older" patients failed to respond and eventually required bilateral adrenalectomy or surgical hypophysectomy (21,36,40). The Cambridge team used Bragg-peak proton beam radiation to treat 175 patients for Cushing's disease. Complete remission, with normal clinical and laboratory findings, was attained in 65% of patients, and another 20% were so improved that they required no further treatment (37). The Moscow team used plateau proton beam radiosurgery. Nearly all (34 of 37) their patients attained partial or total remission (38).

The Berkeley team treated 20 patients with prolactinomas using 50–150 Gy in four fractions over 5 days and followed them for at least 1 year. The serum prolactin level in 12 patients became normal within 1 year; and in 7 patients, the level decreased significantly. In Leningrad, an 85% partial or total remission was obtained, and at Cambridge and Moscow, "excellent results" were reported (39).

Gamma knife radiosurgery has also been used extensively for treating endocrinologically active and inactive pituitary adenomas (Fig. 4). At the Karolinska Hospital, 21 patients with acromegaly and small, growth hormone-producing microadenomas or locally invasive macroade-

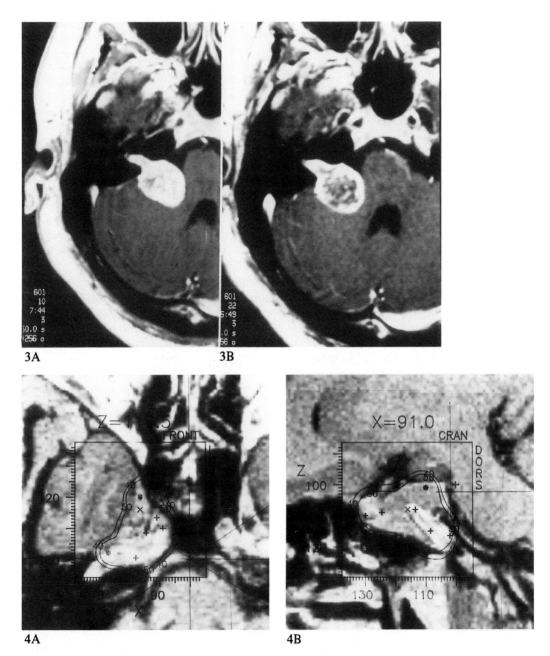

3A   3B

4A   4B

Figure 3 MRI scans of the left acoustic neuroma shown in Figure 2 (A) before and (B) 6 months after radiosurgery. Note decreased signal intensity within tumor in postoperative scan suggesting intratumoral necrosis; Gadolinium-DTPA contast enhancement; axial projection.

Figure 4 Stereotactic MRI of 36-year-old man with acromegaly and persistent growth hormone-secreting macroadenoma after transsphenoidal hypophysectomy. The remaining tumor involves the right cavernous sinus. Eight overlapping isocenters were required to completely cover the tumor. MP-RAGE protocol with gadolinium-DTPA contrast enhancement: (A) axial and (B) sagittal projections.

nomas were treated. Most of these patients had parasellar growth. Radiosurgery was the initial treatment for 7 patients; but 14 had undergone previous microsurgery, and 8 of these had also received external beam radiotherapy. For patients who had not previously received external beam radiotherapy, 40–70 Gy was administered to the tumor for each of up to three treatments. Previously irradiated patients received lower doses (30–50 Gy) each time. These patients were followed for 1–21 years.

Two patients attained complete clinical remission of their acromegaly, and their growth hormone levels came down to near normal levels. In eight patients there was a smaller change in clinical manifestations and growth hormone levels; and in 11, there were only minor changes or none. Only 2 of 13 patients for whom total pituitary function was assessed had developed pituitary insufficiency, and both had had prior external beam radiotherapy (41).

Treatment of patients with Cushing's disease and ACTH-producing tumors has also been reported by the gamma knife team at the Karolinska Hospital. This is a report of some very early work. They treated 35 adults (aged 18–65) (42–44) and 8 children (aged 6–18) (45). These patients all had the usual clinical manifestations, but 23 of 31 adults and all the children had normal sellar anatomy.

The adults were treated with high doses of radiation (70–100 Gy). This was administered in a single treatment and repeated, if needed, two or three times 5–55 months later. The patients were followed for 3–9 years. Fourteen patients (48%) attained complete clinical remission and normal urinary cortisol levels after a single such treatment. Eight patients were given two or three such treatments before they reached full clinical remission with near normal urinary cortisol levels. Five patients failed to respond and required bilateral adrenalectomy, and 12 of 22 adults with clinical remission developed panhypopituitarism.

The radiation dosage was also high for children (50–70 Gy). Seven attained a complete clinical remission with normal urinary cortisol levels. One patient failed to respond, even after a second radiosurgery procedure, required bilateral adrenalectomy, and eventually developed panhypopituitarism. All the children experienced a transient growth spurt and then stopped growing, which the authors suggest apparently reflected postoperative growth hormone deficiency and perhaps even panhypopituitarism.

Eight patients with nonsecreting pituitary tumors were also treated at the Karolinska Hospital. No change in tumor size was seen in four patients, and tumor growth occcurred in one (46).

The complications experienced in these cases of acromegaly and Cushing's disease are probably attributable to the less precise radiographic imaging available at time of treatment and to the high dose of radiation administered. Today, vastly improved imaging and much smaller doses of radiation are being used.

More recent treatment is reported from the University of Pittsburgh. Lunsford's team treated 18 patients with various pituitary tumors (4 acromegaly and growth hormone-secreting, 6 Cushing's disease and ACTH-secreting, 8 endocrinologically inactive) and followed them for up to 32 months. Histological diagnosis was confirmed preoperatively (previous biopsy or transsphenoidal hypophysectomy, 16; neuroradiologic imaging and endocrinological studies, 2). Nine patients had macroadenomas; that is, tumors larger than 1 cm in diameter, and 9 had microadenomas. Preoperative visual acuity and fields were normal in 12 patients, but slightly impaired in 6. Eleven were patients who had developed a recurrence after microsurgery, and five had had adjunctive external beam radiotherapy. For treatment, 28–60 Gy was administered. Individual dosage determination was based on tumor volume, whether blocking patterns were used in dosimetry planning, and whether adjunctive external beam radiation had previously been given (47).

At the time of longest follow-up, eight tumors had become smaller, nine were unchanged in size, and one tumor, a macroadenoma with unilateral extension into a cavernous sinus, showed continued growth. Three of the ten patients with hypersecretion exhibited normal hormonal levels within 3–5 months, and another three had levels that, although still elevated, were substantially reduced. Clinically, the 12 patients with normal visual acuity and fields before surgery were unchanged after treatment, and two of the six with preoperative visual impairment experienced very slight recovery. A sudden severe loss of vision occurred in one patient, a patient who had previously received external beam radiation.

Craniopharyngiomas.   Craniopharyngiomas are usually not treatable with radiosurgery because of their close proximity to the optic nerves and chiasm. However, the occasional one that develops along the lower portions of the pituitary stalk or within the sella itself can be safely treated. Radiosurgery is also often useful to deal with fragments of residual tumor after craniotomy or transphenoidal resection. Because of the proximity to the optic nerve structures, a distance of 3–5 mm between tumor and the overlying optic structures is required, and only the most carefully tailored dosimetry treatment is acceptable. This is best achieved by the gamma knife because of its special multifaceted ability to shape the radiation configuration.

At last count, 78 patients with craniopharyngioma had been treated with the gamma knife. Thirteen of these were patients treated at the Karolinska Hospital, 4 with their prototype model, the Gamma Unit I (9,48) and 9 with the Gamma Unit 2 (49). Nine patients had tumors that were largely cystic and had previously been treated by intracavitary radiation (3 with ^{32}P and 6 with ^{90}Y), and 4 had had prior craniotomy. Doses to the tumor margin of 20–50 Gy were given, which kept doses to the chiasm under 10 Gy. One patient, who received 20 Gy in a single isocenter, died later from an unrelated cause. In all the other patients, tumor growth stopped, and they were able to return to work. Two patients developed "visual impairment," but no loss of endocrine function or other morbidity was observed. Three such patients have also been treated at the University of Pittsburgh. Two had residual solid components after intracavitary radiation of the cystic tumor component with ^{32}P and had then undergone craniotomy and adjunctive external beam radiotherapy for treatment of the solid portion of the tumor. The third had undergone subtotal resection of the tumor within the third ventricle, but required radiosurgery for inactivation of a remnant as well as for tumor at a second site. Tumor growth was arrested in all cases; but, here again, those previously treated with external beam radiotherapy experienced additional visual impairment (50).

Other Skull Base Tumors.   Very little has been reported on the use of radiosurgery to treat such tumors. Seven cases have been treated at University of Pittsburgh with the gamma knife, and five at Stanford University with the modified LINAC.

At the University of Pittsburgh, four chordomas, two chondrosarcomas (51,52), and one squamous cell carcinoma involving the nasopharynx (53) were treated. Five patients (three with chordoma and two with chondrosarcoma) had undergone previous surgical debulking, and one (squamous cell carcinoma) had received adjunctive external beam radiotherapy and chemotherapy [doxorubicin (Adriamycin), pipleomycin, and cisplatin], both initially and at the time of the first tumor recurrence. Gamma knife radiosurgery was used to treat the second recurrence. For all these tumors, 20 Gy was given to the tumor margin at the 50% isodose line. The patients were followed for 7 to 36 months (mean <22 months); and although no recurrence within the treatment volume was observed, evidence of tumor growth was found later at other sites in two patients. Neurological impairments improved in three patients and were stable in the other four.

At Stanford University five patients were treated with the modified LINAC. Three patients had recurrent squamous cell carcinoma, one had recurrent mucoepidermoid carcinoma, and one had adenoidcystic carcinoma with cavernous sinus extension. At the time of radiosurgery, the tumor in four patients was considered unresectable, and the fifth patient rejected microsurgery. Four patients had received adjunctive external beam radiotherapy. For the radiosurgery, the patients were given 17.5–35 Gy to the tumor margin at the 80% isodose line and were followed for 5.5–7 months. In three patients, the tumor became smaller; and in the other two, was unchanged. All five patients improved in one or more of their preoperative symptoms (diplopia, trigeminal dysesthesia, cranial neuropathy, and headache) (54).

4. Pineal Region Tumor

The pineal region is extremely difficult to reach with microsurgery and, therefore, very suitable for treatment with radiosurgery. Many of these tumors, such as pineocytomas, are minimally invasive; and total destruction by radiosurgery can be achieved. For malignant lesions, such as metastases, pineoblastomas, and gliomas, radiosurgery can be used to destroy the solid portion of tumor, and adjunctive external beam radiotherapy can be added to control circumferential tumor cell infiltration. Again, very little has been published in this area.

At the University of Pittsburgh, nine patients were treated with the gamma knife. Four had meningiomas at the falcotentorial junction; two had anaplastic astrocytomas; one had ependymoma; one, a craniopharyngioma; and one, a pineocytoma. All had had their histological diagnosis established before radiosurgery. Six received adjunctive external beam radiotherapy, but three (one meningioma and two pineoblastomas) were treated with radiosurgery alone.

These patients were followed for up to 32 months (mean 20.7 months). Preoperatively, all patients were neurologically normal or nearly normal (KPS rating of 90–100%). Following radiosurgery, two patients had some impairment of extraocular movements; one had a subtle memory deficit; slight preoperative neurological impairments in two of the patients improved; and four others who were normal before treatment remained normal and have required no other treatment. The size of the tumor in six patients decreased after treatment, and in another three was unchanged (55).

At the Karolinska Hospital, two patients with pineocytoma were also treated with the gamma knife and adjunctive external beam radiotherapy, and the tumors reportedly disappeared on follow-up imaging studies (56).

At Vincenza, seven patients with small (<25 mm in diameter) germinomas were treated with the modified LINAC: 10–12 Gy was given with 25–30 Gy of adjunctive external beam radiotherapy. The patients were followed for 26–86 months. In all, the tumor size decreased markedly within a few days. Six patients are neurologically normal; the seventh died of an unrelated cause (57).

5. Other Benign Tumors

Published information is even more limited in this area. Fifteen patients with hemangioblastoma, 14 with glomus jugulare tumors (Fig. 5), and 13 with ocular melanoma, have been treated with the gamma knife. Lunsford et al., described two patients with hemangioblastoma in a review. One tumor developed within the cerebellar hemisphere and the other at the foramen magnum and medulla. Doses of 14 and 16 Gy, respectively, were delivered to the tumor margin (58).

B. Malignant Tumors

1. Metastases

Radiosurgery has been very useful for the treatment of brain metastases. The tumors usually develop within brain parenchyma and are spherical and well circumscribed, so treatment using one to three isocenters can be accomplished with any of the radiosurgery instruments (Fig. 6). So far, the radiosurgery has most often been given as a "boost" to external beam radiotherapy.

More than 400 patients with brain metastases have now been treated with the gamma knife, and the results of treatment of 65 patients with 86 metastases in two series have recently been reported. The histological diagnosis of the primary tumor or of the metastasis was established for all cases, and metastases from a variety of primary sites were treated. Metastases from malignant melanoma, non–small-cell lung carcinoma, and renal cell carcinoma were most common. Pre-

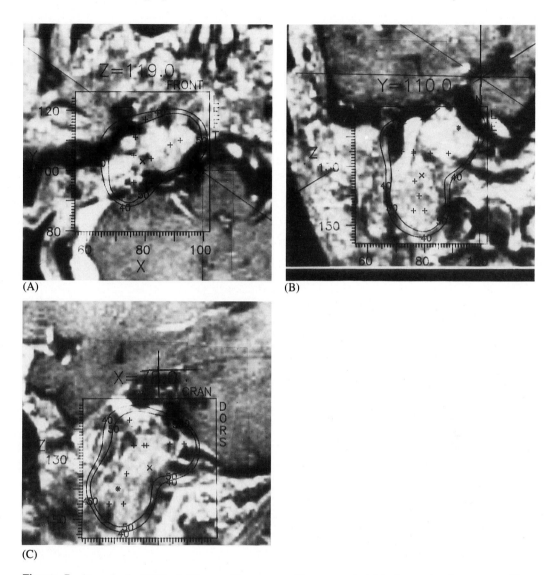

(A)

(B)

(C)

Figure 5 Stereotactic MRI of 68-year-old woman with recurrent right glomus jugulare tumor. Ten overlapping isocenters were required to cover the tumor; MP-RAGE protocol with gadolinium-DTPA contrast enhancement: (A) axial, (B) coronal, and (C) sagittal projections.

operative neurological deficits were observed in one series and were present in 18 of 31 patients, but all 31 patients were ambulatory and capable of self-care (KPS rating above 70). All but 1 patient (renal cell metastasis) received preoperative external beam radiotherapy. For the radiosurgery, most patients were treated at the 50th percentile isodose and received 16.1 Gy to the tumor margin (29.7 Gy to the center).

The patients in these two series were followed for 1–24 months and 6–84 months, and no neurological impairments or new seizure disorders have been observed. The metastases in 53 patients were reduced in size or no longer seen and were unchanged in nine. The tumors enlarged in only five patients, and this was due to continued tumor growth in only three cases. Fourteen of

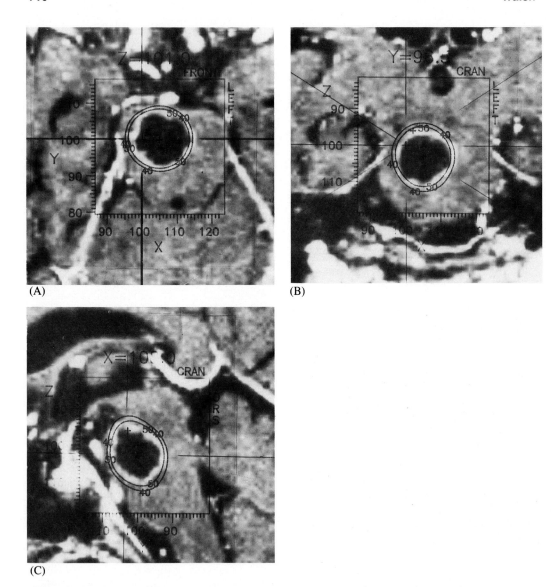

(A)   (B)

(C)

Figure 6 Stereotactic MRI of 85-year-old man with single brain metastasis showing composite isodose distributions used for treatment. Patient has non–small-cell carcinoma of the lung. Three overlapping isocenters were required; MP-RAGE protocol with gadolinium contrast enhancement: (A) axial, (B) coronal, and (C) sagittal projections.

31 patients in one series were clinically improved or stable, and 2 deteriorated. Twelve have now died, all from continued growth of their primary tumor, systemic dissemination of their tumor, or metastases at new brain sites. None had tumor recurrence at the radiosurgically treated site (58,59).

Brain metastases have also been a special target for treatment with the modified LINAC. The results of treatment of more than 220 patients have been reported. Most received preoperative external beam radiotherapy or had undergone craniotomy and tumor resection. In most, the tumor became smaller or remained the same; and clinically, the patients either improved or stabilized. At least 70 of these patients have died, most from uncontrolled growth of their primary tumor, systemic tumor dissemination, or metastasis in a new brain region, but two patients died of progression of tumor in the treated region (60–62).

2. Glial Tumors

The treatment of malignant gliomas (glioblastoma multiform, anaplastic astrocytoma, and low-grade astrocytomas) is more controversial. It has uniformly been performed as a "boost" to external beam radiotherapy or for treatment of a site of tumor recurrence after multimodality treatment.

Approximately 300 patients with gliomas have now been treated with the gamma knife, and the results of treatment of 26 of these patients (10 with glioblastoma, 6 with anaplastic astrocytoma, 5 with low-grade astrocytoma, and 5 with ependymoma) over a 3-year period have recently been reported. All had undergone biopsy or craniotomy and tumor resection or histological diagnosis and had received prior external beam radiotherapy. Some of the patients had received adjunctive chemotherapy or immunotherapy. All but 1 had preoperative neurological deficits, but their KPS scores were greater than 70. For the radiosurgery, 30–40 Gy was administered to the portion of solid tumor seen on a contrast-enhanced CT scan (Fig. 7).

Follow-up data on tumor size is available for 16 patients and on clinical status for 18. The tumor, seen on contrast-enhanced CT or MRI scans, was reduced in size or unchanged in 13; but increased in size in 3. Ten patients were clinically improved or stable and 6 patients were neurologically more impaired. Seven patients (6 with glioblastoma and 1 with anaplastic astrocytoma) have died (59,64).

The results of treatment with the modified LINAC of 76 patients with high-grade glioma (65) (52 glioblastoma, 24 anaplastic astrocytoma) and 16 for low-grade glioma (30) have also recently been reported. For 59 patients, radiosurgery was the primary form of treatment; and for 33, treatment was for tumor recurrence. The histological diagnosis of all tumors was determined by biopsy or craniotomy and tumor resection. The high-grade gliomas received external beam

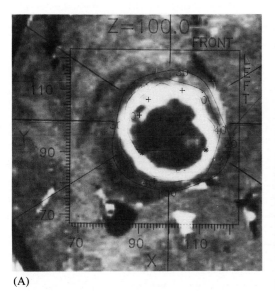
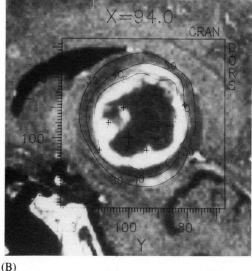

(A)   (B)

Figure 7 Stereotactic MRI of 17-year-old woman with glioblastoma multiforme in the right thalamus showing composite isodose distribution used for treatment. Twelve overlapping isocenters were used to cover the contrast-enhancing portion of tumor; MP-RAGE protocol with gadolinium-DTPA contrast enhancement: (A) axial and (B) sagittal projections.

radiotherapy a median of 14 months before the radiosurgery, and 29 of those with recurrent tumor received adjunctive chemotherapy. The low-grade astrocytomas were treated with radiosurgery alone. Just before radiosurgery, the patients all had a KPS above 60. Twenty-four patients with recurrent tumor are clinically stable. Six patients, with particularly large tumors (tumor volumes greater than 10 cm^3) and in whom multiple radiation isocenters were used, developed radiation-related complications, 2, "mild," and 4, "severe." Three others underwent subsequent craniotomy for tumor progression or radiation necrosis. Twenty-two patients with high-grade gliomas, but none with low-grade astrocytoma, died.

Treatment with the modified LINAC of 21 children with other tumors of glial origin and 1 dysgerminoma has been reported; except for recurrences secondary to tumor dissemination outside the radiosurgical treatment field, the results have been similar (22).

VIII. SUMMARY

Over 6000 tumors have now been treated with radiosurgery. Most of these have been with the gamma knife; but CPBI has been used for over 2700 pituitary adenomas, and small number of various types of tumor have also been treated with modified LINACs. The experience now gathered at the various centers and for a variety of benign and malignant tumors strongly indicates that radiosurgery is effective and remarkably safe. Analysis of this data is difficult because only a small number of studies have been reported; because the larger early studies were performed without the availability of modern neuroradiological and laboratory techniques and without an adequate knowledge about the optimum radiation dose required; and because with more recent studies, there has not been sufficient time for adequate patient follow-up.

Radiosurgery appears to be most effective and is an attractive alternative to microsurgery for the treatment of meningiomas, acoustic neuromas, pituitary adenomas, and brain metastases. Careful patient selection, state-of-the-art imaging, and meticulous dosimetry planning are essential, and a vigorous effort must be made to tailor the shape of the radiation precisely to that of the tumor to avoid exposing adjacent brain structures to the high dose of radiation.

REFERENCES

1. Leksell L. Stereotactic radiosurgery. J Neurol Neurosurg Psychiatry 1983; 46:797–803.
2. Wilson RR. Radiological use of fast protons. Radiology 946; 47:487–491.
3. Leksell L. The stereotaxic method and radiosurgery of the brain. Acta Chir Scand 1951; 12:316–319.
4. Leksell L, Herner T, Liden K. Stereotactic radiosurgery of the brain. Report of a case. Kungl Fysiogr Sallsk Lund Forhandl 1955; 25:1–10.
5. Larsson B, Leksell L, Rexed B, Sourander P, Mair W, Andersson B. The high-energy proton beam as a neurosurgical tool. Nature 1958; 182:1222–1223.
6. Leksell L, Larsson B, Andersson B, Rexed B, Sourander P, Mair W. Lesions in the depth of the brain produced by a beam of high-energy protons. Acta Radiol 1960; 54:251–264.
7. Leksell L, Larsson B, Rexed B. The use of high-energy protons for cerebral surgery in man. Acta Chir Scand 1963; 125:1–7.
8. Leksell L. Cerebral radiosurgery gammathalamotomy in two cases of intractable pain. Acta Chir Scand 1968; 134:585–595.
9. Bachlund EO. Stereotaxic treatment of craniopharyngiomas. In: Hamberger CA, Wersall J, eds. Nobel symposium 10. Disorders of the skull base region. Stockholm: Almqvist & Wiksell 1969:237–244.
10. Arndt J, Backlund EO, Larsson B, Leksell L, Noren G, Rosander K, Rahn T, Sarby B, Steiner L,

Wennerstrand J. Stereotactic radiation of intracranial structures. Physical and biological considerations. INSERM 1979; 12:81–92.

11. Dahlin H, Sarby B. Destruction of small intracranial tumours with ^{60}Co gamma radiation. Acta Radiol 1975; 14:209–227.

12. Lunsford LD, Flickinger JC, Lindner G, Maitz A. Stereotactic radiosurgery of the brain using the first United States 201 cobalt-60 source gamma knife. Neurosurgery 1989; 24:151–159.

13. Kjellberg RN, Koehler AM, Preston WM, Sweet WH. Stereotaxic instrument for use with the Bragg peak of a proton beam. Confin Neurol 1962; 22:183–189.

14. Fabrikant JI, Lyman JT, Hosoguchi Y. Stereotactic heavy-ion Bragg peak radiosurgery: method for treatment of deep arteriovenous malformations. Br J Radiol 1984; 57:479–490.

15. Betti OO, Derechinsky VE. Hyperselective encephalic radiation with linear accelerator. Acta Neurochir [Suppl] (Wein) 1984; 33:385–390.

16. Colombo F, Benedetti A, Pozza F, Avanzo R, Marchetti C, Chierego G, Zanardo A. External stereotactic radiation by linear accelerator. Neurosurgery 1985; 16:154–160.

17. Winston KR, Lutz W. Linear accelerator as a neurosurgical tool for stereotactic radiosurgery. Neurosurgery 1988; 22:454–464.

18. Kjellberg RN, Hanamura T, Davis KR, Lyons SL, Adams RD. Bragg-peak proton-beam therapy for arteriovenous malformations of the brain. N Engl J Med 1983; 309:269–274.

19. Flickinger JC. An integrated logistic formula for prediction of complications from radiosurgery. Int J Radiat Oncol Biol Phys 1989; 17:879–885.

20. Flickinger JC, Lunsford LD, Kondziolka D. Dose prescription and dose–volume effects in radiosurgery. Neurosurg Clin North Am 1992; 3:51–59.

21. Levy RP, Fabrikant JI, Frankel KA, Phillips MH, Lyman JT. Charged-particle radiosurgery of the brain. Neurosurg Clin North Am 1990; 1:955–990.

22. Alexander E III, Loeffler JS. Radiosurgery using a modified linear accelerator. Neurosurg Clin North Am 1992; 3:167–190.

23. Carbini CH, Goodman ML, Jones NH, Ford C. The use of magnetic resonance imaging in performing stereotactic surgery. In: Lunsford LD, ed. Stereotactic radiosurgery update, Proceedings of the international stereotactic radiosurgery symposium. New York: Elsevier Science Publishing, 1992:67–72.

24. Runge VM, Gelblum DY, Wood ML. 3-D imaging of the CBS. Neuroradiology 1990; 32:356–366.

25. Runge VM, Kirsch JE, Thomas GS, Mugler JP III. Clinical comparison of three-dimensional MP-RAGE and FLASH techniques for MR imaging of the head. JMRI 1991; 1:493–500.

26. Steiner L, Lindquist C, Steiner M. Meningiomas and gamma knife radiosurgery. In: Al-Mefty O, ed. Meningiomas. New York: Raven Press, 1991:263–272.

27. Simpson D. The recurrence of intracranial meningiomas after surgical treatment. J Neurol Neurosurg Psychiatry 1957; 20:22–39.

28. Kondziolka D, Lunsford LD, Coffey RJ, Flickinger JC. Stereotactic radiosurgery of meningiomas. J Neurosurg 1991; 74:552–559.

29. Kondziolka D, Lunsford LD. Radiosurgery of meningiomas. Neurosurg Clin North Am 1990; 3:219–230.

30. Colombo F, Pozza F, Chierego G, Casentini L. Linear accelerator radiosurgery: current status and perspectives. In: Lunsford LD, ed. Stereotactic radiosurgery update. Proceedings of the international stereotactic radiosurgery symposium. New York: Elsevier Science Publishing, 1992:37–45.

31. Noren G, Greitz D, Hirsch A, Lax I. Gamma knife radiosurgery in acoustic neuroma. In: Steiner L, Lindquist C, Forster D, Bachlund EO, eds. Radiosurgery: baseline and trends. New York: Raven Press, 1992:141–148.

32. Flickinger JC, Lunsford LD, Coffey RJ, Linskey ME, Bissonette DJ, Maitz AH, Kondziolka D. Radiosurgery of acoustic neurinomas. Cancer 1991; 67:345–353.

33. Linskey ME, Lunsford LD, Flickinger JC. Neuroimaging of acoustic nerve sheath tumors after stereotaxic radiosurgery. AJNR 1991; 12:1165–1175.

34. Linskey ME, Lunsford LD, Flickinger JC, Kondziolka D. Stereotactic radiosurgery for acoustic tumors. Neurosurg Clin North Am 1992; 1:191–205.

35. Friedman WA, Bova FJ, Spiegelmann R. Linear accelerator radiosurgery at the University of Florida. Neurosurg Clin North Am 1992; 3:141–166.

36. Lawrence JH, Linfoot JA. Treatment of acromegaly, Cushing's disease and Nelson syndrome. West J Med 1980; 133:197–202.

37. Kjellberg RN, Kliman B. Lifetime effectiveness—a system of therapy for pituitary adenomas, emphasizing Bragg peak proton hypophysectomy. In: Linfoot JA, ed. Recent advances in the diagnosis and treatment of pituitary tumors. New York: Raven Press, 1979:269–288.

38. Minakova YEI. Review of twenty years proton therapy clinical experience in Moscow. In: Proceedings of the second international charged particle workshop. Loma Linda, Calif, 1987:1–23.

39. Konnov B, Melnikov L, Zargarova O, et al. Narrow proton beam therapy for intracranial lesions. In: International workshop on proton and narrow photon beam therapy. Oulu, Finland: University of Oulu Printing Center, 1989:48–55.

40. Linfoot JA. Heavy ion therapy: alpha particle therapy of pituitary tumors. In: Linfoot JA, ed. Recent advances in the diagnosis and treatment of pituitary tumors. New York: Raven Press, 1979:245–267.

41. Thoren M, Rahn T, Guo W-Y, Werner S. Stereotactic radiosurgery with the cobalt-60 gamma unit in the treatment of growth hormone-producing pituitary tumors. Neurosurgery 1991; 29:663–668.

42. Thoren M, Rahn T, Hall K, Backlund EO. Treatment of pituitary dependent Cushing's syndrome with closed stereotactic radiosurgery by means of Co-60 gamma radiation. Acta Endocrinol 1978; 88:7–17.

43. Rahn T, Thoren M, Hall K. Bachlund EO. Stereotactic radiosurgery in Cushing's syndrome: acute radiation effects. Surg Neurol 1980; 14:85–92.

44. Degerblad M, Rahn T, Bergstrand G, Thoren M. Long-term results of stereotactic radiosurgery of the pituitary gland in Cushing's disease. Acta Endocrinol 1986; 112:310–314.

45. Thoren M, Rahn T, Hallengren B, Kaad PH, Nilsson KO, Ravn H, Ritzen M, Petersen KE, Aarskog D. Treatment of Cushing's disease in childhood and adolescence by stereotactic pituitary radiation. Acta Paediatr Scand 1986; 75:388–395.

46. Backlund EO, Bergstrand G, Hierton-Laurell U, Rosenborg M, Wajnot A, Werner S. Tumor changes after single dose radiation by stereotactic radiosurgery in "non-active" pituitary adenomas and prolactinomas. INSERM 1979; 12:199–206.

47. Stephanian E, Lunsford LD, Coffey RJ, Bissonette DJ, Flickinger JC. Gamma knife surgery for sellar and suprasellar tumors. Neurosurg Clin North Am 1992; 3:207–218.

48. Backlund EO. Solid craniopharyngiomas treated by stereotactic radiosurgery. INSERM 1979; 12:271–281.

49. Bachlund EO. Stereotaxic treatment of craniopharyngiomas. Acta Neurochir [Suppl] (Wien) 1974; 21:177–183.

50. Lunsford LD. Stereotactic treatment of craniopharyngiomas. Intracavitary radiation and radiosurgery. Contemp Neurosurg 1989; 11:1–6.

51. Kondziolka D, Lunsford LD, Flickinger JC. The role of radiosurgery in the management of chordoma and chondrosarcoma of the cranial base. Neurosurgery 1991; 29:38–46.

52. Lunsford LD. Stereotactic methods for diagnosis and treatment of skull base lesions. In: Sekhar LN, Schramm VL, eds. Tumors of the cranial base: diagnosis and treatment. Kisco: Futura Publishing, 1987:151–162.

53. Kondziolka D, Lunsford LD. Stereotactic radiosurgery for squamous cell carcinoma of the nasopharynx. Laryngoscope 1991; 101:519–522.

54. Adler JR, Hicks W Jr, Fuller B, Kaplan I, Goffiner D, Martin D, Fee W Jr. Stereotactic radiosurgery for the treatment of recurrent head and neck cancers of the cranial base. In: Lunsford LD, ed. Stereotactic radiosurgery update. Proceedings of the international stereotactic radiosurgery symposium. New York: Elsevier Science Publishing, 1992:453–456.

55. Dempsey PK, Lunsford LD. Stereotactic radiosurgery for pineal region tumors. Neurosurg Clin North Am 1992; 3:245–253.

56. Backlund EO, Rahn T, Sarby B. Treatment of pinealomas by stereotaxic radiation surgery. Acta Radiol (Ther) 1974; 13:3680376.

57. Casentini L, Colombo F, Pozza F, Benedetti A. Combined radiosurgery and external radiotherapy of intracranial germinomas. Surg Neurol 1990; 34:79–86.

58. Lunsford LD, Kondziolka D, Flickinger JC. Stereotactic radiosurgery: current spectrum and results. Clin Neurosurg 1991; 38:405–444.
59. Coffey RJ, Lunsford LD, Flickinger JC. The role of radiosurgery in the treatment of malignant brain tumors. Neurosurg Clin North An 1991; 3:231–244.
60. Kihlstrom L, Karlsson B, Lindquist C. Gamma knife surgery for brain metastases. In: Lunsford LD, ed. Stereotactic radiosurgery update. Proceedings of the international stereotactic radiosurgery symposium. New York: Elsevier Science Publishing, 1992:429–434.
61. Loeffler JS, Alexander E III, Wen PY, Fine HA, Kooy HM, Black PMcL. Radiosurgery for brain metastases: five year experience at the Brigham and Women's Hospital. In: Lunsford LD, ed. Stereotactic radiosurgery update. Proceedings of the international stereotactic radiosurgery symposium. New York: Elsevier Science Publishing, 1992:383–392.
62. Engenhart R, Romahn J, Gademann G, Muller-Schimpfle M, Jover K-H, Kimmig BN, Wannenmacher M. Indications for radiosurgery in treatment of brain metastases. In: Lunsford LD, ed., Stereotactic radiosurgery update. Proceedings of the international stereotactic radiosurgery symposium. New York: Elsevier Science Publishing, 1992:393–398.
63. Levin AB, Mehta M, Mackie R, Kudsad S. Stereotactic focused radiation in metastatic lesions to the brain. In: Lunsford LD, ed. Stereotactic radiosurgery update. Proceedings of the international stereotactic radiosurgery symposium. New York: Elsevier Science Publishing, 1992:445–451.
64. Dempsey PK, Kondziolka D, Lunsford DL, Coffey RJ, Flickinger JC. The role of stereotactic radiosurgery in the treatment of glial tumors. In: Lunsford LD, ed. Stereotactic radiosurgery update. Proceedings of the international stereotactic radiosurgery symposium. New York: Elsevier Science Publishing, 1992:407–410.

27

Chemotherapy of Brain Tumors: Fundamental Principles

William C. Welch
Albert Einstein College of Medicine, Bronx, New York

Paul L. Kornblith
University of Pittsburgh School of Medicine, Presbyterian
University Hospital, Pittsburgh, Pennsylvania

I. INTRODUCTION

The goal of all health care practitioners is to cure disease and preserve the quality of life. When one is faced with the malignant intracranial mass lesions, adequate control of the disease by any single treatment modality occurs infrequently. Traditionally, therapy has involved the combined techniques of cytoreductive and diagnostic surgery followed by radiotherapy. These combined modalities have increased the median survival of patients in most series from 14–16 weeks with surgery alone, to 36 weeks with surgery and radiotherapy (1–3).

Over the past three decades, therapies have been sought that would increase the duration and quality of life of patients with malignant intracranial lesions. In light of the impressive advances made with chemotherapy in the treatment of malignancies outside of the central nervous system, increased attention has been concentrated on the use of various agents in the adjunctive treatment of patients harboring central nervous system (CNS) malignancies.

The purpose of this chapter is to provide an understanding of the basic scientific principles used in the application of chemotherapeutic agents in the treatment of malignant, intracranial glial tumors. We will provide a select review of the mechanisms of action, delivery, theoretical and practical applications, and limitations of chemotherapeutic agents. We will also discuss factors that govern the effectiveness of various agents and techniques that can be used to influence the choice of chemotherapeutic agents.

II. BLOOD–BRAIN BARRIER

The brain is quite unlike other organ systems in the body in that there exists an effective barrier to the free exchange of components of the vascular system with neuronal cells. This blood–brain barrier is created by tight cellular junctions and lack of fenestrations of the brain capillary endothelial cells and basement membrane (4). Astrocytic foot processes may also play a role in the maintenance of this barrier. Nonionized agents with high lipid solubility are able to cross the vascular barrier and enter the brain with relative ease. Other chemicals may gain access to the brain by crossing vascular endothelial cells through nonspecific adsorptive transcytosis or receptor-mediated transcytosis (5).

Physiological areas exist within the CNS where brain effector organs responsible for endocrine functions and homeostasis have access to the intravascular compartment. These physiological areas of blood–brain barrier breakdown include the pineal body, posterior lobe of the pituitary, tuber cinerum, wall of the optic recess, area postrema, subfornical and commissural organs, and the choroid plexus. Pathological breakdown occurs with trauma, vasculitis, radiation, and infection. Infiltrating tumors, such as gliomas, will often cause a breakdown in proportion to the tumor malignancy (6). Corticosteroids can help improve the integrity of the barrier by stabilizing membranes (7).

All chemotherapeutic agents must reach their target cells (here, either malignant primary central nervous system or secondarily metastatic tumor cells) to be effective. Most effective central nervous system tumor chemotherapeutic agents (the chloroethyl nitrosoureas, in particular) are highly lipid-soluble. This property allows relatively free access to the entire central nervous system and permits the agents to reach not only the tumor mass, but also malignant cells located at a distance from the main mass.

When the use of lipid-soluble agents is not possible or if greater access to the brain parenchyma and tumor is desired, techniques of blood–brain barrier disruption are employed. This usually involves the intra-arterial infusion of mannitol and will be discussed later in the chapter.

III. CELL CYCLE KINETICS

During normal growth and development, a typical eukaryotic cell undergoes several divisions before becoming postmitotic. The processes of cellular division are called the cell cycle. The normal cycle is composed of four stages: G_1 (protein synthesis), S (DNA replication), G_2 (RNA synthesis), and M (mitosis). Post or nonmitotic cells (such as neuronal and glial cells) are said to be in a G_0 phase. Endothelial cells of the cerebral vasculature undergo slow cellular turnover. Transformed and cancerous cells, however, can freely replicate beyond the host's control and form tumors. When these tumors are examined histopathologically, one can appreciate dividing cells in mitosis, reactive cells, multinucleated cells, and necrosis (the latter is a required criterion to establish the diagnosis of glioblastoma multiforme). The pathophysiological correlates of these histological findings are further supported by DNA studies, such as radioactive thymidine DNA labeling. This labeling technique identifies cells in the S phase and enables one to create a labeling index (LI). This provides an estimation of the proliferative activity of the tumor and can correlate with the length of patient survival (8). Similar findings have been found using bromodeoxyuridine labeling of DNA (9). When using these studies, Hoshino and colleagues noted, in 110 glioblastoma multiforme tumors, that the median LI was 7.3% (8). With an S phase duration of 7–13 h, Hoshino calculated that highly malignant tumors would double in size every 5 days. Since this does not occur clinically, he estimated that approximately 85% of the malignant cells die.

The labeling indices also have therapeutic implications. Most tumor cells are not in the S phase at any given time. Unfortunately, most chemotherapeutic agents are effective only during a particular phase of the cell cycle (usually S). Therefore, all tumor cells are not killed uniformly through the administration of a single cycle of chemotherapy. Consequently, chemotherapeutic agents are administered in multiple cycles to kill cells as they enter the correct cell cycle phase.

IV. IN VITRO CHEMOSENSITIVITY TESTING

It is difficult to know if any given patient will respond to a particular chemotherapeutic agent. Most patients receive two or three courses of chemotherapy before conclusions are drawn about the in vivo sensitivity of their tumor to the chemotherapeutic agent. Predictive methods have been devised to help select agents that will arrest tumor growth in vivo. Unfortunately, no method is completely sensitive or specific. Two commonly performed in vitro assessments of drug sensitivity are the human tumor clonogenic assay (HTCA) and the monolayer clonogenic assay (MCA). In the HTCA assay, tumor cells are grown in soft agar and the colonies are counted. Serum and other additives are used to supply the needed nutrients. The MCA assay also uses serum and additives, but the cells are dispersed in a proteolytic solution and allowed to grow in a plastic flask. Whereas the HTCA system usually has a low colony forming efficiency (10), the latter usually has a much higher growth rate.

Both the MCA and the HTCA are capable of being used for in vitro chemosensitivity testing. In both techniques, the cells are collected (usually by removing them with mild trypsination) and counted. Following an exposure to various drugs at differing concentrations, the cells are replated. After a known time interval, the cells are harvested and viable cells (as determined by the ability to exclude vital dyes such as trypan blue, absorb discriminating fluorochromes (11), or incorporate thymidine into DNA) are counted. A graph is then constructed comparing cell survival to drug concentration.

Although obtaining good cell growth can be especially difficult with the HTCA system, there are shortcomings inherent in both systems. These include sample bias, subselection of a population of cells based on their in vitro growth characteristics, and establishing a clinically relevant definition of in vitro responsiveness. Also, as Berens and colleagues have clearly demonstrated, different in vitro cloning assays may yield different chemosensitivities to the same tumor cell lines (10). Despite this, cytotoxicity testing has been shown to be useful clinically. Kornblith and colleagues evaluated 14 patients who met the standard parameters used in evaluating a new chemotherapeutic agent (i.e., they received postoperative radiation therapy and completed at least two courses of a chemotherapeutic agent and had follow-up CT scans) for malignant glioma. Six of nine patients whose tumor cultures were sensitive to carmustine (BCNU) had in vivo responses to lomustine (CCNU), and none of the five patients whose tumor cultures were not sensitive to BCNU had in vivo responses to nitrosoureas (12). Other authors have found increased intervals to tumor recurrence using radioactive methenine uptake assays (13) (Fig. 1).

V. MODES OF DELIVERY

Various routes of delivery are available for the administration of chemotherapeutic agents (see also Chap. 30). The simplest, most readily accessible and most economical delivery process is oral administration. The agent most commonly given in this fashion is CCNU. We have found that patients readily tolerate this route because they can take the agent in the comfort of their home. The vast majority of agents, however, require intravascular access. This includes most of the chloroethyl nitrosoureas as well as cisplatin and diaziquone (AZQ). Patients are often able to receive the appropriate agent in an outpatient setting, but occasionally require brief hospital stays. It may be difficult to obtain intravenous access in oncology patients, and these patients may require the surgical placement of permanent indwelling catheters.

Intra-arterial treatment is an effective means of delivering high concentrations of chemotherapy directly to the region of interest while potentially reducing the risk of systemic toxicity (14). Tumors treated in this fashion have demonstrated acute metabolic changes on phosphorus magnetic resonance spectroscopy (15). Agents given intra-arterially have included BCNU (16,17) numustine (ACNU; 17), PCNU (18), HECNU (19), teniposide (VM-26) and cisplatin (16), etoposide (VP-16; 20), and AZQ (21).

Only BCNU has undergone a Phase III trial for efficacy of intracarotid administration, and it was not proved superior to systemically administered BCNU (22). Intra-arterial therapy has been associated with multiple complications, including depression of consciousness, paresis, loss of

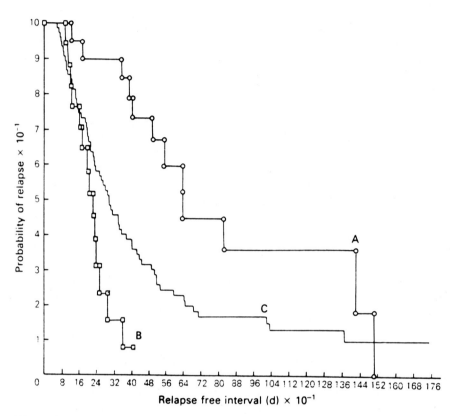

Figure 1 Kaplan–Meier survival plots of the relapse free intervals of patients with malignant gliomas who had been treated with the PCV protocol and were sensitive to PCB or CCNU *in vitro* (group A), those who were insensitive to either of these drugs (group B) and those patients who had not been tested *in vitro* (group C). (From Ref. 13)

visual acuity, aphasia (23), and white matter changes of the brain (24). Retinal injury has led to the acceptance of placement of the catheter above the ophthalmic artery (25). Neurological toxicities may be lessened with diastole-phased pulsatile infusions to reduce drug streamlining (26), and systemic toxicities may be reduced by the removal of the drug from the jugular return (27).

An interesting and innovative route of drug delivery has been the development of the "BCNU wafer" (28). A polyanhydride polymer was combined with BCNU and formed into wafers 1.4 cm in diameter and 1.0 mm thick. This polymer is biocompatible and is able to release diffusable BCNU in a controlled fashion. Patients who had recurrent malignant gliomas underwent surgical resection of their tumors. The wafers were then placed on the resection sites. The maximum patient dose was 102 mg. No patients had laboratory evidence of systemic exposure to BCNU. Ten of the 21 patients underwent reoperation (averaging 17–21 weeks postimplant). Necrotic tissue was found, with occasional remnants of the wafers, none of which had any BCNU remaining. The median survival times were comparable with patients who received surgery with radiation therapy and intravenous BCNU. This mode of therapy provides an extremely local application of BCNU at the site where malignant gliomas are most likely to recur.

The last portion of this chapter will address individual chemotherapeutic agents in more detail. Important clinical information about these agents has been obtained through the use of large prospective studies. Many studies, however, are retrospective, include small numbers of patients, and compare multiple differing drug regimens or adjuvant therapies. This makes evaluating the efficacy of individual agents difficult. Another factor that potentially complicates the interpretation of smaller retrospective studies is that of patient selection bias. Youthfulness, higher Karnofsky performance rating, anaplastic astrocytoma, and complete resection of tumor, all are associated with better patient outcomes. There is a clinical suggestion that tumors with oligodendroglioma components seem particularly sensitive to chloroethyl nitrosourea agents, but this has not been well analyzed.

If patients with these criteria are overrepresented in the treatment group, it is reasonable to expect that their outcomes will be better than those patients who receive similar treatments, but have poor prognostic factors, such as advanced age, poor Karnofsky performance rating, and inability to obtain complete surgical resection. The histological diagnosis of glioblastoma multiforme also confers a poorer prognosis, but in some studies, clear distinctions are not made between glioblastoma multiforme and less aggressive (anaplastic) astrocytomas.

VI. CHEMOTHERAPEUTIC AGENTS: AN OVERVIEW

There are multiple chemotherapeutic agents available to the practitioner interested in treating intracranial tumors. Although patients with brain metastases, medulloblastomas, ependymomas, pineal region tumors, aggressive meningiomas, and other neoplasms receive chemotherapy, most studies of the adult population examine treatment regimens of astrocytic tumors.

The N-(2-chloroethyl)-N–nitrosoureas (CNUs) are compounds that have been used for the past 15 years in the treatment of malignant astrocytic tumors. These compounds have been the mainstay of the chemotherapeutic armamentarium and have been custom-designed to accentuate certain molecular properties. Most of the CNUs share a basic mechanism of action (i.e., DNA interstrand cross-linking, which is probably responsible for the cytotoxic action of the CNUs (29). After entering the vascular system, CNUs decompose into two active components: 2-chloroethyl diazohydroxides (CEDH) and isocyanates. The 2-chloroethyl diazohydroxide component causes an alkylative cross-linking of DNA to occur at an O^6-guanine residue. The cross-linking may begin with the 7 nitrogen of guanine. This N^7-guanine can become alkylated and recognize thymine as complementary (instead of adenine), leading to miscoding of the DNA chain. The alkylated N^7 also renders the DNA chain susceptible to depurination by the excision of guanine residues, again damaging the DNA chain (30). It may also allow the formation of intrastrand cross-links.

The O^6-guanine alkylation allows an ethylene bridge to be then formed to a cytosine residue on the complementary strand of DNA over the course of 6–12 h. This completes the interstrand cross-link. A repair enzyme (O^6-methylguanine-DNA-methyltransferase), which is present in CNU-resistant cells (called Mer$^+$), can prevent this cross-linking from occurring and confers some immunity from this mechanism of CNU cytotoxicity. Nonmetastatic brain tumors have shown a wide range of O^6-methylguanine-DNA-methyltransferase activity (31). This activity may inversely correlate with clinical response to CNUs.

The isocyanate component generated in the breakdown of CNUs reacts with proteins to form carbamoyl derivatives. These isocyanates may interfere with the effectiveness of the CNU and expose the patient to unnecessary toxic effects (32). There is recent in vitro evidence suggesting that the carbamoylation activity may enhance CNU cytotoxicity by inhibiting DNA repair enzymes (33) and esterases (34).

The major toxicity of CNU therapy is the delayed onset of suppression of both bone marrow and lymphoid elements. These hematological elements usually require 4–6 weeks to recover. Unfortunately, the myelosuppressive response may be cumulative and is the single most important factor that limits the frequency that these agents can be given. Recently, factors that stimulate the production of marrow and lymphoid elements have become clinically available through the application of recombinant DNA technology. Granulocyte–macrophage colony-stimulating factor

(GM-CSF) is one such agent. This factor has undergone Phase II trials and reduces the morbidity associated with the administration of myelotoxic agents by raising neutrophil counts (35).

Pulmonary fibrosis and hepatic dysfunction is seen in patients receiving large doses of CNUs. Intra-arterial BCNU has been associated with retinal injury and leukoencephalopathies, which are probably due to its carbamolytic effects. Nausea and vomiting are also common with repeated applications of chemotherapy. In summary, the alkylating CNU agents interfere with DNA at multiple sites. This limits the mitotic processes of rapidly dividing cells and is responsible for both the therapeutic and toxic effects.

VII. CHEMOTHERAPEUTIC AGENTS: SPECIFIC

A. *N*(2-Chloroethyl)-*N*-nitrosoureas

It is useful to divide the CNUs into three clinically significant categories: lipid-soluble CNUs (BCNU, ACNU), water-soluble CNUs (HECNU), and those with an amide group [1-(2-chloro-ethyl)-3-(2,6-dioxy-3-piperidyl)urea PCNU].

1. Carmustine

Carmustine (BCNU) has been the best characterized CNU in clinical use for the treatment of intracranial tumors. It was first used in the 1960s and is the only CNU to have undergone a Phase III trial for intra-arterial use. Most new chemotherapeutic agents for use in CNS tumors are compared with BCNU for efficacy and safety, and many trials of multiple drug regimens use BCNU. A cooperative study in 1978 (37) compared supportive care with BCNU or radiation therapy (RT) or both in 222 patients who had undergone resection of anaplastic astrocytoma or glioblastoma multiforme. Fifty-one patients received BCNU only (median of two doses) and 72 patients received BCNU and radiation therapy (median of three doses). Carmustine alone increased median survival 4.5 weeks ($p = 0.119$) over supportive care (14 weeks). RT increased median survival to 36 weeks ($p = 0.001$). The combination of BCNU and radiotherapy (RT) did not offer significant survival benefits to RT alone. At 18 months, however, a greater survival rate was noted for patients who received BCNU.

A series of more recent studies do demonstrate increased median survival time (MST) in patients receiving BCNU after RT. Walker and colleagues (38) performed a subsequent randomized prospective study of 358 patients and found that the group that received both RT and BCNU had a greater number of long-term survivors (MST of 51 vs 36 weeks for the RT-only group). Chang (39) examined a treatment plan of 535 patients that compared RT versus RT and either BCNU or methyl-CCNU and imidazolcarboxamide. He found a MST of 10 months in the BCNU and RT group (the best survival of all groups). In 1983, Green and colleagues (40) examined 527 patients with malignant gliomas. The treatment groups consisted of RT and various chemotherapeutic regimens. Again, the BCNU plus RT group had the greatest MST. Other large studies have used the RT plus BCNU group as a standard by which various other treatment regimens are compared (41–43).

Carmustine has been used in combination with other chemotherapeutic agents and RT. Most studies have not demonstrated significant improvement in survival times when compared with RT or BCNU alone. One study did show a 67-week MST for patients with glioblastoma multiforme by combining BCNU with ifosfamide (44), but these results will need to be confirmed in future studies.

Carmustine can be given intravenously, intra-arterially, and topically as "wafers." In an effort to further improve the MST of patients with astrocytomas, high doses of BCNU can be given in combination with autologous bone marrow transplantation (ABMT). Researchers at Wilford Hall USAF Medical Center treated 25 patients with 350 mg/m^2 of intravenous BCNU followed by infusion of the patient's cryopreserved marrow 3 days later. Whole-brain RT was administered after the absolute granulocyte count exceeded $1500/\mu l$. Sixty-one percent of patients had a "complete response" (i.e., no identifiable tumor on follow-up CT scans at 12–18 months following transplantation), and 66% demonstrated a decrease in the size of the residual mass (45). Mbidde and colleagues (46) studied 22 patients with glioblastoma multiforme. Each patient received 800–1000 mg/m^2 of BCNU with ABMT and whole-brain irradiation. Historical controls were used. The complication rate (including acute and delayed myleosuppression, lung and liver toxicity) was fairly high, and MST was 17 months.

Clearly, some patients have benefited from this aggressive ABMT/high-dose chemotherapy/whole-brain radiation therapy treatment. In light of the known complications of ABMT, most neuro-oncologists reserve this treatment regimen for those patients who have failed other therapies.

2. Lomustine

Lomustine (CCNU) is another clinically important CNU. It is insoluble in aqueous media and, therefore, is given orally. Its mechanism of action is similar to that of BCNU. Lomustine has undergone multiple clinical trials with good therapeutic results. One of the first trials was published in 1972 (47). In that study, 15 patients with recurrent symptomatic glioblastoma multiforme received CCNU and 5 patients responded (33%). Unfortunately, none of the 4 patients who were previously treated with BCNU responded. This demonstrates that tumor cells can exhibit cross-resistance to CNUs. This in vivo phenomenon may be explained by in vitro studies that show that tumor strains resistant to CNUs produce an enzyme (O^6 methylguanine-DNA-methyltransferase) that reduces DNA cross-linking (31,33). Rosenblum and colleagues (48) treated 26 patients with malignant brain tumors, primarily glioblastoma multiforme, and found a 37% remission rate " . . . for all patients in this study and 43% for all with primary brain tumors regardless of prior radiotherapy." Lomustine has been used in combination with other agents with mixed results (9,50). In light of the 30–40% response rate, oral administration and excellent patient acceptance, it has been our policy to place most patients with either primary or recurrent astrocytomas (who have a good Karnofsky performance score) on a regimen of CCNU as an initial chemotherapeutic agent. Our patients receive 100–150 mg/m^2 every 6 weeks, with close monitoring of red and white blood cell counts. Magnetic resonance imaging (MRI) scans are performed monthly until the pattern of tumor responsiveness is documented. Steroids are tapered whenever possible. Our overall response rate (as determined by tumor regression or by absence of tumor growth) is 30–40% (Figs. 2–6). Whenever possible, we culture the tumor cells and submit them to MCA in vitro chemosensitivity testing.

3. Numustine

Numustine [1-(4-Amino-2-methyl-5-pyrinidimyl)-methyl-3-(2-chloroethyl)-3-nitrosourea; ACNU] is also a lipid-soluble CNU. It has had relatively common use in Europe and Japan. It has good blood–brain barrier penetration, low carbamoylation activity and does not require ethanol as a vehicle. Takakura and colleagues (51) compared 37 patients who received TR alone with 40 patients who received RT and ACNU. Fifty-eight percent of patients had glioblastoma multiforme and 42% had grade III astrocytomas. Although the ACNU–RT group often had reduction in tumor size and clinical improvement, the survival times were not significantly different between the RT and RT–ACNU groups.

Intracarotid BCNU and ACNU with phenobarbital protection has been used with success in oligodendrogliomas and lower-grade gliomas (52). The results were poor with glioblastoma multiforme, but encouraging in lower-grade gliomas.

4. 1-(2-Chloroethyl)-1-nitroso-3-(2-hydroxyethyl)urea

The drug HECNU is a water-soluble CNU that acts primarily as an alkylating agent. Forty patients with recurrent glioma (all of whom received 550–6200 rad of radiation therapy) were entered into a

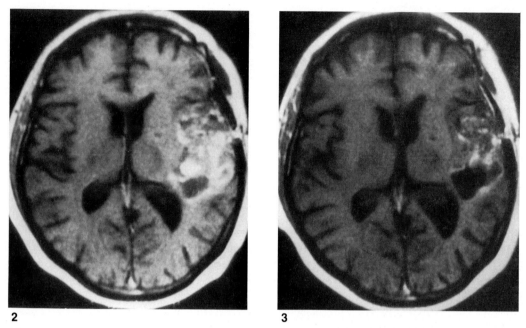

2   3

Figures 2 and 3 A 41-year-old patient with recurrent glioblastoma multiforme following whole-brain radiation therapy. The CT scans were obtained at 10-week intervals following two courses of CCNU.

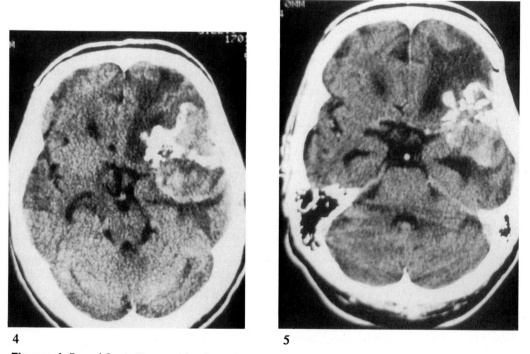

4   5

Figures 4, 5, and 6 A 49-year-old patient who received a craniotomy and whole-brain radiation therapy. His tumor recurred (mixed oligodendroglioma and anaplastic astrocytoma) and he was treated with seven courses of CCNU. The CT scans were performed over 12 months and demonstrate reduction and stabilization of tumor.

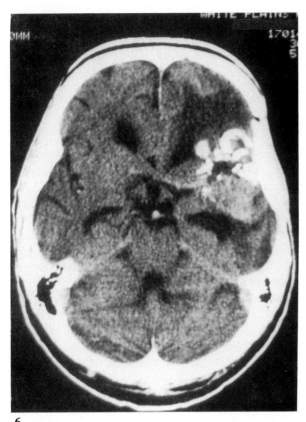

6

prospective trial of intravenous HECNU with a dose of 120–130 mg/m^2 (53). Fifty-five percent of patients showed clinical improvement with chemotherapy and steroids, and 42% of patients deteriorated (17 of 18 of the patients had anaplastic astrocytoma or glioblastoma multiforme). Thirty-two percent of all patients had CT scan evidence of partial or total tumor remission. Toxic effects (including hepatic, myelocytic, and renal) were generally more mild than that seen with BCNU.

Infraophthalmic intracarotid injections of HECNU were performed in 53 patients with recurrent supratentorial gliomas (54). A maximum of 200 mg of HECNU was given to any patient; 49% of patients responded (33% response rate in glioblastoma multiforme, 50% in anaplastic astrocytomas, and 92% in malignant recurrences of low-grade astrocytomas). Complications included monocular blindness in 11% and leukoencephalopathy in 11% of cases. Myelotoxicity was mild and reversible.

5. 1-(2-Chloroethyl)-3-(2,6-dioxy-3-piperidyl)urea

The nitrosourea PCNU, with an amide group, is the last category of CNUs to be considered. It has a short half-life, which lends itself to intra-arterial use. Seventeen patients received up to 110 mg/m^2 in a Phase I study by Stewart et al. (18). The drug was administered by the infraophthalmic route in 16 of these patients who had recurrent gliomas. The response rate was 44%. Although most patients received no more than two doses of PCNU, toxicities included ipsilateral blindness (18%), permanent neurological deficits (12%), transient myelosuppression, and others. The authors felt that intra-arterial PCNU offered no advantage over intravenous PCNU or intracarotid BCNU.

B. Other Adjuvant Chemotherapeutic Agents

Chemotherapeutic agents other than CNUs have been used in the treatment of patients with malignant gliomas. Two of these agents include AZQ and procarbazine.

1. Diaziquone

Diaziquone (AZQ) is a lipophilic, alkylating agent similar to the CNUs with similar toxicities (55). It also possesses the ability to injure mitochondria (56). Multiple Phase II trials have been reported using this agent to treat recurrent CNS neoplasms. Ninety-three patients with recurrent primary CNS neoplasms following RT (including 49 patients who had received prior chemotherapy) were treated with intravenous AZQ (57). A 2-month period to tumor regression was noted in 24 patients and associated with grade IV and gemistocytic cell types. The MST for all patients was 5.6 months (7.3 months for patients who had not received prior chemotherapy and 4.7 months for those who had).

The Southwest Oncology Group studied 15 good-risk patients (i.e., no prior chemotherapy) and 36 poor-risk patients (those who had received prior chemotherapy) with histologically confirmed grade III or IV astrocytoma, ependymoblastoma, medulloblastoma, or oligodendroglioma (58). The MST for 13 of the good-risk patients was 14 weeks, and the MST for 26 of the poor-risk patients was 15 weeks. The authors felt that AZQ administered on an intermittent bolus schedule ". . . is not active in patients with recurrent grades III and IV astrocytomas . . ." Two other studies report 24% tumor regression (59,60). Schold and colleagues compared the combination of AZQ and BCNU with AZQ and procarbazine. No differences in response rates between the two regimens was noted (61). The in vitro responsiveness of AZQ is similar to the in vivo effectiveness found in glioma cell cultures (63).

2. Procarbazine

Procarbazine (PCB) is a cytotoxic agent used frequently in the treatment of Hodgkin's disease. Its mechanism of action is not fully understood, but PCB probably functions as a cytotoxic agent by inhibiting the synthesis of protein, DNA, and RNA. Green and colleagues (40) used a four-arm study to compare (in 527 valid study group patients who received surgery and RT for supratentorial malignant glioma): BCNU; high-dose methylprednisolone; BCNU and methylprednisolone; and procarbazine. After controlling for 16 variables, the authors found that patients receiving either PCB or BCNU alone had similar survival rates (i.e., MST 47 and 50 weeks, respectively), both of which were better than the methylprednisolone groups. Two hundred forty-three patients who had received RT following surgery for malignant glioma were compared in a three-arm study of adjunctive therapy using BCNU, PCB, or dacarbazine (DTIC, a radiosensitizer) (63). Complete and partial response rates were rare in patients receiving PCB (13%), but more common in patients receiving BCNU (39%) or DTIC (38%). Median survival times were 31, 45, and 49 weeks, respectively. Many studies have used PCB in combination with other chemotherapeutic agents, but toxic effects (such as granulocytopenia, gastrointestinal and dermatological problems) have limited its usefulness.

In summary, no single or group of chemotherapeutic agents is ideal for the treatment of malignant gliomas. Most larger clinical trials do support the adjuvant use of a chloroethyl nitrosoureas in patients who have undergone surgical resection of tumor and will receive radiotherapy. Carmustine has been the most widely studied agent and is effective in 30–40% of patients. Our policy has been to use CCNU orally in younger patients who are functioning well, preferably in conjunction with in vitro chemosensitivity testing. We feel that this offers patients a high quality of life and the longest relapse-free interval.

REFERENCES

1. Baglan RJ, Marks JE. Comparison of symptomatic and prophylactic irradiation of brain metastases from oat cell carcinoma of the lung. Cancer 1981; 47:41–47.
2. Salcman M. Survival in glioblastoma: historical perspective. Neurosurgery 1980; 7:435–439.
3. Walker MD, Green SB, Byar DP, et al. Randomized comparisons of radiotherapy and nitrosoureas for the treatment of malignant glioma after surgery. N Engl J Med 1980; 303:1323–1329.
4. Brightman MW, Reese TS. Junctions between intimately opposed cell membranes in the vertebrate brain. J Cell Biol 1969; 40:648–677.
5. Salcman M, Broadwell RD. The blood brain barrier. In: Salcman M, ed. Concepts in neurosurgery: neurobiology of brain tumors. Baltimore: Williams & Wilkins, 1991:145–159.
6. Osborn AG. Introduction to cerebral angiography. Philadelphia: Harper & Row. 1980:276.
7. Marshall LF. Treatment of brain swelling and brain edema in man. Adv Neurol 1980; 28:459–469.
8. Hoshino T. Cell kinetics in brain tumors. In: Salcman M, ed. Concepts in neurosurgery: neurobiology of brain tumors. Baltimore: Williams & Wilkins, 1991:145–149.
9. Yoshii Y, Maki Y, Tsuboi K, Tomono Y, Nakagawa K, Hoshino T. Estimation of growth fraction with bromodeoxyuridine in human central nervous system tumors. J Neurosurg 1986; 65:659–663.
10. Berens ME, Giblin JR, Dougherty DV, Hoifoat HK, Tveit K, Rosenblum ML. Comparison of in vitro cloning assays for drug sensitivity testing of human brain tumors. Br J Neurosurg 1988; 2:227–234.
11. Bowles AP, Pantazis CG, Wansley W, et al. Chemosensitivity testing of human gliomas using a fluorescent microcarrier technique. J Neurooncol 1990; 8:103–112.
12. Kornblith PL, Smith BH, Leonard LA. Response of cultured human brain tumors to nitrosoureas: correlation with clinical data. Cancer 1981; 47:255–265.
13. Thomas DGT, Darling JL, Paul EA, et al. Assay of anticancer drugs in tissue culture: relationship of relapse free interval (RFI) and in vitro chemosensitivity in patients with malignant cerebral gliomas. Br J Cancer 1985; 51:525–532.
14. Fenstermacher JD, Cowles AL. Theoretic limitations of intra-carotid infusions in brain tumor chemotherapy. Cancer Treat Rep 1971; 61:519–526.
15. Arnold DL, Shoubridge EA, Feindel W, Villemure JG. Metabolic changes in cerebral glioma within hours of treatment with intra-arterial BCNU demonstrated by phosphorous magnetic resonance spectroscopy. Can J Neurol Sci 1987; 14:570–575.
16. Stewart DJ, Grahovac Z, Hugenholtz H, Russell N, Richard M, Benoit B. Combined intra-arterial and systemic chemotherapy for intracerebral tumors. Neurosurgery 1987; 21:207–214.
17. Loew F, Papvero L. The intra-arterial route of drug delivery in the chemotherapy of malignant brain tumors. Adv Tech Stand Neurosurg 1988; 16:51–79.
18. Stewart DJ, Grahovac Z, Russell NA, et al. Phase I study of intracarotid PCNU. J Neurooncol 1987; 5:245–250.
19. Poisson M, Chiras J, Fauchon F, Debussche C, Delattre JY. Treatment of malignant recurrent glioma by intra-arterial, infra-ophthalmic infusion of HECNU 1-(2 chloroethyl)-1-nitroso-3-(2-hydroxyethyl) urea—a phase II study. J Neurooncol 1990; 8:255–262.
20. Feun LG, Lee YY, Yung WK, Savaraj N, Wallace S. Intra-carotid VP-16 in malignant brain tumors. J Neurooncol 1987; 4:397–401
21. Greenberg HS, Ensminger W, Layton P, et al. A phase 1–2 evaluation of intra-arterial diaziquone (AZQ) for malignant tumors of the central nervous system [abstract]. Proc Annu Meet Am Soc Clin Oncol 1984; 3:256.
22. Johnson WD, Parkinson D, Wolpert SM, et al. Intra-carotid chemotherapy with 1,3-bis(2-chloroethyl)-1-nitrosourea (BCNU) in 5% dextrose in water in the treatment of malignant glioma. Neurosurgery 1987; 20:577–580.
23. Mahaley MS, Whaley RA, Blue M, Bertsch L. Central neurotoxicity following intra-carotid BCNU chemotherapy for malignant gliomas. J Neurooncol 1986; 3:297–314.
24. Kleinschmidt-DeMaster BK, Geier MJ. Pathology of high dose intra-arterial BCNU. Surg Neurol 1989; 31:435–443.
25. Kapp JP, Vance RB. Supraophthalmic carotid infusion for recurrent glioma: rationale, technique and preliminary results for cisplatin and BCNU. J Neurooncol 1985; 3:5–11.

26. Saris SC, Blasberg RG, Carson RE, et al. Intravascular streaming during carotid artery infusions. J Neurosurg 1991; 74:763–772.
27. Oldfield EH, Dedrick RL, Yeager RL, et al. Reduced systemic drug exposure by combining intra-arterial chemotherapy with hemoperfusion of regional venous drainage. J Neurosurg 1985; 63:726–732.
28. Brem H, Mahaley MS, Vick NA, et al. Interstitial chemotherapy with drug polymer implants for the treatment of recurrent gliomas. J Neurosurg 1991; 74:441–446.
29. McCormik JE, McElhinney RS. Perspectives in cancer research—nitrosoureas from chemist to physician: classification and recent approaches to drug design. Eur J Cancer 1990; 26:208
30. Shaprio R. Chemistry of guanine and its biologically significant derivatives. Prog Nucleic Acid Res Mol Biol 1968; 8:73–112.
31. Yarosh DB. The role of O^6-methylguanine-DNA-methyltransferase in cell survival, mutagenesis and carcinogenesis. Mutat Res 1985; 145:1–16.
32. Kohn KW. Prospects for improved chloroethylnitrosoureas and related haloethylating agents. In: Kornblith PL, Walker MD, ed. Advances in neuro-oncology. Mt Kisco, NY: Futura Publishing, 1988:491–513.
33. Ali-Osman F, Stivengopal K, Berger MS, Stein DA. DNA interstrand cross linking and strand break repair in human glioma cell lines of varying (1,3-bis(2-chloroethyl)-1-nitrosourea resistance. Anticancer Res 1990; 10:677–682.
34. Dive C, Workman P, Watson JV. Inhibition of intracellular esterases by antitumor chloroethylnitrosoureas. Biochem Pharmacol 1988; 37:3987–3993.
35. Hermann F, Schulz G, Wieser M, et al. Effect of granulocyte–macrophage colony-stimulating factor on neutropenia and related morbidity induced by myelotoxic chemotherapy. Am J Med 1990; 88:619–624.
36. McCormick JE, McElhinney RS. Perspectives in cancer research—nitrosoureas from chemist to physician: classification and recent approaches to drug design. Eur J Cancer 1990; 26:207–221.
37. Walker MD, Alexander E, Hunt WE, et al. Evaluation of BCNU and/or radiotherapy in the treatment of anaplastic gliomas. J Neurosurg 1978; 49:333–343.
38. Walker MD, Green JB, Byar DP, et al. Randomized comparisons of radiotherapy and nitrosoureas for the treatment of malignant glioma after surgery. N Engl J Med 1980; 303:1323–1329.
39. Chang CH, Horton J, Schoenfeld D, et al. Comparison of postoperative radiotherapy and chemotherapy in the multidisciplinary management of malignant gliomas. Cancer 1983; 52:997–1007.
40. Green SB, Byar DP, Walker MD, et al. Comparisons of carmustine, procarbazine, and high-dose methylprednisolone as additions to surgery and radiotherapy for the treatment of malignant glioma. Cancer Treat Rep 1983; 67:121–132.
41. Deutsch M, Green SB, Strike TA, et al. Results of a randomized trial comparing BCNU plus radiotherapy, streptozotocin plus radiotherapy, BCNU plus hyperfractionated radiotherapy, and BCNU following misonidazole plus radiotherapy in the postoperative treatment of malignant glioma. Int J Radiat Oncol Biol Phys 1989; 16:1389–1396.
42. Stewart DJ, Benoit B, Richard MT, et al. Treatment of malignant gliomas in adults with BCNU plus metronidozole. J Neurooncol 1984; 2:53–58.
43. Nelson DF, Diener-West M, Weinstein AS, et al. A randomized comparison of misonidazole sensitized radiotherapy plus BCNU and radiotherapy plus BCNU for the treatment of malignant glioma after surgery: final report of an RTOG study. Int J Radiat Oncol Biol Phys 1986; 12:1793–1800.
44. Lange OF, Haase KD, Scheef W. Simultaneous radio- and chemotherapy of inoperable brain tumors. Radiother Oncol 1987; 8:309–314.
45. Johnson DB, Thompson JM, Corwin JA, et al. Prolongation of survival for high grade malignant gliomas with adjuvant high-dose BCNU and autologous bone marrow transplantation. J Clin Oncol 1987; 5:783–789.
46. Mbidde EK, Selby PJ, Perren TJ, et al. High dose chemotherapy with autologous bone marrow transplantation and full dose radiotherapy for grade IV astrocytoma. Br J Cancer 1988; 58:779–782.
47. Fewer D, Wilson CB, Boldrey EB, Enox JK. Phase II study of 1-(2-chloroethyl)-3-cyclohexyl-1-nitrosourea (CCNU; NSC-79037) in the treatment of brain tumors. Cancer Chemother Rep 1972; 56:421–427.

48. Rosenblum ML, Reynolds AF, Smith KA, Rumak BH, Walker MD. Chloroethylcyclohexyl-nitrosourea (CCNU) in the treatment of malignant brain tumors. J Neurosurg 1973; 39:306–314.
49. Rodriguez LA, Prados M, Fulton D, Edwards MSB, Silver P, Levin V. Treatment of recurrent brain stem gliomas and other central nervous system tumors with 5-fluorouracil, CCNU, hydroxyurea, and 6-mercaptopurine. Neurosurgery 1988; 22:691–693.
50. Trojanowski T, Turowski K, Peszynski J, Kozniewski H. Postoperative radiotherapy and radiotherapy combined with CCNU chemotherapy for treatment of brain gliomas. J Neurooncol 1988; 6:285–291.
51. Takakura K, Abe H, Tanaka R, et al. Effects of ACNU and radiotherapy on malignant glioma. J Neurosurg 1986; 64:53–57.
52. Papavero L, Lowe F, Jakeche, H. Intracarotid infusion of ACNU and BCNU as adjuvant therapy of malignant gliomas. Acta Neurochirg (Wein) 1987; 85:128–137.
53. Georges P, Przedborski S, Brotchi J, Chatel M, Gedouin D, Hildebrand J. Effect of HECNU in malignant supratentorial gliomas—a phase II study. J Neurooncol 1988; 6:211–219.
54. Poisson M, Chiras J, Fauchon F, Debussche C, Delattre JY. Treatment of malignant recurrent glioma by intra-arterial infra-ophthalmic infusion of HECNU 1-(2-chloroethyl)-1-nitroso-3-(2-hydroxyethyl)urea. J Neurooncol 1990; 8:255–262.
55. Bender JF, Grillo-Lopez AJ, Posada JG. Diaziquone (AZQ). Invest New Drug 1982; 1:71.
56. Oberc-Greenwood MA, Smith BH. Mitochondrial toxicity of 2,5-diaziridinyl-3, 6-bis(carboethyoxyamino)-1,4-benzoquinone. J Neurooncol 1983; 1:723–733.
57. Eagan RT, Dinapoli RP, Cascino TL, Scherthauer B, O'Neill BP, O'Fallon JR. Comprehensive phase II evaluation of aziridinylbenzoquinone (AZQ, diaziquone) in recurrent human primary brain tumors. J Neurooncol 1987; 5:309–314.
58. Taylor SA, McCracken JD, Eyre HJ, O'Bryan RM, Neilan BA. Phase II study of aziridinylbenzoquinone (AZQ) in patients with central nervous system malignancies: a Southwest Oncology Group study J Neurooncol 1985; 3:131–135.
59. Feun LG, Yung WKA, Leavens ME, et al. A phase II trial of 2,5,-diaziridinyl-3,6-bis(carboethoxyamino)-1,4-benzoquinone (AZQ, NSC 182986) in recurrent primary brain tumors. J Neurooncol 1984; 2:13–17.
60. Decker BA, Al Sarraf M, Kresge C, Austin D, Wilner HI. Phase II study of aziridnylbenzoquinone (AZQ: NSC-182986) in the treatment of malignant gliomas recurrent after radiation. J Neurooncol 1985; 3:19–21.
61. Schold SC, Mahaley MS, Vick NA, et al. Response variability of human brain tumors to AZQ in tissue culture. J Neurooncol 1986; 4:49–54.
62. Kornblith PL, Rosa L, Bon JD, et al. Response variability of human brain tumors to AZQ in tissue culture. J Neurooncol 1986; 4:49–54.
63. Eyre HJ, Eltringham JR, Gehan EA, et al., Randomized comparisons of radiotherapy and carmustine versus procarbazine versus dacarbazine for the treatment of malignant gliomas following surgery: a Southwest Oncology Group study. Cancer Treat Rep 1986; 70:1085–1090.

28

Chemotherapy of Brain Tumors: Clinical Aspects

Kym L. Chandler and Michael D. Prados
University of California, School of Medicine,
San Francisco, California

I. INTRODUCTION

Patients with intracranial tumors were once considered beyond hope, regardless of the type of tumor, and often received supportive care only. Some physicians were reluctant to treat patients with primary or recurrent tumors because the outcome was thought to be unacceptable, and the benefits of therapy were transient. Modern practice, however, dictates that any patient with a brain tumor, whether primary or recurrent, should be considered for surgery, radiation therapy, and chemotherapy. Many patients are successfully treated, and some remain disease-free for years. New approaches to treatment, such as immunotherapy and gene therapy, hold promise for the future.

The era of cancer chemotherapy began in the 1940s, when the nitrogen mustards, originally investigated as prospective agents for chemical warfare, were adapted for the treatment of systemic tumors (1). The first chemotherapeutic drug approved for use in humans was mechlorethamine, the most rapidly acting of the so-called alkylating agents. The first drug shown to be effective against gliomas was the nitrosourea carmustine [1,3-bi(2-chloroethyl)-1-nitrosourea; BCNU]. From these beginnings, the usefulness of cytotoxic therapy in the treatment of intracranial tumors was established. Since then, the most effective drug, combination of drugs, or combination of treatment modalities has been diligently sought through clinical trials.

This chapter summarizes the rationale for chemotherapy and discusses the major chemotherapeutic agents and how they are used alone and with other therapies to treat central nervous system (CNS) tumors. This chapter also describes how chemotherapeutic drugs are evaluated and compared in clinical trials and summarizes the findings of the most important of these studies.

II. RATIONALE FOR CHEMOTHERAPY

In general, the drugs used to treat CNS tumors, like those used to treat systemic tumors, inhibit DNA synthesis and replication. The malignant cell dies during cell division or shortly after the genetic material has been altered. There are, however, several important differences between systemic and CNS malignancies that affect both therapy and outcome.

First, the absence of redundant tissue in the CNS make wide resection with clean margins impossible. "Curative" operations cause permanent neurological disability. Therefore, resection is limited to the removal of obvious tumor, and microscopic tumor is almost invariably left behind. Second, because systemic metastasis from CNS tumors is rare, death is usually due to local recurrence, rather than disseminated disease. This, coupled with the fact that the CNS is contained within the skull, means that the lethal tumor burden, including edema, is approximately 600 g, or less than one-third the lethal burden of systemic tumors. Moreover, the CNS lacks lymphatic drainage; therefore, extracellular fluid products from the tumor cannot be removed rapidly. This edema contributes significantly to the intracranial mass effect as well as to neurological deficit. Third, the blood–brain barrier (BBB), when intact, excludes most drugs from the CNS. In the tumor region, however, the blood–brain barrier is defective or absent. This not only gives rise to the phenomenon of contrast enhancement on radiographic images, it theoretically allows chemotherapeutic agents to act at the site of the tumor, rather than causing toxic neurological damage.

III. TREATMENT DECISIONS

To treat or not to treat a patient with a brain tumor is a decision that must be made case-by-case. It is important to provide the patient and the family with comprehensive, understandable information that allows them to make appropriate treatment decisions and maintain reasonable expectations of the outcome. Multiple factors are considered when evaluating patients for chemotherapy. Each factor must be carefully and thoroughly weighed in each case. A well-informed patient and physician can devise an accurate risk–benefit analysis that will allow the patient to reach the best decision concerning his or her treatment.

The first factor is the pathological diagnosis, including characterization of the growth potential [i.e., the bromodeoxyuridine (BUDR)- or Ki-67-labeling index]. For example, germ cell tumors are remarkably sensitive to chemotherapy, but the role of chemotherapy for glioblastomas multiforme (GM) is less well established. One may surmise that an anaplastic astrocytoma (AA) with a BUDR-labeling index of less than 1% has a lower growth potential and, therefore, is less likely to recur than a histologically similar tumor with a BUDR-labeling index of 15%.

The age and clinical status of the patient are also important considerations. In children younger than 3 years of age, craniospinal radiation has a deleterious effect on developing brain. In such cases, chemotherapy can be used to control tumor growth and "buy time" for the CNS to mature as much as possible. If the tumor subsequently recurs, radiation therapy or additional chemotherapy may be considered. Patients with concomitant medical illnesses or general physical debilitation may elect not to embark on treatment, especially when the prognosis is poor even with available therapeutic options.

Previous therapy must also be reviewed. Patients with high-grade astrocytic tumors are routinely evaluated for chemotherapy after surgery and radiation therapy. The benefit of adjuvant chemotherapy for glioblastoma is questionable, especially in elderly patients; however, glioblastomas treated with chemotherapy at recurrence often stabilize, if only briefly, in some patients. One must also consider the toxicity of a treatment regimen, which correlates directly with a decrease in the quality of life. Thus, if life expectancy is short, even a brief decrease in the quality of life may be unacceptable, and the patient and physician may elect to forgo the treatment.

IV. ROLE OF CHEMOTHERAPY

Rational surgery in conjunction with radiation therapy or chemotherapy provides the best chance of prolonged survival and at least a reasonably good quality of life. The goal of surgery is to obtain tissue for diagnosis, to alleviate symptoms, and to reduce the tumor burden as much as possible. The extent of surgery may affect the overall survival rate (2–6); certain tumors, such as infiltrating astrocytomas, are impossible to remove completely. Although surgery without adjuvant therapy can control some tumors, notably GM, for several months, multimodal therapy, including surgery, is the most effective treatment. Clinical trials have shown that the larger the tumor burden is postoperatively, the shorter the period of survival (2). The postoperative tumor burden was unrelated to age, Karnofsky performance status, or the histopathological findings and diagnosis. A similar trend was noted between survival and tumor burden after radiation therapy. The results of other trials have supported this observation (7), but there have been no randomized prospective trials of biopsy versus resection, and the role of surgery in the management of astrocytomas in adults has been questioned (8). We believe that, unless there are medical contraindications, craniotomy, rather than biopsy, should be performed to remove a surgically accessible lesion. After surgery, radiation therapy is the next most effective treatment for astrocytoma (9–11). Prospective studies have shown that adjuvant radiation therapy prolongs survival more than surgery or chemotherapy alone.

V. ALKYLATING AGENTS

A. Nitrosoureas

Carmustine (BCNU) and lomustine (CCNU) are the only nitrosoureas commercially available in the United States. Other agents in this class are semustine (MeCCNU) and nimustine (ACNU), which are available only in Europe and Japan, and 1-(2-chloroethyl)-3-(2,6-dioxo-3-piperidyl) (PCNU). Of these agents, BCNU and CCNU have the highest and second-highest activities, respectively, against gliomas. Both are lipid-soluble molecules that are small enough to cross the blood–brain barrier and are used separately as first-line treatment for high-grade gliomas. Nitrosoureas have a wide spectrum of activity and are effective against primitive neuroectodermal tumors (PNETs), medulloblastomas, ependymomas, and intracranial metastases from systemic sites.

The nitrosoureas are bifunctional alkylating agents. Their mechanism of action is not completely understood, but they appear to induce cross-linking of two nucleic acid side chains in DNA. The interstrand cross-links are produced by a chloroethyl monoadduct moiety at the guanine (O^6) position in one DNA strand; subsequently, a similar reaction occurs in the alternate strand (12). To a lesser extent, carbamoylation reactions may occur. In any event, the nitrosoureas are not cell cycle-specific agents.

Tumors treated with nitrosoureas often recur, which suggests that some tumors cells are resistant to the cytotoxic effects of the treatment. Resistance to nitrosoureas has been heavily investigated (12–16). Most studies have focused on the ability of tumor cells to prevent cross-linking at the O^6-methylguanine site. The enzyme O^6-methylguanine-DNA-methyltransferase, which is intrinsic to resistant cells, is thought to compete with the formation of BCNU-mediated cross-links. This enzyme does not act on DNA once cross-links have been established; rather, it reacts with the monomeric reaction intermediate and before cross-linking. This mechanism of resistance is similar to that of the nitrogen mustards, except that the pertinent enzyme is different (14).

In humans, the enzymes that make tumor cells resistant to nitrosoureas have not been identified with certainty. However, cells can be phenotypically classified on their ability to repair methylation damage. Human tumor cells incubated with adenovirus cells altered by *in vitro* treatment with *N*-methyl-*N*'-nitrosoguanidine (MNNG) differ in their ability to repair viral DNA sequences inserted into their own DNA. Tumor cells that can incorporate the virus and support its replication are called Mer-positive cells; tumor cells that cannot react with the virus are called

Mer-negative cells. Mer-positive cells can repair O^6-methylguanine damage to their DNA more efficiently than Mer-negative cells (15). The Mer-positive phenotype appears to correlate directly with a paucity of DNA cross-links and, therefore, with increased resistance.

The dose-limiting toxicity of the nitrosoureas is myelosuppression; white blood cell and platelet counts reach their nadir 3–4 weeks after the first dose of the drug, but generally recover within 6–8 weeks. The dosage is adjusted according to the blood counts, which should be monitored at least every 2 weeks. Nausea and vomiting can also occur, reaching their maximum 6 h after treatment. Other side effects include local burning at the intravenous site, diarrhea, and hepatic toxicity, mainly in the form of liver enzyme elevation.

BCNU has one potentially lethal side effect. When the cumulative dose exceeds 1200 mg/m^2, the risk of progressive pulmonary interstitial fibrosis increases, especially in patients with a history of pulmonary disease or exposure to toxins, such as tobacco. Every effort should be made to keep the total dose below 1200 mg/m^2.

CCNU is given orally at a dose of 110 mg/m^2; BCNU is given intravenously at a dose of 200–240 mg/m^2, however, in clinical trials in which autologous bone marrow transplantation is used, BCNU may be administered at doses as high as 600 mg/m^2. Intra-arterial administration of BCNU offers no survival advantage over conventional oral or intravenous therapy and is associated with significant side effects (e.g., ipsilateral blindness and leukoencephalopathy (17–21). For this reason, it has not been used at the University of California, San Francisco (UCSF).

B. Other Alkylating Agents

1. Cyclophosphamide and Ifosfamide

Another frequently used alkylating agent is cyclophosphamide. Ifosfamide, a synthetic analogue of cyclophosphamide, is being evaluated for its efficacy and toxicity. As single agents, both drugs have low activity against glial tumors, but in combination with other drugs both are effective, particularly in the treatment of medulloblastoma. Cyclophosphamide has a broad spectrum of activity and is at least partially effective against low-grade gliomas, PNETs, medulloblastomas, primary CNS lymphomas, and some AAs.

These drugs disturb mechanisms of cell growth, mitotic activity, differentiation, and cell function; therefore, they are most effective against rapidly proliferating cells. Cyclophosphamide and ifosfamide must be activated by the cytochrome P453$_{20}$ (mixed-function oxidase) system. The parent compound is oxidized initially to 4-OH-cyclophosphamide (ifosfamide) and then in two steps to phosphoramide mustard, a reactive electrophile. The toxic side effects of cyclophosphamide are related to the total amount (concentration) of electrophilic metabolites (the moieties that react with DNA) in blood and urine. Particularly in the case of ifosfamide, these electrophilic metabolites are injurious to the bladder epithelium. This can partly be alleviated by the administration of mesna.

Rapidly growing normal cells are most susceptible to the toxic effects of these agents. The dose-limiting side effects are myelosuppression, which is maximal 10–14 days after treatment, and urotoxicity. Other effects include alopecia, somnolence or confusion, nausea and vomiting, sterility, teratogenesis, and oncogenesis. Hemorrhagic cystitis is a unique side effect of cyclophosphamide and ifosfamide.

An oral preparation of cyclophosphamide is available. It is usually given orally for 14–21 days at a dose of 50 mg/m^2 per day, but may be given intravenously at doses of 750–1500 mg/m^2; however, higher dose schedules are being investigated. Ifosfamide is administered intravenously at a usual dose of 1.2 g/m^2 per day for 5 consecutive days every 3–4 weeks. Hydration is essential to reduce renal side effects. When given intravenously, both drugs should be administered by slow infusion over 30–45 min.

2. *Diaziquone (Aziridinylbenzoquinone)*

Diaziquone (Aziridinylbenzoquinone; AZQ), an investigational drug synthesized in the early 1970s, was designed to cross the blood–brain barrier better than other alkylating agents. *In vitro*, as well as in Phase I and II trials, AZQ has shown some efficacy against AA and GM. In a Phase II study, Maral *et al.* (22) found a stabilization rate of 50% and a median time to tumor progression of about 18 weeks in patients with AA and GM.

Diaziquone does not appear to be cross-resistant to the nitrosoureas. The major toxicity is myelosuppression, which occurs 14–21 days after treatment. The usual intravenous dose is 30–40 mg/m^2.

VI. VINCA ALKALOIDS

Vinblastine and vincristine are both derived from the periwinkle plant. Vinblastine is very active against germ cell tumors (23), but has limited activity against most of the common brain tumors and, therefore, will not be discussed further. Vincristine is most often used in combination with other agents. It has some activity against glial tumors and medulloblastomas.

Vincristine's mechanism of action is similar to that of colchicine. It is cell cycle-specific and causes metaphase arrest by specifically binding the intracellular protein tubulin. The cell dies because it cannot segregate chromosomes during cell division.

Unlike previously mentioned agents, vincristine does not cause myelosuppression. The major side effect is a peripheral neuropathy with varied clinical manifestations, including neuritic paresthesia, suppression of deep tendon reflexes, jaw pain, ptosis, and diplopia. Vincristine is a vesicant, and if injected into the extravascular space, may cause skin reactions severe enough to require grafting. It may also contribute to constipation in elderly patients or those taking codeine or other narcotics.

Resistance to vincristine and vinblastine appears to be mediated by the expression of the multiple-drug resistance (*MDR*) gene (24,25). Tumor cells that have the MDR phenotype are cross-resistant to a variety of functionally and structurally unrelated cytotoxic drugs, which are usually lipophilic drugs such as plant alkaloids, to which they have not been exposed. The mechanism of resistance is increased efflux of the drug that reduces the intracellular concentration. Drug efflux can be reduced by calcium channel blockers, most notably verapamil. When the *MDR* gene is amplified and overexpressed, increased amounts of P-glycoprotein, or gp170, a transplasma membrane protein, are found (24). In fact, gp170 may be the transport protein responsible for the drug efflux (24). There is also evidence that previous treatment with agents such as vincristine, daunorubicin (daunomycin), doxorubicin (Adriamycin), colchicine, and etoposide (VP-16) may induce the expression of the *MDR1* gene at low levels; subsequent treatment, even with a structurally unrelated drug, may induce high levels of expression of the gene and, thereby, increase resistance (25).

Vincristine is given intravenously at a dose of 2 mg/week as part of a multiagent drug protocol.

VII. PROCARBAZINE (*N*-METHYLHYDRAZINE)

Procarbazine (PCB) was synthesized as a monoamine oxidase inhibitor; however, the inhibitory effect was not as potent as hoped. It later proved to be active primarily against glial tumors, primary and recurrent PNETs, medulloblastomas, and ependymomas.

Procarbazine's mechanism of action is unknown. It may promote chromosomal breakage, similar to that caused by alkylating agents. There is evidence that PCB has cross-resistance with other drugs. Its antitumor activity is similar to that of the alkylating agents. It is water-soluble and easily crosses the blood–brain barrier.

The toxic side effects of PCB include myelosuppression, nausea and vomiting (especially if an antiemetic is not given beforehand), severe (allergic) rash, and sedation and confusion, especially when PCB is given in combination with other CNS depressants. A disulfiram-like action has been described in patients who drink ethyl alcohol during treatment with PCB.

Procarbazine is administered orally and is excreted almost entirely through the gastrointestinal tract. It can be given at a dose of 60–150 mg/m^2 every day for 3–4 weeks until blood counts are lowered. Recovery from myelosuppression generally takes 3–4 weeks.

VIII. PLATINUM COMPOUNDS

Cisplatin (*cis*-platinum) was first identified as an antitumor agent in 1965 (26,27). It is used almost exclusively in combination with other drugs to treat medulloblastomas, PNETs, ependymomas, and astrocytomas (28,29). Carboplatin, a sister compound, is used alone and in conjunction with other agents against astrocytomas, PNETs, and ependymomas (30).

Platinum compounds enter a cell by diffusion, where their unexposed chloride moities bind to guanosine bases. This facilitates interstrand and intrastrand DNA cross-linking. Platinum compounds are not cell cycle-specific. Carboplatin and cisplatin could conceivably share a final common pathway, yielding the formation of identical platinum adducts.

Despite their structural similarities, cisplatin and carboplatin have quite different toxicities (31–35). The major toxic effect of cisplatin is nausea and vomiting, which can be severe and may lead to electrolyte disturbances. Originally, the dose-limiting toxicity was to the kidney; doses greater than 100 mg/m^2 could not be easily tolerated. Nephrotoxicity can be avoided by hydration (150–200 ml/h before and after infusion) and chloruresis. Now the dose-limiting toxicity is neurotoxicity, which occurs frequently at doses greater than 200 mg/m^2. Cisplatin is also ototoxic and occasionally causes myelosuppression.

Carboplatin has the same spectrum of antitumor activity as cisplatin, but at equivalent doses causes less nausea and vomiting, less nephrotoxicity, and less ototoxicity. Carboplatin does not cause neuropathy at therapeutic doses, but does cause significant myelosuppression, typically affecting the platelet count more than the white blood cell count. Carboplatin is being investigated in a dose-escalating trial to further elucidate its efficacy in the treatment of gliomas. Carboplatin doses range from 350 to 600 mg/m^2. In the setting of autologous bone marrow transplantation with high-dose chemotherapy, doses from 1200 to 1500 mg/m^2 are used. Doz et al. have reported promising experimental strategies for increasing the therapeutic index of carboplatin by pretreatment with WR compounds (36) or a high-zinc diet (37) to protect normal tissues and allow higher doses without increased toxicity. Both drugs are mutagenic and teratogenic (31–35).

IX. RADIATION SENSITIZERS

A. Hydroxyurea

Hydroxyurea (HU) was originally synthesized in 1869. Its oncolytic properties were discovered in the early 1960s (38). Hydroxyurea has some activity against glial tumors; but it also sensitizes cells to radiation and, therefore, is used in combination with radiation therapy. It is water-soluble, readily crosses the blood–brain barrier, and is cell cycle-specific (S phase). Its primary mode of action is to inhibit ribonucleoside diphosphate reductase (RNDR), an enzyme that catalyzes the reductive conversion of ribonucleotides to deoxyribonucleotides. This conversion is likely to be the rate-limiting step in the synthesis of DNA.

The most common side effect of HU is mild myelosuppression. Hydroxyurea is given orally at a dose of 250–300 mg/m^2 four times a day, 3 days a week during external beam radiation therapy.

B. Misonidazole and Metronidazole

Some chemotherapeutic agents render hypoxic tumor cells more susceptible to the cytocidal effects of irradiation. Misonidazole and metronidazole, two nitroimidazoles that are administered during radiation therapy, are electron-affinic and are taken up by hypoxic cells, in which they substitute for oxygen and, thereby, facilitate radiation-induced DNA damage. Unfortunately, this theoretical advantage has not been successful in increasing longevity (39–42). In addition, both drugs have significant clinical toxicity, including myelosuppression, photosensitivity, and allergic rash. No hypoxic cell sensitizer has been shown to increase survival of patients with astrocytomas.

C. Idoxuridine and Bromodeoxyuridine

The halogenated pyrimidines bromodeoxyuridine (BUDR) and iododeoxyuridine; (IUDR) are also administered to sensitize tumor cells to radiation; this effect has been well documented *in vitro*. These agents are investigational drugs and have similar mechanisms of action. Both BUDR and IUDR are thymidine analogues that are incorporated in place of thymidine during the DNA synthesis phase of the cell cycle; nondividing normal cells, such as neurons or normal glia, and tumor cells in the nonproliferating pool do not incorporate these agents. The radiosensitizing effect increases with higher concentration of incorporated IUDR or BUDR.

Both drugs are given as a constant intra-arterial or intravenous infusion during radiation therapy. The side effects of BUDR and IUDR are generally mild and well tolerated. They include myelosuppression, changes in the skin and nail bed, allergic reactions, photosensitization, and hepatic toxicity.

X. OTHER AGENTS

A. Polyamine Inhibitors

In the late 1970s, reduction of intracellular polyamines was shown to decrease the rate of cell proliferation (43,44). Enflornithine (DL-difluoromethylornithine; DFMO) and methylglyoxal bis-(guanylhydrazine (MGBG), a spermidine analogue, are two polyamine inhibitors that have been approved as investigational drugs. They are more effective against AAs than GMs.

Enflornithine is an irreversible inhibitor of ornithine decarboxylase by enzyme activation, whereas MGBG, for which uptake into the cell is facilitated by DFMO, is a competitive inhibitor of *S*-adenosylmethionine decarboxylase and may act by hyperacetylating histones. The mechanism of action *in vivo* has not been fully elucidated.

The most frequent toxic side effects are ototoxicity, nephrotoxicity, and diarrhea, all of which can be reversed by reducing the dosage or stopping the medication altogether. Mild myelosuppression is sometimes noted. Enflornithine is given orally at a dose of 1.8 g/m^2 three times per day; MGBG is given intravenously every 6 weeks at a dose of 200 mg/m^2.

B. Dibromodulcitol

Dibromodulcitol (DBD), a halogenated hexitol compound developed in the early 1970s (45–47), is active against medulloblastomas and malignant ependymomas. It is rapidly hydrolyzed to the active metabolite dianhydrogalactitol, an alkylating agent. The major toxic side effects are myelosuppression, nausea and vomiting, and possibly leukemogenesis. The drug is given orally and has a half-life of days. It is currently being evaluated in investigational protocols.

C. Melphalan

In vitro, melphalan has been effective against astrocytoma and medulloblastoma cell lines. It may have the advantage of lacking cross-resistance with the nitrosoureas. The dosage is 8 mg/m^2 orally for 5 consecutive days every 4 weeks. An intravenous preparation is available only through investigational studies.

D. Etoposide and Teniposide

Etoposide (VP-16, also known as terazanate) and teniposide (VM-26) are epipodophyllotoxins. Similar to vincristine, they are mitotic spindle inhibitors that bind to tubulin and, therefore, are cell cycle-specific. Both drugs are lipid-soluble, but are too large to cross the blood–brain barrier well. They are taken up by passive diffusion. Etoposide and teniposide are active against medulloblastomas, ependymomas, and PNETs. The dose-limiting toxicity is mainly hematological.

E. Methotrexate

Methotrexate has limited use against primary and recurrent gliomas. It has been used to treat leptomeningeal tumors and primary CNS lymphomas. Methotrexate cannot cross the normal blood–brain barrier. To attain therapeutic concentrations in serum, extremely high doses (3–10 g/m^2) must be given, and folinic acid rescue is required.

No controlled trials have been undertaken to evaluate dose schedules. Severe toxicity such as leukoencephalopathy, hepato- and nephrotoxicity, and mucositis are common. This drug is not routinely used at UCSF except in the polypharmacological treatment of primary CNS lymphoma.

XI. CLINICAL TRIALS

Because every patient is unique, each chemotherapeutic agent, or combination of agents, has the potential to control one person's tumor indefinitely. In day-to-day practice, this individuality would make treatment decisions impossible. Clinical trials are designed to efficiently identify therapies that are beneficial to the greatest number of patients for the longest time. Every patient should be informed about these trials and encouraged to participate. This is especially important when there is no established treatment for a patient's tumor, or if the available therapies are only marginally effective.

Clinical trials are conducted sequentially in three phases. Phase I trials define and characterize toxicity to end-organs, such as bone marrow or heart. These studies are reserved for patients whose tumors have not been controlled with conventional therapies. Phase II trials are carried out to define the spectrum of a drug's activity against a specific type of tumor. In these studies, careful attention must be paid to the time between evaluations; if the interval is too long or too short, the effect of treatment could be missed, and a potentially effective therapy would be lost. Phase III trials test the best-known standard therapy against another drug or drug combination previously tested in a Phase II trial. These studies must be carefully designed so that the groups have comparable numbers of patients with similar characteristics. Phase III trials usually require more patients and longer follow-up times than Phase I or II trials and most are multicenter studies. They are important because they define the standard of care.

In 1978, the Brain Tumor Study Group (BTSG) reported the findings of a seminal Phase III trial evaluating postoperative radiation and adjuvant chemotherapy in patients with glial tumors; 90% of the tumors were GM (48). The patients were randomized to four treatment groups: supportive care only; BCNU (80 mg/m^2 iv) given on three successive days every 6 weeks; whole-brain irradiation to a total dose of 5000–6000 rad; and whole-brain irradiation to a total dose of 5000–6000 rad and BCNU (80 mg/m^2 iv) on 3 successive days every 6 weeks. The median durations of survival in these groups were 14, 19, 36, and 35 weeks, respectively; the 1-year survival rates were 3, 12, 24, and 32%, respectively. Surgery and radiation therapy offered notably improved survival over surgery alone or surgery and chemotherapy ($p < 0.05$). The 1-year survival rate was only slightly higher in patients receiving BCNU adjuvantly than in those treated with radiation only. This study was followed by a series of trials conducted by the BTSG (10,49–52), each reaffirming the survival advantage afforded by postoperative irradiation and, in certain subsets of patients, by adjuvant nitrosourea-based chemotherapy.

Currently, clinical trials of multiagent chemotherapy, with or without fractionated radiation schedules, are being proposed. The primary rationale for this approach is that tumors are composed of different cell populations, which have different degrees of resistance to radiation therapy or to single-agent chemotherapy. Polytherapy is the most logical way to approach this complex problem.

In a Phase III trial (53) carried out by the Brain Tumor Research Center (BTRC), treatment with BCNU, radiation therapy, and HU was compared with BCNU and radiation therapy alone in patients with AA and GM. In patients with AA, the median time to tumor progression was longer in patients who did not receive HU than in those who did (72 vs 50 weeks). In patients with GM, however, the opposite was true: the time to tumor progression was longer in patients who received HU than in those who did not (41 vs 31 weeks). These results suggest that adjuvant treatment with HU during radiation therapy may improve tumor control in patients with GM, but not in those with AA.

Deutsch *et al.* (54) participated in a multicenter clinical trial comparing hyperfractionated radiation therapy (with or without a radiation sensitizer) with a conventional radiation therapy schedule (one dose per day) followed in either case by chemotherapy. Five hundred fifty-seven patients, 80% of whom had GM, were randomized to one of four treatment groups: radiation therapy to a total dose of 6000 rad, followed by BCNU; radiation therapy to 6000 rad, followed by streptozocin; hyperfractionated radiation therapy to 6600 rad, followed by BCNU; and hyperfractionated radiation therapy to 6600 rad, in combination with misonidazole, followed by BCNU. The median duration of survival in all arms was approximately 10 months. It was concluded that neither hyperfractionated radiation therapy nor misonidazole offered any survival advantage over conventional radiation therapy followed by BCNU or streptozocin.

The BTSG trial 8001 (55) was a large, multicenter study comparing various forms of radiation and chemotherapy. Eighty percent of patients had GM and were additionally randomized to two radiation therapy regimens. One cohort received whole-brain irradiation to a total dose of 6020 rad; the other cohort received whole-brain irradiation to 4300 rad plus a coned-down boost of 1720 rad to the tumor bed. The three chemotherapy treatment arms were BCNU only, BCNU alternating with the combination of procarbazine and BCNU, and HU alternating with procarbazine and VM-26. The median duration of survival ranged from 11.3–13.8 months; no form of chemotherapy or radiation therapy provided a statistically significant survival advantage. It was concluded that radiation therapy consisting of whole-brain irradiation with a coned-down boost and BCNU was as effective as whole-brain irradiation combined with any other form of chemotherapy.

Adjuvant treatment with BCNU has been the standard therapy for glial tumors after radiation therapy. In 1989, however, the Northern California Oncology Group (NCOG) published the results of a study comparing BCNU and combination therapy with procarbazine, CCNU, and vincristine (PCV) after radiation therapy in patients with AA and GM (56). Patients received 6000 rad of focal radiation therapy plus HU and were then randomized to receive BCNU or PCV. The time to tumor progression and the duration of survival were longer in patients treated with PCV, but only in those with AA was the difference statistically significant; in fact, both times doubled for patients with AAs in the 50th and 25th percentiles of survival. This study was the first to show that any agent or combination of agents after radiation therapy was superior to BCNU alone in the treatment of AAs.

Other radiation sensitizers, most notably the halogenated pyrimidines, have been investigated and scheduled for further trials (57–59). In an uncontrolled trial, Hoshino *et al.* treated 107 patients with continuous arterial BUDR during radiation therapy (60). More than 50% of the patients survived 18 months or longer. Intra-arterial BUDR was also studied in a small cohort by Greenberg *et al.*, who found a survival advantage in patients with grade III and IV gliomas (61). Finally, early findings from the NCOG suggest that there may be a survival advantage in patients with AA, but not in those with GM, when the drug is administered intravenously (62).

Iododeoxyuridine has also been studied to evaluate its efficacy against primary and metastatic intracranial tumors. Preliminary results from a phase I study of continuous intravenous IUDR delivered in a dose-escalating fashion during hyperfractionated radiation therapy (63) indicate that IUDR is less toxic than BUDR and has a higher rate of incorporation into DNA. Both agents have been well tolerated and toxicity has been mild thus far.

Trials are currently underway to attempt to further improve survival with adjuvant chemotherapy as well as other treatment modalities. An example would be high-dose chemotherapy with autologous bone marrow transplantation. Despite its theoretical advantages, this approach has yielded limited success (64). Factors that curtail the success of this regimen are the paucity of effective agents against astrocytoma and the often life-threatening end-organ toxicity caused by larger doses of chemotherapeutic agents.

XII. CONCLUSION

General strategies can be used to treat primary and recurrent brain tumors. A patient with GM would ideally undergo debulking surgery, focal external beam irradiation, and in certain cases, brachytherapy (see Chap. 25). For patients whose tumors are not suitable for brachytherapy, participation in an investigational chemotherapeutic protocol would be appropriate. In patients with AA, rational surgery and focal radiation therapy, followed by the combination of procarbazine, CCNU, and vincristine, would be prudent.

Various treatment possibilities are available for recurrent tumors. First, reoperation should be considered for maximal cytoreduction. Additional radiation therapy should also be considered based on previous radiation dosimetry. Interstitial brachytherapy, radiosurgery, or reirradiation on a hyperfractionated schedule should all be considered. Standard or investigational chemotherapeutic agents may be appropriate during, or in lieu of, radiation therapy. For patients who have not previously received chemotherapy, treatment with nitrosoureas should be considered as first-line therapy. These drugs can be given alone (BCNU or CCNU) or in combination with other agents (e.g., procarbazine, CCNU, and vincristine). If the patient has already undergone nitrosourea-based chemotherapy, procarbazine may be given as a single agent.

With the development and improvement of a wide variety of treatment options, the pessimism once associated with the treatment of primary and recurrent brain tumors can be replaced with cautious optimism. Clinical trials have been invaluable in improving treatment strategies, defining appropriate combinations of therapy, and identifying which patients are likely to benefit most from a given treatment. To test hypotheses in properly designed clinical trials, patient selection and patient motivation are critical. The goal of therapy should be clearly defined before the patient starts treatment. In addition, family members as well as the patient should be as well informed as possible. In any event, attempts to increase the length of survival should never interfere with the quality of survival.

A multimodality approach increases the survival of patients with certain types of tumors. A survey of national trends in the care of patients with malignant brain tumors showed that patients with GM who were treated with investigational protocols had a 5-year survival rate that was nearly three times higher than that in patients who were treated with standard protocols (12% vs 4.5%) (65,66).

Despite the increasing frequency with which patients are referred to centers participating in clinical trials, less than 10% of eligible patients are formally enrolled into such studies. As survival times continue to increase, more emphasis can be placed on reducing the toxicity of therapy and enhancing the quality of life in survivors.

REFERENCES

1. Gilman A. The initial clinical trial of nitrogen mustard. Am J Surg 1963; 105:574–578.
2. Wood JR, Green SB, Shapiro WR. The prognostic importance of tumor size in malignant gliomas: a computed tomographic scan study by the Brain Tumor Cooperative Group. J Clin Oncol 1988; 6:338–343.
3. Andreou J, George AE, Wise A, de Leon M, Kricheff II, Ransohoff J, Foo SH. CT prognostic criteria of survival after malignant glioma surgery. AJNR 1983; 4:488–490.
4. Ammirati M, Vick N, Liao Y, Cerec I, Mikhael M. Effect of the extent of surgical resection on survival and quality of life in patients with supratentorial glioblastomas and anaplastic astrocytomas. Neurosurgery 1987; 21:201–206.
5. Nelson DF, Nelson JS, Davis DR, Chang CH, Griffin TW, Pajak TF. Survival and prognosis of patients with astrocytoma with atypical or anaplastic features. J Neurooncol 1985; 3:99–103.
6. Cairncross JG, Warnick Pexman JH, Rathbone MP, DelMaestro RF. Postoperative contrast enhancement in patients with brain tumors. Ann Neurol 1985; 17:570–572.
7. Salcman M. Resection and reoperation in neurooncology. Rationale and approach. Neurol Clin 1985; 3:831–842.
8. Nazzaro JM, Neuwelt E. The role of surgery in the management of supratentorial intermediate and high-grade astrocytomas in adults. J Neurosurg 1990; 73:331–345.
9. Walker MD, Strike TA, Sheline GE. An analysis of dose–effect relationship in the radiotherapy of malignant gliomas. Int J Radiat Oncol Biol Phys 1979; 5:1725–1731.
10. Salazar OM, Rubin P, Feldstein ML, Pizzutrello R. High dose radiation therapy in the treatment of malignant gliomas: final report. Int J Radiat Oncol Biol Phys 1979; 5:1733–1740.
11. Sheline G. Conventional radiation of primary tumors. Semin Oncol 1975; 2:20–42.
12. Zlotogorski C, Erickson LC. Pretreatment of human colon tumor cells with DNA methylating agents inhibits their ability to repair chloroethyl monoadducts. Carcinogenesis 1984; 5:83–87.
13. Skalski V, Yarosh DB, Batist G, Gros P, Feindel W, Kopriva D, Panasci LC. Accelerated communication: mechanisms of resistance to (2-chloroethyl)-3-sarcosinamide-1-nitrosourea (SarCNU) in sensitive and resistant human glioma cells. Mol Pharmacol 1990; 38:299–305.
14. Robins P, Harris AL, Goldsmith I, Lindahl T. Cross-linking of DNA induced by chloroethylnitrosourea is presented by O(6)-methylguanine-DNA methyltransferase. Nucleic Acids Res 1983; 11:7743–7758.
15. Erickson LC, Laurent G, Sharkey NA, Kohn KW. DNA cross-linking and monoadduct repair in nitrosourea-treated human tumour cells. Nature 1980; 288:727–729.
16. Day RS III, Ziolkowski CHJ, Scudiero DA, Meyer SA, Lubiniecki AS, Girardi AJ, Galloway SM, Bynum GD. Defective repair of alkylated DNA by human tumour and SV40-transformed human cell strains. Nature 1980; 288:724–727.
17. Shapiro WR, Green SB. Reevaluating the efficacy of intra-arterial BCNU. J Neurosurg 1987; 66:313–315.
18. Bashir R, Hochberg FH, Linggood RM, Hottleman K. Pre-irradiation internal carotid artery BCNU in treatment of glioblastoma multiforme. J Neurosurg 1988; 68:917–919.
19. Stewart DS, Grahovac Z, Riding MT. Intracarotid PCNU: an NCI Canada study. Proc Am Soc Clin Oncol 1986; 5:A136.
20. Yamashita J, Handa H, Tokuriki Y, Ha YS, Otsuka S-I, Suda K, Taki W. Intra-arterial ACNU therapy for malignant brain tumors. Experimental studies and preliminary clinical results. J Neurosurg 1983; 59:424–430.

21. Stewart D, Grahovac Z, Hugenholtz H. Combined intraarterial and systemic chemotherapy for intracerebral tumors. Neurosurgery 1987; 21:207–214.

22. Maral J, Poisson M, Pertuiset BF. Phase II evaluation of diaziquone (CI-904, AZQ) in the treatment of human malignant glioma. J Neurooncol 1985; 3:245–249.

23. Allen JD. Management of primary intracranial germ cell tumors of childhood. Pediatr Neurosci 1987; 13:152–157.

24. Matsumoto T, Tani E, Kaba K, Kochi N, Shindo H, Yamamoto Y, Sakamoto H, Furuyama J. Amplification and expression of a multidrug resistance gene in human glioma cell lines. J Neurosurg 1990; 72:96–101.

25. Bourhis J, Goldstein LJ, Riou G, Pastan I, Gottesman MM, Benard J. Expression of a human multidrug resistance gene in ovarian carcinomas. Cancer Res 1989; 49:5062–5065.

26. Rosenberg B, VanCamp L, Grimley EB, Thomson AJ. The inhibition of growth or cell division in *Escherichia coli* by electrolysis products from a platinum electrode. Nature 1965; 205:698–699.

27. Rosenberg B, VanCamp L, Trosko GE, Mansour VH. Platinum compounds, a new class of anti-tumor agents. Nature 1969; 222:385–386.

28. Mahaley MS Jr, Hipp SW, Dropcho EJ, Bertsch L, Cush S, Tirey T, Gillespie GY. Intracarotid cisplatin chemotherapy for recurrent gliomas. J Neurosurg 1989; 70:371–378.

29. Newton HB, Page MA, Junck L, Greenberg HS. Intraarterial cisplatin for the treatment of malignant gliomas. J Neurooncol 1989; 7:39–45.

30. Follezor J-Y, Fauchon F, Chiras J. Intraarterial infusion of carboplatin in the treatment of malignant gliomas: a Phase II study. Neoplasma 1989; 36:349–352.

31. Van Echo DA, Egorin MJ, Aisner J. The pharmacology of carboplatin. Semin Oncol 1989; 16(suppl 5):1–6.

32. Muggia FM. Overview of carboplatin: replacing, complementing and extending the therapeutic horizons of cisplatin. Semin Oncol 1989; 16(suppl 5):7–13.

33. Ozols RF. Optimal dosing with carboplatin. Semin Oncol 1989; 16(suppl 5):14–18.

34. Fillastre JP, Raguenez-Viotte G. Cisplatin nephrotoxicity. Toxicol Lett 1989; 46:163–175.

35. Sridhar KS, Donnelly E. Combination antiemetics for cisplatin chemotherapy. Cancer 1988; 61:1508–1517.

36. Doz F, Berens ME, Spencer DR, Dougherty DV, Rosenblum ML. Experimental basis for increasing the therapeutic index of carboplatin in brain tumor therapy by pretreatment with WR compounds. Cancer Chemother Pharmacol 1991; 28:308–310.

37. Doz F, Berens ME, Deschepper CF, Dougherty DV, Bigornia V, Barker M, Rosenblum ML. Experimental basis for increasing the therapeutic index of *cis*-diaminedicarboxylatocyclobutaneplatinum-(II) in brain tumor therapy by a high-zinc diet. Cancer Chemother Pharmacol 1991; 29:308–310.

38. Beckloff GL, Lerner HJ, Frost D, Russo-Alesi FM, Gitomer S. Hydroxyurea (NSC-32065) in biological fluids: a dose–concentration relationship. Cancer Chemother Rep 1965; 48:57–58.

39. Bleehen NM, Wiltshire CR, Plowman PN, Watson JV, Gleave JR, Holmes AE, Lewin WS, Treip CS, Hawkins TD. A randomized study of misonidazole and radiotherapy for grade 3 and 4 cerebral astrocytoma. Br J Cancer 1981; 43:436–442.

40. Nelson DF, Schoenfeld D, Weinstein AS, Nelson JS, Wasserman T, Goodman RL, Carabell S. A randomized comparison of misonidazole sensitized radiotherapy plus BCNU and radiotherapy plus BCNU for treatment of malignant glioma after surgery: preliminary results of an RTOG study. Int J Radiat Oncol Biol Phys 1983; 9:1143–1151.

41. Hoshino T. Radiosensitization of brain tumors. In: Deely TJ, ed. Modern radiotherapy and oncology: central nervous system tumors. London: Butterworths, 1974:170–183.

42. Jackson D, Kinsella T, Rowland J, Wright D, Katz D, Main D, Collins J, Kornblith P, Glatstein E. Halogenated pyrimidines as radiosensitizers in the treatment of glioblastoma multiforme. Am J Clin Oncol 1987; 10:437–443.

43. Byers TL, Pegg AE. Properties and physiological function of the polyamine transport system. Am J Physiol 1989; 257:C545–C553.

44. Matsui-Yuasa I, Otani S, Yukioka K, Goto H, Morisawa S. Two mechanisms of spermidine/spermine $N(1)$-acetyltransferase-induction. Arch Biochem Biophys 1989; 268:209–214.

45. Andrews NC, Weiss AJ, Ansfield FJ, Rochlin DB, Mason JH. Phase I study of dibromodulcitol (NSC-104800). Cancer Chemother Rep 1971; 55:61–65.

46. Geran RI, Congleton GF, Dudeck LE, Abbott BJ, Cargus JL. A mouse ependymoblastoma as an experimental model for screening potential antineoplastic drugs. Cancer Chemother Rep 1974; 4:53–87.

47. Levin VA, Freeman-Dove MA, Maroten CE. Dianhydrogalactitol (NSC-132313): pharmacokinetics in normal and tumor-bearing rat brain and antitumor activity against three intracerebral rodent tumors. JNCI 1976; 56:535–539.

48. Walker MD, Alexander E Jr, Hunt WE, MacCarty CS, Mahaley MS Jr, Mealey J Jr, Norrell HA, Owens G, Ransohoff J, Wilson CB, Gehan EA, Strike TA. Evaluation of BCNU and/or radiotherapy in the treatment of anaplastic astrocytomas. A cooperative clinical trial. J Neurosurg 1978; 49:333–343.

49. Walker MD, Green SB, Byar DP, Alexander E Jr, Batzdorf U, Brooks WH, Hunt WE, MacCarty CS, Mahaley MS Jr, Mealey J Jr, Owens G, Ransohoff J II, Robertson JT, Shapiro WR, Smith KR Jr, Wilson CB, Strike TA. Randomized comparisons of radiotherapy and nitrosoureas for the treatment of malignant glioma after surgery. N Engl J Med 1980; 303:1323–1329.

50. Green SB, Byar D, Strike TA. Randomized comparisons of BCNU, streptozotocin, radiosensitizer, and fractionation in the postoperative treatment of malignant glioma (study 77-02). Proc Am Soc Clin Oncol 1984; 3:260.

51. Chang CH, Horton J, Schoenfeld D, Salazar O, Perez-Tamayo R, Kramer S, Weinstein A, Nelson JS, Tsukada Y. Comparison of postoperative radiotherapy and combined postoperative radiotherapy and chemotherapy in the multidisciplinary management of malignant gliomas. A joint Radiation Therapy Oncology and Eastern Cooperative Oncology Group study. Cancer 1983; 52:997–1007.

52. Green SB, Byar D, Walker MD. Comparisons of carmustine, procarbazine, and high-dose methylprednisolone as additions to surgery and radiotherapy for the treatment of malignant glioma. Cancer Treat Rep 1983; 67:121–132.

53. Levin VA, Wilson CB, Davis R, Wara WM, Pischer TL, Irwin L. A Phase III comparison of BCNU, hydroxyurea, and radiation therapy to BCNU and radiation therapy for treatment of primary malignant gliomas. J Neurosurg 1979; 51:526–532.

54. Deutsch M, Green SB, Strike TA, Burger PC, Robertson JT, Selker RG, Shapiro WR, Mealey J Jr, Ransohoff J II, Paoletti P, Smith KR Jr, Odom GL, Hunt WE, Young B, Alexander E Jr, Walker MD, Pistenmaa D. Results of a randomized trial comparing BCNU plus radiotherapy, streptozotocin plus radiotherapy, BCNU plus hyperfractionated radiotherapy, and BCNU following misonidazole plus radiotherapy in the postoperative treatment of malignant glioma. Int J Radiat Oncol Biol Phys 1989; 16:1389–1396.

55. Shapiro WR, Green SB, Burger PC, Mahaley MS Jr, Selker RG, VanGilder JC, Robertson JT, Ransohoff J, Mealey J Jr, Strike TA, Pistenmaa DA. Randomized trial of three chemotherapy regimens and two radiotherapy regimens in postoperative treatment of malignant glioma. Brain Tumor Cooperative Group trial 8001. J Neurosurg 1989; 71:1–9.

56. Levin VA, Silver P, Hannigan J, Wara WM, Gutin PH, Davis RL, Wilson CB. Superiority of post-radiotherapy adjuvant chemotherapy with CCNU, procarbazine, and vincristine (PCV) over BCNU for anaplastic gliomas: NCOG 6G61 final report. Int J Radiat Oncol Biol Phys 1990; 18:321–324.

57. Iliakis G, Pantelias G, Kurtzman S. Mechanism of radiosensitization by halogenated pyrimidines: effect of BrdU on cell killing and interphase chromosome breakage in radiation-sensitive cells. Radiat Res 1991; 125:56–64.

58. Iliakis G, Kurtzman S, Pantelias G, Okayasu R. Mechanism of radiosensitization by halogenated pyrimidines: effect of BrdU on radiation induction of DNA and chromosome damage and its correlation with cell killing. Radiat Res 1989; 119:286–304.

59. Iliakis G, Kurtzman S. Application of non-hypoxic cell sensitizers in radiobiology and radiotherapy: rationale and future prospects. Int J Radiat Oncol Biol Phys 1989; 16:1235–1241.

60. Hoshino T, Nagai M, Sano K. Application of BUdR in the radiotherapy of malignant brain tumors. Nippon Acta Neuroradiol 1967; 836–847.

61. Greenberg HS, Chandler WF, Diaz RF, Ensminger WD, Junck L, Page MA, Gebarski SS, McKeever P, Hood TW, Stetson PL, Litchter AS, Tankanow R. Intra-arterial bromodeoxyuridine radiosensitization and radiation in treatment of malignant astrocytomas. J Neurosurg 1988; 69:500–505.

62. Levin V, Wara W, Gutin PH, Wilson CB, Phillips T, Prados MD, Flam M, Ahn D. Initial analysis of NCOG 6G-82-1: bromodeoxyuridine (BUdR) during irradiation followed by CCNU, procarbazine, and vincristine (PCV) chemotherapy for malignant gliomas. Proc Am Soc Clin Oncol 1990; 9:91.
63. Kinsella TJ, Russo A, Mitchell JB, Collins JM, Rowland J, Wright D, Glatstein E. A phase I study of intravenous iododeoxyuridine as a clinical radiosensitizer. Int J Radiat Oncol Biol Phys 1985; 11:1941–1946.
64. Hochberg FH, Parker LM, Takvorian T, Canellos GP, Zervas NT. High-dose BCNU with autologous bone marrow rescue for recurrent glioblastoma multiforme. J Neurosurg 1981; 54:455–460.
65. Prados MD. Treatment strategies for patients with recurrent brain tumors. Semin Radiat Oncol 1991; 1:1–13.
66. Mahaley MS Jr, Mettlin C, Natarajan N, Laws ER Jr, Peace BB. National survey of patterns of care for brain-tumor patients. J Neurosurg 1989; 71:826–836.

29

Chemotherapy of Pediatric Brain Tumors

Arnold I. Freeman

Children's Mercy Hospital, Kansas City, Missouri

I. INTRODUCTION

Each year 1350 primary brain tumors are reported in children younger than 15 years in the United States (1). As such, pediatric brain tumors account for 20% of all childhood cancer. Brain tumors are further subdivided into a number of subtypes (Fig. 1), making any single histological subtype rare in children. The most common are low-grade astrocytomas, medulloblastoma, high-grade gliomas, brain stem gliomas, and ependymomas.

The treatment modalities currently in use are surgery, radiation therapy, chemotherapy, and biological response modifiers.

Surgery remains the first line of therapy in nearly all cases. Surgery alone may be curative for low-grade astrocytomas, especially of the cerebellum, for which resection results in an 80–90% cure rate. Although the cure rate is lower in cerebral tumors, gross total resection may also be curative. When there is gross residual low-grade astrocytoma, there is debate over the role of adjuvant radiation therapy (see Chap. 12). Given the experience with tumors in other locations of the body as well as in the brain, total resection makes biological sense, because there is less tumor burden left for subsequent eradication by radiation or chemotherapy. In fact, total resection in several types of primary brain tumors has led to a better survival than biopsy alone. However, because of the vital nature of the brain, total excision, or even wide resection with margins, commonly employed in other locations of the body is often not feasible.

Radiation has proved to be of great importance in the control and eradication of brain tumors (2). The brain and spine are in an enclosed cavity, and primary brain tumors rarely spread outside the central nervous system (CNS), particularly early in the course of the disease. Hence, at least in theory, this should be an ideal model for radiation therapy. Unfortunately, some brain tumors are not very radioresponsive and require large doses to completely destroy all tumor cells; this must be tempered by the intellectual decline, or even radiation necrosis, that may accompany high-dose radiation. Loss of intelligence is especially prominent in children less than 5 years of age.

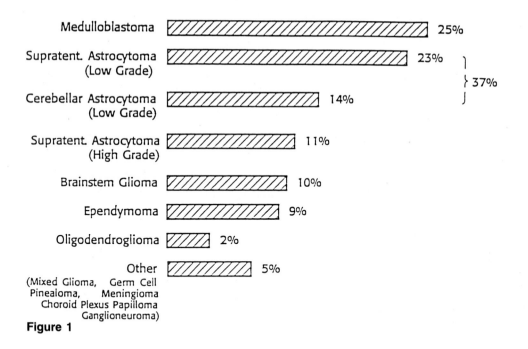

Figure 1

Radiation is curative in 40–60% of medulloblastoma, 20–60% of ependymoma, 20% of brain stem gliomas, and adds to the length of survival in low-grade and high-grade gliomas.

In striving to improve the cure rate and reduce neurotoxicity, chemotherapy and, recently, biological response modifiers continue to be evaluated in brain tumors.

To date, the ability of drugs to enhance survival in children with brain tumors (except for medulloblastoma) has been disappointing. The difficulties in destroying cancer in the CNS are similar to those in other locations in the body, but an additional set of hurdles exist, because of the vital nature of the brain (3).

II. STRUCTURAL CONSTRAINTS TO DRUG DELIVERY

The blood–brain barrier (BBB) forms the basis of the pharmacological sanctuary. It greatly reduces the entry of transmitters, toxins, and other substances into the CNS. Electron microscopic studies have established that the structural basis for the blood–brain barrier are the tight junctions between the capillary endothelial cells. The chemical characteristics that enhance drug entry across this barrier are high lipid solubility, low ionization, and weak protein binding (4).

The corresponding barrier within tumors is termed the blood–tumor barrier (BTB) (5). In contrast with the blood–brain barrier, the capillaries within brain tumors range from structurally normal to grossly abnormal. These abnormalities include thickened capillary walls, surface projections, altered basement membranes, increased pinocytotic vesicles, and fenestrations. Consequently, water-soluble molecules readily permeate the blood–tumor barrier in such areas of the tumor, but there is considerable variation in penetration of water-soluble drugs among different regions within the same tumor. In general, water-soluble drug uptake is small in the central necrotic area of larger tumors, sizably greater in the surrounding tumor bulk, and least in the surrounding normal brain adjacent to tumor where fingerlike projections of tumor growth occur. In humans there is also considerable variation from patient to patient.

The blood–brain barrier and blood–tumor barrier are only one set of obstacles to the delivery of therapeutic amounts of drug to brain tumors. Other problems in drug delivery to the CNS include decreased density of capillaries in the area of tumors and diminished rate of blood flow through these capillaries. When the effects of blood flow are taken into account, the rate of drug transfer across the blood–brain barrier depends on the amount of drug available for exchange within the capillaries, the lipid solubility of the drug, and the surface area of the capillaries perfused by blood (3,6–12). Often, the lipid solubility of a particular antitumor agent is high enough for ready transfer across the blood–brain barrier, but uptake is limited by plasma protein binding or by a relatively short plasma half-life. Differences in perfused capillary surface area among brain loci will affect the distribution of all drugs and yield divergent local rates of drug uptake within the brain and tumor. The implication is that for water-soluble drugs (e.g., methotrexate) the principal limiting factor to drug delivery would be lack of permeability through the blood–brain barrier, whereas, for lipophilic drugs (e.g., BCNU) that readily cross the blood-brain barrier, blood flow would be the limiting factor.

The capillary endothelial wall is highly permeable to water-soluble materials like methotrexate in neuroendocrine areas of the brain such as the neural lobe of the pituitary gland. That is, these structures do not have a blood–brain barrier, and virtually all drugs will readily pass into these areas.

Capillary density blood flow in white matter is approximately 20% that of gray matter. That the brain stem is primarily made up of white matter may account for the poor results of therapy in brain stem gliomas (Fènstermacher J, personal communication), because both radiation therapy and chemotherapy require good perfusion.

Alkylating drugs are particularly important in brain tumors, for which they form the backbone of chemotherapy. Combinations of alkylating agents, such as cisplatin and nitrosoureas, are frequently employed. Interestingly, cross-resistance is lacking between these two agents (13,14). Indeed, therapeutic synergy may be seen among various alkylating agents (14).

Brain tumor resistance to alkylating agents is known to occur. Capillary endothelial cells and normal brain tissue possess enzymes that may inactivate such drugs (8). Two such agents are aldehyde dehydrogenase and glutathione-S-transferase. Aldehyde dehydrogenase inactivates the active metabolite of cyclophosphamide, whereas glutathione-S-transferase activates the formation of glutathione, which is regarded as a xenobiotic or universal detoxicant.

III. THERAPY OF SPECIFIC PEDIATRIC BRAIN TUMORS

A. Medulloblastoma or Primitive Neuroectodermal Tumor (PNET)

Medulloblastoma is an embryonal tumor of neuroectodermal origin primarily seen in the midline of the cerebellum. It likely arises from neuroectodermal cells that are found in the subependymal regions throughout the nervous system. This explains the occurrence of primitive neuroectodermal tumor (PNET)—a tumor that is histologically similar or identical to medulloblastoma that occurs in locations other than the cerebellum. For this reason medulloblastomas are also referred to as PNET of the cerebellum or posterior fossa (15).

Medulloblastomas have a propensity to seed along the cerebrospinal fluid (CSF) pathways (16,17). Therefore, all children with medulloblastoma must be carefully staged with myelograms or magnetic resonance imaging (MRI) of the spine.

Furthermore, a postoperative MRI with gadolinium enhancement should be performed, when feasible, within the first 3 postoperative days to determine the tumor residuum. This, in conjunction with the surgical report, gives a more accurate assessment of what the actual stage is. Unequivocally, patients with tumors that disseminate beyond the posterior fossa have a worse prognosis (18).

Radiation remains the gold standard of therapy in medulloblastomas. Doses of 3500–4000 cGy are commonly administered to the craniospinal axis to eradicate subclinical seeding, and the tumor bed receives approximately 5500 cGy. Unfortunately, this has resulted in a significant loss of intelligence among the survivors (19). Thus, there has been a push to reduce the radiation dose to the craniospinal axis. However, when good-risk (early-stage) medulloblastomas that were treated, in a national study [Children's Cancer Group (CCG) and Pediatric Oncology Group (POG)] with reduced-dose craniospinal radiation were compared with standard dose, there was an unacceptably high incidence of neuraxis failure and overall failures in the former group (20). In neither group was chemotherapy employed. In theory, effective chemotherapy should be able to compensate for reduced-dosage radiation, although this still remains unproved.

A number of agents destroy recurrent medulloblastoma. They include the nitrosoureas, methotrexate (MTX), procarbazine, cyclophosphamide (Cytoxan), the platinum compounds, the vinca alkaloids, and the epipodophylotoxins.

From 1975 to 1982, the Children's Cancer Group (CCG) (21) and Society of International Pediatric Oncology (SIOP) (22) conducted large parallel trials employing lomustine (CCNU) and vincristine (VCR) as adjuvant chemotherapy (Table 1). Chemotherapy showed 59 versus 50% survival advantage over radiation alone. The positive therapeutic benefit of this regimen was evident only in high-stage medulloblastoma (23). This study also confirmed the survival advantage for localized disease (57%) versus metastatic disease (38%) at presentation. By today's standards neither the drugs chosen nor the drug dose was optimal for treating these tumors.

CCG next conducted a study termed "8-in-1" (eight drugs in 1 day) consisting of vincristine, hydroxyurea, prednisone, cisplatin, lomustine, procarbazine, cytarabine (cytosine arabinoside), and cyclophosphamide (24). The CCG first administered 8-in-1 with recurrent brain tumors after surgery, radiation, or chemotherapy. Response was determined by computed tomography (CT) scans after the three courses of chemotherapy. After responses were observed in medulloblastoma, PNET, and malignant gliomas (14/28 or 50%) in the recurrent setting, the study was brought forward (after radiation therapy) to newly diagnosed patients. Fifty-six of 68 newly diagnosed patients were evaluable and, again, 50% (28/56) demonstrated objective responses. Nine of 15 children (60%) with medulloblastoma treated in this fashion had objective responses on neuroimaging.

Next, CCG compared 8-in-1 with vincristine and CCNU in newly diagnosed patients. Both programs were administered after radiation (CCG, unpublished data). Unfortunately, preliminary unpublished results show no survival differences for medulloblastoma between the two treatment arms. It was clearly shown, however, that PNET in the posterior fossa (medulloblastomas) did better than PNET in other locations.

In 1988 Packer et al. (25) conducted an adjuvant trial of vincristine, CCNU, and cisplatin (DDP), following conventional doses of craniospinal radiation, and reported a 90% disease-free survival at 3 years. These results must be tempered by the observation that up to 25% of medulloblastomas can and do relapse late (5–10 years from diagnosis) (26). Nonetheless, the median survival of his patients was prolonged, making it likely that this chemotherapy regimen will improve survival.

The same group of investigators, in attempting to reduce radiation toxicity, decreased the dose of craniospinal radiation to 1800 cGy for children younger than 5 years of age with medulloblastoma (27). The tumor bed received the full dose of radiation. They treated ten children, of whom three relapsed—all outside the primary site. The mean IQ of the group remained unchanged in contrast with earlier studies of full-dose craniospinal radiation for which there were significant declines of IQ.

Table 1 Treatment of Newly Diagnosed PNET (Medulloblastoma)

AUTHOR	DRUGS	SETTING PRE RT	SETTING POST RT	PATIENT NUMBER	RESPONSE RATE (CR OR PR)	SURVIVAL	COMMENT
Evans et al CCG (23)	CCNU, VCR, prednisone		x	233		59% RT + CT 50 RT only high risk {48% RT + CT mets spread {0% RT only	
SIOP (24)	CCNU, VCR		x	286		10 yr overall -45% brain -{54% RT+CT {23% RT stem - 38% RT+CT T3&T4 - 19% RT	significant better survival RT + CT over RT -- in high risk groups
Packer (28)	VCR, CCNU, cisplatin		x	26 "poor risk"		25/26 (96%) alive & disease free median 24 months	results exciting but early
Packer (30)	VCR, CCNU, cisplatin		x	10		7/10	reduced craniospinal RT to 1800 cGy and 3 patients had "drop" mets
Allen (32)	high dose cytoxan + IT ARA-C hydroxyurea	x		5- medulloblast, 3 PNET(cerebral), 1 pinealblastoma	3/8 (37%)		"high risk group"
Pendergrass CCG (26)	"8 in 1" VCR, pred, ARA-C, cytoxan, procarbazine, CCNU, cicplatin, hydroxyurea	x		PNET	9/15 (60%)		
Loeffler (33)	VCR, cisplatin	x		medulloblastoma	4/9 (45.5%)		
Fossanti-Bellani (34)	high dose MTX IV + IT MTX	x		medulloblastoma	(58%)		
Kovnar St. Jude (35)	cisplatin, vp-16	x		medulloblastoma	7/8 (87.5%)		
Mosijczuk POG (36)	VCR, cisplatin, high dose cytoxan	x		PNET	15/32 (47%)		"high risk group"
Freeman (37)	carboplatin, BCNU, streptozotocin	x		PNET 7/8 were medulloblastoma	7/8 (87.5%)		only failure supratentorials PNET

Note: The term medulloblastoma or PNET was used according to the original manuscript.

POG conducted an adjuvant Phase III chemotherapy program comparing MOPP (nitrogen mustard, vincristine, prednisone, and procarbazine) with no MOPP for children with newly diagnosed medulloblastoma who had received radiation, and the results suggested a modest survival benefit for the chemotherapy arm (28).

The use of preradiation chemotherapy in the treatment of newly diagnosed patients with cancer of all types has recently become more commonplace for a number of reasons. In brain tumors, drugs, such as cisplatin and methotrexate, may be less toxic when administered before radiation. Microvascular changes and scarring following radiation may limit drug delivery to the tumor. Also, certain mechanisms of resistance may be shared by radiation and certain alkylating agents. Finally, cisplatin may act as a radiosensitizer when administered before radiation.

Allen et al. employed preradiation chemotherapy and reported a 25% objective response rate in poor-risk patients with PNET: they used high-dose cyclophosphamide, intrathecal cytarabine, and hydroxyurea (29).

Loeffler et al. (30) used preradiation vincristine and cisplatin chemotherapy in children older than 2 years with medulloblastoma. Four of nine (45.5%) showed partial response (PR) or complete response (CR).

Fossati-Bellani used high-dose intravenous and intrathecal methotrexate and observed a 58% response rate in the preradiation setting in medulloblastoma (31).

Kovnar et al., at St. Jude's, treated poor-prognosis medulloblastoma patients before radiation with cisplatin and etoposide (VP-16) and observed seven of eight with objective responses (32).

Mosijczuk et al. evaluated 30 high-risk medulloblastoma patients (33). They used vincristine, cisplatin, and high-dose cyclophosphamide preradiation. There were 9 complete responses (CR), 6 partial responses (PR), 9 with stable disease (SD), 4 with no response (NR), and 4 with progressive disease (PD). In total, 15 of 32 patients (47%) had objective responses.

Freeman used carboplatin, BCNU, and streptozocin in a primary preradiation setting for PNETs (Freeman, et al., unpublished data). There were seven of eight CR or PRs, with the only failure being a PNET of the frontal lobes; the responders were all classic medulloblastomas.

These studies are still too recent to determine their effect on survival. Nonetheless, it appears reasonable that reducing the tumor burden should assist subsequent radiation in achieving total eradication. Interestingly, the survival of patients who responded to preirradiation, neoadjuvant chemotherapy (PR or CR) was superior to that of nonchemotherapy responders (Fig. 2) (Freeman et al., unpublished data).

B. Brain Stem Tumors

Brain stem gliomas account for 10% of childhood brain tumors (1), but brain stem gliomas are not a homogeneous entity (34–40). Those patients presenting with a long-standing history, those with neurofibromatosis, and those with exophytic lesions do better. The latter group may be cured with surgery alone. In contrast, those patients with diffuse intrinsic lesions do poorly (39). Few survive beyond 3 years; this group's lesion is commonly high-grade astrocytoma, although there is frequently no histological diagnosis, since the diagnosis is based on neuroimaging.

Standard therapy is radiation and, for many years, a dose of 5500 cGy was employed. Most children responded with clinical improvement, but this was short-lived, with a median time to recurrence of 6 months and a median survival of 1 year (41–44).

Recently, hyperfractionated radiation has been used to increase the total dose of radiation, without theoretically increasing the toxicity. Initial reports were optimistic, but studies by POG failed to confirm benefit at 6600 cGy (45,46)). At 7020 cGy, there may be a trend to improved survival at 2 years (47).

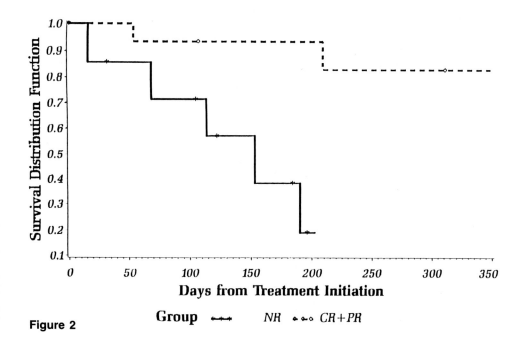

Figure 2

The CCG evaluated 7200-cGy–hyperfractionated RT in the treatment of brain stem tumors. The treatment was well tolerated, but the overall disease-free survival at 3 years was only 20% (CCG, unpublished data). A dose of 7800-cGy–hyperfractionated radiation is now under evaluation by both CCG and POG.

There is a paucity of information concerning single-drug efficacy in the neuroimaging era (48). Even for BCNU, the single most studied drug in brain tumors, there is no published data. By neuroimaging, carboplatin has a 21% objective response rate (3/24) in brain stem tumors (49,50). High-dose cyclophosphamide (at 80 mg/kg), in one report, had an 80% response rate (4/5) (51); but this requires confirmation. Vincristine was reported to be an active drug in brain stem tumors, but this was based on neurological improvement in the preneuroimaging era (52).

To date there is no information that adding adjuvant chemotherapy to radiation improves survival in patients with primary brain stem tumors. Indeed, CCG assessed adjuvant vincristine and CCNU given in addition to radiation and found no survival benefit.

Kretchmer evaluated high-dose cyclophosphamide and cisplatin before radiation for brain stem tumor (22). There were 32 evaluable patients, and only 2 of these had a PR. They noted that preradiation chemotherapy could be safely delivered to this group of patients.

In summary, the role of chemotherapy in brain stem tumors has yet to be demonstrated. In an attempt to identify active agents in these tumors, with the longer-term goal of developing logical and more effective adjuvant Phase III studies, CCG is embarking on a clinical trial testing three pairs of drugs in a preradiation setting. These three pairs are high-dose carboplatin and etoposide (VP-16), high-dose cyclophosphamide and vincristin, and BCNU and streptozocin. Etoposide is a topoisomerase inhibitor and could conceivably overcome resistance to carboplatin. Streptozocin in vitro has overcome BCNU resistance by preventing adduct repair. The CCG is also testing interferon (IFN) at high doses, coupled with hyperfractionated radiation.

C. Malignant Gliomas

Low-grade astrocytomas are termed benign tumors, but this is a poor term, as they frequently result in death, although mostly with a longer survival than malignant gliomas. James and Associates (53), in elegant experiments, showed progressive cytogenetic and molecular derangement and loss of control as tumors progressed from astrocytomas to anaplastic astrocytoma and then to glioblastoma multiforme.

Formerly, many investigators lumped anaplastic astrocytoma with glioblastoma multiforme in evaluating clinical trials. This is unwise because survival rates between these two can vary from 5 to 50%; therefore, stratification is important in designing trials. In the pediatric age range, anaplastic astrocytomas are at least as common as glioblastoma multiforme.

Surgery is the mainstay of therapy, and survival is directly linked to the percentage of tumor resected. After surgery, radiation has improved survival. Following these modalities, chemotherapy is commonly added. In adults, adjuvant BCNU continues to be the standard. However, the influence of adjuvant chemotherapy on survival has been limited.

A large group of drugs result in objective tumor shrinkage. In adults, other approaches have included the use of biological response modifiers. In particular, interferon has shown some antitumor effect. There are current trials that couple biological response modifiers (BRM) with chemotherapy because of their reported synergy. In addition, intra-arterial chemotherapy has been tried; BCNU and cisplatin are most commonly employed, but may be toxic to the brain and retina.

Because high-grade gliomas are uncommon during childhood, most of the Phase II data is extrapolated from adult studies. The number of pediatric trials in high-grade gliomas is limited.

In 1981, CCG embarked upon a study testing the addition of CCNU and vincristine to radiation (54). The group receiving chemotherapy did significantly better than that with radiation alone, with a 5-year event-free survival of 45%, compared with 10% for radiation alone. Unfortunately, patients were not stratified as to whether their tumors were anaplastic gliomas or glioblastoma multiforme; subsequent studies have not confirmed a 45% event-free survival group.

The next study of the CCG compared the vincristine–CCNU arm to 8-in-1 (eight drugs in 1 day) arm. There were no statistical differences in the two groups at 3 years (55).

These generally disappointing results mirror those seen in adult high-grade gliomas and indicate the need for more effective drugs. To that end, CCG is embarking on a study assessing three pairs of drugs given at high doses in a neoadjuvant preradiation setting. These drug pairs are (1) high-dose cyclophosphamide and VP-16; (2) high-dose ifosfamide and VP-16; and (3) high dose carboplatin and VP-16. To determine the efficacy of these pairs when given at high doses the preradiation setting is used, since there is mounting evidence that response rates may be higher before irradiation, thereby enabling the identification of effective agents.

D. Ependymomas

Ependymomas are tumors that arise from the ependymal lining of the ventricles of the brain or central canal of the cord. Approximately two-thirds occur in the posterior fossa, and most of the remainder occur supratentorially (1). There is a peak in childhood at age 2 (1). In teenagers and adults ependymomas of the spinal cord become more prevalent.

Histologically, ependymomas have been graded from I to IV, with grades I and II called benign, and III and IV high-grade or anaplastic (56–59). In addition there is the entity called ependymoblastoma; this is an undifferentiated tumor that behaves much like a primitive neuroectodermal tumor (PNET) and has a high proclivity for dissemination along CSF pathways. A diagnosis of ependymoblastoma mandates PNET-like treatment with craniospinal radiation and chemotherapy. In ependymomas other than ependymoblastomas, it has been extremely difficult to correlate biological behavior and CSF seeding with histological grade (60,61). There is also a lack of correlation of histopathological subtype and survival (62).

Location has been reported to predict CSF spread, with seeding more commonly seen in infratentorial than in the supratentorial tumors.

Afra et al. evaluated 80 "lobar ependymomas" (63). These are supratentorial ependymomas occurring in the paraventricular lobes of the brain. A subset had recurrences after an extremely long time interval (> 10 years). We observed a recurrence of a lobar ependymoma in a 25-year-old woman 19 years after initial presentation at age 6. Most failures that occur in ependymomas are because of inability to eradicate the primary tumors.

Children generally have a poorer prognosis than adults. This may be because infants receive lower-dose radiation to prevent the long-term sequelae to the brain and spinal cord. Until recently, cure rates in infants were less than 20% (1). Ependymomas of the cauda equina region, which occur principally in adults, have a high cure rate (80% or greater) with surgery or localized radiation therapy.

Initial treatment of ependymomas of the brain consists of surgery, followed by radiation. In ependymomas, it has not yet been demonstrated that gross surgical extirpation offers survival advantage over biopsy alone. Radiation to the tumor bed of 5000–5500 cGy is commonly administered. The role of "prophylactic craniospinal radiation" is unclear. In common practice, posterior fossa and high-grade ependymomas receive total CNS irradiation, whereas supratentorial low-grade ependymomas do not. The need for craniospinal radiation is now being tested by the POG.

Adjuvant chemotherapy as yet has not yielded improved survival in ependymomas. The platinum compounds, cisplatin and carboplatin, appear to be the most effective agents for this tumor (64,65).

Treatment with other agents, such as high-dose cyclophosphamide, ifosfamide, methotrexate, vincristine, or nitrosoureas have shown limited benefit.

The "BABY" POG protocol (66) employed cisplatin and VP-16, cycling with high-dose cyclophosphamide and vincristin in children younger than 3 years of age for extended periods prior to radiation. With ependymoma, there were 12 of 25 (48%) (12 CR and 5 PR) objective responses.

A CCG study evaluated adjuvant vincristine and CCNU in addition to craniospinal irradiation in medulloblastoma and posterior fossa ependymomas (21). The prognosis depended heavily on age. Only 5 of 24 (21%) children younger than 9 years at diagnosis with ependymoma were long-term survivors. This may be a falsely high estimate, because the follow-up was curtailed at 3–8 years, and late relapses in ependymoma are not uncommon. For children older than 9 years, 8 of 12 (67%) were long-term survivors. In this group of patients, 18 of 20 failures occurred in the original tumor site (posterior fossa).

Investigators at Children's Hospital of Philadelphia evaluated survival after relapse of ependymoma (67). In their series, relapse occurred in the initial site exclusively in 27 of 52, plus an additional 8 with simultaneous local and distant relapse. Survival was improved for those who had a low-grade histological type at relapse. Responses to chemotherapy were poor, with only a single (1/37) patient showing objective tumor response (PR). Nonetheless, those patients receiving chemotherapy in this setting did better than those who did not, and those who received a cisplatin-based regimen survived longer than those on other chemotherapy regimens.

E. Low-Grade Astrocytomas

Low-grade astrocytomas are the most common brain tumors in childhood. In the posterior fossa region, complete or near complete resection is associated with an 80% or greater event-free survival. When gross residual disease remains, particularly when it infiltrates the brain stem, some surgeons advocate postoperative radiation. In the supratentorium, with incomplete resection, the question of whether or not adjuvant radiation is beneficial has not been resolved. This question is being addressed in a national randomized study by CCG.

The role of chemotherapy in low-grade astrocytomas is unclear. A combination of vincristine, BCNU, and methotrexate was employed, in the mid-1970s, with reported neurological and survival benefit (68), but this was in the pre-CT scan era.

In 1985, the group from Children's Hospital of Philadelphia noted that vincristine and dactinomycin were effective in optic gliomas (69), but those who benefited stabilization of disease and not objective tumor responses of CR or PR.

Friedman evaluated carboplatin in low-grade astrocytomas (70). Nine of 12 patients with clearly progressive disease stabilized following carboplatin, although objective shrinkage (CR or PR by neuroimaging) was not seen.

Thus, the efficacy of chemotherapy in pediatric low-grade gliomas awaits confirmation, since stabilization of disease alone is not sufficient proof of a drug's antitumor efficacy.

F. Infants

Survival in infants and children, younger than 3 years, with brain tumors is bleak. Duffner et al. reviewing the Surveillance, Epidemiology, and End Result (SEER) data found survivals of 20% (1). Furthermore, infants or very young children also suffer the worst treatment-induced neurotoxicity (71), much of which appears to be radiation-related. To this end Baram et al. at M. D. Anderson evaluated MOPP chemotherapy (mechlorethamine, vincristine, prednisone, and procarbazine) in brain tumors in infants and found a high-response rate (72). They also found that some of these infants did not require later radiation therapy.

In 1986, Duffner et al. launched a study employing vincristine, and cyclophosphamide, cycling with cisplatin and VP-16, for infants and young children to age 36 months (66). At the end of chemotherapy, patients were irradiated. They studied 102 patients. Objective responses (CR and PR) were seen in medulloblastoma, 13 of 27 (48%), ependymoma, 12 of 25 (48%), poorly differentiated embryonal tumors, 6 of 21 (29%); and malignant gliomas, 6 of 10 (60%), but not in brain stem gliomas.

Infants with gross total extirpation of their tumor had significantly increased survival ($p = 0.0001$). Poor prognostic factors at diagnosis were tumor dissemination, the presence of brain stem gliomas and, to a lesser extent the presence of an embryonal tumor. At 2 years the overall progeession-free survival was 39%.

Strauss et al. treated eight young children (median 6.5 months) with cisplatin and VP-16 (73). Four of six children with measurable disease had either a CR or a PR.

CCG evaluated an 8-in-1 regimen following surgery in infants younger than 18 months of age (74). There were 78 infants younger in this age group with PNET (including medulloblastoma) or "malignant" ependymoma; and 37 infants younger than 24 months of age with malignant astrocytoma. Treatment consisted of ten cycles of chemotherapy. For the PNET and ependymoma group the 2-year progression-free survival was 25%. None of the 11 infants with pinealblastomas survived, 20% of those with ependymomas survived, and 35% of those with PNETs survived. For the high-grade glioma group (not including those with brain stem glioma) the overall progression-free survival was 33%. There were no recurrences after 2 years in this group. Survival appeared the same whether or not these children received radiation.

The CCG is now embarking on a study retesting the four drugs employed by the POG infant study, but at intensified doses. Infants who experience a CR will be observed without radiation.

G. Pineal Area Tumors

Pineal tumors account for only 2% of childhood brain tumors. Pineal parenchymal tumors make up one-third of the total and germ cell tumors the remainder (75–77).

Pineal parenchymal tumors are subdivided into pinealblastomas and pinealcytomas. Pinealblastomas are undifferentiated tumors that are likely a variant of PNET and should be treated in a like fashion. Chemotherapy as yet has had little or no role in the treatment of pinealcytomas.

Germ cell tumors are divided into germinomas and teratomas. The germinomas appear histologically indistinguishable from their counterpart in the gonads. Dissemination by CSF is not infrequent (77); therefore, classic therapy generally involved field radiation plus craniospinal radiation for subclinical spread. These tumors are also highly sensitive to the same chemotherapy as their gonadal counterparts; accordingly, the platinum compounds are highly effective. Also of use are VP-16 and bleomycin. It has been our practice to treat the germinomas with carboplatin, BCNU, streptozocin and VP-16 for three to six courses, followed by involved field radiation.

Chemotherapy alone is being evaluated for primary CNS germ cell tumors in adults and children (78). Twenty-three patients (14 with germinomas and 9 with nongerminoma germ cell tumors) were treated with carboplatin, VP-16, and bleomycin. All germinomas and 6 of 9 nongerminomas achieved a CR, and they did not receive radiation. This report indicates that it may be feasible to remove radiation from this group of tumor patients who experience a CR.

H. Biological Response Modifiers

There are few studies of biological response modifiers in brain tumors in children. Allen et al., in a CCG pilot study, tested recombinant interferon (IFN) beta at escalating doses to 600 million units/m^2 (79). They observed 4 of 21 (19%) patients with partial responses: two were high-grade gliomas, and 2 were brain stem gliomas. Responses were seen only at doses greater than 100 million units/m^2. It is clear that other pediatric studies with interferon and other biological response modifiers are needed. Synergy has been noted when combining certain modifiers, such as IFN-α and IFN-γ, and synergy has also been noted when combining interferon with certain chemotherapeutic drugs.

I. Bone Marrow Transplantation

Finlay tested high-dose multiagent chemotherapy, followed by bone marrow rescue in ten patients younger than 21 years of age with malignant astrocytoma (80). Seven of ten had recurrent disease. They employed thiotepa and VP-16 or thiotepa, VP-16, and BCNU. There were four CRs and two PRs.

Following this, autologous bone marrow rescue for children younger than 6 years of age was evaluated by CCG (81). Thirty-seven of 39 children had recurrent tumors. Of these children 34 had received prior chemotherapy. The preoperative regimes used thiotepa and VP-16; thiotepa, VP-16, and carboplatin; or thiotepa, VP-16, and BCNU. There were 8 CR and 5 PR for a total of 13 responders (33%) and 6 of 8 CRs are surviving disease-free and may be salvaged.

These results are most encouraging in this very poor-risk group of patients.

IV. NEUROPSYCHOLOGICAL STATUS

The quality of life in children who have been successfully treated and cured of their brain tumors has become an ever-increasing concern. Cured children have a lifetime ahead of them, and their ability to function in society cannot be overstated. Therefore, in recent years, despite the risk, individual investigators and even groups have modified their approaches to treatment to take this into consideration. Recently, Mulhern et al. analyzed 22 reports dealing with the functional status of the survivors (Table 2; 75). In total, 544 children with brain tumors were reviewed. Most of the studies concluded that radiation had a detrimental effect on intelligence. In this review, tumor location did not correlate with loss of intelligence. Also the extent of surgery or the presence of hydrocephalus did not appear to be related. Notable were age—the young child who received whole-brain radiation had a 14-point lower IQ than the older child; although all children who received cranial radiation had lower IQs than their unirradiated counterparts.

Even though there is suspicion that the higher the dose of radiation the greater the deficit, this premise still awaits confirmation. Also unanswered is whether certain drugs may augment radiation toxicity to the brain. Nonetheless, this review confirms many smaller studies.

V. EVALUATION AND SURVEILLANCE

Kramer et al. have suggested a standard format of evaluation for brain tumors, determined by their proclivity for CNS and extra-CNS dissemination (82). Standardization of surveillance techniques and definition of responses are vital to group-wide efforts and interpretation of data (83). The likelihood for CNS subarachnoid spread (SAS) is the major determinant in baseline evalua-

Table 2 Summary of Multistudy Analysis of IQ

Patient group[a]	N	Mean	SE[b]	SD[c]
Overall	403	91.0	2.65	24.1
Age at diagnosis				
<4 yr	48	71.9	3.08	21.4
≥4 yr	135	92.6	1.84	21.4
Tumor region				
3rd ventricle	73	94.2	2.76	23.6
Posterior fossa	101	90.2	2.34	23.6
Cerebral hemisphere	67	89.7	2.88	23.6
Radiation therapy volume				
None	54	101.2	2.85	20.9
Local	98	93.8	2.11	20.9
Cranial (whole brain)	125	82.9	1.87	20.9
Region and age				
Posterior fossa, <4 yr	10	75.0	6.18	18.6
Posterior fossa, ≥4 yr	53	88.9	2.69	18.6
Cerebral hemisphere, ≥4 yr	12	82.0	5.64	18.6
Radiation therapy volume and age				
None, ≥4 yr	10	99.3	6.10	19.3
Local, ≥4 yr	15	85.3	4.98	19.3
Cranial, <4 yr	16	73.4	4.82	19.3
Cranial, ≥4 yr	54	87.0	2.62	19.3
Region and radiation therapy volume				
3rd ventricle, none	24	100.3	4.24	20.8
3rd ventricle, local	45	93.2	3.10	20.8
Posterior fossa, none	24	103.2	4.24	20.8
Posterior fossa, local	17	93.9	5.04	20.8
Posterior fossa, cranial	60	83.9	2.68	20.8
Cerebral hemisphere, local	22	92.2	4.43	20.8

[a]Restricted to those subgroups with n ≥10.
[b]SE, standard error.
[c]SD, standard deviation.

tions and subsequent surveillance testing. Subarachnoid spread varies greatly from tumor type to tumor type and even from investigator to investigator. In children with medulloblastoma, Deutsch reported SAS at diagnosis in 61% of children 5 years old and younger and 38% in those older than 5 years (84). These figures are higher than most series. In ependymoma, an incidence of SAS of 12–15% is common (85,86), and posterior fossa ependymomas are more likely to disseminate. The true incidence of SAS in high-grade gliomas is not fully appreciated, since neuroaxis evaluation is not routinely performed, yet SAS of 18 (87) to 46% (88) has been reported. Germ cell tumors also frequently spread along CSF pathways, and one report noted tumor cells in the CSF in 7 of 20 cases (35%) (89). For low-grade astrocytomas and low-grade oligodendrogliomas, SAS has been observed in 1.2–8.5% (86,90). Brain stem gliomas have been reported with SAS in 5% of cases (91). Thus, initial evaluation in tumors with an appreciable chance of SAS should include an evaluation of not only the brain, but also of the spinal cord.

Kramer also suggested that, for a true baseline evaluation the last MRI should be obtained no longer than 14 days before starting any new form of therapy (82). It has also been noted that neuroimaging, rather than the surgeon's assessment, is the most reliable means to evaluate the degree of surgical resection (92). The MRI scans are most accurate within the first days after surgery before gliosis (93,94); they should be performed with and without gadolinium.

Another area that creates considerable difficulty in interpreting published studies is the wide variation in how responses are reported. Most investigators use the classic oncology definitions that require a 50% shrinkage (a PR) or greater to be termed a response. Others include stable disease (i.e, no change in tumor size). Still others have used volumetric shrinkage as a definition of response. All have valid arguments supporting their position. Thus, differences in results reported by various groups may not reflect important differences in the effectiveness of the therapy. Clearly, a single set of criteria is highly desirable.

Even neuroimaging must be viewed cautiously. Residual tumor may be confused with hemorrhage or gliosis. If chemotherapy is administered soon after radiation, responses may still be due to the radiation and yet be credited to chemotherapy.

VI. PROSPECTS FOR THE FUTURE

Several important factors will aid the design of future drug regimens. Classic neuropathology is often inadequate in predicting which tumor is a "bad actor." The classic example is ependymoma, but some low-grade astrocytomas that appear benign behave like malignant gliomas. The hope is that molecular probes and monoclonal antibodies, currently being evaluated, will cast new light in this area and permit better classification and, consequently, improved stratification of therapy.

Improved drug delivery to brain tumors may be achieved in several ways (3). Intra-arterial therapy may allow delivery of high doses, but only for the first pass. Drugs must also be well tolerated by normal brain tissue. Not all drugs have the desired chemical characteristics for intra-arterial use. There have as yet been no intra-arterial studies specific for pediatrics, perhaps because of technical factors in the young child and perhaps because most tumors are posterior fossa tumors for which the risk factors may be even higher.

Other delivery techniques include (1) monoclonal antibodies bound to radionuclides or toxins, such as ricin (a plant toxin) (95) now being tested in meningeal cancer by intrathecal administration; however, delivery to solid brain tumors through a vascular route may be much more difficult. (2) Liposomes as carriers are showing some limited promise (96). (3) Degradable wafers, impregnated with BCNU and implanted into the tumor bed, are being evaluated for high-grade adult gliomas (97). (4) A novel approach has been suggested by Boder; he linked drugs to a dehydropyridine carrier and injected it intravenously. The drug–carrier complex penetrates the blood–brain barrier readily. Once inside the brain the carrier is oxidized by endogenous enzymes, impeding the exit of the parent drug from the CNS and from the tumor, thereby achieving high levels for prolonged periods.

Expanded trials of bone marrow transplants are also being considered. This would permit much higher doses of chemotherapy to be given.

For more effective drug treatment, clearly more effective drugs must also be developed. We must also learn to use the drugs we have more effectively. This means overcoming resistance. Resistance to alkylating agents is particularly important in brain tumors, since these drugs form the backbone of chemotherapy. Several studies are now addressing resistance to the alkylating drugs, and several clinical studies have been mounted. One example is combining streptozocin with BCNU.

In the more distant future gene therapy and tumor vaccines may lead to the ultimate victory over childhood brain tumors.

REFERENCES

1. Cohen ME, Duffner PK. Trends in treatment, referral patterns and survival statistics of children with brain tumors in the United States. In: Cohen ME, Duffner PK, eds. Brain tumors in children: principles of diagnosis and treatment. New York: Raven Press, 1984:349–352.
2. Bloom HJG. Intracranial tumors: response and resistance to therapeutic endeavors, 1970–1980. Int J Radiat Oncol Biol Phys 1982; 8:1083–1113.
3. Freeman AI, Fenstermacher J, Shapiro W, Kemshead J, Chasin M, Colvin OM, Diksic M, Finley J, Hertler A, Levin V, Mayhew E, Poplack D, Shapiro J, Ushio Y. Forbeck Forum on improved drug delivery to brain tumors. Select Cancer Ther 1990; 6:109–118.
4. Rall DP, Oppelt WW, Patlak CS. Extracellular space of brain as determined by diffusion of insulin from the ventricular system. Life Sci 1962; 2:43.
5. Blasberg RG, Groothuis DR. Chemotherapy of brain tumors: physiological and pharmacokinetic considerations. Semin Oncol 1986; 13:70.
6. Sakurada O, Kennedy C, Jehle J, Brown J, Carbin G, Sokoloff L. Measurement of local cerebral blood flow with iodo[^{14}C]antipyrine. Am J Physiol 1978; 234:H59.
7. Fenstermacher J, Gross P, Sposito N, Acuff V, Pettersen S, Gruber K. Structural and functional variations in capillary systems within the brain. Ann NY Acad Sci 1988; 529:21.
8. Ghersi-Egea JF, Minn A, Siest G. A new aspect of the protective function of the blood–brain barrier: activities of four drug metabolizing enzymes in isolated rat brain microvessels. Life Sci 1988; 42:2515.
9. Levin VA, Landahl H, Freeman-Dove MA. The application of brain capillary permeability coefficient measurements to pathologic conditions and the selection of agents which cross the blood–brain barrier. J Pharmacokinet Biopharm 1976; 4:499.
10. Levin VA, Landahl HD, Patlak CS. Drug delivery to CNS tumors. Cancer Treat Rep 1981; 65:19.
11. Levin VA, Patlak CS, Landahl HD. Heuristic modeling of drug delivery to malignant brain tumors. J Pharmacokinet Biopharm 1980; 8:257.
12. Levin VA. Pharmacokinetics and CNS chemotherapy. In: Hellman K, Carter SK, eds. Fundamentals of cancer chemotherapy. New York: McGraw-Hill, 1986:28–40.
13. Frei E III, Cucchi CA, Rosowsky A, Tantravahi R, Bernal S, Ervin TJ, Ruprecht RM. Alkylating agent resistance: in vitro studies with human cell lines. Proc Natl Acad Sci USA 1985; 82:2158–2162.
14. Schabel FM, Trader MW, Laster WR, Wheeler GP, Witt MH. Patterns of resistance and therapeutic synergy among alkylating agents. Antibiot Chemother 1978; 23:200.
15. Rorke LB. The cerebellar medulloblastoma and its relationship to primitive neuroectodermal tumors. J Neuropathol Exp Neurol 1983; 42:1–15.
16. Kopelson G, Linggood RM, Kleinman GM. Medulloblastoma: the identification of prognostic subgroups and implications for multimodal management. Cancer 1983; 51:312–319.
17. Park TS, Hoffman HJ, Hendrick EB, Humphreys RP, Becker LE. Medulloblastoma: clinical presentation and management. J Neurosurg 1983; 58:543–552.

18. Allen JC, Bloom J, Ertel I, Evans A, Hammond D, Jones H, Levin V, Jenkin D, Sposto R, Wara W. Brain tumors in children: current cooperative and institutional chemotherapy trials in newly diagnosed recurrent disease. Semin Oncol 1986; 13:110–122.

19. Mulhern RK, Hancock J, Fairclough O, Kun LE. Neuropsychological status of children treated for brain tumors: a critical review and integrative analysis. Med Pediatr Oncol 1992; 20:181–191.

20. Kun LE, Constine LS. Medulloblastoma—caution regarding new treatment approaches. Int Radiat Oncol Biol Phys 1990; 20:897–899.

21. Evans AE, Jenkin RDT, Sposto R, Ortega JA, Wilson CB, Wara W, Ertel IJ, Kramer S, Chang CH, Leikin SL, Hammond GD. The treatment of medulloblastoma. Results of prospective randomized trial of radiation therapy with and without CCNU, vincristine, and prednisone. J Neurosurg 1990; 72:572–582.

22. Tait DM, Thorton-Jones H, Blood HJ, Lemerle J, Morris-Jones P. Adjuvant chemotherapy for medulloblastoma: the first multi-centre control trial of the International Society of Pediatric Oncology (SIOP). Eur J Cancer 1990; 26:464–469.

23. Chang CH, Housepian EM, Herbert C. An operative staging system and a megavoltage radiotherapeutic technic for cerebellar medulloblastoma. Radiology 1969; 93:1351–1359.

24. Pendergrass TW, Milstein JM, Geyer JR, Mulne AF, Kosnik EJ, Morris JD, Heideman RL, Ruymann FB, Stuntz JT, Bleyer WA. Eight drugs in one day chemotherapy for brain tumors: experience in 107 children and rationale for preradiation chemotherapy. J Clin Oncol 1987; 5:1221–1231.

25. Packer RJ, Siegel KR, Sutton LN, Evans AE, D'Angio G, Rorke LB, Bunin GR, Schut L. Efficacy of adjuvant chemotherapy for patients with poor-risk medulloblastoma: a preliminary report. Ann Neurol 1988; 24:503–508.

26. Lefkowitz IB, Packer RJ, Ryan SG, Shah N, Alavi J, Rorke LB, Sutton LN, Schut L. Late recurrence of primitive neuroectodermal tumor/medulloblastoma. Cancer 1988; 62:826–830.

27. Packer RJ, Goldwein JW, Sutton LN, Lange B, Rorke LB, Radcliffe J, D'Angio GJ. Low dose craniospinal radiation (CsRT) with chemotherapy for children less than 60 months with posterior fossa (PF) PNET: 2 year survival and intellectual results. J Neurooncol 1992; 12:268.

28. vanEys J, Chen T, Moore T, Cheek W, Sexauer C, Starling C, Starling K. Adjuvant chemotherapy for medulloblastoma and ependymoma using iv vincristine intrathecal methotrexate and intrathecal hydrocortisone: a Southwest Oncology Group study. Cancer Treat Rep 1981; 65:681–684.

29. Allen JC, Helson L, Jereb B. Pre-radiation chemotherapy for newly diagnosed childhood brain tumors. Cancer 1983; 52:2001–2006.

30. Loeffler JS, Kretschmar CS, Sallan SE, LaVally BL, Winston KR, Fischer EG, Tarbell NJ. Pre-radiation chemotherapy for infants and poor prognosis children with medulloblastoma. J Radiat Oncol Biol Phys 1988; 15:177–181.

31. Fossati-Bellani F, Bellegotti L, Tesoro-Tess JD, Ballerini E, Savoiardo M, Lombardi F, Morandi F, Massimino M, Gasparini M. Preradiation chemotherapy for childhood and poor prognosis medulloblastoma [abstract]. International Symposium on Pediatric Neuro-oncology. Seattle, June 1–3, 1989.

32. Kovnar EH, Kellie SJ, Horowitz ME, Sanford RA, Langston JW, Mulhern RK, Jenkins JJ, Douglass EC, Etcubanas EE, Fairclough DL. Pre-irradiation cisplatin and etoposide in the treatment of high-risk medulloblastoma and other malignant embryonal tumors of the central nervous system: a phase II study. J Clin Oncol 1990; 8:330–336.

33. Mosijczuk AD, Nigro MA, Thomas PR, Burger PC, Krischer JF, Morantz R, Kurdunowicz E, Mulne AF, Towbin RB, Freeman AI, Nigro ED, Kun LE, Friedman HS. Preradiation chemotherapy in advanced medulloblastoma: Pediatric Oncology Group pilot 8695 study. (In preparation).

34. Littman P, Jarrett P, Bilaniuk LT, Rorke LB, Zimmerman RA, Bruce DA, Carabell SC, Schut L. Pediatric brainstem gliomas. Cancer 1980; 45:2787–2792.

35. Panitch MS, Berg BO. Brainstem tumors of childhood and adolescence. Am J Dis Child 1970; 119:465–472.

36. Villani R, Gaini SM, Tomei G. Follow-up study of brainstem tumors in children. Childs Brain 1975; 1:126–135.

37. Hoffman HJ, Becker L, Craven MA. A clinically and pathologically distinct group of benign brainstem gliomas. Neurosurgery 1980; 7:243–248.

38. Stroink AR, Hoffman HJ, Hendrick EB, Humphreys RP. Diagnosis and management of pediatric brainstem gliomas. J Neurosurg 1986; 65:745–750.
39. Albright AL, Guthkelch AN, Packer RJ, Price RA, Rourke LB. Prognostic factors in pediatric brainstem gliomas. J Neurosurg 1986; 65:751–755.
40. Berger MS, Edwards MS, LaMasters D, Davis RL, Wilson CB. Pediatric brain stem tumors: radiographic, pathologic and clinical correlations. J Neurosurg 1983; 12:298–302.
41. Bouchard J. Radiation therapy of tumors and diseases of the nervous system. Philadelphia: Lea & Febiger, 1966:119–134.
42. Greenberger JS, Cassady J, Levene MB. Radiation therapy of thalamic midbrain and brainstem gliomas. Radiology 1977; 122:463–468.
43. Hara M, Takeuchi KA. A temporal study of survival of patients with pontine gliomas. J Neurosurg 1977; 216:189–196.
44. Kim TH, Chin HW, Pollan S, Hazel JH, Webster JH. Radiotherapy of primary brainstem tumors. Int J Radiat Oncol Biol Phys 1980; 6:51–57.
45. Edwards MS, Wara WM, Urtasum RC, Prados M, Levin VA, Fulton D, Wilson CB, Hannigan J, Silver P. Hyperfractioned radiation therapy for brain stem glioma: a Phase I–II trial. J Neurosurg 1989; 70:691–700.
46. Freeman CR, Krischer J, Sanford RA, Burger PC, Cohen M, Norris D. Hyperfractionated radiotherapy in brain stem tumors: results of a Pediatric Oncology Group study. Int J Radiat Oncol Biol Phys 1988; 15:311–318.
47. Freeman CR, Krischer J, Sanford RA, Cohen ME, Burger PC, Kan L, Halperin EC, Crocker I, Wharan M. Hyperfractionated radiation therapy in brain stem tumors: results of treatment at the 7020 cGy dose level of Pediatric Oncology Group study 8495. Cancer 1991; 68:474–481.
48. Fulton DS, Levin VA, Wara WM, Edwards MS, Wilson CB. Chemotherapy of pediatric brainstem tumors. J Neurosurg 1981; 54:715–721.
49. Allen JC, Walker R, Luks E, Jennings M, Barfoot S, Tan C. Carboplatin and recurrent childhood brain tumors. J Clin Oncol 1987; 5:459–463.
50. Gaynon PS, Ettinger LJ, Baum ES, Siegel SE, Krailo MD, Hammond GD. Carboplatin in childhood brain tumors. A Children's Cancer study group Phase II trial. Cancer 1990; 66:2465–2469.
51. Allen JC, Helson L. High-dose cyclophosphamide chemotherapy for recurrent CNS tumors in children. Am J Pediatr Hematol Oncol 1990; 12:297–300.
52. Rosenstock JG, Evans AE, Schut L. Response to vincristine of recurrent brain tumors in children. J Neurosurg 1976; 45:135.
53. James CD, Mikkelsen T, Cavenee WK, Collins VP. Molecular genetics aspects of glial tumor evolution. Cancer Surv 1990; 9:631–644.
54. Sposto R, Ertel IJ, Jenkin RD, Boesel CP, Venes JL, Ortega JA, Evans AE, Wara W, Hammond D. The effectiveness of chemotherapy for treatment of high grade astrocytomas in children: results of a randomized trial. J Neurooncol 1989; 7:165–177.
55. Finlay J, Boyett J, Yates A, Turski P, Wisoff J, Milstein J, McGuire P, Bertolone S, Geyer J, Tefft M, Wara W, Epstein F, Edwards M, Berger M, Sutton L, Allen J, Hammond D. A randomized phase III trial of chemotherapy for childhood high grade astrocytoma: report of CCSG trial CCG-945, [abstract]. Proc Am Soc Clin Oncol 1991; 1078.
56. Coulon RA, Till K. Intracranial ependymomas in children: a review of 43 cases. Childs Brain 1977; 3:154–168.
57. Dohrmann GJ, Farwell JR, Flannery JT. Ependymomas and ependymoblastomas in children. J Neurosurg 1976; 45:273–283.
58. Liu HM, Boggs J, Kidd J. Ependymomas of childhood I: histologic survey and clinicopathological correlation. Childs Brain 1976: 2:92–110.
59. Salazar OM, Casto-Vita M, VanHoutte D, Rubin P, Aygun C. Improved survival in cases of intracranial ependymoma after radiation therapy: late report and recommendations. J Neurosurg 1983; 59:652–659.
60. Rorke LB, Gilles FH, Davis RL, Becker LE. Revision of the World Health Organization classification of brain tumors for childhood brain tumors. Cancer 1985; 56:1869–1886.
61. Schnipper LE. Clinical implications of tumor cell heterogeneity. N Engl J Med 1985; 314:1423–1431.

62. Ross GW, Rubinstein LJ. Lack of histopathological correlation of malignant ependymomas with postoperative survival. J Neurosurg 1989; 70:31–36.

63. Afra D, Muller W, Flowik, Wilcke O, Budka H, Turoczy L. Supratentorial lobar ependymomas: reports on the grading and survival periods in 80 cases, including 46 recurrences. Acta Neurochir 1983; 69:243–251.

64. Khan AB, D'Souza BJ, Wharam MD. Cisplatin therapy in recurrent childhood brain tumors. Cancer Treat Rep 1982; 66:2013–2020.

65. Sexauer C, Khan A, Burger P, Krischer J, vanEys J, Vats T, Ragab A. Cis-platinum in recurrent pediatric brain tumors: a POG Phase II study. Proc Am Soc Clin Oncol 1984; C:329.

66. Duffner PK, Horowitz ME, Krischer J, Friedman HS, Burger PC, Cohen ME, Sanford RA, Mulhern RK, Seidel FG, Kun L. Postoperative chemotherapy and delayed radiation in children less than 3 years of age with malignant brain tumors: a Pediatric Oncology Group study. (in preparation).

67. Goldwein JW, Glauser TA, Packer RJ, Finlay JL, Sutton LN, Curran WJ, Laehy JM, Rorke LB, Schut L, D'Angio GJ. Recurrent intracranial ependymomas in children. Cancer 1990; 66:557–563.

68. Sumer T, Freeman AI, Cohen M, Bremer A, Thomas PRM, Sinks LF. Chemotherapy in recurrent non-cystic low grade astrocytomas of cerebrum in children. J Surg Oncol 1978; 10:45–54.

69. Rosenstock JG, Packer RJ, Bilaniuk LT, Bruce DA, Radcliffe JL, Savino P. Chiasmatic optic glioma treated with chemotherapy: a preliminary report. J Neurosurg 1985; 63:862–866.

70. Friedman HS, Krischer JP, Burger P, Oakes WJ, Hockenberger B, Weiner MD, Falletta JM, Norris D, Ragab AH, Mahoney DH, Whitehead MV, Kun LE. Treatment of children with progressive or recurrent brain tumors with carboplatin or iproplatin: a pediatric Oncology Group randomized phase II study. J Clin Oncol 1992; 10:249–256.

71. Mulhern RK, Hancock J, Fairclough D, Kun L. Neuropsychological status of children treated for brain tumors: a critical review and integrative analysis. Med. Pediatr Oncol 1992; 20:181–191.

72. Baram TZ, vanEys J, Dowell RE, Cangir A, Pack B, Bruner JM. Survival and neurological outcome of infants with medulloblastoma treated with surgery and MOPP chemotherapy. Cancer 1987; 60:173–177.

73. Strauss LC, Killmond TM, Carson BS, Maria BL, Wharam MD, Leventhal BG. Efficacy of postoperative chemotherapy using cisplatin plus etoposide in young children with brain tumors. Med Pediatr Oncol 1991; 19:16–21.

74. Geyer R, Zeltzer P, Finlay J, Albright L, Wisoff J, Rorke L, Yates A, Boyett J, Milstein J, Berger M, Shurin S, Allen J, McGuire P, Stehbens J, Stanley P, Stevens J, Tefft M, Bertolone S, Biegel J, Edwards M, Sutton L, Wara W, Hammond D, Arcadia CA. Chemotherapy for infants with malignant brain tumors: report of the Childrens Cancer Study Group trials CCG-921 and CCG-945. Proc Am Soc Clin Oncol 1992; 1259.

75. Packer RJ, Sutton LN, Rosenstock JG, Rorke lb, Bilaniuk LT, Zimmerman RA, Littman PA, Bruce DA, Schut L. Pineal region tumors of childhood. Pediatrics 1984; 74:97–103.

76. Herrick MK. Pathology of pineal tumors. In: Neuwelt EA, ed. Diagnosis and treatment of pineal region tumors. Baltimore: Williams & Wilkins, 1984:31–60.

77. Abay EO II, Laws ER Jr, Grado GL, Bruckman JE, Forbes GS, Gomez MR, Scott M. Pineal tumors in children and adolescents: treatment by CSF shunting and radiotherapy. J Neurosurg 1981; 55:889–895.

78. Finlay J, Walker R, Balmaceda C, Zapater S, Villablanca J, Diez B. Chemotherapy without irradiation (XRT) for primary central nervous system (CNS) germ cell tumors (GCT): report of an international study. Proc Am Soc Clin Oncol, 1992; 420.

79. Allen J, Packer R, Bleyer A, Zeltzer P, Prados M, Nirenberg A. Recombinant interferon beta: a phase I–II trial in children with recurrent brain tumors. J Clin Oncol 1991; 9:783–788.

80. Finlay JL, August C, Packer R, Zimmerman R, Sutton L, Freid A, Rorke L, Bayever E, Kamani N, Kramer E, Cohen B, Sturgill B, Nachman J, Strandjord S, Turski P, Frierdich S, Steeves R, Javid M. High-dose multiagent chemotherapy followed by bone marrow "rescue" for malignant astrocytomas of childhood and adolescence. J Neurooncol 1990; 9:239–248.

81. Garvin J, Finlay J, Walker R, Nachman J, Johnson FL, Cairo M, Cohen B, Harris R, Geyer R, Strandjord S, Chan KW. High-dose chemotherapy and autologous bone marrow rescue for high-risk

central nervous system (CNS) tumors in children under six years of age. Proc Am Soc Clin Oncol 1992; 421.

82. Kramer ED, Vezina LG, Packer RJ, Fitz CR, Zimmerman RA, Cohen MD. Staging and surveillance of children with central nervous system neoplasms. Recommendations of the Neurology and Tumor Imaging Committees of the Childrens Cancer Group.

83. Freeman AI. Introduction to the American Cancer Society workshop. Cancer 1985; 56:1890–1893.

84. Deutsch M, Laurent JP, Cohen ME. Myelography for staging medulloblastoma. Cancer 1985; 56:1763–1766.

85. Goldwein JW, Lefkowitz I. Advances in ependymoma: radiation and chemotherapy. In: Packer RJ, Bleyer WA, Pocedly C, eds. Pediatric neuro-oncology. Harwood Academic Publishers, 1992;242–253.

86. Salazar OM. A better understanding of CNS seeding and a brighter outlook for postoperatively irradiated patients with ependymomas. Int J Radiat Biol Phys 1983; 9:1231–1234.

87. Grabb PA, Albright AL, Pang D. Dissemination of supratentorial malignant gliomas via the cerebrospinal fluid in children. Neurosurgery 1992; 30:64–71.

88. Kandt RS, Shinnar S, D'Souza BJ, Singer HS, Wharam MD, Gupta PK. Cerebrospinal metastases in malignant childhood astrocytomas. J Neurooncol 1984; 2:285–294.

89. Hoffman HJ, Otsubo H, Hendrick B, Humphreys RP, Drake JM, Becker LE, Greenberg M, Jenkin D. Intracranial germ-cell tumors in children. J Neurosurg 1991; 74:545–551.

90. Ludwig CI, Smith MT, Godfrey AD, Armbrustmacher VW. A clinicopathological study of 323 patients with oligodendrogliomas. Ann Neurol 1986; 19:15–21.

91. Packer RJ, Allen J, Nielson S, Petito C, Deck M, Jereb B. Brainstem glioma: clinical manifestations of meningeal gliomatosis. Ann Neurol 1983; 14:177–182.

92. Wood, JR, Green SB, Shapiro WR. The prognostic importance of tumor size in malignant gliomas: a computed tomographic scan study by the Brain Tumor Cooperative Group. J Clin Oncol 1988; 6:338–343.

93. Wakai S, Andoh Y, Ochial C, Inoh S, Nagai M. Postoperative contrast enhancement in brain tumors and intracerebral hematomas: CT study. Compt Assist Tomogr 1990; 14:267–271.

94. Forsting M, Albert FK, Sartor K, Kunze S. Early postoperative CT and MRI in glioblastoma. Neuroradiology 1991; 33[suppl]:25–27.

95. Hertler AA, Schlossman DM, Borowtiz MJ. Poplack DG, Frankel AE. An immunotoxin for the treatment of T-acute lymphoblastic leukemic meningitis: studies in rhesus monkeys. Cancer Immunol Immunother 1989; 28:39.

96. Feng H, Mayhew E. Therapy of central nervous system leukemia in mice by lipsome-entrapped 1-β-D-arabinofuranosylcytosine. Cancer Res 1989; 49:5097.

97. Chasin M, Lewis D, Langer R. Polyanhydries for controlled drug delivery. Biopharm Manuf 1988; 1:33.

30

Chemotherapy of Brain Tumors: Innovative Approaches

Mary Katherine Gumerlock
University of Oklahoma Health Sciences Center,
Oklahoma City, Oklahoma

Edward A. Neuwelt
The Oregon Health Sciences University, Portland, Oregon

I. INTRODUCTION

It is the purpose of this chapter to put brain tumor chemotherapy into clinical perspective, beginning first with the basic principles of anticancer drug therapy, and then discussing a variety of innovative approaches to brain tumor chemotherapy. Perhaps the most unique anatomical aspect of brain tumors from the chemotherapeutic point of view is the blood–brain barrier (BBB), a morphological entity based on the tight junctions of the brain capillary endothelial cells (1,2). This structural barrier serves primarily a protective and regulatory function, constraining diffusion across capillaries in relation to lipid solubility and molecular weight. Brain tumor vascularity and the integrity of the blood–tumor barrier (a similar barrier, between the blood vessels and tumor parenchyma) have long been debated. Suffice it to say that although each specific tumor nodule may have a variably permeable barrier, from the chemotherapeutic point of view, the state of blood–brain and blood–tumor barriers must be factored into each drug delivery equation (3).

II. MODES OF DRUG ADMINISTRATION

As with many aspects of neuro-oncology, therapeutic approaches have been designed along the lines of general oncology. Chemotherapy for systemic disease emphasizes control of metastases, a key part of most malignancies. Thus, adequate tissue exposure against such metastases is required throughout the body. Hence, an emphasis on high-dose intravenous (iv) drug administration. In contrast, extracranial metastases from primary brain malignancy are very rare (0.1% incidence) (3a). Thus chemotherapy against brain neoplasia need not necessarily focus on systemic delivery, except for drug exposure and toxicity.

In an attempt to circumvent the problem of the blood–brain barrier, higher doses of anticancer drugs are given, with attendant increased toxicity. This has generated several unique approaches to maximize the concentration $\times$ time ($C \times T$) parameter, while at the same time minimizing systemic drug toxicity. Current studies also define the role of bolus dosing and continuous infusion. Such novel approaches are particularly justified in primary brain tumor therapy because this disease rarely leaves the central nervous system (CNS).

A. Intra-arterial

The rationale of intra-arterial (ia) chemotherapy infusion involves augmentation of "peak concentration over infusion time." This route of administration offers an advantage over the conventional iv route only during the first passage; thereafter, the ia concentrations are similar to iv levels. If rates of biotransformation, metabolism, and excretion during the first pass are high, a larger amount of drug can be delivered to the brain for a similar level of systemic toxicity. This route of drug administration was pioneered using mechlorethamine in the 1950s, with disappointing results (4). In attempts to decrease toxicity, researchers developed an elaborate method of vessel isolation–perfusion using carotid arteries and jugular veins. Toxicity of the procedure itself with thromboembolic and bleeding complications, as well as increased CNS and ocular toxicity, dampened enthusiasm for this route of drug administration. However, more recently, renewed interest in this approach has led to evaluation of several agents: methotrexate, vincristine, vinblastine, mechlorethamine, melphalan, carmustine (BCNU), cisplatin, etoposide, and tenoposide. Also reminiscent of the past experience is the new discussion of improving therapeutic ratio by ia drug infusion and removal of drug by dialysis, another sound theory, yet to be clinically proved (5,6).

With ia infusions there are several factors that influence drug uptake, toxicity, and effectiveness. The tissue partition coefficient measures the capacity of a given tissue to take up the drug. Drug–tissue interaction is affected by protein binding, membrane transport, and extracellular diffusion (7). A decrease in cerebral blood flow will enhance the effective arterial concentration in that slow blood flow allows higher tissue drug extraction. This extraction fraction measures the rate of blood–brain exchange (3,7,8). Perhaps the most important reason, though, for promoting the possible advantage of ia administration over that of iv is the rate of systemic drug breakdown or clearance; delivery of a more rapidly metabolized or excreted drug will be enhanced by ia administration (8). Certain drugs have the property of rapid intravascular degradation; with ia drug delivery, this property is an advantage in that it limits systemic exposure to the drug and, therefore, leads to decreased systemic toxicity.

In ia injections it is not systemic toxicity, but rather, local toxicity that limits use. Balloon catheterization with superselective arterial drug delivery has the advantage of increased selective drug delivery, but has the attendant risk of thromboembolic complications and cerebral ischemia (7). Slow, continuous infusion may have a therapeutic advantage over rapid bolus in that the latter affords higher drug concentration and, hence, increased toxicity, compared with the former. The concentration $\times$ time ($C \times T$) parameter is not affected by infusion rate (7).

Intracarotid cisplatin has been studied extensively by Stewart (9,10). Neurological toxicity, as well as retinal toxicity with blindness, has been reported. Another major chemotherapeutic agent under study with intracarotid infusion is BCNU, which can produce neurological dysfunction and an associated vasculitis (10). Greenberg described retinal vasculitis in 9 of 36 patients treated with ia BCNU; unexpected white matter necrosis was seen in 7 patients (11). Others noted a higher incidence of symptomatic leukoencephalopathy (12). The associated retinal toxicity was reported less often with supraophthalmic infusion and the use of another drug vehicle. It appears, however, that these two modifications of the BCNU chemotherapy program have not improved the therapeutic ratio. Current randomized Brain Tumor Study Group (BTSG) trials do not look promising. More recent work with flow models suggests that some of the toxicity with ia chemotherapy may result from drug streaming and nonuniform drug delivery (13). Intracarotid plicamycin (formerly mithramycin) has been given as has doxorubicin (14). Etoposide intra-arterially is currently under clinical trial. The drug appears well tolerated; toxicity in 12 patients included transient lethargy in 1 and a grand mal seizure in another (15).

Intra-arterial therapy with a combination of BCNU, cisplatin, and tenoposide has shown some effect, as has each of the agents alone (10,16,17). Problems with diluent toxicity are seen with BCNU and cisplatin. Transient marked cardiorespiratory depression was seen with vertebral artery infusions of BCNU and tenoposide (10).

Stewart has also used intracarotid mitomycin in treating patients with primary and metastatic brain tumors. Although neurotoxicity and ocular side effects were significant at a dose of 18 mg/m^2, further study is underway at a lower dose (18). More recent drug protocols for intracarotid delivery include a combination of plicamycin and vincristine. Other studies combine BCNU with vincristine, followed by oral procarbazine and a combination of BCNU with either cisplatin or etoposide. These combinations have been associated with transient decreased neurological function.

Intra-arterial chemotherapy with the currently available drugs has the potential for substantial local toxicity, although it may limit systemic toxicity. Therefore, it is important to determine which drugs can be used without serious local toxicity, but with a diminution in systemic toxicity. Several methods for further direct arterial catheterization are under investigational trial.

B. Intrathecal

The intrathecal method of chemotherapy administration has developed as an attempt to deliver larger molecular weight or polar drugs past the blood–brain barrier. Initial clinical and experimental work has involved lumbar subarachnoid injection. Such a method may not allow uniform drug distribution, and intraventricular flow is frequently limited. To circumvent the problems of lumbar injection, cisternal or intraventricular installation have been used. The latter, through an Ommaya reservoir, also lends itself to prolonged infusion. Assured cerebrospinal fluid (CSF) administration and more even drug distribution are also advantages of the intraventricular route, in addition to apparent increased drug efficacy (19). Intrathecal agents most commonly used include methotrexate, cytarabine, and thiotepa.

Cerebrospinal fluid pharmacokinetics are sufficiently different to require that each drug should be evaluated independently. For instance, whereas methotrexate has a serum half-life of 45 min, its CSF half-life is approximately 4.5 h (19,20). Drug penetration into the parenchymal is limited, being maximum for methotrexate to a depth of 3.2 mm at 1 h (19,20). Because the depth of drug penetration is somewhat influenced by perfusion time, Wilson conducted a 36-h perfusion study with methotrexate that may have some applicability to treatment of meningeal carcinomatosis (21). Drug distribution in the CSF is influenced by several factors, including bulk CSF flow, diffusion through the extracellular spaces of the brain and spinal cord, transport across the choroid plexus, removal by CSF absorption, and diffusion from the extracellular space into the capillaries of the CNS (19).

To implement the important concentration $\times$ time effect, Poplack has investigated a method to allow minimal, but prolonged, tumoricidal levels of methotrexate into the CSF. With an Ommaya reservoir, instead of the single intraventricular injection, a series of injections every 12 h over a 72-h period maintains a therapeutic level for the 72-h period, as opposed to approximately 32 h with the single injection. This intermittent technique may also be associated with less neurotoxicity (19). Investigation continues with this approach. Another attempt to maintain CSF drug levels would be to decrease CSF clearance. Drug clearance is by CSF reabsorption, diffuse bulk CSF flow, transport across cell membranes, and absorption into capillaries. Probenecid, an inhibitor of the active transport of methotrexate, has been used clinically to prolong CSF levels of this drug, presumably by inhibiting the drug's active transport across the choroid plexus (19). One might also postulate the use of acetazolamide to decrease CSF production and, thereby, reduce the bulk flow and turnover of CSF and intrathecal drugs (19).

The ventriculolumbar CSF perfusion method of drug therapy has been investigated by both Poplack and Wilson (22). The theoretical advantage of this method is that the CSF will be exposed to prolonged high levels of drug, presumably with less systemic absorption and, thus, less systemic toxicity. The latter aspect of systemic/CSF concentration ratios has not yet been well investigated. Although intrathecal therapy and maintenance of CSF drug levels has a certain intellectual appeal, it is well to remember that CSF levels have no correlation with parenchymal and tumor drug levels. This route, then, has limited use, except perhaps in pure carcinomatous meningitis. Even in this situation, though, infiltration of the Virchow–Robin spaces with cancer cells decreases patency, yielding only poor drug penetration in these subarachnoid channels. This may account for the short duration of response to intrathecal treatment in carcinomatous meningitis.

C. Intratumoral

Another method for bypassing the blood–brain barrier is direct installation of chemotherapeutic agents into the tumor bed or into associated tumor cysts. The use of the Ommaya reservoir or an adapted tumor cyst device permits direct installation of several chemotherapeutic agents. If a cyst is part of this tumor complex, access to tumor fluid and ongoing biochemical analysis is possible. Kinetric drug studies can also be performed. The more recent development of the Ommaya tumor cyst device allows the tumor bed cavity to persist. This catheter device remains patent until tumor regrowth essentially engulfs it. Tumor cyst device contents may be aspirated for culture, cytology, and other studies.

Thus far, the agents administered by this route include methotrexate, fluorouracil, and BCNU (19). There are certain technical limitations to such a chemotherapeutic approach. Water-soluble drugs are likely to diffuse slowly throughout the extracellular space. More lipid-soluble agents are likely to diffuse back across the barrier into the systemic circulation. Therefore, either of these limitations will require a large drug dose to overcome the diffusion problem. Avellanosa describes the installation of bleomycin and mitomycin into high-grade gliomas and tumor cavities, without significant success, but showed histopathological evidence of liquefaction necrosis and nonuniform drug distribution (23). Morantz described the use of bleomycin in conjunction with systemic BCNU to be more effective than either modality alone (24).

More recently, Takahashi reported the postoperative intratumor injection of bleomycin in patients with craniopharyngioma (25). He found the drug to be more effective in cystic than in solid or mixed tumors. Craniopharyngiomas, derived from the epithelium, are known to take up bleomycin very well. Intracystic installation of bleomycin is also associated with tumor cell degeneration and decreased secretion of cystic fluid. Systemic exposure and, therefore, toxicity is less with intratumoral bleomycin than with the intravenously administered drug (7). It remains to be seen whether such an approach would be applicable to other tumor types associated with cysts, or with other agents, such as thiotepa, known to have an effect on extracranial tumor-associated malignant effusions. The use of intracyst–intratumoral drugs presupposes a focal disease process and, therefore, is somewhat limited in most primary brain tumors.

Harbaugh has used intratumoral chemotherapy through an external catheter infusion method and has completed a Phase I trial of patients with recurrent glioblastoma having daily methotrexate infusions intratumorally, 30 mg/day for 2 weeks. In one patient, the author was able to demonstrate drug concentrations of 1400 ng/g in tissue 5 cm from the catheter tip. Autopsy specimens also demonstrated detectable methotrexate up to 10 cm from the catheter tip (26). Intratumoral drug infusion with an external catheter allows increased drug delivery within the tumor itself and allows maintenance of drug levels for longer periods, with some potential for diffuse distribution of the drug throughout the CNS.

Kroin et al. used cisplatin and mutiple fixed implanted catheters (27). Bouvier et al. describe a single patient with recurrent glioma in whom they implanted 68 small catheters into the tumor area, with each catheter then being connected to an osmotic minipump for drug infusion to a total daily dose of 0.82 mg/day (28).

D. Liposomes

Another method of achieving an adequate drug concentration over a sufficient time period has been the use of liposomes as drug carriers. This technology first requires the incorporation of antimitotic drugs into the liposomes. *Liposomes* are phospholipid vesicles formed by the dispersion of bilayer lipid lamellae. These micelles can be inverted such that the polar region is inside and the nonpolar phospholipid tails are outside, thereby allowing increased lipid solubility and membrane penetration. These liposomes can be formed in varying sizes. Recent work incorporates such drugs as bleomycin and vincristine into liposomes of 0.1–15 μm diameter (29). Such drug-containing liposomes can then act as a depot for slow drug release. The use of this drug delivery method in rats has demonstrated prolonged levels of bleomycin intracerebally when liposome-entrapped bleomycin is compared with free bleomycin. Additionally, low urine and serum drug levels in the liposome-treated rats were noted (30). Methotrexate entrapped in cholesterol liposomes has been studied in primates, resulting in a higher average brain concentration than injection of the free drug (7). Although this particular method of CNS chemotherapy has not reached the clinical stage, and may be limited by the amount of drug packageable, it represents a unique approach to both penetrating the blood–brain barrier and maintaining prolonged tissue concentrations.

E. Implantable Polymers

Biodegradable polymers are frequently composed of polyanhydrides that have a labile linkage, thereby promoting surface degradation. When these polymers are mixed with a ratio of chemotherapeutic agent, the drug release rate is proportional to the polymer erosion rate. Kubo et al. first described treatment of malignant brain tumors with such polymer composites (31). Brem and colleagues report on 21 patients in whom BCNU incorporated into a polyanhydride polymer was implanted at surgery (32). Several patients underwent reoperation or autopsy between 6 and 23 weeks after polymer implantation. No BCNU nor polyanhydride bonds were present at these time points, although some degrading disk material remained. Some patients demonstrated localized tissue necrosis with increasing mass effect, not dissimilar to radiation necrosis, either clinically, radiographically, or pathologically. This interesting new technology requires further basic and clinical study.

III. BLOOD–BRAIN BARRIER DISRUPTION CHEMOTHERAPY

A. Background

As detailed in the foregoing, multiple methods of enhancing the amount of drug delivered to CNS tumors have been developed, with variable toxicity and varying effect. Also, as mentioned, one of the unique aspects of tumors within the CNS is the presence of the blood-brain barrier, an anatomical and physical barrier to substances within the bloodstream. A unique, though quite rational, approach to the problem of chemotherapeutic drug delivery, therefore, has been drug administration concurrent with transient reversible blood–brain barrier disruption (BBBD).

In the 1940s Broman and Olsson demonstrated reversible opening of the blood–brain barrier with iodinated contrast agents (these are hyperosmolar) (33,34). This observation largely lay dormant until Rapoport began his elaborate studies on rats, rabbits, and monkeys detailing the physicochemical parameters of the blood–brain barrier and its role in the passage of substances from the blood to the CNS extracellular space (2). He has described the methods of using hyperosmolar mannitol, urea, or arabinose to reversibly open this barrier, temporarily opening the tight junctions, thereby precipitating transient unregulated entry of circulating substances into the CNS. Neuwelt subsequently applied these observations and techniques to the clinically relevant problem of chemotherapeutic drug delivery first to animals and then to patients with primary and metastatic CNS tumors (35–45).

How do the basic principles outlined previously apply to this choice of therapeutic modality? First, the concept of a blood–brain barrier in tumors has been debated and studied from various approaches. Suffice it to say that the state of this barrier in tumors differs anatomically and physicochemically *to a varying degree* from tumor nodule to tumor nodule, from tumor type to tumor type, and within any given single focus of tumor. The state of blood–brain barrier in tumors becomes a moot point, because substances diffuse from areas of high concentration, to areas of lower concentration, to the point of equilibrium. Therefore, even if a tumor has complete absence of a blood–brain barrier, because the barrier remains intact in the surrounding brain parenchyma (thus inhibiting drug delivery in the CNS tissue), any immediate increased concentration of drug to the tumor rapidly diffuses out to equilibrate with the remaining CNS (the "sink effect"). Thus any concentration advantage is lost too quickly to be effective. The technique of BBBD provides an increased and more uniform drug delivery, decreases the tendency toward rapid diffusion and, thereby, allows tumor exposure to a higher concentration of drug for a longer period (concentration × time). As this exposes the normal CNS to much higher concentrations of anticancer agents, one must be alert to increased toxicity secondary to this increased drug exposure. One balances the potential morbidity of the BBBD and possible drug toxicity against therapeutic gain.

The technique of reversible osmotic BBBD has been detailed by Neuwelt in both animals and humans, and involves opening the blood–brain barrier in the distribution of one circulation (a carotid or vertebral artery). The exact distribution of disruption, therefore, is dependent on the flow, as determined by these vessels and the circle of Willis. One then selects left carotid, right carotid, or vertebral arterial distribution pertinent to tumor location. For those tumors in the border zone areas, two disruptions may be performed sequentially over 2 days. Attempt at three sequential disruptions has not been described, but all three circulations have been disrupted, two at a time sequentially over 2 days and repeated at monthly intervals.

To obtain reversible disruption of the blood–brain barrier, a hyperosmolar saturated solution of 25% mannitol (lower concentrations are inadequate) is injected at sufficient rate and volume to essentially replace blood flow. Studies have shown that such an infusion must continue for approximately 30 s, at which time the threshold event of disruption occurs (2). Because the degree and extent of barrier disruption can be variable, one must document the disruption. Rapoport describes the use of Evans blue as a marker in animal studies (2). Neuwelt evaluated the use of iodinated contrast agent and radioisotope for BBBD documentation. In clinical studies, whereas CT scanning with contrast is anatomically more sensitive, radionuclide brain scanning is a reproducible and semiquantitative technique, with possibly less toxicity (38), although with the newer nonionic contrast agents for CT, this may no longer be true.

The procedure is performed under general endotracheal anesthesia. Patients undergo retrograde catheterization of the femoral artery (Seldinger technique) and the selected artery is cannulated. The procedure carries the attendant risks of thromboembolic ischemia or infarction, symptomatic in fewer than 0.6% of procedures. Blood–brain barrier disruption allows for nonselective entry (for a period of approximately 30 m) of substances previously excluded from the CNS and tumor. Therefore, monitoring the patient's periprocedure medications is mandatory.

Chemotherapy with BBBD is not yet in widespread clinical use, but several centers are beginning to report their experience. Although protocols at the different institutions vary in terms of mannitol infusion time, documentation of BBBD, and chemotherapeutic agents used (Table 1), these data emphasize the clinical feasibility of such a treatment approach and suggest that this form of adjuvant chemotherapy and hyperosmolar BBBD is associated with a significant advance in the median survival of patients with brain tumors.

B. Malignant Gliomas

In the published series of brain tumor patients treated with BBBD–chemotherapy, 176 patients with malignant gliomas underwent treatment (43,46–57). In 78% (138/176) follow-up data was available, with 53% (73/138) showing clinical and radiographic improvement. Thirty-two patients had stabilization of their disease, and 33 had tumor progression.

In the therapy of malignant brain tumors, it has been standard practice to treat with radiation immediately following surgical diagnosis, with any consideration for chemotherapy following later. Fauchon et al. note that 4 of their 16 patients received BBBD–chemotherapy before radiation treatment, as did 4 of 16 patients in the series of Miyagami et al. (48–51). Although this practice (preradiation chemotherapy) has been gaining popularity in the treatment of pediatric CNS malignancy, its use in adults with glioblastoma has been less common. Three of four patients in the Japanese series remain alive 24–44 months after diagnosis. Our own series of approximately 20 patients receiving BBBD–chemotherapy before radiotherapy demonstrated tumor response to BBBD-chemotherapy, as measured by computed tomography (CT) scan. The question of whether chemotherapy before radiation will offer improved survival or decreased toxicity is currently being evaluated.

In summary, the treatment of patients with high-grade malignant gliomas using adjuvant chemotherapy administered in conjunction with osmotic blood–brain barrier disruption affords a significant chance for improved survival and a stable Karnofsky performance score. The intra-arterial infusion of mannitol before the administration of chemotherapeutic agents is not associated with increased or additional risks beyond those of standard intra-arterial chemotherapy. This route of drug administration offers advantages over standard intravenous, intra-arterial, intrathecal, and intratumoral methods in both the length of time a therapeutic level is achieved in tumor as well as the ability to treat infiltrating tumor cells percolating beyond the defined tumor edge into normal brain tissue. Full quantitation of the possible advantage of BBBD–chemotherapy over more conventional brain tumor chemotherapy still needs to be carried out.

Table 1 BBBD–Chemotherapy Protocols

Author (Ref.)	Mannitol Infusion (ml/s)	Chemotherapeutic agents[a]
Bonstelle (46)	1	5-fluorouracil, doxorubicin
Miyagami (47,48)	1.3–1.6	ACNU
Sato (49,50)	1.0–1.5	None
Fauchon (51,52)	4	Cisplatin, doxorubicin, bleomycin, cytarabine
Neuwelt (43)	5–12	Cyclophosphamide, methotrexate
Heimberger (53)	5.7	Cyclophosphamide, methotrexate
Li (54)	Renograffin	Thiotepa, BCNU
Yamada (55)	0.7	5-fluorouracil, ACNU, interferon beta
Markowsky (56)	5–12	Cyclophosphamide, methotrexate
Gumerlock (57)	5–12	Cyclophosphamide, methotrexate

[a]Drugs given at the time of blood–brain barrier opening. All agents are given intra-arterially except cyclophosphamide (intravenous).

C. Cerebral Lymphoma

The results of BBBD–chemotherapy in the treatment of primary cerebral lymphoma are most impressive, and serve to emphasize that increasing drug delivery to malignant brain tumors improves survival, particularly when the tumors themselves are sensitive to those chemotherapeutic agents used.

Although combination chemotherapy for systemic non-Hodgkin's lymphoma results in long-term remission for most patients, it has had only modest efficacy in the treatment of CNS lymphoma. The best results have been with high-dose methotrexate protocols, resulting in transient responses (58). Administration of high-dose intravenous methotrexate is an attempt to improve drug delivery across the blood–brain barrier. However, methotrexate penetrates the CNS poorly, with resultant subtherapeutic levels, especially in infiltrative brain tumors such as lymphoma. Intraventricular and intrathecal methotrexate infusion also fail to achieve therapeutic levels, except in the superficial CNS parenchyma (59). Animal studies have shown that the tissue level of this agent can be increased in both tumor and surrounding tumor-infiltrated brain if the blood–brain barrier is transiently opened before the drug infusion (39).

Clinical studies have documented the efficacy of chemotherapy in conjunction with osmotic BBBD for patients with primary cerebral lymphoma (40). The most recent report extends observations to include 30 consecutive patients with CNS lymphoma treated with BBBD–chemotherapy using methotrexate, cyclophosphamide, procarbazine, and dexamethasone (42). Group 1 ($n = 13$) patients were initially treated with cranial radiation and, subsequently, received BBBD–chemotherapy for persistent or recurrent tumor. Group 2 ($n = 17$) patients received initial BBBD–chemotherapy and then underwent radiation for persistent or recurrent tumor.

Survival differences between these two groups have been assessed using the Fisher exact test and the logrank method applied to the Kaplan–Meier survival curves. The difference in median survival from diagnosis, 17.8 months for group 1 and 44.5 months for group 2, is statistically significant ($p < 0.04$). One patient in group 1 and eight in group 2 remain alive and disease-free, with a follow-up period of 15–98 months. Morbidity and mortality in these 30 patients undergoing 471 BBBD–chemotherapy procedures include three deaths (two from sepsis and one of disease progression) within 30 days of the last procedure, two cerebral infarctions, three episodes of prolonged obtundation, and a periprocedural seizure incidence of 7%. Neuropsychological testing at 1 year shows stable or improved function in most of the patients tested (60).

IV. PHOTODYNAMIC THERAPY

In this method of treatment, a tumor is exposed to a photosensitizer, such as a hematoporphyrin derivative (HpD), after which the tumor is exposed to light of an appropriate wave length to activate the sensitizer. Photodynamic therapy relies on the selective tumor uptake of hematoporphyrin derivatives by the tumor compared to the surrounding normal brain. The HpD compound is infused preoperatively and at surgery the patient's tumor is exposed to light (630 nm) by an argon dye laser. The mechanism of cell necrosis may be related to activated free radicals, with damage to blood vessels and cell membranes (61–65). The mechanisms of hematoporphyrin localization in the tumor remain to be elucidated. Therapy is usually undertaken with red light (wavelength 630 nm), with a depth of tumor kill of approximately 4–7 mm.

The first attempts at human glioma treatment were by Perria (66,67). Although these initial studies had somewhat disappointing results, improvement in light-producing sources and other technical problems have led to more effective treatment regimens, without significant complications or toxicity (62). There is some suggestion that patients with a round tumor geometry, allowing complete or near complete light distribution to the tumor, have a more favorable response.

Hill et al. describe the selective uptake of hematoporphyrin derivatives in human cerebral glioma in 23 patients with malignant brain tumors (68). The patients received a dose of HpD 5mg/kg 24 h before surgery. Tissue sampling of the tumor and normal brain tissue revealed the highest uptake in glioblastoma, which was 30 times that in normal brain tissue. Low-grade tumors had a HpD uptake of approximately eight times that of normal brain tissue. There was also selective uptake in the brain adjacent to the tumor. Phase II trials have now identified more than 100 patients who have received HpD-sensitized photoradiation therapy (61). There appears to be good control of local tumor growth. Further improvement in light delivery systems and optical dosimetry, as well as the development of sensitizers with better absorbance characteristics and improved light penetration will enhance the effectiveness of photodynamic therapy as adjuvant glioma treatment.

V. BORON NEUTRON CAPTURE THERAPY

Boron neutron capture therapy is predicated on the preferential accumulation of boron (^{10}B) in conjunction with sufficiently high thermal neutron fluences at the tumor site. The disintegration of boron is precipitated by bombarding the boron nucleus with a slow neutron. This nuclear reaction yields ionizing radiation. The slow neturon is, on the average, several thousand times more likely to interact with a boron nucleus than with the nucleus of any element of human tissue. Therefore, this neutron–boron reaction might be useful in radiation therapy. Initial trials of this type of therapy were conducted between 1951 and 1961, with disappointing results. Recently, a resurgence in clinical interest has been noted as many of the original scientific and technical problems have been addressed (69,70).

The sulfhydryl derivative of boron (BSH) has been used more recently as a boron carrier. Hatanaka and co-workers in Japan have used this technique in over 100 patients (71). These investigators employed an intraoperative exposure of the tumor-bearing brain area to slow neutrons from a 100 kw nuclear reactor after intra-arterially infusing BSH over a 1- to 2-h period. Although they report impressive clinical results, they also emphasize the need for a wide field of exposure and have documented recurrence outside of their initial field of treatment. Finkel et al. were able to infuse a terminally ill patient with BSH and subsequently study brain and tumor uptake of boron 19 h following intravenous infusion. There was preferential uptake in the tumor with relatively little boron accumulation in the normal CNS parenchyma (72). Boron neutron capture therapy has resulted in increased survival time in a rat glioma model as well (73). Stragliotto and associates have evaluated several patients undergoing craniotomy for intracranial tumors with BSH pharmacokinetic studies over 5 days (74). Quantitation of boron is a physically challenging procedure; however, magnetic resonance imaging does offer a method of detecting boron nuclei with very short T2 relaxation times (75). We will await the results of clinical studies using this imaging method, as well as further clinical response and patient survival results.

VI. DRUG RESCUE TECHNIQUES

As mentioned earlier, by using the principles of drug delivery one attempts to enhance clinical effect by maximizing the dosage of a cytotoxic drug and the duration of tumor exposure to that drug. Dose limitation is frequently extraneural toxicity. In an effort to provide more effective treatment, the current practice of high-dose chemotherapy has been developed. The rationale for such treatment is to improve drug delivery to relatively protected body areas (i.e., the central nervous system and cerebrospinal fluid) or to improve drug delivery to poorly perfused tumors. Such high-dose chemotherapy may also circumvent or prevent tumor cell resistance. To counter-act increased host toxicity from high-dose chemotherapy, various rescue techniques have been developed. One method available is to alter the drug schedule. Another method is administration of an antidote, either concomitant with or sequential to the administration of the chemotherapeutic agent.

The prototype drug rescue regimen is the use of leucovorin (formyltetrahydrofolate) with methotrexate to reduce this drug's toxicity. The mechanisms of rescue with this regimen include competitive interaction for a common membrane transport carrier, replacement of reduced folate and, thereby, enhanced competition because of increased dihydrofolate pools. Another method of methotrexate rescue is the administration of thymidine and purine (76). Uridine rescue has been used in combination with fluorouracil, as have leucovorin and folinic acid (77). One method of combating cytarabine toxicity is to alter its dosage schedule. One might consider the practice of hydrating patients before cyclophosphamide administration to prevent renal toxicity as another method of "rescue."

Cisplatin administration requires that patients be prehydrated; the drug is given with concomitant mannitol-induced diuresis as prophylaxis against nephrotoxicity. Another rescue involves the administration of systemic thiosulfate in conjunction with intraperitoneal cisplatin in the treatment of ovarian carcinoma and malignant ascites (78,79) The thiosulfate protects against nephrotoxicity, and at a higher dose, reduces thrombocytopenia. The mechanism of such protection is unknown. Recall also the early experience with intracarotid mechlorethamine used with iv thiosulfate for bone marrow protection (80).

Since bone marrow toxicity represents a dose-limiting factor in the use of BCNU for primary brain tumor treatment, neuro-oncologists in the last 10 years have investigated the use of autologous bone marrow transplant (ABMT) rescue in conjunction with chemotherapy. Several studies now report their experience with drugs such as BCNU, thiotepa, and cyclophosphamide (81–83). High-dose etoposide has also been given in conjunction with bone marrow rescue (84). Although there may be some increased survival, toxicity associated with the procedure is not insignificant. Furthermore, even though limiting bone marrow toxicity, such a selective method of rescue allows increased pulmonary and hepatic toxicity (82).

Another attempt to rescue from systemic toxicity involves essentially an "isolated perfusion" approach. Pioneered by the initial investigators in brain tumor chemotherapy, this method, tried recently with BCNU and an extraction hemoperfusion column, results in decreased systemic drug levels and less hematopoietic toxicity in three rhesus monkeys (6).

A novel approach to drug rescue is the use of antibody against a particular chemotherapeutic agent to bind and, one hopes, to inactivate the drug. Such a method is particularly applicable to brain tumor therapy for which systemic toxicity is limiting, and systemically administered antibody can bind peripheral drug, yet has only limited access to CNS drug. Preliminary results in our laboratory, using a rat model and methotrexate with anti-methotrexate antisera, suggests serum drug binding of at least 90%. Such an approach may well be useful with other chemotherapeutic agents used in neuro-oncology.

Another new application of monoclonal antibody (MAb) is the conjugation of the antibody to an enzyme (i.e., alkaline phosphatase), to form a relatively high-molecular-weight molecule (85). The conjugate can be delivered across the blood–brain barrier with osmotic disruption where it binds to surface antigen and the barrier returns to a predisrupted condition. A low-molecular-weight prodrug (i.e., phosphorylated) capable of being activated to the cytotoxic agent by the antibody-bound enzymes is given, resulting in localized drug therapy. This technique is currently being investigated, and preliminary studies are very encouraging.

VII. RADIATION SENSITIZERS

In an effort to improve brain tumor treatment, attempts have been made to potentiate the cytotoxic effects of radiation on tumors, without increasing damage to normal brain. One approach has been an effort to synchronize the cell cycle of tumor cells before radiation using such combinations as numustine (ACNU), epipodophyltotoxin, and vincristine. Described by Takakura, the rationale of this "synchronized chemoradiotherapy" is to potentiate the radiation effect (86).

Bromouridine, a thymidine analogue, is incorporated in DNA and may thus increase radiosensitivity. Tumor cell uptake of bromouridine is enhanced by giving methotrexate or fluorouracil to block the normal thymidine pathway. The bromouridine is given by the intracarotid route because this drug is rapidly dehalogenated by the liver, and intracarotid infusion increases local concentration approximately 11- to 16-fold (87). The Japanese studies describe intrathecal bromouridine administration by an Ommaya reservoir in patients with metastatic brain tumors or carcinomatous meningitis, in conjunction with radiation and systemic antimetabolite (methotrexate or fluorouracil) chemotherapy (86).

Metronidazole acts to radiosensitize hypoxic cells. A clinical trial with this agent showed that its use did not significantly influence the median survival compared to radiation alone. Peripheral neuropathy is a potential side effect of metronidazole. A similar agent, misonidazole, is currently under investigation in patients with high-grade glioma (88). Studied in patients with systemic tumors, the drug had a 12% peripheral neuropathy incidence and a 9% incidence of central neurotoxicity; however, this neurotoxicity rate was less in patients receiving dexamethasone or phenytoin (88).

The most promising agent is hydroxyurea, a chemotherapeutic agent in its own right. This drug figures prominently in several current brain tumor protocols, including the "8-in-1" protocol, in combination with BCNU, and in combination with procarbazine, lomustine (CCNU), and vincristine (89). Used as a single agent with radiation, this drug produced significant tumor necrosis and prolonged survival (90). Cisplatin, also part of the 8-in-1 protocol, has been described to act synergistically with cranial radiation as a "radiosensitizer" (9,91,92).

VIII. CONCLUSION

With some 40 years experience in general antineoplastic chemotherapy and some 30 years experience with chemotherapy for brain neoplasia, where does the neuroclinician stand? We have accumulated a substantial amount of data on malignant cells and tumor cell kinetics with tight experimental constructs that now must be extrapolated to in vivo malignancy. For CNS tumors the methodology must account for the blood–brain barrier and the CSF circulation. General anatomical parameters concerning the infiltrative primary brain tumor and the multifocal metastatic disease have been defined, and yet we have not recognized their importance in treatment protocols. Perhaps the most drastic examples of this are the separate observations of Neuwelt and Stewart of tumor regression in a focally treated CNS circulation with simultaneously observed tumor progression in an adjacent untreated region (18,38).

We have accepted the importance of age and performance status in predicting eventual outcome in glioma patients, and have wrestled with the problem of histological grading as it relates to prognosis and therapeutic response. Little is known about the host's role in treating such neoplasia, let alone the detrimental effect of those *immunosuppressive* agents we call *antineoplastic*. Drug pharmacokinetic clinical observations, previously based on plasma and perhaps CSF concentrations now take into consideration brain tumor and surrounding parenchymal drug levels.

Elaborate drug classifications have been developed based on biochemical definition, metabolic site of action, or tumor susceptibility. Major emphasis is placed on delivering adequate amounts of drug for sufficient lengths of time. We now realize that we have only assumptions at this point concerning these parameters in patients and, furthermore, have no means to account for interpatient metabolic variability, a large enough problem in syngeneic animal studies (let alone patients) to thwart almost all pharmacokinetic conclusions. Given tumor cell population heterogeneity and the propensity to develop drug resistance, we recognize the necessity of multiagent therapy. This at once compounds the metabolic equation requiring consideration of drug synergism and antagonism.

In addition, we are now defining the histological effects of treatment in the face of progressive disease. Is the demyelination or necrosis adjacent to tumor the result of our drugs, previous or concurrent radiation, or the disease itself? Defining toxicity and risk/benefit ratios requires an almost impossible sorting of probably overlapping effects, both clinically and histopathologically.

The specific chemotherapeutic agents are directed against rapidly dividing cells—tumor cells and also normal cells of the bone marrow and gastrointestinal system; hence, their effect and their toxicity. But what about the fact that approximately half of the agents available for brain tumor treatment are associated with some form of neurotoxicity, the mechanisms of which are elusive? Perhaps the potential for drug rescue (currently available for but a few agents) could be expanded.

Can we draw any generalizations from what is currently known about the available drugs and treatment regimens? It seems that although intrathecal methotrexate in association with radiation therapy results in a high incidence of leukoencephalopathy, methotrexate with BBBD is not associated with such. Intracarotid infusion of BCNU has significant toxicity not seen with methotrexate; drug streaming is the implicated mechanism, perhaps accentuated by poor drug solubility. Cisplatin and hydroxyurea are both cytotoxic in their own right and enhance radiation effects. Direct intratumor polymer-associated drug installation is promising for focal disease and may also be beneficial in treating tumor-associated cysts (e.g., with bleomycin); perhaps thiotepa, cisplatin, cytarabine, and mechlorethamine would be useful in this manner too.

Without sufficient success to direct our approach, we have pursued a variety of antineoplastic agents, combinations, and routes of administration, usually based on untestable assumptions. When we discuss drug delivery to tumor, we often do not consider its postimmediate fate, given surrounding normal brain, the blood–brain barrier, and CSF circulation. Previous clinical studies cannot be compared or, in fact, even evaluated owing to a lack of concordance on simple definitions such as response, valid study groups, or data analysis. Current studies have taken these problems into account and are now specific enough to permit more cross-comparison.

Emphasizing the role of the blood–brain barrier in defining adequate drug delivery has resulted in a clinically feasible new approach to brain tumor chemotherapy. Current results with BBBD and subsequent multiagent drug administration establishes this treatment regimen as an alternative to other drug protocols. The use of an etoposide and carboplatin regimen in association with osmotic BBBD is now under study and may add substantially to our therapeutic alternative, as these drugs are more effective against primary CNS tumors.

As safe, adequate, and rational chemotherapy develops, the role of radiation treatment (prominent only by default) must be evaluated by risk–benefit analysis. Advances in molecular biology have established the use of monoclonal antibodies in brain neoplasia diagnosis and treatment. The role of oncogenes in CNS tumorigenesis suggests the more prominent use of such agents as cytarabine and dactinomycin (inhibitors of reverse transcriptase) in tumor chemotherapy.

But where does this leave the neuroclinician? One has the responsibility to avail patients of contemporary therapy, for this is the often unspoken desire of those with such a dreaded futile disease. To justify such a course one must be assured of ongoing improvement in the risk/benefit ratio, of a therapy scientifically based in facts, medically sound, and fiscally responsible.

REFERENCES

1. Bradbury M. The concept of a blood–brain barrier. New York: John Wiley & Sons, 1979.
2. Rapoport SI. Blood-brain-barrier in physiology and medicine. New York: Raven Press, 1976.

3. Groothuis DR, Molnar P, Blasberg RG. Regional blood flow and blood-to-tissue transport in five brain tumor models. Prog Exp Tumor Res 1984; 27:132–153.

3a. Choucair AK, Levin VA, Gutin PH, Davis RL, Silver P, Edwards MS, Wilson CB. Development of multiple lesions during radiation therapy and chemotherapy in patients with gliomas. J Neurosurg 1986; 65:654–658.

4. Ariel IM. Intraarterial chemotherapy for metastatic cancer to the brain. Am J Surg 1961; 102:647–650.

5. Dedrick RL, Oldfield EH, Collins JM. Arterial drug infusion with extracorporeal removal. I. Theoretic basis with particular reference to the brain. Cancer Treat Rep 1984; 68:373–380.

6. Oldfield EH, Dedrick RL, Chatterji DC, Yeager RL, Girton ME, Kornblith PL, Doppman JL. Arterial drug infusion with extracorporeal removal. II. Internal carotid carmustine in the rhesus monkey. Cancer Treat Rep 1985; 69:293–303.

7. Stewart DJ. Novel modes of chemotherapy administration. Prog Exp Tumor Res 1984; 28:32–50.

8. Fenstermacher J, Gazendam J. Intraarterial infusions of drugs and hyperosmotic solutions as ways of enhancing CNS chemotherapy. Cancer Treat Rep 181; 65:27–37.

9. Stewart DJ, Leavens M, Maor M, Feun L, Luna M, Bonura J, Caprioli R, Loo TL, Benjamin RS. Human central nervous system distribution of *cis*-diamminedichloroplatinum and use as a radiosensitizer in malignant brain tumors. Cancer Res 1982; 42:2474–2479.

10. Stewart DJ, Grahovak Z, Benoit B, Addison D, Richard MT, Dennery J, Hygenholtz H, Russell N, Peterson E, Maroun JA, Vandenberg T, Hopkins HS. Intracarotid chemotherapy with a combination of 1,3-bis(2-chlorethyl)-1-nitrosourea (BCNU), *cis*-diamminedichloroplatinum (cisplatin), and 4'-*O*-demethyl-1-*O*-(4,6-*O*-2-thenylidene–D-glucopyranosyl) epipodophyllotoxin (VM-26) in the treatment of primary and metastatic brain tumors. Neurosurgery 1984; 15:828–833.

11. Greenberg HS, Ensminger W, Chandler WF, Layton PB, Junck L, Knake J, Vine AK. Intraarterial BCNU chemotherapy for treatment of malignant gliomas of the central nervous system. J Neurosurg 1984; 61:423–429.

12. Foo S-H, Ransohoff J, Berenstein A, Choy I-S. Intraarterial BCNU chemotherapy for malignant gliomas. J Neurosurg 1985; 62:458–459.

13. Saris SC, Wright DC, Oldfield EH, Blasberg RG. Intravascular streaming and variable delivery to brain following carotid artery infusions in the Sprague–Dawley rat. J Cereb Blood Flow Metab 1988; 8:116–20.

14. Mealey J, Chen TT, Pedlow E. Brain tumor chemotherapy with mithramycin and vincristine. Cancer 1970; 26:360–367.

15. Feun LG, Wallace S, Lee F, Leavens N, Savaraj N, Yung WKA, Chuang V, Burgess MA, Benjamin RS, Fields WS. Phase I trial of intracarotid VP-16-213 (etoposide) in patients with intra-cerebral tumors. Proc Am Soc Clin Oncol 1983; 2:238.

16. Feun LG, Lee YY, Yung KWA, Charnsangavej C, Savaraj N, Tang R, Wallace S. Phase II trial of intracarotid (IC) BCNU and cisplatin in malignant brain tumors (ICT). Proc Am Soc Clin Oncol 1985; 4:C585.

17. Feun LG, Lee YY, Yung WKA. Phase II trial of intracarotid (IC) BCNU and cisplatin (DDP) in malignant brain tumors. Proc Am Soc Clin Oncol 1985; 4:585.

18. Stewart DJ, Grahovac Z, Maroun J, Hugenholtz H, Benoit B, Richard M, Russell N, Dennery J, Peterson E, Luke B, Hopkins H. Intraarterial (IA) chemotherapy (CT) for brain tumors (BT). Proc Am Soc Clin Oncol 1985; 4:C513.

19. Poplack DG, Bleyer WA, Horowitz ME. Pharmacology of antineoplastic agents in cerebrospinal fluid. In: Wood JH, ed. Neurobiology of cerebrospinal fluid I. New York: Plenum Press; 1980:561–578.

20. Greig NH. Chemotherapy of brain metastases: current status. Cancer Treat Rev 1984; 11:157–186.

21. Wilson CB, Levin V, Hoshino T. Chemotherapy of brain tumors. In: Youmans JR, ed. Neurological surgery. Philadelphia: WB Saunders, 1982:3065–3095.

22. Riccardi R, Bleyer WA, Poplack DG. Enhancement of delivery of antineoplastic drugs into cerebrospinal fluid. In: Wood, JH, ed., Neurobiology of cerebrospinal fluid II. New York: Plenum Press, 1983:453–466.

23. Avellanosa A, West C, Barua N, Patel A. Intracavitary combination chemotherapy of recurrent malignant glioma via Ommaya shunt—a pilot study. Proc Am Soc Clin Oncol 1983; 2:234.

24. Morantz RA, Kimler BF, Vats TS, Henderson SD. Bleomycin and brain tumors. J Neurooncol 1983; 1:249–255.
25. Takahashi H, Nakazawa S, Shimura T. Evaluation of postoperative intratumoral injection of bleomycin for craniopharyngioma in children. J Neurosurg 1985; 62:120–127.
26. Harbaugh RE. Novel CNS-directed drug delivery systems in Alzheimer's disease and other neurological disorders. Neurobiol Aging 1989; 10:623–629.
27. Kroin JS, Penn RD. Intracerebral chemotherapy; chronic microinfusion of cisplatin. Neurosurgery 1982; 10:349–354.
28. Bouvier G, Penn RD, Kroin JS, Beique R, Guerard MJ. Direct delivery of medication into a brain tumor through multiple chronically implanted catheters. Neurosurgery 1987; 20:286–291.
29. Firth G, Oliver AS, McKeran RO. Studies on the use of antimitotic drugs entrapped within liposomes and of their action on a human glioma cell line. J Neurosci 1984; 63:153–165.
30. Firth G, Oliver AS, McKeran TO. Studies on the intracerebral injection of bleomycin free and entrapped with liposomes in the rat. J Neurol Neurosurg Psychiatry 1984; 47:585–589.
31. Kubo O, Himuro H, Inoue N, Tajika Y, Tajika T, Tohyama T, Sakairi M, Yoshida M, Kaetsu I, Kitamura K. [Treatment of malignant brain tumors with slowly releasing anticancer drug–polymer composites]. No Skinkei Geka 1986; 10:1189–1195.
32. Brem H, Mahaley MS, Vick NA, Black KL, Schold SC, Burger PC, Friedman AH, Ciric IS, Eller TW, Cozzens JW, Kenealy JN. Interestitial chemotherapy with drug polymer implants for the treatment of recurrent gliomas. J Neurosurg 1991; 74:441–446.
33. Broman T, Olsson O. The tolerance of cerebral blood–vessels to a contrast medium of the diodrast group. Acta Radiol 1949; 31:321–334.
34. Broman T, Olsson O. Experimental study of contrast media for cerebral angiography with reference to possible injurious effects of the cerebral blood vessels. Acta Radiol 1949; 31:321–334.
35. Neuwelt EA, Frenkel EP, Diehl J, Vu LH, Rapoport S, Hill S. Reversible osmotic blood–brain barrier disruption in humans: implications for the chemotherapy of malignant brain tumors. Neurosurgery 1980; 7:44–52.
36. Neuwelt EA, Barnett PA, Frenkel EP. Chemotherapeutic agent permeability to normal brain and delivery to avian sarcoma virus-induced brain tumors in the rodent: observations on problems of drug delivery. Neurosurgery 1984; 14:154–159.
37. Neuwelt EA, Dahlborg SA. Chemotherapy administered in conjunction with osmotic blood–brain barrier modification in patients with brain metastases. J Neurooncol 1987; 4:195–207.
38. Neuwelt EA, Dahlborg SA. Blood–brain barrier disruption in the treatment of brain tumors: clinical implications. In: Neuwelt EA, ed. Implications of the blood–brain barrier and its manipulation. vol 2. New York: Plenum Publishing 1989:195–261.
39. Neuwelt EA, Frenkel E, D'Agostino AN. Growth of human lung tumor in the brain of the nude rat as a model to evaluate antitumor agent delivery across the blood–brain barrier. Cancer Res 1985; 45:2827–2833.
40. Neuwelt EA, Frenkel EP, Gumerlock MK, Braziel R, Dana B, Hill SA. Developments in the diagnosis and treatment of primary CNS lymphoma: a prospective series. Cancer 1986; 58:1609–1620.
41. Neuwelt EA, Glasberg M, Diehl J, Frenkel EP, Barnett P. Osmotic blood–brain barrier disruption in the posterior fossa of the dog. J Neurosurg 1981; 55:742–748.
42. Neuwelt EA, Goldman DL, Dahlborg SA, Crossen J, Ramsey F, Roman-Goldstein S, Braziel R, Dana B. Primary central nervous system lymphoma treated with osmotic blood–brain barrier disruption: prolonged survival and preservation of cognitive function. J Clin Oncol 1991; 9:1580–1590.
43. Neuwelt EA, Howieson J, Frenkel EP, Specht HD, Weigel R, Buchan CG, Hill SA. Therapeutic efficacy of multiagent chemotherapy with drug delivery enhancement by blood–brain barrier modification in glioblastoma. Neurosurgery 1986; 19:573–582.
44. Neuwelt EA, Specht HD, Howieson J. Osmotic blood–brain barrier modification: clinical documentation by enhanced CT scanning and/or radionuclide brain scanning. AJNR 1983; 4:907–913.
45. Neuwelt EA, Specht HD, Barnett PA, Dalhborg SA, Miley A, Larson SM, Brown P, Eckerman KF, Hellstrom KE, Hellstrom I. Increased delivery of tumor-specific monoclonal antibodies to brain after osmotic blood–brain barrier modification in patients with melanoma metastatic to the central nervous system. Neurosurgery 1987; 20:885–895.

46. Bonstelle CT, Kori SH, Rekate H. Intracarotid chemotherapy of glioblastoma after induced blood–brain barrier disruption. AJNR 1983; 4:810–812.

47. Miyagami M, Kagawa Y, Tusbokawa T. [ACNU delivery to malignant glioma tissue by osmotic blood brain barrier modification with intracarotid infusion of hyperosmolar mannitol]. No Shinkei Geka 1985; 13:955–963.

48. Miyagami M, Tsubokawa T, Tazoe M, Kagawa Y. Intra-arterial ACNU chemotherapy employing 20% mannitol osmotic blood–brain barrier disruption for malignant brain tumors. Neurol Med Chir (Tokyo) 1990; 30:582–590.

49. Sato S, Toya S, Otani M. [Barrier opening microcirculation in human brain tumor]. Brain Nerve (Jpn) 1985; 37:109–113.

50. Sato S, Yoshinori A, Kodama R, Fujioka M, Otani M, Inoue H, Toya S. [Blood–brain barrier opening CT]. Prog Comput Tomogr (Jpn) 1985; 7:43–48.

51. Fauchon F, Chiras J, Poisson M, Rose M, Terrier L, Bories J, Guerin RA. Intra-arterial chemotherapy by cisplatin and cytarabine after temporary disruption of the blood–brain barrier for the treatment of malignant gliomas in adults. J Neuroradiol 1986; 13:151–162.

52. Chiras J, Dormont D, Fauchon F, Debussche C, Bories J. Intra-arterial chemotherapy of malignant gliomas. J Neuroradiol 1988; 15:31–48.

53. Heimberger K, Samec P, Podreka I, Binder H, Suess E, Reisner T, Deecke L, Steger G, Hiesmayr M, Dittrich C, Horaczek A, Zimpfer M. [Reversible opening of the blood–brain barrier in the chemotherapy of malignant gliomas]. Wien Klin Wochenschr 1987; 99:385–388.

54. Li V, Levin AB, Turski P. Intra-arterial chemotherapy following blood–brain barrier disruption in patients with recurrent high grade astrocytomas [abstract]. Proc Am Assoc Neurol Surg 1988:404, no 274.

55. Yamada K, Takahama H, Nakai O, Takanashi T, Hosoya T. [Intra-arterial chemotherapy for malignant glioma after osmotic blood–brain barrier disruption]. Jpn J Cancer Chemother 1989; 16:2692–2696.

56. Markowsky SK, Zimmerman CL, Tholl D, Soria I, Castillo R. Methotrexate disposition following disruption of the blood–brain barrier. Ther Drug Monitor 1991; 13:24–31.

57. Gumerlock MK, Belshe BD, Madsen R, Watts C. Osmotic blood–brain barrier disruption and chemotherapy in the treatment of high grade malignant glioma: patient series and literature review. J Neurooncol 1992; 12:33–46.

58. Ervin T, Canellos GP. Successful treatment of recurrent primary central nervous system lymphoma with high-dose methotrexate. Cancer 1980; 45:1556–1557.

59. Blasberg RG, Patlak C, Fenstermacher JD. Intrathecal chemotherapy: brain tissue profiles after ventriculocisternal perfusion. J Pharmacol Exp Ther 1985; 195:73–83.

60. Crossen Jr, Goldman DL, Dahlborg SA, Neuwelt EA. Neuropsychological assessment outcomes of nonacquired immunodeficiency syndrome patients with primary central nervous system lymphoma before and after blood–brain barrier disruption chemotherapy. Neurosurgery 1992; 30:23–29.

61. Kaye AH. Photoradiation therapy of brain tumors. Ciba Found Symp 1989; 146:209–224.

62. Kaye AH, Morstyn G, Apuzzo MLJ. Photoradiation therapy and its potential in the management of neurological tumors. J Neurosurg 1988; 69:1–24.

63. Kaye AH, Morstyn G, Brownhill D. Adjuvant high dose photoradiation therapy in the treatment of cerebral glioma. J Neurosurg 1987; 67:500–505.

64. Laws ER Jr, Cotese D, Kinsey JH, Eagan RT, Anderson RE. Photoradiation therapy in the treatment of malignant brain tumors. Neurosurgery 1981; 9:672–678.

65. Muller PJ, Wilson BC. Photodynamic therapy: cavitary photoillumination of malignant cerebral tumors using a laser coupled inflatable balloon. Can J Neurol Sci 1985; 12:371–373.

66. Perria C. Modified Holter Rickham reservoir: a device for percutaneous photodynamic treatment of cystic malignant brain tumors. J Neurosurg Sci 1988; 32:99–101.

67. Perria C, Capuzzo T, Cavagnaro G, Datti R, Francaviglia N, Rivano C, Tercero VE. First attempts at the photodynamic treatment of human gliomas. J Neurosurg Sci 1980; 24:119–129.

68. Hill JS, Kay AH, Sawyer WH, Morstyn G, Megison PD, Stylli SS. Selective uptake of hematoporphyrin derivative into human cerebral glioma. Neurosurgery 1990; 26:248–54.

69. Barth RF, Soloway AH, Fairchild RG. Boron neutron capture therapy of cancer. Cancer Res 1990; 50:1061–1070.

70. Allen BJ. Epithermal neutron capture therapy: a new modality for the treatment of glioblastoma and melanoma metastatic to the brain. Med J Aust 1990; 153:296–298.

71. Hatanka H. Clinical results of brain tumor treatment with boron neutron capture therapy. In: Allen BJ, Moore DE, Harrington BV, eds. Progress in neutron capture therapy for cancer. New York: Plenum Publishing, 1992:561–568.

72. Finkel GC, Poletti CE, Fairchild RG, Slatkin DN, Sweet WH. Distribution of ^{10}B after infusion of $Na_2{}^{10}B_{12}H_{11}SH$ into a patient with malignant astrocytoma: implications for boron neutron capture therapy. Neurosurgery 1989; 24:6–11.

73. Goodman JH, McGregor JM, Clendenon NR, Gahbauer RA, Barth RF, Soloway AH, Fairchild RG. Inhibition of tumor growth in a glioma model treated with boron neutron capture therapy. Neurosurgery 1990; 27:383–388.

74. Stragliotto G, Biallaz J, Fankhauser H. Pharmacokinetics of boron sulfhydryl (BSH) in patients with intracranial tumors. In: Allen BJ, Moore DE, Harrington BV, eds. Progress in neutron capture therapy for cancer. New York: Plenum Publishing, 1992:561–568.

75. Kabalka SW, Bendel P, Davis M, Berman E. A newborn MRI method for imaging BNCT agents in vivo. In: Allen BJ, Moore DE, Harrington BV, eds. Progress in neutron capture therapy for cancer. New York: Plenum Publishing, 1992:561–568.

76. Grem JL, King SA, Sorensen JM, Christian MC. Clinical use of thymidine as a rescue agent from methotrexate toxicity. Invest New Drugs 1991; 9:281–290.

77. Martin DS, Stolfi RL, Sawyer RC, Spiegelman S, Young CW. Improved therapeutic index with sequential N-phosphonacetyl-L-aspartate plus high-dose methotrexate plus high-dose 5-fluorouracil and appropriate rescue. Cancer Res 1983; 43:4653–4661.

78. Howell SB, Pfeifle CE, Wung WE, Olshen RA. Intraperitoneal cis-diamminedichloroplatinum with systemic thiosulfate protection. Cancer Res 1983; 43:1426–1431.

79. Markman M, Cleary S, Howell SB. Nephrotoxicity of high-dose intracavitary cisplatin with intravenous thiosulfate protection. Eur J Cancer Clin Oncol 1985; 21:1015–1018.

80. Owens G. Intraarterial chemotherapy of primary brain tumors. Ann NY Acad Sci 1969; 159:603–607.

81. Hochberg FH, Parker LM, Takvorian T, Canellos GP, Zervas NY. High-dose BCNU with autologous bone marrow rescue for recurrent glioblastoma mutliforme. J Neurosurg 1981; 54:455–460.

82. Fingert HJ, Hochberg FH. Megadose chemotherapy with bone marrow rescue. Prog Exp Tumor Res 1984; 28:67–78.

83. Saarinen UM, Pihko H, Maikipernaa A. High-dose thiotepa with autologous bone marrow rescue in recurrent malignant oligodendroglioma. J Neurooncol 1990; 9:57–61.

84. Kessinger A. High dose chemotherapy with autologous bone marrow rescue for high grade gliomas of the brain: a potential for impovement in therapeutic results. Neurosurgery 1984; 15:747–750.

85. Senter PD. Activation of prodrugs by antibody–enzyme conjugates: a new approach to cancer therapy. FASEB J 1990; 4:188–193.

86. Takakura K, Sano K, Hojo S, Hirano A. Metastatic tumors of the central nervous system. New York: Igaku-Shoin, 1982.

87. Russo A, Gianni L, Kinsella TJ, Klecker RW Jr, Jenkins J, Rowland J. Glatstein E, Mitchell JB, Collins J, Myers C. Pharmacological evaluation of intravenous delivery of 5-bromodeoxyuridine to patients with brain tumors. Cancer Res 1984; 44:1702–1705.

88. Wasserman TH, Stetz J, Phillips TL. Radiation Therapy Oncology Group clinical trials with misonidazole. Cancer 1981; 47:2382–2390.

89. Allen JC. Childhood brain tumors. Current status of clinical trials in newly diagnosed and recurrent disease. Pediatr Clin North Am 1985; 32:633–651.

90. Irwin L, George F, Pitts F. Hydroxyurea and radiation therapy in primary intracranial malignant glial tumors. Proc Am Assoc Cancer Res 1975; 16:243.

91. Delaney WE, Antoniades J. Combination radiation/cisplatinum for adult malignant gliomas. Proc Am Soc Clin Oncol 1985; 4:522.

92. Herchbergs A, Sahar A, Tadmor R, Brenner HJ. Primary cerebral neoplasia—rapid performance status improvement (up-grading) following hypofractionated radiation combined with cisplatinum. Proc Am Soc Clin Oncol 1985; 4:C516.

31

Immunology and Immunotherapy of Brain Tumors

Frank P. Holladay, Wesley E. Griffitt, and Gary W. Wood
University of Kansas Medical Center, Kansas City, Kansas

I. INTRODUCTION

The combination of surgical debulking and radiation therapy is the standard, currently available treatment for malignant brain tumors. The low cure rate achieved with this approach and the lack of meaningful progress made with alternative treatments, including chemotherapy and immunotherapy, is a cause of frustration for everyone involved in the management of patients with brain tumors. Despite clinical failures, an immunological approach remains theoretically attractive because the immune system should have the potential to distinguish tumor cells from normal cells and be able to eliminate tumor without seriously damaging normal brain tissue.

The rationale for immunotherapy is that tumor cells express molecules (antigens) on their surface that are recognized as foreign by the immune system of the tumor-bearing host. It further presupposes that tumor-associated antigens are able to stimulate B lymphocytes to produce antibodies or activate T lymphocytes to a stage where they can selectively kill tumor cells either directly or by producing factors (cytokines) that stimulate macrophages and natural killer cells to kill tumor cells. The following discussion explores fundamental immunological principles as they apply to tumors, reviews current understanding of the immunology of brain tumors, and reviews the current status of brain tumor immunotherapy.

II. TUMOR IMMUNOLOGY

A. Antigenicity and Immunogenicity of Tumors

The immunology of brain tumors cannot be discussed without first asking whether brain tumor cells are antigenic. A tumor is defined as *antigenic* if it produces molecules that are recognized as foreign by host T lymphocytes. A tumor is defined as *immunogenic*, if, during its progression, a functional immune response is induced. This is an important distinction, because expression of antigens means that the potential for generating an immune response exists, regardless of whether immunity actually develops during tumor progression. Historically, the immunogenicity of experimental tumors was demonstrated by the ability of animals, which, in some way, had been exposed to the tumor, to specifically resist secondary exposure to viable tumor cells.

Tumors arise by malignant transformation of normal cells. A tumor can be antigenic only if it expresses molecules to which the host has not become immunologically tolerant. Presumably, normal individuals are tolerant to all molecules that are expressed on the surface of their own (normal) cells. If malignant transformation leads to expression of new molecules on the surface of tumor cells, such cells would potentially be recognized by the immune system. This definition of tumor antigenicity applies to only self-molecules and should not be confused with stimulation of immune responses against tumor-associated antigens across species barriers. The ability to produce immune responses against tumor cells in another strain or species of animal does not mean that the tumor is antigenic in the sense that the term is used in discussions of tumor immunology.

There are a limited number of ways in which a tumor could be antigenic. Tumor cells in virus-induced tumors express foreign antigens that are encoded by viral genes (1,2). The host would have had no opportunity to develop tolerance to those antigens. Tumors expressing viral antigens would be expected to be more immunogenic than tumors expressing altered self-antigens, and for the most part, that prediction has been supported experimentally. Tumors induced by a particular virus share the same antigenic specificity, because the same viral antigens would be expressed by the tumor regardless of the organ in which the tumor arises.

Generating an explanation for the antigenicity of nonviral tumors (e.g., those that arise spontaneously or that are induced with carcinogens) is considerably more difficult, because very few of those antigens have been identified and characterized. The immune response to chemical or UV-induced tumors appears to be specific for the individual tumor. Tumor cells in non–virus-induced tumors appear to express unique antigenic determinants. In theory, these tumor-associated antigens could be unaltered self-molecules that were not exposed to the immune system during development. One possible example would be products of genes that were activated early in development, but are repressed in the adult. Since immune tolerance to the antigens may not have developed, expression of these antigens by the tumor cell could result in the generation of an immune response. Although tumors can produce these types of oncofetal antigens, currently there is little evidence that immune responses are produced against such molecules during tumor progression.

Products of mutated genes are the most probable source for antigens expressed by nonviral tumors. Malignant transformation is associated with multiple mutations, and the high rate of proliferation exhibited by tumor cells in vivo increases the probability that genes encoding cellular proteins will undergo additional mutations. Changes in the primary structure of cellular proteins can occur without affecting their function. Since T cells recognize differences generated by single amino acid substitutions or deletions, the products of mutated genes could be expected to be recognized by host T cells, as long as the altered self-molecules actually come in contact with T cells in the appropriate format. This hypothesis is most consistent with the nature of immune responses seen in experimental models. Mutations would be expected to occur in a random fashion; thus, the number of altered gene sequences that could arise is nearly unlimited. This would be consistent with the individual specificity of antigens expressed by experimental tumors. Although most experimental tumors are antigenic, the number of antigens that have been identified to date is extremely small. Recently, heat-shocklike proteins were identified as antigens expressed by tumor cells and demonstrated to be responsible for immunogenicity in a chemically induced animal model (3–6). Whether the heat-shock protein genes had undergone point mutations has not yet been determined. In another study, the antigens responsible for tumor-specific immune responses were identified as ribosomal proteins that had undergone mutagen-induced point mutations (7–10). At present, too few tumor-associated antigens have been identified to allow any generalizations to be made about their origin. Nevertheless, considerable work has been done on the general interaction between antigens and the immune system, and understanding these interactions provides insight into immune responses to tumors.

The general question of whether human tumors, including gliomas, are antigenic or immunogenic remains unresolved. Although most carcinogen-induced experimental tumors are immunogenic (11,12), few spontaneous animal tumors are classified as immunogenic by traditional criteria (13). Nevertheless, some nonimmunogenic experimental tumors have been demonstrated to be antigenic (14). Most human tumors arise spontaneously and, consequently, are believed to be nonimmunogenic (15). That general belief has been encouraged by the general difficulty encountered in demonstrating immune responses to tumor-associated antigens in cancer patients. Melanomas and renal cell carcinomas appear to be more immunogenic than other human tumors, because some of them undergo spontaneous regression. There are major technical limitations associated with determining whether human tumors are either immunogenic or antigenic: (1) Transplantation experiments are not possible. (2) Tumor progression is often associated with nonspecific immune suppression (16–18). (3) There are special requirements for demonstration of tumor immunity in vitro that make it technically difficult to demonstrate human tumor-associated antigens, if they exist.

The question of the immunogenicity of experimental brain tumors has not been fully resolved. The main reasons are (1) the brain is not a practical site in which to perform classic immunization experiments, and (2) the large number of cells required to produce brain tumors in extracerebral sites make tumor challenge experiments difficult to perform. Nevertheless, isolated observations have been made that suggest that experimental brain tumors may exhibit a range of immunogenicity that is comparable with that of other experimental tumors. For example, an avian sarcoma virus-induced astrocytoma failed to grow in immunocompetent adult rats and grew, but regressed spontaneously, in immunologically immature newborn rats (19–21). In another study, immunization of rats by multiple intraperitoneal injection of irradiated 9L gliosarcoma cells plus adjuvant yielded populations of cells that conferred immunologically specific protection against 9L in Winn assays (Morantz R, personal communication, 1990). Other investigators produced brain tumor-specific cytotoxic T lymphocytes from both humans and experimental animals that had been exposed to tumors, clearly demonstrating the tumors' antigenicity (22–27).

One observation suggesting that human gliomas are potentially capable in inducing immune responses is that gliomas, as a group, contain higher numbers of macrophages than most other histopathological categories of tumors (28–31) and may contain a higher proportion of $CD8^+$ T cells than do benign brain neoplasms or tumors metastatic to the brain (32–35). There are conflicting correlations between the numbers of those cells and survival (34–37), and there is no compelling evidence that tumor-associated T cells preferentially accumulate because they are directed against tumor antigens. Their presence within the tumor bed does establish, however, that immune cells are able to reach progressing gliomas from the periphery. Although the macrophages could be derived from resident microglia, T lymphocytes are not normally found in the brain (38,39).

Extensive studies designed to determine antigenicity or immunogenicity by identifying tumor-specific or tumor-associated antigens using antibody production or T-cell function assays have been extremely frustrating. It is relatively easy to use hindsight to explain why the studies yielded results that are difficult to interpret and often conflicting. Nevertheless, it is important to realize that those studies were firmly based on the contemporary understanding of immunity. For example, until recently, immunologists believed that when immune responses occur, they almost always include both cellular and humoral components. Thus, if tumors express neoantigens, they should induce both antibody production and cell-mediated immunity. Therefore, it was logical to use antibody production to indicate expression of tumor-specific or tumor-associated antigens. That avenue of investigation was explored in several ways by numerous investigators of brain tumors (40–45). One approach was to assay for antibody production during tumor progression or following surgical excision of the tumor, using the logic that antibody levels might be depressed during tumor progression, but would increase following its removal (16). Antibodies were detected, but titers were never high, and the specificity of the reactivity remained ambiguous. There was little evidence for the existence of individual tumor-specific reactivity patterns (46,47).

In addition, even in experimental models, in which the responses can be manipulated more easily, there was no evidence that classic antibody-type responses occurred in syngeneic animals. Antigens that induce antibody production generate a relatively predictable response. A single injection of antigen will produce a primary response that comprises, almost exclusively, IgM production. Subsequent exposure to antigen produces a greatly amplified antibody response that comprises, almost exclusively, IgG production. This type of antibody response was not seen following immunization of syngeneic hosts with tumor cells.

In view of those types of results, several investigators chose a different approach. It was reasoned that, if glial tumors expressed tumor-specific antigens, one should be able to immunize across species and either produce polyclonal antibodies, from which the background reactivity could be removed by extensive absorption with normal tissue (48,49), or produce monoclonal antibodies that would detect tumor-associated antigens (50). Those studies were extremely important because, theoretically, such antibodies would not only be useful in defining tumor-specific antigens, but potentially could be useful in tumor diagnosis, localization, and therapy. The logic was correct in the sense that tumor-reactive antibodies were produced. However, none of the antibodies exhibited a pattern of specificity that was consistent with current understanding of tumor-associated antigens. For example, monoclonal antibodies directed against antigens derived from avian sarcoma virus-induced tumors did not detect antigens that were restricted to avian sarcoma virus-induced tumors (51), and antibodies directed against nonviral tumors have not detected antigens that were truly tumor-specific (52). Therefore, it must be concluded that the antibodies were directed against components of normal cells that appeared to be tumor-associated because they are expressed at a higher level in tumor cells.

Two general observations have been made concerning T–cell-dependent immune responses in brain tumor patients. First, the progressing glioma produces generalized immunosuppression (16,18). Patients have impaired skin test responses to standard recall antigens, there is a reduced number of circulating lymphocytes with a disproportionate decrease in the number of helper relative to cytotoxic T cells, and the response of peripheral blood T cells to polyclonal mitogens is impaired. Similar immunosuppression is not seen in patients with benign brain tumors and is independent of treatment modality. The immunosuppression may be mediated by a combination of transforming growth factor-beta (TGF-β) and prostaglandin E_2 (PGE$_2$) produced by tumor cells and activated monocytes–macrophages (53). Immunosuppression also is a viable explanation for the general difficulty in demonstrating antiglioma immunity.

The second observation is that cellular immune responses against glioma cells are not detectable in glioma patients' peripheral blood. Extensive studies in animal models demonstrating that immunity to tumors is mediated by T cells led many investigators to try to determine whether T-cell responses to tumor antigens were detectable in humans. Two basic approaches were used. In the first, lymphocytes were removed from tumor-bearing individuals and tested for cytotoxicity against both autologous and allogeneic tumor cell targets (54,55). Like similar studies in numerous other human and nonhuman tumor systems, the results of those studies can be summarized as follows: Sometimes tumor cells were killed, but critical analysis revealed that cytotoxicity was not T–cell-mediated, tumor-specific, or major histocompatibility complex (MHC) gene product-restricted. Most investigators now believe that the reactivity was due to natural killer cells or activated natural killer cells (56). The second approach was to stimulate lymphocytes from tumor-bearing individuals with autologous or allogeneic tumor cells *in vitro* and measure T-cell proliferation as an indicator of an immune response (24–26). Again, as with direct assays of lymphocyte cytotoxicity, those studies failed to indicate the presence of an antitumor T-cell response in the individual bearing a glioma. Although T-cell proliferation assays have the potential for demonstrating whether the test lymphocyte population contains tumor-specific T cells, because the assay detects helper cells, the studies did not reveal convincing evidence for a T-cell immune response by glioma patients against their tumor (54–58). A few studies in which glioma-specific cytotoxic T-lymphocyte (CTL) clones were produced from patients' peripheral blood (22, 25, 59, 60), however, suggested that, although undetectable by conventional means, T cells capable of recognizing glioma-specific antigens are present. These studies also provided evidence that at least some human gliomas are antigenic.

B. Cells and Molecules of the Immune System

There are four major categories of cells involved in generating and mediating immune responses: T lymphocytes, B lymphocytes, antigen-presenting cells, and nonspecific immune effector cells. (1) *T lymphocytes* orchestrate all immune responses; they mediate cellular immune responses, and they provide help for antibody responses. There are at least three functionally distinct subpopulations of T lymphocytes: helper T lymphocytes (helper cells) that mediate delayed hypersensitivity-type responses and provide help for cytotoxic T-lymphocyte (CTL) responses; helper cells that provide help for antibody responses; and CTL. (2) *B lymphocytes* produce antibodies. (3) *Antigen-presenting cells* format antigen for recognition by T lymphocytes. Antigen-presenting cells process externally and internally derived antigen and present antigen-derived peptides to T cells in association with MHC gene product molecules on the cell surface (61). Antigen-presenting cells for helper cell-mediated responses include all class II MHC gene product-positive cells (dendritic cells, macrophages, B lymphocytes). Antigen-presenting cells for CTL responses potentially include all class I MHC gene product-positive cells (all cells). (4) The *nonspecific effector cell* category comprises a heterogeneous group of cells that are functionally enhanced by products of immune system activation and, once stimulated, serve as auxiliary immune effector cells. The functional activity of cells in this category (macrophages, granulocytes, mast cells, and natural killer cells) is increased by interaction with the products of B- and T-cell activation: antibodies and cytokines. Importantly, the specificity of immune responses comes only from T and B lymphocytes. The secondarily activated cells are relatively nonselective in their action; once activated, they destroy tumor cells in a non–antigen-specific, non–MHC-restricted manner.

Informational molecules provide cell-to-cell communication and are involved in the generation and manifestation of immune responses. Antigen-specific stimulation of T cells results in the production of small molecular weight peptide molecules called cytokines or interleukins. For immune responses to tumors, the most important cytokines are interleukin-2 (IL-2), interferon gamma (IFN-γ), and the tumor necrosis factors (TNF-α and TNF-β). Cytokines are responsible for secondary activation of immune cells. For example, in the presence of appropriately presented antigen, IL-2 stimulates the proliferation and differentiation of CTL, and TNF-β and IFN-γ activate macrophages and natural killer cells to kill tumor cells.

Stimulation of a B-lymphocyte response ultimately results in the production of antibodies. *Antibodies* are molecules that specifically bind antigen and act directly (e.g., by neutralizing the antigen) or indirectly through interaction with accessory cells. There are two primary ways that antibodies kill cells. (1) Antibodies bind to the cell surface and activate complement-mediated cell lysis. (2) Antibodies bind to the cell surface and then bind, through the Fc portion of the molecule, to FC receptor-positive accessory cells. The result is phagocytosis or antibody-dependent cellular cytotoxicity. Antibodies that bind to tumor cells can be produced by heteroimmunization or alloimmunization. These antibodies, through rigorous testing, are targeted to antigens that are not restricted to, but are associated with, the tumor (tumor-associated antigens). Many attempts have been made to isolate antigens specific for individual tumors (tumor-specific antigens). No tumor-specific antigen has been reliably and reproducibly identified using antibodies.

C. Antigen Presentation

1. Tumor Antigens

Immunity to tumors is mediated by tumor-specific T lymphocytes (62–66). All mature, functional T lymphocytes express clonally distributed antigen receptors on their surfaces. Both the helper cell and CTL subpopulations comprise numerous clones, each of which contains a variable number of mature T cells, all of which express identical antigen receptors. Each clone expresses a unique receptor that recognizes a unique antigenic specificity. It is this property that imparts specificity to all T–cell-dependent immune responses. T lymphocytes are able to recognize antigen only in association with self class I and class II MHC gene product molecules (67–69). This property is referred to as *MHC restriction*. It is believed that T lymphocytes that are self-reactive (i.e., express receptors that recognize self-antigens) are deleted from the repertoire during T-cell development in the thymus. For deletion to occur, however, immature T cells must encounter the antigen during their maturation.

2. Presentation of Antigen to Helper T Lymphocytes

Antigen is internalized, processed, and presented to helper T lymphocytes by specialized antigen-presenting cells. Macrophages are one example of cells that are able to present antigen. Others include dendritic cells and B lymphocytes, although antigen presentation by B cells probably is restricted to antibody responses. Antigen-presenting cells phagocytose or pinocytose complex antigens (e.g., tumor cells or proteins released from tumor cells). The complex molecules are digested within the cell's lysosomal compartment. Small molecular weight (14–16 amino acids long) peptide digestion products bind to specific sites on class II MHC gene products (61,70). The binding occurs during assembly of the MHC complex before its expression on the surface of the antigen-presenting cell. Class II MHC gene products become integral components of the cell membrane, and antigenic peptides fit into molecular folds or pockets in the MHC molecules (71,72). This is a critical stage in the generation of immune responses, and the need for effective interaction between unstimulated T cells and antigen-presenting cells probably accounts for the fact that adjuvants such as Freund's, BCG, and *Corynebacterium parvum*, all of which nonspecifically activate antigen-presenting cells, greatly enhance immune responses.

Tumor cell-derived antigens are processed and presented by class II MHC gene product-positive antigen-presenting cells to activate helper cells to produce IL-2. Gliomas contain high concentrations of class II MHC-positive macrophages that would be expected to phagocytose dead tumor cells and their products. Those cells could function as antigen-presenting cells, but the afferent phase of the immune response does not occur in the tumor, presumably because high numbers of T cells are not present *in situ* early in tumor development and because the microenvironment is not appropriate for T-cell activation. Tumor-associated macrophages could function as antigen-presenting cells, if, after internalizing tumor cells, they left the tumor and traveled to lymphoid tissue where immune responses are initiated. At present, there is no evidence that macrophages leave tumors. The general view seems to be that, once they have been attracted to the site of tumor progression, they remain there. Another way for antigen presentation to occur is for tumor cells or tumor cell products to be released into blood or lymph and be transported to lymphoid tissue where they would be picked up and processed by antigen-presenting cells. In either event, antigen-presenting cells would present tumor-associated antigens to lymphocytes within organized lymphoid tissue. Despite the fact that the blood–brain barrier does not exist within the neovascularized tumor bed, it is unusual for viable glioma cells to be released into the blood. Unlike metastatic tumors, gliomas remain localized in the brain. Thus, it is unlikely that antigen reaches lymphoid tissue in the form of intact tumor cells. The possibility that glioma-specific antigens reach lymphoid tissue as products of tissue destruction released into the blood has not been addressed adequately in experimental studies. Lack of antigenic stimulation of peripheral lymphoid tissue by glioma-associated antigens remains a viable explanation for our inability to detect responses in the periphery of glioma patients.

Expression of peptides that can be recognized by T cells on the surface of antigen-presenting cells is only part of the antigen presentation process. Helper cells, expressing the appropriate antigen receptors, bind to the surface of a class II MHC-positive antigen-presenting cell, and a stable receptor–ligand complex is formed between T-cell receptors and the peptide–MHC complex. The T cell actually is physically bound to the surface of the antigen-presenting cell. Although a single molecular complex is involved, separate binding events occur between antigenic peptide and the complementary antigen receptor and between the MHC molecule and complementary MHC-binding sites on the T cell. The molecular events that occur subsequent to this interaction generate activation signals that are required for the functional differentiation of helper cells.

3. Presentation of Antigen to Cytotoxic T Lymphocytes

Helper-cell responses are required for immunity to tumors, but that requirement can be eliminated if exogenous IL-2 is provided (64,73,74). This is an extremely important point. During the natural immune response to tumors, it is essential for tumor-associated antigens to activate helper cells to produce IL-2, but helper cells are not required to mediate tumor destruction. Immunity to most tumors is mediated by CTL (15,62,65,75). The CTL do not produce enough IL-2 to sustain their own proliferation, particularly early in the activation phase (76).

Like helper-cell responses, generation of CTL responses involves MHC-restricted antigen presentation (67–69). However, antigen presentation for CTL responses is quite distinct from the process described for helper-cell responses, in that it is class I, not class II, MHC gene product-restricted. The CTLs recognize only a limited range of antigens that are synthesized within antigen-presenting cells (61). Histocompatibility antigens responsible for graft rejection; viruses, certain obligate intracellular parasites, tumor cells, and cellular autoantigens, all are recognized by CTLs. Other antigens that are seen by the immune system only following processing and presentation by class II MHC-positive antigen-presenting cells do not stimulate a CTL response, even though those antigen-presenting cells also are class I MHC gene product-positive (61). As with helper responses, peptides are expressed on the surface of antigen-presenting cells in association with MHC molecules, but a different pathway is involved in the packaging and presentation of the peptides (61). For example, following infection of a cell by virus, viral proteins are synthesized and degraded within the cell. Small peptides (9–10 amino acids long) bind to specific sites on class I MHC gene product molecules and are transported to the cell surface where they are recognized by CTL precursors. Thus, CTL responses are distinct from helper-cell responses in that, in the former, the peptides derived from internal cellular protein synthesis are presented, and presentation is in association with class I MHC molecules.

These requirements strongly suggest that tumor cells function as antigen-presenting cells for CTL responses. Peptides derived from cellular genes bind to class I MHC molecules and are transported to the tumor cell surface. For a peptide to be expressed at the tumor cell surface, it must have the proper structure both to bind to class I MHC molecules and to be recognized by the CTL. At the surface, the peptides are recognized by antigen receptor-positive CTLs and, presumably, a binding event occurs. Unlike helper-cell responses for which interaction between T cell and antigen-presenting cell is a productive one for both types of cells, ultimately CTL recognition of tumor cells leads to death of the antigen-presenting cell.

4. Presentation of Antigen to B Lymphocytes

Antibodies apparently play no role in tumor immunity (25,65), and, in fact, tumor-associated antigens may not even stimulate antibody production in the tumor-bearing host (8). However, antibodies to tumor-associated antigens can be produced by immunizing across species barriers, and extensive studies have been performed using this approach in an attempt to understand brain tumor-associated antigens (40,48,77,78). The relationship, if any, between these antigens and the antigens that are recognized by T lymphocytes and lead to generation of tumor immunity is unclear.

B lymphocytes do not require antigen-presenting cells to "see" antigen. Unlike T cells that express receptors that recognize only peptides, B cells express IgM monomers as integral components of their membrane. Those antibody molecules function as antigen receptors on the surface of B lymphocytes and recognize free antigen in the absence of any MHC restriction. In the presence of T-cell help, antigen directly stimulates B lymphocytes to proliferate and differentiate into antibody-producing plasma cells. B cells themselves are class II MHC gene product-positive and function as antigen-presenting cells to generate T-cell help for their own differentiation.

Antigen presentation requirements may explain many of the negative findings concerning the interaction between tumor cells and antibody. All of the tumor-associated antigens that have been shown to have a role in generating tumor immunity are cytoplasmic or nuclear molecules (1,2,7,8,15,79,80). They are expressed on the surface of tumor cells only as MHC-associated peptides. Even if antibodies were made against the parent molecules (e.g., by cross-species immunization), it is unlikely that the MHC-associated peptides would be accessible for antibody binding. The two most probable explanations for the inability of antibody to recognize tumor cell surface-associated peptides are (1) the amino acid sequences of peptides that are processed and presented on the surface of antigen-presenting cells for T cell recognition are very likely to be different from the amino acid sequences of immunodominant epitopes recognized by antibodies on intact antigens. Even if antibodies were made to the parent molecule, they would be expected to have different specificity than the T cells. This is despite the fact that antibodies are capable of binding to peptide fragments of antigen molecules. (2) It is probable that, even if the antibody were able to recognize the peptide, the peptide would be inaccessible within pockets in the MHC molecules.

The foregoing discussion leaves unanswered the question of why tumor-associated antigens, particularly those derived from highly immunogenic tumors that are spontaneously rejected in immunocompetent hosts, do not induce production of high concentrations of antibody during tumor progression. During the progression of tumors, there is a high degree of cell breakdown. Antigenic proteins released as a result of cell breakdown should produce antibody responses. There are two speculative explanations: (1) Tumor cell-associated molecules occurring as a result of cell breakdown may not reach B lymphocytes in a form that could stimulate antibody production (e.g., as undigested proteins). (2) The modifications in cellular proteins that are generated by single-point mutations may infrequently stimulate B-cell responses.

D.   Activation of Immune Responses

1.   Helper T Lymphocytes

The next stage in the generation of an immune response is the activation of antigen-specific T lymphocytes. Helper cells see antigen in association with specialized class II MHC-positive antigen-presenting cells. When the recognition event occurs, both the antigen-presenting cell and the helper cell are activated. The antigen-presenting cell is stimulated to produce interleukin 1 (IL-1) and possibly other accessory molecules that facilitate helper-cell differentiation. The activated helper cell produces IL-2, which functions as an autocrine signal, stimulating helper-cell proliferation. Helper–cell-derived IL-2 is required for antigen-stimulated differentiation of CTL precursors into activated CTLs. Finally, helper–cell-derived IL-2, IFN-γ, and TNF-β activate natural killer cells and macrophages to become highly proficient nonspecific tumor cell killers.

At the same time that the helper cell is stimulated to produce IL-2, IL-2 receptor expression is increased on the cell's surface. Resting helper cells do not express IL-2 receptors and, therefore, are not responsive to IL-2. This is an important regulatory concept. When an immune response is ongoing, IL-2 production does not activate neighboring T cells unless they coincidentally express IL-2 receptors. This allows the integrity of the immune response to be maintained.

2. Cytotoxic T Lymphocytes

Whereas helper cell activation has been extensively studied, CTL activation against tumors, is less well understood. Because CTL produce little or no IL-2, they are dependent on helper cell activation for their proliferation. At the same time, CTL must be activated by antigen in association with antigen-presenting cells to express IL-2 receptors to be responsive to the helper–cell-derived IL-2. That activation step, which presumably is class I MHC-restricted, is poorly understood. With the exception of CTL against foreign MHC, primary activation of CTL precursors has been observed only *in vivo*, making analysis of the process very difficult.

Full differentiation of primed CTL precursors into functional CTL capable of killing tumor cells occurs only when tumor-associated antigens are presented by tumor cells in association with class I MHC molecules. Such a stringent antigen presentation requirement creates little difficulty during activation of virus-specific CTL responses, because viruses generally infect specialized antigen-presenting cells that are both class I and class II MHC gene product-positive. The same cell is able to function as the antigen-presenting cell for helper and cytotoxic T cells. However, chemically induced, UV-induced, and spontaneously arising tumors generally are not class II MHC-positive. For an effective antitumor CTL response to occur, helper and cytotoxic responses must occur in the same microenvironment. Differentiation of *in vivo* primed CTL into fully functional CTL capable of effective killing of target cells expressing class I-associated antigenic peptides are most efficiently generated following secondary in vitro antigenic stimulation. Differentiation also occurs *in vivo*, but, with tumor cells, it has been documented to occur only within the tumor. These various limitations may explain many of the difficulties associated with generating effective immune responses against tumor antigens and are discussed in greater detail later.

E. Immune Rejection of Tumor

Generation of immunity to tumors can be viewed as follows: The number of activated helper cells and primed CTL in peripheral lymphoid tissue of individuals or experimental animals exposed to tumor should be proportional to tumor antigenicity. Lymphocytes constantly circulate through the peripheral blood and lymph. Therefore, stimulated cells will enter vascularized tumors, probably in a random manner that is dependent primarily on release of chemotactic factors from the tumor. Unless prevented by suppression, a secondary cellular immune response will occur in the tumor. The helper cells will be stimulated to produce IL-2, and the primed CTL precursors will interact with tumor cells and be stimulated to differentiate into CTL. This second stage of differentiation is achieved completely *in vivo* with highly immunogenic tumors (e.g., the few human melanomas that spontaneously regress and some experimental viral and UV-induced tumors). Most immunogenic experimental tumors induce a primary response that will protect the animal from rechallenge with viable tumor cells. The number of CTL precursors that reach the injection site and interact with tumor cells following rechallenge is high enough to produce a local secondary response that rejects the tumor. T cells from the immune animals also will protect against tumor challenge, but, with the exception of a few highly immunogenic tumors, will not affect the progression of established tumors (65,81). However, the number of primed precursors can be increased *in vivo* by immunizing animals with tumor cells mixed with adjuvant. The number of primed CTL precursors that reach the tumor site following rechallenge with weakly antigenic tumors (nonimmunogenic) is not high enough to generate a local secondary response causing tumor rejection, leading to the general impression that such tumors fail to express antigens recognized by the immune system.

The inability of T cells from primed animals to affect tumor progression and the inability of immunization with weakly antigenic tumors to protect against rechallenge can be circumvented by removing primed cells from the animal and exposing them to tumor cells *in vitro* (14,15,66,82–84). *In vivo*, circulation of primed cells from lymphoid tissue to the tumor site dilutes the primed cells. *In vitro*, the dilution effect is eliminated; primed precursors are directly exposed to tumor cells and large numbers of functional CTL are generated. The number of CTL can be expanded by including low levels of exogenous IL-2 in the culture. These *in vitro*-stimulated, expanded populations will reject progressing tumors when adoptively transferred to tumor-bearing hosts (14,22,23,66,82–85).

It is not entirely clear how the process of tumor rejection occurs, but some generalizations based on known functions of T cells can be made. Tumor immunity is mediated by CD8$^+$ T cells in all systems yet tested. Nearly all CTL are CD8$^+$, and CTL directly kill tumor cells in an antigen-specific, class I MHC gene product-restricted manner. Therefore, one possible mechanism for tumor rejection is direct CTL-mediated killing of tumor cells. However, not all CD8$^+$ cells are CTLs, and both CD8$^+$ and CD8$^-$ T cells are able to produce high concentrations of IFN-γ or TNF. Both IFN-γ and TNF activate natural killer cells and macrophages to kill tumor cells. TNF also kills tumor cells directly. Therefore, other mechanisms may be involved in the rejection event. Recent studies with fibrosarcoma-specific CD8$^+$ clones demonstrated that noncytotoxic as well as cytotoxic CD8$^+$ cells could reject tumors (86). Some CD8$^+$ clones rejected tumors in a TNF-dependent manner and others rejected tumors in an IFN-dependent manner. Those studies suggest that tumor rejection is mediated by polyclonal antitumor T-cell populations involving a complex combination of direct and indirect effects.

As noted earlier, the products of T cells—IL-2, IFN-γ, and TNF—activate natural killer (NK) cells to kill a wide spectrum of tumor cells (56). The NK cells are non–antigen-specific, non–MHC-restricted elements of the host natural defense system that play an important, but as yet poorly defined, role in tumor eradication. These cells are present in normal individuals with no known previous exposure to tumor cells and express cytotoxic activity against a restricted range of tumor cells. Exposure of NK cells to high concentrations of IL-2 generates another population of cytotoxic cells, called lymphokine-activated killer (LAK) cells, that kill a wide variety of lymphoid and nonlymphoid tumor cells in a non–antigen-specific and non–MHC-restricted fashion (87–91). The LAK cells are much more potent cytotoxic cells than are their parent NK cells. Although LAK cells are produced both *in vitro* and *in vivo* following exposure to high concentrations of IL-2 (1000 Cetus units/ml), it is unknown whether helper cells generate sufficient IL-2 *in vivo* to activate LAK precursors at sites of tumor rejection. Thus, it is unclear whether lymphokine-activated killer cells play a significant role in natural tumor eradication.

Macrophages are multifunctional cells that are activated to be tumoricidal by products of T-cell activation. Macrophages and T cells exhibit complex interdependence during generation of immune responses to tumors. In their resting state, macrophages do not express class II MHC and are not able to kill tumor cells. However, when activated they are effective antigen-presenting cells and are able to effectively kill tumor cells in an non–antigen-specific, non–MHC-restricted manner. They kill most tumor cells by being stimulated to produce TNF-α, but may also kill tumor cells through production of other metabolites. The brain contains a large population of endogenous macrophages, the microglia. Moreover, progressing gliomas contain large numbers of macrophages (28,29). Endogenous tumor-associated macrophages may play a major role in tumor rejection, but would be expected to do so only following activation by specifically stimulated T cells.

III. IMMUNOTHERAPY OF BRAIN TUMORS

A. Classification

Broadly defined, *immunotherapy* employs the premise that modification of the immune system can alter the course of tumor progression. Unfortunately, a universal classification of immunotherapy subgroups has not been achieved. We have elected to subgroup immunotherapies using a more traditional immunological framework. *Active immunization* is defined as direct stimulation of an individual with antigen. Injecting animals with immunogenic tumor cells, with or without adjuvant, is an example of active immunization. Active tumor immunotherapy includes two subgroups. *Specific active immunotherapy* involves stimulation of tumor bearers with tumor cells or tumor extracts, with or without adjuvant, to enhance T-cell responses. *Nonspecific active immunotherapy* involves stimulation of tumor bearers with nonspecific immune response modifiers such as adjuvants or cytokines.

Passive immunization is defined as transfer of antibodies or immune cells to an individual for the purpose of transferring the associated immune response. The immune factors may be prepared in another individual or *in vitro*. Passive tumor immunotherapy also has been broadened to include two subgroups. *Specific passive immunotherapy* involves transfer of antibodies or immune T cells to the tumor-bearing host. Transferred factors must be specifically reactive with tumor-associated antigens. *Nonspecific passive immunization* involves transfer of cells, such as lymphokine-activated killer cells or macrophages that have nonspecific antitumor activity.

1. Specific Active Immunotherapy

The results of specific active immunotherapies of malignant brain tumors have been uniformly disappointing. Patients injected with their own or allogeneic tumor cells or tumor extracts derived no therapeutic benefit (92–94). Multiple immunizations with autologous tumor cells combined with adjuvant appeared to augment tumor immunity in that skin test responses to autologous tumor were increased, and levels of circulating antibody were increased, but there was no apparent effect on the tumor itself (95). The absence of an effect of immunization with allogeneic tumor cells is not surprising. Although human brain tumors may share antigens, immunity to tumors is almost certainly MHC-restricted. Tumor cells from different humans express individually distinct MHC phenotypes. Therefore, allogeneic tumor cells are unlikely to function as antigen-presenting cells to induce a protective immune response.

There are no apparent conceptual flaws involved in using active immunization with autologous tumor cells plus adjuvant. It is to be anticipated that, if the brain tumor cells are antigenic, active immunization should increase the number of circulating immune precursors. Those cells should be able to get to the tumor, and their local activation should affect its behavior. However, there are few examples of active immunization having an effect on the progression of any tumor. It is possible that the explanation is quantitative. The number of immune cells that are generated may be insufficient to affect the progression of an already-established tumor. However, the explanation may also be qualitative. Injecting patients with tumor cells and adjuvant may increase the number of primed cells, but will have no effect on differentiation of CTL precursors into the tumor-specific CTL that would be the actual mediators of tumor immunity.

Recently, active immunization has been studied from a completely new direction involving gene therapy (96). In several interesting studies, none yet involving brain tumors, cytokine genes (e.g., IL-2, IL-4, and TNF) were transfected into weakly immunogenic tumor cells. Animals were then injected with viable transfectants. The tumors grew and were rejected in an immunologically specific manner (74). Transfection of cells with a cytokine gene converted weakly immunogenic tumors into more highly immunogenic tumors. Production of cytokines by the tumor cells resulted in an amplified immune response, presumably through an adjuvant effect at the priming step. The response was specific for antigens expressed by the original tumor, but exposure of animals to transfected cells had no effect on progression of nontransfected tumor cells. Those studies may hold considerable promise in the active immunotherapy of human tumors.

2. *Nonspecific Active Immunotherapy*

Extensive experimentation has been and continues to be performed using nonspecific active immunization of tumor bearers. Patients have been treated with immune stimulants such as BCG, *C. parvum*, or levamisole (97–101). Unlike surgery, radiation, or chemotherapy, these various agents do not directly impinge on tumor cells. The rationale for their use is complex. The immunological rationale is that, since the agents function as adjuvants when mixed with antigen, exposure of an individual to adjuvant alone should have an enhancing effect on an ongoing immune response. The nonimmunological rationale is that these agents nonspecifically stimulate cells, such as macrophages, to be tumoricidal *in vitro*. Therefore, since macrophages and similar nonspecific effector cells are found in and around tumors, adjuvants may activate their tumoricidal activity *in situ*. Unfortunately, the regulation of immune responses involves an extremely complex balance of positive and negative factors, and it is difficult, if not impossible, to predict how or if introduction of a particular agent will affect that regulatory balance in a particular patient. Although adjuvant therapy has had a beneficial effect in some tumor systems, no significant effect on glioma patients' survival has been observed (102). Moreover, nonspecific immune stimulants often have serious negative effects on normal tissue.

As immunologists became increasingly aware that cell–cell communication during immune responses was mediated by cytokines, it was reasoned that cytokines might have adjuvant effects on antitumor immune responses and that their use would provide a more focused approach than general-purpose adjuvants. Thus, patients were treated with high concentrations of cytokines (e.g., recombinant IFNs or IL-2). Since cytokines mediate informational transfer during immune responses, it was thought that tumor patients may have an immune response defect that could be corrected. More recently, studies have been initiated using immune response effector molecules such as TNF. Here, the rationale simply was that, because TNF kills tumor cells *in vitro*, it might have an antitumor effect *in vivo* as well.

Brain tumors have a special place among tumors in that it is unusual to see metastases. Therefore, antitumor agents may be directly delivered to the tumor, and if the tumor were eradicated, one would not have to be concerned with distant metastases. Interestingly, even though brain tumors contain high numbers of T lymphocytes, direct injection of immunostimulants into progressing tumors or into the area from which most of the tumor has been surgically removed, has had little effect on survival.

3. *Nonspecific Passive Immunotherapy*

The most well-studied example of nonspecific passive immunotherapy for brain tumors involves the use of LAK cells. Extensive studies have been performed in animal models and in humans. The LAK cells are produced by culturing normal peripheral lymphocytes with high concentrations of IL-2 (1000 Cetus units/ml). The cytotoxic cells generated in this manner are highly effective killers of malignant brain tumors *in vitro*, regardless of the antigens that they express or MHC composition of the target (56, 103–105). A combination of LAK cells and systemic IL-2 has been used successfully to treat melanomas and renal cell carcinomas (103,104), but, in extensive trials, has had no apparent effect on the progression of gliomas, despite multiple infusions into the tumor bed or a combination of local and systemic adoptive transfer of lymphocytes (106–109). Despite powerful antitumor activity *in vitro*, LAK cells have had no effect on tumor progression, whether given locally or systemically.

Because LAK cells are extremely effective killers of brain tumor cells, and very large numbers of effector cells can be generated and delivered to the tumor bed, it may be of some value to consider why the therapy failed. One possibility is that, for LAK cells to be effective, they must come in contact with tumor cells. Unlike specific immune cells, there is no evidence that LAK cell numbers or functional activity are increased by exposure to a tumor or that LAK cells amplify secondary effector systems *in situ*. Since gliomas extensively infiltrate brain parenchyma, injection of LAK cells into a the tumor does not guarantee that the cells will be able to infiltrate and act in areas of the tumor away from the injection site. Their injection into the blood stream does not guarantee that they will reach the tumor either, even though gliomas are extensively vascularized. Therefore, even if LAK cells reach the tumor, there are likely to be areas that are unaffected by their cytotoxic activity.

4. Specific Passive Immunotherapy

There are two general ways to perform specific passive immunotherapy. The first is to generate heteroantibodies against glioma cells and inject them into tumor-bearing individuals either alone or coupled to cell toxins. The second is to generate T cells that are specifically directed to tumor-associated antigens and transfer them to the tumor-bearing host.

Initially, polyclonal antibodies, generated by immunizing rabbits with human gliomas, were found to preferentially localize in human gliomas (110,111). The development of hybridoma technology has made possible the development of numerous monoclonal antibodies (MAbs) to tumor-associated antigens. In no instance has there been conclusive evidence that antibodies have been made against antigens that are truly tumor-specific. However, numerous MAbs have been raised against antigens associated with gliomas and neuroectodermal tumors.

Although *in vivo* efficacy of immunotoxins in the treatment of gliomas has not been established, coupling of MAbs against tumor-associated antigens with various toxins produces *in vitro* cytotoxicity. Intrathecal immunotoxin therapy for leptomeningeal neoplasia is efficacious in a guinea pig model (112), and several clinical trials are underway in humans (113). The variety of possible conjugates has made the use of MAbs an active area of investigation (114–116). Radioimmunotherapy, employing ^{131}I-radiolabeled MAbs, is an attempt to target cytotoxic radiation to tumor cells. *In vivo* studies of radioimmunotherapy in the treatment of human tumors have not demonstrated efficacy (117). Bispecific antibodies are hybrid MAbs, consisting of an antibody specific for effector cells (T cells or LAK cells) fused with an antibody specific for a glioma-associated antigen. These bispecific antibodies have been used to target cytotoxic cells (118), with some initial encouraging results (119). The MAbs used in immunocytochemistry, such as antiglial fibrillary acidic protein (GFAP), have revolutionized neuropathological diagnosis (47,120).

There are a few reports that CTL, specifically targeted against glioma-specific antigens, are able to affect tumor progression *in vivo*. This approach has not been tested in humans, but some successes have been achieved in experimental models. Cloned CTL, combined with nontoxic amounts of systemically administered IL-2, slowed the progression and, occasionally, even cured a progressing mouse glioma (22,23,60). More recently, we demonstrated that unfractionated cytotoxic T-cell populations containing both helper cells and CTL, produced by priming rats with tumor cells *in vivo* and restimulating the primed cells with tumor cells *in vitro*, cured a rapidly progressing malignant rat glioma (83). Cytotoxic cells from culture were given intravenously to tumor-bearing rats as late as day 5 of tumor progression when untreated rats generally died between days 12 and 15. Treated rats were cured and exhibited no apparent neurological dysfunction. In the same model, LAK cells, which killed glioma cells very effectively *in vitro*, had no effect on tumors *in vivo* (84). Those studies demonstrated that the progressing gliomas express antigens that make them susceptible to specific passive immunotherapy. They also demonstrated that tumor-associated immunosuppression can be overcome by passive transfer of CTL. Those studies need to be extended to other experimental brain tumor models.

It is important to consider why two populations of cytotoxic cells that exhibit apparently equal ability to kill tumor cells *in vitro* had such different effects *in vivo*. One possibility might be that CTL are able to enter the tumor, but LAKs are not. Although that possibility has not been excluded, preliminary trafficking studies in our laboratory have revealed no apparent differences between the two. The more probable reason rests in the nature of the immune response itself. The effectiveness of LAK cells is not amplified by reexposure to antigen, since they are not generated in response to antigen in the first place. In contrast, interaction of antigen-specific immune cells with antigenic tumor cells *in vivo* would be expected to stimulate their continued proliferation and differentiation. In addition, antigens stimulate antigen-specific effector cells to produce cytokines, such as IFN-γ and TNF-α, that activate macrophages to function as auxiliary effector cells.

IV. SUMMARY

Our understanding of the immunology of brain tumors is increasing. There is some experimental evidence that gliomas are antigenic in the host of origin, and there is some evidence that specifically immune cells are able to affect tumor behavior *in vivo*. This suggests that the immune system has the potential to affect the progression of human brain tumors. Nevertheless, immunotherapy has not yet altered the prognosis of human malignant brain tumors and, as has been pointed out on numerous occasions, rats and mice are not humans. It remains to be determined whether observations obtained under the artifactual conditions operative in experimental models can be used to make meaningful progress in the treatment of human brain tumors.

REFERENCES

1. Kast WM, Offringa R, Peters PJ, Voodouw AC, Meloen RH, Van der Eb AJ, Melief CJM. Eradication of adenovirus E1-induced tumors by E1A-specific cytotoxic T lymphocytes. Cell 1989; 59:603–614.
2. Klarnet JP, Kern DE, Okuno K, Holt C, Lilly F, Greenberg PD. FBL-reactive CD^{8+} cytotoxic and $CD4^+$ helper T lymphocytes recognize distinct Friend murine leukemia virus-encoded antigens. J Exp Med 1989; 169:457–467.
3. Moore SK, Kozak C, Robinson EA, Ullrich SJ, Apella E. Cloning and nucleotide sequence of the murine *hsp*84 cDNA and chromosome assignment of related sequences. Gene 1987; 56:29–40.
4. Srivastava PK, DeLeo AB, Old LJ. Tumor rejection antigens of chemically-induced sarcomas of inbred mice. Proc Natl Acad Sci USA 1986; 83:3407–3411.
5. Srivastava PK, Chen YT, Old LJ. 5' Structural analysis of genes encoding polymorphic antigens of chemically induced tumors. Proc Natl Acad Sci USA 1987; 84:3807–3811.
6. Ullrich SJ, Robinson EA, Law LW, Willingham M, Apella E. A mouse tumor specific transplantation antigen is a heat shock-related protein. Proc Natl Acad Sci USA 1986; 83:3121–3125.
7. Boon T, Van Pel A, de Plaen E, Chomez P, Lurquin C, Szikora JP, Sibille C, Mariame B, van den Eynde B, Lethe B, Brichart V. Genes coding for T-cell-defined tum⁻ transplantation antigens, point mutations, antigenic peptides, and subgenic expression. Cold Spring Harbor Symp Quant Biol 1989; 54:587–596.
8. Boon T, Van Pel A, de Plaen E. Tum⁻ transplantation antigens, point mutations, and antigenic peptides: a model for tumor specific transplantation antigens? Cancer Cells 1989; 1:25–28.
9. De Plaen E, Lurquin C, van Pel A, Mariame B, Szikora JP, Wolfel T, Sibille C, Chomez P, Boon T. Immunogenic (tum⁻) variant of mouse tumor P818: cloning of the gene of a tum⁻ antigen P91A and identification of the tum⁻ mutation. Proc Natl Acad Sci USA 1988; 85:2271–2278.
10. Szikora JP, van Pel A, Brichard V, Andre M, Van Baren N, Henry P, de Plaen E, Boon T. Structure of

the gene of tum⁻ transplantation antigen P35B: presence of a point mutation in the antigenic allele. EMBO J 1990; 9:1041–1050.

11. Foley EJ. Antigenic properties of methylcholanthrene-induced tumors in mice of the strain of origin. Cancer Res 1953; 13:835–837.

12. Prehn RT, Main JM. Immunity to methylcholanthrene-induced sarcomas. JNCI 1957; 18:769–778.

13. Hewitt HB, Blake ER, Walder AS. A critique of the evidence for active host defence against cancer, based on personal studies of 27 murine tumours of spontaneous origin. Br J Cancer 1976; 33:241–259.

14. Shu S, Chou T, Sakai K. Lymphocytes generated by *in vivo* priming and in vitro sensitization demonstrate therapeutic efficacy against a murine tumor that lacks apparent immunogenicity. J Immunol 1989; 143:740–748.

15. Melief CJM. Tumor eradication by adoptive transfer of cytotoxic T lymphocytes. Adv Cancer Res 1992; 58:143–175.

16. Mahaley MS, Brooks WH, Rozman TL, Bigner DD, Dudka L, Richardson S. Immunobiology of primary intracranial tumors. Part 1: studies of the cellular and humoral general immune competence of brain-tumor patients. J Neurosurg 1977; 46:467–476.

17. Thomas DGT, Lannigan CB, Behan PO. Impaired cell-mediated immunity in human brain tumours. Lancet 1975; 1:1389–1390.

18. Wood GW, Morantz RA. Depressed T lymphocyte function in brain tumor patients: monocytes as suppressor cells. J Neurooncol 1983; 1:87–94.

19. Adams DO, Gilbert RW, Bigner DD. Cellular immunity in rats with primary brain tumors: inhibition of macrophage migration by soluble extracts of avian sarcoma virus-induced tumors. JNCI 1976; 6:1119–1123.

20. Anzil AP, Stavrou D. Infection of newborn rat brain cells with a rat glioma associated virus [abstract]. J Neuropathol Exp Neurol 1978; 37:585.

21. Lee YS, Wikstrand CJ, Bigner DD. Glioma-associated antigens defined by monoclonal antibodies against an avian sarcoma virus-induced rat astrocytoma. J Neuroimmunol 1986; 13:183–202.

22. Yamasaki T, Handa H, Yamashita J, Namba Y, Watanabe Y, Kuwata S, Hanaoka M. Establishment of experimental malignant glioma specific cytotoxic T lymphocyte clone by T cell growth factor. J Neurosurg 1984; 60:998–1004.

23. Yamasaki T, Handa H, Yamashita J, Watanabe Y, Namba Y, Hanaoka M. Specific adoptive immunotherapy with tumor-specific cytotoxic T lymphocyte clone for murine malignant gliomas. Cancer Res 1984; 44:1776–1783.

24. Miescher S, Whiteside TL, de Tribolet N, von Fliedner V. In situ characterization, clonogenic potential and antitumor cytolytic activity of T lymphocytes infiltrating human brain cancers. J Neurosurg 1988; 68:438–448.

25. Miyatake S, Handa H, Yamashita J, Yamasaki T, Ueda M, Namba Y, Hanaoka M. Induction of glioma specific cytotoxic T cell lines by autologous tumor stimulation and IL-2. J Neurooncol 1986; 4:55–64.

26. Yoshida S, Tanaka R, Ono M, Takai N, Saito T. Analysis of mixed lymphocyte tumor culture in patients with malignant brain tumor. J Neurosurg 1989; 71:398–402.

27. Holladay FP, Lopez GL, De M, Morantz RA, Wood GW. Generation of cytotoxic immune responses against a rat glioma by *in vivo* priming and secondary in vitro stimulation with tumor cells. Neurosurgery 1992; 30:499–505.

28. Morantz RA, Wood GW, Foster M, Clark M, Gollahon K. Macrophages in experimental and human brain tumors. Part 1: studies of the macrophage content of experimental rat brain tumors of varying immunogenicity. J Neurosurg 1979; 50:298–304.

29. Morantz RA, Wood GW, Foster M, Clark M, Gollahon K. Macrophages in experimental and human brain tumors. Part 2: studies of the macrophage content of human brain tumors. J Neurosurg 1979; 50:305–311.

30. Rossi ML, Hughes JT, Esiri MM, Coakham HB, Brownell DB. Immunohistological study of mononuclear cell infiltrate in malignant gliomas. Acta Neuropathol (Berl) 1987; 74:269–277.

31. Farmer JP, Antel JP, Freedman M, Cashman NR, Rode H, Villemure JG. Characterization of lymphoid cells isolated from human gliomas. J Neurosurg 1989; 71:528–533.

32. Paine JT, Handa H, Yamasaki T, Yamashita J, Miyatake S. Immunohistochemical analysis of infiltrating lymphocytes in central nervous system tumors. Neurosurgery 1986; 18:766–772.

33. Rossi ML, Cruz-Sanchez F, Hughes JT, Esiri MM, Coakham HB, Moss TH. Mononuclear cell infiltrate and HLA-DR expression in low grade astrocytomas. An immunohistological study of 23 cases. Acta Neuropathol 1988; 76:281–286.

34. Rossi ML, Jones NR, Candy E, Nicoll JAR, Compton JS, Hughes JT, Esiri MM, Moss TH, Cruz-Sanchez FF, Coakham HB. The mononuclear cell infiltrate compared with survival in high-grade astrocytomas. Acta Neuropathol 1989; 78:189–193.

35. Sawamura Y, Hiroshi A, Toshimitsu A, Hosokawa M, Kobayashi H. Isolation and in vitro growth of glioma-infiltrating lymphocytes, and an analysis of their surface phenotypes. J Neurosurg 1988; 69:745–750.

36. Brooks WH, Markesbery WR, Gupta GD, Rozman TL. Relationship of lymphocyte invasion and survival of brain tumour patients. Ann Neurol 1978; 4:219–224.

37. Palma L, DeLorenzo N, Guidetti B. Lymphocytic infiltrates in primary glioblastomas and recidivous gliomas: incidence, fate and relevance to prognosis in 228 operated cases. J Neurosurg 1978; 49:854–861.

38. Hanwehr RI, Hofman FM, Taylor CR, Apuzzo MLJ. Mononuclear environment of primary CNS tumors: characterization of cell subsets with monoclonal antibodies. J Neurosurg 1984; 60:1138–1147.

39. Phillips JP, Eremin O, Anderson JR. Lymphoreticular cells in human brain tumors and in normal brain. Br J Cancer 1982; 45:61–69.

40. Coakham HB, Kornblith PL. The humoral immune response of patients to their gliomas. Acta Neurochir [Suppl] 1979; 28:475–479.

41. Eggers AE. Autoradiographic and fluorescence antibody studies in the human host immune response to gliomas. Neurology 1972; 22:245–250.

42. Kornblith PL, Dohan FC, Wood WC, Whitman BO. Human astrocytoma: serum-mediated immunologic response. Cancer 1974; 33:1512–1519.

43. Kornblith PL, Coakham HB, Pollock LA, Wood WC, Green SB, Smith BH. Autologous serologic responses in glioma patients. Correlation with tumor grade and survival. Cancer 1983; 52:2230–2235.

44. Sheikh KMA, Apuzzo MLJ, Kochsiek KR, Weiss MH. Malignant glial neoplasms: definition of a humoral host response to tumor-associated antigen(s). Yale J Biol Med 1977; 50:397–403.

45. Wood WC, Kornblith PL, Quindlen EA, Pollock LA. Detection of humoral immune response to human brain tumors. Specificity and reliability of microcytotoxicity assay. Cancer 1979; 43:86–90.

46. Coakhan HB. Immunology of human brain tumors. Eur J Cancer Clin Oncol 1984; 20:145–149.

47. Coakham HB, Garson JA, Brownell B, Kemshead JT. Monoclonal antibodies as reagents for brain tumour diagnosis: a review. J R Soc Med 1984; 77:780–787.

48. Mahaley MS Jr. Experiences with antibody production from human glioma tissue. Prog Exp Tumor Res 1972; 17:31–39.

49. Schnegg JF, de Tribolet N, Diserens AC, Martin-Achard A, Carrel S. Characterization of a rabbit anti-human malignant glioma anti-serum. Int J Cancer 1981; 28:265–269.

50. Fischer DK, Chen TL, Naratan RK. Immunological and biochemical strategies for the identification of brain tumor-associated antigens. J Neurosurg 1988; 68:165–180.

51. Lee YS, Matthews TJ, Pizzo S, Abernathy JL, Bigner DD. Partial purification and characterization of a murine glioma-associated antigen defined by syngeneic rat monoclonal antibodies. J Neuroimmunol 1986; 13:203–216.

52. Ferracini R, Prat M, Comoglio PM. Dissection of the antigenic determinants expressed on the cell surface of RSV-transformed fibroblasts by monoclonal antibodies. Int J Cancer 1982; 29:477–481.

53. Kuppner MC, Hamou MF, Sawamura Y, Bodmer S, de Tribolet N. Inhibition of lymphocyte function by glioblastoma-derived transforming growth factor $\beta2$. J Neurosurg 1989; 71:211–217.

54. Levy NL. Specificity of lymphocyte-mediated cytotoxicity in patients with primary intracranial tumors. J Immunol 1978; 121:903–915.

55. Sheikh KMA, Apuzzo MLJ, Weiss MH. Preoperative cell-mediated immune status of patients with malignant glial tumors. Neurol Res 1979; 1:133–145.

56. Herberman RB. Natural killer cells. Annu Rev Med 1986; 37:347–352.

57. Sheikh KMA, Apuzzo MLJ, Weiss MH. Specific cellular immune responses in patients with malignant gliomas. Cancer Res 1979; 39:1733–1738.
58. Woosley RE, Mahaley MS, Mahaley JL, Miller GM, Brooks WH. Immunobiology of primary intracranial tumors. Part 3: microcytotoxicity assays of specific immune responses of brain tumor patients. J Neurosurg 1977; 47:871–885.
59. Miyatake S, Kikuchi H, Iwasaki K, Yamasaki T, Ueda M, Namba Y, Hanaoka M. Specific cytotoxic activity of T lymphocyte clones derived from a patient with gliosarcoma. J Neurosurg 1988; 69:751–759.
60. Yamasaki T, Handa H, Yamashita J, Namba Y, Hanaoka M. Characteristic immunological responses to an experimental mouse brain tumor. Cancer Res 1983; 43:4610–4617.
61. Townsend A, Bodmer H. Antigen recognition by class I-restricted T lymphocytes. Annu Rev Immunol 1989; 7:601–624.
62. Rosenberg SA, Terry W. Passive immunotherapy of cancer in animals and man. Adv Cancer Res 1977; 25:323–388.
63. Fernandez-Cruz E, Woda BA, Feldman JD. Elimination of syngeneic sarcomas in rats by a subset of T lymphocytes. J Exp Med 1980; 152:823–841.
64. Cheever MA, Greenberg PD, Fefer A, Gillis. Augmentation of the antitumor therapeutic efficacy of long-term cultured T lymphocytes by *in vivo* administration of purified interleukin-2. J Exp Med 1982; 144:968–980.
65. North RJ. The murine antitumor immune response and its therapeutic manipulation. Adv Immunol 1984; 35:89–155.
66. Shu S, Chou T, Rosenberg SA. In vitro sensitization and expansion with viable tumor cells and interleukin-2 in the generation of specific therapeutic effector cells. J Immunol 1986; 136:3891–3898.
67. Zinkernagel RM, Doherty PC. Restriction of *in vitro* T cell-mediated cytotoxicity in lymphocytic choriomeningitis within a syngeneic or semiallogenic system. Nature 1974; 24:701–702.
68. Zinkernagel RM, Doherty PC. MHC-restricted cytotoxic T cells: studies on the biological role of polymorphic major transplantation antigens determining T-cell restriction-specificity, function, and responsiveness. Adv Immunol 1979; 27:51–177.
69. Bevan MJ. Interaction antigens detected by cytotoxic T cells with the major histocompatibility complex as modifier. Nature 1975; 256:419–421.
70. Neefjes JJ, Stollorz V, Peters PJ, Geuze HJ, Ploegh HL. The biosynthetic pathway of MHC class II but not class I molecules intersects the endocytic route. Cell 1990; 61:171–183.
71. Roche PA, Cresswell P. Invariant chain association with HLA-DR molecules inhibiting immunogenic peptide binding. Nature 1990; 345:615–617.
72. Teyton L, O'Sullivan D, Dickson PW, Lotteau V, Sette A, Fink P, Peterson P. Invariant chain distinguishes between the exogenous and endogenous antigen presentation pathways. Nature 1990; 348:39–44.
73. Donohue JH, Rosenstein M, Chang AE, Lotze MT, Robb RJ, Rosenberg SA. The systemic administration of purified interleukin-2 enhances the ability of sensitized murine lymphocyte lines to cure a disseminated syngeneic lymphoma. J Immunol 1984; 132:2123–2128.
74. Fearon ER, Pardoll DM, Itaya T, Golumbek P, Levitsky HI, Simons JW, Karasuyama H, Vogelstein B, Frost P. Interleukin-2 production by tumor cells bypasses T helper function in the generation of an antitumor response. Cell 1990; 60:397–403.
75. Hellstom I, Hellstrom KE. Cell-mediated reactivity to human tumor-type associated antigens: Does it exist? J Biol Respir Modif 1983; 2:310–320.
76. Kitahara T, Watanabe O, Yamamura A, Makino H, Watanabe T, Suzuki G, Okumura K. Establishment of interleukin-2 dependent cytotoxic T lymphocyte cell line specific for autologous brain tumors and its intracranial administration for therapy of the tumor. J Neurooncol 1987; 4:329–336.
77. Apuzzo MLJ, Mitchell MS. Immunological aspects of intrinsic glial tumors. J Neurosurg 1981; 55:1–18.
78. Coakham HB, Lakshmi MS. Tumour-associated surface antigen(s) in human astrocytomas. Oncology 1975; 31:233–243.
79. Boon T. Antigenic tumor cell variants obtained with mutagens. Adv Cancer Res 1983; 39:121–151.

80. Melief CJM, Vasmel WLE, Offringa R, Sijts EJAM, Matthews EA, Peters PJ, Meloen RH, Van der Eb AJ, Kast WM. Immunosurveillance of virus-induced tumors. Cold Spring Harbor Symp Quant Biol 1989; 54:597–603.

81. North, RJ, Awwad, M, Dunn, PJ. T cell-mediated tumor regression in experimental systems. Progr Immunol 1989; 7:1097–1103.

82. Greenberg PD, Klarnet JP, Kern DE, Cheever MA. Therapy of disseminated tumors by adoptive transfer of specifically immune T cells. Prog Exp Tumor Res 1988; 32:102–127.

83. Holladay FP, Heitz T, Chen Y-L, Chiga M, Wood GW. Successful treatment of a malignant rat glioma with cytotoxic T lymphocytes. Neurosurgery 1992 (in press).

84. Holladay FP, Heitz T, Wood GW. Cytotoxic T lymphocytes, but not lymphokine activated killer cells, exhibit anti-tumor activity against established intracerebral gliomas. J Neurosurg 1992 (in press).

85. Shu S, Chou T, Rosenberg SA. Generation from tumor-bearing mice of lymphocytes with *in vivo* therapeutic efficacy. J Immunol 1987; 139:295–304.

86. Barth RJ, Mule JJ, Spiess PJ, Rosenberg SA. Interferon gamma and tumor necrosis factor have a role in tumor regression mediated by murine CD^{8+} tumor-infiltrating lymphocytes. J Exp Med 1991; 173:647–658.

87. Rosenberg SA, Mule JJ, Spiess PJ, Reichert CM, Schwarz SL. Regression of established pulmonary metastases and subcutaneous tumor mediated by the systemic administration of high dose recombinant interleukin-2. J Exp Med 1985; 161:1169–1188.

88. Mule JJ, Shu S, Schwarz SL, Rosenberg SA. Adoptive immunotherapy of established pulmonary metastases with LAK cells and recombinant interleukin-2. Science 1984; 225:1487–1489.

89. Mule JJ, Shu S, Rosenberg SA. The anti-tumor efficacy of lymphokine-activated killer cells and recombinant interleukin 2 *in vivo*. J Immunol 1985; 135:646–652.

90. Grimm EA, Rosenberg SA. The human lymphokine-activated killer cell phenomenon. Lymphokines 1983; 9:279–311.

91. Grimm EA, Muzumder A, Zhang HZ, Rosenberg SA. Lymphokine-activated killer cell phenomenon: lysis of natural killer-resistant fresh solid tumor cells by interleukin-2 activated autologous human peripheral blood lymphocytes. J Exp Med 1981; 155:1823–1841.

92. Bloom HJG, Peckham MJ, Richardson AE, Alexander PA, Payne PM. Glioblastoma multiforme: a controlled trial to assess the value of specific active immunotherapy in patients treated by radical surgery and radiotherapy. Br J Cancer 1973; 27:253–267.

93. Grace JT, Perese DM, Metzgar RS, Sasabe T, Holdridge B. Tumor autograft responses in patients with glioblastoma multiforme. J Neurosurg 1961; 18:159–167.

94. Mahaley MS, Gillespie GY, Gillespie RP, Watkins PJ, Bigner DD, Wikstrand CJ, MacQueen JM, Defilippo J. Immunobiology of primary intracranial tumors. Part 8: serological responses to active immunization of patients with anaplastic gliomas. J Neurosurg 1983; 59:208–216.

95. Trouillas P. Immunologie et immunotherapie des tumeurs cerebrales. Rev Neurol 1973; 128:23–38.

96. Gutierrez AA, Lemoine NR, Sikora K. Gene therapy for cancer. Lancet 1992; 339:715–721.

97. Mahaley MS, Steinbok P, Aronin P, Dudka L, Zinn D. Immunobiology of primary intracranial tumors. Part 4: levamisole as an immune stimulant in patients and in the ASV glioma model. J Neurosurg 1981; 54:220–227.

98. Mahaley MS, Urso MB, Whaley RA, Williams TE, Guaspari A. Interferon as adjuvant therapy with initial radiotherapy of patients with anaplastic gliomas. J Neurosurg 1984; 61:1069–1071.

99. Mahaley MS, Urso MB, Whaley RA, Blue M, Williams TE, Guaspari A, Selker R. Immunobiology of primary intracranial tumors. Part 10: therapeutic efficacy of interferon in the treatment of recurrent gliomas. J Neurosurg 1985; 63:719–725.

100. Mahaley MS, Bertsch L, Cush S, Gillespie GY. Systemic gamma-interferon therapy for recurrent gliomas. J Neurosurg 1988; 69:826–829.

101. Kennedy JD, Sutton RC, Conley FK. Effect of intracerebrally injected *Corynebacterium parvum* on the development and growth of metastatic brain tumor in mice. Neurosurgery 1989; 25:709–714.

102. Duff TA, Borden E, Bay J, Piepmeier J, Sielaff K. Phase II trial of interferon-β for treatment of recurrent glioblastoma multiforme. J Neurosurg 1986; 64:408–413.

103. Grimm EA, Owen-Schaub L. The IL-2 mediated amplification of cellular cytotoxicity. J Cell Biochem 1991; 45:335–339.
104. Rosenberg SA. Development of new immunotherapies for the treatment of cancer using interleukin-2. Ann Surg 1988; 208:121–135.
105. Ortaldo JR. Comparison of natural killer and natural cytotoxic cells: characteristics, regulation, and mechanism of action. Pathol Immunopathol Res 1986; 5:203–218.
106. Jacobs SK, Wilson DJ, Melin G, Parham CW, Holcomb B, Kornblith PL, Grimm EA. Interleukin-2 and lymphokine activated killer (LAK) cells in the treatment of malignant glioma: clinical and experimental studies. Neurol Res 1986; 8:81–87.
107. McCutcheon IE, Baranco RA, Katz DA, Saris SC. Adoptive immunotherapy of intracerebral metastases in mice. J Neurosurg 1990; 72:102–109.
108. Merchant RE, Merchant LH, Cook SHS, McVicar DW, Young HF. Intralesional infusion of lymphokine-activated killer (LAK) cells and recombinant interleukin-2 (rIL-2) for the treatment of patients with malignant brain tumor. Neurosurgery 1988; 23:725–732.
109. Tzeng JJ, Barth RF, Clendenon NR, Gordon WA. Adoptive immunotherapy of a rat glioma using lymphokine activated killer cells and interleukin 2. Cancer Res 1990; 50:4338–4343.
110. Day ED, Lassiter S, Woodhall B, Mahaley JL, Mahaley MS. The localization of radioantibodies in human brain tumors. I. Preliminary exploration. Cancer Res 1965; 25:773–778.
111. Mahaley MS, Mahaley JL, Day ED. The localization of radioantibodies in human brain tumors. II. Radioautography. Cancer Res 1965; 25:779–793.
112. Zovickian J, Youle RJ. Efficacy of intrathecal immunotoxin therapy in an animal model of leptomeningeal neoplasia. J Neurosurg 1988; 68:767–774.
113. Moseley RP, Benjamin JC, Ashpole RD, Sullivan NM, Bullimore JA, Coakham HB, Kemshead JT. Carcinomatous meningitis: antibody-guided therapy with I-131 HMFG1. J Neurol Neurosurg Psychiatry 1991; 54:260–265.
114. Hall WA, Fodstad O. Immunotoxins and central nervous system neoplasia. J Neurosurg 1992; 76:1–12.
115. Bullard DE, Bigner DD. Applications of monoclonal antibodies in the diagnosis and treatment of primary brain tumors. J Neurosurg 1985; 63:2–16.
116. de Tribolet N, Frank E, Mach JP. Monoclonal antibodies: their application in the diagnosis and management of CNS tumors. Clin Neurosurg 1988; 34:446–456.
117. Rosen ST, Zimmer AM, Goldman-Leikin R, Gordon LI, Kazikiewicz JM, Kaplan EH, Variakojis D, Marder RJ, Dykewicz MS, Piergies A, Silverstein EA, Roenigk HH, Spies SM. Radioimmunodetection and radioimmunotherapy of cutaneous T cell lymphomas using an ^{131}I-labelled monoclonal antibody: an Illinois Cancer Council study. J Clin Oncol 1987; 5:562–573.
118. Perez P, Hoffman RW, Titus JA, Segal DM. Specific targeting of human peripheral blood T cells by heteroaggregates containing ant-T3 cross-linked to ant⁻ target cell antibodies. J Exp Med 1986; 163:166–78.
119. Nitta T, Sato K, Yagita H, Okumura K, Ishii S. Preliminary trial of specific targeting therapy against malignant glioma. Lancet 1990; 335:368–376.
120. Moseley RP, Davies AG, Bourne SP, Popham C, Carrel S, Monro P, Coakham HB. Neoplastic meningitis in malignant melanoma: diagnosis with monoclonal antibodies. J Neurol Neurosurg Psychiatry 1989; 52:881–886.

32

Prognostic Factors in Patients with Brain Tumors

Barton L. Guthrie
University of Alabama School of Medicine, and U.A.B.
Comprehensive Cancer Center, Birmingham, Alabama

Edward R. Laws, Jr.
University of Virginia Health Sciences Center,
Charlottesville, Virginia

I. INTRODUCTION

As is true with any disease, different patients with the same brain tumor may show very different clinical courses. The science and art of medicine demand that physicians not only diagnose the disease, but strive to better understand and identify multifactorial prognostic indicators to allow more effective management planning. Brain tumors are no exception. Overall, 70 per 100,000 patients per year are afflicted by brain tumor, with those between 45 and 75 years of age being most at risk (1). The clinical course for any patient with a brain tumor depends on factors related to the tumor, the patient, and the treatment.

Tumor-related factors known to correlate with prognosis include tumor histology, growth rate, and location of the tumor within the brain. In general, tumors with more malignant histological features result in a poorer prognosis. A patient with a malignant cerebral astrocytoma may live only a few months, despite the best of treatment, whereas the same patient with a low-grade astrocytoma may live many years. Tumors of identical histological type may grow at different rates, resulting in vastly different outcomes. This has been seen time and again in patients with meningiomas. In one patient, this "benign" tumor may grow very little over time, whereas in another, a tumor of similar histological type may grow rapidly, necessitating multiple operations. The location of the tumor within the brain is also an important prognostic factor. Tumors in or near eloquent brain (speech, motor areas, thalamus, and brain stem) result in more rapid disability at the same rate of growth than tumors in other, less vital, brain regions.

Different patients with the same tumor fare differently, indicating that, to the extent that we uniformly classify the tumor, there are patient-related factors acting as determinants of prognosis. Perhaps the most important patient-related factor is the patient's neurological status at the time of diagnosis and treatment. This holds true whether the patient has a meningioma or a malignant astrocytoma. The more normal the neurological examination results, the better the prognosis. Closely related to this is the patient's performance status, rated on the Karnofsky performance scale. Those patients who can care for themselves are rated 70 and higher (100 being normal), and for a given tumor, these patients tend to have a better prognosis. The second most important factor is patient age. For the same disease, younger patients uniformly do better than older patients. Young patients (35–45 years) with grade 4 astrocytoma may survive 2 years, whereas patients older than 65 years of age with the same tumor may survive only several months, under the best of circumstances. Patient sex is not a strong determinant of outcome. Although some tumors tend to affect males or females preferentially, sex is not a strong determinant of prognosis in brain tumor patients. Nevertheless, it is known that symptoms of some tumors (meningioma, pituitary adenoma) may exacerbate during pregnancy, suggesting a hormonal modulation of the tumor.

There is mounting evidence that some brain tumors are associated with host immunodeficiency. Patients who are late in the course of acquired immunodeficiency syndrome (AIDS), with markedly compromised immune responses, are known to have a high propensity for central nervous system (CNS) lymphoma and, once contracted, it is much more aggressive than non-AIDS CNS lymphoma (see Chap. 17) (2). Conversely, there is evidence that gliomas in and of themselves may compromise the patient's immune system, probably by manufacturing a humoral factor that progressively suppresses the helper T-cell response (3). One such factor, transforming growth factor beta (TGF-β), has been identified in human gliomas, and there are data strongly suggesting that grade 4 astrocytoma patients with high serum levels of this molecule do significantly less well than those with lower levels (Gillespi GY, personal communication).

Several prognostic factors are related to the treatment of brain tumors. In general, the best prognosis is rendered by surgical removal of the tumor. The more complete the removal, the better the prognosis. The use of adjuvant therapy, such as radiation therapy, is tremendously beneficial for histologically malignant tumors. Although not as effective as radiation, chemotherapy may favorably influence prognosis, particularly for metastatic lesions or CNS lymphoma.

The following discussion will attempt to delineate a variety of such prognostic factors for the more common brain tumors. The subject is discussed within each tumor type or histological category because, most commonly, management plans are devised after the histological diagnosis is made. Tables 1–3 summarize the prognostic factors for the tumors to be discussed.

II. GLIOMA

Gliomas are very common, constituting 40–60% of all primary brain tumors (1,4). They arise from glial cells within the brain, including astrocytes and oligodendroglial cells. Tumors arising from

Table 1 Prognostic Factors for Patients with Astrocytoma

Parameter	Favorable	Unfavorable
Tumor grade	1,2	3,4
Age	< 40 yr	≥ 40 year
Examination	Normal	Drowsy
KPS[a]	≥ 70	< 70
Seizures	e	d
Increased ICP[b]	Low	High
Tumor cyst	c	d
Extent of resection	Gross total	Partial
Oligodendroglial component	c	d
Necrosis, endothelial proliferation, mitoses, pseudopalisading	c	d
Pilocytic histology, microcysts	c	d

[a]Karnofsky performance scale.
[b]Intracranial pressure.
[c]Present
[d]Absent

Table 2 Prognostic Factors for Patients with Meningioma

Parameter	Favorable	Unfavorable
Atypical histological features	b	c
Extent of resection	Gross total	Partial
Convexity, falcine location	c	b
Age	< 60 yr	≥ 70 yr
Examination	Normal	Drowsy
KPS[a]	≥ 70	< 70
Seizures	c	b
Parasagittal, inner sphenoid, posterior fossa location	b	c

[a]Karnofsky performance scale.
[b]Absent
[c]Present

each tissue type, respectively, are astrocytomas and oligodendrogliomas and show distinctive clinical propensities.

A. Astrocytoma

Astrocytoma, arising from astrocytes, is the most common glioma, constituting over 80% of all gliomas, a proportion that increases with age (5; Fig. 1). For the most part, they are infiltrative tumors such that the tumor edges show varying degrees of tumor cell migration into normal brain. This feature makes them extremely hard to treat. There are several well-known prognostic indicators in a patient with astrocytoma, the most important of which is the grade of the tumor.

1. Histological Features

Grade of Astrocytoma. Astrocytomas are histologically diverse. Their microscopic appearance ranges from atypical infiltrating astrocytic tumor cells to highly cellular tumors with grossly distorted cells of high mitotic activity among tissue with marked vascularity and manifesting necrosis. The extent of abnormality ranges from low (grades 1 and 2; Fig. 2a) to high (grade 4 or glioblastoma multiforme; see Fig. 2b). Survival is directly related to the grade of the tumor (6), and this is the dominant prognostic indicator in patients with glioma. Patients with low-grade astrocytomas (grades 1 and 2) tend to survive longer and in better condition than those with grades 3 and 4. The 5-year survival for low-grade glioma patients can be as high as 68% (7), depending on the

Table 3 Prognostic Factors for Patients with Brain Metastases

Parameter	Favorable	Unfavorable
Number of lesions	1	> 1
Systemic disease	Absent	Present
Age	Young (except melanoma)	Older
Examination	Normal	Altered mental status
KPS[a]	≥ 70	< 70
Increased ICP[b]	No	Yes
Extent of resection	Gross total	Partial
Unknown primary	Yes	No
Posterior fossa	No	Yes
Non–small-cell lung, colon, renal cell carcinoma	Yes	No

[a]Karnofsky performance scale.
[b]Intracranial pressure.

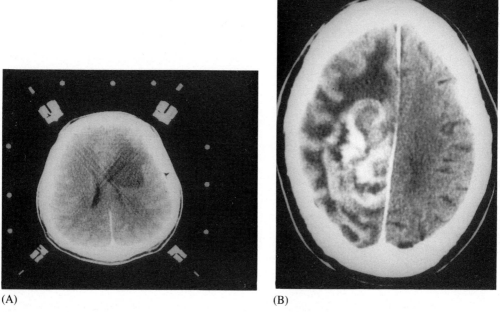

(A)   (B)

Figure 1 (A) Contrast CT scan of a low-grade astrocytoma. Note that there is no contrast enhancement. The tumor is of lower intensity than the brain. (B) Contrast-enhanced scan of a grade 4 astrocytoma. There is irregular, but vigorous uptake of contrast, a poor prognostic sign.

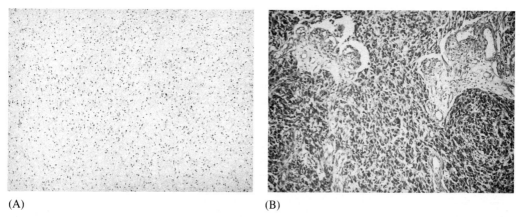

(A)   (B)

Figure 2 (A) Hematoxylin–eosin (H&E)-stained section of the tumor in Figure 1A. Note the benign appearance. This is a grade 2 astrocytoma using the scale of Daumas-Duport. (B) H&E-stained section of the tumor in Figure 1B. This is a grade 4 astrocytoma using the Daumas-Duport scheme.

series and choice of therapy (8). The 5-year survival for patients with a grade 3 or 4 glioma approaches zero. The 2-year survival for patients with a grade 3 astrocytoma is 38–50% and that for grade 4 astrocytoma is 8–12% (9). Figure 3 shows calculated survivals for grades 1 through 4 astrocytoma relative to time. These figures dramatically illustrate the effect of tumor grade on patient survival. In particular, histological elements that correlate with a poor prognosis are necrosis, endothelial proliferation, pseudopalisading, gemistocytic cell type, and sarcomatous degeneration.

Oligodendroglial Component. Astrocytomas are a heterogeneous group of tumors. Among the other histological features involved in tumor grade will be a varying amount of oligodendroglial component. Such tumors are called *mixed gliomas* or *oligoastrocytomas* and are not uncommon. They are without exception low-grade gliomas and are indolent. Data are convincing that the presence of oligondendroglial cells in an astrocytoma improves prognosis (10).

Pilocytic Astrocytoma. Pilocytic astrocytomas are composed of long, thin spindle-shaped glial tumor cells, with a very homogeneous and benign appearance. They generally occur in younger patients, with an average age of 14 years (7). Such a histological type, even for older patients, reflects a very good prognosis, with a 10-year survival of about 80% after resection (7).

2. Neurological Status at Diagnosis

Another extremely important prognostic factor in patients with glioma is the neurological status of the patient at the time of diagnosis. This variable appears to affect each grade of astrocytoma. For example, a neurologically normal patient with a low-grade astrocytoma may have up to a 70% chance of surviving 10 years (7). On the other hand, the same patient, if drowsy or paralyzed by the lesion at the time of diagnosis, can be expected to have a shorter survival time (11). The same is true for higher grades of astrocytoma. A patient with a grade 4 astrocytoma, who is normal at the time of diagnosis, can be expected to survive about 12–18 months with standard therapy (12), whereas the same patient, who has a serious neurological deficit from the tumor, will survive a much shorter period, often only a matter of weeks. Of all the neurological signs, state of

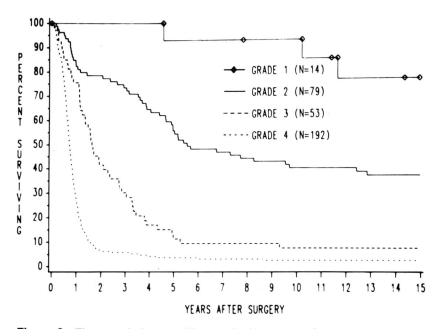

Figure 3 These survival curves illustrate the importance of tumor grade on prognosis in patients with astrocytoma. The prognosis worsens from grade 1 to grade 4. (From Ref. 6)

consciousness seems to be the most important prognostic factor (11,13). A drowsy patient has a much worse prognosis than one who is alert. This may be directly related to increased intracranial pressure, which is a poor prognostic indicator (13). Patients who present with seizures tend to have a better prognosis than those who do not (13). Slow-growing, infiltrative lesions may be more epileptogenic than their faster-growing, more malignant counterparts. In addition, the presence of seizures may allow a tumor diagnosis to be made earlier than it would be otherwise.

3. Patient Age

In most disease processes that affect all age groups, younger patients fare better than older patients, and astrocytoma is no exception. Patients with low-grade astrocytomas tend to be younger than those with higher grades; however, even within the grade 1 and 2 astrocytomas, younger patients survive longer than older patients (7,13). Age is especially a factor with higher-grade astrocytomas. Young patients with grade 4 astrocytoma (glioblastoma multiforme) can expect to survive 12–24 months with aggressive therapy (12,14). In general, the older the patient, the worse the prognosis. Patients older than 60 years of age with grade 4 astrocytomas survive at a median of 16 weeks with aggressive therapy (15).

4. Tumor Size and Location

In general, patients with larger tumors do worse than those with smaller tumors. In the days before computed tomography (CT) and magnetic resonance imaging (MRI) scanning, tumors tended to grow to a larger size before diagnosis. In these pre-CT series, the median survival of such patients with low-grade gliomas was 4–5 years (13; for tabulation see Ref. 16). In modern series, tumor size is generally smaller at the time of diagnosis and survival of patients appears to be better, with a median survival of 7–8 years (16,17). Although these are not controlled studies on tumor size, the role of earlier diagnosis (at a smaller size) is obvious in extending the apparent survival. The location of the tumor is also important. In general, patients with tumors in less eloquent areas of brain (anterior frontal lobes, temporal lobes, occipital lobes) do better than those with tumor in more vital brain regions (posterior frontal, parietal lobes, thalamus, and brain stem). For example, a patient with a grade 4 astrocytoma in the right anterior frontal lobe may live 2 years, whereas the same patient with a glioblastoma in the brain stem will live only a matter of weeks after diagnosis. The effect of location is obviously related to the fact that tumors in vital brain areas tend to disable the patient earlier.

5. Treatment

The efficacy of any treatment modality is measured by how it improves the course of the disease against the natural history of the disease. Because most patients with astrocytomas are treated, the natural history remains a bit vague, but we may assume that the course of minimally treated patients reflects the natural history of the disease. Patients with untreated or minimally treated low-grade astrocytomas have a 5- and 10-year survival of near 20 and 5%, respectively (11,18). Similar patients with grade 4 astrocytomas live 4–6 months.

Surgery alone for patients with low-grade astrocytomas may extend survival, resulting in a 5- and 10-year survival of up to 38 and 11%, respectively (10,19). Surgery alone for patients with grade 4 astrocytomas results in rather short survivals, in the range of 3–4 months (20).

Surgery, followed by radiation therapy, appears to extend survival of patients with larger low-grade astrocytomas to a 5- and 10-year rate of approximately 30 and 10%, respectively (10). Similar therapy is standard for all patients with grade 4 astrocytomas, with postoperative radiation therapy extending survival to over 9 months (20).

The extent to which the tumor is removed (gross total versus subtotal removal) appears to correlate relatively well with survival in the year after surgery. One series of patients with malignant gliomas reports an approximately 60% 1-year survival for those with gross total resection versus a 30% 1-year survival for those with a subtotal removal (21). In the same series, the only 2-year survivors were those patients who received a gross total resection. In addition, there is ample evidence that patients who remain healthy at the time of recurrence are benefited by reoperation (14,22).

To date, no chemotherapeutic agent has been significantly effective against astrocytomas. A large cooperative trial suggests that carmustine (BCNU) added to standard therapy adds 2–4 weeks to survival (20).

B. Oligodendrogliomas

Patients with oligodendrogliomas of a pure histological type are not as common as those with astrocytomas. These patients average 35–40 years of age (discussed in Ref. 8). Their lower numbers and long survival preclude definitive survival data. The best current information suggests an average survival at 5 and 10 years that may be as high as 83 and 55%, respectively (23,24), which is somewhat better than low-grade astrocytomas and mixed gliomas. Relative to prognostic factors, it appears that tumor histological type is a factor. Patients with oligodendrogliomas with benign-appearing histological features have a 5-year survival of over 60%, whereas those whose tumor shows malignant features (necrosis, pseudopalisading, pleomorphism) do much worse (25,26). In addition, all other parameters outlined in the foregoing discussion on astrocytoma pertain to the prognosis of the patient with oligodendroglioma.

III. MENINGIOMA

Meningiomas constitute 19–24% of all primary intracranial tumors (4,27). They arise from arachnoid cap cells within the arachnoid layer of the meninges. Not being truly "brain tumors," they are referred to as extra-axial or outside the neuraxis and compress the brain as they grow. Very few actually invade the brain. This, combined with their generally benign histological character, makes surgery an excellent mode of therapy for these tumors. When discussing prognostic factors in patients with meningioma, it must be realized that many of these tumors (diagnosed presumptively by CT or MRI) lie dormant for years without growing; thus, one obvious prognostic factor is the tumor's rate of growth, and the following discussion involves only those patients with meningioma who exhibit symptomatic tumor growth.

A. Histology

Meningiomas have three gross histological patterns that seem to be related to prognosis: the typical meningioma, the atypical meningioma, and the angioblastic meningioma or hemangiopericytoma.

1. Typical Meningioma

Meningiomas with typical histological characteristics are considered benign tumors. Typical meningiomas are grouped into three major histological patterns: meningotheliomatous, transitional, and fibrous. All yield similar prognoses. After diagnosis and surgery, the recurrence rate at 5 years is approximately 15%, at 10 years is 22%, and at 15 years is 34%. The 5-, 10- and 15-year survival is approximately 83, 77, and 63%, respectively (see Ref. 28 for review). From these numbers, it is readily apparent that prognosis for meningioma is markedly better than for glioma.

2. Atypical Meningioma

Atypical meningiomas resemble their typical counterparts, except for increased cellularity, the presence of nuclear pleomorphism, occasional mitotic figures, and papillary patterns (29). Although they generally grow slowly, there are data to suggest that their clinical course is more aggressive than typical meningiomas. The recurrence-free postsurgical interval and survival are shorter for these patients than for patients with ordinary meningioma (29).

3. Angioblastic Meningioma or Meningeal Hemangiopericytoma

The angioblastic meningioma also arises within the meninges, but is felt to be derived from pericytes around meningeal vessels, rather than from arachnoid cells. The histological pattern is that of swirling spindle-shaped cells, with frequent mitotic figures. They often resemble meningioma neurodiagnostically, and the diagnosis often rests with the neuropathologist. The clinical course is quite aggressive when compared with typical meningioma, with a 5-, 10-, and 15-year recurrence rate of 65, 76, and 87%, respectively (30). Survival at these time intervals is 67, 40, and 23%, respectively (30).

An ominous feature of this tumor is its propensity to metastasize. The common sites of metastasis are lung, bone, and liver. The 5-, 10-, and 15-year rate of metastasis is 13, 33, and 64%, respectively, and the average time to metastasis is 7–8 years (30). The importance of metastasis as a prognostic factor is evidenced by the fact that after metastasis, the average survival is 24 months, marking a relatively rapid deterioration in the patient's condition (30).

B. Tumor Location

The location of the tumor is an important prognostic determinant. Patients with tumors in difficult surgical regions (sphenoid, near the foramen magnum) had a 15–year survival of 53–57%, whereas those with more accessible tumors (convexity, falcine) survived at a rate of 74–86% at 15 years (31). Thus, meningiomas located in difficult surgical areas have a worse prognosis, not only because of the sensitivity of the area within which they are located, but because of their surgical inaccessibility.

C. Extent of Surgical Removal

In patients who have been surgically treated for meningioma of the typical histological type, perhaps the most important prognostic factor is the extent of the surgical removal. This was realized as early as 1957, when meningioma surgery was becoming widespread (32). Patients who have had a complete surgical removal of their tumor have a 10–20% recurrence rate at 10 years, whereas those with an incomplete tumor removal have a 33–70% recurrence rate at 10 years (33,34). Patients with gross residual tumor have a 5- and 10-year survival of 53 and 25%, respectively (32). It is evident from these figures that extent of removal (related to tumor location and accessibility) is an extremely important prognostic factor.

D. Other Factors

There are several other factors that are predictive of outcome. As with other tumors, patients with poor neurological status at the time of diagnosis and treatment do worse than healthier patients. Long-standing symptoms suggest a slow-growing tumor as opposed to the rapid onset of symptoms, which correlates with a more aggressive tumor and poorer prognosis (29,30). Patients with seizures tend not to have aggressive meningiomas (30) and, thus, do better. In general, younger patients fare better than older patients; however, old age does not seem to be a negative factor until the seventh or eighth decade (31).

IV. METASTASES

Metastatic brain tumors constitute a growing percentage of all brain tumors. In a neurosurgical practice, 10–20% of brain tumors will be metastatic (1). On the other hand, the number of systemic cancer patients dying with brain metastases is as large or larger than patients dying with primary brain tumors (35). In general, the development of a cerebral metastasis in patients with systemic cancer is an extremely poor prognostic sign, with a median survival of 8–9 months (35). However, given that a patient has been diagnosed with this malady, there are certain indicators of varying prognoses. Patients with no active systemic disease may do well if the brain lesion is treated. A single metastasis is a good prognostic sign, and survival is significantly prolonged if the lesion is removed (36). Patients with metastatic non–small-cell lung cancer, renal cell cancer, or colon cancer generally do better than those with other types of metastatic tumors (median survival 10–14 months) (35). As with other tumors, younger patients and those with good neurological function do better than those with older patients or those with significant deficits. In general, the patient faring best is a young, neurologically intact patient free of systemic disease with a single metastasis that is removed surgically. These patients will have a median survival time of 22 months (35).

V. SUMMARY

In summary, the primary prognostic determinant in patients with brain tumor is the type of tumor. Patients with histologically malignant tumors (metastases, high-grade gliomas) do much worse than those with benign tumors. Other, rather constant, predictors of favorable outcome for brain tumor patients include: young age, good neurological status at the time of treatment, single lesion that is surgically accessible, complete (or near complete) surgical removal, and effective adjuvant therapy (primarily radiation therapy).

REFERENCES

1. Butler AB, Brooks, WH, Netsky MG. Classification and biology of brain tumors. In: Youmans JR, ed. Neurological surgery. vol 2. Philadelphia. WB Saunders, 1982:2686–2687.
2. Chappell ET, Guthrie BL, Orenstein J. The role of stereotactic biopsy in the management of HIV-related focal brain lesions. Neurosurgery 1992; 30:825–829.
3. Bullard DE, Gillespie GY, Mahaley MS, Bigner DD. Immunology of human gliomas. Semin Oncol 1986; 13:94–109.
4. Mahaley MS Jr, Mettlin C, Natarajan N, Laws ER Jr, Peace BB. National survey of patterns of care for brain-tumor patients. J Neurosurg 1989; 71:826–836.
5. Butler AB, Brooks WH, Netsky MG. Classification and biology of brain tumors. In: Youmans JR, ed. Neurological surgery. vol 2. Philadelphia: WB Saunders, 1982:2685.
6. Daumas-Duport C, Scheithauer BW, O'Fallon JR, et al. Grading of astrocytomas: a simple and reproducible method. Cancer 1988; 62:2152–2165.
7. Shaw EG, Daumas-Duport C, Scheithauer BW, et al. Radiation therapy in the treatment of low-grade supratentorial astrocytomas. J Neurosurg 1989; 70:853–861.
8. Guthrie BL, Laws ER Jr. Supratentorial low-grade gliomas. Neurosurg Clin North Am 1990; 1:37–48.
9. Burger PC, Vogel FS, Green SB, Strike TA. Glioblastoma multiforme and anaplastic astrocytoma: pathologic criteria and prognostic implications. Cancer 1985; 56:1106–1111.
10. Shaw E, Earle J, Scheithauer BW, et al. Postoperative radiation for supratentorial low grade gliomas. Radiat Oncol Biol Phys 1987; 13(suppl 1):148.
11. Soffietti R, Chio A, Giordana MT, et al. Prognostic factors in well-differentiated cerebral astrocytomas in the adult. Neurosurgery 1989; 24:686–692.
12. Cooper JS, Borok TL, Ransohoff J, Carella R. Malignant glioma: results of combined modality therapy. JAMA 1982; 248:62–65.
13. Laws ER Jr, Taylor WF, Clifton MB, et al. Neurosurgical management of low-grade astrocytoma of the cerebral hemisphere. J Neurosurg 1984; 61:665–673.
14. Salcman M. Malignant glioma management. Neurosurg Clin North Am 1990; 1:49–61.

15. Whittle IR, Denholm SW, Gregor A. Management of patients aged over 60 years with supratentorial glioma: lessons from an audit. Surg Neurol 1991; 36:106–112.

16. Vertosik FT, Seiker RG, Arena VC. Survival of well-differentiated astrocytomas diagnosed in the era of computed tomography. Neurosurgery 1991; 28:496–501.

17. Piepmeier JM. Observations on the current treatment of low-grade astrocytomas of the cerebral hemispheres. J Neurosurg 1987; 67:177–181.

18. Liebel SA, Sheline GE, Wara WM, et al. The role of radiation therapy in the treatment of astrocytoma. Cancer 1975; 35:1551–1557.

19. Bouchard J, Pierce CB. Radiation therapy in the management of neoplasms of the central nervous system with a special note in regard to children: twenty year's experience, 1930–1958. AJR 1960; 84:610–628.

20. Waker MD, Alexander E Jr, Hunt WE, MacCarty CS, Mahaley MS, Mealey J, Norrell HA, Owens G, Ransohoff J, Wilson CB, Gehan EA, Strike TA. Evaluation of BCNU and/or radiotherapy in the treatment of anaplastic gliomas. A cooperative clinical trial. J Neurosurg 1978; 49:333–343.

21. Ammirati M, Vick N, Liao Y, Ciric I, Mikhael M. Effect of the extent of surgical resection on survival and quality of life in patients with supratentorial glioblastomas and anaplastic astrocytomas. Neurosurgery 1987; 21:201–206.

22. Harsh GR IV, Levin VA, Gutin PH, Seager M, Silver P, Wilson CB. Reoperation for recurrent glioblastoma and anaplastic astrocytoma. Neurosurgery 1987; 21:615–621.

23. Chin HW, Hazel JJ, Kim TH, et al. Oligodendrogliomas: I. A clinical study of cerebral oligodendrogliomas. Cancer 1980; 45:1458–1466.

24. Sheline GE, Boldey E, Karlsberg P, et al. Therapeutic considerations in tumors affecting the central nervous system: oligodendrogliomas. Radiology 1964; 82:84–89.

25. Burger PC, Rawlings CE, Cox EB, et al. Clinicopathologic correlations in ologiodendroglioma. Cancer 1987; 59:1345–1352.

26. Snith MT, Ludwig CL, Godfrey AD, et al. Grading of oligodendrogliomas. Cancer 1983; 52:2107–2114.

27. Cushing H, Eisenhardt L. Meningiomas: their classification, regional behavior, life history and surgical end results. Springfield: Charles C Thomas, 1938.

28. Guthrie BL, Eberasold MJ, Scheithauer BW. Neoplasms of the intracranial meninges. In: Youmans, JR, ed. Neurological surgery. Philadelphia: WB Saunders, 1990.

29. Jaaskelainen J, Haltia M, Servo A. Atypical and anaplastic meningiomas: radiology, surgery, radiotherapy and outcome. Surg Neurol 1986; 25:233–242.

30. Guthrie BL, Ebersold MJ, Scheithauer BW, Shaw EG. Meningeal hemangiopericytoma: histopathological features, treatment and long-term followup of 44 cases. Neurosurgery 1989; 25:514–522.

31. MacCarty CS, Taylor WF. Intracranial meningiomas: experiences at the Mayo Clinic. Neurol Medico-Chir 1979; 19:569–574.

32. Simpson D. The recurrence of intracranial meningiomas after surgical treatment. J Neurol Neurosurg Psychiatry 1957; 20:22–39.

33. Adegbite AB, Khan MI, Paine KWE, Tan LK. The recurrence of intracranial meningioma after surgical treatment. J Neurosurg 1983; 58:51–56.

34. Chan RC, Thompson GB. Morbidity, mortality and quality of life following surgery for intracranial meningiomas: a retrospective study in 250 cases. J Neurosurg 1984; 60:52–60.

35. Galicich JH, Arbit E. Metastatic brain tumors. In: Youmans JR, ed. Neurological surgery. Philadelphia: WB Saunders, 1990.

36. Patchell RA, Tibbs PA, Walsh JW, Dempsey RJ, Maruyama Y, Kryscio RJ, Markesbery WR, Young B. Randomized trial of surgery in the treatment of single metastases to the brain. N Engl J Med 1990; 322:494–500.

33

The Psychological Care of the
Brain Tumor Patient and Family

Peggy Ward Smith
The Brain Tumor Institute of Kansas City, Research Medical
Center, Kansas City, Missouri

James G. Lemons
Research Medical Center, Kansas City, Missouri

I. INTRODUCTION

An interest in the psychological care of the cancer patient has heightened over the last several years. Lederberg and associates (1) attribute this to three sources. First, psychiatrists have begun to focus on the problems of patients with cancer and have begun defining cancer patients' emotional problems as well as understanding the difficulties of their families and the staff who care for them. Second, the social climate in the United States has changed such that most patients demand more knowledge about their diagnosis and more participation in decisions about their treatment. Finally, the specialty of oncology has developed rapidly from the time 30 years ago when little was known about the cause or cures of cancer. Today, research in cancer is providing new insights into basic patterns of both abnormal and normal cell growth; consequently, cancer patients are surviving longer than previously.

II. HISTORICAL BACKGROUND

Literature on the effect of a cancer diagnosis on the patient is both varied and extensive. It has been well documented that the discovery of cancer is a stressful and traumatic event with responses ranging from anger to guilt, from anxiety to disbelief, and from self-pity to bitterness and hostility (2–5). Despite the abundance of literature available, few empirical studies are available that document the actual physiological effect on the patient and family (6). Available literature does enable us to discuss known psychological reactions of individuals who received the diagnosis of cancer, as well as to predict, to a certain degree, their responses to the diagnosis. The diagnosis of cancer causes an individual to experience stress related to the actual symptoms of the disease and to the psychological meaning attached to cancer. Any given patient's ability to manage these stresses depends on his or her prior level of emotional adjustment, the threat the cancer poses to their age-appropriate goal (career, family, or other), the presence of emotional support from persons in the environment, and variables determined by the disease (disabling symptoms, site, treatment re-

809

quired, prognosis and so forth). Age may be a factor in how an individual responds emotionally and psychologically to a diagnosis of cancer. Younger patients appear to experience more frequent or severe psychological and treatment-related problems than older patients, particularly in relation to work and chemotherapy. Ganz states that younger patients have a greater difficulty in dealing with the health care setting (7). They generally have had less experience with illness and more family and career responsibilities and thus experience a poor adjustment. They are also unable to tolerate short-term discomfort for long-term benefit. In young adults, cancer is disruptive of the attainment of roles and important life tasks not yet carried out. The struggle with disengagement from work and dependency on others is the greatest cause of concern for this age group.

Cassileth and colleagues found that mental health was better in clients with advancing age, regardless of their diagnosis (8). Elderly people considered themselves more vulnerable to disease and view illness of any sort as more serious than those in other age groups. Older individuals view illness as a premonition of death or shortened life. The fear of extended life with deterioration that would make life itself unwanted is also the fear of an older adult. Illness at any age produces anxiety, but this is particularly true for older people. Most health care systems are geared toward curing, rather than caring, and as such, a sick elderly person may have less social value than a sick younger person. Newgarten contends that most older people, aware of this fact, either speak up for themselves, or live with an expressed rage and become demanding in hostile ways (9). Many of these same attributes can be found in younger patients, although they seem to be magnified in older individuals. Cancer is seen as an acceleration of the aging process that results in a rapid disengagement from the work setting and an increased dependency on others. Edlund and Sneed studied the oldest patients (i.e., those older than 70), and reported that they experienced significantly less psychological disruption in the period after learning of their diagnosis (10).

III. PSYCHOLOGICAL EFFECTS OF CANCER

Magnes and Mendelsohn identified three variables that are predictive of psychosocial adjustment in cancer patients in general as well as in long-term survivors (11): the severity of the illness, the psychological stability of the patient, and the presence of social supports. The presence of another person in the home, regardless of the relationship correlates highly (positively) with optimal psychosocial functioning.

Recently, greater attention has turned to the emotional, physical, and behavioral consequences of rigorous treatment regimens—especially in young people. Quality of life and delayed treatment effects in long-term survivors have become important issues. Patients no longer accept the statement "You should be grateful just to be alive." Their concerns about long-term sequelae of treatment on psychological and physical functions needs to be addressed. When the cancer patients' emotional distress exceeds what seems reasonable for the circumstances, the psychiatric symptoms must be evaluated.

To meet the increasing demand for information concerning significant psychiatric disorders among cancer patients, the Psychosocial Collaborative Oncology Group (PSYCOG) studied 215 randomly selected hospitalized and ambulatory patients at three major cancer centers (12). Clinical interviews that revealed a psychiatric disorder, as defined by the *Diagnostic and Statistical Manual of Mental Disorders*, 3rd ed. (*DSM-III*) were present in 47% of patients. Sixty-eight percent had an adjustment disorder with a depressed, anxious, or mixed mood; 13% had a major depression; 8% had an organic mental disorder; 7% had a personality disorder; and 4% had an anxiety disorder. In another study (13), the prevalence of depression in hospitalized cancer patients was explored. It was found that 24% were severely depressed, 18% were moderately depressed, and 14% had depressive symptoms of sadness. The remaining 44% showed no depression at all, despite their cancer illness. The fact most significantly related to the presence of severe depression was a level of impaired physical functioning; 77% of those who were most depressed were also the most physically impaired. Separation of cancer symptoms from vegetative signs of depression is almost impossible in the very ill—making interpretation of such studies difficult. However, the finding that 24% of cancer patients have severe depression is similar to that of Plumb and Holland (14). This study reports that approximately 23% of cancer patients are significantly depressed. Two studies of patients on a general medical floor found similar prevalence of depression, suggesting the cancer patients were no more or less depressed than equally physically ill patients with other diseases (15,16). Up to a quarter of all cancer patients may thus be experiencing substantial emotional distress, most often of a depressive nature. In a study of psychiatric consultations (17), patients who were referred and found to be depressed constituted less than 3% of the patient population hospitalized for cancer. A PSYCOG survey of psychotropic drugs ordered by physicians for cancer patients over an 8-month period found that only 1% of the prescriptions were for antidepressive medications (18). Taken together the studies of depression and of psychiatric consultation in cancer patients suggest that although 20–25% of cancer patients are depressed, many depressions go unrecognized and untreated. The most common psychiatric disorders encountered in cancer patients are major depressive disorders, delirium and dementia, and anxiety disorders (19).

The range of human responses documented in other situations of threatened or actual loss (20–22) are seen with similar symptoms in cancer patients at times of crisis. When individuals are told of their diagnosis of cancer, they are transiently distressed and reactions may vary from minimal to major disruptions of emotions and activities. The psychological symptoms seen are initially shock and disbelief, followed by anxiety symptoms, depressive symptoms, anger, and a disruption of appetite and sleep. The ability to concentrate and to carry out the normal daily patterns of work and home life may be impaired, and intrusive thoughts about the diagnosis and fear for the future may be uncontrollable. Psychiatric consultation should be requested when the acute symptoms of distress last longer than a week, when they worsen rather than improve, or when they interfere with the patient's ability to cooperate with the planned treatment. Short-term support psychotherapy (four to six sessions) based on a crisis intervention model is usually sufficient to reduce symptoms to a tolerable level. The sessions should deal with the "here-and-now" process of adaptation to the diagnosis and treatment. Sadness and grief are normal responses to painful life events associated with threatened or actual loss. They are to be expected in instances of life-threatening illness—especially cancer. The frequency of these responses makes it important to establish criteria for distinguishing between normal and abnormal degrees of depression in such patients. To identify those with clinical and depressive syndromes, the physician must consider the prevalence of depression in a noncancerous population for comparison purposes.

Estimates of the prevalence of depressive symptoms among cancer patients have been made from consultations and select patient samples. Worden and Weisman approached preventive mental health in those with cancer by trying to identify, in advance, those with serious distress (23). The goal was to identify those who were at high risk and to offer help before serious emotional distress and poor coping develop. The advantages to this system are great from an economic standpoint, since only those at most risk are treated. Within 10 days of initial diagnosis, patients are screened by interview. The issues recorded include church attendance, marital status, socioeconomic status, mental health history, health and religious concerns, as well as family, existential, and friendship concerns. Those felt to be in a high-risk category were given four sessions with a therapist.

IV. NEUROLOGICAL MALIGNANCIES

Many patients with other cancers can be cured. The patient with a malignant glioma will not be cured. The brain tumor patient experiences many losses over varying lengths of time. Most patients with a primary brain tumor undergo a neurosurgical procedure, and surgical removal of primary or metastatic brain tumors can usually achieve worthwhile palliation (24). Sooner or later, major neurological disabilities complicate the course of most patients. Initially, defects may be minimal, family and friends attentive, denial high, and hope for cure real. Often professionals look at these patients with disdain, wondering if they have actually heard what their diagnosis was. As the patient deteriorates, it becomes increasingly difficult to reestablish a sense of equilibrium. They grieve these losses and frequently become angry at their inability to perform the simplest of tasks (25).

Clinical signs of a brain tumor may arise from generalized manifestation of increased intracranial pressure, from secondary focal effects caused by displaced intracranial structures, and from direct focal effects caused by the local damage produced by the tumor or edema. The most common symptom of increased intracranial pressure is headache. Usually the patient is awakened in the morning with a headache, which may be accompanied by nausea and vomiting. Malaise, somnolence, ataxia, and incontinence may eventually develop.

The most common manifestations of tumors within the cerebral hemispheres are seizures, impairment of memory and intellect, dysphasia, visual field defects, and hemiparesis. Focal motor seizures, which are common with tumors located in the cerebral hemispheres, may become generalized. Every effort should be made to control seizures, for they are frightening to both the patient and their family, as well as possibly causing temporary or permanent worsening of neurological deficits. Progressive loss of brain function leads to personality changes, deterioration in judgment, and the inability to conceptualize a host of more subtle phenomena, which often arise before the development of the frank speech and cognitive disturbances (26). The impairment of memory and intellect does not make patients oblivious to what is being said in their presence. To avoid misapprehension, explanations given to the patient should be as simple as possible to enable them to participate in their own care as much as feasible. Any attainable remaining cognitive function should be used. Tumors that affect the dominant hemisphere may result in expressive aphasia, wherein the patients' comprehension exceeds their ability to speak. Speaking slowly, using hand gestures, and allowing them adequate response time decreases their frustrations. Partial or complete hemiparesis may accompany lesions involving any part of the visual pathways from the optic tract to the occipital cortex. If these are present, patients need to learn to compensate. Hemiparetic patients benefit from physical and occupational therapies, to maintain muscle function as long as possible, as well as to prevent contractures.

Patients have many fears—including the fear of prolonged suffering and disability, fear of becoming a burden to their family, and fear of death—and they often find these fears difficult to express. Outlining realistic goals and organizing a treatment plan can help ally the patients' apprehension about the future. The patients' dignity and self-esteem can be maintained by encouraging them to care for themselves and by recognizing their individual needs and wishes (27).

Hochberg and Slotnick selected 13 patients with primary astrocytic tumors and examined them by neuropsychiatric testing (28). In the absence of tumor regrowth or other neurological disorders, each patient documented difficulty with problem-solving or coping with novel situations psychometrically measured intelligence appeared consistent with their premorbid levels. The diffuse difficulties appeared unrelated to tumor type or location, but did explain, in part, why their patients failed to resume active social lives or their premorbid employment.

The psychological problems of long-term survivors constitutes a new area of concern (29). Common psychological problems include fears associated with termination of treatment, fears of recurrence or secondary malignancy, adaptation to or anticipated late effects (infertility, CNS dysfunction, organ failure), chronic stress experienced by patients and families, development of a survivor syndrome (guilt), and adaptation to negative social responses (job, friends). Massie and

Holland observed that patients finishing radiation therapy revealed an unexpected and significant increase in psychological distress at the end of treatment (30). This distress seemed to be related to fear that the tumor might recur when treatment was stopped. Loss of daily supportive contact with staff and the security provided by close physical monitoring caused heightened distress. The even more difficult question of when maintenance therapy should end was also a source of fear. Patients continued years later to experience anxiety when they developed minor symptoms that earlier they would have ignored.

V. PATIENT–PHYSICIAN RELATIONSHIP

Physicians' attitudes in dealing with cancer have also changed over the last several decades. Pessimism in both physician and patient has given way to cautious optimism, as radiation therapy and chemotherapy have begun to cure several common neoplasms in children and young adults. Although in many countries an open discussion of cancer diagnosis is viewed as cruel and inhuman, in the United States concealing the diagnosis is regarded as both unethical and illegal. In an effort to carry out these required conversations, and yet to soften the psychological blow of delivering the diagnosis, physicians frequently substitute other words for the word "cancer" in their initial conversations with patients. Despite the use of substitute words, one study found that over 90% of their physician respondents revealed the cancer diagnosis (31). This trend is attributed to the complex nature of the tests and treatments involved that require the patient's cooperation, increasing legal and ethical concerns about informed consent, patients' greater information and expectations, and the individual physician's own comfort with discussions about cancer. Patients, in general, will do better with complex treatment plans if they understand the goal. A knowledge of what side effects will occur makes them a little easier to live with. The physicians in the previous survey felt that disclosing the diagnosis of cancer to a patient has a positive effect 68% of the time. The positive effect was manifested in increased patient coping, compliance, communication, tolerance of treatment, and planning for the future. Negative changes were seen by 12% of the oncologists responding to the survey. These were related to the patients affect, with transient depression, anger, and anxiety.

Weisman describes the way a physician should act when working with the cancer patient as *safe conduct* (32). Safe conduct can best be described as candor with hope when telling one of his or her diagnosis. Safe conduct is that dimension beyond diagnosis, treatment, and relief that refers to the manner in which a physician will conduct a patient through a maze of uncertain, perplexing, and distressing events. It means to behave prudently while guiding a patient, such as one with cancer, through a perilous unknown. It does not mean that the physician is always adherent to a script of convention, caution, and rigid routine. Good behavior is taken for granted. Safe conduct should not be confused with rehabilitation or psychotherapy. Even though a primary physician cannot reduce all danger and distress, she or he can be consistently cool, courteous, and courageous. The latter is not a universal trait. Physicians can be apprehensive themselves. It takes more than intellectual integrity to say "I do not know, but will try to find out." For the cancer patient, safe conduct is assured when the physician is accessible, not necessarily at all times, but at times of need. Accessibility can relieve anguish and make uncertainty tolerable. Good treatment does not mean treatment by a committee of anonymous technicians. There is no safe conduct without individualization.

Vulnerable patients are those with physical symptoms, advanced staging, and rapid proliferation. They are patients who are "born losers" and expect the future to be no different than the past. Their pessimism may be justified, but they also may have current concerns and past regrets that increase distress. Support from others is minimal, or at best, questionable. Lasting loyalty is simply not present. In fact, people who have previously been confirmed loners cope better than those with shabby support systems. The least psychologically vulnerable cancer patients are those who are optimistic, expecting support from others, and getting it. Communication is always open. If it is not, then such a patient demands attention and will not submit without question. As redundant as it is, resourceful people have ample resources to draw upon. They are usually amicable, but firm and articulate when necessary, and accustomed to success. They may live longer with the same disease. If not, the quality of their life will be better than that of the more marginal person.

Cancer does not confer emotional immunity. Patients with a history of psychiatric problems also tend to be more vulnerable to the emotional complications of cancer. The diagnosis of emotional vulnerability in newly diagnosed cancer patients is not solely due to pessimism, marital problems, and lack of expected support. People like to put themselves in the best light, especially when talking with the professional whose respect they want. Consequently, the more vulnerable the cancer patients seems to be, the more difficult it is to get direct confirmation of distress. Safe conduct not only demands that the warning signs of vulnerability be recognized early, but that firm alliances be established and continue throughout the course. Helping a vulnerable cancer patient cope better requires help that is optimistic, resourceful, and realistic. If physicians negativistically believe that cancer is a deadly disease, they cannot offer safe conduct. The patient who copes best and the most effective interviewers are themselves optimists who believe that the future can be better, regardless of the prognosis. Such people tend to confront problems directly, redefine salient issues constructively, seek competent assistance when needed, and selectively address themselves to problems that are most alarming and disconcerting.

Antidepressants, tranquilizers, narcotics, or combinations of drugs are often necessary and should not be withheld; neither should they replace compassionate care and safe conduct. Safe conduct never ends. This implies that the physician who has been in charge throughout the illness does not desert the cancer patient once there is no longer any surgery to be done or medicine to be given. If the physician is not going to personally render care, there is still the moral obligation to see that the patient has the necessary support systems in place. Hospice and other health care agencies may be employed. Most terminally ill patients do not require hospitalization and would rather die in the comfort of their own home. The physician also has the moral obligation to allow the cancer patient the choice in determining the course of their life in the late stages of their disease. This is not euthanasia, but the opportunity to choose a dignified, peaceful death, without exposure to the seemingly relentless application of medical technology. The physician must take the opportunity and initiative to discuss this with the patient. Anxiety is the most common feeling of the dying individual. The medical professionals must overcome their own anxiety, so that they do not compound it in the cancer patient.

Quality-of-life issues are equally important for the patient whose treatment is only palliative. When patients have advanced disease and cure is no longer possible, the physician must carefully weigh the likely benefits of a given treatment versus toxicity. These issues become complex when conventional treatments have failed and the physician, patient, and family must decide between supportive care with maximum comfort and participation in a clinical investigation of new, unproved anticancer treatments. Candid discussions with both the patient and their support system should assist the physician in the delivery of proper care. The range and intensity of psychological and social needs of cancer patients and their families have led many oncologists to make use of multidisciplinary teams. To be effective, the team approach requires a high level of communication among team members and with the patient. Patients presenting with recurrent disease require the same handling as those people entering with initial disease, except that they are even more uncertain about their outcome. They usually require more time and additional explanation. The interval for follow-up appointments should be inversely proportionate to the amount of fear the patient is expressing. It is safe conduct that physicians and other health care professionals pledge to those patients who are obliged to surrender their autonomy as time goes on and must yield essential control of their lives to someone else.

VI. TERMINAL CARE

Terminal care begins at the unspecified point when the aim of treatment is no longer to cure, but to preserve life and relieve distress as long as possible. Terminal care should begin in the preterminal period, just before the patient begins the descent into death. Terminal care rightly includes the family, close friends, and colleagues. Therapeutically, people who stand to lose the most by the patient's death must be those who can give the most and contribute to a dignified, harmonious exodus. Significant psychological problems may occur at any stage of a fatal illness, and we must realize that such problems not only differ from stage to stage, but also from person to person, depending on the diagnosis, age, social and cultural resources, economic independence, and ethnic customs of the patient.

Weisman defines three stages patients pass through while dealing with their cancer (33). Stage 1 is the period from onset of symptoms until the diagnosis is made. Few people are under medical observation when stage one begins. They may need family and friends to encourage them to seek help. Most of the psychosocial problems related to stage 1 are related to delay, denial and postponement. Stage 2 is the interval between diagnosis and the onset of terminal decline. Most treatment is given during this stage, but from a psychological standpoint, few people pass directly from stage 1 to stage 2. Regardless of the treatment given during stage 2, the psychological problems are recognized by the changes in equilibrium of denial and acceptance. Stage 3 starts when active treatment begins to have a diminishing value. Therapeutic emphasis shifts from cure, to control, to symptomatic relief. Doctors are likely to begin withdrawing during this decline. Patients are faced with having to yield personal control to someone else and of coming to terms with their mortality. Stage 3 is sickness until death.

At each stage, the psychosocial problems of the patient's potential survivors should be anticipated. Not only are there general problems of bereavement, but also highly practical issues, such as the disruption of households, financial problems, and whether to tell or not to tell the children. Planning must be both short- and long-range. Bereavement does not start at the moment of death, but at the moment when a significant person realizes that loss is inevitable and that drastic changes cannot be avoided. Psychosocial management is intended to prevent and control secondary suffering from a terminal illness. Patients feel annihilation and alienation, and specifically fear dying less than they fear being deserted. Patients fluctuate between denial and acceptance during the course of their illness, but, as a rule, the tendency is to surrender denial and replace it with acceptance. Unusual persistence of denial is often brought on by fear of alienation and endangerment. Efforts to encourage denial may have an opposite effect; alienation is heightened, people withdraw more and more, and communication becomes more and more remote and ritualized.

Given a chance, dying people are willing to talk about their plight. Conscious efforts to deny reality may silence a terminal patient, but this does not mean that they have been helped toward a significant and dignified death. Even experienced therapists find themselves withdrawing from the presence of death. The threat of alienation may be too great. Many well-meaning people feel a natural revulsion when faced with death. Some are put off by the sights and smells of the disease, others are distraught by the atmosphere of hopelessness and helplessness that affects all who are present. Psychosocial interventions must be honestly and realistically planned and carried out. A guiding principle here is that global reassurance of the patient is seldom reassurance for the patient, but rather a denial of the reality at hand. Accept the terminal patient according to what *they* would like to be like without the illness. Otherwise one may fall victim to a tendency to confuse the patient with the disease or illness. One should make allowances for the deterioration and disability caused by the illness. This does not mean to support regressive defenses. One should permit and encourage the patient to talk about how illness has changed them.

The one who cares for the cancer patient is not immune to denial, antipathy, and fears of personal annihilation. Caring for the dying is exposure to endangerment. One should enlist the assistance of others to obtain support. Safe conduct requires acceptance, clarity, candor, compassion, and mutual accessibility. One should not rush to talk about death or underscore the gloomier side of the illness, nor should one persist with empty optimism when the facts no longer justify it. Unless the patients' physical and mental condition justifies it, one should not exclude them from decisions and information about their illness. One should not allow the family to make decisions for the patient, but rather ensure that all decisions are made with the patient present, so that all are aware of the patients' desires as their illness progresses.

Assess the specific changes that will occur when death happens within the family. The optimal attitude is compassionate objectivity. Remain sufficiently detached to be the intermediary between the family and other professional staff, without usurping the prerogatives of either. One should help survivors accept the inevitable death, but do not force a theory of bereavement on anyone. In addition to bereavement, the family may need help with the practical problems of readjustment to an altered life. An appropriate death, if such a thing exists, is not an ideal death. An appropriate death is a death a person might choose had they a choice.

The question of whether or not patients with cancer are different from those with other chronic or fatal illnesses has been raised. We believe the answer is, yes, for two reasons: First, there is the constant anxiety for the patient because of the threatening fatal illness, which they cannot alter. The heart patient, through rest and medication, can be stabilized, and the diabetic can control his or her illness through diet and medications. Second, these are the attitudes of family members and professional people in charge of their care. The family is usually doubtful of a cure and remains fearful of a fatal outcome. The professional people adopt a guarded attitude. Perhaps it is this that increases apprehension and mental anxieties, such that highly defensive, markedly anxious, inhibited patients run a more rapid course from carcinoma than do relaxed patients (34). Regardless of the actual relationship that might have existed before death, the tendency is to idolize the relationship once death has occurred. The task of dying is not simply a polite exchange of confidences or expression of concern or affection. Dying involves the person having to take leave of all those who have been important to them. The array of questions pertaining to this range from the education of grandchild, the marriage of a daughter or niece, to the disposal of a favorite ring to a favorite cousin.

VII. COMMUNICATION PROCESS

One of the very common themes reported is the very important role that the communication process plays. The communication between doctor and patient, the patient and allied health staff, and patient and family is the primary vehicle through which the patient tries to cope with the cognitive as well as emotional aspects of their medical condition. In our day-to-day experience in working with the patients' family members and medical support system, we have found the communication process to be either a vehicle that may help the patient cope with the medical condition or an obstacle that will hamper the process of coping. In light of the importance of the communication process, it is felt necessary to focus on this theme to provide some insights and guidelines into providing more effective communication between all of the parties involved.

A very brief overview of some very basic communication patterns will be discussed and then specific application to brain tumor patients will be presented. Most of the comments made will refer to verbal communication processes, as this is the primary vehicle through which patients communicate with their doctor and family members.

In the verbal communication process, one of the most frequently used techniques is that of using questions in an attempt to communicate. It has been pointed out by various authors in the communication skills area that questions are not an effective or efficient way of communicating.

Some of the most basic reasons for this are that questions can be very easily closed off, and that questions tend to arouse defensiveness or guardedness in the party being spoken to. A very common example of the first of these processes is when the doctor may speak to the patient, but using a question form as follows: "How are you feeling today?" which will be responded to very frequently by the patient as "fine." This illustrates how easy it is for the question to be responded to with a "dead-end" or closed-off answer, which does not facilitate good communication. Another example is often seen when the family members come to visit the patient in the hospital environment. They come attempting to provide a show of support for the patient, but communicate through a series of questions to which the patient often ends up feeling intruded upon. This dialogue often goes as follows: "How are you feeling today, what did the doctor say, did you eat your lunch, have you taken your medicine, when will you get to come home . . . ?" After a series of questions similar to these, the patient often feels intruded upon and even after having given very closed-end responses to most of them, will often feel guarded or defensive rather than feeling the emotional support the family has been trying to provide.

Questions are a very common form of communication and some literature suggests that questions are used over three-fourths of the time in persons' attempts to communicate with one another. With the high prevalence of this verbal pattern, it suggests that the communication process will end up being quite inefficient or, in fact, may be producing stress, as opposed to the support that the communication process has strived to provide.

A second very common form of communication is the use of the *you* messages. These are two reasons why the *you* statement may not be an efficient or effective method of communicating. One is that the you statement is invariably a form of judgment about the other person. An example of this type of message may be from family to patient where the family will communicate messages such as the following: "You look better today, you are making good progress, you seem to be feeling good, you are going to make it. . . ." All of these are illustrative of judgments that are positive in nature, and these may go reasonably well. However, many of the judgments are of a negative type, as would be indicated by the following examples: "You don't look good today, you seem upset, you're angry, you're down, you're not cooperating with the doctor. . . ." In these examples the judgments are very negative. These types of you messages will very quickly arouse a defensive or guarded posture on the part of the person being spoken to.

The second reason that *you* messages are not effective or efficient is that they may be a command. Examples of you messages as commands would be as follows: "You do what the doctor told you to do, you eat your lunch, you calm down, you take it easy. . . ." Even though all of these messages may be correct in the sense of their content, many patients have a tendency to feel uncomfortable after being commanded or directed to do things. Such directions from the physicians are often received appropriately, but when the family members issue such commands or directives the patients often will become resistant, and the communication process will tend to break down.

In lieu of using questions or *you* messages it has been our experience that a more effective communication pattern is to learn how to use more of the *I* message. In the use of I messages we are not advocating talking about oneself, but we are asking that family members as well as medical staff learn to communicate with the patients by using I messages to indicate their own feelings, thoughts or, needs. The I messages do not have as much of a tendency to be "dead-ended" or closed-off as the questions do, nor do they present a commanding or judgmental approach. When the speaker becomes more used to and proficient in the use of I messages, it is often found that the respondent will begin to use I messages of their own, and this sets up a much more efficient and effective dialogue than the question process or the you process. Some examples of how the I messages may be used, rather than the previously mentioned question or you statement format, are as follows: "I am sure glad to see you, I would like to know what the doctor has said, I am concerned about the medication that is being taken, I would like to know more about the physical therapy program, I am concerned about the sadness that seems to present. . . ." When the speaker is able to rephrase their thoughts, feelings, or needs in the I format, the respondent has much less tendency to feel defensive or guarded.

The verbal part of the communication process is important and often facilitated by the previously mentioned suggestion. However, the listening part of the pattern is equally important; therefore, some thoughts and suggestions about different listening techniques need to be reviewed as well. The ideal communication process is one during which the speaker uses the I message format and the listener also has learned how to use the appropriate type of listening skills.

Out of many types of listening patterns, there are two that seem to be particularly important in dealing with health issues. One pattern of listening that is frequently seen in the hospital environment and also between patient and family members is the pattern of listening defined as *passive listening*. Passive listening occurs when an individual is listening to the speaker, but is doing something else at the same time. For example, in the hospital environment passive listening is being used when the doctor is listening to the patient, but also examining the patient at the same time. The nurse is using passive listening when she is listening to what the patient is saying, but is taking vital signs or giving the patient a bath. The family members are involved in passive listening when they are listening to the patient, but watching television or reading the newspaper at the same time. It should be pointed out that passive listening is an appropriate type of communication process when the speaker is talking about general knowledge or information, trivia, gossip, weather, sports, politics, religion, and such. However, when the speaker begins to express any of their emotional responses to situations, the passive listening format will be quite inefficient and often detrimental. The reason for this is that passive listening gives the message back to the speaker that the listener is just as interested in doing vital signs, making the bed, or watching television, as in the content that the speaker is revealing. If the person talking is sharing their feelings, which are of vital importance to them, it leaves the speaker with the impression that his feelings are no more important than the television story, the vital signs the nurse is taking, or whatever else the listener is doing at the same time the patient is speaking.

The result of this type of dialogue usually is one of two different patterns. The most common result of passive listening to the emotional expressions of the patient is that the patient will stop talking. In the hospital environment the medical staff often becomes concerned about the withdrawn or noncommunicative state of the patient. At times this is a result of the passive listening format that is all too prevalent in the communication process. The second pattern that is seen, but less often, is that, when the patient does not feel that they are really being heard, they will become more demanding and more aggressive in their attempt to get the full undivided attention of the staff or family members. Such patients are often identified as demanding, hard to get along with, uncooperative, or whiny. In fact, many of these people are really responding to the passive listening pattern that they are receiving.

To alleviate this type of situation one needs to understand and use more often the second type of listening, which is defined as *active listening*. Active listening is the process whereby the listener will give the speaker his or her full and undivided attention. This means that the listener will not be doing other tasks at the same time, but will be responding only to the patient's communication. Most medical staff do not feel that they have time to provide active listening to the patients because they are required to do numerous other things in addition to trying to hear our patients. What is often found, however, is that the old idea of "a little dab will do" applies to active listening. For many patients, a little bit of full, undivided attention when they are expressing their feelings will provide them with a great deal of help. It would be helpful to learn that to be able to sit and listen to the patient and not do something else at the same time, even for a very short period will provide more emotional support to the patient than if one is with them for a much longer period, but busy doing other things at the same time.

Active listening is a very powerful form of communication. By giving the person your full, undivided attention when he or she is expressing his or her feelings, you are communicating back to the speaker that you truly do care about what is being said.

This same process is equally important to the family system. In working with those who are trying to provide support to the patient, it is important to help them learn that they need to just listen to the patients when they are expressing their feelings, rather than to give them a lot of questions or give them a lot of the judgmental answers. Active listening communicates to patients a great deal of concern, support, and care, and makes them more likely to be willing to open up and share the feelings that they are experiencing as they go through their medical situation.

VIII. EMOTIONAL RESPONSES

As noted in previous comments, patients definitely experience emotional responses to their medical condition. However, family members also will go through a variety of emotional responses to the medical situation. In our experience, there are four negative emotions that almost universally seem to be part of the process of dealing with brain tumors. These four negative emotions are characterized as mad, sad, scared, and guilt. Even though there are a variety of other labels that may be used to describe each of these four basic negative emotions, in working with the patients, it is advised to use terms that are very familiar to them. All patients who are facing a brain tumor will go through different emotional responses. To come to a successful resolution of these negative emotional states, however, good communication is not enough.

Whenever a patient and the family system around him or her is facing a brain tumor, this needs to be identified as the "medical problem." It is important for the patients as well as the professional staff to realize that there is a difference between the "problem" and the emotional responses that come with the medical problem. In communicating about the medical problem, the patients will often require much direct educational and informative feedback. In dealing with the informational part of the situation, they will often use the questioning format—to which the family or medical staff appropriately can give as much information as the patient can understand. The *emotional* aspect of the same situation, however, requires a different communication process. When it comes to working more effectively with the feelings or emotions that come with the medical problem, the patients must be encouraged to express their feelings in an *I* format when they express their feelings of fear, worry, anger, sadness, or guilt. When this is happening, it then is also important for the staff and family system to be active listeners. One of the biggest mistakes made by the person responding to another person's feelings is to feel that they need to try to solve their problem or carry their burden. In reality, this is not an effective response and leaves the patient feeling as if she or he has not been heard or understood. What works far more effectively for the family or medical staff is to recognize that the patient is expressing emotion, rather than a problem.

It is very important to help the medical staff as well as the family system realize and come to an acceptance that their patients will undergo these negative emotional responses. The family members undergo the same emotional responses, and the difficulty is that the patient and family members may be going through different feelings at different times. This makes the situation very complex and requires very good communication skills for it to be handled effectively. For example, if the patient may be going through a period of sadness in association with a brain tumor, the family member at the same time may be going through a period of anger. What works best is for both parties to have learned that these feelings are normal and natural.

To help avoid the process of making an immediate judgment about a negative emotion, it is helpful to remember that a feeling is just a feeling. There is nothing wrong with having angry feelings about getting a brain tumor, or being frightened because of this medical condition, or at some point of going through a sense of sadness or guilt. These are normal, natural emotional responses to a negative situation. We need to teach the patients and their family members this fact, and this, in turn, will facilitate their being able to more effectively and adaptively communicate these emotional responses, rather than keeping them bottled up inside.

IX. STRESS SYMPTOM CYCLE

Those patients who do not know how to communicate their feelings in an appropriate way end up either bottling them up inside or finally expressing them in inappropriate ways. Either path is going to produce a stress response that brings along with it certain physiological and biochemical changes that may not be conducive to their ability to effectively cope with their medical condition. In helping patients and family members to adeptly cope with the medical condition, it is important to focus on some stress management concepts. The stress management model does indeed help patients, family members, and medical staff people understand the interplay between stress and the patients' medical condition.

The stress symptom cycle is a pattern whereby we know that the occurrence and the presence of medical symptoms act as a stressor to the patient and family. There has been much data collected on the effect of stress on a person's physiological and biochemical status. Because of this interaction, this pattern may turn into a "vicious cycle." If it is not successfully dealt with on both the symptom management side as well as the stress management side, deleterious effects will occur.

Much has been written recently concerning the effect of stress upon health. In our experience over the past 10 years, a stress management model has been employed that has proved to be effective in helping the patients and their families cope with the stress part of the cycle. This model is one that presents to patients and families the importance of four basic stress management tools: (1) knowledge and awareness; (2) relaxation training; (3) communication skills; (4) pacing skills. In working with patients with brain tumors and their family systems, this concept is presented to them, and they are given several sessions of didactic information to help them begin developing stress management skills.

REFERENCES

1. Lederberg MS, Holland JC, Massie MJ. Psychological aspects of patients with cancer. In: Holland JC, Rowland JH, eds. Psycho-oncology: the psychological care of the patient with cancer. New York: Oxford University Press, 1989.
2. Kubler-Ross E. On death and dying. New York: Macmillan, 1969.
3. Peck A. Emotional reactions to having cancer. Cancer 1972; 22:284–291.
4. Aitken-Susan J, Ecissin E. Reactions of cancer patients on being told their diagnosis. Br J Med 1959; 779–783.
5. Holland J. Coping with cancer: a challenge to the behavioral sciences. In: Cuyllen JW, Fox BH, Isom RN, eds. Cancer: the behavioral dimension. New York: Raven Press, 1976.
6. Friedenbergs I, Gordon W, Hubband M, Levine L, Wolf C, Diller L. Psychosocial aspects of living with cancer: a review of the literature. Int J Psychiatry Med 1981–1982; 11:303–329.
7. Gary P, Schag C, Henrich R. The psychosocial impact of cancer in the elderly: a comparison with younger patients. J Am Geriat Soc 1985; 331:429–435.
8. Cassileth R, Lush EJ, Strouss TB. Psychosocial status in chronic illness: a comparative analysis of six diagnostic groups. N Engl J Med 1984; 311:506–511.
9. Newgarten B. Psychological aspects of aging and illness. Clin Issues Geriat Psychiatry 1984; 25:123–125.

10. Edlund B, Sneed NV. Emotional responses to the diagnosis of cancer: age-related comparisons. Oncol Nurs Forum 1989; 16:691–697.
11. Magnes N, Mendelsohn G. Effects of cancer on patient's lives: a personological approach. In: Stone GC, Cohen F, Adlery NE, eds. Health psychology. San Francisco: Jossey-Bass, 1979.
12. Derogatis LR, Morrow GR, Fegging J, Penman D, Piasetsky S, Schmale AM, Hendrich SM, Carnicke CL. The prevalence of psychiatric disorders among cancer patients. JAMA 1983; 249:751–757.
13. Bukberg J, Penman D, Holland JC. Depression in hospitalized cancer patients. Psychosom Med 1984; 46:199–212.
14. Plumb MU, Holland J. Comparative studies of psychological function in patients with advanced cancer-1: self reported depressive symptoms. Psychosom Med 1977; 39:264–276.
15. Schwab JJ, Bialow M, Brown JM, Holzer CE. Diagnosing depression in medical inpatients. Ann Intern Med 1967; 67:695–707.
16. Moffic TT, Paykel ES. Depression in medical inpatients. Br J Psychiatry 1975; 126:346–353.
17. Levine P, Silberfarb PM, Lipowski ZJ. Mental disorders in cancer patients. Cancer 1978; 42:1385–1391.
18. Derogatis LR, Morrow GR, Fetting J, et al. A survey of psychotropic drug prescriptions in an oncology population. Cancer 1979; 44:1919–1929.
19. Massie MJ, Holland JC. Psychiatry and oncology. In: Greenspoon L, ed. Psychiatry update: the american psychiatric association annual review. vol 3. Washington, DC: American Psychiatric Press, 1984.
20. Hamburg D, Hamburg B, deGoZa S. Adaptive problems and mechanisms in severely burned patients. Psychiatry 1953; 16:1–20.
21. Lindemann E. Symptomatology and management of acute grief. Am J Psychiatry 1944; 101:141–148.
22. Lifton RJ. Death in life: survivors of Hiroshima. New York: Random House, 1967.
23. Worden JW, Weisman AD. Preventive psychosocial intervention with newly diagnosed cancer patients. Gen Hosp Psychiatry 1984; 6:243–249.
24. Wilson, CB. Brain metastasis: the basis for surgical selection. Int J Radiat Oncol Biol Phys 1977; 2:169–172.
25. Amato CA. Malignant glioma: coping with a devastating illness. J Neurosurg 1991; 23:20–22.
26. Ransohoff J. Death, dying and the neurosurgical patient. J Neurosurg 1978; 10:198–201.
27. Wilson CB, Fulton DS, Seager ML. Supportive management of the patient with malignant brain tumor. JAMA 1980; 244:1249–1251.
28. Hochberg FH, Slotnick B. Neuropsychologic impairment in astrocytoma survivor. Neurology 1980; 30:172–177.
29. Holland J, Rowland J. Emotional effects of cancer and cancer therapy. In: Greenspoon L, ed. Psychiatric update. Proc XIII Int Cancer Congr. 1982; abstr. 2069:363.
30. Massie MJ, Holland JC. Psychiatry and Oncology. In: Greenspoon L, ed. Psychiatry update. vol 3. Washington, DC: American Psychiatry Press, 1984.
31. Holland JC, Geary N, Marchini A, Tross S. An international survey of physician attitudes and practice in regard to revealing the diagnosis of cancer. Cancer Invest 1987; 5:151–154.
32. Weisman AD. Coping with cancer. New York: McGraw-Hill, 1979.
33. Weisman AD. Psychosocial considerations in terminal care. In: Schoenberg B, Carr AC, Peretz D, Kutscher AH, eds. Psychosocial aspects of terminal care. New York: Columbia University Press, 1972.
34. Abrams RD. The responsibility of social work in terminal cancer. In: Schoenberg B, Carr AC, Peretz D, Kutscher AH, eds. Psychosocial aspects of terminal care. New York: Columbia University Press, 1972.

Index

823

About the Editors

ROBERT A. MORANTZ is Clinical Associate Professor of Neurosurgery at the University of Kansas School of Medicine, and University of Missouri—Kansas City, and Clinical Professor of Radiation Oncology at the University of Kansas School of Medicine, Kansas City, Kansas. The author or coauthor of over 50 journal articles and book chapters dealing with various aspects of neuro-oncology, Dr. Morantz is a Fellow of the American College of Surgeons and a member of the American Association of Neurological Surgeons and the Congress of Neurological Surgeons. He received the A.B. degree (1963) in philosophy from Columbia University and the M.D. degree (1967) from New York University School of Medicine, both in New York City.

JOHN W. WALSH is a Professor in the Department of Neurosurgery at the University of Texas Health Sciences Center at Houston and Staff Neurosurgeon at Hermann Hospital, Houston, Texas. The author or coauthor of numerous professional papers and book chapters, Dr. Walsh is a Fellow of the American College of Surgeons and a member of the American Association of Neurological Surgeons, the Congress of Neurological Surgeons, the American Society for Pediatric Neurosurgeons, and the American Association of Neuropathologists, among others. He received the B.S. degree (1959) in chemistry and the B.A. degree (1959) in mathematics and microbiology from San Diego State College, California, and the M.D. degree (1966) and the Ph.D. degree (1969) in medical microbiology and immunology from the University of California, Los Angeles.